CHRONIC DISEASE EPIDEMIOLOGY, PREVENTION, AND CONTROL 4TH EDITION

CHRONIC DISEASE EPIDEMIOLOGY, PREVENTION, AND CONTROL 4TH EDITION

Edited by
Patrick L. Remington, MD, MPH
Ross C. Brownson, PhD
Mark V. Wegner, MD, MPH

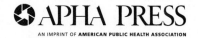

AN IMPRINT OF **AMERICAN PUBLIC HEALTH ASSOCIATION**

American Public Health Association
800 I Street, NW
Washington, DC 20001-3710
www.apha.org

Georges C. Benjamin, MD, FACP, FACEP (Emeritus), Executive Director

Printed and bound in the United States of America
Book Production Editor: Maya Ribault
Typesetting: The Charlesworth Group
Cover Design: Alan Giarcanella
Printing and Binding: Sheridan Books

Library of Congress Cataloging-in-Publication Data

Names: Remington, Patrick L., editor. | Brownson, Ross C., editor. | Wegner,
   Mark V., 1972- editor. | American Public Health Association, issuing body.
Title: Chronic disease epidemiology, prevention, and control / edited by
   Patrick L. Remington, Ross C. Brownson, Mark V. Wegner.
Other titles: Chronic disease epidemiology and control.
Description: 4th edition. | Washington, DC : American Public Health
   Association, [2016] | Preceded by: Chronic disease epidemiology and
   control / [edited by] Patrick L. Remington, Ross C. Brownson, Mark V.
   Wegner. 3rd ed. c2010. | Includes bibliographical references and index.
Identifiers: LCCN 2016028216 (print) | LCCN 2016028866 (ebook) | ISBN
   9780875532776 (softcover : alk. paper) | ISBN 9780875532783 (e-book)
Subjects: | MESH: Chronic Disease--epidemiology | Chronic Disease--prevention
   & control | Risk Factors | Epidemiologic Methods
Classification: LCC RA644.6 (print) | LCC RA644.6 (ebook) | NLM WT 500 | DDC
   614.4/273--dc23
LC record available at https://lccn.loc.gov/2016028216

TABLE OF CONTENTS

Foreword   ix
John Auerbach, MBA, and James S. Marks, MD, MPH

Preface   xiii
*Patrick L. Remington, MD, MPH, Ross C. Brownson, PhD,
and Mark V. Wegner, MD, MPH*

PART I. PUBLIC HEALTH APPROACHES   1

1.   Current Issues and Challenges in Chronic Disease   3
     Prevention and Control
     *Ursula E. Bauer, PhD, MPH, and
     Peter A. Briss, MD, MPH, CAPT USPHS*

2.   Chronic Disease Epidemiology   35
     *Robert Redwood, MD, MPH,
     Patrick L. Remington, MD, MPH, and
     Ross C. Brownson, PhD*

3.   Chronic Disease Surveillance   77
     *Mark V. Wegner, MD, MPH, Ousmane Diallo, MD, PhD,
     and Patrick L. Remington, MD, MPH*

4.   Community-Based Interventions   109
     *Robert J. McDermott, PhD, Carol A. Bryant, PhD,
     Alyssa B. Mayer, PhD, MPH,
     Mary P. Martinasek, PhD, MPH,
     Julie A. Baldwin, PhD, and Sandra D. Vamos, EdD*

5.   The Role of Health Care Systems in Chronic   165
     Disease Prevention and Control
     Karina A. Atwell, MD, MPH, and
     Maureen A. Smith, MD, PhD, MPH

PART II. UPSTREAM RISK FACTORS   199

6.   The Social Determinants of Chronic Disease   201
     Carlyn M. Hood, MPH, MPA, Parvathy Pillai, MD, MPH,
     and Paula Lantz, PhD, MS

7.   Tobacco Use   243
     Corinne G. Husten, MD, MPH, and
     Benjamin J. Apelberg, PhD, MHS

8.   Diet and Nutrition   331
     Cassandra Greenwood, BS, Rachel Sippy, MPH,
     Bethany Weinert, MD, MPH, and
     Alexandra Adams, MD, PhD

9.   Physical Activity   391
     Barbara E. Ainsworth, PhD, MPH, FACSM, and
     Caroline A. Macera, PhD, FACSM

10. Alcohol Use   431
     Karly Christensen, BS, Matthew Thomas, MD,
     Jordan Mills, DO, PhD, Brienna Deyo, MPH,
     Brittany Hayes, MA, and
     Randall Brown, MD, PhD, FASAM

PART III. MIDSTREAM CHRONIC CONDITIONS   483

11. Obesity   485
     Deborah A. Galuska, PhD, MPH, and
     Heidi M. Blanck, PhD, CAPT USPHS

12. Diabetes   519
     Donald B. Bishop, PhD,
     Patrick J. O'Connor, MD, MA, MPH,
     Renée S.M. Kidney PhD, MPH, and
     Debra Haire-Joshu, PhD

13.   High Blood Pressure   581
          Leonelo E. Bautista, MD, DrPH, MPH

14.   Dyslipidemia   633
          Carla I. Mercado, PhD, MS, and
          Fleetwood Loustalot, PhD, FNP

PART IV. DOWNSTREAM CHRONIC DISEASES   671

15.   Cardiovascular Disease   673
          Longjian Liu, MD, PhD, MSc, Craig J. Newschaffer, PhD,
          and Julianne Nelson, MPH

16.   Cancer   743
          Maria Mora Pinzon, MD, MS,
          Corinne Joshu, PhD, MPH, MA, and
          Ross C. Brownson, PhD

17.   Chronic Respiratory Diseases   795
          Henry A. Anderson, MD, Carrie Tomasallo, PhD, MPH,
          and Mark A. Werner, PhD

18.   Mental Disorders   857
          Elizabeth Stein, MD, MS, and Ron Manderscheid, PhD

19.   Neurological Disorders   895
          Edwin Trevathan, MD, MPH

20.   Arthritis and Other Musculoskeletal Diseases   965
          Huan J. Chang, MD, MPH, Daniel J. Finn, MPH,
          Dorothy D. Dunlop, PhD, Diego Tamez, MD, and
          Rowland W. Chang, MD, MPH

21.   Chronic Liver Disease   1017
          Adnan Said, MD, MSPH

22.   Chronic Kidney Disease   1065
          Sana Waheed, MD, and Jonathan B. Jaffery, MD, MS

Contributors   1097

Index   1103

FOREWORD

Decades from now people will likely look at this period of time and reflect in awe at both the significance and the rapidity of the health system changes that occurred. It is difficult for those of us who are living through it to fully appreciate the transformation. Will the health and well-being of the American people improve? Will the inequity of health outcomes among different populations decrease? Will health care costs continue to increase or level off? In large part, the answers to these questions will depend upon how successfully the evolving health system can prevent and control chronic disease.

The 4th edition of *Chronic Disease Epidemiology, Prevention, and Control* is timely during this era of transition and uncertainty and namely serves as a useful and informative guide to get us from where public health is to where public health needs to be.

Chronic diseases are already common and costly but are becoming increasingly so due in part to the fact that older adults are a rapidly growing proportion of the U.S. population. By 2030, the number of Americans over 65 is expected to reach 72 million, up from 40 million in 2010 (Colby and Ortman 2015). Those aged 65 years and older are members of the fastest-growing age group in the United States (US Census Bureau 2011). Virtually all older adults will develop one or, more likely, multiple chronic diseases. With chronic diseases growing in significance, it is vital that public health learns how to better control and prevent these diseases, perhaps by learning from the successes of emergency response as public health (in spite of the alarming Ebola and Zika outbreaks) has been able to effectively control infectious disease domestically and abroad.

This is not to say that public health hasn't made progress in preventing, diagnosing, and controlling chronic disease. Public health has. Perhaps most noteworthy has been the expanded access to care resulting from the Affordable

Care Act (ACA). Millions more people are likely to receive care that will diminish their risks and their symptoms. Furthermore, the dramatic shift from fee-for-service to value-based contracting and other reimbursement innovations that reward health care providers for improving health outcomes among their patient population is opening new possibilities for effective chronic disease prevention and treatment services. These services include coverage for the community-based National Diabetes Prevention Program and home-based asthma risk reduction counseling and medical equipment support. And perhaps what is even more transformative is that the ACA explicitly supports prevention and community programs, directly with specific new resources such as requirements for community health needs assessment and in the new accountability for community benefit commitments of health systems. Elements like these had not been included in earlier health care reform efforts. Implicitly, the ACA signaled the common purpose of health care and public health and laid the foundation for future health reform, which will routinely address both clinical and community solutions.

Yet in spite of the progress in reducing and controlling certain chronic diseases, we often still struggle to understand and implement the best approaches. Cigarette use is down, but teens are increasingly using other tobacco-related products. Consciousness of the dangers of obesity is higher than ever, but obesity and its health consequences remain major issues. It seems that every year there are new pharmaceutical or clinical interventions promising to reduce the onset or progression of chronic diseases. But we can't seem to adequately apply the effective medications we already have; for example, the percentage of people with hypertension who have their condition under control still hovers around 54% (Farley et al. 2010).

As this book highlights, tackling chronic disease prevention requires a sophisticated approach to the contributions that can be made by both the health care and the public health sectors. While we need high quality, effective clinical care, health education, and counseling, we also need interventions that address socioeconomic factors that can change the conditions in people's lives.

Unfortunately, funding for the public health system—a key sector in mobilizing a multifaceted approach—was dramatically reduced during the recession and those budget cuts have not been restored (NACCHO 2013). What funding it receives is usually disease specific. These limitations have inhibited a broader public health approach, one that may help a community to address its most serious health problems. We need a public health system that is able to demonstrate how risk factors that contribute to chronic disease can be mitigated, that has up-to-date tools including more real-time data and evidence-based approaches, that can build authentic partnerships with health care and other sectors, and that can draw upon and nurture the strengths of local residents and institutions in reshaping their own communities.

The foreword of the third edition noted that

> Lifestyle risks such as tobacco use and poor nutrition are defined in large part by how communities are designed—with sidewalks and markets . . . with safe places to play . . . where jobs are available and accessible by affordable public transportation . . . where schools ensure a high graduation rate and promote health. Simply put, societal policies and practices are fundamental causes of good or ill health.

What makes this current period so hopeful is that there is both a growing recognition of this truth and a widespread commitment to address it.

This awareness is reflected in insightful and comprehensive new chapters in the 4th edition, on the innovative reimbursement approaches of the ACA's Center for Medicare and Medicaid Innovation, and on the centrality of addressing the social determinants of health. This edition rightly draws attention to the social, economic, and behavioral factors that play a major role in causing and exacerbating or, alternatively, preventing the development of chronic illness. These factors ultimately contribute to the disparities in life expectancy between minority and majority populations and between the rich and the poor. The authors and editors richly deserve credit for their crisp overview of the current knowledge and best practices, provided in such frank detail and in a time—an exciting time—of transition and change.

Reducing disease, decreasing disparities, and bending the cost curve will not come easily. We need to make these goals a top priority, to adapt both the health care and the public health systems and integrate them into a single health-oriented system, and to accept the necessity of working outside the walls of our clinical settings to promote health equity.

This volume points the way to the future and is a useful summary and an influential framework for our challenges. Now more than ever, the best audiences and highest uses of this edition may come from those partners outside of traditional public health who receive and use this book as they work together to promote public health. The ability to embrace this challenge is within our power. Future generations should judge us harshly if we fail to take advantage of the opportunities in this transformative period to reduce chronic disease.

They will note that we had the knowledge and an emerging societal will for this to be a—if not the—turning point in reducing the heartbreaking illnesses, premature deaths, and extraordinary costs associated with chronic disease.

John Auerbach, MBA
James S. Marks, MD, MPH

Acknowledgment

The conclusions in this Foreword are those of the contributors and do not necessarily represent the official positions of the Centers for Disease Control and Prevention and the Robert Wood Johnson Foundation.

References

Colby SL, Ortman JM. US Census Bureau. Current Population Reports, P25-1143, Projections of the size and composition of the US population: 2014 to 2060. Washington, DC: US Government Printing Office; 2015.

Farley TA, Dalal MA, Mostashari F, Frieden TR. Deaths preventable in the US by improvements in the use of clinical preventive services. *Am J Prev Med*. 2010;38(6):600–609.

National Association of County & City Health Officials (NACCHO). Local health department job losses and program cuts: finds from the 2013 profile study. 2013. Available at: http://archived.naccho.org/topics/infrastructure/lhdbudget/upload/Survey-Findings-Brief-8-13-13-2.pdf. Accessed June 29, 2016.

US Census Bureau. 2010 census shows 65 and older population growing faster than total US population. 2011. Available at: https://www.census.gov/newsroom/releases/archives/2010_census/cb11-cn192.html. Accessed June 29, 2016.

PREFACE

Since the publication of the first edition of *Chronic Disease Epidemiology and Control* almost 25 years ago, our understanding of the causes and consequences of chronic diseases has continued to progress. More importantly, researchers have continued to identify effective programs and policies to reduce the risk of chronic disease, or to control their consequences. The addition of "prevention" to the title of this 4th edition—now *Chronic Disease Epidemiology, Prevention, and Control*—reflects an increasing focus in public health and health care on the prevention of chronic diseases and their related risk factors.

The 2002 report by the Institute of Medicine, *The Future of the Public's Health in the 21st Century*, pointed to the multiple determinants of disease with a call to action for nontraditional public health partners, such as health care, business, media, academia, and community groups, to engage in community health improvement efforts. The Affordable Care Act has a number of policies and has added significant funding to promote chronic disease prevention and control. Furthermore, some health care systems are responding to this call with efforts to not only increase health care coverage and improve quality but also to develop incentives to reward population health improvement rather than simply rewarding more high-cost treatments.

In addition, information technology has continued to evolve and is now able to provide an overwhelming amount of information, which has become increasingly accessible with the near ubiquity of smart phones and other mobile devices. However, conflicting with the promise of better information for public health are concerns about patient privacy, confidentiality, and propriety rights to health information technology.

With the changing landscape, this edition has been updated to help students and practitioners keep abreast of advances in chronic disease prevention and control by providing up-to-date and practical information about the leading chronic diseases, conditions, and risk factors. This book is intended to support a broad range of chronic disease prevention and control activities; it is designed to serve as a quick reference guide for students or practicing public health and health care professionals who need to locate critical background information or develop appropriate interventions.

This book is intended for several audiences. First, it will be useful to professionals involved in the practice and teaching of chronic disease epidemiology, prevention, and control at all levels. In state public health agencies, the book will be helpful to staff involved in primary and secondary prevention of chronic diseases, including epidemiologists, physicians, nurses, health educators, and health promotion specialists. In local public health agencies, administrators, physicians, nurses, health educators, and sanitarians will find the text of value.

In academic institutions, the book will provide helpful background information on chronic diseases for students taking beginning and advanced public health courses. Although the book is intended primarily for a North American audience, there is literature drawn from all parts of the world, and we believe that much of the information covered will be applicable in any developed or developing country.

Finally, the book will provide health care systems with important information about chronic disease prevention, especially as these systems seek to achieve the "Triple Aim" of health care—by improving quality, reducing costs, and improving population health. Accountable care organizations are beginning to extend care into the community, using many of the evidence-based interventions described in this book.

The authors of the various chapters were selected for both their scientific expertise and their practical experience in carrying out chronic disease control programs at the community level. The new edition now includes 22 chapters and is organized into four major parts: Part I. Public Health Approaches; Part II. Upstream Risk Factors; Part III. Midstream Chronic Conditions; and Part IV. Downstream Chronic Diseases. In the new edition, we reflect feedback we have received informally from colleagues and have added two new chapters (The Social Determinants of Chronic Disease and The Role of Health Care Systems in Chronic Disease Prevention and Control).

Chapter 1 provides a historical review of chronic disease control, a brief explanation of the current status of chronic disease control programs, and a discussion of the prospects and challenges for chronic disease control during the next decade and beyond. Chapters 2 and 3 briefly review the methods used in chronic disease epidemiology and surveillance and provide a framework for the interpretation of the information in the following chapters. Chapter 4 provides an overview of chronic disease intervention methods, providing a theoretical grounding for interventions that address the diseases and risk factors discussed in later chapters. It also summarizes some of the important features of successful interventions and provides practical examples. Finally, Chapter 5 provides an overview of approaches that can be used in the health care system to not only better manage chronic diseases but also to prevent them, focusing on health behaviors and even social and economic determinants.

In Part II, Chapters 6 through 10 focus on upstream and potentially modifiable risk factors for chronic diseases. The chapters in this section examine the important areas of tobacco use, diet and nutrition, physical inactivity, and alcohol use. In Part III, Chapters 11 through 14 focus on those chronic disease conditions that often result from high risk behaviors and substantially increase the risk of chronic diseases. These conditions include obesity, diabetes, high blood pressure, and high blood cholesterol. In Part IV, Chapters 15 through 22 describe major downstream chronic diseases: cardiovascular disease, cancer, chronic lung diseases, mental disorders, chronic neurological disorders, arthritis and other musculoskeletal diseases, liver disease, and kidney disease.

A standard format has been used for all chapters that focus on specific risk factors and chronic diseases to allow the reader quick and easy access to information. Each chapter begins with a brief introduction, reviewing the significance of the chronic disease, condition, or risk factor, and the underlying biological or physiological processes. The next section addresses descriptive epidemiology by examining high-risk groups (person), geographic variation (place), and secular trends (time). The third section describes the causes of the disease, condition, or risk factor under consideration. The final section discusses evidence-based interventions for prevention and control. When available, specific examples of practical and effective public health interventions are described as well as recommendations for future research and demonstration. A bibliography and list of resources are also included to facilitate access to additional information.

This book is not intended to provide a complete and final review of chronic disease epidemiology, prevention, and control. Because the field is so broad, with overlapping issues, any division of the topic becomes somewhat arbitrary.

There are literally thousands of different chronic diseases. We have chosen to focus on those that account for a large proportion of morbidity and mortality in the adult population and to emphasize risk factors that can be modified through public health interventions.

Future research will continue to expand our understanding of chronic disease epidemiology, prevention, and control. Epidemiological studies will identify new risk factors and quantify their effects. Intervention studies underway will expand the array of interventions available for public health practitioners.

Chronic disease epidemiology, prevention, and control is a rapidly expanding field, and much has changed in the six years since the 3rd edition was published. We are indebted to the contributors of this 4th edition for volunteering their time and talents as scholars in field and to Cassandra Greenwood for help coordinating all aspects of the work.

There is a compelling and increasing need for health professionals with knowledge and expertise in chronic disease prevention and control. We hope this book will become a useful resource for public health and health care professionals as they are called on to meet new public health challenges.

Patrick L. Remington, MD, MPH

Ross C. Brownson, PhD

Mark V. Wegner, MD, MPH

PART I. PUBLIC HEALTH APPROACHES

CURRENT ISSUES AND CHALLENGES IN CHRONIC DISEASE PREVENTION AND CONTROL

Ursula E. Bauer, PhD, MPH, and Peter A. Briss, MD, MPH, CAPT USPHS

Introduction

In the first quarter of the 20th century, major public health advances transformed communities and initiated a remarkable increase in life expectancy for Americans. At the same time, the distribution and demographic composition of the American population was undergoing a major shift, growing rapidly and becoming more urban, older, and more diverse. One hundred years later, public health again is taking innovative steps to strengthen environments to support health and healthful behaviors and nudge the movement to transform health care delivery in the direction of population health. And, again, major demographic shifts in the composition of the American population are well underway, with an aging population and several states—California, Hawaii, and New Mexico—and the District of Columbia becoming "majority 'Minority'" (Hobbs and Stoops 2002). Nearly a century ago, an epidemiologic transition, instigated in part by advances in public health, resulted in heart disease becoming the leading cause of death by 1933, overtaking infectious causes. Although heart disease remains the leading cause of death in the first quarter of the 21st century, incidence, prevalence, and mortality rates of heart disease have declined dramatically. As was the case a century earlier, these changes in the distribution of diseases are driven in part by public health and health care improvements across the nation.

The epidemiologic transition (Omran 2005; McKeowan 2009) from primarily infectious disease causes of death to primarily chronic disease causes of death and the demographic transition from a predominantly young to an older and even very old population both continue into the 21st century in the United States and continue to shape the practice of public health and the demands on clinical care. The two transitions are related and are driven, historically, by economic development and technological advances leading to improvements in nutrition, education, sanitary conditions, safety, housing, perinatal and newborn survival, and other factors that reduce death rates and increase life expectancy. These changes lead to lower birth rates and alter the characteristics of the population, including the age distribution (Figure 1-1). As of 2014, the median age of the U.S. population was 37.7 years, compared to 29.5 years in 1960, and just 22.9 years in 1900. In addition, 40 million adults—13% of the population—are aged 65 years or older, compared to just three million adults (less than 4% of the population) in 1900. Of those 40 million, about 5.5 million are aged 85 years or older (Federal Interagency Forum on Aging-Related Statistics 2012). Age is a leading nonmodifiable risk factor for chronic disease. As the population ages, even if incidence, prevalence, and mortality rates decline, the number of people living with (and dying from) these diseases increases. Thus, the age structure of the population has a large impact on the burden of chronic diseases.

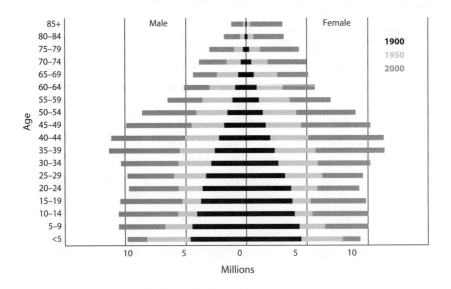

Source: Adapted from Hobbs and Stoops (2002).

Figure 1-1. Total U.S. Population by Age and Sex: 1900, 1950, and 2000

Definition of Chronic Disease

There is not a single universally accepted definition of "chronic disease." Many definitions have been proposed (Bernstein et al. 2003; USDHHS 2010; NCHS 2011; WHO 2016a; Goodman et al. 2013). Definitions typically share characteristics including a long course (months to lifelong, generally longer than a year), but vary on other characteristics including whether they are noninfectious, reversible, result in functional limitations, or produce a need for medical care.

For the purpose of this chapter, we will adopt the U.S. Department of Health and Human Services (USDHHS) definition of a chronic condition: one that lasts a year or more and requires ongoing medical attention and/or limits activities of daily living (USDHHS 2010). Although, for public health practice, a distinction is often made between infectious and chronic diseases, this boundary is increasingly blurry. Many infections (e.g., HIV, hepatitis C, *Helicobacter pylori*) can cause chronic diseases and many chronic diseases (e.g., cervical and other cancers) have infectious etiologies (O'Connor et al. 2006).

Significance

Life expectancy at birth for Americans in 2015 was 79 years. Although Americans are living longer than ever before, they are not living as long as their peers in countries including Japan (84 years), Norway (82 years), Germany (81 years), and the United Kingdom (81 years), and are just keeping pace with lower-income countries such as Cuba (79 years) and Costa Rica (79 years) (WHO 2016b). Americans spend more per capita on health care services than any other country in the world (Mossialos et al. 2015)—fully 50% more than the next highest spender (Switzerland)—and yet our health outcomes are worse than those in dozens of peer nations (WHO 2016c). At the same time, the United States lags considerably behind other high-income countries in investments in health promotion and disease prevention, and other public health and social services interventions that keep people well (Bradley and Taylor 2013).

The same economic and technological advances that improved quality of life and helped usher in longer lives brought with them new threats to health including tobacco use, overconsumption of calories, and reduced physical activity. These, along with excessive alcohol use, are the leading "actual" causes of death (McGinnis and Foege 1993; Mokdad et al. 2004) in the 20th and 21st centuries, contributing to all the major killers: heart disease, cancer, stroke, chronic obstructive lung disease, and diabetes. These so-called lifestyle behaviors contribute to nearly 40% of all deaths in the United States (Mokdad et al. 2004) and are part of the reason that life expectancy in the United States lags behind that of other countries and chronic diseases affect such a large portion of the population. Although debate continues about precise contributions of key risk behaviors to mortality (Flegal et al. 2005), the contribution of these behaviors to morbidity and diminished quality of life is unquestioned, confirming the important role of "lifestyle behaviors" in producing chronic diseases (McGinnis and Foege 1993; Mokdad et al. 2004; Ford et al. 2009).

Chronic diseases, including heart disease, cancer, and diabetes, and chronic conditions, such as obesity, nicotine addiction, and high blood pressure, are among the most common, costly, and preventable health problems in the United States. How common? Seven of the top-10 causes of death in 2014 were chronic diseases, with heart disease and cancer accounting for almost half (46%) of all deaths (Table 19 in USDHHS 2016a).

Every year, about 610,000 people die of heart disease and almost half of Americans have one or more of the three major risk factors for heart disease: uncontrolled high blood pressure, high cholesterol, or smoking (Fryar et al. 2012). Almost 600,000 Americans die of cancer each year, with nearly 1.6 million cases diagnosed annually (US Cancer Statistics Working Group 2016). In 2014, 1.4 million American adults were diagnosed with diabetes, a stunning number despite five straight years of declines following a peak in the incidence rate in 2009. Currently about 29 million Americans (9.3%) are living with diabetes and another 86 million Americans have prediabetes, a condition that puts them at high risk of developing diabetes (Tabak et al. 2012). More than one third of adults, or about 78 million people, are obese (defined as body mass index [BMI] ≥ 30 kg/m^2) and nearly one in five youths aged 2 to 19 years is obese (BMI $\geq$ 95th percentile; Ogden et al. 2014). Cigarette use peaked in the United States in the 1960s and prevalence of cigarette smoking has steadily declined, but 15.2% of adults in the United States continue to smoke (CDC 2015) including more men than women (Figure 24 in USDHHS 2016a). Arthritis is the most common cause of disability. Of the 53 million adults with doctor-diagnosed arthritis, more than 22 million have trouble with usual activities because of the condition (Hootman et al. 2009; Barbour et al. 2013). About half of U.S.

adults—117 million people—have one or more chronic conditions, and one in four adults have two or more chronic conditions (Ward et al. 2014). Indeed, "multiple chronic conditions" is the most common chronic condition in the United States today.

Chronic diseases, conditions, and risk factors are very common, even as prevalence rates of many are on the decline. In contrast, the economic costs of these diseases, conditions, and risk factors continue to increase; the economic costs are as staggering as the conditions are common. How costly? Noncommunicable diseases are estimated to account for fully 86% of the nation's $2.7 trillion per year health care expenditures (Gerteis et al. 2014), including the leading causes of death, substance use, and mental health. Annual health care costs in 2010 for heart disease, cancer, diabetes, and tobacco, and in 2008 for obesity have been estimated at $234 billion, $116 billion, $126 billion, $170 billion, and $147 billion, respectively (Dunn et al. 2015; Xu et al. 2014; Finkelstein et al. 2009); the annual costs of excessive alcohol use in 2006 were estimated at $1.90 per alcoholic drink consumed (Bouchery et al. 2011). Total health care expenditures for the elderly in 2011 were $414.3 billion (Mirel and Carper 2014). These costs are largely borne by private and public health insurers, governments, and businesses, which means we all pay these costs, through taxes, health care insurance premiums, employer health insurance contributions, and out-of-pocket payments.

Economic costs are just one kind of cost. Individual and family suffering, lost wages and employment, disability, premature death, reduced productivity on the job, and lack of economic competitiveness are other kinds of costs that result from the high burden of chronic diseases in the United States. For excessive alcohol use, other additional costs include violence, injury, and harm to others (e.g., family dysfunction, adverse childhood events, and motor vehicle fatalities).

Prevention Models

Common. Costly. And preventable. As McGinnis and Foege first noted in 1993, and Mokdad et al. (2004) updated, the leading actual causes of death in the United States are the behaviors that give rise to the diseases that lead to premature death. These are tobacco use, poor nutrition and lack of physical activity (and associated obesity), and excessive alcohol use. But what causes these behaviors? They often reflect the easiest, most accessible choices in our society and may even be the choices that are most aggressively promoted through advertising and marketing. As a society, it often seems as if we are designed for disease, designed in a way that makes the disease-promoting behaviors the easiest, most affordable or most desirable choices to make. All too often, the unhealthy choice is the default choice or even the only choice. Advertising, marketing, and promotion; community design; readily available prepared, packaged, and restaurant foods; and the lack of safe public spaces in which to be physically active all shape the choices we make and the behaviors we are most likely to adopt.

The factors that influence health (Figure 1-2) were described by Frieden (2010) as falling into five categories, or levels of a pyramid, organized from greatest to least impact. The base of the pyramid includes income, education, housing, and inequality (among other factors), often called "socioeconomic factors" or "social determinants." These factors affect large numbers of people, contribute powerfully to poor health, and, if ameliorated or mitigated, can dramatically improve the health of large numbers of people.

At the next level, "environmental" or "community" factors, such as community water fluoridation, smoke-free indoor air, the availability of nutritious

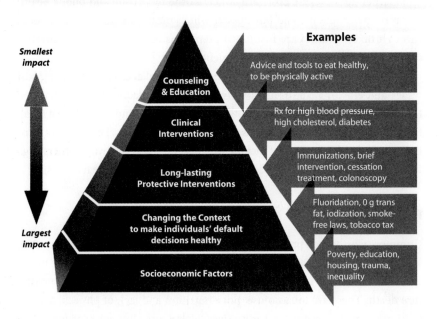

Source: Adapted from Frieden (2010).

Figure 1-2. Health Impact Pyramid

foods, community walkability, and the density of alcohol and tobacco outlets and the prices of these products, each shape the context within which people live and strongly influence whether people have the wherewithal to adopt and maintain healthful behaviors. Improving these environmental or community factors—changing the context to make healthy choices the easy, or default, choice—are the public health strategies that have typically delivered the greatest health impact and with which chronic disease prevention and health promotion efforts will have the greatest reach and greatest return on investment.

The next level of the Health Impact Pyramid, termed "long-lasting protective interventions," can be described as the intersection of public health and health care, where outreach is critical to engage large populations for delivery of one-time or long-acting interventions such as childhood and adult immunizations and cancer-screening services including colonoscopy. These interventions can prevent diseases from developing in the first place (e.g., polyp removal to prevent colon cancer), detect diseases early when they can be treated and often cured more cheaply and effectively (e.g., screening Papanicolaou test for cervical cancer early detection), and effectively manage risk factors to avert disease (e.g., smoking cessation).

To have a population health impact, long-lasting protective interventions must reach widely into the population, even as interventions are delivered to individuals. "Clinical interventions" and "counseling and educational interventions" (the fourth and fifth levels of the pyramid) require the greatest investment of resources and the greatest commitment on the part of individuals to obtain the interventions and follow through on the treatment or education. Although they can be highly effective on a case-by-case basis, these interventions are often squarely in the medical sphere and can present enormous obstacles to individuals as they need to access the intervention, complete treatment, and follow through on recommended behavioral change.

Chronic disease prevention, and public health more generally, work most effectively in the "context changing" and "long-acting" levels, where population impact is great, fewer resources are required, and individuals are more strongly supported in achieving and maintaining behaviors that keep them well. Nonetheless, public health also has a role in monitoring and addressing the socioeconomic factors that have such a profound impact on health status, and in strengthening the effective delivery of quality health care services where the existing burden of disease must be treated cost-effectively. The levels of the pyramid are not in competition with one another; work at all levels is necessary to improve the health of the population.

Mental health and substance use disorders, often referred to collectively as "behavioral health disorders," are increasingly recognized as intertwined with the prevention and control of chronic diseases. In 2014, an estimated 43.6 million U.S. adults (18.1%) had any mental health disorder in the past year, including 9.8 million adults with serious mental illness (SAMHSA and CBHSQ 2015). Fully 21.5 million Americans aged 12 years and older (8.1%) had a substance use disorder in the past year, with alcohol being the predominant substance, affecting 14.4 million Americans who had problems with alcohol only and another 2.6 million who had problems with both alcohol and other drugs (SAMHSA and CBHSQ 2015). In addition, about 38 million Americans binge drink, most of whom would not be defined as having an alcohol disorder (Kanny et al. 2012), but whose binge drinking contributes to injury, violence, and premature death. Nearly eight million Americans aged 18 years and older had both a mental health disorder and a substance use disorder.

People with mental health disorders or substance use disorders, whether occurring alone or in combination, have higher mortality and lower life expectancy than people without these disorders (Laursen et al. 2007; Colton and Manderscheid 2006; Druss et al. 2011). They often have chronic diseases or chronic disease risk factors along with their behavioral health conditions. People with mental health disorders are more likely to smoke cigarettes and have obesity, diabetes, or heart disease than people without these disorders, and an estimated 50% of people with chronic physical diseases have comorbid behavioral health conditions (Mandersheid and Kathol 2014).

Our highly specialized health care system serves people with comorbid physical and behavioral health conditions poorly (Lawrence and Kisely 2010). Half of patients who have both and are under care for the physical condition do not receive care for the behavioral health condition. This gap results in poor management and persistence of the physical condition, greater likelihood of disability, higher health care utilization and costs, and premature death (Manderscheid and Kathol 2014). The additional cost of treating chronic diseases (e.g., diabetes and heart disease) among people who also have a behavioral health condition—not including the cost of treating the behavioral health condition—was estimated to be $290 billion in 2012 (Melek et al. 2014).

Mental health disorders and substance use disorders challenge the ability of public health and health care to effectively prevent, treat, and manage chronic (and other) diseases. These challenges reinforce the need to more effectively address socioeconomic factors to prevent and control chronic diseases, conditions, and risk factors across the entire population; to "change the context" to support healthful behaviors for all people; and, within the health care system, to integrate medical and behavioral health services to improve management of chronic diseases among those with behavioral health conditions (and to improve the management of behavioral health conditions among those with chronic diseases).

Given the prevalence, burden, and costs imposed by chronic diseases, a broad range of actors and institutions is required to take part in preventing and controlling chronic diseases, conditions, and risk factors, and improving health outcomes. A diverse set of stakeholders will play an expanded role in developing and implementing effective programs, policies, systems, and environmental improvements, and mobilizing community demand to prevent and control chronic diseases. This book provides all of those people with an up-to-date overview of the major chronic diseases, conditions, and risk factors, and the scientific and programmatic principles related to chronic disease prevention and control, including current challenges and opportunities.

Goals of Chronic Disease Prevention and Control

The goals of chronic disease prevention and control are to improve health, life expectancy, and quality of life, so people live longer, healthier lives, free of disability, with final morbidity, if it occurs, compressed into a very brief period of time before death (Fries et al. 1993). Such improvements would off-load considerable burden from the health care delivery system, reducing both utilization and costs of health care services. However, there is currently a substantial burden of disease requiring medical intervention, and many health care services that work effectively to prevent and control chronic diseases. Thus, parallel goals, advanced in partnership with the health care system, are to (1) increase the effective delivery of quality clinical preventive, management, and treatment services; (2) reduce the costs of health care delivery; and (3) improve population health (Berwick et al. 2008). These goals become easier as public health achieves success in improving the overall health of the population and as health care payment models move from paying for large numbers of services to be delivered to paying for the value of the services delivered, measured in terms of health outcomes (Miller 2009).

Defining Chronic Disease Prevention and Control

With these goals in mind, chronic disease prevention and control focuses on preventing the development of risk behaviors (e.g., cigarette smoking and excessive alcohol use), promoting the development of healthful behaviors (e.g., regular physical activity and adequate sleep), identifying and eliminating modifiable risk behaviors and factors when they do occur (e.g., tobacco use cessation and exposure to secondhand smoke), screening for and reducing disease risks (e.g., screening for high blood pressure and cancers of the breast, cervix, and colon), community delivery of structured lifestyle interventions to help people manage disease once it occurs and prevent progression and complications, and treatment of disease to prevent progression, disability, and premature death. A commonly used taxonomy names these levels of interventions health promotion, primary prevention, secondary prevention, and tertiary prevention, based on the populations targeted by the interventions (healthy people, those with risk factors, asymptomatic people with adverse biologic changes, and those with frank disease, respectively). This classification scheme is not unique to chronic disease prevention, but applies to disease prevention more generally.

Strategies to prevent and control chronic disease fall into a four-part domain framework (epidemiology and surveillance, environmental approaches, health systems interventions, and linking community and clinical services; Bauer et al. 2014) and continue to require attention to improve the upstream conditions that set the stage for chronic disease development (i.e., the socioeconomic factors at the base of the pyramid in Figure 1-2). Upstream conditions include poverty, low education, and adverse childhood events, and may also include more traditional areas of public health work, such as lack of access to tobacco-free environments, healthful foods, and opportunities for physical activity, and rampant promotion of alcohol and tobacco use. The four-part domain framework, which incorporates and goes beyond traditional disease prevention and control strategies, is described in the next paragraphs.

Epidemiology and Surveillance

Epidemiology and surveillance involve monitoring the occurrence and distribution of diseases, conditions, and risk factors across a population. They require expertise to collect data and information and to develop and deploy effective interventions, identify and address gaps in program delivery, and monitor and evaluate progress in achieving program goals. Work in these areas provides essential data and information to define and prioritize public health problems, identify populations most affected, guide solutions, and monitor progress. Information and insights can be used to educate decision-makers and the public about the high rates of disease, disability, and death and the high health care costs associated with chronic diseases, evidence-based interventions, and other actions that can be taken to prevent and control chronic diseases, successes in preventing and controlling chronic diseases, and unmet needs and priorities to more effectively address chronic diseases.

Environmental Approaches

Environmental approaches promote health and support and reinforce healthful behaviors across the nation, in states and communities, and in settings such as schools, child care and senior programs, worksites, and businesses. This strategic area works to expand access to and availability of healthy foods and beverages, promote increased physical activity, reduce availability and affordability of tobacco, eliminate exposure to secondhand smoke, and increase the proportion of the U.S. population served by community water systems with optimally fluoridated water, among many other environmental improvements. These kinds of approaches are often advanced through policy and regulatory processes that change the environment and therefore change the context in which people live, work, and play; they reach more people, are more cost-efficient, and are more likely to have a lasting effect on population health.

Health Systems Interventions

Health systems interventions increase the effective use and improve the quality of clinical and other preventive services within the health care system to prevent disease, detect diseases early, reduce or eliminate risk factors, and mitigate or manage complications. Interventions that increase access to and build demand for quality preventive services can also reduce disparities in access to care and care-related health outcomes. This is particularly true in an era of health care reform that facilitates system improvements in the service of improving population health. These include improvements in the way care is organized, such as accountable care organizations (Berwick 2011) or Accountable Communities for Health (Alley et al. 2016), and the way care is paid for to reward value rather than volume (Miller 2009).

Although health care interventions can be powerful drivers of population health, and have, for example, driven much progress in cardiovascular outcomes (Ford et al. 2007), they typically generate smaller health improvements than policies and environmental changes (Frieden 2010) and are complements to and not replacements for more upstream and community approaches. Nonetheless, clinical and other preventive services that detect diseases early and better manage risk factors play a critical role in chronic disease prevention and health promotion and offer the promise of improving quality of life and reducing health care costs.

Linking Community and Clinical Services

Strategies that link community and clinical services help ensure that people with or at high risk of chronic diseases have access to the resources they need to prevent or manage these diseases. With community-delivered programs linked to clinical services and reimbursed by health plans, employers, and insurers, people can improve their quality of life, delay or avert the onset or progression of disease, avoid complications, and reduce the need for more health care. Community programs that provide these benefits include chronic disease self-management programs, the National Diabetes Prevention Program, and a variety of falls prevention, arthritis self-management, and diabetes self-management programs. To be most effective, these programs must be linked to clinical services and reimbursed by health plans and insurers.

Chronic disease prevention and control is an "all-in" enterprise, working most effectively when there is broad buy-in to the goals; involvement from multiple sectors, actors, and institutions at the local, state, and federal level; and the political and social will to undertake the most effective strategies.

Approaches to Prevention: Priorities and Strategies

Chronic diseases have major negative effects on morbidity, mortality, and quality of life, and yet they can be prevented or delayed and their effects ameliorated at every stage with simple, cost-effective strategies and interventions.

Although some gains can be realized quickly, chronic disease prevention and control generally take time and a persistent, long-term approach. Effective strategies implemented in both community and clinical settings have resulted in substantial progress on many diseases, conditions, and risk behaviors. For example, smoking prevalence among adults in the United States has declined by nearly two thirds from 42.4% in 1965 (Xu et al. 2016) to 15.2% in the first quarter of 2015 (CDC 2015). Coronary heart disease death rates have sharply declined since the 1960s, from a peak of 483 deaths per 100,000 population in 1968 to 169.8 per 100,000 in 2013 (NHLBI 2012; Xu et al. 2016). Overall death rates from cancer have shown gradual declines since 1993 (Xu et al. 2016), with similar gradual declines in cancer incidence, from 484 cases per 100,000 population in 1999 to 440 per 100,000 in 2012 (CDC 2016a).

The British epidemiologist Geoffrey Rose contrasted general population-wide and high-risk approaches to disease prevention. The former attempts to move the distribution of risk factors to healthier levels in the whole population whereas the latter attempts to reduce risk among the most affected. Rose and others have argued that the population-wide approach has important advantages. The common risk factors for chronic diseases are usually distributed among a large proportion of the population and the largest number of the cases of chronic disease arises from the populations that possess intermediate- and low-risk profiles (because that is where the bulk of the population is). The implication for prevention is that small changes in risk in the total population will result in a greater overall disease reduction than will greater changes in a specified and relatively smaller high-risk group (Rose 1992).

High-risk approaches also require correct classification of people at high risk (Murray et al. 1999), but can allow efficiently targeting people with highest need. For example, targeting Diabetes Prevention Program activities to people at highest risk improves the efficiency and cost-effectiveness of that program (Zhuo et al. 2013). In general, health professionals select from a menu of interventions that address major chronic diseases, conditions, and risk behaviors based on a range of factors including effectiveness, cost-effectiveness, preventable burden, and feasibility, among others. For the major chronic diseases, both population-wide and high-risk approaches are warranted.

Even as chronic diseases, conditions, and risk behaviors are broadly disseminated in the U.S. population, some population subgroups bear a greater burden than others. These include groups that are more heavily affected by "bottom of the pyramid" conditions such as poverty, low education, adverse childhood events, and other factors. Thus, prevention approaches would be more efficient and effective if better coordinated. The Centers for Disease Control and Prevention's (CDC's) four-part domain framework, discussed previously, helps coordinate efforts across populations and topical disease areas and thus more efficiently deploy resources while reaching populations with the greatest need (Bauer et al. 2014).

Key Information Sources to Support Decision-Making

Program planning involves assessing the community, setting priorities and objectives, selecting interventions that address community conditions and priorities, implementing interventions, and evaluating results (Zaza et al. 2005). Key information sources are now available (Table 1-1) that assist with documenting the burden of disease, prioritizing health issues and interventions, establishing appropriate goals and targets, and understanding the effectiveness and sometimes cost-effectiveness of programs, policies, and interventions (Briss 2012).

Current Opportunities and Challenges

Perhaps the greatest opportunities to accelerate progress in chronic disease prevention and control are the transformations currently under way in the U.S. health care system (Shortell et al. 2000; CMS 2016a) and the emerging attention to what the Robert Wood Johnson Foundation terms "a culture of health" (RWJF 2016a). With the enactment of the Patient Protection and Affordable Care Act of 2010, numerous approaches are being tested to improve the quality of clinical care, reduce health care costs, and improve health outcomes. While many models and approaches are being tested, a central theme is improving population health. Health care system transformation has drawn the attention of health care providers and payers to population health. Seeking to contain and even reduce health care costs, and simultaneously deliver better outcomes, the health care delivery system is newly interested in public health strategies that improve the health of people in a community.

Because individuals spend most of their time outside the health care system and health is greatly influenced by what happens outside the health care setting, public health and health care—community and clinic—are collaborating to improve the community conditions that improve health. Improving the community conditions that support health is part of what the movement toward a culture of health seeks to achieve, such that all individuals have an equal opportunity to live the healthiest lives possible (RWJF 2016a; RWJF 2016b). Because of initiatives such as the Culture of Health, Communities Putting Prevention

Table 1-1. Sources of Evidence to Support Decision-Making

Source	Comments
Burden of disease	
CDC and NCHS (2016)	Regularly summarizes information on U.S. causes of death.
Behavioral Risk Factor Surveillance System (CDC 2016b)	Regularly provides information on risk behaviors, including the "actual" causes of death, and other issues at the state level.
State (UHF 2016) and county (RWJF 2016b) health rankings	Published annually by the United Health Foundation and the Robert Wood Johnson Foundation, respectively.
The Global Burden of Disease study (Institute for Health Metrics and Evaluation 2016)	Provides information on leading causes of morbidity, mortality, and disability for more than 100 countries worldwide.
Setting goals and targets	
Healthy People (USDHHS 2016b)	Sets health goals (~600) and objectives (~1200) for the nation that are frequently adapted for use in individual states.
	Also provides a shorter list of 26 leading health indicators, most of which are related to chronic diseases, conditions and risk factors.
Health care quality data for	Can be used for benchmarking and goal setting on a range of health care issues.
Health plans (NCQA 2016)	
Hospitals (The Joint Commission 2016)	
Group practices and providers (CMS 2016b)	
Intervention selection	
Cochrane Collaboration (Cochrane Collaboration 2016)	Provides good-quality systematic reviews, primarily related to medicine.
	A Cochrane Public Health Group has done some reviews related to the social determinants of health and health equity.
Campbell Collaboration (Campbell Collaboration 2016)	Provides good quality systematic reviews, primarily in education, criminal justice, and social welfare.
National Registry of Effective Programs and Practices (SAMHSA 2016)	Provide information on specific programs thought to have good supporting evidence and promoted as
Research Tested Intervention Programs (NCI 2016)	models for other communities on topical areas related to behavioral health and cancer, respectively.
Links evidence and recommendations	
The US Preventive Services Task Force (USPSTF 2016)	Link systematic reviews to practice recommendations:
	The USPSTF provides reviews and recommendations for clinical prevention in the United States.
National Institute for Health and Clinical Excellence (NICE 2016)	NICE provides reviews and recommendations related to health care for the United Kingdom.
The Guide to Community Preventive Services (The Community Preventive Services Task Force 2016)	The Community Guide provides recommendations for community prevention in the United States.

(Continued)

Table 1-1. (Continued)

Source	Comments
Other high-quality general evidence resources	
The US Surgeon General (USDHHS 2014; USDHHS 2016c)	Periodically issues reports summarizing evidence and making recommendations on the prevention of tobacco use and a broad range of other topics.
The National Academies (National Academies of Science, Engineering, Medicine: Health and Medicine Division 2016)	Issues reports summarizing evidence and making recommendations on a broad range of health and medical topics. Recently changed name from Institute of Medicine to reflect a broader health agenda.

to Work (Soler et al. 2016), Let's Move (Bumpus et al. 2015), Complete Streets (Smart Growth America 2016), and dozens more, Americans are increasingly demanding the conditions that promote health. From walkable communities to farmers' markets, tobacco-free environments, and sustainable food systems, there is renewed interest in expanding access to the things that promote health and a valuing of those things as part of our quality of life. Health care system transformation and community health are important opportunities for chronic disease prevention and control. Nonetheless, challenges remain.

Surveillance

Surveillance is needed to support policy and environmental change, health systems interventions, and community–clinical linkages. Many factors are currently driving the need for improvements in surveillance. First, high and increasing burden and cost related to chronic disease and its behavioral and other risk factors increases pressure for timely surveillance data to support decision-making and monitoring the effectiveness of interventions at federal, tribal, state, and local levels. Next, sources of data are regularly asynchronous and untimely. Third, there are perceived and real redundancies in some of the data systems used for surveillance or in results generated by those systems.

There are also emerging solutions that will help achieve integrated and timely surveillance of prevalent and incident chronic diseases and conditions for analysis, visualization, and action at national, tribal, state, and local levels. Over time, there will be greater use of the wealth of chronic disease information available in electronic health records and other clinical data sources, although health care data are not the whole solution. Next, there will be an increasing use of private-sector (e.g., marketing) data sources. Finally, federal data sources will continue to become faster, more efficient, and more coordinated.

Information Gaps and Translation Gaps

There are many remaining knowledge gaps that need to be filled to allow more and faster progress toward preventing and controlling chronic disease. For example, there remain many important knowledge gaps impeding progress in promoting physical activity, improving diets, and reducing obesity (IOM 2010). On the other hand, many chronic disease areas such as tobacco-use prevention and cardiovascular disease prevention and control have numerous known effective interventions that are inadequately resourced (e.g., state tobacco funding relative to CDC-recommended levels; CDC 2014) or inadequately delivered (e.g., effective clinical and community prevention for cardiovascular disease such as hypertension and cholesterol control is under-delivered; CDC 2011). Much more work is needed to find effective ways to fill these and other translation gaps.

Reach and Impact

Even the most effective public health efforts and programs fail to reach many people who could benefit from them. Examples include the more than 50% of the population who are still not covered by comprehensive smoke-free air laws (ANRF 2016), the still small numbers of the 86 million Americans with prediabetes who are currently reached by the Diabetes Prevention Program, and the 23.5 million people who have been estimated to live in food deserts (Ver Ploeg et al. 2009).

Much more work is needed to continue to expand the reach of programs, services, and health-promoting environments, both in the general population and in the most affected groups. Better coordination of public health programs is likely to help improve reach and efficiency. In addition, movement of individually oriented efforts outside clinical contexts (e.g., the Diabetes Prevention Program and tobacco quitlines), and delivery of such programs in ways other than one-on-one and face-to-face, are also likely to improve reach and efficiency.

Aging and Increasingly Diverse Population

Because of the public health successes of longer lives and lower birth rates, average ages of the population are increasing in the United States and worldwide (CDC 2003). For example, the proportion of adults aged older than 65 years has been projected to increase from 13% in 2010 to 20.2% in 2050 (Vincent and Velkoff 2010). Because older people use more health care and social services than younger people (CDC 2003), the public health successes that led to an aging population have resulted in strains on public health, health care, and social service resources. Public health efforts to address these challenges will need to particularly focus on moving services from clinic to community settings and from highly trained to lay providers, where appropriate, and on improving the behaviors that extend healthy life, thus facilitating high-value health care, linking people to needed services outside the clinic setting, improving efficiencies in health care delivery, and ultimately reducing the need for health care.

Without major shifts in the way health care is delivered in the United States, the increasing diversity of the U.S. population will likewise increasingly tax the public health and health care systems. Racial and ethnic minorities experience poorer health status, because of a variety of factors including upstream conditions such as lower income and education and downstream conditions and such as reduced access to quality health care. With the U.S. racial and ethnic minority population expected to reach 35% by 2020 (up from 28% in 2010; Hobbs and Stoops 2002), challenges to public health and health care will include growing a culturally diverse workforce, expanding team care (including community health workers and traditional healers), understanding and accommodating cultural attitudes toward health and disease, overcoming linguistic barriers, and improving overall cultural humility (Hook et al. 2013) and competency (Health Policy Institute 2004).

Disparities

Death and disability rates remain elevated among socioeconomically disadvantaged populations, for some racial and ethnic populations (particularly African Americans, Hispanics, and American Indians), and vary widely by geographic location (Minkler et al. 2006; Isaacs and Schroeder 2004; CDC 2013a). Woolf and colleagues have demonstrated that during the last decade of the 20th century, 886,202 premature deaths could have been averted in the United States by eliminating the disparity in death rates between blacks and whites (Woolf et al. 2008). Other investigators have noted the gaps between the poorest and richest Americans are much greater than the disparities in mortality between races at each level of income or education (Isaacs and Schroeder 2004). Recently, deaths have been increasing among some populations of poor and less educated whites, particularly from suicide, poisoning, and cirrhosis (Case and Deaton 2015).

Poverty has been associated with higher rates of morbidity, disability, and mortality for centuries. Possible explanations for these higher rates include the disproportionate burden of individual risk factors associated with poverty, but also a constellation of social conditions including inadequate or crowded housing, poor education, substandard medical care, exposures to hazardous environments, racial discrimination, and stressful life events (Murray et al. 2006). In the United States, there are also substantial disparities by geography. For example, in 2007, life expectancy at birth for American men and women was 75.6 and 80.8 years, respectively, with variations by county from 66 to 81 years for men and 74 to 86 years for women. The lowest life expectancies for both sexes were concentrated in the Southeast and Appalachia (Kulkarni et al. 2011). These high rates of morbidity and mortality in the south and Appalachia also are apparent for specific diseases, including heart disease (CDC 2013a; CDC 2013b).

Reducing and eliminating disparities in health status based on race, ethnicity, income, education, geography, and other factors is a critical step to ensure that all persons have the opportunity to achieve an optimal level of health. Multicomponent approaches—that reach people in different settings, from different vantage points, and with different messages, all converging on the same health problem—are generally most effective. Often, these will include whole-population and targeted strategies to increase the likelihood that as jurisdiction-wide trends improve, gaps between individuals based on race/ethnicity, gender, geography, and other factors actually narrow simultaneously. For example, tobacco-control policies that increase price, reduce exposure to secondhand smoke, provide support for cessation services, and educate the population on the dangers and consequences of tobacco use all work together to reduce tobacco use and are effective in a variety of populations, with intensive interventions as appropriate in particular jurisdictions or with particular populations. Targeted efforts such as CDC's Racial and Ethnic Approaches to Community Health (REACH) have served racial and ethnic populations with higher rates of disease and shown that disparities in risk factors and conditions can be reduced or eliminated with concentrated effort and effective interventions (Giles and Liburd 2006). A key challenge is how to scale and sustain such programs to achieve large and lasting impacts.

Global Health and Chronic Diseases

The changes described in the opening of this chapter in the major sources of disease and death seen in the United States and other high-income countries during the 20th century are now being seen throughout the world. Infections and other acute conditions continue to exact a tremendous toll on the health of persons living in low- and middle-income countries. However, these countries are simultaneously experiencing the emergence of chronic disease epidemics. The World Health Organization (WHO) estimated that, in 2012, chronic diseases—especially cardiovascular disease, cancer, and chronic respiratory diseases—caused 68% of all the deaths worldwide (up from 60% in 2000), and about 75% of these deaths occurred in low-income and middle-income countries (WHO 2016c; Mendis 2014). It is not just the large population size in many of these countries that accounts for this disproportionate burden. The age-standardized rates for chronic diseases in low- and middle-income countries exceed those observed in wealthier nations. This documents an enormous toll in premature mortality that will continue to increase unless there are major changes in health policy, training, and resource allocation.

Just as the traditional public health infrastructure in the United States still devotes disproportionate resources to infectious diseases, the international donor community has predominately focused on communicable conditions (Dear et al. 2007). To raise awareness about the burden and preventability of the chronic disease epidemic in the developing world, in 2014, the WHO set voluntary goals with the intent of reducing chronic disease death rates from cardiovascular diseases, cancer, and diabetes: to reduce sodium intake, the prevalence of inadequate physical activity, tobacco use, and inadequately treated high blood pressure; to halt the rise of obesity and diabetes; to increase treatment intended to prevent heart attacks and strokes; and to increase the availability of essential medicines and basic technologies to treat major chronic diseases (WHO 2014).

In addition to developing policies and health systems priorities that address these health problems, there will also need to be improvements in the training received by health care and public health workers. The current medical and public health workforce in developing countries is inadequate in terms of numbers, and has also been primarily trained to address acute health problems. Effective care for older patients and populations requires ongoing attention to lifestyle behaviors and coordinated care for complex, chronic conditions that often require multiple specialties and interventions across a variety of settings (Pruitt and Epping-Jordan 2005). Although the science, strategies, and public health approaches described in this book are based on evidence from high-income nations, they are relevant to current challenges in global health (Koplan et al. 2009).

Ongoing work on chronic diseases internationally provides reason for optimism. In addition to the work of WHO noted previously and work in countries to achieve public health goals, initiatives such as the Bloomberg Initiative to Reduce Tobacco Use (2016), and the Bill & Melinda Gates Foundation Tobacco Control in Africa project (Bill and Melinda Gates Foundation 2016) are also stimulating high-quality work and bringing much-needed resources to bear on a major cause of disease, disability, and premature death.

Workforce and Training

The skills required for the successful public health professional continue to broaden. For some time, skills have been required in epidemiology, public health management, and community organization, but new skills are always being added. Current examples include traditional and new communication, informatics, and the ability to bridge health care and public health to improve population health. In addition, the ability to work across sectors and with a broadening range of professionals is essential. However, assessments of the workforce engaged in institutional public health routinely identify major deficiencies in the education, training, and experience of the practitioners in this workforce (Thacker 2005; Coronado et al. 2014).

In 2002, the Institute of Medicine (IOM) published a report, "Who Will Keep the Public Healthy? Educating Public Health Professionals for the 21st Century," which identified the training needs of the public health workforce now and into the future (Gebbie et al. 2003). This report called for greater funding and support for training and developing the public health workforce to meet current and emerging skill needs. Some progress is being made, including creative approaches to using distance learning and relatively new undergraduate training in public health (Coronado et al. 2014). However, critical barriers remain, including providing continuing education and training for current public health professionals and matching governmental hiring systems to workforce needs. In spite of important progress in some areas, achieving progress in initial and ongoing training of the public health workforce will continue to be a challenge for the foreseeable future.

Coordinating Multisector Approaches

Chronic disease prevention and control is never accomplished by one actor alone. Success is achieved when interventions occur at multiple levels (e.g., local, state, and federal), involve multiple sectors (e.g., health, health care, housing, education, transportation, agriculture, and justice), and are implemented in multiple settings (e.g., schools, child care and early learning, workplaces, and public places). Building, strengthening, and activating these multisectoral coalitions and coordinating work across a variety of sectors is an essential component of population health improvement. As has been noted by IOM,

> . . . in a society as diverse and decentralized as that of the United States, achieving population health requires contributions from all levels of government, the private business sector, and the variety of institutions and organizations that shape opportunities, attitudes, behaviors, and resources affecting health (IOM 2003).

The National Prevention, Health Promotion, and Public Health Council, established under the Patient Protection and Affordable Care Act of 2010, is a federal-level multisectoral coalition comprising 21 federal departments and agencies joined together to implement the National Prevention Strategy (National Prevention Council 2014), focused on increasing the number of Americans who are healthy at every stage of life, by advancing seven strategic priorities, through action by each council member. Members as diverse as Departments of Interior, Defense, Housing, and Agriculture are adopting tobacco-free policies, improving nutritional quality of foods offered, increasing opportunities for physical activity, and identifying opportunities to improve mental and emotional well-being—all foundational actions to prevent and control chronic diseases. The remaining three strategic priorities are preventing drug abuse and excessive alcohol use, reproductive and sexual health, and injury- and violence-free living.

Conclusions

Further progress in chronic disease prevention and control will require sustained effort to make communities healthier, strengthen environments to better support health and healthful behaviors, and increase access to and quality of health care services. It will require hard work in the public and private sectors, at all levels of civil society, and with the active engagement of employers and businesses, planning and economic development, and multiple sectors embracing health goals from multiple perspectives. It will require people in the United States and the world valuing health, and making individual and collective changes to help people live longer, healthier, more productive, and more connected lives. It will not be easy, but it is a challenge worth taking on.

Acknowledgment

The findings and conclusions in this chapter are those of the authors and do not necessarily represent the official position of the Centers for Disease Control and Prevention.

Resources

Guide to Community Preventive Services, http://www.thecommunityguide.org

Health system transformation and improvement resources for health departments, https://www.cdc.gov/stltpublichealth/program/transformation/index.html

Healthy People 2020, https://www.healthypeople.gov

Suggested Reading

Berwick DM, Nolan TW, Whittington, J. The triple aim: care, health, and cost. *Health Aff (Millwood).* 2008;27(3):759–769.

Eaton WW. *Public Mental Health.* Oxford, UK: Oxford University Press; 2012.

Institute of Medicine. *The Future of the Public's Health in the 21st Century.* Washington, DC: National Academy Press; 2003.

Marmot M, Wilkenson RG. *Social Determinants of Health.* 2nd ed. Oxford, UK: Oxford University Press; 2008.

Rose G. *The Strategy of Preventive Medicine.* New York, NY: Oxford University Press; 1992.

World Health Organization. *Preventing Chronic Diseases: A Vital Investment.* Geneva, Switzerland: World Health Organization; 2005.

References

Alley DE, Asomugha CN, Conway PH, Sanghavi DM. Accountable health communities—addressing social needs through Medicare and Medicaid. *N Engl J Med.* 2016;374(1):8–11.

American Nonsmokers' Rights Foundation (ANRF). Summary of 100% smokefree state laws and population protected by 100% US smokefree laws. 2016. Available at: http://www.no-smoke.org/goingsmokefree.php?id=519. Accessed May 25, 2016.

Barbour KE, Helmick CG, Theis KA, et al. Prevalence of doctor-diagnosed arthritis and arthritis-attributable activity limitation—United States, 2010–2012. *MMWR Morb Mortal Wkly Rep.* 2013;62(14):869–873.

Bauer UE, Briss PA, Goodman RA, Bowman BA. Preventing chronic disease in the 21st century: eliminating the leading preventable causes of premature death and disability in the United States. *Lancet.* 2014;384(9937):45–52.

Bernstein AB, Hing E, Moss AJ, Allen KF, Siller AB, Tiggle RB. *Health Care in America: Trends in Utilization.* Hyattsville, MD: National Center for Health Statistics; 2003.

Berwick DM, Nolan TW, Whittington J. The triple aim: care, health, and cost. *Health Aff (Millwood).* 2008;27(3):759–769.

Berwick DM. Launching accountable care organizations—the proposed rule for the Medicare Shared Savings Program. *N Engl J Med.* 2011;364(16):e32.

Bill and Melinda Gates Foundation. Tobacco control strategy overview. 2016. Available at: http://www.gatesfoundation.org/What-We-Do/Global-Policy/Tobacco-Control. 2016. Accessed May 25, 2016.

Bloomberg Initiative to Reduce Tobacco Use. Bloomberg Initiative to Reduce Tobacco Use grants program: about the Bloomberg Initiative. 2016. Available at: http://tobaccocontrolgrants.org/Pages/44/About-the-Bloomberg-Initiative. Accessed May 25, 2016.

Bouchery EE, Harwood HJ, Sacks JJ, Simon CJ, Brewer RD. Economic costs of excessive alcohol consumption in the United States, 2006. *Am J Prev Med.* 2011;41(5):516–524.

Bradley EH, Taylor LA. *The American Health Care Paradox: Why Spending More Is Getting Us Less.* New York, NY: Public Affairs Books; 2013.

Briss PA. *The Guide to Community Preventive Services*. Oxford Bibliographies Online. 2012. Available at: http://www.oxfordbibliographies.com/view/document/obo-9780199756797/obo-9780199756797-0024.xml. Accessed May 25, 2016.

Bumpus K, Taqtow A, Haven J. Let's Move! celebrates 5 years. *J Acad Nutr Diet.* 2015;115(3):338–341.

Campbell Collaboration. The Campbell Collaboration: What helps? What harms? Based on what evidence? 2016. Available at: http://www.campbellcollaboration.org. Accessed May 25, 2016.

Case A, Deaton A. Rising morbidity and mortality in midlife among white non-Hispanic Americans in the 21st century. *Proc Natl Acad Sci U S A.* 2015;112(49):1–6.

Centers for Disease Control and Prevention (CDC). Trends in aging—United States and worldwide. *MMWR Morb Mortal Wkly Rep.* 2003;52(6):101–104, 106.

Centers for Disease Control and Prevention (CDC). Million hearts: strategies to reduce the prevalence of leading cardiovascular disease risk factors—United States, 2011. *MMWR Morb Mortal Wkly Rep.* 2011;60(36):1248–1251.

Centers for Disease Control and Prevention (CDC). CDC health disparities and inequalities report—United States, 2013. Foreword. *MMWR Suppl.* 2013a;62S(3):S1–S187.

Centers for Disease Control and Prevention (CDC). Vital signs: avoidable deaths from heart disease, stroke, and hypertensive disease—United States, 2001–2010. *MMWR Morb Mortal Wkly Rep.* 2013b;62(35):721–727.

Centers for Disease Control and Prevention (CDC). *Best Practices for Comprehensive Tobacco Control Programs—2014*. Atlanta, GA: National Center for Chronic Disease Prevention and Health Promotion, Office on Smoking and Health; 2014.

Centers for Disease Control and Prevention (CDC), National Center for Health Statistics (NCHS). Early release of selected estimates based on data from the National Health Interview Survey, January–March 2015. 2015. Available at: https://www.cdc.gov/nchs/data/nhis/earlyrelease/earlyrelease201509_08.pdf. Accessed May 25, 2016.

Centers for Disease Control and Prevention (CDC). US cancer statistics: an interactive cancer atlas. 2016a. Available at: https://nccd.cdc.gov/DCPC_INCA. Accessed April 16, 2016.

Centers for Disease Control and Prevention (CDC). Behavioral Risk Factor Surveillance System. 2016b. Available at: http://www.cdc.gov/brfss. Accessed May 25, 2016.

Centers for Medicare and Medicaid Services (CMS). CMS quality strategy. 2016a. Available at: https://www.cms.gov/medicare/quality-initiatives-patient-assessment-instruments/qualityinitiativesgeninfo/downloads/cms-quality-strategy.pdf. Accessed May 26, 2016.

Centers for Medicare and Medicaid Services (CMS). About Physician Compare. 2016b. Available at: https://www.medicare.gov/physiciancompare/staticpages/about physiciancompare/about.html. Accessed May 26, 2016.

Cochrane Collaboration. 2016. Available at: http://www.cochrane.org. Accessed May 26, 2016.

Colton CW, Manderscheid RW. Congruencies in increased mortality rates, years of potential life lost, and causes of death among public mental health clients in eight states. *Prev Chronic Dis.* 2006;3(2):A42.

Community Preventive Services Task Force. *The Guide to Community Preventive Services: What Works to Promote Health?* 2016. Available at: http://www.thecommunityguide.org. Accessed May 26, 2016.

Coronado F, Koo D, Gebbie K. The public health workforce: moving forward in the 21st century. *Am J Prev Med.* 2014;47(5 suppl 3):S275–S277.

Dear AS, Singer PA, Persad DL, et al. Grand challenges in chronic non-communicable disease. *Nature.* 2007;450(7169):494–496.

Druss BG, Zhao L, Von Esenwein S, Morrato EH, Marcus SC. Understanding excess mortality in persons with mental illness: 17-year follow up of a nationally representative US survey. *Med Care.* 2011;49(6):599–604.

Dunn A, Rittmueller L, Whitmire B. The New BEA Health Care Satellite Account. US Department of Commerce, Bureau of Economic Analysis. 2015. Available at: http://www.bea.gov/national/health_care_satellite_account.htm. Accessed April 16, 2016.

Federal Interagency Forum on Aging-Related Statistics. *Older Americans 2012: Key Indicators of Well-Being. Federal Interagency Forum on Aging-Related Statistics.* Washington, DC: US Government Printing Office; 2012.

Finkelstein EA, Trogdon JG, Cohen JW, Dietz W. Annual medical spending attributable to obesity: payer-and service-specific estimates. *Health Aff (Millwood)* 2009;28(5): w822–w831.

Flegal KM, Graubard BI, Williamson DF, Gail MH. Excess deaths associated with underweight, overweight, and obesity. *JAMA.* 2005;293(15):1861–1867.

Ford ES, Ajani UA, Croft JB, et al. Explaining the decrease in US deaths from coronary disease, 1980–2000. *N Engl J Med.* 2007;356(23):2388–2398.

Ford ES, Bergmann MM, Kroger J, Schienkiewitz A, Weikert C, Boeing H. Healthy living is the best revenge. *Arch Intern Med.* 2009;169(15):1355–1362.

Frieden TR. A framework for public health action: the Health Impact Pyramid. *Am J Public Health.* 2010;100(4):590–595.

Fries JF, Koop CE, Beadle CE, et al. Reducing health care costs by reducing the need and demand for medical services. The Health Project Consortium. *N Engl J Med.* 1993;329(5):321–325.

Fryar CD, Chen T, Li X. Prevalence of uncontrolled risk factors for cardiovascular disease: United States, 1999–2010. Hyattsville, MD: National Center for Health Statistics; 2012. NCHS Data Brief, no. 103.

Gebbie K, Rosenstock L, Hernandez LM, eds. *Who Will Keep the Public Healthy? Educating Public Health Professionals for the 21st Century.* Washington, DC: National Academies Press; 2003.

Gerteis J, Izrael D, Deitz D, et al. *Multiple Chronic Conditions Chartbook.* Rockville, MD: Agency for Healthcare Research and Quality; 2014. AHRQ publications no. Q14-0038.

Giles WH, Liburd L. Reflections on the past, reaching for the future: REACH 2010—the first 7 years. *Health Promot Pract.* 2006;7(suppl 3):179S–180S.

Goodman RA, Posner SF, Huang ES, Parekh AK, Koh HK. Defining and measuring chronic conditions: imperatives for research, policy, program, and practice. *Prev Chronic Dis.* 2013;10:e66.

Health Policy Institute. Cultural competence in health care: is it important for people with chronic conditions? 2004. Available at: https://hpi.georgetown.edu/agingsociety/pubhtml/cultural/cultural.html. Accessed May 24, 2016. Issue Brief no. 5.

Hobbs F, Stoops D. Demographic trends in the 20th century: Census 2000 special reports. 2002:10. Available at: https://www.census.gov/prod/2002pubs/censr-4.pdf. Accessed May 24, 2016.

Hook JN, Davis DE, Owen J, Worthington EL, Utsey SO. Cultural humility: measuring openness to culturally diverse clients. *J Couns Psychol.* 2013;60(3):353–366.

Hootman JM, Brault MW, Helmick CG, Theis KA, Armour BS. Prevalence and most common causes of disability among adults—United States, 2005. *MMWR Morb Mortal Wkly Rep.* 2009;58(16):421–426.

Institute for Health Metrics and Evaluation. Global Burden of Disease (GBD). 2016. Available at: http://www.healthdata.org/gbd. Accessed May 26, 2016.

Institute of Medicine (IOM). *The Future of the Public's Health in the 21st Century.* Washington, DC: National Academy Press; 2003:17.

Institute of Medicine (IOM). *Bridging the Evidence Gap in Obesity Prevention: A Framework to Inform Decision Making.* Washington, DC: The National Academies Press; 2010.

Isaacs SL, Schroeder SA. Class—the ignored determinant of the nation's health. *N Engl J Med.* 2004;351(11):1137–1142.

The Joint Commission. America's hospitals: improving quality and safety—The Joint Commission's Annual Report 2015. 2016. Available at: https://www.jointcommission. org/annualreport.aspx. Accessed August 4, 2016.

Kanny D, Liu Y, Brewer RD, Garvin WS, Balluz L. Binge drinking prevalence, frequency, and intensity—United States, 2010. *MMWR Morb Mortal Wkly Rep.* 2012; 61(1):14–19.

Koplan J, Bond TC, Merson M, et al. Towards a common definition of global health. *Lancet.* 2009;373(9679):1993–1995.

Kulkarni SC, Levin-Rector A, Ezzati M, Murray CJ. Falling behind: life expectancy in US counties from 2000 to 2007 in an international context. *Popul Health Metr.* 2011;9(1):16.

Laursen TM, Munk-Olse T, Nordentoft M, Mortensen PB. Increased mortality among patients admitted with major psychiatric disorders: a register-based study comparing mortality in unipolar depressive disorder, bipolar affective disorder, schizoaffective disorder, and schizophrenia. *J Clin Psychiatry.* 2007;68(6):899–907.

Lawrence D, Kisely S. Inequalities in healthcare provision for people with severe mental illness. *J Psychopharmacol.* 2010;24(suppl 4):61–68.

Manderscheid R, Kathol R. Fostering sustainable, integrated medical and behavioral health services in medical settings. *Ann Intern Med.* 2014;160(1):61–65.

McGinnis JM, Foege WH. Actual causes of death in the United States. *JAMA.* 1993;270(18):2207–2212.

McKeowan RE. The epidemiologic transition: changing patterns of mortality and population dynamics. *Am J Lifestyle Med.* 2009;3(suppl 1):S19–S26.

Melek SP, Norris DT, Paulus J. *Economic Impact of Integrated Medical-Behavioral Healthcare: Implications for Psychiatry.* Denver, CO: Milliman Inc; 2014.

Mendis S. *Global Status Report on Noncommunicable Diseases.* Geneva, Switzerland: World Health Organization; 2014.

Miller HD. From volume to value: better ways to pay for health care. *Health Aff (Millwood).* 2009;28(5):1418–1428.

Minkler M, Fuller-Thomson E, Guralnik JM. Gradient of disability across the socioeconomic spectrum in the United States. *N Engl J Med.* 2006;355(7):695–703.

Mirel LB, Carper K. Trends in health care expenditures for the elderly, age 65 and over: 2001, 2006, and 2011. Agency for Healthcare Research and Quality. 2014. Statistical Brief no. 429. Available at: http://www.meps.ahrq.gov/mepsweb/data_files/publications/st429/ stat429.pdf. Accessed August 4, 2016.

Mokdad AH, Marks JS, Stroup DF, Gerberding JL. Actual causes of death in the United States, 2000. *JAMA*. 2004:291(10):1238–1245.

Mossialos E, Wenzl M, Osborn R, Anderson C. 2014 international profiles of health care systems: Australia, Canada, Denmark, England, France, Germany, Italy, Japan, the Netherlands, New Zealand, Norway, Singapore, Sweden, Switzerland, and the United States. New York, NY: The Commonwealth Fund; 2015.

Murray CJ, Gakidou EE, Frenk J. Health inequalities and social group differences: what should we measure? *Bull WHO*. 1999:77(7):537–543.

Murray CJ, Kulkarni SC, Michaud C, et al. Eight Americas: investigating mortality disparities across races, counties, and race-counties in the United States. *PLoS Med*. 2006:3(9):e260.

National Academies of Science, Engineering, Medicine. Health and Medicine Division. 2016. Available at: http://www.nationalacademies.org/hmd. Accessed May 26, 2016.

National Center for Health Statistics (NCHS). *Health, United States, 2010: With Special Feature on Death and Dying*. Hyattsville, MD: National Center for Health Statistics; 2011.

National Cancer Institute (NCI). Research-tested intervention programs (RTIPs): RTIPs—moving science into programs for people. 2016. Available at: http://rtips.cancer.gov/rtips/index.do. Accessed May 26, 2016.

National Committee for Quality Assurance (NCQA). *HEDIS and Performance Measurement*. 2016. Available at: http://www.ncqa.org/hedis-quality-measurement. Accessed May 26, 2016.

National Heart, Lung, and Blood Institute (NHLBI). *Morbidity and Mortality: 2012 Chart Book on Cardiovascular, Lung, and Blood Diseases*. 2012. Available at: http://www.nhlbi.nih.gov/research/reports/2012-mortality-chart-book. Accessed May 25, 2016.

National Institute for Health and Care Excellence (NICE). Improving health and social care through evidence-based guidance. 2016. Available at: https://www.nice.org.uk. Accessed May 26, 2016.

National Prevention Council. *Annual Status Report*. Washington, DC: US Department of Health and Human Services, Office of the Surgeon General; 2014. Available at: http://www.surgeongeneral.gov/priorities/prevention/about/annual_status_reports.html. Accessed May 25, 2016.

O'Connor SM, Taylor CE, Hughes JM. Emerging infectious determinants of chronic diseases. *Emerg Infect Dis*. 2006;12(7):1051–1057.

Ogden CL, Carroll MD, Kit BK, Flegal KM. Prevalence of childhood and adult obesity in the United States, 2011–2012. *JAMA*. 2014;311(8):806–814.

Omran AR. The epidemiologic transition: a theory of the epidemiology of population change. *Milbank Q.* 2005;83(4):731–757.

Pruitt SD, Epping-Jordan JE. Preparing the 21st century global healthcare workforce. *BMJ.* 2005;330(7492):637–639.

Robert Wood Johnson Foundation (RWJF). About a Culture of Health: a new vision of health in America. 2016a. Available at: https://www.cultureofhealth.org/en/about.html. Accessed August 4, 2016.

Robert Wood Johnson Foundation (RWJF). County Health Rankings and Roadmaps. 2016b. Available at: http://www.countyhealthrankings.org. Accessed May 26, 2016.

Rose G. *The Strategy of Preventive Medicine.* New York, NY: Oxford University Press; 1992.

Shortell SM, Gillies RR, Anderson DA, Erickson KM, Mitchell JB. *Remaking Health Care in America: The Evolution of Organized Delivery Systems.* San Francisco, CA: Jossey-Bass; 2000.

Smart Growth America. Complete Streets: A to Z. 2016. Available at: http://www.smartgrowthamerica.org/complete-streets/a-to-z. Accessed May 26, 2016.

Soler R, Orenstein D, Honeycutt A, et al. Community-based interventions to decrease obesity and tobacco exposure and reduce health care costs: outcome estimates from communities putting prevention to work for 2010–2020. *Prev Chronic Dis.* 2016;13:E47.

Substance Abuse and Mental Health Services Administration (SAMHSA), Center for Behavioral Health Statistics and Quality (CBHSQ). *Behavioral Health Trends in the United States: Results From the 2014 National Survey on Drug Use and Health.* Rockville, MD: Center for Behavioral Health Statistics and Quality; 2015. HHS publication no. SMA 15-4927, NSDUH Series H-50.

Substance Abuse and Mental Health Services Administration (SAMHSA). SAMHSA's National Registry of Evidence-Based Programs and Practices. 2016. Available at: http://www.nrepp.samhsa.gov/01_landing.aspx. Accessed May 26, 2016.

Tabak AG, Herder C, Rathmann W, Brunner EJ, Kivimaki M. Prediabetes: a high risk state for developing diabetes. *Lancet.* 2012;379(9833):2279–2290.

Thacker SB. How do we ensure the quality of the public health workforce? *Prev Chronic Dis.* 2005:2(2):A06.

United Health Foundation (UHF). America's Health Rankings. 2016. Available at: http://www.americashealthrankings.org. Accessed May 26, 2016.

US Cancer Statistics Working Group. United States Cancer Statistics: 1999–2013. Incidence and mortality Web-based report. US Department of Health and Human

Services, Centers for Disease Control and Prevention, National Cancer Institute. 2016. Available at: https://nccd.cdc.gov/uscs. Accessed September 14, 2016.

US Department of Health and Human Services (USDHHS). *Multiple Chronic Conditions—A Strategic Framework: Optimum Health and Quality of Life for Individuals With Multiple Chronic Conditions.* Washington, DC: US Department of Health and Human Services; 2010.

US Department of Health and Human Services (USDHHS). *The Health Consequences of Smoking–50 Years of Progress: A Report of the Surgeon General.* Atlanta, GA: US Department of Health and Human Services, Centers for Disease Control and Prevention; 2014.

US Department of Health and Human Services (USDHHS). *Health, United States, 2015: With Special Feature on Racial and Ethnic Health Disparities.* Atlanta, GA: Centers for Disease Control and Prevention, National Center for Health Statistics; 2016a. DHHS publication no. 2016-1232.

US Department of Health and Human Services (USDHHS), Office of Disease Prevention and Health Promotion. *Healthy People 2020.* 2016b. Available at: https://www.healthypeople.gov. Accessed May 26, 2016.

US Department of Health and Human Services (USDHHS). Reports of the Surgeon General, US Public Health Service. 2016c. Available at: http://www.surgeongeneral.gov/library/reports. Accessed May 26, 2016.

US Preventive Services Task Force (USPSTF). US Preventive Services Task Force: Home. 2016. Available at: http://www.uspreventiveservicestaskforce.org. Accessed May 26, 2016.

Ver Ploeg M, Breneman V, Farrigan T, et al. Access to affordable and nutritious food—measuring and understanding food deserts and their consequences: report to Congress. 2009. Administrative publication no. AP-036. Available at: http://www.ers.usda.gov/publications/ap-administrative-publication/ap-036.aspx. Accessed May 25, 2016.

Vincent GK, Velkoff VA. *The Next Four Decades, the Older Population in the United States: 2010 to 2050.* Washington, DC: US Census Bureau; 2010. Current Population Reports, P25-1138.

Ward BW, Schiller JS, Goodman RA. Multiple chronic conditions among US adults: a 2012 update. *Prev Chronic Dis.* 2014;11:E62.

Woolf SH, Johnson RE, Fryer GE Jr, Rust G, Satcher D. The health impact of resolving racial disparities: an analysis of US mortality data. *Am J Public Health.* 2008;98 (suppl 9):S26–S28.

World Health Organization (WHO). NCD global monitoring framework: ensuring progress on noncommunicable diseases in countries. 2014. Available at: http://www.who.int/nmh/global_monitoring_framework/en. Accessed May 28, 2016.

World Health Organization (WHO). Noncommunicable diseases. 2016a. Available at: http://www.who.int/topics/noncommunicable_diseases/en. Accessed May 24, 2016.

World Health Organization (WHO). Global Health Observatory data repository. Life expectancy data by country. 2016b. Available at: http://apps.who.int/gho/data/view. main.SDG2016LEXv. Accessed May 24, 2016.

World Health Organization (WHO). Global Health Observatory data: NCD mortality and morbidity. 2016c. Available at: http://www.who.int/gho/ncd/mortality_morbidity/ en. Accessed May 24, 2016.

Xu JQ, Murphy SL, Kochanek KD, Bastian BA. *Deaths: Final Data for 2013*. Hyattsville, MD: National Center for Health Statistics; 2016. National Vital Statistics Reports, vol. 64(2).

Xu X, Bishop EE, Kennedy SM, Simpson SA, Pechacek TF. Annual healthcare spending attributable to cigarette smoking: an update. *Am J Prev Med*. 2014;48(3):326–333.

Zaza S, Briss P, Harris, K, eds. *The Guide to Community Preventive Services*. New York, NY: Oxford University Press; 2005.

Zhuo X, Zhang P, Kahn HS, Gregg EW. Cost-effectiveness of alternative thresholds of the fasting plasma glucose test to identify the target population for type 2 diabetes prevention in adults aged ≥ 45 years. *Diabetes Care*. 2013;36(12):3992–3998.

2

CHRONIC DISEASE EPIDEMIOLOGY

Robert Redwood, MD, MPH, Patrick L. Remington, MD, MPH, and
Ross C. Brownson, PhD

Introduction

As noted in Chapter 1, chronic diseases are distinguished from other health
problems by their multiple and interrelated causes often rooted in early life
and related to multiple health factors, including individual behaviors, health
care, social and economic factors, and the environment. As public health
advances have reduced the burden from infectious diseases, chronic diseases
have become the leading causes of death and disability in the United States. In
addition, many people are surviving with chronic diseases, as most are controlled through health care or lifestyle interventions, rather than being cured
or rapidly fatal.

The field of epidemiology has been invaluable in understanding the causes
of chronic diseases and measuring the effects of interventions to prevent
chronic diseases. Each of the chapters in this book, which describe chronic
diseases, conditions, and risk factors, is organized to address these two basic
questions:

1. What is the epidemiology of this problem? That is, what do we know
   about the burden of chronic diseases, their distribution in populations,
   and their causes?
2. What can be done to control this problem in the population? That is,
   what are effective strategies to prevent, detect, and treat this problem in
   populations?

The purpose of this chapter is to provide a brief overview of the methods that
can be used to answer this first question, by summarizing the methods used to
understand the epidemiology of chronic diseases, conditions, and risk factors.

Breast cancer and tobacco use will be used to illustrate the various methods used in chronic disease epidemiology and control. The next chapter (Chapter 3, Chronic Disease Surveillance) provides additional information about how public health surveillance can be used to measure and monitor chronic diseases and their risk factors in populations. And the following two chapters describe what can be done to prevent or control chronic diseases in communities (Chapter 4, Community-Based Interventions) and health care systems (Chapter 5, The Role of Health Care Systems in Chronic Disease Prevention and Control).

Definition of Epidemiology

Epidemiology is considered the "science of public health." The word comes from the Greek terms *epi* (upon), *demos* (people), and *logos* (study); thus, it is literally the study upon people. Traditionally, epidemiology was defined as the "study of the distribution and determinants of disease in populations." Over time, this definition broadened to include the study of other health states, such as injury, disability, risk factors, and health-related quality of life.

More than 40 years ago, William Foege coined the term "consequential epidemiology" to further broaden the definition of the term to include the use of epidemiology in disease control (Koplan and Thacker 2001). He stated that "the reason for collecting, analyzing, and disseminating information on a disease is to control that disease. Collection and analysis should not be allowed to consume resources if action does not follow" (Foege et al. 1976).

The Centers for Disease Control and Prevention (CDC) currently defines epidemiology as "the study of the distribution and determinants of health-related states or events in specified populations, and the application of this study to the control of health problems." The key words include the following (CDC 2016):

- Study: Epidemiology is a quantitative discipline based on principles of statistics and research methods.
- Distribution: Epidemiologists study the distribution of health events within groups in a population, characterizing health events in terms of person, place, and time. This type of epidemiology is referred to as "descriptive epidemiology."
- Determinants: Epidemiologists also search for determinants (i.e., causes or factors) that are associated with increased risk or probability of disease. This type of epidemiology, where we move from questions of

who, what, where, and when and start trying to answer how and why, is referred to as "analytical epidemiology."

- Health-related states: Whereas infectious diseases were clearly the focus of much of the early epidemiological work, the field is no longer limited in this way. Epidemiology as it is practiced today is applied to the whole spectrum of health-related events, which includes chronic diseases, conditions, and risk factors. Although not addressed in this chapter, some forward-thinking epidemiologists are further expanding the concept of health-related states, applying epidemiologic methods to broader social ills (e.g., drug addiction, firearm violence, homelessness).

- Populations: One of the most important distinguishing characteristics of epidemiology is that it deals with groups of people rather than with individual patients.

- Control: Finally, although epidemiology can be used simply as an analytical tool for studying diseases and their determinants, it can also play a more active role. Epidemiological data and methods steer public health decision-making and aid in developing and evaluating interventions to control and prevent health problems. This is the primary function of applied, field, or consequential epidemiology.

Brownson and Petitti (2006) defined "applied epidemiology" according to the intended purpose. In their view, the field can be defined on the basis of five core purposes: (1) the synthesis of the results of etiologic studies as input to practice-oriented policies; (2) the description of disease and risk factor patterns as information to set priorities; (3) the evaluation of public health programs, laws, and policies; (4) the measurement of the patterns and outcomes of health care; and (5) the communication of epidemiological findings effectively to health professionals and the public.

The Chronic Disease Continuum

For diseases of known infectious origin, such as AIDS, measles, and influenza, the presence of a single, known, necessary cause (e.g., the microorganism) helps to focus epidemiological research and intervention strategies. For injuries, the cause is often acute and leads to immediate health consequences, such as drinking and driving or a child drowning.

In contrast, the wide variety of chronic diseases lacks such unifying causal agents and often develops over the life course. Research has demonstrated that many chronic diseases have their origins early in the life course (Felitti et al. 1998). These early life experiences and exposures to social and economic factors increase the risk of unhealthy behaviors later in life. Unhealthy behaviors eventually lead to conditions such as hypertension, obesity, or high blood cholesterol. Finally, individuals with these conditions are at increased risk for developing chronic diseases, such as heart disease, cancer, or diabetes.

This model of a chronic disease continuum is shown in Figure 2-1 and has been used to organize this text, with different parts for chronic disease risk factors, chronic disease conditions, and chronic diseases. The chronic disease continuum also requires special methods for chronic disease epidemiology and control. Because the causal process is prolonged and typically complex, many modest influences, rather than a single predominant cause, contribute to the probability of developing disease. The prolonged duration of these diseases, which often includes a presymptomatic phase and subsequent development of chronic disease conditions, provides numerous overlapping opportunities for intervention. For most chronic diseases, the large number of modest risk factors and the diverse opportunities for

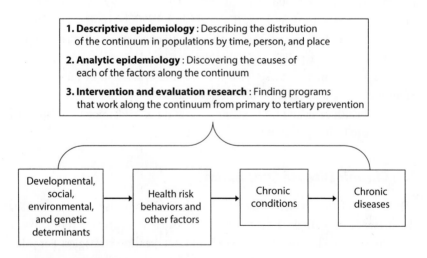

Figure 2-1. Methods Used in Chronic Disease Epidemiology, Prevention, and Control, Applied along the Chronic Disease Continuum

intervention make their control difficult and typically require a multifaceted approach.

Because disease is the end result of a continuum, it is sometimes difficult to determine whether "disease" is even present at all. For example, the large increase in mammography over the late 1980s and 1990s has led to a large increase in the incidence of a pathological lesion known as ductal carcinoma in situ (DCIS). Although DCIS is not invasive breast cancer and many women with DCIS will not develop invasive breast cancer, DCIS is often treated in the same way as invasive cancer—that is, by surgical excision. Many women with DCIS consider themselves to have "breast cancer." Similarly, many men with "prostate cancer" actually have a pathological lesion that would never have progressed to clinical disease. In general, as our ability to detect earlier and earlier stages of the disease process improves, the point at which disease truly begins becomes increasingly unclear (Fryback et al. 2006).

Another important consideration for chronic disease is the meaning of "control" or what it is we are trying to prevent. Chronic disease often affects the quality of life long before it affects the duration of life, if it affects duration at all. People with diabetes, for example, do have higher mortality, but only many years after diagnosis. In the interim, however, they may experience blindness, kidney failure, painful feet ulcers, leg amputation, or premature heart disease, all as a direct result of having diabetes. "Controlling" diabetes implies not only prolonging life, but also, as importantly, improving the quality of life while one is living with diabetes. Both disease-specific and general measures of quality of life have been developed and validated (McDowell and Newell 2006), and these measures are being used increasingly to describe the course ("natural history") of disease as well as the effect of various methods of control.

There is a need to pay careful attention to methodological principles in many areas of the study and control of chronic disease. The need for clarity of terminology and thought is enhanced by the advancements that have been made and the expansion of options for tackling chronic disease through public health measures. In this chapter, we provide some basic terms and concepts common in epidemiological literature on the etiology (i.e., causes), consequences, and control of chronic diseases. We also describe how epidemiology has been used to better understand the factors that increase (or decrease) a person's risk of progressing along the chronic disease continuum shown in Figure 2-1.

Building on this continuum, each chapter in Parts II through IV of this text has the following sections:

1. Significance: The first section of each chapter provides an overview of the "significance" of the disease, condition, or risk factor in populations. This section measures the burden to public health by estimating the number of people affected, rates, and economic costs.

2. Pathophysiology: The second section of each chapter describes the biology and pathophysiology of the disease, condition, or risk factor. This information is important to understand when one is interpreting epidemiological information or designing interventions.

3. Descriptive epidemiology: The third section of each chapter provides an overview of the "distribution" of the disease, condition, or risk factor in populations. This section uses "descriptive epidemiology" to identify high-risk groups (person), geographic variation (place), and secular trends (time).

4. Causes: The fourth section of each chapter provides an overview of the "causes" of the disease, condition, or risk factor in populations. This section uses "analytic epidemiology" to identify those factors that increase the risk of an individual developing a chronic disease, condition, or risk factor. Special techniques, described in the "Analytic Epidemiology" section, are used to go beyond finding associations to finding factors that are causally related to the outcome of interest.

5. Evidence-based interventions: The final section of each chapter provides an overview of the interventions that may be used to prevent or control the chronic disease, condition, or risk factor. These methods go beyond the use of epidemiology to determine the causes to finding programs that affect the disease course, along the continuum from primary prevention to secondary and tertiary prevention. The final section of this chapter describes methods that can be used to move from descriptive and analytic epidemiological research to developing effective interventions. Intervention methods are described in detail in Chapter 4.

The epidemiology of each chronic disease, condition, or risk factor is summarized in a figure in each chapter of Parts II through IV, as shown in Figure 2-2. This figure shows the "upstream causes" on the left side, the "high-risk groups" in the middle, and the "downstream consequences" on the right side. The next sections will provide a brief overview of the methods used to measure the

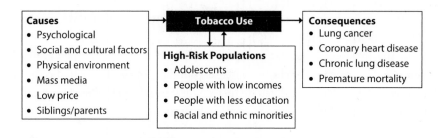

Figure 2-2. Tobacco Use: Causes, Consequences, and High-Risk Groups

burden, describe high-risk groups and trends in the population, and identify modifiable risk factors.

Descriptive Epidemiology

The first step in developing approaches to chronic disease control is to understand the nature and extent of the problem. Echoing the Institute of Medicine's (1988) landmark report on the future of public health, the director of the CDC (Frieden 2015) stressed the importance of epidemiology in carrying out public health assessment—one of the core functions of public health. Frieden and the Institute of Medicine report emphasize the governmental role in public health and affirm that every public health agency should regularly and systematically collect, analyze, interpret, and disseminate information on the health of the community, including statistics on health status, community health needs, and epidemiological and other studies of health problems.

The type of epidemiological studies used to support this assessment function varies, depending on the nature of the public health program. Descriptive epidemiology makes use of available data to examine the distribution of diseases in populations by time, person, or place. This type of information can be used to assess the burden of disease, identify high-risk groups, or monitor trends over time. The public and health policymakers frequently underestimate the health and economic burden from chronic diseases. Research has demonstrated that the public is more concerned about diseases and exposures that are unknown or out of one's individual control. For example, although social determinants of health (tobacco use, poor nutrition, and physical inactivity) account for nearly two thirds of preventable deaths in the United States (Mokdad et al. 2004; Galea et al. 2011), the public often perceives much greater risk from AIDS, homicide, and environmental pollution (Tinker and Vaughan 2002; so-called involuntary risks).

In the first section of each chapter of Parts II through IV, the authors describe the burden of the chronic disease, condition, or risk factor in the population and how it is distributed by "person, place, and time." For example, in Chapter 16, the following questions are addressed for breast cancer:

1. Significance: What are the "downstream consequences" of this problem? This is addressed through measures of disease occurrence: incidence rate, cumulative incidence, and prevalence. Both incidence rate and cumulative incidence indicate the risk of newly acquiring the disease, whereas prevalence is the number of people who have the disease at a point in time. Mortality rates are often used when incidence rates are unavailable.

2. High-risk populations: What groups have the highest risk? This question is addressed by comparing the risk or incidence of disease among people within the population who have some characteristic (e.g., older age) with those who do not have the characteristic. To do this, we use measures of association—rate ratio—and difference measures.

3. Geographic distribution: How does the burden of disease in one area compare with that in other areas? In calculating statistics that quantify the disease burden in one area versus other areas, consider the potential for distortion attributable to such factors as differing age, sex, and race in your population. To avoid distortion, you may need to divide measures of disease occurrence into categories to make them age-, sex-, or race-specific or standardize (adjust) them to make the populations comparable.

4. Time trends: What are the trends in the disease over time? Monitoring trends over time can provide insight on the etiology of chronic diseases (e.g., increases in lung cancer followed increases in smoking), burden (e.g., increasing rates of obesity), and control (e.g., declines in breast cancer mortality). The methods used to answer these questions are described in more detail in the following sections.

Measuring the Burden of Disease

Several measures are used to quantify the magnitude of disease occurrence, each one valid for a slightly different purpose. The number or actual count of persons affected by a chronic disease, condition, or risk factor is often used as the most fundamental measure of burden in the population. This measure is useful when one is assessing the need for health care or public health services as a direct measure of the burden on these systems. The actual burden of cancer is described in Chapter 16 (American Cancer Society 2015):

- Cancer is the leading cause of death among persons aged younger than 85 years and the second leading cause of death overall in the United States.
- Cancer accounted for an estimated 1.5 million new cases and 560,000 deaths in the United States in 2012.
- Breast cancer is the most common cancer type among women in the United States and the second leading cause of cancer death.
- The American Cancer Society expects 249,260 new cases of breast cancer and 40,890 breast cancer deaths in the United States in 2016.
- Worldwide, breast cancer is the second most common cancer and the fifth among cancer deaths.
- Breast cancer rarely occurs in men, with only 2,600 new cases and 440 deaths expected in the United States in 2016.

The actual number of people with a chronic disease or the number of deaths is an easy way to communicate burden to the general public and to policymakers. However, the absolute number of people affected is almost entirely dependent on the size of the population under consideration. Therefore, other measures must be used when one is making comparisons across populations and over time.

Calculating Rates in Populations

Rates must be calculated to compare populations of various sizes and characteristics. The principal rates used in chronic disease epidemiology are incidence and prevalence. Measures such as rate ratios and rate differences are then used to compare these different measures of risk across populations.

Incidence (or incidence rate) refers to the number of new cases over a defined period divided by the "person-time experience of the population"—that is, the number of persons multiplied by the period over which they were monitored; this is often called "person-years." However, in practice, the incidence rate is typically used to describe the number of new cases that develops in a year in a specified population. For example, if 500 women develop breast cancer in a year in a population of 342,000 women, the incidence rate would be 146 cases of breast cancer per 100,000 population of women. For many chronic diseases, such as coronary heart disease and diabetes, mortality rates are calculated because incidence data are unavailable.

Cumulative incidence is defined as the probability or risk of developing a disease over a defined period. It ranges from 0 to 1 and indicates the probability that the disease will develop in a population that is monitored over a set period. For example, according to a 2012 report from the National Cancer Institute (Howlader et al. 2012), a woman's lifetime risk of developing breast cancer is 0.127, or about 1 in 8. Thus, we can estimate that a girl born today has a 12.7% chance of eventually being diagnosed with breast cancer, although such estimates ignore any competing causes of mortality and are based on the somewhat unrealistic assumption that the present incidence rates will persist over time.

Prevalence also is measured as a proportion—that is, existing cases of disease divided by total population—but the occurrence of disease is measured at a point in time rather than over some interval. At the time of a disease survey, prevalence is defined as the number of existing cases divided by the population count. The prevalence of disease is influenced by the incidence (more new cases yield more existent cases) and persistence of the disease (rapid recovery or rapid death reduces the number of affected individuals at any point in time). For breast cancer, for example, the prevalence greatly exceeds the annual incidence because most women diagnosed with breast cancer survive for at least five years.

Because it is influenced by survival and recovery, prevalence is less valuable than incidence for identifying etiologic factors. For assessing public health needs, however, prevalence may be exactly the measure of interest. For example, women diagnosed with breast cancer are at a higher risk of a second breast cancer. Therefore, a prevalence estimate of the number of breast cancer survivors in a given area may be useful in targeting limited public health resources to women in high-risk groups.

Comparing Rates across Populations

Many local, state, and federal health agencies now calculate incidence rates for various conditions. Likewise, mortality rates (which can be viewed as incidence rates of death) are also published, often for such geographic areas as counties or cities. Public health officials have a natural interest in comparing incidence or mortality rates from other areas with their own to determine which areas have a greater problem.

Once rates have been calculated for various populations or population subgroups, these rates can be compared by using rate ratios or relative risks. For example, data from the Surveillance, Epidemiology, and End Results (SEER) program of the National Cancer Institute provide breast cancer incidence rates for men and women. We will use a hypothetical example that approximates actual SEER data, in which the age-adjusted incidence rate for women is 120 per 100,000 person-years and the comparable incidence rate for men is 1.2 cases per 100,000 person-years. Having determined the incidence rate in each of the two groups we wish to compare, our next challenge is to determine how that comparison should be summarized.

The ratio of the incidence rate in one group to that in another is referred to as a rate ratio. Likewise, the ratio of the cumulative incidence or risk in two groups is termed the "risk ratio" or "relative risk." Considering the incidence rate in men as the reference, we can calculate the rate ratio for women compared with men as 120 divided by 1.2 equals 100. Thus, we can say that women have an incidence rate 100 times that of men: breast cancer is predominantly a disease of women, although it does occur infrequently in men.

One advantage of such ratio measures is the ease of intuitive understanding (i.e., disease occurrence is increased about 100-fold among the women). Also, this ratio is independent of the absolute incidence rates in the two groups and, therefore, is directly interpretable: there is a strong association between gender and breast cancer.

Other risk factors besides gender can be discussed in similar terms. For example, research has demonstrated that the risk of breast cancer increases as the age of first birth increases. The five-year risk of breast cancer among women who have their first child before the age of 20 years is 0.7%, compared with a risk of 1.3% for women who have their first child after the age of 30 years (Table 2-1). In this instance, the relative risk for developing breast cancer in the next five years is 1.86 times (1.3/0.7 = 1.86).

An alternative to the ratio measure is the rate difference, calculated by subtracting the rates from one another. For example, the rate difference between women who have their first child after the age of 30 years, compared with women who have their first child before the age of 20 years, is calculated as follows: 1.3% minus 0.7% equals 0.6%, or 0.6 more cases per

Table 2-1. Five-Year Breast Cancer Risk, Rate Ratios, and Rate
Differences for Women Based on Age of First Pregnancy

Age at First Birth	Rate, %[a]	Rate Ratio	Rate Difference
<20	0.7	Reference group	Reference group
20-24	0.9	0.9/0.7=1.29	0.9−0.7=0.2%
25-29	1.1	1.1/0.7=1.57	1.1−0.7=0.4%
30+	1.3	1.3/0.7=1.86	1.3−0.7=0.6%
No births	1.1	1.1/0.7=1.57	1.1−0.7=0.4%

Source: NCI (2016b).
Note: Based on women aged 50 years with no family or personal history of breast cancer and age at menarche of 12 to 13 years.
[a]Rate=percentage who will develop breast cancer in the next 5 years.

100 women (or six cases per 1,000 women) over the next five years. This difference indicates how much, in absolute rather than relative terms, the risk differs depending on childbearing histories. The advantage of this measure is that the actual amount by which the disease has increased in one group as opposed to another has public health importance beyond the ratio of the two rates.

A doubling or even tripling of rate of a disease (e.g., the incidence or mortality rate) may not indicate an important public health problem if the baseline rate is extremely low. That is, the increment in disease burden from doubling a very small number would be very small. The difference in incidence rates, however, provides direct information about the public health effects of a particular exposure. A large difference indicates an important problem, regardless of the size of the baseline rate.

The difference between rate ratios and rate differences is shown in Table 2-2. If one compares smokers with nonsmokers, the relative risk is much greater for developing lung cancer than for coronary heart disease. However, the rate difference for heart disease (the rate in smokers minus the rate in nonsmokers) is actually greater than the rate difference for lung cancer because the baseline mortality rate of heart disease is so much greater than that for lung cancer. The public health impact attributable to increasing heart disease risk twofold is similar to the impact of increasing lung cancer risk tenfold. Both ratio and difference measures contribute to our understanding of the effect of an exposure on disease occurrence, and both measures should be examined when the data permit.

Table 2-2. Smoking-Related Rate Ratio and Rate Difference Estimates for Coronary Heart Disease and Lung Cancer among Women

| | Mortality Rate | | | |
| | Smokers (a) | Nonsmokers (b) | Rate Ratio (a/b) | Rate Difference (a−b) |
Disease				
Lung cancer	131	11	11.9	120
Coronary heart disease	275	153	1.8	122

Source: Adapted from Thun et al. (1997).

Finally, rates can be used to identify subgroups at need for program targeting. For example, identifying factors associated with compliance with cancer screening (Boehm et al. 2013; Shelby et al. 2012) helps program planners and managers to select subpopulations at greater risk for negative outcomes. Also, identifying these associations simultaneously with that of health-related behaviors (Liang et al. 2006; Coughlin et al. 2007; Ward et al. 2014) and other screening practices provides managers with practical information on whom and how to offer joint interventions.

Controlling for Differences in Age When Comparing Populations

Perhaps the most important issue to consider when one is comparing rates across populations is the potential that the two populations differ in average age. The risk of most chronic diseases increases dramatically with increasing age. For example, a retirement community may have a higher rate of breast cancer because they have a greater proportion of older women. Thus, this higher rate might not be attributable to some risk factors (e.g., genetics, childbearing practices). How then could we compare the rates in one area with those in another area, accounting for the differing ages, to determine whether some other factors are influencing the rate of breast cancer?

Two approaches are possible. First, age-specific rates can be calculated. That is, incidence rates may be given only for people in a specific age range. If the incidence rate of breast cancer for women aged 50 through 59 years is much greater in one area than in another, the difference could not have been caused by differences in age distributions between the two groups. A drawback with such calculations is that the problem of precision may be worsened: fewer cases are diagnosed (therefore, the numerator for the incidence rate is smaller) in a narrow age range than in the entire population. Such age-specific calculations typically require cases diagnosed over longer periods or from larger populations.

A second way to ease comparison of incidence rates is to adjust the rate to a standard population. This, in effect, combines many age-specific rates into a single age-adjusted rate. For example, the breast cancer incidence rate given in the previous example (110 cases per 100,000 women) is age-adjusted to the 1970 U.S. standard population. This means that statistical adjustments were made to the initial calculations to provide the rate that would be expected in the area's population if it had the same age distribution as did the U.S. population in 1970. Rates adjusted to the same standard population can be compared directly.

Small Area Analyses

Once differences in the ages of populations have been taken into account (either by comparing age-specific rates or through age adjustment), the problem of precision must be addressed by considering the statistical precision of the incidence or mortality rate. When rates are calculated for small areas such as a county, the numerator of the rate will usually be small. When a numerator is smaller than 20, rates are "unstable" and may vary by chance alone. If only a few cases are detected a year early or a year late, the incidence rate calculated for a particular year may appear much higher or much lower than it is on average over a longer period.

For example, if the incidence rate for breast cancer is 110 new cases per 100,000 women, a county with 25,000 women would be expected to have about 27 new cases each year (27/25,000 = 110 cases per 100,000). If only four cases were diagnosed too late to be counted for a particular year, the rate would decrease to 23 cases that year (23/25,000 = 92 cases/100,000), yielding an incidence rate ratio of 92 divided by 110 or 0.84. If only six cases from the next year were diagnosed a bit early, the rate would appear to increase dramatically to 33 cases per year (33/25,000 = 132 cases/100,000 women), for an incidence rate ratio of 1.20 and an apparent 20% increase in breast cancer incidence.

Thus, rates calculated from cases diagnosed in a single year from an area with a small population are subject to a large amount of variation from year to year and are said to be imprecise. For this reason, one should calculate rates from cases diagnosed over several years to increase the number of cases in the numerator of the incidence rate, thereby increasing the precision of the calculated rate.

The use of these methods can be seen in the maps of breast cancer mortality for white women and lung cancer mortality for white men for the United States (produced by the authors; NCI 2016a). These maps (Figures 2-3 and 2-4) compare the breast cancer mortality rates for white women and lung cancer mortality for white men for 1995 to 2004. First, notice that rates are presented by grouping counties into "state economic areas" and that many years of data were combined to produce more reliable rates. In addition, these rates are age-adjusted (to the 1970 U.S. population) to account for differences in the ages of the populations, not only among counties but also over time.

These maps provide insight into the epidemiology of breast and lung cancer. First, the mortality rates for breast cancer are higher in the northeastern United States. Research has shown that differences in cancer incidence and survival explain some, but not all, of these geographic differences (Kohler et al. 2015). Considerable interest remains in the possibility that environmental exposures contribute to these differences (Reynolds et al. 2005). In contrast, the reasons for the higher rates of lung cancer mortality among white men are almost entirely due to higher rates of smoking among men living in the southeastern United States.

Analytic Epidemiology

The second major function for epidemiology in chronic disease prevention and control is to understand the "determinants" (i.e., causes) of chronic diseases—with a focus on those determinants that can be modified. In the second section of each of the chapters in Parts II through IV, authors describe the modifiable factors for each of the major chronic diseases, conditions, and, when possible, chronic disease risk factors.

One of the most important and challenging roles for epidemiology is to differentiate between factors that are simply *associated* with chronic diseases and those factors that actually *cause* those chronic diseases. Criteria have been established to help epidemiologists determine which associations are truly causal and which are not, such as the Bradford Hill criteria (Hill 1965). Experimental evidence provides the strongest evidence for a causal association, but it is most useful in examining the effects of drugs and clinical interventions,

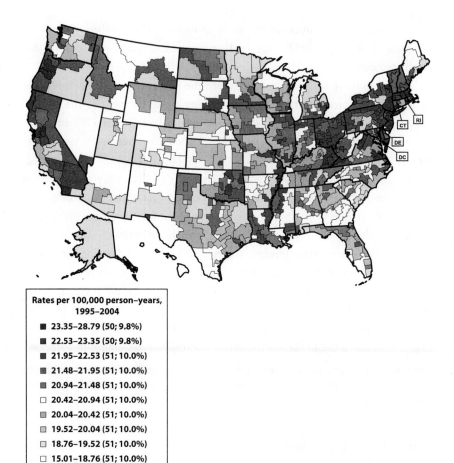

Rates per 100,000 person–years, 1995–2004

- 23.35–28.79 (50; 9.8%)
- 22.53–23.35 (50; 9.8%)
- 21.95–22.53 (51; 10.0%)
- 21.48–21.95 (51; 10.0%)
- 20.94–21.48 (51; 10.0%)
- 20.42–20.94 (51; 10.0%)
- 20.04–20.42 (51; 10.0%)
- 19.52–20.04 (51; 10.0%)
- 18.76–19.52 (51; 10.0%)
- 15.01–18.76 (51; 10.0%)
- Sparse data (0)

Source: Maps were calculated on the Cancer Mortality Maps website (NCI 2016a).
Note: Rates are age-adjusted to the 1970 U.S. population.

Figure 2-3. Breast Cancer Mortality Rates for White Women by State Economic Area, United States, 1995–2004

rather than the complex associations between environmental, social, or lifestyle factors and chronic diseases. Ultimately, subjective judgments must be made.

Epidemiology can not only be used to identify modifiable risk factors for chronic diseases, but it can also be used to estimate the morbidity and mortality that might be prevented by interventions. Although interventions such as education and screening programs often seem valuable, many have little

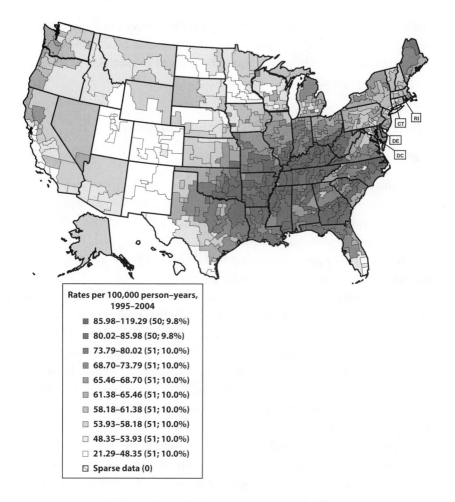

Rates per 100,000 person–years, 1995–2004

■ 85.98–119.29 (50; 9.8%)
■ 80.02–85.98 (50; 9.8%)
■ 73.79–80.02 (51; 10.0%)
■ 68.70–73.79 (51; 10.0%)
■ 65.46–68.70 (51; 10.0%)
■ 61.38–65.46 (51; 10.0%)
▨ 58.18–61.38 (51; 10.0%)
▧ 53.93–58.18 (51; 10.0%)
□ 48.35–53.93 (51; 10.0%)
□ 21.29–48.35 (51; 10.0%)
⊠ Sparse data (0)

Source: Maps were calculated on the Cancer Mortality Maps website (NCI 2016a).
Note: Rates are age-adjusted to the 1970 U.S. population.

Figure 2-4. Lung Cancer Mortality Rates for White Men by State Economic Areas, United States, 1995–2004

effect on the number of people with the disease. Therefore, we need to evaluate the effects of intervention programs and use those results to design new and better programs for controlling chronic diseases. Even when there are strong theoretical reasons to expect benefit, a determination is needed that the intervention reduces mortality or improves quality of life when applied in a real setting. Every intervention, even those that reduce the burden of disease, has a "downside," both through undesired consequences and by consuming resources. Calculating the proportion of a disease that is attributable to a particular risk factor may help to quantify the effect of its reduction or elimination (i.e., the population-attributable risk).

Study Designs in Chronic Disease Epidemiology

Experimental Studies

Randomized controlled trials (RCTs) are considered the most scientifically rigorous type of epidemiological study. In an RCT, participants are randomly assigned to either receive or not receive a preventive or therapeutic procedure, such as a clinical smoking cessation intervention or a new drug. The disease course or mortality patterns are then observed over time to assess the effectiveness of the preventive or therapeutic procedure.

The advantage of using a clinical trial, when possible, was best demonstrated by an RCT of the health effects of estrogen replacement therapy among women, called the Women's Health Initiative. This study was halted in 2002, when, contrary to its original hypothesis, the estrogen replacement therapy actually increased risk of breast cancer and heart disease (Writing Group for the Women's Health Initiative Investigators 2002). These results were definitive and conflicted with results that had been obtained from observational research decades before.

In practice, however, RCTs are either impossible or impractical when one is studying many interventions, especially those based outside clinical settings and in the community focusing on policy change. For example, it may be impractical to design a study to examine the effects of a community-wide educational intervention encouraging women to get a mammogram. In these situations, interventions can be tested in "quasi-experimental studies," in which a program (e.g., education program, screening program, new treatment regimen) is systematically offered to a population and the effect on health is measured. One key objective of such a study is to draw specific conclusions about the intervention. If the health of the population receiving the intervention improves, the investigators must demonstrate that a similar population that did not receive the intervention did not improve, at least to the same extent. This implies that to clearly interpret the results, such studies require comparison groups, which, unfortunately, are often lacking.

Comparison groups vary in their appropriateness for disease intervention studies. Least convincing are comparisons with national data or populations in other studies. Previous data on the same population are most appropriate if the disease can be shown to have been stable for a long period and if there are no other reasons for a change in disease incidence. The best control groups are those that can be shown to be similar to the intervention population and from which disease information is collected concurrently.

Despite certain limitations, quasi-experimental studies have shown that low-cost interventions can significantly improve the population's health. In one such study, low-cost community-based information campaigns were conducted in four low-income rural counties to encourage women to get routine breast and cervical cancer screening examinations. The rates of screening from baseline to follow-up were significantly higher among women living in these counties, compared with the trends among women living in four similar rural counties in Wisconsin (Eaker et al. 2001; Jaros et al. 2001). The strengths and limitations of the different types of experimental studies are summarized in Table 2-3.

Observational Studies

Randomized controlled trials or quasi-experimental interventions are either impossible or impractical when one is studying many of the causes of chronic diseases in the population. In some cases, it would be unethical or impossible to randomly assign the exposure (e.g., asbestos exposure, cigarette smoking, hypertension). In other cases, it is impractical to design a study to examine the effects of a randomly assigned exposure (e.g., effects of exercise during adolescence on the risk of postmenopausal breast cancer). In these instances, investigators must use observational methods. In observational studies, in contrast to RCTs (which are considered experimental studies), the risk factor or disease process is allowed to take its course without intervention from the researcher.

The observational study that is closest to an experiment is the prospective cohort design. In this approach, exposed and unexposed participants are identified and then observed over time for the development of disease. Unlike a true experiment, however, the exposures are observed rather than randomly assigned. Exposures are implicitly "assigned" on the basis of physician recommendations (e.g., x-ray use), genetic heritage (e.g., family history of breast cancer), or individual behavior (e.g., dietary fat intake). Having obtained measures of disease occurrence (incidence rates or cumulative incidence) for both exposed and unexposed groups, the influence of

Table 2-3. Summary of Strengths and Limitations of Various Study Designs

Study Type	Strengths	Limitations
Experimental studies		
Randomized clinical trial	Controls for bias by random assignment	High cost
		Not practical for many exposures (e.g., lifestyle, environmental, social/economic)
		Not practical for long latency periods
Randomized community trial	Can examine population-wide exposures	Very high cost
	Multicomponent interventions may be more effective	Often involves small number of study groups
Quasi-experimental studies	Can be used to study real-world program and policy interventions	Potential for bias in comparison groups
	Can use multiple comparison groups, repeated baseline measures to strengthen design	Lack of control of confounding factors
Observational studies		
Prospective cohort	Opportunity to measure risk factors before disease occurs	Often expensive
	Can study multiple disease outcomes	Requires large number of participants
	Can yield incidence rates as well as relative risk estimates	Requires long follow-up period
Case–control	Useful for rare diseases	Possible bias in measuring risk factors after disease has occurred
	Relatively inexpensive	Possible bias in selecting control group
	Relatively quick results	Identified cases may not represent all cases

exposure can be quantified as either the ratio of exposed to unexposed (the relative risk) or the difference between exposed and unexposed (the rate difference), as discussed earlier.

The primary advantage of a true prospective study over other observational designs is the opportunity to actively and intensively measure the exposures of interest before the period of disease induction. For example, instead of having participants recall dietary fat intake over many years, intake could be calculated more accurately if periodic direct measurements were made. For rare diseases and those with a prolonged period between exposure and the manifestation of adverse effects (typical of chronic diseases), however, true prospective studies must be extremely large and prolonged and, therefore, are very expensive.

One way to overcome these problems is to study exposures that occurred in the past and to monitor disease either up to the present or into the future. The ability to conduct these historical (or retrospective) cohort studies depends on the availability of exposure records that can be linked to disease outcomes. For example, in a study of the effect of chest x-ray and the subsequent rate of breast cancer occurrence, Andrieu et al. (2006) were able to identify a roster of exposed and unexposed participants from an earlier study of women with a gene that increases the risk of breast cancer (*BRCA1* and *BRCA2*). This study demonstrated that women who had a chest x-ray were 1.5 times more likely to develop breast cancer compared with women who had not had a previous chest x-ray.

A case–control study is another type of observational study that can be used to investigate the causes of chronic diseases. Case–control studies study participants on the basis of their health outcomes (e.g., disease); this design intentionally oversamples persons who have developed the disease of interest. In case–control studies, researchers identify a sample of people with the disease, or case patients (often, all available case patients), and a sample of people without the disease, or control participants, from the same population that yielded the case patients.

The historical exposures that may have influenced disease risk are ascertained for all participants, and the frequency of exposure among case patients is compared with that among control participants. Such studies cannot yield incidence rates or cumulative incidence because the population at risk is not comprehensively defined; the control participants are typically a sample of that source population, but the sampling fraction is unknown. An estimate of the ratio of incidence rates or risks can be obtained, however, by calculating the ratio of the odds of exposure among cases (the number exposed divided by the number not exposed) to the odds of exposure among controls, referred to as the odds ratio. The odds ratio is intended to approximate the relative risk. No estimate of the risk difference can be obtained from a case–control study.

The obvious advantages of case–control studies are the relative speed with which they can be conducted, because the latent period is all in the past, and the small number of participants who have to be enrolled. In contrast to a cohort study, in which many participants who never develop the disease must be monitored, a case–control study includes only a small but adequate fraction of the nondiseased population. The principal weakness is the study's vulnerability to some forms of bias that arise from the fact that the disease has usually occurred before risk factor information was ascertained. The strengths and limitations of prospective and case–control studies are summarized in Table 2-3.

To evaluate the potential causes of breast cancer mortality, the National Cancer Institute has supported an ongoing case–control study of breast cancer among residents of Wisconsin, Massachusetts, and New Hampshire since 1988 (Sprague et al. 2015). These studies compare the exposures (e.g., physical activity patterns during adolescence, childbearing history) of women diagnosed with breast cancer (i.e., cases) with the exposure histories of women of the same age, who have not had breast cancer (i.e., controls). These studies have led to the identification of potentially modifiable risk factors for breast cancer, including a long menstrual history (early menarche and late menopause), having no children or not having breastfed, previous chest irradiation, postmenopausal hormone therapy use, obesity (particularly postmenopausal), and moderate to heavy alcohol intake.

How Do We Measure Associations between Exposures and Outcomes?

The "relative risk" is the primary measure used to determine whether there is an association between an exposure (e.g., cigarette smoking) and a health outcome (e.g., lung cancer). As described previously, the ratio of the risk in two groups is termed the "relative risk." Associations can be assessed anywhere along the continuum shown in Figure 2-1. For example, the risk of lung cancer mortality among smokers is 131 deaths per 100,000 persons who smoke, compared with only 11 deaths per 100,000 persons who do not smoke—yielding a relative risk of 11.9.

Similarly, studies have shown that the risk of becoming a smoker is higher among children who view smoking in the movies versus children who do not view smoking in the movies (Charlesworth and Glantz 2005). For example, if 34% of children who view smoking become smokers, compared with only 20% of children who do not view smoking in the movies, the relative risk of smoking would be 34% divided by 20% equals 1.7. If this association is causal, one could say that children who view smoking in the movies are 1.7 times more likely to become smokers, compared with children who do not view smoking in the movies.

How Do We Evaluate Whether the Study Results Are Valid?

Despite the increasing sophistication of research studies, uncertainty continues to exist in our understanding of the causes and consequences of chronic diseases. As most chronic disease epidemiology studies use observational methods, it is possible that errors in measurement or in selection of study participants lead to spurious results. For example, there may be uncertainty in epidemiological studies about a measure of association, such as relative risk. If we obtain an odds ratio or relative risk of 2.0, are we fully confident that becoming exposed will truly double the risk of disease or that removing exposure will cut the risk in half?

Considerable expertise is needed to address uncertainty in research and to determine the quality of a research study. Riegelman uses an organizing framework to evaluate whether results from a research study are valid (Riegelman 2013). Two of the most important factors to consider include "confounding" and "bias."

Confounding

One reason for uncertainty is the possibility for confounding, in which the influence of an exposure of interest is mixed with the effect of another. This arises when a risk factor for the disease of interest is also associated with the exposure of interest. For example, people who drink alcohol are also more likely to drink coffee. When a study is conducted to examine alcohol use and breast cancer, the possible confounding role of coffee and caffeine must be taken into consideration. The estimated effect of alcohol on breast cancer will be confounded by caffeine intake if (1) caffeine and alcohol use are correlated and (2) caffeine use independently influences the risk of breast cancer.

In an experiment or RCT, these potential confounders can be balanced among the study groups through the design of the study and the random manner in which the exposure is assigned. Conversely, in an observational study, potential confounders must be measured and adjusted statistically. The strategy involves creating groups that are similar with respect to the potential confounder and examining the impact of the exposure of interest within each of those groups. For example, we could measure caffeine consumption and create strata of nonconsumers, low caffeine consumers, and high caffeine consumers and assess the role of alcohol use on breast cancer within each of those strata. As long as the potential confounder can be measured, the adjustments will be effective; however, some potential confounders, such as psychological stress, health consciousness, or dietary intake, may be difficult to measure, or we simply may be unaware of the risk factors that should be considered for adjustment.

Selection and Information Bias

A different source error comes from bias regarding how the participants enter the study or how information is collected from study participants. A faulty sampling mechanism, caused by such problems as nonresponse or refusal to participate, could produce a sample that has a higher or lower disease risk. Note that the only kind of sampling distortion that matters is the selection that influences disease risk. Similarly, in a case–control study, the selected case patients should reflect the exposure distribution of all case patients of interest, and the selected control participants should reflect exposure in the overall population that produced the cases. The potential for a poorly constituted control group is a major threat to the validity of case–control studies. For example, when we choose control participants from a hospital, health problems that led to their hospitalization may be associated with the exposure of interest. Similarly, when we choose control participants by telephone screening, omitting households without telephones could introduce a bias.

Another category of bias that can occur in epidemiological studies is the result of errors in classification of exposure or disease; this is referred to as information bias. Although efforts should be made to minimize such bias, errors in classification of exposure are unavoidable. Past exposures such as dietary intake, alcohol use, or physical activity are impossible to measure perfectly, even if we know what aspect of such exposures was the most relevant to disease causation. In many instances, the errors in exposure classification can be assumed to be similar for those who do and do not develop disease. This situation, referred to as nondifferential misclassification of exposure, results in a predictable bias in which the measure of association (such as odds ratio or relative risk) will be biased toward the null value of no association (1.0 for ratio measures, 0 for difference measures). This means that virtually all reported associations between exposure and disease will be diluted to some degree or missed entirely.

When the patterns of misclassification are different for the study groups, this is referred to as differential misclassification. This can occur when exposure is classified differently for diseased and nondiseased participants or when disease is classified differently for exposed and unexposed participants. Now the distortion in the measure of association can be in either direction (exaggerated or understated), depending on the precise pattern of error. A particular worry in case–control studies is the possibility of recall bias, which is a particular type of differential misclassification. Recall bias exists when the recall of exposure information is different for case patients than for control participants, presumably because the illness experience of the case patients has in some way altered their memory or reporting of past events. Intuitively, one might expect case patients to overreport exposures that did not occur in an effort to explain their illness. Also, studies suggest that case patients may report accurately (presumably because their memory search is more thorough), whereas control participants tend to underreport past exposures. In either situation, the reported exposures of case patients are artificially greater than the reported exposures of control participants, and the relative risk is falsely elevated.

Information bias was thought to be responsible for the apparent association between breast cancer and abortion. Case–control studies demonstrated that women with breast cancer were more likely to report having had an abortion in the past, compared with similar women who did not have breast cancer. In contrast, prospective studies comparing the future risk of breast cancer among women who had an abortion with women who had not had an abortion did not find an association. Researchers suspect that information bias in the case–control studies led to a spurious association, as women may underreport having had an abortion. This underreporting may be more common among controls, as women diagnosed with breast cancer may have provided a more accurate history (Rookus and van Leeuwen 1996). A review of the literature a decade later confirmed that researchers have not found a cause-and-effect relationship between abortion and breast cancer (Kitchen et al. 2005).

How Do We Assess Whether Associations between Potential Etiologic Factors and Disease Are Causal?

Any intervention program or public health action is based on the presumption that the associations found in epidemiological studies are causal rather than arising through bias or for some other spurious reason. Unfortunately, in most instances in observational epidemiology, such as the research showing an association between viewing smoking in the movies and becoming a smoker, there is no opportunity to absolutely prove that an association is causal. Nonetheless, some principles are helpful when one must make this judgment.

The Bradford Hill criteria (Hill 1965) are often cited as a checklist for causality in epidemiological studies. These criteria have value but only as general guidelines. Most of Hill's nine criteria relate to particular cases of refuting biases or drawing on nonepidemiological evidence.

1. Strength of association: Stronger associations are less likely to be the result of some subtle confounding or bias, presuming that major distorting influences would be more readily recognized than small ones.

2. Consistency of association: The association is observed across diverse populations and circumstances, making a particular bias unlikely to explain a series of such observations.

3. Specificity of association: The exposure causes one rather than many diseases, and the disease is associated with one rather than many exposures, suggesting that the association is not the result of bias. This is the weakest of the criteria for chronic diseases and might as well be eliminated because we now know that many, perhaps most, exposures that influence one health outcome affect others (e.g., tobacco, radiation, diet) and that virtually all diseases have multiple causes.

4. Temporality: The exposure must precede the disease. This is the only absolute criterion for causality. Prospective study design helps establish the case for temporality.

5. Biological gradient: A dose–response curve, in which the risk of disease increases with increasing exposure, indicates that an association probably is not the result of a confounder or other bias. This criterion is generally valid, but the absence of a perfect dose–response pattern does not negate the possibility of a causal explanation because true thresholds or ceilings of effects may exist. Conversely, the presence of a dose–response gradient may be the result of a strong confounder that closely tracks the exposure.

6. Plausibility: Evidence from other disciplines suggests that the agent is biologically capable of influencing the disease. This is useful supportive evidence when it is available, but the lack of advancements in the other

biological sciences should not be used to negate an epidemiological observation.

7. Coherence: The evidence should not be contradictory to the known biology and natural history of the disease (similar to the plausibility criterion).

8. Experimental evidence: When attainable, experimental evidence for causality—obtained by removing or randomly assigning exposure—is very strong because both known and unknown confounders are controlled when exposure is randomly allocated.

9. Analogy: When other similar agents have been established as causes of disease, then the credibility of theories regarding a new disease operating in a similar manner is enhanced. This is the epidemiological counterpart to plausibility; however, the supportive evidence comes from other areas of epidemiology rather than from other disciplines.

In practice, the establishment of evidence for causality is largely through the elimination of noncausal explanations for an observed association. Consider, for example, the evidence that alcohol use may increase the risk of breast cancer. A series of further studies might confirm that this relationship is valid and not a result of confounding or other biases such as detection bias (in which disease is more thoroughly diagnosed among alcohol users) or nonresponse bias. By whittling away alternative explanations, the hypothesis that asserts that alcohol use causes breast cancer becomes increasingly credible. It is the job of critics to propose and test noncausal explanations, so that when the association has withstood a series of such challenges, the case for causality is strengthened.

The danger of formalizing the process of declaring causality on the basis of a checklist or any other mechanistic process is that it can only lead to endless debates about the degree of certainty and can impede needed public health actions. Those who argue that causality must be established with absolute certainty before interventions can begin fail to appreciate that their two alternatives—action and inaction—each have risks and benefits. Decisions must therefore be based on evidence that exposure causes diseases and must take into account the costs of intervention, the potential for the intervention to produce adverse side effects, and the potential costs of failing to act.

For example, the tobacco companies have argued, until recently, that the association between smoking and disease is uncertain. In a technical sense, we will always have some degree of uncertainty, especially with no definitive data from large numbers of participants randomly assigned to be smokers and nonsmokers. We have no doubt, however, that the evidence indicates a need to intervene because smoking has no clear health benefits and scientists have exhausted all reasonable noncausal explanations for the strong associations observed between smoking and a number of diseases. Nonetheless, to the extent that tobacco companies continue to argue that the evidence for causality is not definitive, they create enough controversy to distract some policymakers from supporting needed interventions. Establishing causality is an important goal for epidemiological research, but absolute proof is not needed to justify action.

How Much Morbidity and Mortality Might Be Prevented by Interventions?

In each chapter in Parts II through IV, authors report the relative risk (discussed previously) and the "population-attributable risk." The population-attributable risk is particularly useful in evaluating the potential benefits of intervention. When presented with an array of potential causal factors for disease, we need to evaluate how much might be gained by reducing or eliminating each of the hazards. Relative risk estimates indicate how strongly exposure and disease are associated, but this measure does not indicate directly the benefits that could be gained through modifying the exposure.

Attributable Risk

The attributable risk is a measure of how much of the disease burden could be eliminated if the exposure were eliminated. The attributable risk represents the proportion of disease among exposed people that actually results from the exposure. This issue might arise in a court case in which an exposed individual claims that the agent to which he or she was exposed caused the disease. Note that we are presuming that the associations reflect causality for the purposes of estimation. The attributable risk among exposed individuals is calculated as follows:

[relative risk–1]/relative risk

Thus, a relative risk of 2.0 (risk is doubled by exposure) yields an attributable proportion among exposed people of 0.5. This suggests a 50% chance that the disease resulted from the exposure in this study population.

Population-Attributable Risk

Of still greater potential value is the incorporation of information on how common the exposure is. Although some exposures exert a powerful influence on individuals (i.e., a large relative risk), they are so rare that their public health impact is minimal. Conversely, some exposures have a modest impact but are so widespread that their elimination could have great benefit. To answer the question, "What proportion of disease in the total population is a result of the exposure?" the population-attributable risk or etiologic fraction is used. The population-attributable risk can be calculated in two ways. First, if the rate in the exposed and unexposed population is known, then the population-attributable risk is

$$[\text{rate (total population)} - \text{rate (unexposed)}]/[\text{rate (total population)}]$$

The population-attributable risk can also be calculated with information only about the relative risk (usually obtained from research studies) and exposure in the population (often obtained from surveys). It is calculated as follows:

$$[P_e \text{ (relative risk} - 1)]/[1 + P_e \text{ (relative risk} - 1)]$$

where P_e represents the proportion of the population that is exposed.

The population-attributable risk is used most commonly to estimate the proportion of disease caused by a certain risk factor, such as the proportion of lung cancer caused by smoking. Assuming that the relative risk of lung cancer attributable to cigarette smoking is 15 and that 30% of the population are smokers, the population-attributable risk is 0.81, or 81%. This would suggest that 81% of the lung cancer burden in the population is caused by cigarette smoking and could be eliminated if the exposure were eliminated.

Population-attributable risk could also be used to estimate the proportion of a risk factor attributable to various "upstream" determinants. As described previously, research has shown that children exposed to smoking in the movies are at increased risk of becoming regular smokers (Charlesworth and Glantz 2005). If one assumes that this is a causal relationship, about 35% of smoking among adolescents could be attributed to exposure to smoking in the movies. Intuitively, the 35% figure sounds very high, which would cast doubt on the assumption of a casual relationship. It is also important to note that, because of the effects of interactions between various risk factors, population-attributable risk estimates for a given disease can sometimes add up to more than 100%.

The relationship between risk, relative risk, and population-attributable risk is illustrated in Figure 2-5 as a hypothetical example for 100 children:

- Risk (e.g., 34% of children exposed to smoking in the movies become smokers, compared with only 20% of children not exposed to smoking in the movies).
- Relative risk (e.g., children exposed to smoking in the movies are 1.7 times more likely to become smokers).
- Population-attributable risk (e.g., 35% of smoking among adolescents is because of smoking in the movies).

Although population-attributable risk estimates provide a useful estimate of the public health burden, they may be unrealistic as absolute goals because only rarely can a risk factor be completely eliminated.

Interactions among exposures, also known as effect modification, in the causation of disease are of particular importance in fully understanding etiology. Effect modification occurs when the effect of one exposure on disease risk is modified by the presence of another exposure. In the purest form, which is rarely observed, each of two exposures alone may have no effect on disease, but when the two are combined, a synergism occurs, causing an increase in disease. Conversely, two exposures that each can influence disease risk independently may be antagonistic, so that in combination they have a smaller effect on disease risk.

In epidemiological studies, interaction is measured as a combined effect of exposures that is larger than would be expected by simply adding the effects

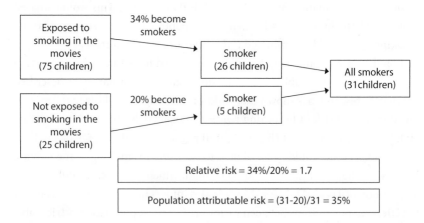

Figure 2-5. Risks of Becoming a Smoker among 100 Children Exposed or Not Exposed to Smoking in the Movies

of the two separate exposures. Interaction is most easily detected by comparing the disease risk in groups with all combinations of exposure to the group exposed to neither agent. For example, cigarette smoking and asbestos exposure have been demonstrated to multiply the risk of lung cancer (Table 2-4). The risk of lung cancer among nonsmokers who are exposed to asbestos (relative risk = 5.2) is approximately half that of smokers who are not exposed to asbestos (relative risk = 10.8). However, a multiplicative effect is observed among smokers who are exposed to asbestos (relative risk = 53.2).

This measure of interaction has direct implications for developing intervention and prevention programs. If two factors interact, then the benefit of removing a given exposure will be greater if the other exposure is also present. For example, eliminating smoking has even more benefit for a group of workers exposed to asbestos than for individuals who are not exposed to asbestos.

Obviously, many factors enter into decisions about interventions, including certainty of causality, amenability to intervention, and social and political issues. However, in the traditional role of epidemiology as the basic science of public health, quantitative considerations of preventable disease can help us make a rational choice. How can we predict what benefits one or more of these interventions might yield in the community? This is where estimates of population-attributable risk may be particularly useful. If one considers the earlier example of smoking and lung cancer, it is apparent that lung cancer incidence could be reduced by more than 80% if cigarette smoking were eliminated.

Additional Uses of Epidemiology in Chronic Disease Prevention and Control

Although descriptive epidemiology is necessary, it is not sufficient to prevent and control chronic diseases in populations. Developing evidence-based

Table 2-4. Example of Relative Risk Estimates for Lung Cancer Associated with Smoking and Asbestos Exposure

Smoking Category	Relative Risk Estimate	
	No Asbestos Exposure	Asbestos Exposure
Nonsmoker	1	5
Smoker	10	50

Source: Data from IARC (2004).

interventions requires going beyond epidemiology to use other disciplines, such as behavioral and social sciences, environmental health sciences, health management, and policy analysis. This section briefly describes a set of questions and issues to be considered when one is interpreting data in chronic disease epidemiology. It also describes several analytic tools and processes of interest to practitioners (e.g., meta-analysis, expert panels).

Why Should Action Not Be Taken on the Basis of a Single Epidemiological Study?

Scientists and practitioners committed to improving the public's health have a natural tendency to scrutinize the epidemiological literature for new findings that would serve as the basis for prevention or intervention programs. In fact, application to public health practice is a principal motive for conducting such research. Adding to this inclination to intervene may be claims from investigators regarding the critical importance of their findings, media interpretation of the findings as the basis for immediate action, and even community support for responding to the striking new research findings with new or modified programs or elimination of existing programs. John Oliver, a television satirist who blends investigative journalism with slapstick humor, scrutinized the misuse and misinterpretation of scientific studies by the media on his program *Last Week Tonight*. The program illustrates how the misuse of science can lead to erroneous and often bizarre conclusions such as a news anchor's assertion that "women are more open to romance when they are full instead of hungry" (Last Week Tonight 2016). The statement is presented as fact, and may indeed be true; however, it originated from a pilot study with a sample size of 20 that was published in a niche journal (Ely et al. 2015). Oliver points out these necessary disclaimers, which the news anchor failed to do. Although it is presented in a humorous fashion, Oliver's satire highlights an important concept: a single study is never sufficient for making such assertions. This is particularly true for epidemiological research, in which an appreciation of epidemiological methods applied to chronic disease prevention and control leads to the inevitable conclusion that multiple studies are required to ascertain the truth behind the statistical noise. Well-designed and carefully conducted research adds evidence to assist in setting policy, but the stakes are so high in economic terms and public credibility that cautious interpretation of research findings that have not been replicated is required.

We have already discussed the validity of epidemiological research and criteria for causality, but a more direct consideration of why a single study is insufficient for action should be helpful. Breast cancer had rarely been considered a disease that might be affected by environmental pollutants, in contrast, for example, to lung or bladder cancer. However, a paper published by Wolff et al. (1993) changed that perception. This study, which was well designed, carefully conducted, and certainly worthy of publication, reported that pesticide residues from dichlorodiphenyltrichloroethane (DDT) in the blood were positively associated with the risk of breast cancer, with relative risks on the order of 3.0. Media interest was high, and the notion that a common, life-threatening disease could be related in part to environmental agents was both terrifying and promising of the potential for intervention. Although these exposures had been accrued over a lifetime, if found to be related to breast cancer, interventions to reduce body burden of DDT would be worthy of consideration. For other reasons, largely based on adverse effects on wildlife, DDT was banned more than 40 years ago.

How could a study be methodologically sound, published in a reputable journal, generate substantial media and public interest, and yet not be worthy of any action on the part of public health practitioners? First, despite the talents of the investigators and quality of the resulting study, its findings may simply be wrong or misleading. That is, for reasons discussed earlier, even within the population studied, there may well be no causal association between DDT residues and breast cancer. One critical concern is whether the measured levels of DDT residues were affected by early stages of breast cancer rather than the reverse. Also, potential confounding by lactation was examined but produced rather anomalous results, and the number of cases available for analysis was small.

Second, even if valid for the population under study, the generalizability of the findings has to be examined. Can results from women in the New York area be applied to other populations with different exposure histories, ethnic backgrounds, and risk factor profiles? Although we look for universal explanations for disease and occasionally find strong causal factors that account for most of the disease in most populations (e.g., smoking and lung cancer), these successes are rare. More often, there is a multitude of interacting factors that must be considered for extrapolating findings from one population to apply to another.

Finally, even if findings are valid and generalizable, thus making a contribution to public health decision, what action should be taken for an agent that was banned long ago? At the margins, in evaluating costs and benefits, this research would (if valid) add to the evidence of health harm from exposure, but in this case, there is not a clear decision to be made. If we had two comparably effective pesticides, one of which was associated with health harm and one that was not, such evidence might tip the balance. Public health decisions must integrate the full array of considerations regarding risks and benefits of different courses of action, as discussed in the following section.

How Do We Assess a Series of Epidemiological Studies and Integrate the Evidence to Make Decisions?

Several important methods and tools are available to epidemiologists and practitioners to assist in determining when public health action is warranted. It is often necessary to use these because exposure–disease relationships in chronic disease epidemiology typically show relatively weak associations, in which the relative risk estimate is not too different from the null value of 1.0. Most accepted risk factors for breast cancer are associated with relative risks of less than 5.0, and often less than 3.0, considered by some to be weak (Wynder 1987; Boffetta 2010). The closer a relative risk estimate comes to unity (i.e., 1.0), the more likely that it can be explained by methodological limitations such as confounding, misclassification, and other sources of bias. Yet, as noted earlier in the description of population-attributable risk, even when a risk factor is weak, if highly prevalent in the population, the public health impact can be large. Therefore, we have great interest in determining when even relatively weak associations provide the basis for public health intervention, which can only come from a series of well-designed studies.

Although it is tempting to intervene rather than conduct yet more studies in the face of a serious health problem, in the long run, evaluation of all major interventions is essential. To conduct such an evaluation, investigators must study a comparison group and rule out other factors as the cause of any observed change. The diagnosis of breast cancer in a prominent local citizen, for example, could be the main cause of increased breast cancer screening, rather than a community education program. In programs that combine several interventions, investigators may be able to determine which intervention(s) actually produced the health benefits and whether the results of an evaluation are generalizable to a different population. The debate continues, for example, as to whether the results of studies of reduced serum cholesterol in men can be applied to women. Thus, determining whether a proposed intervention will actually bring about more good than harm can be difficult.

It is important to note that even ostensibly useful interventions may not have positive effects and that almost all programs may have unintended negative effects. An education program to increase breast cancer screening, for example, could have no effect on women who need screening, yet it could raise anxiety among younger women at low risk who do not need screening. The usefulness of a particular screening test is based on several characteristics, including its accuracy, reproducibility, sensitivity, and specificity.

This section provides an overview of three related methods that have proven useful in assimilating large bodies of evidence in chronic disease epidemiology. In turn, the summarized evidence can be useful in shaping public health interventions and policies. Because this consideration is necessarily brief, readers are referred to other sources for more detail.

Systematic Reviews and Meta-analyses

The volume of information published about chronic diseases and their risk factors in journals every day is far beyond that which any person can remain current on. To address this problem, researchers conduct "systematic reviews" to consolidate all the information from studies addressing a single clinical or public health question. Systematic reviews use explicit and comprehensive (systematic) methods to identify, select, and critically assess all relevant research on the issue under consideration. To avoid bias, all Cochrane reviews start as a published protocol stating in advance how the review will be carried out (searching for data, appraising and combining study data). Over the past two decades, systematic reviews have been increasingly using "meta-analysis" to provide a more quantitative approach for integrating the findings of individual studies (Petitti 2000). Petitti describes four steps in undertaking a meta-analysis.

1. Identify relevant studies: Relevant studies must first be identified for inclusion in the meta-analysis. These can be identified through computerized sources such as MEDLINE, review articles, other journal articles, doctoral dissertations, and personal communications with other researchers.

2. Inclusion and exclusion criteria: Explicit criteria distinguish a meta-analysis from a qualitative literature review. Criteria for inclusion should specify the study designs to be included; the years of publication or of data collection; the languages in which the articles are written (e.g., English only or English plus other specified languages); the minimum sample size and the extent of follow-up; the treatments and/or exposures; the

manner in which the exposures, treatment, and outcomes were measured; and the completeness of information. Study quality should also be considered. As a minimum, studies whose quality falls below some specified rating criteria should be excluded. Rating scales may be developed to assess the quality of the included studies, although the basis for rating can be controversial and it may be preferable to consider the actual study attributes rather than a summary quality score.

3. Data abstraction: In this step, important features of each study are abstracted such as design, number of participants, and key findings. The abstraction summary should produce findings that are reliable, valid, and free of bias. Blinding of abstractors and reabstraction of a sample of studies by multiple abstractors may be beneficial.

4. Statistical analysis and exploration of heterogeneity: The data are combined to produce a summary estimate of the measure of association along with confidence intervals. Data are also examined to determine if the effect across studies was homogeneous and, if not, the reasons for heterogeneity.

Meta-analysis is most useful for combining the results of multiple, small RCTs whose results are generally consistent yet imprecision is a problem in each individual trial. The method is less useful in situations in which intervention trials have found truly heterogeneous results through different methods or because the relationship of interest varies across populations. Partly for that reason, one must be careful not to be overwhelmed by the impressively large numbers that can be accrued in a meta-analysis. Although the improved precision is a strength, one must also consider the validity of combining results across studies and whether the estimated size of the effect is large enough to warrant action.

Risk Assessment

Quantitative risk assessment is a widely used term for a systematic approach to characterizing the risks posed to individuals and populations by environmental pollutants and other potentially adverse exposures. Risk assessment has been described as a "bridge" between science and policy-making. In the United States, its use is either explicitly or implicitly required by a number of federal statutes, and its application worldwide is increasing. There has been considerable debate over the U.S. risk-assessment policies, and the most widely recognized difficulties in risk assessment are because of extrapolation-related uncertainties (i.e., extrapolating low-dose effects from higher exposure levels). Risk assessment has become an established process through which expert scientific input is provided to agencies that regulate environmental or occupational exposures.

Four key steps in risk assessment are hazard identification, risk characterization, exposure assessment, and risk estimation (USEPA 2005). An important aspect of risk assessment is that it frequently results in classification schemes that take into account uncertainties about exposure–disease relationships. For example, the U.S. Environmental Protection Agency has developed a five-tier scheme for classifying potential and proven cancer-causing agents, which includes the following: (1) group A, carcinogenic to humans; (2) group B, probably carcinogenic to humans; (3) group C, possibly carcinogenic to humans; (4) group D, not classifiable as to human carcinogenicity; and (5) group E, evidence of noncarcinogenicity for humans.

Sources of Evidence

Most government agencies, in both executive and legislative branches, and voluntary health organizations, such as the American Cancer Society, use expert panels when examining epidemiological studies and their relevance to health policies and interventions (Brownson 2006). Ideally, the goal of expert panels is to provide peer review by scientific experts of the quality of the science and scientific interpretations that underlie public health recommendations, regulations, and policy decisions. If conducted well, peer review can provide an important set of checks and balances for the regulatory process. Optimally, the expert review process has the following common properties: experts are sought in epidemiology and related disciplines (e.g., clinical medicine, biomedical sciences, biostatistics, economics, ethics); panels typically consist of 8 to 15 members and meet in person to review scientific data (written guidance is provided to panel members); panel members should not have financial or professional conflicts of interest; and draft findings from expert panels are frequently released for public review and comment before final recommendations.

The Community Guide is a source of information about the effectiveness of chronic disease prevention and control interventions, based on the findings of the Community Preventive Services Task Force and the related systematic reviews. The Community Guide is a credible resource with many uses because it is based on a scientific systematic review process and answers questions critical to almost everyone interested in community health and well-being such as

- What interventions have and have not worked?
- In which populations and settings has the intervention worked or not worked?
- What might the intervention cost?
- What should I expect for my investment?
- Does the intervention lead to any other benefits or harms?
- What interventions need more research before we know if they work or not?

The goal of the Community Guide is to promote the use of interventions that have been shown to work, discourage the use of interventions that have been shown not to work, and promote research on interventions for which there is not enough evidence to say whether or not they work (Community Preventive Services Task Force, 2016).

Conclusions

In this chapter, we have discussed the issues that help to determine whether associations are causal, the role of intervention research in disease control, and the uses of epidemiological evidence to make public health decisions. We have also outlined several types of epidemiological study designs and the biases that can complicate interpretation of results. We have discussed issues that help to determine whether associations are causal, as well as the role of intervention research in disease control. Such information serves as a foundation that will help readers address the more complex issues of chronic disease etiology and control. Some of the key epidemiological concepts that the reader will encounter in other chapters are summarized in Table 2-5.

The final section in each chapter of Parts II through IV describes the evidence that exists for effective programs and policies. Epidemiological, behavioral, social science, and other research methods have been used to identify effective intervention strategies that can be implemented at the individual and community level (Zaza et al. 2005). These methods are described in more detail in the following two chapters.

Table 2-5. Key Concepts in Chronic Disease Epidemiology

Term	Definition
	A = Number of new events in a specified time period
Incidence rate = A/B	B = Number of persons exposed to risk during this period
	C = Risk of disease or death in the exposed population
Relative risk = C/D	D = Risk of disease or death in the unexposed population
Population-attributable risk[a] = E/F	E = Rate of a disease in a population that is associated
	with (attributed to) a certain risk factor
	F = Total rate of a disease in the population

[a]This concept implies causality and should be used with caution.

Suggested Reading

Brownson, RC, Petitti DB, eds. *Applied Epidemiology.* 2nd ed. New York, NY: Oxford University Press; 2006.

Cochran Collaboration and Library. Available at: http://www.cochrane.org.

Friss RH, Sellers TA. *Epidemiology for Public Health Practice.* Frederick, MD: Aspen; 1996.

Gordis L. *Epidemiology.* 2nd ed. Philadelphia, PA: W. B. Saunders; 2000.

Riegelman RK. *Studying a Study and Testing a Test: How to Read the Medical Evidence.* 6th ed. Philadelphia, PA: Lippincott Williams & Wilkins; 2013.

Szklo M, Nieto FJ. *Epidemiology: Beyond the Basics.* Gaithersburg, MD: Aspen; 2000.

References

American Cancer Society. *Breast Cancer Facts & Figures 2015–2016.* Atlanta, GA: American Cancer Society Inc; 2015.

Andrieu N, Easton DF, Chang-Claude J, et al. Effect of chest X-rays on the risk of breast cancer among BRCA1/2 mutation carriers in the international BRCA1/2 carrier cohort study. *J Clin Oncol.* 2006;24(21):3361–3366.

Boehm JE, Rohan EA, Preissle J, DeGroff A, Glover-Kudon R. Recruiting patients into the CDC's colorectal cancer screening demonstration program: strategies and challenges across 5 sites. *Cancer.* 2013;119(suppl 15):2914–2925.

Boffetta P. Causation in the presence of weak associations. *Crit Rev Food Sci Nutr.* 2010;50(suppl 1):13–16.

Brownson RC. Epidemiology and health policy. In: Brownson RC, Petitti DB, eds. *Applied Epidemiology: Theory to Practice.* 2nd ed. New York, NY: Oxford University Press; 2006:361–363.

Brownson RC, Petitti DB, eds. *Applied Epidemiology.* 2nd ed. New York, NY: Oxford University Press; 2006.

Charlesworth A, Glantz SA. Smoking in the movies increases adolescent smoking: a review. *Pediatrics.* 2005;116(6):1516–1528.

Centers for Disease Control and Prevention (CDC). *Principles of Epidemiology.* 3rd ed. 2016. Available at: http://www.cdc.gov/ophss/csels/dsepd/ss1978/lesson1/section1. html. Accessed May 20, 2016.

Community Preventive Services Task Force. *The Guide to Community Preventive Services: What Works to Promote Health?* 2016. Available at: http://www.thecommunityguide. org. Accessed August 4, 2016.

Coughlin SS, Berkowitz Z, Hawkins NA, Tangka F. Breast and colorectal cancer screening and sources of cancer information among older women in the United States: results from the 2003 Health Information National Trends Survey [erratum in: *Prev Chronic Dis.* 2007;4(4):A114]. *Prev Chronic Dis.* 2007;4(3):A57.

Eaker ED, Jaros L, Vierkant RA, Lantz P, Remington PL. Women's Health Alliance Intervention Study: increasing community breast and cervical cancer screening. *J Public Health Manag Pract.* 2001;7(5):20–30.

Ely AV, Childress AR, Jagannathan K, Lowe MR. The way to her heart? Response to romantic cues is dependent on hunger state and dieting history: an fMRI pilot study. *Appetite.* 2015;95:126–131.

Felitti VJ, Anda RF, Nordenberg D, et al. Relationship of childhood abuse and household dysfunction to many of the leading causes of death in adults. The Adverse Childhood Experiences (ACE) study. *Am J Prev Med.* 1998;14(4):245–258.

Foege WH, Hogan RC, Newton LH. Surveillance projects for selected diseases. *Int J Epidemiol.* 1976;5(1):29–37.

Frieden TR. Shattuck lecture: the future of public health. *N Engl J Med.* 2015;373(18): 1748–1754.

Fryback DG, Stout NK, Rosenberg MA, Trentham-Dietz A, Kuruchittham V, Remington PL. The Wisconsin Breast Cancer Epidemiology Simulation Model. *J Natl Cancer Inst Monogr.* 2006;(36):37–47.

Galea S, Tracy M, Hoggatt KJ, Dimaggio C, Karpati A. Estimated deaths attributable to social factors in the United States. *Am J Public Health.* 2011;101(8):1456–1465.

Hill AB. The environment and disease: association or causation? *Proc R Soc Med.* 1965;58(5):295–300.

Howlader N, Noone AM, Krapcho M, et al., eds. *SEER Cancer Statistics Review, 1975–2009 (Vintage 2009 Populations).* Bethesda, MD: National Cancer Institute; 2012.

Institute of Medicine. *The Future of Public Health.* Washington, DC: National Academy Press; 1988.

International Agency for Research on Cancer (IARC). Tobacco smoke and involuntary smoking. In: *Monographs on the Evaluation of Carcinogenic Risks to Humans.* 2004;83:913–972. Available at: https://monographs.iarc.fr/ENG/Monographs/vol83/mono83-6B-4.pdf. Accessed August 25, 2016.

Jaros L, Eaker ED, Remington PL. Women's Health Alliance Intervention Study: description of a breast and cervical cancer screening program. *J Public Health Manag Pract.* 2001;7(5):31–35.

Kitchen AJ, Trivedi P, Ng D, Mokbel K. Is there a link between breast cancer and abortion: a review of the literature. *Int J Fertil Womens Med.* 2005;50(6):267–271.

Kohler BA, Sherman RL, Howlader N, et al. Annual report to the nation on the status of cancer, 1975–2011, featuring incidence of breast cancer subtypes by race/ethnicity, poverty, and state. *J Natl Cancer Inst.* 2015;107(6):djv048.

Koplan JP, Thacker SB. Fifty years of epidemiology at the Centers for Disease Control and Prevention: significant and consequential. *Am J Epidemiol.* 2001;154(11):982–984.

Last Week Tonight. John Oliver discusses how and why media outlets so often report untrue or incomplete information as science. May 8, 2016. Available at: https://www.youtube.com/watch?v=0Rnq1NpHdmw. Accessed August 4, 2016.

Liang SY, Phillips KA, Nagamine M, Ladabaum U, Haas JS. Rates and predictors of colorectal cancer screening. *Prev Chronic Dis.* 2006;3(4):A117.

McDowell I, Newell C. *Measuring Health: A Guide to Rating Scales and Questionnaires.* 3rd ed. New York, NY: Oxford University Press; 2006.

Mokdad AH, Marks JS, Stroup DF, Gerberding JL. Actual causes of death in the United States, 2000. *JAMA.* 2004;291(10):1238–1245.

National Cancer Institute (NCI). Cancer mortality maps. 2016a. Available at: http://ratecalc.cancer.gov/ratecalc/index.jsp. Accessed August 29, 2016.

National Cancer Institute (NCI). Breast Cancer Risk Assessment Tool. 2016b. Available at: http://www.cancer.gov/bcrisktool/Default.aspx. Accessed August 4, 2016.

Petitti DB. *Meta-Analysis, Decision Analysis, and Cost-Effectiveness Analysis: Methods for Quantitative Synthesis in Medicine.* 2nd ed. New York, NY: Oxford University Press; 2000.

Reynolds P, Hurley SE, Gunier RB, Yerabati S, Quach T, Hertz A. Residential proximity to agricultural pesticide use and incidence of breast cancer in California, 1988–1997. *Environ Health Perspect.* 2005;113(8):993–1000.

Riegelman RK. *Studying a Study and Testing a Test: How to Read the Medical Evidence.* 6th ed. Philadelphia, PA: Lippincott Williams and Wilkins; 2013.

Rookus MA, van Leeuwen FE. Induced abortion and risk for breast cancer: reporting (recall) bias in a Dutch case–control study. *J Natl Cancer Inst.* 1996;88(23):1759–1764.

Shelby RA, Scipio CD, Somers TJ, Soo MS, Weinfurt KP, Keefe FJ. Prospective study of factors predicting adherence to surveillance mammography in women treated for breast cancer. *J Clin Oncol.* 2012;30(8):813–819.

Sprague BL, Gangnon RE, Hampton JM, et al. Variation in breast cancer–risk factor associations by method of detection: results from a series of case–control studies. *Am J Epidemiol.* 2015;181(12):956–969.

Thun MJ, Myers DG, Day-Lally C, et al. Age and the exposure–response relationships between cigarette smoking and premature death in Cancer Prevention Study II. In: *Monograph 8: Changes in Cigarette-Related Disease Risks and Their Implications for Prevention and Control.* National Cancer Institute. 1997:383–413. Available at: http://cancercontrol.cancer.gov/brp/tcrb/monographs/8/m8_5.pdf. Accessed August 4, 2016.

Tinker T, Vaughan E. Risk communication. In: Nelson DE, Brownson RC, Remington PL, Parvanta C, eds. *Communicating Public Health Information Effectively: A Guide for Practitioners.* Washington, DC: American Public Health Association; 2002:185–203.

US Environmental Protection Agency (USEPA). Guidelines for Carcinogen Risk Assessment. Risk Assessment Forum. PA/630/P-03/001F. Washington, DC: US Environmental Protection Agency; 2005.

Ward BW, Schiller JS, Goodman RA. Multiple chronic conditions among US adults: a 2012 update. *Prev Chronic Dis.* 2014;11:E62.

Wolff M, Toniolo P, Lee E, Rivera M, Bubinn N. Blood levels of organochlorine residues and risk of breast cancer. *J Natl Cancer Inst.* 1993;85(8):648–652.

Writing Group for the Women's Health Initiative Investigators. Risks and benefits of estrogen plus progestin in healthy postmenopausal women. Principal results from the Women's Health Initiative randomized controlled trial. *JAMA.* 2002;288(3):321–333.

Wynder EL. Workshop on guidelines to the epidemiology of weak associations. *Prev Med.* 1987;16(2):139–141.

Zaza S, Briss PA, Harris KW, eds. *The Guide to Community Preventive Services: What Works to Promote Health?* New York, NY: Oxford University Press; 2005:431–448.

3

CHRONIC DISEASE SURVEILLANCE

Mark V. Wegner, MD, MPH, Ousmane Diallo, MD, PhD,
and Patrick L. Remington, MD, MPH

Introduction

Public health surveillance is the systematic, ongoing collection, management, analysis, and interpretation of data followed by the dissemination of these data to public health programs to stimulate public health action (CDC 2012a). The final link in the surveillance chain is the application of surveillance findings to disease prevention and health promotion programs (Figure 3-1). A public health surveillance "system" includes a functional capacity for data collection, analysis, and dissemination linked to public health programs (CDC 2012a). In addition, public health surveillance serves as an early warning system for emergencies, evaluates the impact of health interventions, and sets priorities to inform public health policies and strategies (WHO 2016).

Public health surveillance evolved during the 20th century as the health burden from chronic diseases increased. In the early 1900s, surveillance described the practice of monitoring people who had been in contact with patients with certain infectious diseases, such as plague, smallpox, or typhus (Table 3-1). In the 1950s, practitioners began using surveillance to describe the practice of monitoring populations for the occurrence of specific infectious diseases, such as polio, measles, or tetanus (Langmuir 1963). By the 1970s, surveillance techniques were being applied to a broader array of diseases, including cancer, childhood lead poisoning, and congenital malformations (Thacker and Berkelman 1988).

After the events of September 11, 2001, surveillance in the United States again became strongly associated with infectious diseases, as bioterrorism preparedness and surveillance became national priorities, prompting more widespread use of syndromic surveillance methods and monitoring programs such

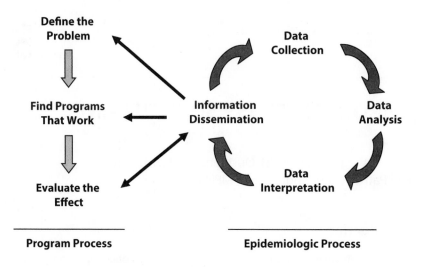

Source: Wegner (2010).

Figure 3-1. Conceptual Model for Public Health Surveillance (Epidemiologic Process) and Its Link to the Program Planning Process

as BioSense (Henning 2004; Loonsk 2004). However, at the same time, partly because of the increased cost of health care attributable to the impact of chronic diseases, interest in chronic disease surveillance continued to grow to include monitoring trends in behavioral, occupational, and environmental risk factors and other health conditions, such as disabilities (Perdue et al. 2003). Use of the established surveillance systems that monitor the health of individuals in the context of the communities in which they live helps draw attention to the complex interaction of health determinants, health outcomes, physical measurements, biological samples, policies, and the built environment.

Unlike infectious diseases, which are the focus of the overwhelming majority of the national surveillance systems, chronic diseases do not have an established integrated national surveillance system that can deliver data to stakeholders at a national, regional, and local level. Providing guidance on chronic disease surveillance to the National Institutes of Health (NIH) and the Centers for Disease Control and Prevention (CDC), the Institute of Medicine (IOM) identified the key characteristics of a national surveillance system. Among other functionalities, the system should be able to provide data on incidence and prevalence longitudinally, to identify adequate prevention measures, to determine health and quality-of-life outcomes, and to provide

Table 3-1. Trends in the Application of Surveillance to Public Health, 1900 to Present

Period	Application	Examples
1900s	Individual contacts of infected patients	Surveillance of individuals who came in contact with a case of smallpox is conducted.
1950s	Communicable diseases	Cases of polio are reported to the public health agency as part of a communicable disease control program.
1970s	Selected chronic diseases	Cancer registries are established as part of the Surveillance, Epidemiology, and End Results Program.
1990s	Behavioral, occupational, and environmental risk factors	Trends in the prevalence of cigarette smoking, determined through telephone surveys, are used to plan tobacco control programs.
2000s	Bioterrorism and preparedness	Syndromic surveillance for early detection of outbreaks is conducted.
	The built environment	Surveillance programs look at both health status and the communities in which individuals live.
2010s	Electronic health records and meaningful use	Surveillance is enhanced with more real-time data and data on results of clinical procedures.

representative data to support local public health actions to address health disparities (IOM 2011, IOM 2012).

The need for improved chronic disease surveillance systems gained even greater importance after the Affordable Care Act (ACA) was signed into law on March 23, 2010. The comprehensive set of health insurance reforms that aimed to help cover 17 million Americans who did not currently have health insurance (CMS 2014) will likely increase the number of health care events and services related to chronic conditions (Carman et al. 2015). The ACA's promotion of payment-based value models led to an increased importance for documentation through electronic health records (EHRs). This resulted in the "meaningful use" concept introduced in the Health Information Technology for Economic and Clinical Health Act, which required hospital systems to demonstrate that they "meaningfully used" EHRs in a way that would make a difference to patient care (ONC 2014).

This chapter describes the three basic elements of a chronic disease surveillance system: (1) data sources, (2) analysis and interpretation, and (3) dissemination to public health programs and other important constituents. The chapter concludes by emphasizing the importance of linking these data to chronic disease prevention and control efforts.

Data Sources

Important changes in how health data are collected occurred within the recent decades ranging from the classical data repository systems to new applications such as interoperable systems of health data allowing exchange of real-time data among clinicians, researchers, and public health practitioners (Lee and Thacker 2011). These data systems include notifiable diseases, vital statistics, sentinel surveillance, registries, health surveys, administrative data collection systems (claims), EHRs, prescription drug monitoring systems, and the U.S. Census (Table 3-2). Chronic disease surveillance may use data from one or more of these systems. For example, surveillance of the health effects of prescription drugs relies on data from vital statistics, administrative claims, telephone surveys about use of prescription drugs, and pharmacy reporting of dispensing events to the Department of Public Safety.

Public health researchers need access to most data systems to draw a comprehensive picture of the burden of chronic disease. Health departments who are the custodian of those data systems differ in the scope and structure of their data governance structure. In some health departments, access to those data is regulated by policies requiring researchers to go through an application process explaining their research or analytical needs. In others, researchers only need to sign data-use agreements or confidentiality statements certifying that they will not use the data except as intended. Data governance and data access policies represent an important part of Public Health Accreditation Standards (PHAB 2014). Therefore, public health departments should use their chronic disease data collection systems, analytics, and data sharing and dissemination plan to help secure accreditation.

Notifiable Disease Systems

The Council of State and Territorial Epidemiologists (CSTE), an organization consisting of public health epidemiologists working in states, territories, and local agencies in the United States, recommends modifications to the list of notifiable diseases annually, with input from the CDC. This list of reportable diseases and illnesses (numbering 77 illnesses and disease types in 2016)

Table 3-2. Selected Chronic Disease Data Sources and Surveillance Systems

Data System	Example	Strengths	Limitations
Notifiable diseases[a,b,c]	State-based lead poisoning reporting systems	Data are available at the local level. Usually coupled with a public health response (e.g., lead paint removal). Detailed information can be collected to aid in designing control programs.	Requires participation by community-based clinicians. Clinician-based systems have low reporting rates. Active reporting systems are time-consuming and expensive.
Vital statistics[a,b,c]	Death certificates	Laboratory-based systems are inexpensive and effective. Data are widely available at the local, state, and national levels. Population-based. Can monitor trends in age-adjusted disease rates. Can target areas with increased mortality rates.	Cause of death information may be inaccurate (e.g., lack of autopsy information). No information about risk factors.
Sentinel surveillance[b,c]	Sentinel Event Notification System for Occupational Risks (SENSOR)	Low-cost system to monitor selected diseases. Usually coupled with a public health response (e.g., asbestos removal following report of mesothelioma). Provides information on risk factors and disease severity.	Requires motivated reporting providers. May not be representative.
Disease registries[b,c]	Cancer registries	Data are increasingly available throughout the United States. Includes accurate tissue-based diagnoses. Provides stage-of-diagnosis data.	Systems are expensive. Data are affected by patient out-migration from one geographic unit to another. Risk factor information is seldom available.
Health surveys[b,c]	Behavioral Risk Factor Surveillance System telephone surveys	Monitors trends in risk factor prevalence. Can be used for program design and evaluation.	Information is based on self-reports. May be too expensive to conduct at the local level. May not be representative because of nonresponse (e.g., telephone surveys).

(Continued)

Table 3-2. (Continued)

Data System	Example	Strengths	Limitations
Administrative data collection systems[b,c]	Hospital discharge systems	Reflects regional differences on disease hospitalization rates. Can capture cost information. Data are readily available. One of the few sources of morbidity data.	Often lacks personal identifiers. Rates may be affected by changing patterns of diagnosis based on reimbursement mechanisms. Difficult to separate initial from recurrent hospitalizations.
U.S. Census[a,b,c]	Poverty rates by county	Required to calculate rates. Important predictors of health status. Available to all communities and readily available online.	Collected infrequently (every 10 years). May undercount certain populations (e.g., the poor, homeless persons).
Electronic health records	Diabetes care	Monitoring of hemoglobin A1c.	Mostly used within the health system because of the lack of integrated and interoperable systems. Social determinants not always available.

[a]Data are available from most local public health agencies.

[b]Data are available from most state departments of health.

[c]Data are available from many U.S. federal health agencies (e.g., Centers for Disease Control and Prevention, National Cancer Institute, Health Care Financing Administration).

includes primarily infectious diseases, such as measles, salmonella, and HIV infection (CDC 2016a), with five noncommunicable diseases: cancer, lead poisoning, acute carbon monoxide poisoning, silicosis, and acute pesticide-related illness and injury. Although there is a national disease surveillance list, because states are by statute responsible for collecting the data, they may chose to add reportable conditions to their lists.

In 1996, the CSTE voted to include the prevalence of cigarette smoking as an indicator for nationwide surveillance. This was the first time that a behavior, rather than a disease or illness, had been considered for national surveillance. The goals of this addition included monitoring the trends in tobacco use, guiding intervention resources, and evaluating public health interventions. Furthermore, a survey—the state-based Behavioral Risk Factor Surveillance System—was identified as the source of data for trends in smoking.

A uniform set of indicators for chronic disease surveillance has also been constructed by the CDC, the CSTE, and the Association of State and Territorial Chronic Disease Program Directors (CDC 2004a). The 2014 revision of this list includes 124 indicators organized in 18 health topic areas including cancer, cardiovascular disease, diabetes, alcohol, nutrition, tobacco, oral health, physical activity, renal disease, asthma, osteoporosis, and immunizations, as well as 22 indicators related to environmental and system changes (CDC 2016b). The Chronic Disease Indicators website provides access to state-level data and definitions of all indicators.

Vital Statistics

Information collected at the time of birth and death are often used for chronic disease surveillance to monitor prevalence of disease and overall health status, develop programs to improve public health, and evaluate the effectiveness of those interventions. Vital statistics measure the impact of health insurance, access to care, and prenatal care on birth outcomes, and monitor deaths attributable to injury, cancer, heart disease, diabetes, and other conditions (NAPHSIS 2013). Mortality records are the records most often used for chronic disease surveillance and constitute the oldest data systems used for disease surveillance.

In the United States, mortality data are collected through the vital registration system. After a person dies, a physician or coroner completes the death certificate. He or she lists the immediate cause of death (e.g., pneumonia), the sequence of events that led to the death (e.g., lung cancer), other contributing causes (e.g., tobacco use), and the manner of death, which specifies the context surrounding the death, such as accidents, suicide, homicide, or natural causes. The disease or condition that triggered the chain of events that eventually caused the death is considered to be the "underlying cause of death" (Kirscher and Anderson 1987; CDC 2003). In the example cited previously, lung cancer would be listed as the underlying cause, tobacco use and pneumonia would be listed as contributing causes, and the manner of death would be natural cause.

One important limitation of using mortality data for surveillance is that death certificates are occasionally incomplete. Physicians do not receive extensive training in completing death certificates, and the physician or coroner who is completing the certificate may not know the entire clinical history of the deceased person, or may not take the time to properly complete the certificate. States register the death certificates and transmit the files to the National Center for Health Statistics (NCHS) for processing, and in return the states receive their files coded (using *International Classification of Disease* codes). The NCHS uses SuperMICAR, a coding software, to sift through the text fields the coroner or medical examiner provide to the state (NCHS 2016a). With the advent of electronic reporting, the text in the fields is typed; however, the clinical information from the physician establishing the cause of death might not be. In cases in which the event could not be coded by SuperMICAR, professional coders are used. The NCHS manual showed evidence of how difficult it is for coders to read doctors' handwriting, yet most attestations that doctors provide are handwritten and faxed into the reporting system. Finally, the manner of death often may not be determined even after autopsy and forensic investigation (NCHS 2016b).

In most states, mortality data are readily accessible for chronic disease surveillance. State-specific data are collected and maintained by vital statistics departments in a standard format. The CDC has developed guidelines for the use of mortality data for chronic disease surveillance (Office of Surveillance and Analysis 1992). In addition, these mortality data are easily accessible online (CDC 2016c). Birth certificate data can be used to identify the presence of some chronic conditions during pregnancy, such as hypertension, diabetes, and cardiac disease; however, hospital discharge or other data sources may perform better than vital statistics for identifying some chronic diseases in pregnancy (Devlin et al. 2009).

In addition to death and birth certificates, State Vital Records Systems collect marriage, divorce, and abortion data. Although state registrars are mandated to report on death and birth data (e.g., State of Wisconsin 2016) for surveillance purposes, depending on data governance disposition, those systems are available for research scientists and analysts to report on disease processes.

The maternal and birth screening is another important feature of national and state public health surveillance. At birth, all babies are screened before they leave the hospital with a heel stick (blood card), hearing test, and pulse oximetry. Newborn screening began in the early 1960s when Dr. Robert Guthrie developed a blood test for the metabolic disorder phenylketonuria, which causes devastating brain damage and death if left untreated (Holt 1997). Ever since, more tests have been developed to screen newborns for a variety of severe conditions. Currently, there are more than 60 disorders for which a test is available. Although there are commonly accepted tests across the United States, each state may mandate different newborn screening panels according to the state department of health (CDC 2015).

Sentinel Surveillance

The term *sentinel surveillance* encompasses a wide range of activities that focus on key health indicators in the population. A sentinel event could be a particular symptom or constellation of symptoms, preventable disease, disability, or untimely death whose occurrence serves as a warning that prevention may need to be improved, or steps need to be taken to prevent a widespread outbreak. This type of surveillance lends itself well to communicable disease issues, such as monitoring the spread of influenza-like illness (CDC 2016d), and has also been proposed as a method for early identification of symptom patterns that may be indicative of a naturally occurring outbreak or a bioterrorist attack.

When applied to chronic diseases, sentinel surveillance most often focuses on occupational-related health conditions. The National Institute for Occupational Safety and Health has developed the Sentinel Event Notification System for Occupational Risks, which depends on sentinel providers to report detailed information about people diagnosed with diseases such as silicosis, lead poisoning, or carpal tunnel syndrome (Baker 1989).

Chronic Disease Registries

Chronic disease registries are essential for monitoring trends in diseases. Collection of chronic disease information for surveillance is often mandated under state law, and the chronic disease registry is usually the entity charged with fulfilling that mandate. Detailed information about each disease can be collected, such as patient demographics, stage at diagnosis, or types of treatment provided. Given the scope and complexity of the data collection and processing, these registries require considerable financial resources to implement and maintain.

Cancer registries are the most common type of disease registry used for chronic disease surveillance. Hospitals, pathology laboratories, physician offices, and clinics collect data on patients after they have been diagnosed with or treated for cancer. Those data are then reported to a cancer registry. These data include demographic information, tumor information (primary site, histology, diagnostic confirmation, stage of disease at diagnosis, distant metastases at time of diagnosis, date of diagnosis, patient's residence at diagnosis, behavior, and grade), and treatment information (date and type of cancer-directed first-course treatment).

The type of cancer registry varies according to the population on which data are collected, the standards followed for collection, and the extent of follow-up performed. Hospital-based registries collect information on patients diagnosed or treated at that facility; they are often able to collect follow-up information on their patients from time of diagnosis to death. In contrast, population-based registries collect information on all people residing in a specific geographic area, such as a county, region, or state. These registries are more appropriate for epidemiological analysis and research covering a particular population group because the data collected can be tailored to the defined population at risk; thus, cancer incidence rates can be calculated over time and among geographic regions, and for a variety of patient demographic groups. However, patient migration out of the area covered by a population-based registry for care can often limit the accuracy of these systems, necessitating follow-up work to improve completeness of the data (Walsh et al. 2006). Many population-based registries do not have sufficient funds to conduct such follow-up. Hospital-based registries have the ability, more often, to conduct patient follow-up, making it possible to calculate survival statistics.

Population-based cancer registries were established to identify regional differences in cancer incidence rates and to better understand the reasons for these differences (Austin 1983). The first population-based cancer registry was established in Connecticut in 1936. The Surveillance, Epidemiology, and End Results program of the National Cancer Institute, established in

1972, is composed of individual population-based registries in 18 separate geographic areas, covering approximately 26% of the U.S. population. This program provides data on national trends in both cancer incidence and mortality and is used by researchers to conduct epidemiologic studies of cancer (NCI 2016).

In October 1992, Congress established the National Program of Cancer Registries by enacting The Cancer Registries Amendment Act (1992). As a result of this law, the CDC provides annual financial support to state and territorial health departments and some universities to establish and improve population-based cancer registries. As of the writing of this text, 45 states, the District of Columbia, Puerto Rico, and the U.S. Pacific Island Jurisdictions receive CDC support for cancer registries, representing 96% of the U.S. population (CDC 2016e).

Other chronic disease registries include traumatic brain injury, stroke, and birth defects registries. Since the 1990s, with the development of "sentinel injuries" surveillance systems, states have developed statewide registries for traumatic brain injury to identify individuals and facilitate and coordinate their rehabilitation and other needed services (Langlois and Rutland-Brown 2005). For example, the Iowa Department of Public Health funds the Brain Injury Alliance of Iowa to maintain the Iowa Brain Injury Resource Network, which provides information and support to meet the needs of Iowa families experiencing brain injury and the providers that assist them (BIAA 2016).

After Georgia Senator Paul Coverdell died suddenly from a stroke in 2000, the U.S. Congress directed the CDC to implement state-based registries of all acute strokes. The CDC funded and provided technical assistance to nine states to develop, implement, and enhance systems for collecting data on patients experiencing an acute stroke. As of 2015, there were more than 550,000 stroke patients in the Paul Coverdell National Acute Stroke Registry (CDC 2016f).

Health Surveys and Surveillance Systems

Health surveys may be used to collect information about self-reported behaviors and health practices in the general population. In the United States, surveys such as the National Health Interview Survey are important sources of information for monitoring trends in the prevalence of health conditions and risk factors in the general population. These surveys, conducted annually since 1957, provide information on self-reported chronic conditions, health behaviors, and use of health services.

To obtain comparable information at the state or local level, CDC has developed an ongoing telephone surveillance system called the Behavioral Risk Factor Surveillance System. These data are collected with standardized methods and questionnaires, thus permitting comparison of the prevalence of behavioral risk factors, such as smoking and alcohol use, between states, over time, and for various sociodemographic groups.

Data are collected monthly, with more than 400,000 adults interviewed each year by a stratified random-digit-dial telephone sampling. Each interview takes about 15 to 20 minutes to complete and addresses a variety of conditions and risk factors, including cardiovascular disease, asthma, cancer, tobacco use, alcohol consumption, exercise, diet, and the use of preventive health services. States may choose to include topical modules relevant to their local health issues in addition to core questions used by all states. These data are usually entered directly into a computer and are summarized annually by CDC and state health departments. Data quality concerns include validity and reliability of the questions, sample bias, reporting accuracy, and changing trends in telephone surveys, such as decreasing landline coverage and increasing use of cellular telephones (Kempf and Remington 2007; Blumberg and Luke 2009). Recognizing the increased use of cellphones and the decrease in landline coverage in households, the CDC added cellular telephone lines to the BRFSS sampling in 2010 (CDC 2012b). The change in the sampling and the calculation of the sampling weights had a significant impact on the prevalence estimates, which limits the value of any trend analyses before 2011.

The CDC also supports the Youth Risk Behavior Surveillance System (Brener et al. 2004). Anonymous surveys are administered to a representative sample of 9th to 12th grade students in many states, territories, and cities across the United States. This surveillance system monitors six categories of priority chronic disease risk behaviors, including tobacco use, alcohol and other drug use, sexual behaviors, unhealthy dietary behaviors, and physical inactivity. Health and education officials use these data to improve national, state, and local policies and programs designed to reduce risks associated with the leading causes of mortality and morbidity.

Some health surveys go beyond self-reported risk factors and conditions to include additional information collected through physical examinations and biologic samples. The National Health and Nutrition Examination Survey (NHANES) was created in the late 1950s to monitor the health status of the U.S. population. Data collection for NHANES has focused on different population age groups over time, but today it operates continuously and includes all ages. Mobile examination centers are used to conduct interviews and physical examinations, collecting information on prevalence of chronic conditions, risk factors, body measurements, and blood samples. Because of the extensive amount of data collected on each individual, NHANES is most valuable for providing national information. One of the first state- and local-level adaptations of this approach was started in Wisconsin in 2008 (Survey of the Health of Wisconsin; University of Wisconsin School of Medicine and Public Health 2016).

Administrative Data Collection Systems

Many data on chronic diseases are collected as part of routine administration, such as hospital discharge and Medicaid and Medicare claims. Hospital discharge data—hospitalizations, emergency department visits, and outpatient visits—are the most widely available of these types of data. In particular, hospital discharge data are often used to characterize morbid conditions associated with chronic diseases and to predict short-term and long-term mortality (Quail et al. 2011). Information is collected from the medical abstracts and billing records of each patient discharged from the hospital. After a number of delays, the United States officially switched to *International Classification of Diseases, Tenth Revision, Clinical Modification* (NCHS 2016b) for coding of patient diagnoses and procedures.

Unfortunately, the usefulness of administrative databases is limited by incomplete records, unreliable or invalid coding, and missing important clinical variables. Measurement errors associated with hospital discharge data arise chiefly in the coding process, which requires coders to know clinical diagnoses and the organization of the *International Classification of Diseases* coding scheme. Thus, misclassification may occur either unintentionally if providers lack understanding of diagnostic coding and grouping, or if providers code with an eye toward maximizing reimbursement via particular diagnosis-related groups (NORC 2005). Also, although diagnoses are often listed on the face sheet of the medical record, the principal diagnoses may not be cited accurately when the hospital discharge form is completed.

Another limitation is inherent in the fact that these data only capture events that occur in a hospital. Thus, the growing number of procedures that historically required hospitalization, but that now can be performed in outpatient settings, would not be captured. In addition, information on injuries may be missed by this system if the injury is either serious enough that the patient dies before being admitted to a hospital, or is not serious enough to warrant a hospital stay (Schoenman et al. 2007).

The principles of surveillance can also be applied by state and national agencies to monitor the quality of health care (Chassin et al. 1996). For example, consumers and purchasers of health care use Healthcare Effectiveness Data and Information Set (HEDIS) data to assess the performance of managed health care plans (Iglehart 1996). Developed and maintained by the National Committee for Quality Assurance, HEDIS addresses eight performance domains: effectiveness of care, access or availability of care, satisfaction with the experience of care, cost of care, health plan stability, informed health care choices, use of services, and health plan descriptive information. It is one of the most widely used sets of health care performance measures in the United States.

With the increased use of EHRs, public health will have an opportunity to improve its surveillance capabilities. Some states have piloted surveillance based on automated data feed from hospitals and providers to their surveillance systems and found improved efficiency and timely data reporting, as well as including clinical information related to the reported disease. In Boston, the Electronic Medical Record Support for Public Health system detects notifiable diseases by scanning ambulatory encounter data for combinations of laboratory test results, diagnostic codes, medication prescriptions, and vital signs suggestive of reportable conditions. The system is configured as an independent data repository consisting of flat file extracts from a clinical practice's EHRs (Klompas et al. 2007).

The use of EHRs can be extended to serve as a venue of providing data to many data systems, such as birth—collecting parental information and the data needed for the birth certificates—and chronic disease registries. In addition, in health care settings, patients fill out questionnaires collecting behavioral, socioeconomic, cultural, and environmental information.

Census Data

Every 10 years, the U.S. government conducts a census of the entire U.S. population. In addition to counting the population, the census collects detailed information on individual and household characteristics, such as age, race, education, occupation, insurance coverage, income, and disability. These census data are essential for calculating rates in populations, to compare disease burden and trends among regions or over time, and to generate geographic characteristics associated with social determinants of health.

Despite efforts to enumerate the entire population, however, the census misses some people. In an effort to improve the timeliness of population information, the U.S. Census has instituted the American Community Survey (ACS). The ACS uses monthly samples, combining data over multiple years when necessary, to create small-area data on topics such as educational attainment, income, ancestry, and housing. This information was previously collected in the "long form" of the decennial census. More timely small area population estimates are especially important for population groups whose numbers are changing rapidly and for areas that may experience large, sustained population changes because of natural disasters, economic changes, or other causes (see Chapter 2, Chronic Disease Epidemiology, for more information on small-area analyses). With declining response rates, ACS started to combine computer-assisted telephone interviews and computer-assisted personal interviews to the mailed data collection strategy. Although the ACS provides housing-unit data, it also includes group quarters, which consist of military barracks and school dormitories. The strength of the ACS data resides more in its capabilities to estimate sociodemographic characteristics (percentage, means, or median estimates) of geographical areas than for population total for rate calculation (U.S. Census Bureau 2014). However, it is standard practice to use the ACS single age, sex, and race estimates to compute age-adjusted rates over time.

Health Policy Surveillance

Because the core functions of public health include assessment, assurance, and policy development, identifying and supporting policies enacted to protect the health of the people is as important as collecting and analyzing health data and enforcing laws and regulations. Policies consist of any laws, regulations, or procedures from federal, state, and local health departments that influence health either by reducing the disease burden and risk factors or by promoting environmental and social determinant changes. The development of policy surveillance systems helps keep track of policies and offers a venue for impact and outcome evaluation. In addition, policy surveillance systems can help conduct more sophisticated research on the determinants of health based on hypotheses that can be tested in intervention studies. A few efforts are under-way to develop public health policy surveillance systems. For example, a group of federal and voluntary agencies has developed policy surveillance systems for tobacco, alcohol, and, more recently, school-based nutrition and physical edu-cation (Brownson et al. 2009).

The analysis of the impact of health policies can be quantitative or qualita-tive. Measures based on policies are diverse as they can range from "yes or no" questions to more sophisticated measures. Time- and location-based varia-tions may be necessary "policy inputs" in analytics to address needed behavior changes (Chriqui et al. 2011).

In conclusion, chronic disease surveillance can be conducted by using a wide variety of existing data sources. When using these data, public health practitioners must understand the advantages and limitations inherent in each system. Despite these limitations, a comprehensive surveillance system—using a wide variety of chronic disease data—can serve as a resource to improve the health of the entire population (Roos et al. 1993).

Data Analyses and Interpretation

Chronic disease surveillance systems must have the capacity to analyze data. Data analysis and interpretation require knowledge about chronic diseases, epi-demiology, and the relationship among risk factors, conditions, morbidity, and death. In addition, interpretation of analyses should include a thorough under-standing of the data systems and statistical techniques used in all analyses. Because of the large number of cases involved, analysis at one time required the use of mainframe computers; however, today, large data sets can be easily accommodated on personal computers, and powerful laptops have made data entry, surveillance, and analysis highly portable. Data are also frequently avail-able in an online or electronic format. Internet-based query systems provide quick access to national (e.g., CDC WONDER, http://wonder.cdc.gov), state (e.g., Wisconsin Interactive Statistics on Health, http://dhs.wisconsin.gov/ wish), and local (e.g., the Chicago Health Atlas, http://www.chicagohealthatlas. org) data.

Chronic disease surveillance uses descriptive epidemiology to examine the distribution of diseases in the population by person, place, and time. On the basis of needs and priorities, public health agencies usually develop a set of indicators to monitor change in their communities and evaluate programs in the long term (Rogers et al. 2011). Moving forward, researchers need to envision using advanced analytics to better understand disease outcomes and associated risk factors. Brief descriptions of these important analyses follow.

Person Analyses

Descriptive studies begin by examining how the distribution of a disease or condition varies in the population according to personal characteristics, such as age, race, or gender. Survey data also provide useful information at the population level. When reporting on prevalence estimates such as risky behaviors, researchers need to pay attention to the survey sampling frame and use appropriate statistical methods for analyzing survey data, including using the right stratification and weighting procedures. For example, Table 3-3 shows the prevalence estimates of obesity by race in Alabama. Overall, there were fewer than 3,000 adults aged 18 years and older who responded to the body mass index categories. This sample represented three million Alabama adult residents among whom 69% were white, 26% were black, and 4% were Hispanic. Because of the low sample size among Hispanics and other racial groups, the 95% confidence intervals of the race-specific prevalence estimates are much wider for Hispanics and other groups than for whites and blacks (CDC 2014).

Place Analyses

A second type of analysis involves comparing the occurrence of a disease, condition, or risk factor between one geographic region and another. Typically,

Table 3-3. Obesity Prevalence in Alabama by Race/Ethnicity, 2014 Behavioral Risk Factor Surveillance System

Race/Ethnicity	Sample, No.	% (95% CI)
White, non-Hispanic	1729	31.4 (29.7, 33.1)
Black, non-Hispanic	954	41.9 (38.7, 45.0)
Hispanic	18	22.9 (11.3, 34.5)
Other, non-Hispanic	48	21.7 (12.9, 30.5)
Multiracial, non-Hispanic	37	39.3 (25.6, 53.0)

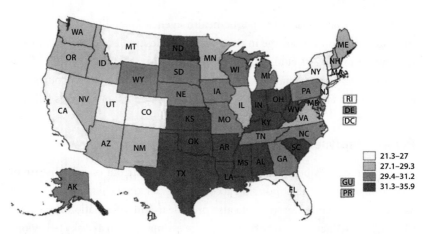

Source: Reprinted from CDC (2014).

Figure 3-2. Obesity Prevalence in the United States, 2014 Behavioral Risk Factor Surveillance System

the rate in a city or county is compared with rates for the rest of the state or the nation. This information may be used to target a specific intervention in a region (Brownson et al. 1992). Figure 3-2 shows the differences in obesity prevalence between states in the United States.

Regional analyses must account for differences in age structure between and among regions by using age-standardized rates. In addition, regional differences in disease rates may result from differences in diagnostic practices or disease definitions. Finally, these analyses are often limited because of the small number of cases typically occurring in small regions, such as cities, villages, or towns. See Chapter 2 for a more detailed discussion of the challenges created by working with small numbers of cases, and how to handle these types of analyses.

A specialized form of regional analysis involves the analysis of diseases that appear to "cluster" in a geographic area, such as a cluster of cancer cases that occur in a neighborhood. The investigation of these disease clusters poses a continuing challenge to state and local public health officials. Most often, these disease clusters are reported by members of the public or by clinicians who are looking for explanations for the apparent increase in the incidence of a disease.

Public health agencies have developed systematic protocols to aid in the investigation of these apparent disease clusters (Fiore et al. 1990; Devier et al. 1990). These procedures involve defining the population at risk, ascertaining all cases, estimating rate ratios (i.e., observed vs. expected), and assessing exposure and biological plausibility. With this approach, few investigations identify specific environmental exposures responsible for the disease cluster. A major difficulty in studying such clusters involves the small number of disease cases available for analysis. In fact, Rothman (1990) states that, with very few exceptions, there is little scientific or public health purpose in investigating individual disease clusters at all.

Time Analyses

Finally, and perhaps most importantly, chronic disease surveillance systems must monitor the trends in chronic disease rates over time. The epidemic curve has traditionally been used to detect outbreaks, to better characterize transmission patterns, and to determine appropriate intervention strategies. Similarly, trends in variables such as per capita cigarette sales can be used to monitor the effectiveness of interventions following the implementation of a statewide tobacco control program (Bandi et al. 2006).

Temporal trend analyses must consider changes in the age structure of the population over time, usually by using age standardization with a standard reference population. In addition, changes in diagnostic practices and disease definitions may cause apparent trends in disease incidence over time. Both temporal trend and regional analyses may be conducted for specific subgroups of the population. For example, as mammography began to be widely implemented in the mid- to late 1980s, and improvements in treatment were achieved in the 1990s, a significant gap developed in breast cancer mortality between white women and black women in the United States (Figure 3-3). Although more recently the rates of breast cancer appear to be declining among both white women and black women in the United States, the rate decline for black women began later and has been less pronounced than the decline for white women, and a large disparity gap continues to exist. These findings have important implications in the development of programs to ensure that all demographic groups have equal access to advances in public health knowledge.

Data Dissemination

The final step in chronic disease surveillance is to disseminate the information that has been collected. The increasing amount of surveillance data described previously provides a wealth of information to public health agencies. However, too often these agencies simply analyze the data and report the results in agency reports or occasionally in state or national publications. These reports

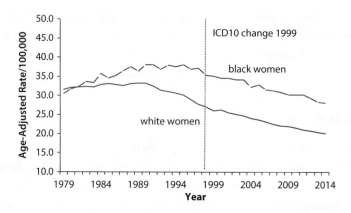

Source: Adapted from CDC (2016c).

Figure 3-3. Trends in Age-Adjusted Breast Cancer Mortality in the United States by Race, 1980–2014

are often long and contain technical jargon. In addition, the information is seldom linked to program priorities, and the reports are seldom used to promote public health practice or as a vehicle for setting priorities for action.

In the past, communicable disease surveillance systems typically produced surveillance reports and distributed them to health care providers. Today's chronic disease programs address a broader constituency, including policymakers, voluntary health organizations, professional organizations, and the general public. Thus, the information must be communicated through several channels by using different strategies to ensure that it reaches the appropriate target groups.

Epidemiologists working in public health agencies are frequently asked to disseminate the results of a surveillance report, often by publishing the information in a health department report. To increase application of surveillance findings to disease prevention and health promotion programs, a basic framework for communicating surveillance information can be used (Remington 1998; Goodman and Remington 1993; Table 3-4). Once the analysis has been completed, this framework has five additional steps:

Establish the Message

This is perhaps the most important step in disseminating health and surveillance information. Like businesses, public health agencies have a product (i.e., information) that they need to sell (i.e., communicate). An epidemiologist

Table 3-4. Steps in Communicating Public Health Surveillance Information

Step	Question	Action
1	What are the results?	Conduct the analysis.
2	What should be accomplished?	Set an objective.
3	Who needs to hear the message?	Define the audience.
4	What is the key take-away point?	Establish the message.
5	What is the best way to deliver the message?	Select the channel.
6	Was the communication successful?	Evaluate the impact.

Source: Based on Remington (1998).

must convince the audience that it is worth their time to read, understand, and act on the information. An important adage in marketing the message is "less is more."

Many reports produced by public health agencies are long, technical, and full of information. These reports might be mailed to the media, policymakers, or health care providers who, in turn, rarely take the time to read through the report to find the important information. To capture their attention, the main point of the report must be obvious and simple to understand.

Population health rankings are an effective, yet sometimes controversial, approach to call attention to differences in population health data, including mortality rates and chronic disease risk factors. Implementations of this concept, such as the America's Health Rankings and the County Health Rankings, are often used as a catalyst for the improvement of health by drawing attention to the areas that need improvement through an easily interpretable synthesis of objectively measured community health data (Remington et al. 2015). Ranking the health of places increases interest in the results, enabling organizations reporting the information to craft messages to not only explain the observed differences, but also to suggest ways to improve health through community action.

Set an Objective

Why is the information being reported? Public health agencies often report information without any specific goal, but simply "because it is there." Other times, the purpose is to educate the general public about a health issue. This is a worthwhile but challenging goal given the complexity of the message and the inability to shape the message for the intended audience.

Define the Audience

Once the objective for communicating the information has been established, one can define the appropriate target audience. Local health departments and health care providers have been the long-standing audience of communicable disease surveillance information, as these professionals have been responsible for implementing disease control strategies. In addition, physicians were the source of these reports, and reporting back to them showed the usefulness of the system and helped maintain their continued reporting.

The audience for public health surveillance information is much broader today and includes policymakers, voluntary health organizations, professional organizations, and the general public. A report that breast cancer death rates are increasing among minorities, or low-income women, or women who are uninsured or underinsured in a state could be communicated to the general public, or to women specifically. This would increase awareness of the importance of mammography and early detection. It might also be targeted to policymakers, such as legislators considering developing a breast cancer detection program focused on reducing breast cancer deaths among racial/ethnic minority, low-income, or uninsured women. Finally, the report could be given to an advocacy organization, such as a statewide minority health council, to use in its efforts to advocate minority health.

Select the Channel

A "channel" can be considered the medium through which messages must travel to reach the intended audience. Examples of channels include professional journals, direct mail, television, radio, newspapers, blogs, and other Internet sources. Public health agencies traditionally report surveillance information in newsletters or statistical bulletins. These reports are routinely mailed to local public health agencies, physicians, health care institutions, the media, and other interested individuals in the community or the state. A press release is occasionally used to increase the media interest in the story.

Careful selection of a proper communication channel increases the likelihood that the information will reach the target audience. This requires a thorough understanding, based on market research, of how those individuals obtain their information. For example, children and teachers might best be reached through the school system newsletter. Policymakers might be reached through a direct mailing to their offices or via a constituent organization. Doctors might be reached through a state medical society journal. For most target groups, it is also helpful in disseminating a message through an effective presence on the Internet, as Internet access has become nearly universal and, with the rise of smartphones and social media, is often the most accessible and first source individuals turn to for information.

Creative presentation of information can also increase the media coverage of a health issue. For example, in support of a comprehensive smoking ban in Wisconsin, it was pointed out that in Wisconsin in a given year, the number of people who die from secondhand smoke exposure (a harm viewed by many as an insignificant risk not requiring government intervention) and the number of people who die in motor vehicle accidents (a cause of death well recognized as a significant public health issue requiring government regulation) is approximately the same at about 800 individuals per year.

Evaluate the Impact

The final step in a communication plan is to evaluate how widely the information was disseminated and whether the information led to the intended outcome. The dissemination can be measured by determining the number of reports distributed, the readership of a journal, coverage in the media, or the number of hits on a particular website. Web searches can be an effective means of finding all articles on a particular topic in a defined geographic area. These articles can be reviewed by the program staff to assess the geographic distribution and extent of the media coverage. In addition, the content can be reviewed to assess both the accuracy and appropriateness of the messages as they were picked up by the media.

These methods can provide early indicators of success of public health campaigns. However, one major drawback of evaluating interventions aimed at reducing chronic disease is that as a consequence of the slow progression from risk factors to physiologic changes to symptoms to eventual disease development, demonstrating definitive proof of disease reduction may take decades, whereas the typical political cycle is only every 2 to 6 years. Thus, if the political winds shift, potentially effective programs may be cut before they have had a chance to demonstrate their impact. In addition, evaluations of societal change and impact on disease are often expensive, time consuming, and difficult to interpret.

Conclusion

Data collection, analysis, and dissemination are vital components of a chronic disease surveillance system. The final link in surveillance is the application of the data to prevention and control (Thacker and Berkelman 1988). Unfortunately, the long latency period of most chronic diseases often results in a perceived lack of urgency in developing and implementing control measures. For example, at the onset of a potential influenza pandemic or an outbreak of an illness new to the world or a particular region of the world such as the Zika virus or Ebola, media attention is intense and considerable amounts of resources are deployed within hours, days, and weeks to implement control measures and contain disease spread. In contrast, it has been more than 50 years since the First Surgeon General's Report on Smoking and Health was released, definitively linking smoking to cancer and other serious chronic diseases. However, about half of the states in the United States still lack comprehensive smoke-free laws. In those states where legislation has passed, it has come only after heavy sustained effort and occasionally compromises on issues for which the strong weight of the evidence rests on the side of public health. This demonstrates that building up a definitive library of evidence and scientific data in support of a public health issue does not in and of itself constitute a "public health surveillance system" unless these data are disseminated in such a way that they can have an impact on public health policies aimed at controlling chronic disease.

With the recent emergence of chronic disease program integration as a priority (Ogino et al. 2012), chronic disease surveillance has played an even bigger role at state departments of health. An integrated approach requires innovative new methods for tracking and reporting chronic diseases, with specific emphasis on how chronic disease risk factors and certain chronic diseases are interrelated. The link between clinical medicine and public health also must continue to be strengthened, and enhanced monitoring systems that take advantage of EHRs must continue to be developed. As links among chronic diseases and risk factors are more clearly demonstrated to policymakers, there is significant potential to reframe the health care reform debate from a focus on access to a focus on prevention, and in the process increase the amount of state and federal resources allocated to addressing the important chronic disease issues that exist in our society.

Resources

Information on the availability of routinely collected chronic disease surveillance data is available from a variety of federal agencies and other sources:

Agency for Health Care Research and Quality, http://www.ahrq.gov

Behavioral Risk Factor Surveillance System, http://www.cdc.gov/BRFSS

Centers for Disease Control and Prevention (CDC), including the National Center for Health Statistics, the National Center for Chronic Disease Prevention and Health Promotion, and the Epidemiology Program Office, http://www.cdc.gov

CDC WONDER, http://wonder.cdc.gov

Centers for Medicare and Medicaid Services, http://www.cms.hhs.gov

Chronic Disease Indicators—CDC, http://www.cdc.gov/cdi

National Birth Defects Registry—CDC, http://www.cdc.gov/ncbddd/birthdefects/index.html

National Institute for Occupational Safety and Health/Sentinel Event Notification System for Occupational Risks (SENSOR), http://www.cdc.gov/niosh/topics/pesticides/overview.htm

National Institutes of Health, including the National Cancer Institute, the National Heart, Lung, and Blood Institute, and the National Institute on Drug Abuse, https://www.nih.gov

National Notifiable Diseases Surveillance System, https://wwwn.cdc.gov/nndss

U.S. Census Bureau, http://www.census.gov

Youth Risk Behavior Surveillance System, http://www.cdc.gov/HealthyYouth/yrbs/index.htm

Additional surveillance information and data can be obtained from state health departments and many local public health agencies.

Suggested Reading

Centers for Disease Control and Prevention. Indicators for chronic disease surveillance. *MMWR Recomm Rep.* (2004):53(RR11):1–6.

Centers for Disease Control and Prevention. Surveillance for certain health behaviors among states and selected local areas—Behavioral Risk Factor Surveillance System,

United States, 2004. Indicators for chronic disease surveillance. *MMWR Surveill Summ.* 2006;55(SS07):1–124.

Choi BC, McQueen DV, Puska P, et al. Enhancing global capacity in the surveillance, prevention, and control of chronic diseases: seven themes to consider and build upon. *J Epidemiol Community Health.* 2008:62(5):391–397.

Institute of Medicine. Surveillance and assessment. In: *Living Well With Chronic Illness: A Call for Public Health Action.* Washington DC: National Academies of Science; 2012.

Lee LM, Teutsch SM, St Louis ME, Thacker SB, eds. *Principles and Practice of Public Health Surveillance.* 3rd ed. New York, NY: Oxford University Press; 2010.

Pelletier AR, Siegel PZ, Baptiste MS, Maylahn C. Revisions to chronic disease surveillance indicators, United States, 2004. *Prev Chronic Dis.* 2005:2(3):1–5.

Remington PL, Simoes E, Brownson RC, Siegel PZ. The role of epidemiology in chronic disease prevention and health promotion programs. *J Public Health Manag Pract.* 2003:9(4):258–265.

Remington P, Flood T. *Public Health Surveillance.* Oxford Bibliographies; 2014. ISBN: 9780199756797.

References

Austin DF. Cancer registries: a tool in epidemiology. In: Lillienfeld AM, ed. *Reviews in Cancer Epidemiology.* Vol. 2. New York, NY: Elsevier North Holland; 1983:118–140.

Baker EL. Sentinel Event Notification System for Occupational Risks (SENSOR): the concept. *Am J Public Health.* 1989;79(suppl):18–20.

Bandi P, Remington PL, Moberg DP. Progress in reducing cigarette consumption: the Wisconsin tobacco control program, 2001–2003. *Wis Med J.* 2006;105(5):45–49.

Blumberg SJ, Luke JV. Reevaluating the need for concern regarding noncoverage bias in landline surveys. *Am J Public Health.* 2009;99(10):1806–1810.

Brain Injury Alliance of Iowa (BIAA). Support, information and education. 2016. Available at: http://www.biaia.org/support.htm#Tote. Accessed April 16, 2016.

Brener ND, Kann L, Kinchen SA, et al. Methodology of the Youth Risk Behavior Surveillance System. *MMWR Recomm Rep.* 2004b;53(RR-12):1–13.

Brownson RC, Smith CA, Jorge NE, Deprima LT, Dean CG, Cates RW. The role of data-driven planning and coalition development in preventing cardiovascular disease. *Public Health Rep.* 1992;107:32–37.

Brownson RC, Chriqui JF, Stamatakis KA. Understanding evidence-based public health policy. *Am J Public Health*. 2009;99(9):1576–1583.

Cancer Registries Amendment Act, Pub L No. 102-515, 106 Stat 3372 (1992). Available at: http://www.cdc.gov/cancer/npcr/pdf/publaw.pdf. Accessed April 26, 2016.

Carman KG, Eibner C, Paddock SM. Trends in health insurance enrollment, 2013–15. *Health Aff (Millwood)*. 2015;34(6):1044–1048.

Centers for Disease Control and Prevention (CDC). *Physicians' Handbook on Medical Certification of Death*. Atlanta, GA: CDC; 2003. DHHS Publication no. (PHS) 2003-1108.

Centers for Disease Control and Prevention (CDC). Indicators for chronic disease surveillance. *MMWR Recomm Rep*. 2004a;53(RR-11):1–6.

Centers for Disease Control and Prevention (CDC). CDC's vision for public health surveillance in the 21st century. *MMWR Suppl*. 2012a;61(3):1–40.

Centers for Disease Control and Prevention (CDC). Methodologic changes in the Behavioral Risk Factor Surveillance System in 2011 and potential effects on prevalence estimates. 2012b. Available at: http://www.cdc.gov/surveillancepractice/reports/brfss/brfss.html. Accessed March 26, 2016.

Centers for Disease Control and Prevention (CDC). BRFSS prevalence and trends data. 2014. Available at: http://www.cdc.gov/brfss/brfssprevalence. Accessed April 10, 2016.

Centers for Disease Control and Prevention (CDC). National birth defects registries: United States. 2015. Available at: http://www.cdc.gov/ncbddd/birthdefects/index.html. Accessed April 10, 2016.

Centers for Disease Control and Prevention (CDC). Nationally notifiable infectious diseases: United States. 2016a. Available at: https://wwwn.cdc.gov/nndss/conditions/notifiable/2016/infectious-diseases. Accessed April 26, 2016.

Centers for Disease Control and Prevention (CDC). Chronic disease indicators. 2016b. Available at: http://www.cdc.gov/cdi/index.html. Accessed April 19, 2016.

Centers for Disease Control and Prevention (CDC). Wide-ranging ONline Data for Epidemiologic Research (WONDER). 2016c. Available at: http://wonder.cdc.gov. Accessed August 8, 2016.

Centers for Disease Control and Prevention (CDC). Overview of influenza surveillance in the United States. 2016d. Available at: http://www.cdc.gov/flu/weekly/overview.htm. Accessed April 26, 2016.

Centers for Disease Control and Prevention (CDC). National Program of Cancer Registries (NPCR): about the program. 2016e. Available at: http://www.cdc.gov/cancer/npcr/about.htm. Accessed April 29, 2016.

Centers for Disease Control and Prevention (CDC). CDC state heart disease and stroke prevention programs. 2016f. Available at: http://www.cdc.gov/dhdsp/programs/stroke_registry.htm. Accessed May 17, 2016.

Centers for Medicare and Medicaid Services (CMS). Report to Congress on the impact on premiums for individuals and families with employer-sponsored health insurance from the guaranteed issue, guaranteed renewal, and fair health insurance premiums provisions of the Affordable Care Act. 2014. Available at: https://www.cms.gov/Research-Statistics-Data-and-Systems/Research/ActuarialStudies/Downloads/ACA-Employer-Premium-Impact.pdf. Accessed March 19, 2016.

Chassin MR, Hannan EL, DeBuono BA. Benefits and hazards of reporting medical outcomes publicly. *N Engl J Med*. 1996;334(6):394–398.

Chriqui JF, O'Connor JC, Chaloupka FJ. What gets measured, gets changed: evaluating law and policy for maximum impact. *J Law Med Ethics*. 2011;39(suppl 1):21–26.

Devier JR, Brownson RC, Bagby JR, Carlson GM, Crellin JR. A public health response to cancer clusters in Missouri. *Am J Epidemiol*. 1990;132(suppl 1):S23–S31.

Devlin HM, Desai J, Walaszek A. Reviewing performance of birth certificate and hospital discharge data to identify births complicated by maternal diabetes. *Matern Child Health J*. 2009;13(5):660–666.

Fiore BJ, Hanrahan LP, Anderson HA. State health department response to disease cluster reports: a protocol for investigation. *Am J Epidemiol*. 1990;132(suppl 1):S14–S22.

Goodman R, Remington PL. Disseminating surveillance information. In: Teutsch SM, Churchill RE, eds. *Principles and Practice of Public Health Surveillance*. New York, NY: Oxford University Press; 1993.

Henning KJ. Overview of syndromic surveillance: what is syndromic surveillance? *MMWR Suppl*. 2004;53:5–11.

Koch J. *Robert Guthrie—The PKU Story: A Crusade Against Mental Retardation*. Pasadena, CA: Hope Publishing House; 1997.

Iglehart JK. The National Committee for Quality Assurance. *N Engl J Med*. 1996; 335(13):995–999.

Institute of Medicine (IOM). *A Nationwide Framework for Surveillance of Cardiovascular and Chronic Lung Diseases*. Washington, DC: The National Academies Press; 2011.

Institute of Medicine (IOM). Surveillance and assessment. In: *Living Well With Chronic Illness: A Call for Public Health Action*. Washington DC: National Academies of Science; 2012.

Kempf AM, Remington PL. New challenges for telephone survey research in the twenty-first century. *Annu Rev Public Health*. 2007;28:113–126.

Kirscher T, Anderson RE. Cause of death: proper completion of the death certificate. *JAMA*. 1987;258(3):349–352.

Klompas M, Lazarus R, Daniel J, et al. Electronic medical record support for public health (ESP): automated detection and reporting of statutory notifiable diseases to public health authorities. *Adv Dis Surveill*. 2007;3:3.

Langlois JA, Rutland-Brown W. *Traumatic Brain Injury in the United States: The Future of Registries and Data Systems*. Atlanta, GA: Centers for Disease Control and Prevention, National Center for Injury Prevention and Control; 2005.

Langmuir AD. The surveillance of communicable diseases of national importance. *N Engl J Med*. 1963;268:182–192.

Lee LM, Thacker SB. Public health surveillance and knowing about health in the context of growing sources of health data. *Am J Prev Med*. 2011;41(6):636–640.

Loonsk JW. BioSense—a national initiative for early detection and quantification of public health emergencies. *MMWR Suppl*. 2004;53:53–55.

National Association for Public Health Statistics and Information Systems (NAPHSIS). Strategies for improving the timeliness of vital statistics. 2013. Available at: http://www.naphsis.org/Documents/NAPHSIS_Timeliness%20Report_Digital%20(1).pdf. Accessed April 10, 2016.

National Cancer Institute (NCI). Surveillance Epidemiology and End Results (SEER). 2016. Available at: http://seer.cancer.gov/about. Accessed April 26, 2016.

National Centers for Health Statistics (NCHS). SuperMICAR. 2016a. Available at: http://www.cdc.gov/nchs/nvss/mmds/super_micar.htm. Accessed August 8, 2016.

National Centers for Health Statistics (NCHS). *International Classification of Diseases, Tenth Revision, Clinical Modification (ICD-10-CM)*. 2016b. Available at: http://www.cdc.gov/nchs/data/icd/10cmguidelines_2016_final.pdf. Accessed August 8, 2016.

National Opinion Research Center (NORC). *The Value of Hospital Discharge Databases*. Bethesda, MD: NORC; 2005.

Office of Surveillance and Analysis. *Using Chronic Disease Data: A Handbook for Public Health Practitioners*. Atlanta, GA: National Center for Chronic Disease Prevention and Health Promotion, Centers for Disease Control and Prevention; 1992.

Office of the National Coordinator for Health Information Technology (ONC). Update on the adoption of health information technology and related efforts to facilitate the electronic use and exchange of health information. Report to Congress October 2014. Available at: https://www.healthit.gov/sites/default/files/rtc_adoption_and_exchange 9302014.pdf. Accessed August 8, 2016.

Ogino S, King EE, Beck AH, Sherman ME, Milner DA, Giovannucci E. Interdisciplinary education to integrate pathology and epidemiology: towards molecular and population-level health science. *Am J Epidemiol.* 2012;176(8):659–667.

Perdue WC, Stone LA, Gostin LO. The built environment and its relationship to the public's health: the legal framework. *Am J Public Health.* 2003;93(9):1390–1394.

Public Health Accreditation Board (PHAB). *Standards and Measures.* Version 1.5. 2014. Available at: http://www.phaboard.org/wp-content/uploads/SM-Version-1.5-Board-adopted-FINAL-01-24-2014.docx.pdf. Accessed August 8, 2016.

Quail JM, Lix LM, Osman BA, Teare GF. Comparing comorbidity measures for predicting mortality and hospitalization in three population-based cohorts. *BMC Health Serv Res.* 2011;11:146.

Remington PL. Communicating epidemiologic information. In: Brownson RC, Petitti DB, eds. *Applied Epidemiology: Theory to Practice.* New York, NY: Oxford University Press; 1998:323–348.

Remington PL, Catlin BB, Gennuso KP. The county health rankings: rationale and methods. *Popul Health Metr.* 2015;13(11):1–12.

Rogers T, Chappelle EF, Wall HK, Barron-Simpson R. *Using DHDSP Outcome Indicators for Policy and Systems Change for Program Planning and Evaluation.* Atlanta, GA: Centers for Disease Control and Prevention; 2011.

Roos LL, Mustard CA, Nicol JP, et al. Registries and administrative data: organization and accuracy. *Med Care.* 1993;31(3):201–212.

Rothman KJ. A sobering start for the cluster buster's conference. *Am J Epidemiol.* 1990;132(suppl 1):S6–S13.

Schoenman J, Sutton J, Elixhauser A, Love D. Understanding and enhancing the value of hospital discharge data. *Med Care Res Rev.* 2007;64(4):449–468.

State of Wisconsin. Chapter 69—Collection of Statistics. 2016. Available at: http://docs. legis.wisconsin.gov/statutes/statutes/69.pdf. Accessed August 8, 2016.

University of Wisconsin School of Medicine and Public Health. Survey of the Health of Wisconsin (SHOW). 2016. Available at: http://www.show.wisc.edu. Accessed April 26, 2016.

Thacker SB, Berkelman RL. Public health surveillance in the United States. *Epidemiol Rev.* 1988;10:164–190.

US Census Bureau. Design and methodology report. American Community Survey. 2014. Available at: https://www.census.gov/programs-surveys/acs/methodology/design-and-methodology.html. Accessed August 8, 2016.

Walsh MC, Stephenson L, Strickland J, Trentham-Dietz A. Enhancing the completeness of the Wisconsin Cancer Reporting System—the Border County Pilot Project. Surveillance Brief. Madison, WI: University of Wisconsin Comprehensive Cancer Center; 2006:2–3.

Wegner MV, Rohan AM, Remington PL. Chronic disease surveillance. In: Remington PL, Brownson RC, Wegner MV, ed. *Chronic Disease Epidemiology and Control.* 3rd ed. Washington, DC: American Public Health Association; 2010:96.

World Health Organization (WHO). Public health surveillance. 2016. Available at: http://www.who.int/topics/public_health_surveillance/en. Accessed April 10, 2016.

4

COMMUNITY-BASED INTERVENTIONS

Robert J. McDermott, PhD, Carol A. Bryant, PhD,
Alyssa B. Mayer, PhD, MPH, Mary P. Martinasek, PhD, MPH,
Julie A. Baldwin, PhD, and Sandra D. Vamos, EdD

Introduction

When one speaks of chronic diseases in the United States, one is likely to be referring to heart disease, stroke, cancer, type 2 diabetes, obesity, and arthritis, as these conditions represent the most common and economically threatening of all health problems (CDC 2016a; see Parts III and IV). Fortunately, these problems are largely preventable or can have their severity markedly reduced. Whereas the risk factors for most of these chronic diseases and conditions are well-known, preventing their occurrence is an arduous task for public health authorities. This challenge stems from the fact that many chronic diseases have their origins in social, cultural, environmental, and behavioral factors, thereby making their causes (and potential interventions) both complex and multilevel (see Part II of this text). Social and cultural factors influencing the development, dissemination, and consequences of chronic diseases include, but are not limited to, social and economic status, race, education, income, and access to health care (CDC 2014a).

Interventions to prevent or control chronic diseases can address the individual level, the system level, or the community level, where both system- and individual-level strategies are organized to become multilevel, comprehensive programs. Moreover, interventions can address primary prevention (e.g., reducing the risk of disease through exercise, healthy eating, nonsmoking), secondary prevention (e.g., early detection of breast cancer through mammograms for women, colon cancer screening for men and women aged 50 years or older, blood pressure checks for persons of all ages), or tertiary prevention (e.g., management of disease to minimize confounding complications through carefully monitored insulin intake for diabetes management, adherence to a prescribed diet, or moderate-to-vigorous exercise several days per week for patients who have had a heart attack).

Interventions for altering a health risk profile may address behaviors at the individual level—such as poor diet, tobacco use, excessive alcohol consumption, physical inactivity, and so on. Health-promoting messages can be presented through print and electronic media, including Internet and social media, or from health care providers and prevention specialists, teachers, employers, members of the faith-based community, or a host of other individuals.

Other chronic disease interventions focus on system-level changes, including policy development or change, economic incentives, and specific actions within the health care system. Examples of these interventions include food product labeling of nutrition content, enactment of tobacco excise taxes to reduce purchases by new users, and insurance coverage for physical examinations and early detection screening, among other actions.

Multilevel interventions seek to change many aspects of the environment that contribute to development of chronic diseases. These interventions include a combination of activities that prioritize change at the individual level as well as the system level. Comprehensive interventions also may address the root causes of some chronic diseases, such as poverty, low literacy, or limited education. In addition, they may attempt to garner social support for positive health behaviors. These interventions often involve health advocacy groups and empower coalitions comprising individuals or whole communities to take action.

Multiple Determinants of Chronic Disease

To be effective, chronic disease prevention and control efforts must consider the multiple determinants of chronic disease, including lifestyle and health risk behaviors, the health care system, the physical environment, and social and economic factors. The influence of these determinants on chronic disease is described in the next paragraphs.

Behavioral Determinants

Approximately half of all American adults, nearly 117 million people, had one or more chronic disease conditions in 2012, and about one fourth had two or more co-occurring chronic conditions (Ward et al. 2014). Many chronic disease conditions can be prevented, have their onset delayed, or have their symptoms significantly reduced through modest changes in individual behaviors. Four behaviors in particular—physical inactivity, poor nutrition, smoking, and drinking too much alcohol—account for much of the illness and early death caused by chronic illness. Despite this, more than half of adults do not meet the recommendations for physical activity (CDC 2015a), nearly 40% eat less than one serving of fruits and vegetables per day (CDC 2013a), 20% report smoking cigarettes (USDHHS 2014), and 38 million Americans, or nearly 12%, report binge drinking an average of 4 times a month (Kanny et al. 2012).

Many chronic illnesses are associated with overweight and obesity, and Americans have experienced significant increases in obesity during the past three decades. According to the CDC (2016a), one third of American adults— more than 78 million people—are obese and at increased risk of developing associated chronic diseases, including hypertension, dyslipidemia (e.g., high total cholesterol or high levels of triglycerides), type 2 diabetes, coronary heart disease, stroke, gallbladder disease, osteoarthritis, sleep apnea, respiratory problems, and several cancers, notably cancers of the endometrium, breast, and colon (CDC 2016a).

Adults are not alone in experiencing obesity. Despite modest declines in obesity rates among preschool-aged children in recent years, overall obesity among children remains high. Based on 2011–2012 data, 8.4% of children aged 2 to 5 years, 17.7% of children aged 6 to 11 years, and 20.5% of youths aged 12 to 19 years were obese (defined as a body mass index [BMI] in the 95th percentile for age and sex). In addition, 31.8% of all children were at risk for being overweight or obese (i.e., had a BMI ≥ 85th percentile but < 95th percentile for age and sex; CDC 2015b).

Many Americans do not follow a healthy diet. The American Cancer Society (ACS) reports that more than 85% of adults eat fewer than three servings of fruits and vegetables a day. A large proportion of Americans are physically inactive, with nearly one third of adults not engaged in any form of physical activity during a typical week (ACS 2015a). Annual medical costs for people who are obese are $1,429 higher than for people of normal weight (Finkelstein et al. 2009). Research indicates that the direct medical costs associated with obesity totaled nearly $147 billion in 2008 (CDC 2016a). Medical costs for heart disease and stroke are even higher, estimated at $315 billion for 2010 (Go et al. 2014). Smoking and drinking too much alcohol are also expensive, costing $289 billion and $223 billion a year in medical costs, respectively (USDHHS 2014). Taken together, these risk behaviors and resulting chronic disease conditions accounted for 86% of all health care spending in 2010 (Gerteis et al. 2014).

Health Care Determinants

Access to high-quality health care is an important determinant of health at the individual and community level. Medicare, the federal health insurance program for people aged 65 years and older and people with permanent disabilities, contributes to the reimbursement for hospital and physician visits, prescription drugs, and other services. Medicare spending in 2014 accounted for 14% of the federal budget. Medicare reimbursements to the health care system accounted for 22% of total national health spending in 2013, 26% of spending on hospital care, and 22% of spending on physician services (Henry J. Kaiser Family Foundation 2016). The cost of treating chronic diseases contributes significantly to these costs.

Since 2015, the Affordable Care Act (ACA) requires that every health plan cover all costs related to preventive services. Under Section 2713 of the ACA, private health plans must provide coverage for a range of preventive services and may not impose cost-sharing (such as copayments, deductibles, or co-insurance) on patients receiving these services (Henry J. Kaiser Family Foundation 2015). Among the adult-targeted preventive services for chronic disease covered under the ACA are ones related to screening for breast, cervical, colorectal, and lung cancer, as well as skin cancer counseling, and screenings related to cardiovascular disease (including hypertension and hyperlipidemia), type 2 diabetes, obesity, and osteoporosis (Henry J. Kaiser Family Foundation 2016).

Environmental Determinants

The environment can affect health, not only from traditional exposures in the air, water, or food, but also as a result of how we design and build our communities. Americans have witnessed many discussions during the past few years, in both scholarly literature and the popular press, about the obesity epidemic. One cause attributed to the rise in obesity is the role of the so-called "built environment"—those aspects of a person's surroundings that contribute favorably or unfavorably to his or her individual health initiatives. These elements broadly encompass not only one's local environment (e.g., inside the home and school), but also one's surroundings, such as neighborhoods, urban development, land use, transportation, industry, and agriculture.

An environment that has accessible and safe sidewalks, nearby parks, and such entities as bike trails and community swimming pools will encourage people to engage in physical activity. Likewise, aesthetically pleasing stairways at work, signs reminding people to use the stairs, and such amenities as showers and facilities for changing clothes at work after exercising are pro-health surroundings. In contrast, an environment that lacks aesthetics and is dangerous (e.g., sidewalks in need of repair, no sidewalks, heavy vehicular traffic, poor lighting) will discourage people from being physically active. A person's home environment also has an important influence on activity level—a point that has become more evident with the presence of multiple-television households, desktop and laptop computers as well as tablets, and video games—all of which contribute to sedentary behavior.

The built environment also influences what one chooses nutritionally. Menu choices in schools, restaurants, and worksite cafeterias may offer healthy choices, but perhaps too often, less-healthy alternatives. Neighborhoods lacking grocery stores or convenient farmers' markets may be devoid of fresh fruit and vegetable options, thereby forcing people to purchase what is cheap or available, regardless of its nutritional value. The many linkages between the built environment and obesity have resulted in diverse considerations for health promotion programming (Singh et al. 2010).

Social Determinants

For the past three decades, public health professionals have viewed individual behaviors (e.g., smoking, alcohol and other substance abuse, sexual activity, physical activity, nutrition) as contributing to most of the suboptimal health of Americans. As a consequence, most interventions have been focused on change at the individual level. Although individual behaviors are clearly determinants of health status, focusing on the individual presents a limited and inefficient view of change on a population scale.

According to Garg and Dworkin (2016),

Social determinants—the circumstances in which people live and work—powerfully affect health. In fact, social and environmental factors are estimated to have twice the impact of quality health care on the overall health of an individual. Research in such diverse fields as epidemiology, neuroscience, genomics, and molecular and developmental biology is advancing our understanding of how social risk factors, manifesting as toxic stress, get "under the skin" of vulnerable children via epigenetic changes and disruptions to key physiological and neurocognitive pathways.

Population health is the science of variations in health status among segments within a society or culture. Population health scientists study the indicators of health behavior and health status as they relate to a social determinants' perspective. These indicators encompass social, economic, political, and environmental factors. Therefore, issues such as level of education, level of social or economic stressors, access to health care, transportation, housing, income inequality, or social inclusion or exclusion stemming from sex, race, or age are relevant matters. Policymakers and health professionals often blame persons at high risk for poor health on their own "lifestyles" or "choices" when, in fact, their available lifestyle choices are limited, and their behaviors are strongly influenced by their social, economic, cultural, or physical environment (CDC 2015c). The many observed health disparities are largely a result of these social determinants.

If the United States is to achieve the goal of reducing the burden of chronic disease and eliminating health disparities, there will need to be a better understanding of the relationship between individual health behaviors and social context. Advertising, pricing, and retail practices of the food, alcohol, and tobacco industries that target particular population segments strongly influence health choices. In addition, the lack of public transportation may deter persons with less income and people on fixed incomes from meeting health care appointments. Whereas improvement in school graduation rates could reduce disparities in health, especially among the most disadvantaged, public health agencies, legislatures, and policymakers rarely make the school dropout problem a priority for altering the status quo in health matters. Stronger alliances among public health authorities, policymakers, and educators may favorably influence population health.

Levels of Intervention: A Social-Ecological Perspective

A social-ecological perspective takes into consideration the fact that health decisions are influenced by numerous factors (Figure 4-1). Therefore, this perspective addresses individual as well as social and environmental factors as the foci of chronic disease interventions. Whereas individual health behaviors are

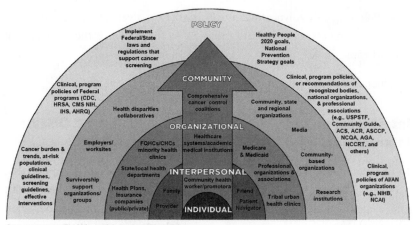

Some groups may fit within multiple levels of this model.

Source: Reprinted from CDC (2016c).

Figure 4-1. Social Ecological Model

popular targets of interventions, they often result in a "victim blaming" culture that fails to take into account the influence of the social and physical environment that may also need to be modified. Use of an ecological approach acknowledges the interaction of an individual and the environment and takes into account the following elements that influence health behavior:

- Intrapersonal factors: Altering knowledge, attitudes, skills, and future behavioral intentions at the level of the individual person.
- Interpersonal factors: Understanding and accessing the relationships that people have with other individuals in their social network such as friends, peers, coworkers, family members, neighbors, and others from whom behavioral patterns and behavioral norms are acquired.
- Organizational factors: Using organizations such as schools, faith-based groups, worksites, or health care facilities to direct, influence, or support health behavior change and help to define health behavior norms.
- Community factors: Catalyzing interest within an area having geographic or political boundaries to leverage power structures to achieve a particular set of health objectives, perhaps to address the most serious health problems among persons typically in the weakest position to advocate on their own behalf (e.g., the rural poor, members of underrepresented minorities, less educated, physically or mentally challenged).

- Policy factors: Advocating, organizing, and analyzing policies and proce-dures, regulations, and laws that favorably influence the fight against chronic diseases.

These factors are examined further in this chapter.

Intrapersonal (Individual) Approaches to Chronic Disease Intervention

Intrapersonal models or theoretical frameworks draw on the assumption that people can be motivated to take individual action that changes their health knowledge, attitudes, skills, behavioral intentions, and eventual behavior. Although there are many such approaches, the potential usefulness of four popular theoretical approaches are presented here for their potential utility for chronic disease prevention and intervention.

Health Belief Model

The Health Belief Model was one of the first attempts of behavioral scientists to use theory to study preventive health behaviors. The model was developed by a group of social psychologists at the U.S. Public Health Service in the 1950s to explain the failure of people to participate in programs designed to prevent or detect disease (Hochbaum 1958). According to the original model, the likeli-hood of someone taking a preventive action to avoid disease is enhanced if they perceive themselves to be susceptible to the disease, perceive the consequences of contracting the disease to be at least of moderate severity, recognize the ben-efits of choosing a preventive action, view the benefits as being superior to the costs and barriers of adopting the behavior, and receive cues to action—the cumulative internal or external messages that affect their readiness to take action. In the 1980s, another component was added to the Health Belief Model—self-efficacy, the belief that one can perform the activity of interest.

The American Cancer Society (2015b) recommends that women with aver-age risk of developing breast cancer have a baseline screening mammogram at age 45, with annual mammograms thereafter until age 55, and then at least a biennial procedure until age 70. A simple application of the Health Belief Model can be seen in the following example of a 45-year-old woman with average breast cancer risk deciding whether to seek a baseline mammogram, a health behavior in the category of secondary prevention. She may see herself as susceptible (e.g., past her 44th birthday, no previous baseline mammogram). She may see breast cancer as being severe (e.g., in the event of disease, possible mastectomy, physical disfigurement, loss of self-esteem, and even death). She may perceive the benefits of mammography (e.g., early detection of disease, and consequently, easier intervention if disease is present, and peace of mind if there is no disease) to outweigh any perceived costs or barriers (e.g., fear of disease, fear or embarrassment related to the procedure). Her motivation may be inspired by cues to action (e.g., reminder postcard received in the mail, recommendation by a physician, message seen or heard through mass media, learning that an acquaintance just had a mammogram or recently received a breast cancer diagnosis). Finally, her likelihood of following through is enhanced if she possesses the confidence and ability (i.e., self-efficacy) to ask her physician about receiving a baseline mammogram, to know where to obtain one, to feel comfortable with calling for an appointment, and to know she can get herself to the facility.

Whereas the Health Belief Model has been used largely to explain the failure of people to adopt preventive behaviors, the model can be useful for intervening at points along the way to develop targeted messages and other intervention strategies (i.e., changing perceptions of susceptibility and severity, assessing benefits and costs or barriers accurately, creating effective cues to action to which women will respond, and increasing women's confidence to follow through in receiving the procedure).

Transtheoretical Model and Stages of Change

The Transtheoretical Model, often referred to as the Stages of Change Model, was developed by Prochaska and DiClemente (1983) through their work on understanding how people quit smoking. The essence of the model is that not everyone is at an equivalent stage of readiness to change health behavior and, thus, interventions need to take on different characteristics to be responsive to these various stages.

The model is comprised of a series of stages, the exact number of which may vary. In the *precontemplation stage*, there is no intention to change behavior, perhaps not even any awareness that change is an alternative or something that can result in an improvement of health or lifestyle. In the *contemplation stage*, an individual may recognize that change is a possibility but is still thinking about making the change or adaptation and has not fully committed to doing so.

In the *preparation stage*, people may gather information about the consequences of altering their lifestyle, affirming the need to change, and, possibly, making a plan to do so at a specified time in the future—usually, in the next 30 days. At the *action stage*, the person actually implements the change, shifting the plan from one that is theoretical to one that is operational—a period that may last up to 6 months. If the action stage becomes routinized, one moves on into the *maintenance stage*—the consolidation of the behaviors initiated previously into one's typical lifestyle. At this point, people can go in one of two possible directions—enter the *termination stage*, in which the former problem behavior is no longer perceived as being acceptable, or the *relapse stage*, in which there is recidivism and a resumption of former, less healthy behavior.

With respect to planning and designing interventions, taking a person's stage of readiness to change into account can enhance the likelihood of moving them along the behavioral continuum, and ultimately improving success. For example, addressing the needs of a person who has a long history of physical inactivity and is contemplating change is quite different than intervening with someone who is in the preparation stage or who has moved back and forth between that stage and the action stage. Whereas the contemplative individual may require encouragement to evaluate the pros and cons of behavior change and identification of positive outcomes and expectations, the person who has already "tested the waters" instead may need to find social support, receive specific suggestions for overcoming obstacles to cementing the change, and seek satisfaction from small, incremental successes in the direction of the desired behavior. It is important to realize that this model is more circular or spiral in nature than linear. People may advance a stage but then fall back. Moreover, individuals may go through multiple cycles of contemplation, preparation, and action before reaching a terminal stage or exiting the system altogether. Understanding what stage people are in will assist intervention efforts.

Theory of Planned Behavior

The Theory of Planned Behavior posits that individual behavior is driven by behavioral intentions (Ajzen 1985; Ajzen 1991). Behavioral intentions are influenced by a person's collective attitudes about the behavior in question, the subjective norms with respect to carrying out the behavior, and the person's perception of the ease with which the behavior can be carried out (behavioral control). This theory has its roots in Fishbein's model of behavioral intentions

Fishbein (1967) and the theory of reasoned action (Ajzen and Fishbein 1973; Fishbein and Ajzen 1975).

With the Theory of Planned Behavior, one's attitude toward a behavior (e.g., daily exercise) is the sum of all the positive feelings (e.g., doing something good for one's health, feeling better about one's self, exercise is a popular activity) or negative feelings (e.g., exercise wears me out, exercise is inconvenient, exercise will make me sore) about performing a behavior. This sum comes from determining one's beliefs about the consequences arising from a behavior and an evaluation of the desirability of these consequences. A person's overall attitude is the sum of the individual consequences and the desirability assessments for all expected consequences of the behavior.

The beliefs underlying a person's subjective norms are called normative beliefs. The subjective norm is defined as a person's perception of whether people important to him or her value a behavior and think the person should engage in it. The opinion of any significant other is weighted by the motivation that the person has to comply with the wishes of that significant other. The overall subjective norm is the sum of the individual perceptions and the motivation assessments for all significant others who may influence the person considering a behavior.

Behavioral control is a person's perception of the difficulty of carrying out the behavior (e.g., skills, available time, sacrifice of other activities for this particular behavior). In the Theory of Planned Behavior, the control that people have over their behavior is a continuum of behaviors from ones that are easily carried out to ones requiring much time, effort, resources, and so on. The link between behavior and behavioral control in this model should be between behavior and actual behavioral control rather than perceived behavioral control. However, the difficulty of assessing actual behavioral control has resulted in behavioral scientists using perceived control as a proxy measure.

Health Locus of Control Model

Locus of control refers to a person's expectations about where control over events in life resides. In a health context, it means who or what is responsible for that which happens to one's health. Expectancy, which concerns future events, is an important part of the locus of control construct. Locus of control is grounded in expectancy value theory; that is, if a person values a particular outcome and believes that carrying out a particular behavior will result in that outcome, then they are more likely to pursue that behavior.

Rotter (1966) classified beliefs concerning who or what influences things along a continuum from completely internal control to completely external control. Whereas internal control is the expectancy that future events are largely under the control of the individual, external control refers to the belief that future events are outside individual control—such as under the control of others or attributable entirely to fate or chance.

Since its introduction in the 1960s, the locus of control construct has seen many permutations and iterations through the work of behavioral scientists in numerous fields. However, health behavior researchers have used the locus of control idea extensively. Among the most widely used health-specific measure is the Multidimensional Health Locus of Control Scale (Wallston et al. 1978).

In practice, people who believe that their health status is largely within their own control are more likely to embrace preventive, positive health behaviors. Persons perceiving their locus of control to be more external are less inclined to take on preventive actions, concluding that a higher power, fate, luck, or other influences beyond their control ultimately will determine their health outcomes. Public health workers attempting to influence health behavior choices may have better success with a target group that possesses more of an internal locus of control perspective. Conversely, changing policies or using a systems approach may be more effective for individuals who perceive an external locus of control.

Interpersonal Approaches to Chronic Disease Intervention

Models of interpersonal health behavior assume that the interpersonal environment is one of the most powerful sources of influence for health-related behavior and health status. Moreover, mechanisms that link individuals' social contexts with health effects revolve around two social processes—social support and social influence. The next section describes the interactions of individuals, environments, and corresponding health behaviors.

Social Cognitive Theory

Social cognitive theory is one interpersonal-level theory that has been used readily in a number of chronic disease prevention and control studies. Social cognitive theory addresses both the psychosocial dynamics influencing health behavior and methods for promoting behavioral change. Within this theory, human behavior is explained in terms of a triadic, dynamic, and reciprocal model in which behavior, personal factors (including cognitions), and environmental influences all interact (Bandura 1977). Critical factors include the individual's ability to monitor behavior, to anticipate the outcomes of behavior (including overcoming the obstacles in performing a given behavior), to self-determine or self-regulate behavior, and to reflect on and analyze experiences (Bandura 1977).

Social cognitive theory emphasizes the importance of enhancing a person's behavioral capability (knowledge and skills) and self-confidence (self-efficacy) to engage in a particular health behavior. Self-efficacy, one of the most important constructs in this theory, has been demonstrated to predict the initiation of a new health behavior, the continuation of the target behavior, and the maintenance of complex health behaviors. The most powerful and consistent way of enhancing self-efficacy is through mastery of a task. Successful social cognitive theory interventions engage participants in small steps of an enacted behavior, with self-monitoring as well as feedback from others. Bandura (1977; 1986) also developed a number of other theory constructs that are important to understand and intervene in health behavior. These constructs include reciprocal determinism, environments and situations, observational learning, behavioral capability, reinforcement, outcome expectations, outcome expectancies, self-control of performance, and managing emotional arousal. Case studies and examples of how these constructs might be translated into intervention strategies are described in detail by Kelder et al. (2015).

Social cognitive theory has wide applicability for different audiences and has been used successfully in disaster and emergency preparedness (Ejeta et al. 2015), in physical activity promotion interventions (e.g., Young et al. 2014), in health education campaigns for people with chronic medical conditions such as arthritis (Coleman et al. 2012), and in cardiovascular disease prevention programs for children and adults (Bandura 1986; Farquhar et al. 1990; Phillips and Klein 2012; Puska and Uutela 2000). One estimate is that there have been at least 52 studies of cardiovascular disease prevention programs that have employed this theory (Winter et al. 2016). By recognizing the importance of the environment, people, and behavior, social cognitive theory provides a framework for designing, implementing, and evaluating comprehensive behavioral change programs.

Family-Based Interventions

Family-based interventions draw upon the enhancement of existing close social network linkages and often entail education and interventions that can have a direct impact on the somatic health and self-care behavior of those with chronic disease. Family interventions affect not only the patient, but also the family and its environment. Interventions can be utilized to improve coping, communication, and problem-solving skills of the involved family members; in turn, they can aid in decreasing relationship stress around a chronic illness (Hartmann et al. 2010).

Martire and Schulz (2007) used a heuristic model of three domains of functioning (emotional, health behaviors, and family), and found that interventions with a family orientation may provide greater benefits over patient-only oriented interventions. In their systematic review, Meis et al. (2013) demonstrated that family involvement reduced substance use in individuals with mental health issues. In addition, self-efficacy, knowledge, self-care, and social support were shown to have improved across studies involving family interventions and diabetes (Baig et al. 2015). Family-based approaches to chronic disease emphasize the context of the disease to include the physical environment, relationships, education, and personal needs in a more comprehensive care program. Two systematic reviews on the effects of family interventions in diabetes outcomes found that both glycemic control and disease-related knowledge increased with the implementation of family interventions (Armour et al. 2005) and influenced psychosocial and familial dimensions (Torenholt et al. 2014).

The family environment can contribute to childhood obesity as children assimilate the behaviors and beliefs of their parents. Ethical family interventions focused on sound nutrition and physical activity practices can have an impact on the entire family and serve to reduce childhood obesity (Perryman 2011).

Social Support and Social Networks

The powerful influence that social relationships have on health has elicited a great deal of interest among public health researchers and practitioners. An understanding of the impact of social relationships on health status, health behaviors, and health decisions has the potential to influence the design of interventions for more effective chronic disease prevention and health promotion.

One important function of social relationships is the provision of social support, a concept that has been defined and measured in numerous ways.

According to House (1988), social support is the functional aspects of relationships that can be defined as four broad types of supportive behaviors: (1) emotional support, (2) instrumental support, (3) informational support, and (4) appraisal support. A social network, in comparison, is the web of relationships surrounding individuals. Whereas the provision of social support is one important function of these networks, not all social networks are supportive (Ferlander 2007). Social networks can be described by the following characteristics (Glanz et al. 2008):

- Homogeneity: How alike network members are in terms of demographic characteristics such as age, race, and socioeconomic status.
- Geographic dispersion: The extent to which network members live in close proximity to each other.
- Density: How well network members know each other and how often they interact.
- Intensity: The emotional closeness of people within a network.
- Formality: The extent to which relationships are embedded in organizational structures within a social network.
- Complexity: How many functions are served by relationships within a network.
- Reciprocity: Whether or not resources and support are both given and received among members in a network.

Several types of social network and social support interventions involving neighborhood environments and peer influence have been advanced (Gordon-Larsen et al. 2006; Smith and Christakis 2008). These interventions leverage existing social linkages while developing new linkages and strengthening social networks at the community level through participatory community capacity development and problem-solving processes.

Friends and Social Networks

Another type of social network intervention entails developing new social network linkages through mentor programs, buddy systems, and self-help groups. Groups such as Alcoholics Anonymous, Overeaters Anonymous, and Weight Watchers provide access to new social networks designed to provide cognitive, instrumental, and emotional support for lifestyle change (Medline Plus 2016).

Peer groups are particularly important for interventions focused on adolescents. Studies of adolescent friendship networks show peer influence to play an important role in risk behaviors associated with chronic disease development (Shoham et al. 2012; Simpkins et al. 2013). Specifically, Christakis and Fowler (2007) documented a phenomenon wherein obesity moved through immediate peer groups as well as second- and third-degree contacts among adolescents, suggesting a diffusion of peer influence greater than originally thought. In addition, Oman et al. (2004) found that having peer role models, family communication, spiritual beliefs, good health practices, and future aspirations result in lowered risk of alcohol and drug use. Positive orientation to school and academic achievement are also consistently protective factors for health; on the other hand, poor health behaviors are linked to lower academic achievement among children and adolescents (Michael et al. 2015). This connection between health and academic achievement has been formalized into a framework that acknowledges the reciprocal influences among children, school, and the broader community and the impact these connections have on health-related behaviors and risk factors for chronic disease (Lewallen et al. 2015).

Community Health Workers

Community health workers are lay members of communities who perform volunteer or compensated work for the local health care system and in the indigenous community. Community health workers usually share ethnicity, language, socioeconomic status, and life experiences with the community members they serve. They have been identified by many titles such as community health advisors, lay health advocates, *promotores(as)*, outreach educators, community health representatives, peer health promoters, and peer health educators (USDHHS 2007).

Community health workers are respected and trusted members of social networks to whom individuals turn for advice, support, and other types of aid. These workers are able to access underserved communities impacted by health and economic disparities and, therefore, are a valuable asset to public health education and chronic disease prevention efforts. Community health workers provide direct support to members within a network as well as link people within the network to each other and to outside resources. They have collaborated with researchers on numerous and diverse community-based interventions in urban neighborhoods, rural counties, residential institutions for the elderly, migrant farmworker communities, and churches (USDHHS 2007), but are especially recognized for their work in Latino communities, where they are typically called *promotores* (Berthold et al. 2009; O'Brien et al. 2009; USDHHS 2007).

Promotores have engaged in educational movements and social activism in the United States and Latin America since the 1960s, and in recent decades have moved into health promotion and disease prevention interventions within some of the hardest to reach and most underserved communities in the United States. For example, *promotores* in one migrant farmworker program conducted eye safety programs and distributed safety eyewear to the workers (Monaghan et al. 2011; Monaghan et al. 2012; Tovar-Aguilar et al. 2014). Community health workers in another intervention were responsible for implementing a standardized program for pediatric asthma diagnosis and management based on the National Asthma Education and Prevention Program (Peterson-Sweeney et al. 2003). These community health workers also have been instrumental in providing language translation in clinical settings to improve access to health care within immigrant and ethnic communities (USDHHS 2007). In summary, community health workers have emerged as an effective resource in chronic disease prevention programs.

Examples of Interpersonal-Level Interventions

Interpersonal interventions frequently use social cognitive theory as the basis for program design. Social cognitive theory is appealing for health promotion programs because it both addresses the causal mechanisms of individual behavior and guides the design of intervention approaches. Reiterating the earlier discussion about social cognitive theory, with respect to interpersonal-level interventions, among the 52 interventions for cardiovascular disease prevention, this theory has been used in focused research for promoting weight loss, glucose monitoring, healthy eating, and tobacco cessation (Winter et al. 2016).

Social cognitive theory was used in the implementation of a randomized control trial of a weight loss program called Project SMART (Patrick et al. 2014). This project was aimed at college-aged students who are in a vulnerable time period for unhealthy eating and potential weight gain. The SMART intervention was informed by the social cognitive theory and focused on technology commonly used by college students. In particular, the intervention included

Facebook, mobile apps, blogs, e-mails, and text messaging. Having focused and theory-based interventions that resonate with the target audience is important for engagement and, therefore, for outcome assessment.

Organizational-Level Venues for Intervention

Health Care System

The health care setting is an effective venue for providing screening and follow-up services that help to control chronic diseases (see Chapter 5). Historically, the health care setting has been used for blood pressure monitoring, diabetes control, cardiovascular health assessment, cancer screening, and various other secondary prevention measures. However, the health care setting is an ideal, although often underutilized, venue for patient education, including primary prevention. Research firmly establishes that physician advice given in the health care setting provides a powerful and motivational message for cardiovascular disease risk reduction (CDC 1999; CDC 2013b); weight loss, dietary change, and physical activity improvement among adolescents (Kant and Miner 2007); tobacco control (Lancaster and Stead 2005); and alcohol consumption (Grossberg et al. 2004). In a review of published literature (1949–2008) involving 106 correlational studies and 21 experimental interventions, Zolnierek and DiMatteo (2009) showed that patients with physicians who were poor communicators had a 19% lower likelihood of adhering to their advice than patients with physicians who were good communicators.

An intervention that has shown effectiveness without being especially burdensome on health care providers or patients is known as the "brief intervention." Brief interventions usually last for 5 to 60 minutes and consist of counseling and education. Sometimes there are multiple sessions, perhaps initiated by a primary care provider, and then transitioned to a health education specialist to carry on the intervention. However, a brief intervention can be as limited as 30 seconds and consist of just one "teachable moment" session conducted by an alert and opportunistic health care provider. The content, duration, and number of sessions may depend on the provider, the patient's receptivity and readiness to change, the setting, and previous patient–provider rapport. The brief intervention can be leveraged at any point in the health promotion–disease prevention–treatment continuum depending on the patient's readiness to change.

Table 4-1. Examples of Brief Interventions for Health Promotion

- When taking a blood pressure reading: Sharing information about the causes and problems of high blood pressure, and talking about exercise and proper diet as ways to reduce blood high pressure.
- When taking a medical history or conducting a routine physical examination: Encouraging a patient at risk of developing diabetes to talk about the foods they eat, offering nutrition advice, and talking about practical ways to shop for food and prepare healthy meals.
- When taking a medical history or conducting a routine physical examination: Mentioning that just 150 minutes of brisk walking per week can reduce one's risk of obesity and several chronic disease conditions compounded by obesity.
- When treating an infant or child with a respiratory infection: Talking to the mother who smokes to find out if she knows about passive smoking, recommending ways of reducing the child's exposure to smoking, and asking if she is thinking about quitting.
- When taking a medical history or conducting a routine physical examination: Urging adults to obtain a screening mammogram, prostate examination, colonoscopy, etc. as recommended for women or men in selected age groups.
- When taking a medical history or conducting a routine physical examination: Finding out from patients who drink alcohol if they are drinking in a harmful way, and if they are addressing the need to adjust their drinking to a healthier level, perhaps conveying factual information about the health effects of alcohol.

There are a number of circumstances that lend themselves to brief interventions such as the ones listed in Table 4-1. However, a creative and alert health care provider will be able to note many other opportunities to intervene.

Schools

Schools are excellent venues for primary and secondary prevention. Philosophically, schools ought to convey health education along with the many other essential subjects that comprise responsive education. Youths attend school for 12 or more years and are a captive audience for educators and health professionals to convey prevention messages and for health care providers to conduct selective health screenings. Moreover, establishing healthy habits in youths can help prevent many chronic health problems later in life that are attributable to unhealthy eating, sedentary lifestyle, sexual risk taking, and other health-related issues. In addition to teaching health education, schools can offer services that promote health and monitor key health indicators in children and youths (e.g., height, weight, BMI, blood pressure, immunizations).

The Whole School, Whole Community, Whole Child (WSCC) model depicted in Figure 4-2 (Lewallan et al. 2015) expands upon the coordinated or

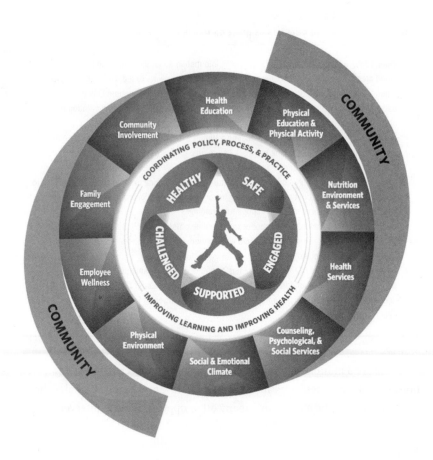

Source: Reprinted from CDC (2016d).

Figure 4-2. Whole School, Whole Community, Whole Child Model

comprehensive school health program model developed by Allensworth and Kolbe (1987). This model includes 10 components and illustrates a multitude of health-promoting opportunities within the school setting for youths as well as adults. Many public health care providers work with school systems, thereby offering an opportunity for an effective partnership.

Prevention research focused on children and youths has yielded a number of evidence-based interventions that have applicability in school health education curricula. Several initiatives have emanated from the CDC's Prevention Research Centers (PRCs), a national network of community–academic research partnerships situated in either a school of public health or a medical school

(CDC 2014b). These centers are funded by CDC in five-year cycles to engage in community-based participatory prevention research and translate this research into public health policy and practice. Each PRC comprises academic and community partners who develop chronic disease prevention initiatives that fit the local context (CDC 2014b). Community partners include health departments, school boards, and community-based organizations and residents who collaborate with the PRC to form long-term partnerships engaged in community-based research and action (CDC 2014b). Three programs especially worth noting include one aimed at smoking cessation among adolescents (Not-On-Tobacco [N-O-T]) and two targeting physical activity and healthy eating for elementary- and middle-school children (Coordinated Approach to Child Health [CATCH] and Reading, Writing, and Reducing Obesity; CDC 2015d). Shared features of these three programs (CDC 2015d) include

- Focus on chronic disease prevention and health promotion.
- Identification of staff and resources that facilitate program implementation and dissemination.
- Stakeholder involvement (e.g., teachers, students, other school personnel, parents, nonprofit organizations, professional organizations) during all phases of program development and dissemination.
- Planning for dissemination of programs.
- Rigorous evaluation.

The Workplace

The workplace provides a ready channel for health promotion interventions as a large proportion of the U.S. population typically spends 7.8 hours working each weekday (Goetzel and Ozminkowski 2008; Person et al. 2010; Bureau of Labor Statistics 2015). A report by the Congressional Research Service indicated that in 2014, 136 million U.S. residents were employed by public or private employers (Mayer 2014). According to the RAND Employer Survey, a national survey of employers with at least 50 employees, approximately half of employers provided some form of health promotion initiative (Mattke et al. 2013). Worksite health promotion programs are characterized by 72% of employers as a combination of both screenings and activities (Mattke et al. 2013).

With chronic diseases collectively comprising the leading cause of death in the United States, worksite wellness programs can reach a large population of employed individuals with a focus on addressing risk factors for chronic disease in the individual, supporting individual and family stressors, and providing health protection benefits such as occupational safety and health interventions (Sorensen et al. 2011). A Total Worker Health model is supported by the Institute of Medicine, the CDC, and the National Institute for Occupational and Safety Health. Total Worker Health is defined as "a strategy integrating occupational safety and health protection with health promotion to prevent worker injury and illness and to advance health and well-being (CDC 2015e; Lessin 2014). These combined organizational efforts are designed to develop comprehensive and essential elements of effective workplace programs and policies (CDC 2015e).

Employers feel confident in the programs they implement and report reduced cost, absenteeism, and health-related productivity losses; however, only half of the employers conduct an evaluation of the programs (Mattke et al. 2013). The Total Worker Health model provides guidance from program initiation to program evaluation of worksite wellness programs. The model encompasses four overarching areas, with key elements in each area. The four areas include organizational culture and leadership, program design, program implementation, and resources and program evaluation (CDC 2015e). Although programs may differ across worksites, there are time-tested guiding principles that should be taken into consideration with any promotion program (Sparling 2010). Effective worksite health promotion programs

- Have multiple components and strive to be comprehensive and integrated.
- Demonstrate visible and unequivocal commitment to employee health through the actions for the top leadership of the organization.
- Are open to all employees.
- Provide systematic health assessments, timely and meaningful feedback, and assistance in setting and monitoring individual health goals.
- Tailor health promotion activities to the needs of the employees.
- Attain high participation by using creative and appealing incentive-based programs.
- Implement and sustain environmental and policy changes that support healthy behaviors.
- Link health promotion services to occupational safety and job performance at all employee levels.
- Extend health promotion services to spouses and family members.
- Evaluate employees' health needs and the effectiveness of health promotion services and activities in meeting these needs.

Clearly, the economic burden of chronic disease conditions has an impact on workers, their families, and the worksites themselves. There is a distinct link between health risks associated with chronic disease and productivity and health-related costs (Partnership for Prevention 2009). To lower health care costs from diseases resulting from modifiable behaviors such as smoking, poor diet, and lack of physical activity, the ACA provides for employers to use up to 30% (and in some cases 50%) of their employees' health insurance premiums for wellness initiatives (Volpp et al. 2011).

Employees with multiple risk factors for chronic disease (e.g., smoking, poor dietary habits, sedentary behaviors) require interventions independent of the individuals with established chronic disease (Partnership for Prevention 2009). Between 25% and 50% of employee annual medical costs are associated with modifiable health risk factors such as poor nutrition, lack of exercise, excess stress, and other lifestyle factors (Wellness Councils of America 2012). There is a direct correlation between unhealthy lifestyle risk factors and loss of productivity (Mitchell and Bates 2011). America's aging workforce is showing increased prevalence of chronic diseases, such as chronic obstructive pulmonary disease, which also contributes to lost productivity, as well as disability and loss of mobility (Patel et al. 2014).

With the increased desire by public health professionals to mitigate chronic disease development and employers to decrease costs, there is a surge of interest in businesses adopting wellness programs. Using a meta-analysis of the scholarly literature, researchers found that for every dollar spent on wellness programs, associated medical costs were reduced by approximately $3.27, and absenteeism costs were reduced by approximately $2.73 (Baicker et al. 2010). A separate systematic review supported these cost-saving findings (Soler et al. 2010). The positive return on investment may motivate employers' interest in wellness programs, especially those with a large employee base.

Numerous benefits that can be garnered through interventions that serve to prevent risk factors associated with chronic disease, help to mitigate chronic disease through screening and intervention, and aim to control chronic diseases, include the following:

- Improved employee productivity: Employees with multiple health risk factors are less productive than employees with fewer risk factors (Partnership for Prevention 2009).
- Reduced employee health risks: In two years, high-risk employees for chronic disease based on obesity, tobacco use, and physical activity

metrics reduced their risk by 15% at Dow Chemical by participating in a comprehensive worksite wellness program guided by the Community Prevention Services Task Force (Community Guide 2012).

- Reduced health care costs: An analysis of 56 worksite wellness programs showed an average 26% reduction in health care costs (Partnership for Prevention 2009).
- Improved corporate image: Dow Chemical learned that through the institution of a culture of health in the workplace, employees valued the organization's commitment to health (Community Guide 2012).

Despite worksite wellness program initiation, employees may choose not to participate. Behavioral economists suggest that, in general, individuals are more attracted to immediate than to delayed benefits and more deterred by immediate than delayed costs (Volpp et al. 2011).

Other primary barriers to participation include insufficient incentives, time constraints and schedules, inconvenient locations, and general lack of interest (Person et al. 2010). Social marketing strategies may help to understand the priority audience and to determine which benefits could overcome these barriers to participation.

Faith-Based Organizations

Faith-based organizations have a long history of supporting health promotion programs in areas such as general health education, screening for and management of high blood pressure and diabetes, weight loss, smoking cessation, cancer prevention and control, geriatric care, nutritional guidance, and mental health care (CDC 2015f). Lumpkins et al. (2013) studied pastors of churches with predominantly African-American memberships and determined that African-American clergy see themselves as health promoters in the church and believe that this communication (i.e., pastor-endorsed health information materials) has an impact on health behavior among underserved and minority populations.

Community-Level Interventions

The term "community" gets defined in numerous ways, but in public health it is used to describe a group of people with diverse characteristics who are linked by social ties, share common perspectives, and engage in joint action (Yuen et al.

2015; Wallerstein et al. 2015; MacQueen et al. 2001). Communities may be bounded geographically (e.g., a neighborhood, city, or other place); by shared issues and characteristics (e.g., sexual orientation, language, ethnic heritage); or virtually through social media and networks. In all cases, a shared identity and interdependency are extremely important. Neighborhoods and other social groups that do not share a sense of identity, norms and values, and common activities are not considered communities. This section examines community intervention strategies, including community-level activities, involvement of community members, and community-based participatory research (CBPR).

Community interventions are designed to educate the entire community instead of individual members, enhance their ability to tackle problems, and modify the community environment or structure to make it easier for people to adopt healthy practices. Physical activity promotion programs, for instance, may rely on a variety of strategies—classes and neighborhood walking programs offered through local organizations; information channels employed to motivate large numbers of its members to be more active and use program services; and modification of the environment to make it easier for people to be active (e.g., by creating outdoor walking paths, purchasing exercise equipment for worksites or community centers, making staircases safer and more pleasant to walk; Kerr et al. 2012).

Guiding actions for improving community intervention effectiveness (Savage et al. 2015; Wallerstein et al. 2015) include

- Assessing community needs and priorities.
- Acknowledging and building on community partners' skills and assets.
- Aligning goal setting and intervention activities with community members' perceived needs, knowledge, attitudes, values, and constraints.
- Integrating activities within the community structure (e.g., by offering programs through local businesses, faith-based organizations, or other community-based organizations).
- Offering a broad range of activities to reach large numbers of community members, build community capacity, and modify the community to facilitate change.
- Implementing the intervention for a sufficient period of time and with adequate resources to make change realistic and sustainable (i.e., providing an adequate intervention dose).
- Monitoring activities to identify and remedy problems quickly.

As we shall see in greater detail in the next paragraphs, it also is essential to involve community members in all phases of the intervention.

Community Engagement

Many public health organizations (e.g., CDC, National Institutes of Health, and Institute of Medicine) have endorsed community engagement as a way to increase intervention effectiveness (O'Mara-Eves et al. 2015; Hicks et al. 2012). Involving community members in goal setting, program design, and program implementation has been shown to improve health and psychosocial outcomes (O'Mara-Eves et al. 2015). In a meta-analysis of more than 9,000 primary studies, O'Mara-Eves et al. (2015) found that community engagement improved program impact on health behaviors, health consequences, self-efficacy, and perceived social support. Interventions were especially effective when community members were engaged in delivering the intervention.

Community engagement can take many forms, ranging from asking community members for information and advice to equal sharing of all program decisions. A full partnership between public health professionals and local community members can lead to empowerment of individuals, enhance the community's capacity to identify and solve its own problems, and result in more effective management of health issues and economic, social, and political forces in the community (Wallerstein et al. 2015). Community participation also increases its sense of ownership of the intervention. This, in turn, may provide better access to community leaders, lead to changes in community norms, enhance local problem-solving skills, and increase the likelihood that the intervention will be sustained. Community members' help tailoring the intervention to fit the norms and values of the community ensures that it will be culturally sensitive and relevant.

Community-Based Participatory Research

One form of community engagement that has gained recognition over the past two decades or so is CBPR, a collaborative process in which community members and public health researchers work together as equal partners in the research process to tackle community health problems (Wallerstein et al. 2015). The fundamental principles of CBPR include that it is participatory, engages community members and researchers in a collaborative process to which each contributes equally, is a co-learning process, involves local capacity building and systems development, empowers participants, and results in a balance between research and action (Israel et al. 2005; Smith et al. 2015).

Community-based participatory research offers public health researchers and their community partners many benefits. A review of 23 CBPR partnerships described in 276 publications (Jagosh et al. 2012) found that this approach can

- Ensure culturally and logistically appropriate research.
- Enhance recruitment capacity.
- Generate professional capacity and competence in stakeholder groups.
- Result in productive conflicts followed by useful negotiation.
- Increase the quality of outputs and outcomes over time.
- Increase the sustainability of project goals beyond funded time frames and during gaps in external funding.
- Create system changes and new unanticipated projects and activities.

Despite these benefits, CBPR is also challenging to carry out (Hicks et al. 2012; Mayer 2014). Of special importance is trust and mutual commitment between public health researchers and community members. Trust is subject to overall power relations in the community and the larger society, members' previous experience with research and researchers, the immediate issues facing the community, and the ability to negotiate relationships between the CBPR researchers and community participants (Wallerstein et al. 2015). Community members engaged in CBPR report difficulty understanding the research language, protocols, and rules (e.g., institutional review board approval of study enrollment and study design issues). Thus, time is needed to develop both trust and understanding to support it.

Unfortunately, relatively few chronic disease prevention and control programs have taken advantage of community-level interventions and strategies (Golden and Earp 2012; Savage et al. 2015). A review of in-depth descriptions of 157 health promotion programs published in the journal *Health Education and Behavior* between January 1989 and December 2008 revealed that only 20% of the programs included community-level activities compared to 95% that targeted individual-level activities and 67% that included interpersonal activities. Programs designed to promote smoking cessation and physical activity were among the most common to include community-level activities. Even fewer programs, just 6%, attempted to promote or change public policy (Golden and Earp 2012).

Community Coalitions

Community coalitions with public health–related missions are formal, semi-permanent, action-oriented partnerships typically comprising community members, representatives of government agencies, policymakers, and academic partners that focus primarily on health promotion, disease prevention, and relevant local social issues (Butterfoss et al. 1993; Feinberg et al. 2008a; Motley et al. 2013). Coalitions identify specific community-level health problems, assess existing needs and resources, develop and implement formal strategies for addressing these problems, and, ultimately, work to improve the health and well-being of the community (Butterfoss et al. 1993; McLeroy et al. 1994; Motley et al. 2013; Whitt 1993).

Community coalitions evolved from the experiences of civic engagement and community building in the 1960s and 1970s and now encompass a diverse array of community-based partnerships tasked with improving local health and social conditions (Bracht 1990; Butterfoss et al. 2006). Evolving in structure and scope over the past 30 years, coalitions have formed around issues as diverse as smoking cessation, prevention of sexually transmitted infections, and childhood obesity, using different strategies and approaches to make a local impact; at times, these efforts have been disseminated to other coalitions statewide and even across regions of the United States (Butterfoss et al. 2006; Butterfoss et al. 2003; Feinberg et al. 2008b). Several studies have shown the community coalition approach to health promotion to be effective when best practices, often referred to as evidence-based programs or policies, are implemented (Feinberg et al. 2008a; Feinberg et al. 2008b; Gloppen et al. 2012). Both governmental and nongovernmental organizations have recognized the potential of coalitions by promoting them to address many public health issues (Feinberg et al. 2008a; Feinberg et al. 2008b).

The theoretical basis for coalition functioning was formalized by Butterfoss and Kegler (2009) in the Community Coalition Action Theory (CCAT). The CCAT builds on ideas from inter-organizational relations, as well as community development, community participation, citizen participation, political science, and group processes (Hage and Alter 1993; Butterfoss and Kegler 2009; Gray 1989). The CCAT is based on several models of partnership building that focus on community building and community development, as well as those that focus more on the structure of these types of organizations (Butterfoss et al. 1993; Lasker and Weiss 2003; Minkler and Wallerstein 2008; Prestby et al. 1990). Whereas these models address some aspects of coalition structures and processes, none encompasses all the factors and characteristics of a community coalition.

The CCAT was developed for the purpose of integrating the relevant characteristics of these models into a comprehensive picture of coalition structure and function (Butterfoss and Kegler 2009). The CCAT is comprised of 14 constructs that exist within three stages—formation, implementation, and maintenance—formalizing how coalitions function as they plan, implement, and monitor community-based initiatives (Butterfoss and Kegler 2009; Motley et al. 2013). The theory's propositions emphasize the need for coalition building that is focused on community assets rather than deficiencies, participation of stakeholders, a holistic approach to community improvement, and skill building within the community, all elements of effective community partnerships (McLeroy et al. 1994; Minkler 1994; Goodman et al. 1998; Zakocs and Guckenberg 2007).

The increasing use of coalitions as a health promotion strategy parallels the growth of large-scale community-level health promotion and chronic disease prevention efforts over the past two decades, such as the National Heart, Lung, and Blood Institute's demonstration projects (Powell-Wiley et al. 2015). These projects, which include the Stanford Three Community and Five City Projects and the Minnesota and Pawtucket Heart Health Programs, utilized community advisory boards to plan and implement cardiovascular disease prevention efforts (NHLBI 2015). In addition, the CDC supported formation of community coalitions in the Planned Approach to Community Health, which was widely adopted by state and local health departments in the late 1980s and early 1990s (Green and Kreuter 2005; USDHHS 2015).

Media Advocacy

Media advocacy is "the strategic use of mass media in combination with community organizing to advance healthy public policies" (Wallack 2000). Whereas most communication strategies address individuals as consumers by delivering focused information to help people decrease their risks of injury and illness, media advocacy focuses on raising the voices of populations for systems change from a policy level with the policymakers as the audience (Dorfman and Krasnow 2014). By learning to use media to address system-level factors, communities are empowered to participate in the political process.

Like other forms of advocacy, a variety of tasks are used to create a shift in public opinion and bring about policy change—agenda setting, framing, and working with groups to reach opinion leaders to change public policies and address social inequities. Agenda setting refers to activities that shine the "spotlight on a particular issue and hold it there" (Wallack et al. 1993). Media coverage is used to bring the policy issue to the public's attention and onto the official public agenda. News coverage is of special importance in this process because it can lend credibility to an issue. Media advocates also use paid advertising and other forms of media coverage to shape the nature of the debate.

How an issue is framed is of critical importance. Framing uses symbols, metaphors, and stories to define an issue, to suggest who is responsible for the problem, and to propose solutions. Media advocates try to frame public health issues in ways that direct attention to environmental or system-level factors responsible for the problem, and suggest policy solutions rather than hold individual "victims" responsible for it.

Mass media also are used to place pressure on decision makers (Wallack et al. 1993). As with media coverage designed to garner public support, media advocates frame policy positions to make them attractive to policymakers and use a variety of techniques to keep their issue in the news (e.g., by framing an event as a milestone, a breakthrough, or a controversial topic). Because policy battles often wage for years, media advocates must identify new opportunities to reintroduce an issue and keep it in the media spotlight over long periods of time (Wallack 2000).

Media advocacy in public health dates back to the 1980s when it was used by public health groups working to control tobacco and alcohol abuse. Tobacco control advocates, for instance, have used media advocacy to stop the distribution of Uptown cigarettes in Philadelphia, Pennsylvania, and to defuse a national public relations event organized by Phillip Morris. Since then, media advocacy has been applied to a variety of public health topics, such as decreasing salt intake and alcohol consumption (Katikireddi et al. 2014; Webster et al. 2014). The major advantage of using media advocacy to address these issues is "escaping a traditional, limited focus on disease conditions and instead, promote a greater understanding of the conditions that will support and improve the public's health" (Wallack 2005).

The growth in popularity of social media sites such as Facebook, Twitter, and others has provided additional platforms for advocacy and political pressure. In 2012, the nonprofit Susan G. Komen Foundation's decision to discontinue funding for breast cancer screening for Planned Parenthood because of a congressional investigation resulted in a social media campaign by Planned

Parenthood to raise awareness and funds. The campaign garnered more than 10,000 "likes" on Facebook and raised more money than the Susan G. Komen Foundation planned to cut in funding (Dorfman and Krasnow 2014).

Health Policy and Legal Interventions

Effective health policies can have a substantial impact on the public's health (CDC 2016b). Public health policies include laws, regulations, written standards, ordinances, resolutions, and organizational and institutional practices designed to guide individual and group behavior that have an impact on population health (CDC 2016b). Examples include economic incentives, taxes, business regulations, and other laws that protect the public or special population groups, such as workers. Laws requiring drivers to wear seatbelts, sanctions for illegal drug use, and environmental protection standards are well-known examples.

Policy changes have been deemed more effective than behavior change programs and more easily sustained for long periods of time when external funding has ended (Moreland-Russell and Brownson 2015). In fact, policy initiatives have brought about some of the most important public health victories in the United States in the past century. Declining lead exposure rates, reduced rates of smoking, improvements in motor vehicle safety, and increased vaccination rates, have resulted from legislation, regulation, litigation, or a combination of these three actions (CDC 1999).

Federal policies, in particular, can have a significant population impact. Consider, for example, the impact of the ACA on health care access, especially for chronic disease prevention and control services. Unfortunately, many promising public health policies have yet to be enacted. For instance, one analysis of federal obesity policies (Kristensen et al. 2014) showed that policies to offer afterschool physical activity programs, to ban fast food advertising on television to children, and to tax sugar-sweetened beverages by just 1 cent would have a small (5.1%) but clinically significant impact on childhood obesity rates.

In light of public health's embrace of policy change as an intervention to reduce chronic diseases and other health problems, it is not surprising that many tools are available to help public health professionals identify, tailor, and promote policy change and evaluate its impact (see Resources listed at the end of this chapter).

Multilevel Approaches to Chronic Disease Control

Comprehensive interventions for controlling chronic diseases require primary, secondary, and tertiary prevention approaches. Moreover, these strategies must be directed at the individual, interpersonal, organizational, community, and policy levels. A relevant example is tobacco use, still one of the leading causes of death among Americans. Because of tobacco's important negative health consequences, a multilevel or comprehensive intervention to control tobacco must involve

- Primary prevention education programs for youths in school settings.
- Education programs for physicians, dentists, and other health care providers to inspire patient education in care settings through brief interventions and other mechanisms.
- Free or low-cost cessation programs for smokers before the onset of disease (secondary prevention).
- Health insurance cost reductions for nonsmokers as an economic incentive to eliminate tobacco use.
- Tobacco excise taxes to bring an economic disincentive to continue use and raise revenue to finance care for affected individuals (tertiary prevention).
- Rigorous enforcement of age restriction for purchase of cigarettes.
- Partnering with national and local voluntary organizations (e.g., American Heart Association, American Lung Association, American Cancer Society) for advocacy of anti-tobacco programs and policies.
- Clean indoor air legislation.
- Restriction of smoking in public places.

Whereas each one of these initiatives may have a modest influence on smoking and tobacco consumption, none is as singularly effective as a comprehensive program. Arguably, multilevel anti-tobacco programs have changed the cultural norm in the United States in the more than five decades since the Surgeon General's first report on smoking and health and are beginning to do so in other countries that have had a history of high tobacco consumption.

Given the demographic transition of age distribution, population growth and the dynamics of chronic diseases, coordinated chronic disease prevention strategies are gaining momentum from state health departments (Allen et al. 2014). The purpose of coordinated approaches is to work with state and community partners to efficiently and effectively implement chronic disease prevention and health promotion strategies (CDC 2015g). These multipronged approaches are warranted given the increased prevalence of multiple chronic conditions in the population (Goodman et al. 2013).

Examples of Community-Level Health Planning Approaches

The frameworks used in chronic disease prevention and control can provide structure to the planning process for an overall cohesive plan and a foundation for critical analysis (Community Toolbox 2015a). Although various intervention planning frameworks exist, most comprise similar principles. Successful program planning in the community involves time and resources for identifying key stakeholders, understanding the "culture" of the community, and gathering necessary data. Program planning processes to combat chronic diseases need to be carried out for ongoing implementation and interventions need to address agreed-upon priorities. Having both short-term and long-term goals is important; accomplishing short-term goals demonstrates small "wins" that can inspire continued effort, and having long-term goals helps to maintain focus and direction. A logic model can be utilized for the process to keep the community members aligned and offer a reminder of where we are in the process (Community Toolbox 2015b).

One innovative approach to monitoring health status and planning health interventions at the community level was represented by the Mobilizing Action Toward Community Health project (Kindig et al. 2010), an initiative that

- Used relevant criteria to calculate county-level health rankings for each of the 50 states.
- Developed partnerships and models for increasing involvement and accountability for population health improvements.
- Developed incentive-based models to encourage implementation of community-level programs and policies to improve population health.

The criteria (physical and mental health measures) used for determining county health rankings provide estimates of a community's overall health-related quality of life and enable public health authorities to assess priorities for intervention. This initiative led to the development of the County Health Ranking and Roadmaps, an initiative that ranks the health of all 3,000 counties in the United States, and provides an "Action Model" for community health improvement (see http://www.countyhealthrankings.org; Robert Wood Johnson Foundation 2016).

Numerous planning models provide frameworks for implementing community-level interventions for chronic disease prevention and control through behavioral change. The following ones illustrate popular or emerging strategies: PRECEDE-PROCEED, Mobilizing Action through Planning and Partnerships (MAPP), Intervention Mapping, and Community-Based Prevention Marketing (CBPM). Interventions that are grounded in behavior change theory are likely to produce a greater return on investment (Goetzel and Ozminkowski 2008).

PRECEDE-PROCEED Framework

The PRECEDE-PROCEED framework reflects an ecological and educational approach to intervention planning that respects both the real and perceived needs of the community of interest while following a systems approach to improving health and quality of life (Green and Kreuter 2005). The PRECEDE-PROCEED framework comprises two main components, each having a series of phases. The first component is referred to as PRECEDE (predisposing, reinforcing, and enabling constructs in educational/Ecological diagnosis and evaluation) and comprises four phases:

- Phase 1, social assessment and situational analysis: During this phase, one assesses the real and perceived needs of the community of interest. Data include both social indicators and subjective problems and priorities reflective of the community of interest.
- Phase 2, epidemiological assessment: During the epidemiological assessment, one specifies and prioritizes health issues in addition to the etiologic genetic, behavioral, and environmental risk factors.
- Phase 3, educational and ecological assessment: Once the key health issue and etiologic factors have been prioritized and selected, the educational and ecological assessment explores and prioritizes the predisposing, enabling, and reinforcing factors that influence the selected behavioral and environmental risk factors.
- Phase 4, administrative and policy assessment and intervention alignment: During this phase, one identifies the program components, interventions, and policy, organizational, and administrative resources needed to effect changes determined in phases 1 through 3.

The second component referred to as PROCEED (policy, regulatory, and organizational constructs in educational and environmental development) comprises of the following phases:

- Phase 5, implementation: During this phase, one assesses organizational readiness and capacity before program implementation.
- Phase 6, process evaluation: One assesses that the intervention is implemented according to plan and makes any necessary midcourse adjustments.
- Phase 7, impact evaluation: One assesses the immediate effects of the intervention on factors related to the health problem of interest.
- Phase 8, outcome evaluation: Phases 6 through 8 pertain to intervention evaluation. During these phases, the planning team determines the evaluation plan and design taking into account program processes (phase 6), short-term impacts (phase 7), and longer-term outcomes (phase 8).

Mobilizing Action through Planning and Partnerships

Mobilizing Action through Planning and Partnerships is a planning framework developed in 2000 by the National Association of County and City Health Officials (NACCHO) in cooperation with the Public Health Practice Program Office at CDC (NACCHO 2016). The guiding principles in the MAPP planning model include systems thinking, dialogue, shared vision, data, partnerships and collaboration, strategic thinking, and celebration for success. The MAPP planning model consists of four core assessments that drive the planning process (Figure 4-3). The main purposes of these four assessments are to provide insight concerning gaps between community wants and current circumstances, to provide information for identifying strategic issues, and to provide information for developing goals and strategies. These assessments are

- Community themes and strengths: This assessment provides the planning team with an understanding of the perceived strengths and needs of the selected community.
- Local public health system: Assessment of the local public health system comprises a capacity assessment in addition to an overview of how essential services are being provided to the community.
- Community health status: Similar to the previously described planning models, the community health status assessment provides the planning

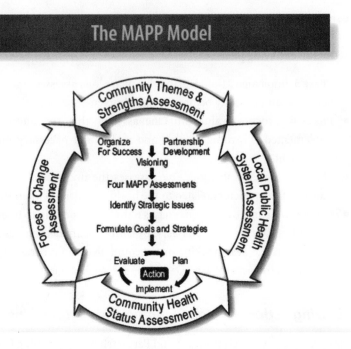

Source: Reprinted from NACCHO (2016).

Figure 4-3. Mobilizing for Action through Planning and Partnerships Planning Model

team with the community health and quality-of-life status for determining health priorities.

- Forces of change: The forces of change assessment provides the planning team with information on legislation, technology, and other issues that may affect the priority health issue, the community functioning, or the operations of the public health system.

Intervention Mapping

Bartholomew and Mullen (2011) describe intervention mapping as a systematic and cumulative process for developing, implementing, and sustaining public health interventions. The steps and procedures within the intervention mapping framework facilitate the development of theory-based interventions based on the literature and population-specific data. Intervention mapping is a tool that can serve as a blueprint for the design, implementation, and evaluation of an intervention once the planners have identified the health issue, behavioral and environmental risk factors, and associated determinates. The six core steps in the intervention mapping framework are

1. Needs assessment: The first step in the intervention mapping process entails performing a needs assessment to describe the individuals that have or are at risk for a health problem needing intervention within a community.

2. Preparing matrices of change objectives: This stage requires stating expected program outcomes for health-related behavior and environmental conditions. Behavioral and environmental conditions are then subdivided into performance objectives, and ranked by importance and changeability. This information informs the creation of a matrix of change objectives for each level of the intervention.

3. Selecting theory-informed intervention methods and practical applications: Once program ideas are developed, the theoretical methods that influence change are identified, informing the creation of intervention strategies.

4. Producing program components and materials: Working with intended program participants, program components, including delivery channels, themes, and program materials, are developed. Program materials are then pretested.

5. Planning program adoption, implementation, and sustainability: Program outcomes and performance objectives are stated; determinants of program adoption, implementation, and sustainability are specified; and matrices of change objectives are developed to ensure that interventions are aligned with program adoption, implementation, and sustainability.

6. Planning for evaluation: The research team writes evaluation questions about performance objectives and determinants based on the matrices developed in step 2. Indicators and measures are developed on the basis of these questions, and the team writes an evaluation plan.

Community-Based Prevention Marketing

Community-based prevention marketing is a community-directed, social change planning framework that employs marketing techniques to design, implement, and evaluate health promotion and disease prevention programs, policies, or system-wide changes (Bryant et al. 2007; Bryant et al. 2014). It draws from community organization principles and practices and marketing concepts and methods to create a social change planning framework.

From community organizing, CBPM borrows the principles of community participation, community capacity building and empowerment, and participatory research (Wallerstein et al. 2015). Community members select the issue to address and direct program planning, implementation, and evaluation activities, working with academic researchers to conduct formative research and create a marketing plan. Participatory research is used by CBPM in formative, pretesting, and evaluation research. Community partners provide academic researchers with a new perspective on local problems and present new research questions to explore. Academicians teach community members to develop research objectives, collect data, and interpret results.

The primary objective of CBPM is to build the community's capacity to apply marketing principles, to set goals, and to solve problems. Academic-based researchers provide training and technical assistance as community members use marketing principles and techniques to analyze problems and design effective change strategies. During the process, local leaders are developed who can direct problem-solving activities and guide prevention activities.

The social marketing component refers to the application of commercial marketing concepts and techniques to promote social change. Social marketing provides the conceptual framework that guides strategy development—the use of formative research to gain input from the people the intervention plans to reach, analytical techniques for segmenting market audiences, and monitoring to identify ineffective activities that require modification and effective activities worthy of sustaining. Community-based prevention marketing has been used to promote behavior change programs (Bryant et al. 2009), policy changes (Bryant et al. 2014), and, combined with system modeling, to design multi-level interventions.

Community-based prevention marketing follows an eight-step process:

1. Mobilizing the community: The first step is devoted to building a community structure to guide the CBPM process. A readiness checklist is used to assess the coalition's assets and identify resource gaps that need to be filled for the group to be successful.
2. Identify the problem and changes required to remedy it: The coalition prioritizes problems and determines the type of interventions needed to resolve it—behavior change programs, policy change at the local or organizational level, or for complex or "wicked" problems, a system-wide intervention that targets multiple levels.
3. Select a subgroup or segment to give the greatest priority in program planning: A community coalition identifies distinct segments within

the population of interest and uses marketing's "return on investment" concept to identify subgroups that will benefit most from an intervention and also be likely to respond to the type of intervention activities the coalition has resources to implement. This step results in the selection of one or more "priority populations" that will be the foci of planning and implementation activities.

4. Conduct research: A systematic review of existing literature of evidence-based interventions is combined with primary research to gain insights into the factors that will motivate and constrain the priority population from making the desired change. Data also are assembled to determine the most effective communication channels, spokespersons, and opportunities for mobilizing people to change.

5. Develop a marketing plan strategy: A marketing plan organized around the "4 P's" (product, price, place, and promotion) and an implementation plan with timeline and organizational assignments are created to guide intervention development.

6. Develop and pretest intervention materials and strategies: Intervention materials, advocacy tools, communication, and training materials are designed and pretested before mass production. The community coalition mobilizes resources needed for intervention activities and creates the institutional foundation for sustaining the program.

7. Tracking and evaluation: An evaluation and monitoring plan is created so that intervention activities can be assessed as they are launched and results used to make program enhancements and identify new problems that require further attention.

8. Implementing the program: A local program leader works closely with the community coalition to coordinate intervention launch and implementation.

Enhancing Health Literacy—The Key to All Chronic Disease Interventions

Low health literacy constitutes a significant challenge for public health. Health literacy includes a broad range of skills needed in everyday settings, whereby communication and decision-making coupled with an understanding of health and medical concepts and context across the life course are all important (Vamos and Frankish 2013). Reading a medicine or nutrition label, using an asthma inhaler, or managing diabetes represent a few examples in which health literacy skills are both relevant and required to function. Given the complexity of chronic disease, health literacy is an important lens for understanding health promotion constructs (Vamos and Rootman 2013).

Many definitions of health literacy have been advanced since the World Health Organization introduced the concept in its 1998 glossary of health promotion terms (Nutbeam 1998). Health literacy has expanded from a narrow medical concept to a much broader multidimensional concept associated with skills and factors contributing to individual and social empowerment. Health literacy refers not only to the abilities or traits of individuals, but also to the health-related systems and providers of information and services within those systems (Vamos and Rootman 2013). As a complex concept needed in chronic disease prevention, self-management, and treatment, it comprises the application to access, comprehend, evaluate, communicate, and act on health information (Poureslami et al. 2016). A definition put forth in the *National Action Plan to Improve Health Literacy* (USDHHS 2010) refers to health literacy as "the degree to which individuals have the capacity to obtain, process, and understand basic health information and services needed to make appropriate health decisions."

The Institute of Medicine (IOM 2004) reports that almost half of Americans have difficulty understanding and acting on health information. Persons with lower health literacy and chronic disease have less knowledge of their illness management than those with higher levels (Kalichman et al. 2000; Schillinger et al. 2002; Rootman and Gordon-El-Bihbety 2008) summarize that people with limited health literacy may

- Have reduced access to services and information (e.g., free cancer screening clinics, community health services).
- Be less likely to act on important public health alerts (influencing health outcomes).
- Make less use of secondary prevention and diagnostic services (e.g., mammograms, Papanicolaou tests).
- Be more likely to misunderstand instructions about prescription medication and make medication errors.
- Be unable to manage chronic conditions (e.g., diabetes, high blood pressure, asthma).
- Overuse hospitals and emergency rooms.

Greater health literacy has been associated with reductions in risk behaviors linked to chronic disease (Canadian Public Health Association 2006), decreased rates of hospitalizations (Cho et al. 2008; Nielsen-Bohlman et al. 2004), and higher self-reported health status (OECD 2013). Lower health literacy is linked to poorer health outcomes and higher health care costs. It is estimated that low health literacy costs the U.S. economy between $106 billion and $238 billion annually in the form of additional health care and sick days pay (Eichler et al. 2009). Chronic disease interventions that targeted low health literacy have been shown to be cost-effective. For example, one study revealed that implementing a health literacy–focused intervention to promote breast and cervical cancer screenings among Korean American women overdue for these tests saved on average $236 per patient, when compared to usual care (Schuster et al. 2015). A program to teach low-income parents how to treat common childhood illnesses at home resulted in significant decreases in emergency department visits, days off school for children, and days off work for the caregivers (Herman and Jackson 2010).

The relevance of health literacy for the complex dimensions of chronic diseases is evident for prevention, self-management, and treatment efforts. Health literacy plays many roles and at the individual, provider, and system levels. For example, to manage long-term conditions on a daily basis, individuals must be able to understand the diagnoses, instructions for self-care, and medical regimens; interpret and translate health information often for multiple outputs and often for multiple comorbidities; plan and make lifestyle adjustments for comorbidities; know when and where to access screenings, health care, services, and products when necessary; and communicate any health needs, concerns, and questions.

Health literacy is also a function of the complexity of the health care system consisting of providers and organizations. It is also important for health-related personnel to have a range of skills and strategies to respond to patients with varying health literacy needs (Batterham et al. 2016) and to reduce the complexity of medical care and related situational factors to protect the safety and promote the health of the patients. More specifically, those who provide information and services require health literacy skills to help people find what they need, decide which information and services are appropriate for different situations, understand how to provide the appropriate information and services, and communicate effectively with others (CDC 2015h). Furthermore, "systems can be health literate by providing equal, easy, and shame-free access to and delivery of health care and information" (Centre for Literacy 2011). The Calgary Charter on Health Literacy (Centre for Literacy 2011) outlines the key principles to support the development of curricula, initiatives, and tools to improve the health literacy of the public and of those who work in any capacity in health care or related systems.

Health literacy as an emerging field of research and practice has the potential to increase understanding of both chronic diseases and health promotion in the global context (Vamos and Frankish 2013). Increasing health literacy levels of the population is an effective health intervention (Mitic and Rootman 2012). Health literacy can be seen as an intervention in emerging strategies, initiatives, specific policies, and through an increasing number of national action plans around the world. The Intervention Research on Health Literacy for Aging project, a European research project on health literacy for older people, analyzed many of these documents to see how countries envision the development of health literacy interventions. Among other commonalities, countries that see health literacy as a priority often link their health literacy efforts to initiatives addressing chronic diseases, such as diabetes, cardiovascular diseases, and mental health (Health Literacy Centre Europe 2015). Moreover, several organizations have created toolkits and trainings, which provide recommendations to help address health literacy issues (Brach et al. 2012; CDC 2013c; Dewalt et al. 2010; The Joint Commission 2007; National Patient Safety Foundation 2016; Weiss 2003). The scope of promising health literacy research, policy, and practice developments continues to expand throughout the United States and around the globe.

Conclusions

Chronic diseases financially burden the American health care system and reduce the overall quality of life for many Americans. Intervention science for chronic disease prevention has increased its precision, making it possible for many of these disease threats to be prevented, delayed, or have their overall impact lessened. Today, there is excellent surveillance of diseases and an improved understanding of the interrelationships involving individual, social, environmental, and political factors. Moreover, there are sophisticated models, theories, and frameworks for intervening at the individual, interpersonal, organizational, community, and policy levels. The most promising of these interventions are multilevel ones that simultaneously address the complex disease causes. More case studies and applications of interventions are necessary to test the adaptability of previous findings in diverse settings. However, the evidence base gained to date through an abundance of demonstration projects can now be manifested and enlarged in scale to translate and disseminate these findings to broader audiences and address the major chronic disease issues facing Americans.

Resources

The Community Guide: What Works to Promote Health, http://www.thecommunityguide.org

A summary of state legislative bills throughout nation, http://www.ncsl.org

The American Public Health Association's policy statements, webinars, legislative updates, and a media advocacy manual, http://apha.org/policies-and-advocacy and http://nyspha.roundtablelive.org/Resources/Documents/2013%20APHA%20Affiliate%20Mtg/Policy%20Framework%20and%20Tools/APHA%20Media%20Advocacy%20Manual.pdf

The Community Tool Box, http://ctb.ku.edu/en/table-of-contents

The Harvard Family Resource Project's Guide to Measuring Advocacy and Policy, http://www.hfrp.org/evaluation/the-evaluation-exchange/issue-archive/advocacy-and-policy-change/a-guide-to-measuring-advocacy-and-policy

A set of metrics that can be used to assess public health policies (Brownson et al. 2010), http://www.cdc.gov/pcd/issues/2010/jul/09_0249.htm

References

Ajzen I. From intentions to actions: a theory of planned behavior. In: Kuhl J, Beckmann J, eds. *Springer Series in Social Psychology*. Berlin, Germany: Springer; 1985:11–39.

Ajzen I. The theory of planned behavior. *Organ Behav Hum Decis Process*. 1991;50(2):179–211.

Ajzen I, Fishbein M. Attitudinal and normative variables as predictors of specific behavior. *J Pers Soc Psychol*. 1973;27(1):41–57.

Allen P, Sequeira S, Best L, Jones E, Baker EA, Brownson RC. Perceived benefits and challenges of coordinated approaches to chronic disease prevention in state health departments. *Prev Chronic Dis*. 2014;11:E76.

Allensworth D, Kolbe LJ. The comprehensive school health program. *J Sch Health.* 1987;57(10):409–412.

American Cancer Society (ACS). Cancer prevention and early detection facts and figures 2015–2016. Atlanta, GA: ACS; 2015a.

American Cancer Society (ACS). Breast cancer screening for women at average risk. *JAMA.* 2015b;314(15):1599–1614.

Armour TA, Norris S, Jack L, Zhang X, Fisher L. The effectiveness of family interventions in people with diabetes mellitus: a systematic review. *Diabet Med.* 2005;22(10):1295–1305.

Baicker K, Cutler D, Song Z. Workplace wellness programs can generate savings. *Health Aff (Millwood).* 2010;29(2):304–311.

Baig AA, Benitez A, Quinn MT, Burnet DL. Family interventions to improve diabetes outcomes for adults. *Ann N Y Acad Sci.* 2015;1353(1):89–112.

Bandura A. *Social Learning Theory.* Englewood Cliffs, NJ: Prentice Hall; 1977.

Bandura A. *Social Foundations of Thought and Action.* Englewood Cliffs, NJ: Prentice Hall; 1986.

Bartholomew LK, Mullen PD. Five roles for using theory and evidence in the design and testing of behavior change interventions. *J Public Health Dent.* 2011;71:S20–S33.

Batterham RW, Hawkins M, Collins PA, Buchbinder RH, Osborne RH. Health literacy: applying current concepts to improve health services and reduce health inequalities. *Public Health.* 2016;132:3–12.

Berthold T, Miller J, vila-Esparza AA. *Foundations for Community Health Workers.* San Francisco, CA: Jossey-Bass; 2009.

Brach C, Keller D, Hernandez LM, et al. Ten attributes of a health-literate care organization. 2012. Available at: http://www.ahealthyunderstanding.org/Portals/0/Documents1/IOM_Ten_Attributes_HL_Paper.pdf. Accessed April 23, 2016.

Bracht N. *Health Promotion at the Community Level.* Newbury Park, CA: Sage; 1990.

Brownson RC, Seiler R, Eyler AA. Measuring the impact of public health policy. *Prev Chronic Dis.* 2010;7(4):A77.

Bryant CA, Courtney A, McDermott RJ, et al. A social marketing approach for increasing community coalitions' adoption of evidence-based policy to combat obesity. *Soc Mar Q.* 2014;20(4):219–246.

Bryant CA, McCormack Brown K, McDermott RJ, et al. Community-based prevention marketing: a new planning framework for designing and tailoring health promotion interventions. In: DiClemente R, Crosby RA, Kegler MC, eds. *Emerging Theories in*

Health Promotion Practice and Research: Strategies for Improving Public Health. 2nd ed. San Francisco, CA: Jossey-Bass; 2009.

Bryant CA, McCormack Brown K, McDermott RJ, et al. Community-based prevention marketing: a framework for facilitating health behavior change. *Health Promot Pract.* 2007;8(2):154–163.

Bureau of Labor Statistics. American Time Use Survey. 2015. Available at: http://www.bls.gov/tus/charts/work.htm. Accessed March 21, 2016.

Butterfoss FD, Goodman R, Wandersman A. Community coalitions for prevention and health promotion. *Health Educ Res.* 1993;8(3):315–330.

Butterfoss FD, Kegler MC. The community coalition action theory. In: DiClemente RJ, Crosby RA, Kegler MC, eds. *Emerging Theories in Health Promotion Practice and Research.* San Francisco, CA: Jossey Bass; 2009:451–510.

Butterfoss FD, LaChance LL, Orians CE. Building allies coalitions: why formation matters. *Health Promot Pract.* 2006;7(2 suppl):23S–33S.

Butterfoss FD, Morrow AL, Webster JD, Crews C. The coalition training institute: training for the long haul. *J Public Health Manag Pract.* 2003;9(6):522–529.

Canadian Public Health Association. Low health literacy and chronic disease prevention and control—perspectives from the health and public sectors. 2006. Available at: http://www.cpha.ca/uploads/portals/h-l/kl_summary_e.pdf. Accessed April 23, 2016.

Centers for Disease Control and Prevention (CDC). Ten great public health achievements—United States, 1900–1999. *MMWR Morb Mortal Wkly Rep.* 1999;48(12):241–243.

Centers for Disease Control and Prevention (CDC). *State Indicator Report on Fruits and Vegetables, 2013.* Atlanta, GA: CDC; 2013a.

Centers for Disease Control and Prevention (CDC). Prevention: what you can do. 2013b. Available at: http://www.cdc.gov/heartdisease/what_you_can_do.htm. Accessed April 20, 2016.

Centers for Disease Control and Prevention (CDC). Health Literacy for Public Health Professionals. 2013c. Available at: http://www.cdc.gov/healthliteracy/training. Accessed April 23, 2016.

Centers for Disease Control and Prevention (CDC). NCHHSTP social determinants of health. 2014a. Available at: http://www.cdc.gov/nchhstp/socialdeterminants/faq.html. Accessed April 20, 2016.

Centers for Disease Control and Prevention (CDC). Prevention Research Centers. 2014b. Available at: http://www.cdc.gov/prc/about-prc-program/index.htm. Accessed April 20, 2016.

Centers for Disease Control and Prevention (CDC). Exercise or physical activity. 2015a. Available at: http://www.cdc.gov/nchs/fastats/exercise.htm. Accessed April 20, 2016.

Centers for Disease Control and Prevention (CDC). Childhood obesity facts. 2015b. Available at: http://www.cdc.gov/obesity/data/childhood.html. Accessed April 20, 2016.

Centers for Disease Control and Prevention (CDC). Social determinants of health: know what affects health. 2015c. Available at: http://www.cdc.gov/socialdeterminants. Accessed April 21, 2016.

Centers for Disease Control and Prevention (CDC). Prevention Research Centers: stories and highlights of notable accomplishments. 2015d. Available at: http://www.cdc.gov/prc/program-research/index.htm. Accessed April 20, 2016.

Centers for Disease Control and Prevention (CDC). *Essential Elements of Effective Workplace Programs and Policies for Improving Worker Health and Wellbeing.* 2015e. Available at: http://www.cdc.gov/niosh/twh/essentials.html. Accessed March 21, 2016.

Centers for Disease Control and Prevention (CDC). Faith-based organizations. 2015f. Available at: http://www.cdc.gov/minorityhealth/resources/faith.html. Accessed April 21, 2016.

Centers for Disease Control and Prevention (CDC). About coordinated chronic disease prevention. 2015g. Available at: http://www.cdc.gov/coordinatedchronic/about-coordination.html. Accessed March 21, 2016.

Centers for Disease Control and Prevention (CDC). Learn about health literacy. 2015h. Available at: http://www.cdc.gov/healthliteracy/learn. Accessed April 23, 2016.

Centers for Disease Control and Prevention (CDC). Chronic disease overview. 2016a. Available at: http://www.cdc.gov/chronicdisease/overview. Accessed April 21, 2016.

Centers for Disease Control and Prevention (CDC). Public health policy. 2016b. Available at: http://www.cdc.gov/stltpublichealth/policy. Accessed March 18, 2016.

Centers for Disease Control and Prevention (CDC). Social ecological model. 2016c. Available at: http://www.cdc.gov/cancer/crccp/sem.htm. Accessed August 9, 2016.

Centers for Disease Control and Prevention (CDC). Whole School, Whole Community, Whole Child. 2016d. Available at: http://www.cdc.gov/healthyyouth/wscc/index.htm. Accessed August 10, 2016.

Centre for Literacy. The Calgary Charter on Health Literacy: rationale and core principles for the development of health literacy curricula. 2011:3. Available at: http://www.centreforliteracy.qc.ca/sites/default/files/CFL_Calgary_Charter_2011.pdf. Accessed April 23, 2016.

Cho YI, Arozullah AM, Crittenden KS, Lee SYD. Effects of health literacy on health status and health service utilization amongst the elderly. *Soc Sci Med.* 2008;66(8):1809–1816.

Christakis NA, Fowler JH. The spread of obesity in a large social network over 32 years. *N Engl J Med.* 2007;357(4):370–379.

Coleman S, Briffa NK, Carroll G, Inderjeet C, Cook N, McQuade J. A randomised controlled trial of a self-management education program for osteoarthritis of the knee delivered by health care professionals. *Arthritis Res Ther.* 2012;14(1):R21.

Community Guide. Investing in worksite wellness for Dow employees. 2012. Available at: http://www.thecommunityguide.org/CG-in-Action/worksite-Dow.pdf. Accessed March 24, 2016.

Community Toolbox. PRECEDE–PROCEED model. 2015a. Available at: http://ctb. ku.edu/en/table-contents/overview/other-models-promoting-community-health-and-development/preceder-proceder/main. Accessed March 24, 2016.

Community Toolbox. Developing a logic model. 2015b. Available at: http://ctb.ku.edu/en/table-of-contents/overview/models-for-community-health-and-development/logic-model-development/main. Accessed March 24, 2016.

DeWalt DA, Callahan LF, Hawk VH, et al. *Health Literacy Universal Precautions Toolkit.* Rockville, MD: Agency for Healthcare Research and Quality; 2010.

Dorfman L, Krasnow ID. Public health and media advocacy. *Annu Rev Public Health.* 2014;35:293–306.

Eichler K, Wieser S, Bruegger U. The costs of limited health literacy: a systematic review. *Int J Public Health.* 2009;54(5):313–324.

Ejeta LT, Ardalan A, Paton D. Application of behavioral theories to disaster and emergency health preparedness: a systematic review. *PLoS Curr.* 2015;7.

Farquhar J, Fortmann S, Flora J, et al. Effects of community-wide education on cardiovascular disease risk factors: the five-city project. *JAMA.* 1990;264(3):359–365.

Feinberg ME, Bontempo DE, Greenberg MT. Predictors and level of sustainability of community prevention coalitions. *Am J Prev Med.* 2008a;34(6):495–501.

Feinberg ME, Ridenour TA, Greenberg MT. The longitudinal effect of technical assistance dosage on the functioning of communities that care prevention boards in Pennsylvania. *J Prim Prev.* 2008b;29(2):145–165.

Ferlander S. The importance of different forms of social capital for health. *Acta Sociol.* 2007;50(2):115–128.

Finkelstein EA, Trogdon JG, Cohen JW, Dietz W. Annual medical spending attributable to obesity: payer- and service-specific estimates. *Health Aff (Millwood)*. 2009;28(5): w822–w831.

Fishbein M. Attitude and the prediction of behavior. In: Fishbein M, ed. *Readings in Attitude Theory and Measurement*. New York, NY: Wiley; 1967:477–492.

Fishbein M, Ajzen I. *Belief, Attitude, Intention, and Behavior: An Introduction to Theory and Research*. Reading, MA; Don Mills, ON: Addison-Wesley; 1975.

Garg A, Dworkin PH. Surveillance and screening for social determinants of health: the medical home and beyond. *JAMA Pediatr*. 2016;170(3):189–190.

Gerteis J, Izrael D, Deitz D, et al. *Multiple Chronic Conditions Chartbook*. Rockville, MD: Agency for Healthcare Research and Quality; 2014. AHRQ Publications no. Q14-0038.

Glanz K, Rimer B, Viswanath K. *Health Behavior and Health Education: Theory, Research, and Practice*. 4th ed. San Francisco, CA: Jossey-Bass; 2008.

Gloppen KM, Arthur MW, Hawkins JD, Shapiro VB. Sustainability of the Communities That Care prevention system by coalitions participating in the Community Youth Development Study. *J Adolesc Health*. 2012;51(3):259–264.

Go AS, Mozaffarian D, Roger VL, et al. American Heart Association Statistics Committee and Stroke Statistics Committee. Heart disease and stroke statistics—2014 update: a report from the American Heart Association. *Circulation*. 2014;129(3):399–410.

Goetzel RZ, Ozminkowski RJ. The health and cost benefits of work site health-promotion programs. *Annu Rev Public Health*. 2008;29:303–323.

Golden SD, Earp JAL. Social ecological approaches to individuals and their contexts: twenty years of health education and behavior health promotion interventions. *Health Educ Behav*. 2012;39(3):364–372.

Goodman RA, Posner SF, Huang ES, Parekh AK, Koh HK. Defining and measuring chronic conditions: imperatives for research, policy, program, and practice. *Prev Chronic Dis*. 2013;10:E66.

Goodman RM, Speers M, McLeroy K, et al. Identifying and defining the dimensions of community capacity to provide a basis for measurement. *Health Educ Behav*. 1998;25(3):258–278.

Gordon-Larsen P, Nelson MC, Page P, Popkin BM. Inequality in the built environment underlies key health disparities in physical activity and obesity. *Pediatrics*. 2006;117(2): 417–424.

Gray B. *Collaboration: Finding Common Ground for Multiparty Problems*. San Francisco, CA: Jossey-Bass; 1989.

Green LW, Kreuter M. *Health Program Planning: An Educational and Ecological Approach.* 4th ed. Columbus, OH: McGraw Hill; 2005.

Grossberg PM, Brown DD, Fleming MF. Brief physician advice for high risk drinking among young adults. *Ann Fam Med.* 2004;2(5):474–480.

Hage C, Alter J. *Organizations Working Together.* Newbury Park, CA: Sage; 1993.

Hartmann M, Bäzner E, Wild B, Eisler I, Herzog W. Effects of interventions involving the family in the treatment of adult patients with chronic physical diseases: a meta-analysis. *Psychother Psychosom.* 2010;79(3):136–148.

Health Literacy Centre Europe. National health literacy policies and what we can learn from them. 2015. Available at: http://healthliteracycentre.eu/national-health-literacy-policies. Accessed April 23, 2016.

Henry J. Kaiser Family Foundation. The facts on Medicare spending and financing. 2015. Available at: http://kff.org/medicare/fact-sheet/medicare-spending-and-financing-fact-sheet. Accessed April 21, 2016.

Henry J. Kaiser Family Foundation. Preventive services covered by private health plans under the Affordable Care Act. 2016. Available at: http://kff.org/health-reform/fact-sheet/preventive-services-covered-by-private-health-plans. Accessed April 21, 2016.

Herman A, Jackson P. Empowering low-income parents with skills to reduce excess pediatric emergency room and clinic visits through a tailored low literacy training intervention. *J Health Commun.* 2010;15(8):895–910.

Hicks S, Duran B, Wallerstein N, et al. Evaluating community-based participatory research to improve community-partnered science and community health. *Prog Community Health Partnersh.* 2012;6(3):289–299.

Hochbaum GM. *Public Participation in Medical Screening Programs: A Socio-Psychological Study.* Washington, DC: US Government Printing Office; 1958. Public Health Service Publication no. 572.

House JS, Umberson D, Landis KR. Structures and processes of social support. *Ann Rev Sociol.* 1988;14:293–318.

Institute of Medicine (IOM). *Health Literacy—A Prescription to End Confusion. Committee on Health Literacy, Board on Neuroscience and Behavioral Health.* Nielsen-Bohlman L, Panzer AM, Kindig DA, eds. Washington, DC: The National Academies Press; 2004.

Israel BA, Schulz AJ, Parker EA, Becker AB. Review of community-based research: assessing partnership approaches to improve public health. *Annu Rev Public Health.* 2005;19(1):173–202.

Jagosh J, Macaulay AC, Pluye P, et al. Uncovering the benefits of participatory research: implications of a realist review for health research and practice. *Milbank Q.* 2012;90(2): 311–346.

The Joint Commission. *What Did the Doctor Say? Improving Health Literacy to Protect Patient Safety.* 2007. Available at: http://www.jointcommission.org/What_Did_the_ Doctor_Say. Accessed April 23, 2016.

Kalichman SC, Benotsch E, Suarez T, Catz S, Miller J, Rompa D. Health literacy and health-related knowledge among persons living with HIV/AIDS. *Am J Prev Med.* 2000;18(4):325–331.

Kanny D, Liu Y, Brewer RD, Garvin WS, Balluz L. Vital signs: binge drinking prevalence, frequency, and intensity among adults—United States, 2010. *MMWR Morb Mortal Wkly Rep.* 2012;61(1):14–19.

Kant AK, Miner P. Physician advice about being overweight: association with self-reported weight loss, dietary, and physical activity behaviors of US adolescents in the National Health and Nutrition Examination Survey, 1999–2002. *Pediatrics.* 2007;119(1): e142–e147.

Katikireddi SV, Bond L, Hilton S. Changing policy framing as a deliberate strategy for public health advocacy: a qualitative policy case study of minimum unit pricing of alcohol. *Milbank Q.* 2014;92(2):250–283.

Kelder SH, Hoelscher D, Perry CL. How individuals, environments, and health behaviors interact. In: Glanz K, Rimer BK, Viswanath K, eds. *Health Behavior Theory, Research, and Practice.* 5th ed. San Francisco, CA: Jossey-Bass; 2015:159–181.

Kerr J, Rosenberg DE, Nathan A, et al. Applying the ecological model of behavior change to a physical activity trial in retirement communities: description of the study protocol. *Contemp Clin Trials.* 2012;33(6):1180–1188.

Kindig DA, Booske BC, Remington PL. Mobilizing Action Toward Community Health (MATCH): metrics, incentives, and partnerships for population health. *Prev Chronic Dis.* 2010;7(4):A68.

Kristensen AH, Flottenmesch TJ, Maciosek MJ, et al. Reducing childhood obesity through U.S. federal policy: a microsimulation analysis. *Am J Prev Med.* 2014;47(5):604–612.

Lancaster T, Stead LF. Individual behavioural counselling for smoking cessation. *Cochrane Database Syst Rev.* 2005;(2):CD001292.

Lasker RD, Weiss ES. Broadening participation in community problem solving: a multidisciplinary model to support collaborative practice and research. *J Urban Health.* 2003;80(1):48–60.

Lessin N. *Promising the Best Practices in Total Worker Health: Workshop Summary.* 2014. Available at: http://www.ncbi.nlm.nih.gov/books/NBK268671. Accessed April 23, 2016.

Lewallen TC, Hunt H, Potts-Datema W, Zaza S, Giles W. The whole school, whole community, whole child model: a new approach for improving educational attainment and healthy development for students. *J Sch Health.* 2015;85(11):729–739.

Lumpkins CY, Greiner KA, Daley C, Mabachi NM, Neuhaus K. Promoting healthy behavior from the pulpit: clergy share their perspectives on effective health communication in the African American church. *J Relig Health.* 2013;52(4):1093–1107.

MacQueen KM, McLellan E, Metzger DS, et al. What is community? An evidence-based definition for participatory public health. *Am J Public Health.* 2001;91(12):1929–1938.

Martire LM, Schulz R. Involving family in psychosocial interventions for chronic illness. *Curr Dir Psychol Sci.* 2007;16(2):90–94.

Mattke S, Liu H, Caloyeras JP, et al. Workplace Wellness Programs Study: final report. RAND Corporation. 2013. Available at: http://www.rand.org/pubs/research_reports/RR254.html. Accessed August 9, 2016.

Mayer G. Selected characterisitics of private and public sector workers. Congressional Research Service. 2014. Available at: https://www.fas.org/sgp/crs/misc/R41897.pdf. Accessed August 10, 2016.

McLeroy KR, Kegler M, Steckler A, Burdine JM, Wisotzky M. Editorial. Community coalitions for health promotion: summary and further reflections. *Health Educ Res.* 1994;9(1):1–11.

Medline Plus. Living with a chronic illness—reaching out to others. 2016. Available at: https://www.nlm.nih.gov/medlineplus/ency/patientinstructions/000602.htm. Accessed April 21, 2016.

Meis LA, Griffin JM, Greer N, et al. Couple and family involvement in adult mental health treatment: a systematic review. *Clin Psychol Rev.* 2013;33(2):275–286.

Michael SL, Merlo CL, Basch CE, Wentzel KR, Wechsler H. Critical connections: health and academics. *J Sch Health.* 2015;85(11):740–758.

Minkler M. Ten commitments for community health education. *Health Educ Res.* 1994;9(4):527–534.

Minkler M, Wallerstein N. *Community-Based Participatory Research for Health: From Process to Outcomes.* 2nd ed. San Francisco, CA: Jossey-Bass; 2008.

Mitchell RJ, Bates P. Measuring health-related productivity loss. *Popul Health Manag.* 2011;14(2):93–98.

Mitic W, Rootman I. *Inter-Sectoral Approach to Improving Health Literacy for Canadians*. Vancouver, BC: Public Health Association of British Columbia; 2012.

Monaghan PF, Forst LS, Tovar-Aguilar JA, et al. Preventing eye injuries among citrus harvesters: the community health worker model. *Am J Public Health*. 2011;101(12):2269–2274.

Monaghan PF, Forst LS, McDermott RJ, Bryant CA, Luque JS, Contreras RB. Adoption of safety eyewear among citrus harvesters in rural Florida. *J Immigr Minor Health*. 2012;14(3):460–466.

Moreland-Russell S, Brownson R. *Prevention, Policy, and Public Health*. New York, NY: Oxford University Press; 2015.

Motley M, Holmes A, Hill J, Plumb K, Zoellner J. Evaluating community capacity to address obesity in the Dan river region: a case study. *Am J Health Behav*. 2013;37(2):209–217.

National Association of County and City Health Officials (NACCHO). Mobilizing for Action Through Planning and Partnerships. 2016. Available at: www.naccho.org/mapp. Accessed August 10, 2016.

National Heart, Lung, and Blood Institute (NHLBI). NACI strategic partnership program. 2015. Available at: http://www.nhlbi.nih.gov/health-pro/resources/lung/naci/naci-in-action/partners.htm. Accessed April 23, 2016.

National Patient Safety Foundation. Ask me 3: good questions for your good health. 2016. Available at: http://www.npsf.org/?page=askme3. Accessed April 23, 2016.

Nielsen-Bohlman L, Panze AM, Kindig DA, eds. *Health Literacy: A Prescription to End Confusion*. Washington, DC: National Academies Press; 2004.

Nutbeam D. Health promotion glossary. *Health Promot Int*. 1998;13(4):349–364.

O'Brien MJ, Squires AP, Bixby RA, Larson SC. Role development of community health workers: an examination of selection and training processes in the intervention literature. *Am J Prev Med*. 2009;37(6 suppl 1):S262–S269.

Oman R, Vesel S, Aspay C, McLeroy KR, Rodine S, Marshall L. The potential protective effect of youth assets on adolescent alcohol and drug use. *Am J Public Health*. 2004;94(8):1425–1430.

O'Mara-Eves A, Brunton G, Oliver S, Kavanagh J, Jamal F, Thomas J. The effectiveness of community engagement in public health interventions for disadvantaged groups: a meta-analysis. *BMC Public Health*. 2015;15:129.

Organisation for Economic Co-operation and Development (OECD). *OECD Skills Outlook 2013: First Results from the Survey of Adult Skills*. Washington, DC: OECD Publishing; 2013.

Partnership for Prevention. *Healthy Workforce 2010 and Beyond.* 2009 Available at: http://www.oecd-ilibrary.org/education/oecd-skills-outlook-2013_9789264204256-en. Accessed August 10, 2016.

Patel JG, Nagar SP, Dalal AA. Indirect costs in chronic obstructive pulmonary disease: a review of the economic burden on employers and individuals in the United States. *Int J Chron Obstruct Pulmon Dis.* 2014;9:289–300.

Patrick K, Marshall S, Davila E, et al. Design and implementation of a randomized controlled social and mobile weight loss trial for young adults (Project SMART). *Contemp Clin Trials.* 2014;37(1):10–18.

Perryman ML. Ethical family interventions for childhood obesity. *Prev Chronic Dis.* 2011;8(5):A99.

Person AL, Colby SE, Bulova JA, Eubanks JW. Barriers to participation in a worksite wellness program. *Nutr Res Pract.* 2010;4(2):149–154.

Peterson-Sweeney K, McMullen A, Yoos HL, Kitzman H. Parental perceptions of their child's asthma: management and medication use. *J Pediatr Health Care.* 2003;17(3): 118–125.

Phillips JE, Klein WM. Socioeconomic status and coronary heart disease risk: the role of social cognitive factors. *Soc Personal Psychol Compass.* 2010;4(9):704–727.

Poureslami I, Nimmon L, Rootman I, Fitgerald M. Health literacy and chronic disease management: drawing from expert knowledge to set an agenda. *Health Promot Int.* 2016; epub ahead of print February 11, 2016.

Powell-Wiley TM, Cooper-McCann R, Ayers C, et al. Change in neighborhood socioeconomic status and weight gain: Dallas Heart Study. *Am J Prev Med.* 2015;49(1): 72–79.

Prestby J, Wandersman A, Florin P, Rich R, Chavis DM. Benefits, costs, incentives management and participation in voluntary associations. *Am J Community Psychol.* 1990;18(1):117–149.

Prochaska JO, DiClemente CC. Stages and processes of self-change of smoking: toward an integrative model of change. *J Consult Clin Psychol.* 1983;51(3):390–395.

Puska P, Uutela A. Community intervention in cardiovascular health promotion: North Karelia, 1972–1999. In: Schneiderman N, Speers MA, Silva JM, Tomes H, Gentry JH, eds. *Integrating Behavioral and Social Sciences With Public Health.* Arlington, VA: American Psychological Association; 2000:73–96.

Robert Wood Johnson Foundation. County health rankings and roadmaps. 2016. Available at: http://www.countyhealthrankings.org. Accessed August 6, 2016.

Rootman I, Gordon-El-Bihbety D. *A Vision for a Health Literate Canada: Report of the Expert Panel on Health Literacy.* Ottawa, Ontario: Canadian Public Health Association; 2008.

Rotter JB. Generalized expectancies for internal versus external control of reinforcement. *Psychol Monogr.* 1966;80(1):1–28.

Savage C, Aboul-Enein BH, Bernstein J. Perspectives of health promotion and primary prevention of cardiovascular disease: revisiting the social ecological model. *Evid Based Med Public Health.* 2015;2:e911.

Schillinger D, Grumbach K, Piette J, et al. Association of health literacy with diabetes outcomes. *JAMA.* 2002;288(4):475–482.

Schuster AL, Frick KD, Huh B-Y, Kim KB, Kim M, Han H-R. Economic evaluation of a community health worker-led health literacy intervention to promote cancer screening among Korean American women. *J Health Care Poor Underserved.* 2015;26(2):431–440.

Shoham DA, Tong L, Lamberson PJ, et al. An actor-based model of social network influence on adolescent body size, screen time, and playing sports. *PLoS One.* 2012;7(6):e39795.

Simpkins SD, Schaefer DR, Price CD, Vest AE. Adolescent friendships, BMI, and physical activity: untangling selection and influence through longitudinal social network analysis. *J Res Adolesc.* 2013;23(3):537–549.

Singh GP, Siahpush M, Kogan MD. Neighborhood socioeconomic conditions, built environments, and childhood obesity. *Health Aff (Millwood).* 2010;29(3):503–512.

Smith KP, Christakis NA. Social networks and health. *Annu Rev Sociol.* 2008;34:405–429.

Smith SA, Whitehead MS, Sheats JQ, Ansa BE, Coughlin SS, Blumenthal DS. Community-based participatory research principles for the African American Community. *J Ga Public Health Assoc.* 2015;5(1):52–56.

Soler RE, Leeks KD, Razi S, et al. Systematic review of selected interventions for worksite health promotion: the assessment of health risks with feedback. *Am J Prev Med.* 2010;38(2):S237–S262.

Sorensen G, Landsbergis P, Hammer L, et al. Preventing chronic disease in the workplace: a workshop report and recommendations. *Am J Public Health.* 2011;101(suppl 1): S196–S207.

Sparling PB. Worksite health promotion: principles, resources, and challenges. *Prev Chronic Dis.* 2010;7(1):A25.

Torenholt R, Schwennesen N, Willaing I. Lost in translation—the role of family in interventions among adults with diabetes: a systematic review. *Diabet Med.* 2014;31(1):15–23.

Tovar-Aguilar JA, Monaghan P, Bryant C, et al. Improving eye safety in citrus harvest crews through the acceptance and use of personal protective equipment, community-based participatory research, social marketing, and community health workers. *J Agromedicine.* 2014;19(2):107–116.

US Department of Health and Human Services (USDHHS). *2007 Community Health Worker National Workforce Study.* Atlanta, GA: USDHHS; 2007.

US Department of Health and Human Services (USDHHS). *National Action Plan to Improve Health Literacy.* Washington, DC: USDHHS; 2010: 5.

US Department of Health and Human Services (USDHHS). *The Health Consequences of Smoking—50 Years of Progress: A Report of the Surgeon General.* Atlanta, GA: USDHHS; 2014.

US Department of Health and Human Services (USDHHS). *Planned Approach to Community Health: Guide for the Local Coordinator.* Atlanta, GA: USDHHS; 2015.

Vamos S, Frankish J. Health literacy and non-communicable diseases. In: McQueen D, ed. *Oxford Bibliographies in Public Health.* New York, NY: Oxford University Press; 2013.

Vamos S, Rootman I. Health literacy as a lens for understanding non-communicable diseases and health promotion. In: McQueen D, ed. *Global Handbook on Non-Communicable Diseases and Health Promotion.* New York, NY: Springer Business-Science Media Publishing; 2013.

Volpp KG, Asch DA, Galvin R, Loewenstein G. Redesigning employee health incentives—lessons from behavioral economics. *N Engl J Med.* 2011;365(5):388–390.

Wallack L. The role of mass media in creating social capital: a new direction for public health. In: Smedly BD, Syme SL, eds. *Promoting Health: Intervention Strategies From Social and Behavioral Research.* Washington, DC: National Academy Press; 2000:337–365.

Wallack L. Media advocacy: a strategy for empowering people and communities. In: Minkler M ed. *Community Organizing and Community Building for Health.* 2nd ed. New Brunswick NJ: Rutgers University Press; 2005:430.

Wallack L, Dorfman L, Jernigan D, Themba M. *Media Advocacy and Public Health: Power for Prevention.* Thousand Oaks, CA: Sage Publications; 1993:61.

Wallerstein N, Minkler M, Carter-Edwards L, Avila M, Sanchez V. Improving health through community engagement, community organization, and community building. In: Glanz K, Rimer B, Viswanath K, eds. *Health Behavior: Theory, Research, and Practice.* San Francisco, CA: John Wiley and Sons; 2015:277–300.

Wallston KA, Wallston BS, DeVellis R. Development of the multidimensional health locus of control (MHLC) scales. *Health Educ Monogr.* 1978;6(2):160–170.

Ward BW, Schiller JS, Goodman RA. Multiple chronic conditions among US adults: a 2012 update. *Prev Chronic Dis.* 2014;11:E62.

Webster J, Dunford E, Kennington S, Neal B, Chapman S. Drop the salt! Assessing the impact of a public health advocacy strategy on Australian government policy on salt. *Public Health Nutr.* 2014;17(1):212–218.

Weiss BD. *Health Literacy: Help Your Patients Understand.* Chicago, IL: American Medical Association Foundation and American Medical Association; 2003.

Wellness Councils of America. Current medical expenditures and lost productivity costs. 2012. Available at: http://www.welcoa.org/store/resources/documents/econohealthroi-bannack-labs-sample-ch1.pdf. Accessed March 21, 2016.

Whitt M. *Fighting Tobacco: A Coalition Approach to Improving Your Community's Health.* Lansing, MI: Michigan Department of Public Health; 1993.

Winter SJ, Sheats JL, King AC. The use of behavior change techniques and theory in technologies for cardiovascular disease prevention and treatment in adults a comprehensive review. *Prog Cardiovasc Dis.* 2016;58(6):605–612.

Young MD, Plotnikoff RC, Collins CE, Callister R, Morgan PJ. Social cognitive theory and physical activity: a systematic review and meta-analysis. *Obes Rev.* 2014;15(12):983–995.

Yuen T, Park AN, Seifer SD, Payne-Sturges D. A systematic review of community engagement in the US environmental protection agency's extramural research solicitations: implications for research funders. *Am J Public Health.* 2015;105(12):e44–e52.

Zakocs RC, Guckenberg S. What coalition factors foster community capacity? Lessons learned from the fighting back initiative. *Health Educ Behav.* 2007;34(2):354–375.

Zolnierek KBH, DiMatteo MR. Physician communication and patient adherence to treatment: a meta-analysis. *Med Care.* 2009;47(8):826–834.

THE ROLE OF HEALTH CARE SYSTEMS IN CHRONIC DISEASE PREVENTION AND CONTROL

Karina A. Atwell, MD, MPH, and Maureen A. Smith, MD, PhD, MPH

Introduction

A rapidly aging population in the United States, combined with advances in medicine and public health leading to increased life expectancy, are key contributors to the growing burden of chronic disease on health systems and communities. In 2010, 86% of all health care spending was for people with one or more chronic medical condition(s) (Gerteis et al. 2014). One quarter of individuals with chronic disease live with multiple chronic conditions (Ward et al. 2014). This number reaches two thirds of all Medicare beneficiaries (Nash et al. 2015). People with multiple or complex chronic conditions have more complicated health needs, including frequent monitoring and evaluation, and multiple care providers across different health environments. As an individual's number of chronic conditions increases, that individual's risk for dying, incurring avoidable hospitalizations, and experiencing poor day-to-day functioning also rise. In addition, these conditions contribute to frailty and disability, which often complicate access to health care, interfere with self-management, and necessitate reliance on caregivers (Anderson 2010). Many chronic diseases act synergistically, such as diabetes and depression, compounding the risk for poor outcomes (Parekh et al. 2011).

These extra layers of complexity bring with them more challenges and costs to caring for chronic disease populations. Increased spending on chronic diseases among Medicare beneficiaries is a key factor driving the overall rise in spending in the traditional Medicare program. In 2010, almost all (93%) of the $300 billion in total spending for the Medicare patients was to support

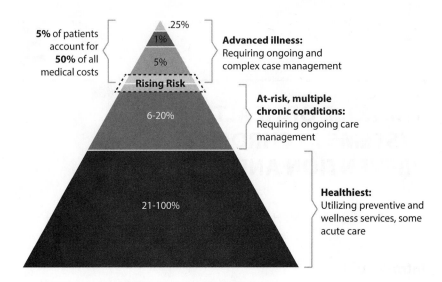

Source: Reprinted with permission from Marks (2015).

Figure 5-1. Population Pyramid Depicting How a Health System Might Characterize Its Population of Patients as It Relates to Chronic Disease Status, Risk, Health Care Needs, and Costs

people with two or more chronic conditions (DeVol and Bedroussian 2007). Most nations across the globe are strategizing ways to address the growing burdens of chronic disease in their populations, but this chapter will focus on U.S. health care system approaches, despite our ability to learn much from other countries who are ahead of the United States in this feat.

The disproportionate distribution of costs and opportunities for chronic disease management and prevention across a population serviced by a health care system can be outlined in a population pyramid (Figure 5-1). At the top of the pyramid are those 5% of patients with the most complex and advanced disease, highest risk, and highest costs. They have multiple chronic conditions, typically at least one of which is under poor control or at end stages for which acute care and tertiary prevention measures are the mainstay of management. This subset of the population requires the most intensive and frequent care, often through specialized complex case management. They can consume 50% or more of total cost of care within the health system.

The next 15% of the pyramid is the chronic care population; they usually have at least one chronic condition, often under suboptimal control. These patients require frequent monitoring and are at risk for progression and complications of their chronic disease(s). This subgroup also requires ongoing care management, albeit less intense than the most complex 5% of the population.

The bottom 80% of the pyramid represents the generally "well" or "still healthy" share of the population. They tend to interact with the health system only for acute care and preventive services, but may be at risk for development of chronic diseases because of one or a combination of lifestyle, hereditary, socioeconomic, and environmental factors. This group presents opportunities for primary and early secondary prevention through timely evidence-based screening and health promotion counseling.

As health care systems shoulder the current, and anticipated growing, strain of chronic disease care for the top 20% of this pyramid, there is a recognized need to transform the ways in which this care is delivered to achieve better and equitable outcomes at lower costs (Nash 2012). As a majority of chronic conditions and their subsequent complications are preventable, there is also expanding interest in health care system approaches that target health promotion and disease prevention (the bottom 80% of the pyramid), activities once considered mainly in the arena of public health.

This broader reach demands a true population health perspective. Population health refers to the "distribution of health outcomes within a population, the health determinants that influence distribution, and the policies and interventions that impact the determinants" (Kindig and Stoddart 2003). It spans the breadth of wellness and prevention, management of chronic disease, care of the frail and elderly, and end-of-life transitions. Population health rests on four pillars (Figure 5-2): chronic care management, quality and safety, public health, and health policy (Nash 2012). As its own pillar, the model acknowledges the critical role chronic disease plays in population health. It also reinforces the opportunities health care systems have to have an impact on all four pillars of population health.

This population health lens expands the scope of health care systems beyond their historical reactionary "sick care" delivery models targeting the individual patient, which have proven ineffective, fragmented, and poorly incentivized for preventing and managing chronic disease. To meet the goals of successful population health management, health care systems must not only better manage their chronic disease patients, but also invest in strategies to preserve wellness and minimize the impact of illness for their entire cohort of consumers. Health care leaders see population health as an essential element of health reform. Provisions of the Affordable Care Act (ACA)

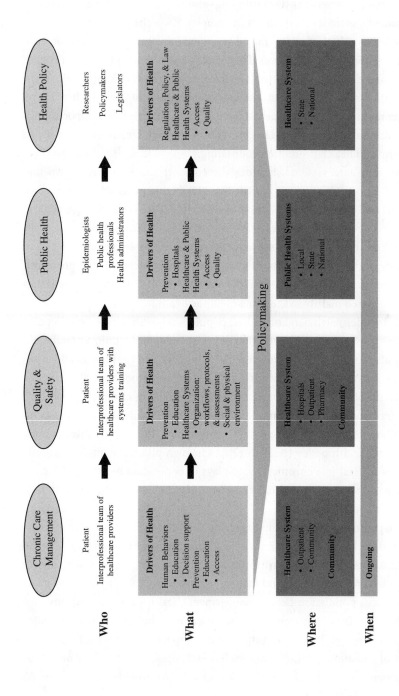

Source: Reprinted with permission from Nash (2012).

Figure 5-2. The Four Pillars of Population Health

encouraging transformative models of care delivery and "value over volume" have motivated health systems to broaden their scope for how to best manage and prevent chronic disease and its complications at the population level (Abrams et al. 2015).

Collaboration among health care systems, public health, and communities in tackling chronic disease has also been prioritized within heath care reform and within other leading national health improvement initiatives, including *Healthy People 2020* and the Centers for Disease Control and Prevention's (CDC's) four domains of chronic disease prevention (epidemiology and surveillance, environmental approaches, health care system interventions, and community–clinical links; Bauer et al. 2014). This call for partnership signals the recognition that health is dependent on many factors beyond the walls of the health care system. Among the various contributing health factors that affect an individual's and community's health, the County Health Rankings Model of Population Health attributes only approximately 20% to the health care system (Remington et al. 2015). To effectively and equitably address the chronic disease burden, health care systems need to deploy integrated approaches with public–private partnerships and other stakeholders that bundle strategies and interventions, address many risk factors and conditions simultaneously, create population-wide changes, and target the population subgroups most affected (Bauer et al. 2014).

Health Care Reform: Incentives for Improved Chronic Disease Control and Prevention

In addition to its more familiar health insurance coverage reforms, the ACA contains numerous provisions that directly target how health care is organized, delivered, and paid for in the United States. These provisions directly and indirectly affect chronic disease prevention and management. Building on existing reform models in the both the private and public sectors, the law takes multiple, complementary approaches to addressing the health system's long-standing issues in effectively tackling chronic disease.

Centers for Medicare and Medicaid Services Innovation Center

The ACA created a number of new resources to establish a foundation for accelerated public- and private-sector innovation in health care delivery.

One example is the Centers for Medicare and Medicaid Services (CMS) Innovation Center. This center was established to identify, test, and spread new payment and service delivery models to reduce expenditures while maintaining or improving quality of care for beneficiaries of Medicare, Medicaid, and the Children's Health Insurance Program. The U.S. Secretary of Health and Human Services has been granted authority to expand innovations if evidence shows actual cost reductions or improvements in outcomes.

When the ACA was enacted, the Congressional Budget Office estimated that the Innovation Center, with its $10 billion of direct funding over 10 years, would save $1.3 billion between 2010 and 2019. Since 2010, the center has launched an array of initiatives that together reach more than 2.5 million patients and 60,000 clinicians across the nation. Recognizing the critical role of states in providing, purchasing, and regulating health care services, the CMS Innovation Center established the State Innovation Models Initiative to help states achieve better health outcomes at lower cost. These grants provide federal dollars and technical assistance for a wide range of health system transformation efforts. Thirty-nine states have received State Innovation Model grants thus far (Abrams et al. 2015).

Accountable Care Organizations

One of the most notable incentives to shift toward population health–minded systems is the promotion of accountable care organizations (ACOs), led by CMS Innovation Center initiatives. An ACO is an entity formed by health care providers across various practice settings who agree to collectively take responsibility for the quality and total costs of care for a population of patients. Beginning in 2012, the ACA established the Medicare Shared Savings Program to encourage the development of ACOs. If participating ACOs meet quality benchmarks, such as with diabetes care or depression screening, and keep spending for their attributed patients below budget, they receive half the savings that result, with the rest going to the CMS, which administers the program. Effective chronic disease care and prevention is a cornerstone to achieving benchmarks and realizing cost savings within an ACO structure.

In 2015, there were more than 400 shared savings ACOs serving nearly 7.2 million beneficiaries (14%) of the Medicare population (CMS 2016a). Participation by health care systems in ACOs is promising; however, results from the program's first year of operation were mixed. Of the 220 shared savings

ACOs that year, only 52 were able to meet quality-of-care benchmarks and keep spending below budget targets. These ACOs generated $700 million in total savings and roughly $315 million in shared-savings bonuses (CMS 2016b). The ACOs in the Shared Savings Program showed some improvement on most of the 33 quality measures compared with other Medicare providers. The ACOs that have proved successful from the start tend to make investments in information technology systems, data analytic tools, and the necessary staff to identify high-risk patients (typically those with poorly controlled and multiple chronic conditions) and closely monitor their care (Abrams et al. 2015).

Primary Care Transformation through Implementation of Medical Homes

Although primary care is fundamental to a well-functioning health system, the United States has undervalued and underinvested in it for decades. The disregard of primary care is largely a consequence of the prevailing fee-for-service reimbursement approach in which providers have inherent financial incentives to provide more care and procedures over care management and other cost-saving services targeting chronic disease.

There is considerable evidence that comprehensive, coordinated, and well-targeted primary care can improve outcomes and reduce costs (Nielsen et al. 2015). These characteristics are embodied in the patient-centered medical home (PCMH), a model of care that emphasizes more comprehensive care coordination, care teams, patient engagement, and population health management. A number of the ACA's reforms seek to transform primary care by way of the medical home model across various care environments. The ACA is also supporting health care systems and states to experiment with ways to improve quality by testing models that integrate primary care more seamlessly with other health care services, such as behavioral health and long-term care. This integration is key to successful management of chronic disease, in particular for the most costly and complex patients. Examples of primary care transformation initiatives include

- The Comprehensive Primary Care Initiative, which is testing a new way to deliver and pay for care that is designed to improve access, coordination, and chronic disease management while engaging patients and their caregivers.

- Health homes targeting low-income patients with complex needs, such as chronic conditions, mental health, or substance abuse problems. Under this optional new benefit, state Medicaid programs can designate certain providers to serve as health homes. Building on the PCMH, health homes integrate physical and behavioral health care, as well as long-term services and supports for high-need, high-cost patients. The federal government pays 90% of the costs of these additional services for two years with the expectation that the state will sustain the program thereafter. More than one million Medicaid beneficiaries have been enrolled in a health home as of 2015 (Abrams et al. 2015).

A major theme emerging from this work to transform primary care is the critical role of technical and financial support in building the capacity of physician practices to function as medical homes. Each of the ACA-supported transformation initiatives includes some level of support for practices to address common challenges, including the timely collection, reporting, and use of data for care management and quality improvement; shifting the practice culture to enable effective teamwork; and acquiring information about patients from settings outside the clinical setting. Overall, federal investments have stimulated extraordinary collaboration and dialogue among payers, both private and public, and providers on how to reorganize primary care to achieve the aims of improved population health and decreased costs (Abrams et al. 2015).

Provider Payment Reform

In addition to these ACO programs and PCMH initiatives, the CMS Innovation Center is also testing a payment approach known as bundled payment—a single reimbursement for all of the services required for a given medical condition or procedure (e.g., physician, hospital, or post-acute services). Ideally, this should incentivize the various providers involved in a given patient's care to collaborate and strive for efficient and effective outcomes, including prevention of complications and disease progression. As of 2015, nearly 7,000 organizations have signed up to participate in bundled-payment demonstrations, which represent a further step toward shared accountability for quality and costs of health care delivery (Abrams et al. 2015).

Most of the new payment models are still in their early phases, and evidence of their impact is far from conclusive. Many initiatives have adopted a gradual approach to financial accountability. This approach recognizes that the type of structural change required to be successful under risk-based payment models takes time. The momentum for these transitions has picked up recently, with the U.S. Secretary of Health and Human Services announcing a goal to have at least 90% of traditional Medicare payments linked to some form of ACO, medical home, bundled payment, or other value-related approach by 2018 (Burwell 2015).

Other Affordable Care Act Provisions Related to Chronic Disease Prevention and Management

Beyond care delivery and payment reform, multiple other ACA activities support chronic disease management and prevention and health promotion at the health care system and community level. Examples include

- Medicaid Incentives for the Prevention of Chronic Diseases Model Grants awarded to states to help Medicaid beneficiaries with evidence-based healthy lifestyle programs. Most states are targeting multiple conditions and health behaviors, often using patient and provider incentives.
- The Prevention and Public Health Fund provides sustained national investment in preventive care and public health. Through 2015, it has awarded more than $5 billion to local community efforts (NACCHO 2013). Among other things, the fund supports diabetes prevention, immunization programs, tobacco use prevention, and heart disease and stroke prevention. Community Transformation Grants provide resources to state and local governmental agencies and local organizations to address chronic disease; grantees must reduce rates of obesity, tobacco-related death and disability, heart disease, or stroke by 5% within five years. More than $370 million has been awarded—20% to rural areas— benefiting nearly 130 million Americans.
- The Accountable Health Communities Model is a CMS Innovation Center initiative that addresses a critical gap between clinical care and community services in the current health care delivery system. It aims to test whether systematically identifying and addressing the health-related social needs of beneficiaries reduces total health care costs, improves health, and improves quality of care. Emerging evidence shows that addressing health-related social needs, such as food insecurity and inadequate or unstable housing, through enhanced clinical–community linkages, can improve health outcomes and reduce costs. Unmet health-related social needs may increase the risk of developing chronic conditions,

reduce an individual's ability to manage these conditions, increase health care costs, and lead to avoidable health care utilization (CMS 2016b).

- Community benefit is a requirement of nonprofit hospitals to provide benefits to the communities they serve to keep a tax-exempt status. Nationwide, about 2,900 hospitals (60% of hospitals) are nonprofit, and the financial benefit to these hospitals from being tax-exempt is estimated to be worth $12.6 billion annually (RWJF 2012). Historically, much of hospitals' community benefit activities were charity care and other forms of uncompensated care. A lack of transparency and wide variations in how, and how much, hospitals spend for community benefits led to increased oversight by the Internal Revenue Service and Congress. The ACA added new requirements to the community benefit including community health needs assessments and improvement plans. The benefits of the new requirements go beyond improving health through more accountability for hospitals, effective use of resources, and building community capacity and engagement in addressing health issues. Assessing community health needs and adopting a strategy to address those needs provides hospitals with a valuable opportunity to work together with community partners to identify strategies for improving health, quality of life, and the community's vitality (RWJF 2012).

There is widespread agreement that fee-for-service health care should no longer be the norm, and that fundamental shifts are needed to produce affordable, high-quality, value-based care. The ACA has stimulated activity in both the public and private sectors, contributing to the accelerated pace of state and local innovations across the country, as well as recognition that there is no single solution. Although implementation of new programs has not been without delays and hiccups, the culture change occurring across the health care sector is laying the groundwork for greater strides in population health and health care systems improvements that support chronic disease prevention and control.

Three Levels of Involvement for Health Care Systems in Chronic Disease Prevention and Control

The spectrum of prevention introduced in Chapter 1 is a helpful framework for exploring the ways in which health care systems influence chronic disease management and prevention. Health promotion (primary prevention) activities encourage healthy living and limit the initial onset of chronic diseases. Early detection efforts (secondary prevention) include screening at-risk populations and applying strategies for proactive management of existing diseases to prevent complications. Complex care management and care coordination approaches for high-risk populations with multiple comorbidities or complications of chronic disease encompass tertiary prevention. These three levels of health care system activities will subsequently be explored further, starting with tertiary prevention efforts and moving upstream.

Level 1: Chronic Disease Management—The Chronic Care Model

Discussed earlier, the management of chronic diseases and their complications makes up a significant portion of a health care system's activities and spending. Effectively managing disease and minimizing complications requires a well-coordinated, interdisciplinary approach. One well-recognized framework for achieving comprehensive chronic disease management is the Chronic Care Model (CCM; Wagner 1998; Figure 5-3). The basis for the CCM stemmed from a review of interventions to improve care for various chronically ill populations.

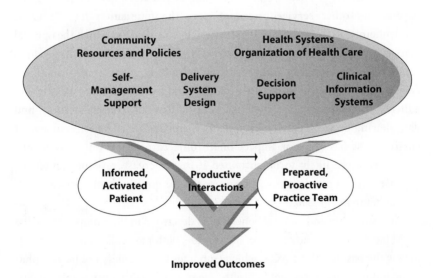

Source: Reprinted with permission from Wagner (1998).

Figure 5-3. The Chronic Care Model

This review concluded that multicomponent practice changes in four categories led to the greatest improvements in health outcomes: increasing providers' expertise and skill, educating and supporting patients, making care delivery more team-based and planned, and making better use of registry-based information systems (Wagner 1998).

The CCM's six interrelated components are health care organization, clinical information systems, delivery system redesign, decision support, self-management support, and community resources. Whereas the first four concepts in the CCM address practice strategies, the final two are specifically patient-centered (Fiandt 2006). In the CCM, improved functional and clinical outcomes for disease management are the result of productive interactions between informed, activated patients and the prepared, proactive practice team of clinicians and other health care professionals (Bodenheimer et al. 2002). Each of the components of CCM will be explored further, and they are summarized in Table 5-1.

Components of the Chronic Care Model

One component of the CCM is *organization of health systems*. The structure, goals, and values of a health care system and its relationships with purchasers, payers, and other service providers form the foundation for the CCM (Bodenheimer et al. 2002). The ideal system has a culture in which the optimal management of chronic disease and practice improvement are key values. Leadership is committed and visibly involved, supports transformational change, and creates incentives for providers and patients to improve care and adhere to evidence-based practice. Facilitation of communication and data-sharing between care environments is emphasized. The reimbursement environment has a major impact on chronic care delivery improvements, which are more likely to be sustained if they increase revenues or reduce expenses, and if purchasers and insurers reward quality chronic disease care (Bodenheimer et al. 2002).

The leadership and cultural benchmarks described in this component of the CCM have gained steady traction nationwide, with particular momentum following the passage of the ACA, which embodies these values. The new emphasis on linking reimbursement to health care system performance within quality, safety, and health outcome measures has ignited new investments by health care system leadership in assessing how their systems are managing chronic disease, and adopting improvement strategies to address identified gaps.

Table 5-1. The Chronic Care Model Components

Model Component	General Examples
Health system: Create a culture, organization, and mechanisms that promote safe, high-quality care.	Visibly support improvement at all levels of the organization, beginning with the senior leader. Promote effective improvement strategies aimed at comprehensive system change. Encourage open and systematic handling of errors and quality problems to improve care. Provide incentives based on quality of care. Develop agreements that facilitate care coordination within and across organizations.
Delivery system design: Ensure the delivery of effective, efficient clinical care and self-management support.	Define roles and distribute tasks among team members. Use planned interactions to support evidence-based care. Provide clinical case management services for complex patients. Ensure regular follow-up by the care team. Give care that patients understand and that fits with their cultural background.
Decision support: Promote clinical care that is consistent with scientific evidence and patient preferences.	Embed evidence-based guidelines into daily clinical practice. Share evidence-based guidelines and information with patients to encourage their participation. Use proven provider-education methods. Integrate specialist expertise and primary care.
Clinical information systems: Organize patient and population data to facilitate efficient and effective care.	Provide timely reminders for providers and patients. Identify relevant subpopulations for proactive care. Facilitate individual patient care planning. Share information with patients and providers to coordinate care. Monitor performance of practice team and care system.
Self-management support: Empower and prepare patients to manage their health and health care.	Emphasize the patients' central role in managing their health. Use effective self-management support strategies that include assessment, goal-setting, action planning, problem-solving and follow-up. Organize internal and community resources to provide ongoing self-management support to patients.
The community: Mobilize community resources to meet needs of patients.	Encourage patients to participate in effective community programs. Form partnerships with community organizations to support and develop interventions that fill gaps in needed services. Advocate policies to improve patient care.

Source: Compiled from ICIC (2016).

Another component of the CCM is *delivery system design*. Improving the health of people with chronic illness requires a shift from systems that are essentially reactive—responding mainly once a person is sick—to one that is proactive and focused on maintaining health. This requires determining what care is needed; having clear roles and tasks on a care team to ensure that the patient gets the care; making sure that everyone taking care of a patient has centralized, up-to-date information; and making follow-up a part of standard procedure. Patients with complex or multiple problems may need more intensive management (care or case management) to optimize clinical care and self-management. Health literacy and cultural sensitivity are two important emerging concepts in health care, and systems must respond effectively to the diverse cultural and linguistic needs of their patients as they perform these functions.

The PCMH described previously is one example of an effort to become proactive and team-based in caring for patients with chronic disease. This transformation is in response to health care systems that have tended to be disjointed, variable in processes across practice settings, and poorly designed for clear communication between primary care and specialty providers (AHRQ 2015a). Ideally, the medical home model focuses on a person's overall health and provides coordinated, comprehensive care, in particular for those whose needs are complex, such as people with chronic conditions. Care coordination involves deliberately organizing patient care activities and sharing information among all of the participants concerned with a patient's care to achieve safer and more effective services. This requires that the patient's needs and preferences are known ahead of time and communicated at the right time to the right people (AHRQ 2015b). Medical homes attempt to better coordinate care across health, behavioral, community, and long-term services.

Health care systems taking on financial risk for the overall costs of care through ACOs are developing complex care management programs to improve care, and thereby control costs, for the highest-need, highest-cost patients. These programs perform four essential activities:

1. Identifying and engaging patients who are at high risk for poor outcomes and unnecessary utilization.
2. Performing comprehensive health assessments to identify problems that, if addressed through effective interventions, will improve care and reduce the need for expensive services.

3. Working closely with patients and their caregivers as well as primary care, specialty, behavioral health, and social service providers.

4. Rapidly and effectively responding to changes in patients' conditions to avoid use of unnecessary services, particularly emergency department visits or hospitalizations (Hong et al. 2014).

Complex care management extends beyond medical issues, attempting to address how patients' psychosocial circumstances affect their ability to follow treatment recommendations and achieve a healthy lifestyle (Goodell et al. 2009). The goals are to maintain or improve functional status, increase the capacity to self-manage conditions, eliminate unnecessary clinical testing, and reduce the need for acute care services.

To date, there is scant evidence of the effectiveness of primary care–integrated complex care management in reducing overall health care costs. Many programs demonstrate improved quality or reduced acute care utilization, but their effects on net costs have been inconsistent across programs (Peikes et al. 2009). In a recent review of the operational approaches of 18 successful complex care management programs, it was found that effective programs customize their approach to their local contexts and caseloads, use a combination of qualitative and quantitative methods to identify patients with complex care needs, consider care coordination one of their key roles, focus on building trusting relationships with patients as well as their primary care providers, match team composition and interventions to patient needs, offer specialized training for team members, and use technology to bolster their efforts (Hong et al. 2014).

Decision support is another component of the CCM. An important problem in health care is the significant gap between optimal evidence-based medical practice and the care actually performed. Clinical decision support provides timely information, usually at the point of care, to help inform decisions about a patient's care backed by evidence and guidelines. Examples include order sets created for particular conditions or types of patients, practice guidelines accessible at the point of care, databases that can provide information relevant to particular patients, reminders for preventive screening, and alerts about potentially dangerous situations such as medication interactions. Health care organizations can creatively integrate these functions into the day-to-day practice of providers in an accessible and easy-to-use manner. Providers should receive ongoing education to stay up to date on the latest evidence, and guidelines should also be discussed with patients, so they can understand the principles behind their care. Clinical decision support can potentially lower costs, improve efficiency, and reduce patient inconvenience (AHRQ 2015b).

In the past, many clinical decision support systems were stand-alone and not well integrated with other electronic systems, or into clinical workflow. With the passage of the Health Information Technology for Economic and Clinical Health (HITECH) Act of 2009, which provides the Department of Health and Human Services with the authority to establish programs to improve health care quality, safety, and efficiency through the promotion of health information technology, much work has been done to integrate decision support tools into electronic health records (EHRs; AHRQ 2016). Electronic health records with integrated decision support and chronic care management tools help providers manage patient information and monitor health outcomes. Early adopters of this technology have found that it supports the PCMH and CCM models by allowing redistribution of patient care tasks to non-physician support personnel. Integrated laboratory and pharmacy information systems can further bolster decision support functions, promote coordinated care, and reduce errors and duplication (AHRQ 2015b).

Advances in this arena have not been without obstacles. Significant investments of time and resources are required to transition practice settings to EHRs and configure clinical decision support tools to meet the needs and clinical workflows of practice environments. Usability in the midst of busy clinical schedules is key to successful adoption and functionality. Ultimately, these systems must prove return on investment through better clinical management of chronic disease and cost savings to maintain financial support from health care system leadership, insurers, and grant-based sources. Findings thus far point toward evidence that incorporating health information technology in chronic disease management efforts can yield improved quality of care and significant cost savings (AHRQ 2008).

Another component of the CCM is *clinical information systems*. Effective chronic disease management is virtually impossible without information systems that guarantee ready access to key data on individual patients, as well as populations served by a health care system. A comprehensive clinical information system, or registry, can enhance care by providing timely reminders for needed services such as laboratory tests and immunizations, with the summarized data helping to track and plan care and outreach. At the population level, the registry can identify groups of patients overdue for services or who might benefit from outreach, and facilitate performance monitoring and quality improvement efforts. Most disease registries are used to support care management for groups of patients with one or more chronic diseases, and are the foundation for successful integration of all the elements of the CCM. Similar to decision-support tools, patient registries are increasingly being integrated into EHRs to allow for more streamlined disease management and communication among care teams. Some registries with more advanced features may even include clinical decision support functionality that can prompt users with care recommendations.

A promising area for further development and implementation of computerized disease registries, also supported by the HITECH Act, is the establishment of electronic health information exchanges. Health information exchanges share clinical and administrative data across the boundaries of health care institutions, health data repositories, and states. Many stakeholder groups (e.g., health care systems, insurers, patients) realize that if such data are shared, health care processes would improve with respect to safety, quality, cost, and other indicators. As it relates to chronic disease, a health information exchange offers the ability to effectively identify and manage patients with a particular condition across a region, both for the individual patient who may have multiple chronic conditions managed by a variety of providers and settings, and to guide prevention and management initiatives for a population of interest (AHRQ 2015b).

Sharing such data from a cultural and technical standpoint is not easy. Competing priorities, financial concerns, issues related to data ownership, and privacy and security are among some of the most difficult barriers to overcome. Regional health information organizations and other groups that facilitate health information exchange must combat how to support interfacing from different providers' health IT systems. The few currently operating registries have limited real-time data feeding capabilities, or integration into clinicians' workflows at the point of care (AHRQ 2015b). Nonetheless, the implementation of computerized disease registries by health information exchange organizations poses promising opportunity to better manage chronic diseases.

Self-management support is another component of the CCM. All patients with chronic illness make decisions and engage in behaviors that affect their health. Disease control and outcomes depend to a significant degree on the effectiveness of this self-management. The greatest contributor to premature death from preventable chronic illness is patient behavior (Nash et al. 2015). The degree to which patients are informed and active in their care is, therefore, critical.

Effective self-management support by heath care systems requires not only counseling patients on what to do in their care, but also acknowledging their central role, and fostering a sense of responsibility for their own health. It includes the use of proven programs that provide basic information, emotional support, and strategies for living with chronic disease. Five self-management skills that form the core of self-management support programs have been identified and tested: problem solving, decision-making, resource utilization, the patient–provider relationship, and taking action (Lorig and Holman 2003). Using a collaborative approach and evidence-based techniques that emphasize patient activation or empowerment, providers and patients can work together to enhance these skills. Care teams must also be sensitive to the role that families, caregivers, and communities play in these activities.

One of the most widely recognized and studied self-management initiatives is the Stanford Chronic Disease Self-Management Program. Developed at Stanford University in the early 1990s in collaboration with the National Council on Aging (2015) and CDC, this community-based program provides in-person and online courses in which individuals with chronic diseases, such as heart disease, hypertension, cancer, stroke, arthritis, and diabetes, learn and practice problem-solving, coping, and communication skills to deal with their condition. They discover lifestyle strategies for good health, including diet, exercise, medications, managing pain and fatigue, living with disability, social support for change, and overcoming depression. The Stanford Chronic Disease Self-Management Program has been studied extensively, with results showing significant, measurable improvements in the health, quality of life, and communication with providers for people living with chronic conditions. The program also appears to save enough through reductions in health care expenditures to pay for itself within the first year. Studies have indicated fewer outpatient and emergency department visits and fewer hospitalizations, and a health care cost savings of approximately $590 per participant (Ory et al. 2013).

Patient activation, or engagement, is the knowledge, skills, and confidence persons have in managing their own health and health care (Hibbard and Gilbert 2014), and is now recognized as a crucial element to successful management of chronic disease. Multiple studies show that an individual's level of activation is predictive of most health behaviors, including preventive behaviors (e.g., obtaining screenings and immunizations), healthy behaviors (e.g., healthy diet and regular exercise), self-management behaviors (e.g., medication management), and health information seeking (Greene et al. 2015).

Higher activated individuals also have better health outcomes and lower rates of costly utilization, such as emergency department use and hospitalizations. Furthermore, there is evidence that with support and appropriate interventions it is possible to increase activation levels in patients. These interventions focus on the gaining of new skills and encouraging a sense of ownership over one's health. Health care systems are also increasingly applying measures of patient activation to help inform population risk stratification and distribution of appropriate levels of support, and as a measure of performance and effectiveness of interventions (Hibbard and Gilbert 2014).

Another component of the CCM is *the community*. Health care systems can enhance care for patients, make strides in population health improvement, and avoid duplication of efforts by reaching out to form powerful alliances and partnerships with state and local agencies, nonprofit organizations, schools, and businesses to share resources and collaborate on chronic disease initiatives. Local and state health policies, insurance benefits, and other health-related regulations also play a critical role in chronic disease care. Health care systems can make a difference for their patients by advocating on their behalf at the policy level (ICIC 2016).

This collaboration signals a recognition that factors beyond the walls of clinical care must be recognized and addressed to effect positive change in chronic disease management, and that individuals, social support systems, community resources, health care systems, and public policy leaders must be engaged and working together. The role of clinical–community linkages in chronic disease prevention and management will be explored further later in this chapter.

These six components of the CCM are interdependent, and build upon one another. For instance, community resources can support patients with self-management skills. For chronic disease registries to be successful, redesigning delivery systems is necessary so that a designated team member can manage the registry and perform indicated patient outreach, order placement, and data management. Clinical practice guidelines are the evidence upon which physician reminder systems and performance feedback are based. Chronic care model elements are unlikely to be introduced or maintained without an organizational environment featuring innovative leadership and favorable reimbursement structures (Bodenheimer et al. 2002).

Accumulated evidence appears to support the CCM as an integrated framework to guide practice redesign that leads to improved patient care and better health outcomes for a variety of chronic diseases (Coleman et al. 2009; Ory et al. 2013; Stock et al. 2014). Although work remains to be done in areas such as cost-effectiveness, the CCM, or adaptations of the model, have become a standard for health care delivery and performance measurement as it relates to chronic disease care. This includes several state programs in the United States, national certification agencies for chronic disease programs, and new models of primary care proposed by the American Academy of Family Physicians and American College of Physicians, as well as by the U.K. National Health Service, the World Health Organization, and several Canadian provinces (ICIC 2016).

At the national level, and prompted by increased support from the ACA, the U.S. Department of Health and Human Services developed a Strategic Framework on Multiple Chronic Conditions, building on elements of the CCM. This framework aims to convert the CCM into a set of specific, actionable, national-level strategies to "provide a foundation for realizing the vision of optimum health and quality of life for individuals with multiple chronic conditions" who frequently suffer suboptimal health outcomes and incur significant health care expenses (USDHHS 2010). The framework comprises four overarching goals:

1. Foster health care and public health system changes to improve the health of individuals with multiple chronic conditions.
2. Maximize the use of proven self-care management and other services by individuals with multiple chronic conditions.
3. Provide better tools and information to health care, public health, and social services workers who deliver care to individuals with multiple chronic conditions.
4. Facilitate research to fill knowledge gaps about, and interventions and systems to benefit, individuals with multiple chronic conditions.

Each of these goals includes several key objectives and strategies that the health care system, in conjunction with stakeholders and partners, should use to guide its efforts. Although this framework addresses those individuals with multiple chronic conditions, many of the strategies also apply to persons with only one chronic disease, or those with no chronic conditions (USDHHS 2010).

Level 2: Chronic Disease Screening Approaches

Moving along the prevention spectrum to more upstream approaches, chronic disease screening is a cornerstone of secondary prevention activities performed by health care systems. Screening aims to reduce the impact of chronic disease by detecting and treating it early to halt or slow its progress, and encouraging personal behaviors to restore wellness and prevent long-term problems.

Primary care clinics, as the ideal site of a patient's medical home, are an effective and efficient setting to provide evidence-based chronic disease screening. However, it can be challenging to optimally carry out recommended practices, because of, in part, the competing care demands on primary care providers. One study found that the time required to provide all recommended preventive services to a typical family practice is 7.4 hours per working day, which would leave little time for any other patient care activities (Yarnall et al. 2003). Patients with multiple chronic conditions or other complexities to their health care needs can experience even larger gaps between recommended screening practices and receipt of these services because of the many other issues that must be addressed during clinical encounters. The challenge for health care systems is to develop strategies for improving rates of evidence-based recommended chronic disease screening that can be incorporated into workflows without undue provider burden or compromised quality and efficiency of care.

The PCMH model, now implemented broadly across a variety of practice settings, emphasizes the core primary care function of providing clinical preventive services including chronic disease screening within its comprehensive approach to care over a patient's life course. Increased use of recommended preventive services is considered a key indicator for evaluating the success of the PCMH (Rosenthal et al. 2012). Early evaluations have shown consistent evidence of a positive association between implementation of the PCMH and cancer screening (Jackson et al. 2013). Findings also suggest that the effects of the PCMH model on cancer screening rates vary depending on the socioeconomic context of the practice, with greater effects occurring in lower socioeconomic contexts (Markovitz et al. 2015). Thus, the PCMH model could also contribute to reductions in disparities in screening rates across socioeconomic contexts. The model may be especially effective in lower socioeconomic status areas by overcoming some of the challenges that drive disparities through improved access to care, care coordination, and health literacy. Although this research focused on cancer screening, one might hypothesize that similar impact could be observed for other chronic disease screening.

Concurrent with the adoption of the PCMH is the integration of health information technology capacity that can support chronic disease screening activities. Outlined earlier, the use of patient registries can identify those who are overdue for recommended screening services, for which a designated member of the care team can perform outreach. Evidence-based reminders at the point of care, triggered on the basis of patient characteristics, and prevention-focused hubs within the EHR are two methods of clinical decision support tools that allow for increased delivery of screening services. Online "patient wellness portals" have also been created that focus on wellness, prevention, and longitudinal health, alerting patients when they are due for screening. A significantly greater proportion of patients who used these portals received all recommended preventive services compared with controls (Nagykaldi et al. 2012).

One example of an approach that embodies team-based care, clinical decision support tools, and patient engagement and self-management skill support outlined in the CCM is the Building on Existing Tools to Improve Chronic Disease Prevention and Screening in Family Practice (BETTER) trial (Grunfeld et al. 2013). This study, based in Canada, was able to significantly improve chronic disease prevention and screening through a new skilled role of a "prevention practitioner." These clinicians (e.g., licensed practical nurse, nurse, dietitian, nurse practitioner) had appointments with patients aged 40 to 65 years focusing on primary prevention activities and screening of cancer (breast, colorectal, cervical), type 2 diabetes, and cardiovascular disease, and associated lifestyle factors. To ensure that high-level evidence guidelines were used, existing clinical practice guidelines and tools were reviewed and integrated into blended BETTER tool kits. The tools emphasized shared decision-making, and provided the patient with an individualized "prevention prescription" that included actionable goals.

The BETTER trial not only proved effective in increasing the use of clinically important chronic disease prevention and screening activities within primary care, but it was also cost-effective (Grunfeld et al. 2013). This evidence garnered further funding to improve the approach and broaden the reach of the BETTER program through revisions to the toolkits and formats of delivery that could be used across a diverse range of primary care settings (Manca et al. 2015).

As the health demands of populations grow, there is more interest in how health care systems can use the skills and competencies of other allied health professionals outside the walls of the examination room to increase access to care and decrease burden on physician workload. One such profession is pharmacists, who are increasingly performing activities around health promotion and disease prevention in addition to their medication dispensing roles. The nature and frequency of contact between patients and pharmacists provides significant opportunities for chronic disease screening and healthy lifestyle counseling, as well as assisting patients with monitoring and management of their chronic condition(s). Community pharmacists can play a key role in population-based screening programs or initiatives targeting populations with certain risk behaviors. Close collaboration with other primary care and public health professionals is essential to avoid duplication of work and to ensure continuity of patient care. To realize the potential of pharmacists and other allied health professionals as a resource for chronic disease screening and prevention efforts, they must be allowed the time, training, and regulatory and policy support to perform these functions within the health care system (George and Zairina 2016).

A notable signal of increased investment in chronic disease screening is the ACA mandates that eliminate consumer cost sharing (e.g., co-payments and deductibles) for selected preventive services in marketplace plans and many other individual health plans. States are also encouraged to extend preventive health services in their Medicaid programs, paid for in large part by increased federal payments for Medicaid. This elimination of cost sharing helps overcome the financial barriers that deter people from getting the screenings and preventive services that are recommended for them (Shearer 2010).

Level 3: Chronic Disease Prevention and Health Promotion

The third level of chronic disease prevention activities targets primary prevention of chronic diseases and the promotion of wellness, which can deter the development of chronic diseases from the outset. The economic argument for investing in this prevention is compelling. It is estimated that 25% of all direct medical costs are attributable to a small number of excess risk factors such as smoking, obesity, physical inactivity, and poor nutrition; however, less than 1% of health care dollars are spent on scientifically proven, effective prevention strategies (Koh 2011). A report by Trust for America's Health estimated that investments in community-based initiatives that address such factors can yield an overall $5.60 return in health cost savings for every $1 spent toward prevention (Levi et al. 2008).

Individual- and population-level improvements in chronic disease prevention require primary prevention actions targeting the multiple determinants of health, including medical care, health behaviors, and the social and physical environment (Remington et al. 2015). Although a health care organization's core responsibility is to improve population health through the delivery of clinical services, they can also work beyond this core mission to address other determinants of health. Unfortunately, health care systems have traditionally had little success in tackling such factors. Without concerted efforts to link clinical services with socio-environmental and political efforts, success will continue to be elusive in health care system efforts to prevent disease and improve the overall health of their populations. Acknowledging that no single entity can be held accountable for achieving improved outcomes, Kindig and Isham proposed a "community health business model," forming a new generation of partnerships among health care systems, government, schools, businesses, and community organizations (Kindig and Isham 2014). In this model, all of these entities are tasked with making substantial changes in how they approach health, allocate resources, and work together collectively on disease prevention and population health efforts.

An overarching theme within this call for partnership is the important foundation of primary care as a location and vehicle for both delivering preventive services and catalyzing engagement with the community and public health (Koo et al. 2012). The fields of primary care and public health in the United States have, for the past century, tended to function independently of each other despite both having chronic disease prevention objectives. In an attempt to foster collaboration of efforts, the Institute of Medicine released a report in 2012 titled "Primary Care and Public Health: Exploring Integration to Improve Population Health," which reviewed promising models of primary care and public health integration. From this report came a set of principles deemed essential for successful integration of primary care and public health: (1) a shared goal of population health improvement; (2) community engagement in defining and addressing population health needs; (3) aligned leadership; (4) sustainability, including shared infrastructure; and (5) sharing and collaborative use of data and analysis (IOM 2012a; IOM 2012b).

Examples of this integration include a joint referral system for services provided by a community health center and local public health department, and the use of trained health department representatives within primary care offices in medically underserved areas to promote clinical preventive services and chronic disease management targeted by the health department (Koo et al. 2012). Bridging not only primary care and public health, but also school systems, the San Diego Healthy Weight Collaborative exemplifies partnership in chronic disease prevention. Recognizing a growing trend in obesity and related diseases including hypertension, diabetes, and liver disease in their pediatric patients, local clinics reached out to schools with the highest obesity rates to engage in education and wellness activities with support from the local public health department. This work blossomed into a larger community-wide collaborative through national funding targeting childhood obesity. Early outcomes have shown a 3.2% reduction in obese or overweight range for all students in the target population (Duke and CDC 2016). These partnerships must overcome the obstacles of varied training backgrounds and perspectives; the isolation in which each sector operates, which contributes to a general lack of awareness of each other's activities and resources; and funding limitations. The ACA contains certain provisions aimed at alleviating this last hurdle, encouraging combined efforts and a leveraging of resources between public health and health care systems to achieve common goals (Elliott et al. 2014).

The CCM explored earlier was geared mainly toward clinically oriented systems and is difficult to apply for broader prevention and health promotion practices such as these. In 2003, Barr and colleagues proposed the Expanded Chronic Care Model (ECCM), which includes elements of the population health promotion field so that broadly based prevention efforts, recognition of the social determinants of health, and enhanced community participation could also be integrated into the work of health system teams as they seek to address chronic disease issues. The ECCM includes three additional components in terms of community resources and policies: building healthy public policy, creating supportive environments, and strengthening community action. These interrelated components and relationships are shown in Figure 5-4.

The ECCM represents the shift from health care systems focused on illness and disability to community-oriented services that focus on primary prevention. Working on both the prevention and treatment ends of the continuum from such a broad perspective offers the best potential for improved health outcomes in the long term (Barr et al. 2003). This change is a vital element of responsible, accountable, and population-focused health care management in today's climate of health care reform and innovation.

One example of evolving mechanisms for community-based chronic disease prevention efforts is the integration of community health workers into clinical care teams. Known by a variety of names (community health advisor, outreach worker, *promotora/promotores de salud* [health promoter/promoters], patient navigator, and lay health advisor) these are frontline public health workers

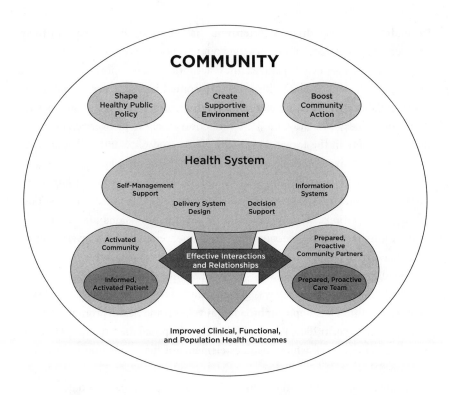

Source: Based on Barr et al. (2002).

Figure 5-4. The Expanded Chronic Care Model

who are trusted members of or possess an unusually close understanding of the community served. This relationship enables community health workers to be a liaison between health and social services and the community. This both facilitates access to services and improves the quality and cultural competence of service delivery. Community health workers also build individual and community capacity by increasing health knowledge and self-sufficiency through activities such as outreach, community education, informal counseling, social support, and advocacy (Brownstein et al. 2011).

In addition, they can educate health care providers and administrators about the community's health needs and the cultural relevancy of interventions. Using their unique position, skills, and knowledge base, community health workers can help reduce system costs for chronic disease management. Mechanisms for these savings include linking patients to community resources, helping avoid unnecessary hospitalizations and other forms of more expensive care through improved and proactive disease management, and having an impact on the upstream determinants of disease (Brownstein et al. 2011).

Using an even more robust concept for community–clinical linkages, Vermont's Blueprint for Health is an example of the ECCM in action. This state-wide public–private initiative incorporates community health teams as a key aspect of their model to transform care delivery, improve health outcomes, and enable everyone in the state to receive seamless, well-coordinated care. These teams, supported by medical homes, comprise locally based, multidisciplinary members (e.g., nurse coordinators, community health workers, behavioral health counselors, dietitians, and social workers) that provide a link between primary care and community-based services, connecting patients to medical, social, and economic support. Community health teams offer individual care coordination and disease management support, behavioral health counseling, health and wellness coaching, health system navigation, and teaching of self-management skills. In addition, they perform community outreach to support public health initiatives such as screening campaigns. Community health teams can effectively expand the capacity of primary care practices by providing patients direct support and individualized follow-up.

The Vermont initiative actually grew out of a chronic care project to make the CCM come alive across the state, evolving into a "true transformation of the delivery system with broad, multidisciplinary care support for the general population, not just a targeted population" (Bielaszka-DuVernay 2011). The Blueprint model is one example of health care delivery innovation incorporating various approaches to effective chronic disease management and prevention highlighted in this chapter. Although every health care system will have unique variables to consider when crafting effective approaches to address chronic disease according to their populations, resources, and operational climate, the Vermont experience can help inform these efforts at a local and national scale.

Conclusion

It is now evident that health care systems will need creative and collaborative strategies to address chronic disease prevention and management at all levels of the prevention spectrum—from primary, to secondary, to tertiary prevention—if they are to make any noticeable impact on the concerning trends of chronic diseases in their populations. With proven frameworks as a guide, bolstered by health care reform incentives and innovative new models of care delivery, health care systems now have a robust toolkit for crafting strong prevention and care management systems to tackle chronic diseases, which can lead to significant cost-savings and improved population health outcomes.

Resources

Centers for Disease Control and Prevention, National Center for Chronic Disease Prevention and Health Promotion, http://www.cdc.gov/chronicdisease

The Centers for Medicare and Medicaid Services Innovation Center, http://www.cdc.gov/chronicdisease

Improving Chronic Illness Care—The MacColl Center for Health Care Innovation, http://www.improvingchroniccare.org

Suggested Reading

Barr V, Robinson S, Marin-Link B, et al. The expanded chronic care model: an integration of concepts and strategies from population health promotion and the chronic care model. *Hosp Q.* 2003;7(1):73–82.

Bauer UE, Briss PA, Goodman RA, Bowman BA. Prevention of chronic disease in the 21st century: elimination of the leading preventable causes of premature death and disability in the USA. *Lancet* 2014;384(9937):45–52.

Institute of Medicine. Living well with chronic illness: a call for public health action. Washington, DC: National Academies Press; 2012. Available at: http://www.nationalacademies.org/hmd/~/media/Files/Report%20Files/2012/Living-Well-with-Chronic-Illness/livingwell_chronicillness_reportbrief.pdf. Accessed August 7, 2016.

Kindig D, Isham G. Population health improvement: a community health business model that engages partners in all sectors. Frontiers of Health Services Management. 2014. Available at: https://uwphi.pophealth.wisc.edu/publications/other/frontiers-of-health-services-management-vol30-num4.pdf. Accessed August 7, 2016.

US Department of Health and Human Services. Multiple chronic conditions—a strategic framework: optimum health and quality of life for individuals with multiple chronic conditions. 2010. Available at: http://www.hhs.gov/ash/initiatives/mcc/mcc_framework.pdf. Accessed August 7, 2016.

References

Abrams MK, Nuzum R, Zezza MA, et al. The Affordable Care Act's payment and delivery system reforms: a progress report at five years. The Commonwealth Fund. 2015. Available at: http://www.commonwealthfund.org/publications/issue-briefs/2015/may/aca-payment-and-delivery-system-reforms-at-5-years. Accessed April 3, 2016.

Ackermann RT, Marrero DG, Hicks KA, et al. An evaluation of cost sharing to finance a diet and physical activity intervention to prevent diabetes. *Diabetes Care.* 2006;29(6):1237–1241.

Agency for Healthcare Research and Quality (AHRQ). AHRQ decisionmaker brief—chronic disease management. 2008. AHRQ Publication no. 08-0084. Available at: https://healthit.ahrq.gov/sites/default/files/docs/page/08-0084_cdm_0.pdf. Accessed April 10, 2016.

Agency for Healthcare Research and Quality (AHRQ). Care coordination. 2015a. Available at: http://www.ahrq.gov/professionals/prevention-chronic-care/improve/coordination/index.html. Accessed April 2, 2016.

Agency for Healthcare Research and Quality (AHRQ). Clinical decision support. 2015b. Available at: http://www.ahrq.gov/professionals/prevention-chronic-care/decision/clinical/index.html. Accessed April 2, 2016.

Agency for Healthcare Research and Quality (AHRQ). Health information exchange. 2016. Available at: https://healthit.ahrq.gov/key-topics/health-information-exchange#projects. Accessed April 10, 2016.

Anderson G. *Chronic Care: Making the Case for Ongoing Care.* Princeton, NJ: Robert Wood Johnson Foundation; 2010.

Barr V, Robinson S, Marin-Link B, et al. The expanded chronic care model: an integration of concepts and strategies from population health promotion and the chronic care model. *Hosp Q.* 2003;7(1):73–82.

Bauer UE, Briss PA, Goodman RA, Bowman BA. Prevention of chronic disease in the 21st century: elimination of the leading preventable causes of premature death and disability in the USA. *Lancet.* 2014;384(9937):45–52.

Bielaszka-DuVernay C. Vermont's blueprint for medical homes, community health teams, and better health at lower cost. *Health Aff (Millwood).* 2011;30(3):383–386.

Bodenheimer T, Wagner EH, Grumbach K. Improving primary care for patients with chronic illness. *JAMA.* 2002;288(15):1909–1914.

Brownstein JN, Hirsch GR, Rosenthal EL, Rush CH. Community health workers "101" for primary care providers and other stakeholders in health care systems. *J Ambul Care Manage.* 2011;34(3):210–220.

Burwell SM. Setting value-based payment goals—HHS efforts to improve U.S. Health Care. *N Engl J Med.* 2015;372(10):897–899.

Centers for Medicare and Medicaid Services (CMS). Shared Savings Program. 2016a. Available at: http://www.cms.gov/medicare/medicare-fee-for-service-payment/sharedsavingsprogram/index.html. Accessed April 12, 2016.

Centers for Medicare and Medicaid Services (CMS). Accountable Health Communities Model. 2016b. Available at: https://innovation.cms.gov/initiatives/AHCM. Accessed April 13, 2016. Coleman K, Austin BT, Brach C, Wagner EH. Evidence on the chronic care model in the new millennium. *Health Aff (Millwood).* 2009;28(1):75–85.

DeVol R, Bedroussian A. *An Unhealthy America: The Economic Burden of Chronic Disease Charting a New Course to Save Lives and Increase Productivity and Economic Growth.* Milken Institute. 2007. Available at: http://www.milkeninstitute.org/publications/view/321. Accessed August 10, 2016.

Duke University Medical Center (Duke) and Centers for Disease Control and Prevention (CDC). Practical Playbook. Success story—San Diego School System and local medical residents jumpstart health habits in students: primary care, public health, and school district partner to address obesity. de Beaumont Foundation. 2016. Available at: https://www.practicalplaybook.org/success/story/san-diego-school-system-and-local-medical-residents-jumpstart-healthy-habits-students. Accessed May 1, 2016.

Elliott L, Mcbride TD, Allen P, et al. Health care system collaboration to address chronic diseases: a nationwide snapshot from state public health practitioners. *Prev Chronic Dis.* 2014;11:E152.

Fiandt K. The chronic care model: description and application for practice. *Top Adv Prac Nurs eJ.* 2006;6(4).

George J, Zairina E. The potential role of pharmacists in chronic disease screening. *Int J Pharm Pract.* 2016;24(1):3–5.

Gerteis J, Izrael D, Deitz D, et al. *Multiple Chronic Conditions Chartbook.* Agency for Healthcare Research and Quality. 2014. AHRQ Publications no. Q14-0038. Available at: http://www.ahrq.gov/sites/default/files/wysiwyg/professionals/prevention-chronic-care/decision/mcc/mccchartbook.pdf. Accessed April 12, 2016.

Goodell S, Bodenheimer T, Berry-Millett R. *Care Management of Patients With Complex Health Care Needs.* Princeton, NJ: Robert Wood Johnson Foundation; 2009.

Greene J, Hibbard JH, Sacks R, Overton V, Parrotta CD. When patient activation levels change, health outcomes and costs change, too. *Health Aff (Millwood).* 2015;34(3):431–437.

Grunfeld E, Manca D, Moineddin R, et al. Improving chronic disease prevention and screening in primary care: results of the BETTER pragmatic cluster randomized controlled trial. *BMC Fam Pract.* 2013;14(1):175.

Hibbard J, Gilbert H. *Supporting People to Manage Their Health: An Introduction to Patient Activation.* London, UK: The King's Fund; 2014.

Hong CS, Siegel AL, Ferris TG. Issue Brief: Caring for high-need, high-cost patients: what makes for a successful care management program? Vol. 19. A Commonwealth Fund Pub. 1764. 2014. Available at: http://www.commonwealthfund.org/~/media/files/publications/issue-brief/2014/aug/1764_hong_caring_for_high_need_high_cost_patients_ccm_ib.pdf. Accessed April 9, 2016.

Improving Chronic Illness Care (ICIC). The Chronic Care Model. The MacColl Center for Health Care Innovation. 2016. Available at: http://www.improvingchroniccare.org/index.php?p=Model_Elements&s=18. Accessed September 8, 2016.

Institute of Medicine (IOM). Living well with chronic illness: a call for public health action. Washington, DC: National Academies Press; 2012a. Available at: http://www.nationalacademies.org/hmd/~/media/Files/Report%20Files/2012/Living-Well-with-Chronic-Illness/livingwell_chronicillness_reportbrief.pdf. Accessed March 30, 2016.

Institute of Medicine (IOM). Report Brief—Primary care and public health: exploring integration to improve population health. 2012b. Available at: https://www.nationalacademies.org/hmd/~/media/Files/Report%20Files/2012/Primary-Care-and-Public-Health/Primary%20Care%20and%20Public%20Health_Revised%20RB_FINAL.pdf. Accessed April 6, 2016.

Jackson GL, Powers BJ, Chatterjee R, et al. Improving patient care: the patient centered medical home: a systematic review. *Ann Intern Med.* 2013;158(3):169–178.

Kindig D, Isham G. Population health improvement: a community health business model that engages partners in all sectors. Frontiers of Health Services Management. 2014. Available at: https://uwphi.pophealth.wisc.edu/publications/other/frontiers-of-health-services-management-vol30-num4.pdf. Accessed March 25, 2016.

Kindig D, Stoddart G. What is population health? *Am J Public Health.* 2003;93(3):380–383.

Koh H. Statement to the Committee on Health, Education, Labor and Pensions, United States Senate. The state of chronic disease prevention. 2011. Available at: http://www.hhs.gov/asl/testify/2011/10/t20111012b.html. Accessed April 2, 2016.

Koo D, Felix K, Dankwa-Mullan I, Miller T, Waalen J. A call for action on primary care and public health integration. *Am J Public Health.* 2012;102(S3):S307–S309.

Levi J, Segal L, Juliano C, et al. Prevention for a healthier America: investments in disease prevention yield significant savings, stronger communities. Trust for America's Health; 2008. Available at: http://www.rwjf.org/content/dam/farm/reports/reports/2008/rwjf29920. Accessed April 11, 2016.

Lorig K, Holman HR. Self-management education: history, definition, outcomes, and mechanisms. *Ann Behav Med.* 2003;26:1–7.

Manca DP, Campbell-Scherer D, Aubrey-Bassler K, et al. Developing clinical decision tools to implement chronic disease prevention and screening in primary care: the BETTER 2 program (Building on Existing Tools to Improve Chronic Disease Prevention and Screening in Primary Care). *Implement Sci.* 2015;10(1):107.

Markovitz AR, Alexander JA, Lantz PM, Paustian ML. Patient-centered medical home implementation and use of preventive services. The role of practice socioeconomic context. *JAMA Intern Med.* 2015;175(4):598–606.

Marks S, Levin D; Amatihealth. Population health methodology, step 2: stratification. 2015. Available at: http://amatihealth.com/blog/2015/6/3/population-health-methodology-step-2-stratification. Accessed March 30, 2016.

Nagykaldi Z, Aspy CB, Chou A, Mold JW. Impact of a wellness portal on the delivery of patient-centered preventive care. *J Am Board Fam Med.* 2012;25(2):158–167.

Nash DB. The population health mandate: a broader approach to care delivery. The Boardroom Press. The Governance Institute. 2012. Available at: http://www.populationhealthcolloquium.com/readings/Pop_Health_Mandate_NASH_2012.pdf. Accessed August 10, 2016.

Nash DB, Reifsnyder J, Fabius RJ, Skoufalos A, Clarke JL. *Population Health: Creating a Culture of Wellness.* Burlington, MA: Jones and Bartlett Publishers; 2015:1–15.

National Association of County and City Health Officials (NACCHO). Public health and prevention provisions of the Affordable Care Act. 2013. Available at: http://archived.naccho.org/advocacy/upload/PH-and-Prevention-Provision-in-the-ACA-Revised.pdf. Accessed April 3, 2016.

National Council on Aging. Chronic disease self-management. 2015. Available at: https://www.ncoa.org/wp-content/uploads/Chronic-Disease-Fact-Sheet_Final-Sept-2015.pdf. Accessed April 10, 2016.

Nielsen M, Gibson A, Buelt L, Grundy P, Grumbach K. The patient-centered medical home's impact on cost and quality: annual review of evidence 2013–2014. Patient-Centered Primary Care Collaborative, Milbank Memorial Fund. 2015. Available at:

http://www.milbank.org/uploads/documents/reports/PCPCC_2015_Evidence_ Report.pdf. Accessed April 13, 2016.

Ory MG, Ahn S, Jiang L, et al. Successes of a national study of the chronic disease self-management program. *Med Care.* 2013;51(11):992–998.

Parekh AK, Goodman RA, Gordon C, Koh HK; The HHS Interagency Workgroup on Multiple Chronic Conditions. Managing multiple chronic conditions: a strategic framework for improving health outcomes and quality of life. *Public Health Rep.* 2011;126(4):460–471.

Peikes D, Chen A, Schore J, Brown R. Effects of care coordination on hospitalization, quality of care, and health care expenditures among Medicare beneficiaries. *JAMA.* 2009;301(6):603–618.

Remington PL, Catlin BB, Gennuso KP. The County Health Rankings: rationale and methods. *Popul Health Metr.* 2015;13:11.

Robert Wood Johnson Foundation (RWJF). Health Policy Snapshot Issue Brief: What's new with community benefit? 2012. Available at: http://www.rwjf.org/content/dam/ farm/reports/issue_briefs/2012/rwjf402124. Accessed April 2, 2016.

Rosenthal M, Abrams M, Bitton A; Patient-Centered Medical Home Evaluators' Collaborative. Recommended core measures for evaluating the patient-centered medical home: cost, utilization, and clinical quality. Commonwealth Fund. 2012. Available at: http:// www.commonwealthfund.org/~/media/files/publications/data-brief/2012/1601_rosenthal_recommended_core_measures_pcmh_v2.pdf. Accessed April 11, 2016.

Shearer G. Prevention provisions in the Affordable Care Act. APHA Issue Brief. 2010. Available at: https://www.apha.org/~/media/files/pdf/topics/aca/prevention_aca_final. ashx. Accessed April 12, 2016.

Stock S, Pitcavage JM, Simic D, et al. Chronic care model strategies in the United States and Germany deliver patient-centered, high-quality diabetes care. *Health Aff (Millwood).* 2014;33(9):1540–1548.

US Department of Health and Human Services (USDHHS). Multiple chronic conditions —a strategic framework: optimum health and quality of life for individuals with multiple chronic conditions. 2010. Available at: http://www.hhs.gov/ash/initiatives/ mcc/mcc_framework.pdf. Accessed April 11, 2016.

US Department of Health and Human Services (USDHHS). Prevention and Public Health Fund. Available at: http://www.hhs.gov/open/prevention/index.html. Accessed April 3, 2016.

Wagner E. Chronic disease management: what will it take to improve care for chronic illness? *Eff Clin Pract.* 1998;1(1):2–4.

Ward BW, Schiller JS, Goodman RA. Multiple chronic conditions among US adults: a 2012 update. *Prev Chronic Dis.* 2014;11:E62.

Yarnall KSH, Pollak KI, Østbye T, Krause KM, Michener JL. Primary care: is there enough time for prevention? *Am J Public Health.* 2003;93(4):635–641.

PART II. UPSTREAM RISK FACTORS

6

THE SOCIAL DETERMINANTS OF CHRONIC DISEASE

Carlyn M. Hood, MPA, MPH, Parvathy Pillai, MD, MPH, and Paula Lantz, PhD, MS

Introduction

Conditions in the places where people live, learn, work, pray, and play affect a wide range of health risks and outcomes (WHO 2008). These conditions are known as social determinants of health and include an individual's socioeconomic status (SES)—including income, employment, and education—in addition to multiple other factors such as social cohesion, social support, community safety, affordable housing, and food security.

As described in Chapter 1, the underlying determinants of health are grouped into four main categories: (1) healthy behaviors, (2) clinical care, (3) social and economic (SES) determinants, and (4) physical environment (Remington et al. 2015). According to a recent research, social determinants constitute roughly 47% of health outcomes alone (Hood et al. 2016). This model highlights the importance of recognizing the underlying determinants of health, or risk factors, and their powerful and sustained influence on health and on the distribution of chronic disease, illness, and premature death in the population.

It is well documented that achieving optimum health and minimizing the risk of chronic disease occurs through such health-promoting behaviors as eating well, staying physically active, and avoiding smoking and excessive alcohol consumption (CDC 2016). Yet the ability to adhere to behavioral recommendations is largely influenced by individual and contextual social factors.

Previous research has observed that social determinants—income, education, and occupation—are powerful determinants of health; they do not necessarily have a direct effect but fundamentally shape other determinants

(Angell 1993). Therefore, what appears to be a direct impact of socioeconomic inequality may instead primarily be operating through differential exposure to conditions that have more immediate effects on health (Adler and Newman 2002) such as access to healthy foods, a safe and clean place to live, and the ability to get routine physical exercise. Those with less education and less income are more likely to smoke (Hiscock et al. 2012), less likely to engage in physical activity and less physically fit than their higher-income peers (Jin and Jones-Smith 2015), and are less likely to consume fiber and fresh fruits and vegetables (Darmon and Drewnowski 2008). Research has clearly demonstrated that education promotes knowledge and life skills, which increase access to information and resources that promote health (Adler and Newman 2002). In addition, education builds occupational opportunities and earning potential, which in turn can lead to better nutrition, housing, schooling, and recreation (Adler and Newman 2002). The documented links between SES and health are consistent across time and geography and a variety of outcomes (Marmot 2010).

This chapter addresses the social determinants of health, with a focus on the factors that play a major role in chronic disease risk and development, and the pathways by which social factors lead to differential health outcomes. It will be helpful to review these concepts within the framework used throughout this text, considering the causes of social determinants, the health consequences of social determinants, and the high-risk groups (Figure 6-1).

Figure 6-1 is similar to the conceptual model developed by the World Health Organization (WHO), showing how upstream socioeconomic and political context can affect the social determinants; which in turn affect the downstream outcomes such as one's material conditions, health behaviors, access to health services, and increased risk of disease, disability, and premature death. By applying what is known about the social determinants of health, improvements in individual and population health can be realized along with advancements in health equity (Williams et al. 2008; Marmot 2007).

Significance

The Downstream Health Consequences of the Social Determinants

The ways in which SES influences the intermediary or more "downstream" determinants of health and creates health inequities within populations are multiple and interrelated (WHO 2008). These intermediary determinants can

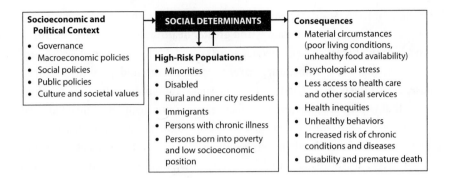

Source: Based on Solar and Irwin (2010).
Note: Social determinants include one's education, income, and occupation, as well as other factors such as social cohesion, social support, community safety, affordable housing, and food security.
Figure 6-1. Social Determinants of Health: Causes, Consequences, and High-Risk Groups

be categorized as (1) exposures that work through material living conditions, which are the basic material resources related to well-being; (2) health-promoting and health-risk behaviors; and (3) psychosocial risk factors. In addition, these exposures and risk factors work at both the individual and contextual levels, including at the neighborhood level.

Exposures Related to Material Living Conditions

There is ample evidence within and across societies that SES is highly correlated with the material conditions needed for individual and community well-being, including financial resources, food, shelter, transportation, health care, and safe environments (WHO 2008; Braveman et al. 2011b; Adler 2013). Adults with lower levels of income and education and their children have higher rates of nearly every major health risk factor or health-damaging process, creating health inequities over the entire life course. In addition, extreme events such as natural disasters, war, and famine also have a disproportionate negative impact on individuals and communities that are already experiencing socioeconomic challenges (Juntunen 2005).

Material deprivation, which is the inability of individuals or households to afford basic consumption goods and activities, leads to food insecurity and poor nutrition and to housing insecurity and a higher risk for homelessness. Lower socioeconomic position is also associated with unemployment (in a bi-directional relationship), and with jobs that come with lower pay, fewer benefits including health insurance, and greater health risks (Benach et al. 2014). In addition, there is strong evidence across countries that the use of health care services, including ambulatory care, hospitalization, and prescription drug use, is positively associated with lower socioeconomic positions, a relationship that is primarily driven by higher rates of poor health and medical need (Regenstein and Lantz 2015). Research also suggests, however, that persons with fewer socioeconomic resources underuse health care services relative to their needs, are more likely to delay or forgo diagnostic and treatment services because of financial concerns, and are less likely to receive clinical preventive services, including immunizations, teeth cleaning, cancer screening, and behavioral counseling (Regenstein and Lantz 2015).

Another critically important part of material conditions is the physical environment, including air, water, and housing quality. A large and growing literature has documented that neighborhoods or communities with higher levels of poverty and unemployment are significantly more likely to experience air pollution, water pollution, and other environmental hazards (Kruize et al. 2014). The unequal and disproportionate exposure of poor, minority, and marginalized populations to environmental hazards has been labeled "environmental injustice" and is viewed as a contributing factor to socioeconomic and racial/ethnic health status inequities (Brender et al. 2011). As one of many examples, a governor-appointed task force declared in March 2016 that the high level of lead poisoning among children that occurred in Flint, Michigan, after the municipal water source was switched without implementing corrosion controls in pipes was attributable to "government failure, intransigence, unpreparedness, delay, inaction and environment injustice" (Flint Water Advisory Task Force 2016).

Having higher levels of education and income affords individuals not only with the material conditions that are essential for health (e.g., security in income, healthy food, clothing, clean and safe shelter, and health care), but also with a number of other resources that are fundamental to the production of health (Link and Phelan 1995). This includes knowledge (through education), power, prestige, access to health-promoting technology, and beneficial social relationships. This also includes the resources to be mobile and to select neighborhood, school, and employment contexts that bring individual benefits and that also build social capital (Phelan et al. 2010).

In addition to absolute deprivation, relative deprivation in the form of income inequality has been associated with increased adult mortality, infant mortality, heart disease, diabetes, respiratory disease, mental health, and violence in dozens of studies across and within a number of countries (Pickett and Wilkinson 2014). Although some researchers have raised concerns about causal inference, meta-analyses and literature reviews have come to the conclusion that the large income disparities within populations produce social mechanisms with damaging health consequences (Pickett and Wilkinson 2014; Diez-Roux and Mair 2010).

People living in poverty struggle to pay their rent, buy food, bear the costs of transportation, purchase education-related supplies for their children, pay for health care, and other material necessities for well-being, and they often have to make difficult trade-offs (Edin and Shaefer 2015). Food insecurity is a serious problem in low-income families, even in high-income countries. Adults who experience food insecurity have higher rates of physical and mental health problems, and lower self-reported health (Stuff et al. 2004). The monthly "pay cycles" of both employment and public assistance often produce cycles of deprivation toward the end of each month when money runs outs, with consequences for both mental and physical health. For example, in a population-based study in California, the risk of a hospital admission for hypoglycemia was significantly higher for low-income patients at all times, but 27% higher in this group during the last week of the month, ostensibly when food budgets were exhausted (Seligman et al. 2014).

Deprivation in regard to specific material conditions—such as safe housing—leads to specific types of chronic health conditions and outcomes, with myriad negative interactions from multiple exposures (Braveman et al. 2011a; Braveman and Gottlieb 2014; Marmot et al. 2012). For example, it is estimated that 7 million children aged younger than 18 years in the United States have asthma, with much higher rates among poor and minority children in urban areas, because of both air pollution and triggers such as dust and mold within the home environment (Akinbami et al. 2012). Poor-quality housing is associated with a number of additional health risks including lead poisoning, respiratory infections, injuries, and mental health (Krieger and Higgins 2002).

A growing body of research underscores the importance of the prenatal period and early childhood for health over the entire life course (Schickedanz et al. 2015). Furumoto-Dawson et al. (2007) claim that the "impact of material and psychological stresses imposed by social inequities and marginalization is felt most intensely during perinatal/early childhood and puberty/adolescent periods, when developmental genes are expressed and interact with social-physical environments."

Health-Promoting and Health-Risk Behaviors

The majority of health-related behavioral risk factors are patterned by income and educational attainment (Pampel et al. 2010). An inverse relationship between individual SES and health-risk behaviors (i.e., as SES increases, the prevalence of risky behavior decreases) has been observed for a wide variety of behaviors including but not limited to tobacco use, illicit drug use, obesity, physical inactivity, sexual risk taking, driving while intoxicated, and wearing a helmet on a bicycle or motorcycle.

For example, although there are some differences in the epidemiology of tobacco use across countries, a prominent pattern is higher rates of cigarette smoking and other forms of tobacco use among people of lower socioeconomic position (Garrett et al. 2015). Jha et al. (2006) estimates that cigarette smoking produces almost half of the excess mortality experienced by the lowest SES stratum in a number of countries. It is also recognized, however, that personal risk behavior does not happen in a vacuum. The socioeconomic background of individuals and the contexts in which they live, work, and age play a major role in creating the underlying disparities in the risk factors and exposures and are challenging to modify (Phelan et al. 2010). As information regarding the health risks of tobacco has been disseminated, and as policies, technologies, and resources for smoking prevention and cessation have been implemented and supported, socioeconomic disparities in tobacco use have been widening over time (Ding et al. 2015). This is an important illustration of how the deployment of resources (e.g., money, knowledge, expertise, access to technology, and positive policy attention) is a critical component of how SES influences, maintains, and sometimes exacerbates health disparities beyond simply the differential prevalence of risk behavior across social strata (Phelan et al. 2010; Garrett et al. 2015).

In addition, several studies across countries have shown that the higher prevalence of major health-risk behaviors in lower-SES populations explains only a proportion of their higher rates of morbidity and mortality (Lantz et al. 2001; Marmot 2006; Avendano and Kawachi 2014). Pampel et al. (2010) argue that the relationship between social position and health behavior is multifaceted, and posit that a number of broad mechanisms underlie this phenomenon, including the relationship among deprivation, inequality, and stress; the use of health behaviors for class members to set themselves apart from other groups and to provide social support, social cohesion, and peer dynamics; the association of lower SES with lower knowledge and information access; and the ways in which the socioeconomic conditions of communities influence the health behaviors of their members.

Psychosocial Risk Factors

Psychosocial factors are social phenomena that influence health through psychological mechanisms. Because most psychosocial circumstances and characteristics are patterned by socioeconomic position, these factors play a critical role in producing social disparities in health outcomes. A major psychosocial risk factor for poor health outcomes is stress in both its acute and chronic forms. Lower-income people and families experience significantly higher rates of stress, including stress from material deprivation such as financial pressures and concerns, food insecurity, housing insecurity and homelessness, neighborhood safety threats, and transportation challenges (Adler and Newman 152002; Edin and Shaefer 2015).

In addition to stress, several other psychosocial factors are associated with socioeconomic position including psychosocial and personality factors that exist primarily within individuals, such as the psychological effects of exposure to traumatic life events, coping and resilience, self-efficacy, self-esteem, cynical hostility, and hopelessness. Psychosocial factors also include things that reflect social relationships and structural conditions, such as social support, social networks, sense of job control, experiences of discrimination, and the use of risky behaviors as a form of self-medication (Braveman et al. 2011b; WHO 2008; Marmot et al. 2012).

Neighborhood Factors

Neighborhood factors, which are driven in large part by the socioeconomic resources within neighborhoods and allocated to them through economic and policy decisions, can be both health-promoting and health-damaging. Macintyre et al. (2002) identified five main features of neighborhoods that are related to health: (1) the physical infrastructure and environment shared by residents, including water, air, and street and sidewalk conditions; (2) the level of risk in the environments in which people work, play, and rest; (3) the quality of public and private services provided to residents, such as garbage removal, police protection, and social services; (4) sociocultural features of neighborhoods, including norms, values, social cohesion, social networks, and civic engagement; and

(5) the reputation of a neighborhood, which signals how it is perceived by residents and nonresidents, and involves shared community morale.

A growing body of neighborhood effects research has shown that neighborhood context plays a critically important role in producing disparities in major health risk behaviors and their related outcomes (Diez-Roux and Mair 2010). For example, many features of the built environment and urban design (including land-use patterns, sidewalks, transportation systems, and street connectivity) are associated with physical activity and other features of mobility important to health (Diez-Roux and Mair 2010). Similarly, neighborhood features such as the absence of grocery stores and the types of food available are associated with dietary features and obesity rates across communities. One U.S. study found that features of urban food deserts, such as distance between stores and prices, were associated with obesity, and that price was the main driver of this relationship (Ghosh-Dastidar et al. 2014).

In the past 20 years, there has been a significant increase in research attempting to link neighborhood socioeconomic, cultural, institutional, and physical conditions with health outcomes and as an explanation for persistent social inequalities in health (Diez-Roux and Mair 2010). A number of studies have concluded that, above and beyond the individual characteristics of residents, neighborhood characteristics produce both positive and negative impacts on health behaviors, health status outcomes, and health inequities (Wilkinson and Pickett 2006). Neighborhood effects research, however, is challenging both conceptually and methodologically, including that it is difficult to control for neighborhood selection processes and to take into account cumulative exposures, lagged effects, and the dynamic nature of neighborhood contexts (Diez-Roux 2007).

Reverse Causality

Thus far, this chapter has focused on poor health as the outcome or result of upstream social determinants, including exposures to material living conditions, behavioral risk factors, and psychosocial processes at the individual and contextual levels. However, the reverse is also possible: health status can causally influence socioeconomic position and other more proximate determinants of health. For example, the quantity and quality of educational attainment is negatively affected by serious childhood health conditions. Also, the inability to work because of physical or mental health problems has a negative impact on income and all associated material conditions.

Chronic disease and social epidemiologists should be extremely careful about causal inference. Causality and reverse-causality in the relationship between socioeconomic position and health is especially challenging to sort out in most population-based research studies. Nonetheless, the bulk of existing evidence strongly suggests that, although causality works in both directions, the dominant direction is that the socioeconomic position of individuals and the social conditions in which they live precede and are the fundamental causes of subsequent health outcomes and health inequities across sociodemographic groups in society (Braveman et al. 2011b; Herd et al. 2007).

The Impact of Downstream, More Proximate Determinants of Health on Chronic Disease

The preceding section described four main types of downstream, more proximate social determinants of health and health disparities (material conditions, behavioral risk factors, psychosocial risk factors, and neighborhood context) that are primarily influenced by the socioeconomic position of individuals and their mezzo and macro environmental contexts. This strong and enduring social patterning of a large set of interrelated precursors of and risk factors for health leads to social inequities in most types of health outcomes, especially morbidity and mortality from chronic disease (Avendano and Kawachi 2014).

The burden of chronic disease is large and growing in every country and is a serious global public health problem. In the United States, the majority of adults have more than one chronic condition (notably hypertension, arthritis, diabetes, depression, some type of cardiovascular disease, asthma, and chronic pulmonary disease), with significant disparities in prevalence by race, ethnicity, income, and education (Bodenheimer et al. 2009). Research that attempts to distinguish the effects of education and income suggests that education is more strongly related to the onset of illness and chronic conditions, and income is more predictive of health trajectories and mortality after illness onset (Herd et al. 2007).

Pathophysiology

The landmark Whitehall study demonstrated an inverse relationship between social status and coronary heart disease (CHD) mortality among middle-aged British men with stable employment, such that those with lower social status based on occupation had higher rates of mortality; this association remained even after controlling for potential behavioral and laboratory-based confounders (Marmot et al. 1978). A 10-year follow-up of the same cohort again demonstrated the inverse association between grade of employment and not only CHD mortality, but also non-CHD mortality and all-cause mortality (Marmot et al. 1984). There have been multiple additional reports noting the inverse relationship between SES and morbidity and mortality associated with various health outcomes (Adler et al. 1994; Adler and Rehkopf 2008; Braveman et al. 2010; Evans et al. 2012).

In addition, the socioeconomic gradient of health cannot be explained away by lack of material goods, health behaviors, illiteracy, or access to quality health care (Lantz et al. 1998; McEwen and Gianaros 2010). Thus, in the past few decades, there has been a great deal of effort in demonstrating not only the potential pathways through which the social determinants of health can have an impact on health on a macro-level and through behavioral factors, but also through direct biological mechanisms, including the theory that life experiences associated with SES could have an impact on health through stress-related pathways (Adler et al. 1994; McEwen and Gianaros 2010).

Hans Selye described "general adaptation syndrome" and the role of stress in defending and restoring the body from injury, as well as recognizing the role that stress can play in damaging the body during this process (Selye 1950). Subsequently, the concept of allostatic load, the long-term effect of the physiologic response to stress, was developed (McEwen 1993; McEwen 1998). Allostasis refers to fluctuations in physiologic systems within the body to meet the demands of external stressors (Taylor et al. 1997). Allostatic systems allow individuals to respond to a broad range of stressors, not only biologic, such as infection or injury, but also to those stressors that may fall into the category of social determinants of health. The body's response to any stressor should involve both turning on an allostatic response and turning off the response once the stressor has passed (McEwen 1998).

Over time, the "wear and tear" that accumulates as a result of the chronic overactivity or underactivity of allostatic systems is referred to as the allostatic load (McEwen 1998). The hypothalamic–pituitary–adrenal (HPA) axis, the autonomic nervous system, the metabolic system, the gut, the kidneys, and the immune system are all involved in promoting adaptation (McEwen and Gianaros 2010). The biomediators associated with this system operate in a complex, interactive network, and are further modulated by unique individual characteristics, including one's psychological and genetic make-up, developmental history, behaviors, and experiences (McEwen 1998; McEwen and Gianaros 2010). Allostatic load can occur in the setting of frequent stressors, lack of adaptation to a repeated stress, continued allostatic response after stressor has resolved, or an inadequate response leading to a compensatory hyperactivity of other mediators (McEwen 1993; McEwen 1998).

The brain is thought to be central in allostasis and adaptation, processing information (including perceived stressors), and regulating functions involved in both adaptation and pathophysiology (McEwen 1998; McEwen and Gianaros 2010). The limbic brain, comprising areas of the prefrontal cortex, hippocampus, and amygdala, regulates allostatic control through neuroendocrine, autonomic, and immune systems; these systems are involved in the bidirectional regulation of central and peripheral physiology (McEwen and Gianaros 2010).

The areas in the limbic brain are targets for stress hormones; thus, childhood stressors during development, including those caused by lower socioeconomic environments, can potentially affect neuroplasticity (McEwen and Gianaros 2010). Subsequently, the resultant changes in the structure and function of the limbic brain can affect patterns of emotional expression and regulation, stress reactivity, recovery, coping, and perhaps even bodily aging (McEwen and Gianaros 2010). Specifically, the hippocampus has an important function in supporting aspects of memory and regulating the HPA axis (McEwen and Gianaros 2010; McEwen 1998). Repeated stress has been shown to result in altered hippocampal circuitry, although this change can be reversible (McEwen and Gianaros 2010; McEwen 1998). Changes in the structure or function may affect an individual's ability to process new information and make decisions on how best to approach challenges; in addition, given the hippocampal role in terminating the HPA stress response, stress-induced changes could potentially lead to elevated HPA activity and repeated stresses through a glucocorticoid cascade (McEwen and Gianaros 2010; McEwen 1998). Changes in brain development, structure, and function secondary to allostatic load can not only result in changes to the HPA axis and the sympathetic nervous system, but can also result in a SES gradient across other major regulatory system parameters, including cardiovascular, metabolic, and inflammatory system parameters (Seeman et al. 2010).

A population-based, longitudinal study in the United States found that negative life events and other types of stressors were more common in lower socioeconomic strata, that higher financial stress was associated with future reports of lower self-rated health and physical functioning, and that having a large number of negative life events, including being the victim of violence, was positively associated with future mortality (Lantz et al. 2005). Other psychosocial characteristics that have been shown to be linked with chronic disease mortality and other outcomes such as depression and decreased ability to change risk behaviors include "low control beliefs" such as helplessness, hopelessness, fatalism, low self-esteem, alienated labor, hostility, anger, and passive coping (Bosma 2006; Adler 2013; Bleich et al. 2012). Such psychosocial factors are viewed as "mediators" in the relationship between socioeconomic position and health because they are "rooted and shaped by adverse socio-economic conditions during upbringing and adulthood, and . . . are related to adverse health outcomes through complex psychological, behavioral and biological pathways" (Bosma 2006).

The life course perspective on poverty and health suggests that early childhood stress and exposure to disadvantage establishes a health trajectory that is difficult for an individual to change despite subsequent upward social mobility (Evans et al. 2012). Independent of adult SES, childhood SES has been shown to predict blood pressure (Hardy et al. 2003; Lehman et al. 2009). There has also been a suggested association with low SES in childhood and diminished cortisol-mediated signaling through adulthood, which in turn facilitates excessive inflammatory responding in cells of immune system and excessive cortisol release by the HPA axis (Miller et al. 2009; Evans et al. 2012). Inflammatory markers were found to be higher among adults who had low SES as children, even after controlling for adult SES (Tabassum et al. 2008). In addition, among British adult women, parent's occupation status more was found to have a greater impact on insulin resistance, dyslipidemia, and obesity than adult occupation status (Lawlor et al. 2002).

Discrimination and Stress

A growing amount of research regarding self-reported experiences of discrimination on the basis of on race, ethnicity, and social class demonstrates significant associations with a number of health outcomes (Williams 2012; Bleich et al. 2012). The research literature is most developed in the case of perceived racial/ethnic discrimination and mental health disorders (i.e., depression, anxiety disorders) and the physical health outcomes of hypertension and low birth weight (Gee and Ford 2011; Dolezsar et al. 2014;

Priest et al. 2013). Strong associations between perceived discrimination and some health outcomes have been observed in longitudinal studies after adjusting for psychosocial and other potential confounders (Lewis et al. 2015). Nonetheless, causal inference is a significant challenge, along with inconsistent definitions of discrimination, measurement challenges, and the difficulty of observing institutional or structural discrimination (Lewis et al. 2015; Priest et al. 2013; Williams 2012).

Population-based studies of attempts to address structural discrimination through public policy provide compelling evidence of the impact of such discrimination on health outcomes. For example, after the civil rights movement and Civil Rights Act of 1964 forced the integration of hospitals in Mississippi, racial disparities in infant mortality were reduced by 50% in only six years (Almond et al. 2006). Similarly, a time-series analysis of the timing of the abolition of Jim Crow laws across states revealed that this change in public policy led to significant decrease in black infant mortality rates and racial disparities in infant death (Krieger et al. 2013).

Case Study—Racial Disparities in Breast Cancer

Given the myriad ways in which individual and community socioeconomic conditions interact to produce health-promoting and health-damaging exposures and risk factors, it is not surprising that putative causal pathways and patterns play out differently across populations and diseases or conditions. The complex interrelationships that exist between upstream and more proximate determinants of health can be seen in the phenomenon of racial disparities in breast cancer mortality in the U.S. context. Although African-American women in the United States have a lower incidence of breast cancer than white women, their mortality rates are higher and survival is lower, even with controlling for later stage at diagnosis (Ademuyiwa et al. 2011).

Material factors explain some of the mortality disparity, including differential access to screening and diagnostic services, accurate disease staging, and state-of-the-art treatment (Aizer et al. 2014). Racial differences in economic resources also appear to be driving some differences in treatment compliance and completion, especially in regard to hormonal therapy (Hershman et al. 2015). African-American women also have higher rates of comorbid conditions, such as diabetes and hypertension, which could be influencing treatment tolerance and survival.

In addition, Griggs and colleagues uncovered a type of "statistical discrimination" in the first breast cancer chemotherapy dose for African-American women, which should be based on an algorithm derived from a patient's height and weight with subsequent doses calibrated with patient tolerance. Griggs et al. (2005) discovered that African-American women are significantly more likely to be underdosed for their first chemotherapy treatment, compared to white women. This is partly but not fully explained by the higher prevalence of obesity within the African-American population, as obesity is associated with lower doses of chemotherapy than indicated (Griggs et al. 2007). There are also some questions about the role of biology in persistent racial disparities in breast cancer mortality in younger women (McCarthy et al. 2015). In summary, understanding racial disparities in breast cancer mortality involves consideration of a large number of competing phenomena with complex interrelationships that are challenging to observe and measure.

Descriptive Epidemiology

High-Risk Populations

With poverty used as a proxy indicator, certain population groups have a significantly higher risk of socially driven exposures and experiences that threaten health status. Data collected through the U.S. Census Bureau (2016) through the 2015 Current Population Survey (CPS) Annual Social and Economic Supplement (ASEC) estimates the official 2014 poverty rate at 14.8% (46.7 million) among U.S. residents (DeNavas-Walt and Proctor 2015). However, there is marked variation when one examines poverty rates by race, ethnicity, age, gender, family status, sexual orientation, nativity, employment, education, and disability status (Table 6-1). Furthermore, the ASEC sample does not include the homeless population.

The ASEC data demonstrate that 2014 poverty rates among blacks and Hispanics exceed the national average, in contrast to the poverty rates among Asians and non-Hispanic whites (DeNavas-Walt and Proctor 2015; Table 6-1). Estimates of the poverty rates based on 2010–2014 ACS 5-year estimates demonstrate similar trends but also demonstrate the highest poverty rates among American Indians and Alaska Natives, with a rate of 28.8% compared with rates of 10.8% among non-Hispanic whites and 15.6% among the total population (U.S. Census Bureau 2016).

When one examines poverty rates by age, children are disproportionately affected by poverty (DeNavas-Walt and Proctor 2015; Table 6-1). Furthermore,

Table 6-1. People Living in Poverty by Selected Characteristics, United States, 2014

Characteristic	Total No. × 1,000	In Poverty, No. × 1,000 (%)	Margin of Error,[a] ±
Total	315,804	46,657 (14.8)	0.3
Race[b] and Hispanic origin			
White	244,253	31,089 (12.7)	0.3
White, not Hispanic	195,208	19,652 (10.1)	0.3
Black	41,112	10,755 (26.2)	0.9
Asian	17,790	2,137 (12.0)	1.2
Hispanic, any race	55,504	13,104 (23.6)	0.8
Sex			
Male	154,639	20,708 (13.4)	0.3
Female	161,164	25,949 (16.1)	0.3
Age, years			
Younger than 18	73,556	15,540 (21.1)	0.5
18 to 64	196,254	26,527 (13.5)	0.3
65 and older	45,994	4,590 (10.0)	0.4
Nativity			
Native-born	273,628	38,871 (14.2)	0.3
Foreign-born	42,175	7,786 (18.5)	0.6
Naturalized citizen	19,731	2,347 (11.9)	0.7
Not a citizen	22,444	5,439 (24.2)	0.9
Work experience			
Total, aged 18 to 64 years	196,254	26,527 (13.5)	0.3
All workers	147,712	10,155 (6.9)	0.2
Worked full-time, year-round	103,379	3,091 (3.0)	0.1
Worked less than full-time, year-round	44,332	7,064 (15.9)	0.5
Did not work at least 1 week	48,542	16,372 (33.7)	0.7
Disability status[c]			
Total, aged 18 to 64 years	196,254	26,527 (13.5)	0.3
With a disability	15,429	4,403 (28.5)	1.1
With no disability	179,905	22,055 (12.3)	0.3
Educational attainment			
Total, aged 25 years and older	212,132	25,163 (11.9)	0.2
No high-school diploma	24,582	7,098 (28.9)	0.8
High school, no college	62,575	8,898 (14.2)	0.4

(Continued)

Table 6-1 (Continued)

Characteristic	Total No. × 1,000	In Poverty, No. × 1,000 (%)	Margin of Error,[a] ±
Some college, no degree	56,031	5,719 (10.2)	0.4
Bachelor's degree or higher	68,945	3,449 (5.0)	0.2

Source: Adapted from DeNavas-Walt and Proctor (2015).

[a]The 90% confidence interval. For more information, see "Standard errors and their use" at US Census (2015c).

[b]Federal surveys now give respondents the option of reporting more than one race. Therefore, two basic ways of defining a race group are possible. A group such as Asian may be defined as those who reported Asian and no other race (the race-alone or single-race concept) or as those who reported Asian race regardless of whether they also reported another race (the race-alone-or-in-combination concept). This table shows data using the first approach (race alone). The use of the single-race population does not imply that it is the preferred method of presenting or analyzing data. The U.S. Census Bureau uses a variety of approaches. Information on people who reported more than one race, such as White *and* American Indian and Alaska Native or Asian *and* Black or African American, is available from Census 2010 through American FactFinder (U.S. Census Bureau 2016). About 2.9% of people reported more than one race in Census 2010. Data for American Indians and Alaska Natives, Native Hawaiians and other Pacific Islanders, and those reporting two or more races are not shown separately.

[c]The sum of those with and without a disability does not equal the total because disability status is not defined for individuals in the Armed Forces.

there is additional variation in poverty rates among children by age; rates are 24% among children aged younger than 3 years, 23% among children aged 3 to 5 years, 22% among children aged 6 to 11 years, and 19% among children aged 12 to 17 years (Jiang et al. 2016).

The ASEC poverty rate tends to be higher among female than among male U.S. residents (DeNavas-Walt and Proctor 2015; Table 6-1). However, these gender differences in poverty rates vary by age, with differences being more marked with increasing age (Table 6-1). In addition, the overall poverty rates among families with children was 17.6%, but this rate was 8.2% among married couples with children, 22% among single male–householder families with children, and 39.8% among single female–householder families with children (Hess and Román 2016).

Data based on the ACS suggest that disparities in poverty also occur on the basis of sexual orientation, with a poverty rate of 5.7% among married different-sex couples, 14.1% among unmarried different-sex couples, 4.3% among male same-sex couples (with rates as high as 18.8% among black men in same-sex couples), and 7.6% among female same-sex couples (with rates as high as 17.9% among black women in same-sex couples; Badgett et al. 2013).

The ASEC 2014 data showed that poverty rates were lower for the U.S. population who are native-born, compared with those who are foreign-born (DeNavas-Walt and Proctor 2015; Table 6-1). However, among the foreign-born population, these rates are not uniform (DeNavas-Walt and Proctor 2015; Wight et al. 2011). The poverty rate of naturalized citizens is lower than that of the native-born population, whereas the poverty rate among the non-citizen foreign-born population is roughly 1.7 times higher than that of the native-born population (DeNavas-Walt and Proctor 2015; Table 6-1). When one examines poverty rates among children of immigrant parents, rates were highest among children of recently immigrated (living in the United States less than 10 years) compared with children of established immigrants and children of native-born individuals, with rates of 38.5%, 27.2%, and 18.2%, respectively (Wight et al. 2011). A 2009 report from the Pew Hispanic Center estimated that, although undocumented immigrants and their U.S.-born children comprised 5.5% of the total U.S. population, they accounted for 11% of the population living in poverty (Passel and Cohn 2009).

Among adults, poverty rates are inversely related to employment status and educational attainment (DeNavas-Walt and Proctor 2015; Table 6-1). Furthermore, more stable employment and higher levels of education among parents have both been shown to decrease the likelihood that children will live in poverty (Jiang et al. 2016).

In 2014, adults with a disability were disproportionately affected by poverty (DeNavas-Walt and Proctor 2015; Table 6-1). In addition, a report prepared by the National Center for Veterans Analysis and Statistics highlighted that among those aged 17 years and older, disabled Veterans have lower poverty rates than disabled non-Veterans, and that disabled male Veterans have lower poverty rates compared to disabled female Veterans at 9.4% and 15.3%, respectively (NCVAS 2016).

Geographic Distribution

According to the 2015 ASEC report, poverty rates vary across the United States by geographic regions and population density (DeNavas-Walt and Proctor 2015). The poverty rate (and number in poverty) was greatest in the South at 16.5% (19.5 million people), followed by the West, Midwest, and Northeast at

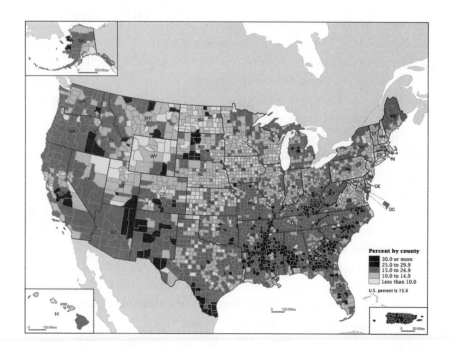

Source: Reprinted from U.S. Census Bureau (2015b).

Figure 6-2. U.S. Percentage of Population in Poverty 2010–2014

15.2% (11.4 million people), 13.0% (8.7 million people), and 12.6% (7.0 million people), respectively (DeNavas-Walt and Proctor 2015).

In addition, within metropolitan statistical areas (MSAs), the poverty rate and number of people in poverty is 14.5% and 38.4 million, respectively; this can be further divided into those living inside MSAs but not in principal cities (poverty rate 11.8%; 19.7 million people) and those in principal cities (18.9% and 18.7 million people). Among those living outside MSAs, the poverty rate and number of people in poverty is 16.5% and 8.2 million, respectively (DeNavas-Walt and Proctor 2015). Data based on the U.S. Census Bureau 2010–2014 ACS 5-year estimates can provide poverty rates at the county level (U.S. Census Bureau 2015b; Figure 6-2).

Time Trends

Following a marked decrease in U.S. poverty rates from 19.0% in 1964 to 11.1% in 1974, the poverty rate has since remained within a relatively narrow range

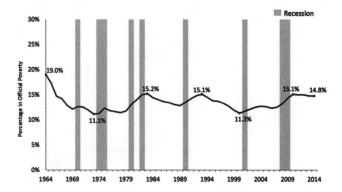

Source: Reprinted from U.S. Census Bureau (2015a).
Figure 6-3. U.S. Percentage of Population in Official Poverty, 1964–2014

(Figure 6-3). Nevertheless, there is a clear relationship between economic cycles and poverty rates in the United States, with poverty rates rising during periods of recession and decreasing during economic upturns (Chaudry et al. 2016).

Causes and Evidence-Based Interventions

The "causes" of the social determinants of health—such as poverty, lower educational attainment, low-paying jobs, or unemployment—are inextricably related to broad social and economic policies and the political context of communities, states, and the nation. A comprehensive analysis of the root causes of inequities in social determinants is beyond the scope of this chapter. However, the following section describes evidence-based approaches to improving the social determinants of health. It is ultimately up to society to invest in these proven programs and policies to improve the social determinants and reduce the associated downstream health disparities.

Despite an increasing awareness about the social determinants of health, many people still believe that health is largely improved by reducing unhealthy behaviors and increasing access to health care (Robert et al. 2008). In fact, the United States is the only developed country that spends more on the diagnosis and treatment of health issues than on providing social care programs (Squires and Anderson 2015). In 2010, Thomas Frieden, the director of the Centers for Disease Control and Prevention, developed a model to consider the broader factors that affect health. The Health Impact Pyramid (as seen in Figure 6-4)

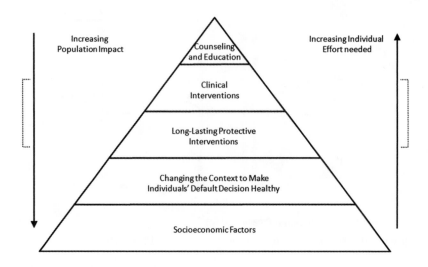

Source: Reprinted from Frieden (2010).

Figure 6-4. Health Impact Pyramid

is a five-tier pyramid showing varying health interventions that occur at various aspects of society and gauges the potential impact of the interventions. This model shows the increasing reach of population-based interventions focused on the upstream social determinants of health compared to a focus on individual counseling, personal education, or even clinical interventions (Frieden 2010).

Achieving health improvement not only requires promoting healthy behaviors and access to high-quality medical care, but also demands a focus on the broader set of factors that lie outside an individual and beyond the traditional spheres of both medical care and public health (Koltun and Swain 2013). Improving the conditions in which we live, learn, work, and play and the quality of our relationships will create a healthier population, society, and workforce. Table 6-2 indicates several examples of education, income, and housing research that have shown an evidence base for improving population health (UW-Madison 2016). These particular policies and programs are those that have been tested in multiple robust studies with consistently positive results, and are "scientifically supported" as most likely to make a difference (UW-Madison 2016).

Education

Education and income are closely interwoven determinants of health—as one's educational attainment increases, so do opportunities for higher-paying

Table 6-2. Policies and Programs with Scientific Evidence of Health Impact

Determinant	Program or Policy	Detail
Education	Career Academies	Establish small learning communities in high schools focused on fields such as health care, finance, technology, communications, or public service.
	[Chicago] Child Parent Centers	Provide preschool education and comprehensive support to low-income families, including small classes, student meals, and home visits with referrals for social service support as needed.
	Dropout prevention programs	Provide services such as remedial education, vocational training, case management, and life skills training to help students complete high school.
	Dropout prevention programs for teen mothers	Provide teen mothers with services such as remedial education, vocational training, case management, health care, and transportation assistance to support high-school completion.
	Early Head Start	Provide child care, parent education, physical health and mental health services, and other family supports to pregnant women with low incomes and children aged 0 to 3 years.
	Families and Schools Together	Convene small groups of families for facilitated weekly meetings that include a family meal, structured activities, parent support time, and parent–child play therapy.
	Full-day kindergarten	Offer kindergarten programs for children aged 4 to 6 years five days per week for at least five hours per day.
	Health career recruitment for minority students	Recruit and train minority students for careers in health fields via information about health careers, classes, practicum experiences, advising about college or medical school admissions, etc.
	Incredible Years	Support young children who exhibit or are at risk for behavioral problems with interpersonal relationship training and parents and teachers who are trained to meet their needs.
	Knowledge is Power Program in Middle Schools	Emphasize high expectations for all students, parent and student commitment, empowered principals, and regular student assessments that inform continuous improvement in a lengthened school-year.
	Mentoring programs for high-school graduation	Establish programs that connect at-risk students with trained adult volunteers who provide ongoing guidance for academic and personal challenges

(Continued)

Table 6-2. (Continued)

Determinant	Program or Policy	Detail
	No Excuses charter school model	Focus heavily on reading and math achievement, enforce high behavioral expectations through a formal discipline system, lengthen instructional time, and increase feedback on teacher performance.
	Preschool education programs	Provide center-based programs that support cognitive and social–emotional growth among children who are not old enough to enter formal schooling.
	Preschool programs with family support services	Provide center-based programs that support cognitive and social–emotional growth among young children from low-income families, usually with supports such as home visiting or parental skills training.
	Reach Out and Read	Partner with doctors, nurse practitioners, and other medical professionals to incorporate literacy support into regular well-child visits, especially in lower-income communities.
	School-based social and emotional instruction	Implement focused efforts to help children recognize and manage emotions, set and reach goals, appreciate others' perspectives, and maintain relationships; also called social and emotional learning.
	School-based violence and bullying prevention programs	Address students' disruptive and antisocial behavior by teaching self-awareness, emotional self-control, self-esteem, social problem-solving, conflict resolution, team work, social skills, etc.
	School breakfast programs	Partner with doctors, nurse practitioners, and other medical professionals to incorporate literacy support into regular well-child visits, especially in lower-income communities.
	School-wide Positive Behavioral Interventions and Supports (SWPBIS; Tier 1)	Teach positively stated behavior expectations to all students, often reinforced with prizes or privileges and supported with coaching and data; SWPBIS is Tier 1 of Positive Behavioral Interventions and Supports.
	Summer learning programs	Provide academic instruction to students during the summer, often along with enrichment activities such as art or outdoor activities.
	Targeted programs to increase college enrollment	Help students prepare academically for college, complete applications, and enroll, especially first-generation applicants and students from low-income families.

(Continued)

Table 6-2. (Continued)

Determinant	Program or Policy	Detail
	Targeted truancy interventions	Support interventions that provide chronically truant students with resources to improve self-esteem, social skills, etc., as well as familial and school-related factors that can contribute to poor attendance.
	Technology-enhanced classroom instruction	Incorporate technology into classroom instruction via computer-assisted instruction programs, computer-managed learning programs, use of interactive white boards, etc.
	Universal pre-kindergarten	Provide pre-kindergarten (pre-K) education to all 4-year-olds, regardless of family income.
Employment and income	Child care subsidies	Provide financial assistance to working parents, or parents attending school, to pay for center-based or certified in-home child care.
	Earned Income Tax Credit	Expand refundable Earned Income Tax Credits for low- to moderate-income working individuals and families.
	Flexible scheduling	Offer employees control over an aspect of their schedule through arrangements such as self-scheduled shift work, flex time, and compressed work weeks.
	Full child support pass-through and disregard	Adopt policies that allow custodial parents who receive Temporary Assistance for Needy Families to collect all child support paid by the non-custodial parent; no portion is retained by the state.
	Transitional jobs	Establish time-limited, subsidized, paid job opportunities to provide a bridge to unsubsidized employment.
	Vocational training for adults	Support acquisition of job-specific skills through education, certification programs, or on-the-job training, often with personal development resources and other supports.
Housing access and quality	Housing choice voucher program (Section 8)	Provide eligible low- and very-low-income families with vouchers to help cover the costs of rental housing.
	Housing First	Provide rapid re-housing and support (e.g., crisis intervention, needs assessment, case management), usually for individuals who are chronically homeless and have persistent mental illness or problems with substance abuse.
	Housing rehabilitation loan and grant programs	Provide funding, primarily to low- or median-income families, to repair, improve, or modernize dwellings and remove health or safety hazards.

(Continued)

Table 6-2. (Continued)

Determinant	Program or Policy	Detail
	Integrated pest management for indoor use	Support a four-tiered approach to indoor pest control that minimizes potential hazards to people, property, and the environment.
	Moving to Opportunity	Provided housing vouchers, counseling, and assistance to low-income families in various parts of the country to help them move to low-poverty neighborhoods.

Source: Adapted with permission from UW-Madison (2016).
Note: Included are all education, employment, income, and housing programs or policies with "scientifically supported" evidence that the policy or program has an impact on health.

employment, access to resources such as better housing, and healthy food, improving overall quality of life (Dahlgren and Whitehead 2006; DeNavas-Walt et al. 2011). However, while educational success generally translates into higher incomes, higher levels of education may also confer knowledge and cognitive assets that are health protective in and of themselves. Some research indicates that individuals who have not graduated from high school are more than twice as likely to have poorer self-reported health as those who graduated, even after adjustment for age, income, and other sociodemographic characteristics (Lantz et al. 2001).

From a life course perspective, the period of formal education may be important in the development, adoption, and maintenance of certain health-protective and health-risk behaviors and may be more strongly linked to functional and self-rated health status through behavioral mechanisms than are earnings in later life (Lantz et al. 2001). Early childhood education has strong and consistent evidence for positively influencing health over the life course, and the WHO's Commission on Social Determinants of Health has identified early childhood education as a priority area, urging governments to put resources into the area (WHO 2008). Children who attend high-quality early learning programs see gains later in life including improved graduation rates and earnings, as well as decreased rates of crime and teen pregnancy (Ahmad and Hamm 2013). In addition, randomized controlled preschool intervention trials have shown that early childhood education is associated with improved adult health status, lower behavioral risk factors, and lower criminal activity (Muennig et al. 2009; Muennig et al. 2011). Other educational policies and programs can be seen in Table 6-2.

Employment and Income

Employment and working conditions have powerful effects on health. With employment comes improved financial security, social status, personal development, social relations, and self-esteem, and protection from physical and psychosocial hazards (WHO 2008). There are many pathways by which this gradient operates (Marmot 2010). One is that those with lower income usually have poorer access to health care. Income also influences whether or not people can live in safe houses and neighborhoods, have access to healthy and affordable foods, and have time and safe space for physical activity.

Increasing employment rates and income levels typically requires broader systems-level policy change, and although income- and employment-based policies often do not have health improvement as a primary goal, they often have major health effects. A rigorous analysis by the Urban Institute and Milwaukee's Community Advocates Public Policy Institute has shown that a five-component policy package could substantially reduce poverty (Cherry et al. 2015)—and therefore improve population health outcomes. Research has shown that many such policies, from an expanded Earned Income Tax Credit and minimum wage laws to various job training and job creation policies, are effective in improving health outcomes (Cherry et al. 2015). A list of such policies can be found in Table 6-2.

Housing

The daily conditions in which people live have a strong influence on health and, in particular, three important and interrelated aspects of residential housing as seen in Figure 6-5: the physical conditions within homes, conditions in the neighborhoods surrounding homes, and housing affordability, which not only shapes home and neighborhood conditions but also affects the overall ability of families to make healthy choices (Braveman et al. 2011a).

Poor indoor air quality, lead paint, lack of home safety devices, and other housing hazards often coexist in homes, placing children and families at great risk for multiple health problems. Families with fewer financial resources are most likely to experience unhealthy and unsafe housing conditions and

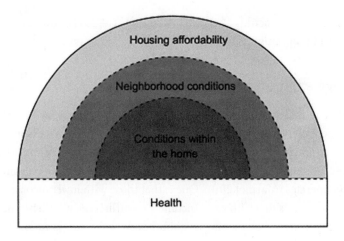

Source: Reprinted with permission from Braveman et al. (2011a).
Figure 6-5. Housing and Health

typically are least able to remedy them, contributing to disparities in health across socioeconomic groups in this country (Braveman et al. 2011a).

Along with conditions in the home, conditions in the neighborhoods where homes are located also can have powerful effects on health (Braveman et al. 2011a). A neighborhood's physical characteristics may promote health by providing safe places for children to play and for adults to exercise that are free from crime, violence, and pollution. Access to grocery stores selling fresh produce—as well as having fewer neighborhood liquor and convenience stores and fast-food outlets—can make it easier for families to find and eat healthful foods. Social and economic conditions in neighborhoods may improve health by affording access to employment opportunities and public resources including efficient transportation, an effective police force, and good schools (Braveman et al. 2011a).

Finally, the affordability of housing has clear implications for health. The shortage of affordable housing limits individuals' choices about where they live, often leaving lower-income families to substandard housing in unsafe, overcrowded neighborhoods. Furthermore, the financial burden of unaffordable housing can prevent families from meeting other basic needs including nutrition and health care (Braveman et al. 2011a).

Historically, housing and health-related efforts have included addressing fire hazards, sanitation, ventilation, and crowding to reduce injuries and certain infectious diseases (Braveman et al. 2011a). With the increasing understanding of how neighborhood infrastructure and affordability also affect health, it is clearer that strategies must be multifaceted to include not only efforts targeting the physical quality of housing, but also those strengthening neighborhoods and increasing access to affordable housing. Table 6-2 includes a number of housing-focused programs or policies that have been shown to affect health. Beyond rehabbing houses to ensure internal safety and cleanliness, these programs may include

- Providing housing choice vouchers to low-income families.
- Supporting chronically homeless individuals with rapid re-housing support.
- Counseling and assistance to help low-income persons move neighborhoods (UW-Madison 2016).

Other evidence-based policies include

- Strengthening enforcement of fair housing laws, including the Federal Fair Housing Act and other state and local regulations prohibiting racial discrimination in housing markets (Squires and Kubrin 2005; Flournoy and Yen 2004).
- Implementing state and local land use and zoning policies to promote fair housing choice in communities (Katz et al. 2003).
- Improving banking and lending procedures of the private sector to create equal opportunities for credit (Braveman et al. 2011a).
- Exploring private initiatives—such as Habitat for Humanity—to create more affordable, healthy housing (Braveman et al. 2011a).

Given the complexity of these policies and programs, a wide range of partners from local to national government, nongovernmental agencies, and community groups should be engaged to be most effective.

Case Study—How Health Departments Can Address the Social Determinants

One effort increasingly being considered and used by local and state health departments is a "health in all policies" framework. This is a collaborative approach to improving the health of all people by incorporating health considerations into decision-making across sectors and policy areas (Rudolph et al. 2013). Governments, at all levels, are challenged by declining revenues and shrinking budgets. Collaboration across sectors—such as through a "health in all policies" approach—can promote efficiency by identifying cross-agency issues and fostering communication regarding how agencies can share resources and reduce redundancies, thus potentially decreasing costs and improving performance and outcomes (Rudolph et al. 2013). In 2013, the American Public Health Association and Public Health Institute wrote a "health in all policies" guide for state and local governments to help professionals working in such settings respond to complex and inextricable population health problems. The following are examples of initiatives that have been created to support a formal structure to incorporate this approach in a government agency:

- Legislation: The Governor's Interagency Council on Health Disparities in Washington State was established by the state legislature in 2006, and was assigned "the primary responsibility of creating an action plan for eliminating health disparities by race/ethnicity and gender." The council is chaired by a representative of the governor's office and is staffed by the Washington State Board of Health (Governor's Interagency Council on Health Disparities 2013).
- City, county, and school partnership: As of 2013, the City of Richmond, California, was developing a strategy document to support "health in all policies" approaches through a partnership between the city manager's office (which coordinates input from city agencies), the county health agency, one of the two school districts in the county, a local university, and local community groups and residents. The partnership has worked on institutionalizing "health in all policies" goals and objectives and assigning responsibility for implementation, monitoring, and reporting (Rudolph et al. 2013).
- County ordinance: In 2010, Ordinance 16948 established an Inter-Branch Team (IBT) in King County, Washington, to implement the county's "fair and just principle" in the countywide strategic plan. This IBT is made up of the directors of all county branches, departments, agencies, and offices; meets monthly; and sits within the Office of the Executive. The IBT develops tools, engages the public and communities, and creates trainings and work plans (King County 2013).
- Incorporating health into existing government processes: The 2002 Québec Public Health Act (Section 54) specifies that the Minister of

Health and Social Services should act as an advisor to the government on any public health issue and "shall be consulted during the development of measures provided for in Bills and Regulations that could have significant impact on population health." As a result, a mechanism was developed for incorporating health impact assessments and other less formal methods into a process of inter-ministerial consultation that already exists within the provincial government's structure (Gagnon et al. 2008).

Areas of Future Research

The inclusion of a chapter on the social determinants of health in this most recent edition reflects the growing recognition that social determinants of health cannot simply be viewed as a descriptive characteristic. Rather, social determinants of health represent a modifiable risk factor across many health outcomes. Future research in this area can help delineate how best to meaningfully address the social determinants of health to reduce health inequities and improve health outcomes.

In terms of future areas of research, a top priority necessitates strengthening the basis for causal inference between upstream social determinants of health and downstream mediating or moderating factors and health outcomes. As it is impossible to randomly assign people or communities to socioeconomic conditions, the vast majority of scholarship in this area suffers from research designs with significant threats to internal validity. Selection processes, endogeneity concerns, omitted variable bias, lack of temporal ordering of exposures and outcomes, long lag periods, measurement issues, and bi-directional relationships are just some of the challenges that researchers face when trying to establish causation between the potential benefits of social and economic policies and programs, and health outcomes.

The increased use of longitudinal studies, natural experiments, regression discontinuity designs, sophisticated simulation modeling, and other research designs that are better able to identify causal relationships is needed. In all cases, researchers need to be extremely careful to not overinterpret significant associations as causal relationships. In addition, more research on the pathology of the social determinants of health is needed, including increased understanding of the cumulative impact of stressors on health, the role of social determinants of health in epigenetics, and the multiple, biological pathways by which social determinants of health "get under one's skin" (Seeman et al. 2010).

Another priority area for future work in social determinants of health is the need for a better data system. Numerous indicators relevant to the social determinants of health have been identified and could have a role in surveillance and evaluation (Hillemeier 2004). In practice, physicians and other health care professionals can address the social determinants of health at both the individual and population levels (Swain et al. 2014). Today, four in five physicians believe that unmet social needs are leading to worse health among Americans, yet the same percentage also feel unable to address health concerns caused by the unmet social needs of their patients (Goldstein 2011). On the individual patient-care level, clinicians can implement broader and deeper screening for social determinants using tools such as the Income, Housing, Education, Legal Status, Literacy, Personal Safety tool (Kenyon et al. 2007) and the Institute of Medicine's recommended core set of social determinants to be captured in the electronic health record (IOM 2014).

Collecting high-quality electronic health data on a core set of social determinant health indicators could be used to supplement population health surveillance data, further the understanding of the causal pathway between social determinants and health, and improve patient care by considering the social determinants of health when developing treatment plans. However, given the complex nature of the social determinants of health, using single indicators as a proxy for a multifaceted issue may not allow for a holistic picture of the issue. Therefore, the identification of a core set of social determinants of health data elements that were routinely collected, high-quality, inclusive of multiple sectors, and could be paired with other public health surveillance systems could be a valuable tool in better understanding the role of social determinants of health in specific health conditions (Beltran et al. 2011).

More recently, there has been a greater focus on addressing social determinants of health within bigger health care systems, with a growing number of initiatives emerging to aim at addressing some of the social issues faced by patients and developing integrated solutions within the context of the health care delivery system (Heiman and Artiga 2015). Many of these efforts are being developed in the context of accountable care organizations, payment reform, and other innovations being led by the Centers for Medicare and Medicaid Services (Heiman and Artiga 2015). In addition, there is recognition that considerations of social determinants of health should be more routinely incorporated into the clinical encounter, and that health care providers should be further educated with regard to addressing social determinants of health at the clinical level. The Institute of Medicine recommended a core set of social determinants of health be captured in the electronic health record (IOM 2014; Phase 2). In proposing these recommendations, the report recognized the associated implementation challenges, not only with modification of technologies, but also with regard to the ways clinical teams typically work and patients engage in their own care (IOM 2014; Phase 2).

As there has been a call for physicians to incorporate consideration of the social determinants of health into treatment plans, there has been a gradual increase in the routine inclusion of teaching the social determinants of health in the undergraduate and graduate medical education curricula (Oandasan and Barker 2003). How best to integrate this curriculum with the standard basic and sciences curriculum is yet to be determined, as is the best way to assess medical student and physician capacity to address social determinants of health. In addition, at a population level, health care professionals can advocate pro-health socioeconomic policies, work collectively with peers and professional organizations, and be persistent in advocating policy change (Swain et al. 2014), recognizing that what physicians and other health care professionals bring to the table is unparalleled credibility and expertise in the area of health (Swain et al. 2014).

At the same time, however, there is growing concern about the medicalization of "population health" by the health care system and the conflation of "population health" with "population medicine" or efforts to improve the health of a specific population of people covered by a health plan or managed care organization (Kindig 2015). The majority of efforts to address the social determinants of health within the medical care system remain focused on health care access and behavioral health (substance abuse and mental health issues) at the individual patient level.

Even with increased exposure to the social determinants of health in clinical training (IOM 2016), the fact is that the health care system and clinicians that work within it have the primary mission to diagnose and treat individual patients. Expecting the health care system to identify and address upstream social determinants of health will further medicalize population health and continue to conflate health status and health status disparities with health care and health care disparities (Lantz et al. 2007). Striking a balance that ensures that medical professionals are able to continue diagnosing patients while taking individual patient context into consideration when developing a treatment plan is essential in ensuring that practitioners are able to realistically and effectively improve health outcomes, particularly for their most vulnerable patients.

Finally, at the community, program, and policy level, there is a need to establish an evidence base for programs and policies addressing the social determinants of health and a better understanding of the relative impacts of various programs these on health outcomes, thus allowing both maximum efficiency and effectiveness when allocating resources and guiding social policies (Braveman et al. 2011c). This research could further be extended to determine the role public health agencies can play in effectively addressing the social determinants of health.

Resources and Suggested Readings

Association of Academic Health Centers: Social Determinants of Health Toolkit for Collaboration, http://wherehealthbegins.org

Centers for Disease Control and Prevention, Social Determinants of Health, http://www.cdc.gov/socialdeterminants

Health Affairs, Health Policy Brief: The Relative Contribution of Multiple

Determinants to Health Outcomes, http://healthaffairs.org/healthpolicybriefs/brief_pdfs/healthpolicybrief_123.pdf

Health Begins: Making "Upstreamists": Healthcare professionals and innovators equipped to transform care and the social and environmental conditions that make people sick, http://www.healthbegins.org

Healthy People 2020, Social Determinants of Health, http://www.healthypeople.gov/2020/topics-objectives/topic/social-determinants-of-health#five

Woolf SH, Aron LY. The US health disadvantage relative to other high-income countries: findings from a National Research Council/Institute of Medicine Report. *JAMA*. 2013;309(8):771–772.

National Association of City and County Health Officials, Roots of Health Inequity online course, http://rootsofhealthinequity.org

Policy Link, http://www.policylink.org

Robert Wood Johnson Foundation, Social Determinants of Health, http://www.rwjf.org/en/topics/search-topics/S/social-determinants-of-health.html

Unnatural Causes, http://www.unnaturalcauses.org

Wellesley Institute, Advancing Urban Health, http://www.wellesleyinstitute.com

World Health Organization Commission on Social Determinants of Health, http://www.who.int/social_determinants

References

Ademuyiwa FO, Edge SB, Erwin DO, Orom H, Ambrosone CB, Underwood W III. Breast cancer racial disparities: unanswered questions. *Cancer Res.* 2011;71(3): 640–644.

Adler NE. Health disparities: taking on the challenge. *Perspect Psychol Sci.* 2013;8(6): 679–681.

Adler NE, Boyce T, Chesney MA, et al. Socioeconomic status and health: the challenge of the gradient. *Am Psychol.* 1994;49(1):15–24.

Adler NE, Newman K. Socioeconomic disparities in health: pathways and policies. *Health Aff (Millwood).* 2002;21(2):260–276.

Adler NE, Rehkopf DH. U.S. disparities in health: descriptions, causes, and mechanisms. *Annu Rev Public Health.* 2008;29(1):235–252.

Ahmad FZ, Hamm K. The school-readiness gap and preschool benefits for children of color. Center for American Progress. 2013. Available at: https://www.americanprogress.org/issues/education/report/2013/11/12/79252/the-school-readiness-gap-and-preschool-benefits-for-children-of-color. Accessed March 17, 2016.

Aizer AA, Wilhite TJ, Chen M, et al. Lack of reduction in racial disparities in cancer-specific mortality over a 20-year period. *Cancer.* 2014;120(10):1532–1539.

Akinbami LJ, Moorman JE, Bailey C, et al. *Trends in Asthma Prevalence, Health Care Use, and Mortality in the United States, 2001–2010.* Atlanta, GA: Centers for Disease Control and Prevention, National Center for Health Statistics; 2012.

Almond DV, Chay KY, Greenstone M. Civil rights, the war on poverty, and black–white convergence in infant mortality in the rural South and Mississippi. Cambridge, MA: Department of Economics, Massachusetts Institute of Technology; 2006. Working paper no. 07-04.

Angell M. Privilege and health: what's the connection? *N Engl J Med.* 1993;329(2):126–127.

Avendano M, Kawachi I. Why do Americans have shorter life expectancy and worse health than do people in other high-income countries? *Annu Rev Public Health.* 2014;35:307–325.

Badgett MVL, Durso LE, Schneebaum A. New patterns of poverty in the lesbian, gay and bisexual community. The Williams Institute. 2013. Available at: http://williamsinstitute. law.ucla.edu/wp-content/uploads/LGB-Poverty-Update-Jun-2013.pdf. Accessed April 1, 2016.

Beltran VM, Harrison KM, Hall HI, et al. Collection of social determinant of health measures in U.S. National Surveillance System for HIV, viral hepatitis, STDs and TB. *Public Health Rep.* 2011;126(3):41–53.

Benach J, Vives A, Amable M, Vanrolelen C, Tarafa G, Muntaner C. Precarious employment: understanding an emerging social determinants of health. *Ann Rev Public Health.* 2014;35:229–253.

Bleich SN, Jarlenski MP, Bell CN, LaVeist TA. Health inequalities: trends, progress, and policy. *Ann Rev Public Health.* 2012;33:7–40.

Bodenheimer T, Chen E, Bennett HD. Confronting the growing burden of chronic disease: can the U.S. health care workforce do the job? *Health Aff (Millwood).* 2009;28(1):64–74.

Bosma H. Socio-economic differences in health: are control beliefs fundamental mediators? In: Marmot M, Siegrist J, eds. *Social Inequalities in Health: New Evidence and Policy Implications.* New York, NY: Oxford University Press; 2006:153–166.

Braveman PA, Cubbin C, Egerter S, Williams DR, Pamuk E. Socioeconomic disparities in health in the United States: what the patterns tell us. *Am J Public Health.* 2010; 100(suppl 1):S186–S196.

Braveman P, Dekker M, Egerter S, Sadegh-Nobari T, Pollack C. Housing and health. Exploring the Social Determinants of Health Series: Issue Brief no. 7. Robert Wood Johnson Foundation. 2011a. Available at: http://www.rwjf.org/content/dam/farm/ reports/issue_briefs/2011/rwjf70451. Accessed March 17, 2016.

Braveman P, Egerter S, Williams DR. The social determinants of health: coming of age. *Annu Rev Public Health.* 2011b;32:381–398.

Braveman PA, Egerter SA, Woolf SH, Marks JS. When do we know enough to recommend action on the social determinants of health? *Am J Prev Med.* 2011c;40(1):S58–S66.

Braveman P, Gottlieb L. The social determinants of health: it's time to consider the causes of the causes. *Public Health Rep.* 2014;129(suppl 2):19–31.

Brender JD, Maantay JA, Chakraborty J. Residential proximity to environmental hazards and adverse health outcomes. *Am J Public Health.* 2011;101(suppl 1):S37–S52.

Centers for Disease Control and Prevention (CDC). Core functions of public health and how they relate to the 10 essential services. 2016. Available at: http://www.cdc.gov/nceh/ehs/ephli/core_ess.htm. Accessed March 16, 2016.

Chaudry A, Wimer C, Macartney S, et al. Poverty in the United States: 50-year trends and safety net impacts. US Department of Health and Human Services, Office of Human Services Policy, Office of the Assistant Secretary for Planning and Evaluation. 2016. Available at: https://aspe.hhs.gov/poverty-united-states-50-year-trends-and-safety-net-impacts. Accessed April 5, 2016.

Cherry R, Reimer D, Williams C, Kerksick J. Working our way out of poverty. Community Advocates Public Policy Institute and Urban Institute. 2015. Available at: http://ppi.communityadvocates.net/content/publicationspublications_3_link_to_pdf.pdf. Accessed March 17, 2016.

Dahlgren G, Whitehead M. *Levelling Up (Part 2): A Discussion Paper on European Strategies for Tackling Social Inequities in Health.* World Health Organization. 2006. Available at: http://www.euro.who.int/__data/assets/pdf_file/0018/103824/E89384.pdf. Accessed April 1, 2016.

Darmon N, Drewnowski A. Does social class predict diet quality? *Am J Clin Nutr.* 2008;87(5):1107–1117.

DeNavas-Walt C, Proctor B, Smith J. *U.S. Census Bureau, Current Population Reports, P60-239, Income, Poverty, and Health Insurance Coverage in the United States: 2010.* US Census Bureau. 2011. Available at: http://www.census.gov/prod/2011pubs/p60-239.pdf. Accessed March 17, 2016.

DeNavas-Walt C, Proctor B. *U.S. Census Bureau, Current Population Reports, P60-252, Income and Poverty in the United States: 2014.* 2015. Available at: https://www.census.gov/content/dam/Census/library/publications/2015/demo/p60-252.pdf. Accessed April 1, 2016.

Diez-Roux A. Neighborhoods and health: where are we and where do we go from here? *Rev Epidemiol Sante Publique.* 2007;55(1):13–21.

Diez-Roux A, Mair C. Neighborhoods and health. *Ann N Y Acad Sci.* 2010;1186:125–145.

Ding D, Do A, Schmidt HM, Bauman AE. A widening gap? Changes in multiple lifestyle risk behaviours by socioeconomic status in New South Wales, Australia, 2002–2012. *PLoS One.* 2015;10(8):e0135338.

Dolezsar CM, McGrath JJ, Herzig AJ, Miller SB. Perceived racial discrimination and hypertension: a comprehensive systematic review. *Health Psychol.* 2014;33(1):20–34.

Edin KJ, Shaefer HL. *$2.00 a Day: Living on Almost Nothing in America.* New York, NY: Houghton Mifflin Harcourt Publishing Company; 2015.

Evans GW, Chen E, Miller G, Seeman T. *How Poverty Gets Under the Skin: A Life Course Perspective*. Oxford Handbooks Online; 2012.

Flint Water Advisory Task Force. *Flint Water Advisory Task Force: Final Report*. 2016:5. Available at: https://www.michigan.gov/documents/snyder/FWATF_FINAL_REPORT_21March2016_517805_7.pdf. Accessed March 21, 2016.

Flournoy RE, Yen IH. *The Influence of Community Factors on Health: An Annotated Bibliography. Policylink Report*. Oakland, CA: PolicyLink; 2004.

Frieden T. A framework for public health action: the Health Impact Pyramid. *Am J Public Health*. 2010;100(4):590–595.

Furumoto-Dawson A, Gehlert S, Sohmer D, Olopade O, Sacks T. Early-life conditions and mechanisms of population health vulnerabilities. *Health Aff (Millwood)*. 2007;26(5):1238–1248.

Gagnon F, Turgeon J, Dallaire C. Health impact assessment in Quebec: when the law becomes a lever for action. National Collaborating Centre for Healthy Public Policy. 2008. Available at: http://www.ncchpp.ca/docs/GEPPS_HIAQu%C3%A9becANoct2008.pdf. Accessed April 21, 2016.

Garrett BE, Dube SR, Babb S, McAfee T. Addressing the social determinants of health to reduce tobacco-related disparities. *Nicotine Tob Res*. 2015;17(8):892–897.

Gee G, Ford C. Structural racism and health inequities: old issues, new directions. *Du Bois Rev*. 2011;8(1):115–132.

Ghosh-Dastidar B, Cohen D, Hunter G, et al. Distance to store, food prices, and obesity in urban food deserts. *Am J Prev Med*. 2014;47(5):587–595.

Goldstein D. Physicians' daily life report. Harris Interactive. Prepared for the Robert Wood Johnson Foundation. 2011. Available at: http://www.rwjf.org/content/dam/web-assets/2011/11/2011-physicians--daily-life-report. Accessed on August 11, 2016.

Washington State Board of Health. Governor's Interagency Council on Health Disparities. 2013. Available at: http://healthequity.wa.gov. Accessed August 11, 2016.

Griggs JJ, Culakova E, Sorbero MS, et al. The effect of patient socioeconomic status and body mass index on the quality of breast cancer adjuvant chemotherapy. *J Clin Oncol*. 2007;25(3):277–284.

Griggs JJ, Sorbero MES, Lyman GH. Under treatment of obese women receiving breast cancer chemotherapy. *Arch Intern Med*. 2005;165(11):1267–1273.

Hardy R, Kuh D, Langenberg C, Wadsworth ME. Birthweight, childhood social class, and change in adult blood pressure in the 1946 British birth cohort. *Lancet*. 2003;362(9391):1178–1183.

Heiman HJ, Artiga S. Beyond health care: the role of social determinants in promoting health and health equity: Issue Brief. Kaiser Family Foundation and the Satcher Health Leader Institute. 2015. Available at: http://files.kff.org/attachment/issue-brief-beyond-health-care. Accessed April 1, 2016.

Herd P, Goesling B, House JS. Socioeconomic position and health: the differential effects of education versus income on the onset versus progression of health problems. *J Health Soc Behav.* 2007;48(3):223–238.

Hershman DL, Tsui J, Wright JD, Coromilas EJ, Tsai WY, Neugut AI. Household net worth, racial disparities, and hormonal therapy adherence among women with early-stage breast cancer. *J Clin Oncol.* 2015;33(9):1053–1059.

Hess C, Román S. Poverty, gender, and public policies. Vol. D505. Institute for Women's Policy Research. 2016:1–14. Available at: http://www.iwpr.org/initiatives/poverty. Accessed April 1, 2016.

Hillemeier M. *Data Set Directory of Social Determinants of Health at the Local Level.* Atlanta, GA: US Department of Health and Human Services, Centers for Disease Control and Prevention; 2004.

Hiscock R, Bauld L, Amos A, et al. Socioeconomic status and smoking: a review. *Ann N Y Acad Sci.* 2012;1248:107–123.

Hood CM, Gennuso KP, Swain GR, Catlin BB. County health rankings: relationships between determinant factors and health outcomes. *Am J Prev Med.* 2016;50(2):129–135.

Institute of Medicine (IOM). *Capturing Social and Behavioral Domains and Measures in Electronic Health Records: Phase 2.* Washington, DC: The National Academies Press; 2014.

Institute of Medicine (IOM). *A Framework for Educating Health Professionals to Address the Social Determinants of Health.* Washington, DC: The National Academies Press; 2016.

Jha P, Peto R, Zatonski W, Boreham J, Jarvis MJ, Lopez AD. Social inequalities in male mortality, and in male mortality from smoking: indirect estimation from national death rates in England and Wales, Poland, and North America. *Lancet.* 2006;368(9533):367–370.

Jiang Y, Ekono M, Skinner C. *Basic Facts About Low-Income Children: Children Under 6 Years, 2014.* New York, NY: National Center for Children in Poverty, Mailman School of Public Health, Columbia University; 2016.

Jin Y, Jones-Smith JC. Associations between family income and children's physical fitness and obesity in California, 2010–2012. *Prev Chronic Dis.* 2015;12:E17.

Juntunen L. Addressing social vulnerability to hazards. *Disaster Saf Rev.* 2005;29(5): 676–698.

Katz B, Turner MA, Brown KD, et al. *Rethinking Local Affordable Housing Strategies: Lessons From 70 Years of Policy and Practice.* Washington DC: The Brookings Institution Center on Urban and Metropolitan Policy and the Urban Institute; 2003.

Kenyon C, Sandel M, Silverstein M, Shakir A, Zuckerman B. Revisiting the social history for child health. *Pediatrics.* 2007;120(3):e734–e738.

Kindig D. What are we talking about when we talk about population health? *Health Affairs Blog.* April 6, 2015. Available at: http://healthaffairs.org/blog/2015/04/06/what-are-we-talking-about-when-we-talk-about-population-health. Accessed on August 11, 2016.

King County. King County Equity and Social Justice. The Inter Branch Team (IBT). 2013. Available at: http://www.kingcounty.gov/exec/equity/team.aspx. Accessed April 21, 2016.

Koltun R, Swain G. Social, economic, and educational factors that influence health. *Healthiest Wisconsin 2020*: Focus Area Profile. 2013. Available at: http://www.wche. org/uploads/8/8/9/8/8898682/hw2020_see_profile_20131101b_finalforweb.pdf Accessed August 11, 2016.

Krieger J, Higgins DL. Housing and health: time again for public health action. *Am J Public Health.* 2002;92(5):758–768.

Krieger N, Chen JT, Coull B, Waterman PD, Beckfield J. The unique impact of abolition of Jim Crow laws on reducing inequities in infant death rates and implications for choice of comparison groups in analyzing societal determinants of health. *Am J Public Health.* 2013;103(12):2234–2244.

Kruize H, Droomers M, van Kamp I, Ruijsbroek A. What causes environmental inequalities and related health effects? An analysis of evolving concepts. *Int J Environ Res Public Health.* 2014;11(6):5807–5827.

Lantz PM, House JS, Lepkowski JM, Williams DR, Mero RP, Chen J. Socioeconomic factors, health behaviors, and mortality. *JAMA.* 1998;279(21):1703–1708.

Lantz PM, House JS, Mero RP, Williams DR. Stress, life events, and socioeconomic disparities in health: results from the Americans Changing Lives study. *J Health Soc Behav.* 2005;15:17–50.

Lantz PM, Lichtenstein RL, Pollack HA. Health policy approaches to population health: the limits of medicalization. *Health Aff (Millwood).* 2007;26(5):1253–1257.

Lantz PM, Lynch JW, House JS, et al. Socioeconomic disparities in health change in a longitudinal study of US adults: the role of health-risk behaviors. *Soc Sci Med.* 2001;53(1):29–40.

Lawlor DA, Ebrahim S, Davey Smith G. Socioeconomic position in childhood and adulthood and insulin resistance: cross sectional survey using data from British Women's Heart and Health Study. *BMJ.* 2002;325(7368):805–805.

Lehman BJ, Taylor SE, Kiefe CI, Seeman TE. Relationship of early life stress and psychological functioning to blood pressure in the CARDIA study [erratum in *Health Psychol.* 2009;28(4):413]. *Health Psychol.* 2009;28(3):338–346.

Lewis TT, Cogburn CD, Williams DR. Self-reported experiences of discrimination and health: scientific advances, ongoing controversies, and emerging issues. *Annu Rev Clin Psychol.* 2015;11:407–440.

Link BG, Phelan JC. Social conditions as fundamental causes of disease. *J Health Soc Behav.* 1995;35(extra issue):80–94.

Macintyre S, Ellaway A, Cummnins S. Place effects on health: how can we conceptualise, operationalize and measure them? *Soc Sci Med.* 2002;55(1):125–139.

Marmot M, Allen J, Bell R, Bloomer E, Goldblatt P. Social determinants of health and the health divide. *Lancet.* 2012;380(9846):1011–1029.

Marmot M, Shipley M, Rose G. Inequalities in death—specific explanations of a general pattern? *Lancet.* 1984;323(8384):1003–1006.

Marmot M. Smoking and inequalities. *Lancet.* 2006;368(9533):341–342.

Marmot M. Commission on Social Determinants of Health. Achieving health equity: from root causes to fair outcomes. *Lancet.* 2007;370(9593):1153–1163.

Marmot M. *Fair Society, Healthy Lives: The Marmot Review.* Institute of Health Equity. 2010. Available at: http://www.instituteofhealthequity.org/Content/FileManager/pdf/fairsocietyhealthylives.pdf. Accessed March 16, 2016.

Marmot MG, Rose G, Shipley M, Hamilton JP. Employment grade and coronary heart disease in British civil servants. *J Epidemiol Community Health.* 1978;32(4):244–249.

McCarthy AM, Yang J, Armstrong K. Increasing disparities in breast cancer mortality from 1979 to 2010 for US black women aged 20 to 49 years. *Am J Public Health.* 2015;105(suppl 3):S446–S448.

McEwen BS. Stress and the individual. *Arch Intern Med.* 1993;153(18):2093.

McEwen BS. Protective and damaging effects of stress mediators. *N Engl J Med.* 1998;338(3):171–179.

McEwen BS, Gianaros PJ. Central role of the brain in stress and adaptation: links to socioeconomic status, health, and disease. *Ann N Y Acad Sci.* 2010;1186(1):190–222.

Miller GE, Chen E, Fok AK, et al. Low early-life social class leaves a biological residue manifested by decreased glucocorticoid and increased pro-inflammatory signaling. *Proc Natl Acad Sci USA*. 2009;106(34):14716–14721.

Muennig P, Robertson D, Johnson G, Campbell F, Pungello EP, Neidell M. The effect of an early education program on adult health: the Carolina Abecedarian Project randomized controlled trial. *Am J Public Health*. 2011;101(3):512–516.

Muennig P, Schweinhart L, Montie J, Neidell M. Effects of a prekindergarten educational intervention on adult health: 37-year follow-up results of a randomized controlled trial. *Am J Public Health*. 2009;99(8):1431–1437.

National Center for Veterans Analysis and Statistics (NCVAS). Profile of Veterans in poverty: 2014 report. 2016. Available at: http://www.va.gov/vetdata/docs/SpecialReports/Profile_of_Veterans_In_Poverty_2014.pdf. Accessed April 1, 2016.

Oandasan IF, Barker KK. Educating for advocacy: exploring the source and substance of community responsive physicians. *Acad Med*. 2003;78(10 suppl):S16–S19.

Pampel FC, Krueger PM, Denney JT. Socioeconomic disparities and health behaviors. *Annu Rev Sociol*. 2010;36:349–370.

Passel JS, Cohn V. A portrait of unauthorized immigrants in the United States. Washington, DC: The Pew Hispanic Center, Pew Research Center; 2009. Available at: http://www.pewhispanic.org/files/reports/107.pdf. Accessed on April 5, 2016.

Phelan JC, Link BG, Tehranifar P. Social conditions as fundamental causes of health inequalities: theory, evidence and policy implications. *J Health Soc Behav*. 2010; 51(suppl 1):S28–S40.

Pickett KE, Wilkinson RG. Income inequality and health: a causal review. *Soc Sci Med*. 2014;128:316–326.

Priest N, Paradies Y, Trenerry B, Truong M, Karlsen S, Kelly Y. A systematic review of studies examining the relationship between reported racism and health and wellbeing for children and young people. *Soc Sci Med*. 2013;95:115–127.

Regenstein M, Lantz PM. Socioeconomic status and health care. In: Wright JD, ed. *International Encyclopedia of the Social and Behavioral Sciences*. Oxford, UK: Elsevier Ltd; 2015:937–941.

Remington PL, Catlin BB, Gennuso KP. The county health rankings: rationale and methods. *Popul Health Metr*. 2015;13(11):1–12.

Robert SA, Booske BC, Rigby E, Rohan AM. Public views on determinants of health, interventions to improve health, and priorities for government. *WMJ*. 2008;107(3):124–130.

Rudolph L, Caplan J, Ben-Moshe K, Dillon L. *Health in All Policies: A Guide for State and Local Governments*. Washington, DC; Oakland, CA: American Public Health Association and Public Health Institute; 2013.

Schickedanz A, Dreyer BP, Halfon N. Childhood poverty: understanding and preventing the adverse impact of a most-prevalent risk to pediatric health and well-being. *Pediatr Clin North Am*. 2015;62(5):1111–1135.

Seeman T, Epel E, Gruenewald T, Karlamangla A, Mcewen BS. Socio-economic differentials in peripheral biology: cumulative allostatic load. *Ann N Y Acad Sci*. 2010;1186(1):223–239.

Seligman HK, Bolger AF, Guzman D, López A, Bibbins-Domingo K. Exhaustion of food budgets at month's end and hospital admissions for hypoglycemia. *Health Aff (Millwood)*. 2014;33(1):116–123.

Selye H. Stress and the general adaptation syndrome. *BMJ*. 1950;1(4667):1383–1392.

Solar O, Irwin A. A Conceptual Framework for Action on the Social Determinants of Health. World Health Organization. 2010. Social Determinants of Health Discussion Paper 2 (Policy and Practice). Available at: http://www.who.int/sdhconference/resources/ConceptualframeworkforactiononSDH_eng.pdf. Accessed August 17, 2016.

Squires D, Anderson C. U.S. health care from a global perspective: spending, use of services, prices, and health in 13 countries. The Commonwealth Fund. 2015. Available at: http://www.commonwealthfund.org/publications/issue-briefs/2015/oct/us-health-care-from-a-global-perspective. Accessed April 7, 2016.

Squires GD, Kubrin CE. Privileged places: race, uneven development and the geography of opportunity in urban America. *Urban Stud*. 2005;42(1):47–68.

Stuff JE, Casey PH, Szeto KL, et al. Household food insecurity is associated with adult health status. *J Nutr*. 2004;134(9):2330–2335.

Swain GR, Grande KM, Hood CM, Tran Inzeo P. Health care professionals: opportunities to address social determinants of health. *Wis Med J*. 2014;113(6):218–222.

Tabassum F, Kumari M, Rumley A, Lowe G, Power C, Strachan DP. Effects of socioeconomic position on inflammatory and hemostatic markers: a life-course analysis in the 1958 British Birth Cohort. *Am J Epidemiol*. 2008;167(11):1332–1341.

Taylor SE, Repetti RL, Seeman T. Health psychology: what is an unhealthy environment and how does it get under the skin? *Annu Rev Psychol*. 1997;48(1):411–447.

University of Wisconsin-Madison (UW-Madison), Population Health Institute. What Works for Health: Policies and Programs to Improve Wisconsin's Health. 2016. Available at: http://www.whatworksforhealth.wisc.edu. Accessed February 26, 2016.

US Census Bureau. *Current Population Survey, Annual Social and Economic Supplement*. Historical poverty tables. 2015a. Available at: http://www.census.gov/hhes/www/poverty/data/historical/people.html. Accessed April 4, 2016.

US Census Bureau. Percentage of population in poverty: 2010–2014. 2014 American Community Survey 5-year estimates. 2015b. Available at: https://www.census.gov/content/dam/Census/newsroom/releases/2015/percent_poverty.pdf. Accessed April 4, 2016.

US Census Bureau. *Current Population Survey, 2015 Annual Social and Economic (ASEC) Supplement*. 2015c. Available at: http://www2.census.gov/programs-surveys/cps/techdocs/cpsmar15.pdf. Accessed August 18, 2016.

US Census Bureau. 2010–2014 American Community Survey 5-Year Estimates. American FactFinder. 2016. Available at: http://factfinder.census.gov. Accessed April 5, 2016.

Wight VR, Chau M, Aratani Y. Who are America's poor children? The official story. New York, NY: National Center for Children in Poverty, Columbia University, Mailman School of Public Health; 2011. Available at: http://www.nccp.org/publications/pdf/text_1001.pdf. Accessed April 5, 2016.

Wilkinson RG, Pickett KE. Income inequality and population health: a review and explanation of the evidence. *Soc Sci Med*. 2006;62(7):1768–1784.

Williams DR, Costa MV, Odunlami AO, Mohammed SA. Moving upstream: how interventions that address the social determinants of health can improve health and reduce disparities. *J Public Health Manag Pract*. 2008;14(suppl):S8-S17.

Williams DR. Miles to go before we sleep: racial inequities in health. *J Health Soc Behav*. 2012;53(3):279–295.

World Health Organization Commission on the Social Determinants (WHO). *Closing the Gap in a Generation: Health Equity Through Action on the Social Determinants of Health*. 2008. Available at: http://www.who.int/social_determinants/thecommission/finalreport/en. Accessed February 12, 2016.

7

TOBACCO USE

Corinne G. Husten, MD, MPH, and Benjamin J. Apelberg, PhD, MHS

Introduction

Surgeon General's reports (USDHHS 2014) have established a long list of serious health consequences of tobacco use, and it has been estimated that since the first Surgeon General's Report in 1964, there have been more than 20 million premature deaths from tobacco smoke and secondhand smoke. As far back as 1988, the Surgeon General concluded that nicotine met the primary criteria for drug dependency, and cigarettes and other forms of tobacco (including smokeless tobacco) are addicting (USDHHS 1988). In 1996, the Council of State and Territorial Epidemiologists added prevalence of cigarette smoking to the list of conditions designated as reportable by states to the Centers for Disease Control and Prevention (CDC 1996). Decades of research have elucidated the causes, consequences, and groups at high risk of tobacco use (Figure 7-1). This chapter summarizes this information, as well as effective interventions to reduce tobacco use in children and adults and eliminate exposure to secondhand smoke.

Significance

The Surgeon General (USDHHS 2004; USDHHS 2014) has concluded that cigarette smoking harms nearly every organ of the body causing myriad diseases (Figure 7-2) such as

- Cardiovascular diseases, including coronary heart disease, atherosclerosis, abdominal aortic aneurysm, and cerebrovascular disease.
- A variety of cancers, including lip, mouth, pharynx, esophagus, stomach, pancreas, liver, colon, larynx, trachea, lung, cervix, kidney, bladder, and acute myeloid leukemia.

- Respiratory problems, including chronic obstructive pulmonary disease, pneumonia, active tuberculosis, reduced lung function in infants, impaired lung growth during childhood and adolescence, lung function decline in adolescents and young adults, respiratory symptoms in children and adolescents, asthma-related symptoms in childhood and adolescence, premature onset and accelerated age-related decline in lung function among adults, major respiratory symptoms in adults (coughing, phlegm, wheezing, shortness of breath), and poor asthma control.
- Reproductive disorders, including reduced fertility, fetal death, stillbirth, low birthweight, and pregnancy complications.
- Other diseases, such as diabetes, rheumatoid arthritis, periodontitis, congenital defects such as orofacial clefts, sudden infant death syndrome (SIDS), blindness, cataracts, age-related macular degeneration, adverse surgical outcomes related to wound healing and respiratory complications, low bone density in postmenopausal women, hip fractures, altered immune function, peptic ulcer disease in persons who are *Helicobacter pylori*–positive, and overall diminished health.

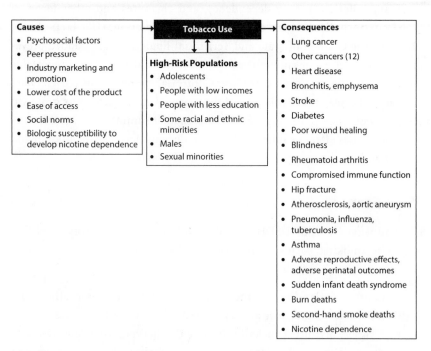

Figure 7-1. Tobacco Use: Causes, Consequences, and High-Risk Groups

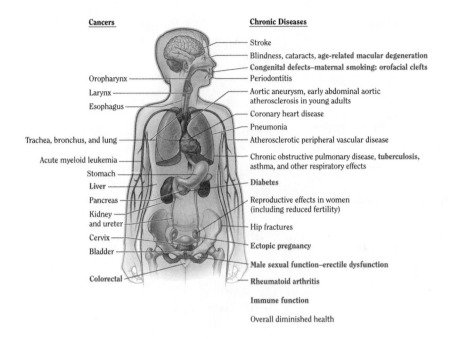

Cancers

Oropharynx
Larynx
Esophagus
Trachea, bronchus, and lung
Acute myeloid leukemia
Stomach
Liver
Pancreas
Kidney and ureter
Cervix
Bladder
Colorectal

Chronic Diseases

Stroke
Blindness, cataracts, age-related macular degeneration
Congenital defects–maternal smoking: orofacial clefts
Periodontitis
Aortic aneurysm, early abdominal aortic atherosclerosis in young adults
Coronary heart disease
Pneumonia
Atherosclerotic peripheral vascular disease
Chronic obstructive pulmonary disease, tuberculosis, asthma, and other respiratory effects
Diabetes
Reproductive effects in women (including reduced fertility)
Hip fractures
Ectopic pregnancy
Male sexual function–erectile dysfunction
Rheumatoid arthritis
Immune function
Overall diminished health

Source: Reprinted from USDHHS (2014).

Figure 7-2. The Health Effect of Cigarette Smoking on the Human Body

The Surgeon General (USDHHS 2006; USDHHS 2014) has also concluded that secondhand smoke (a mixture of sidestream smoke given off by a smoldering cigarette and the mainstream smoke exhaled by the smoker) causes lung cancer, stroke, coronary heart disease, odor annoyance, and nasal irritation in adults, and reduced birthweight, reduced lung function, lower respiratory infections (pneumonia, bronchitis), middle-ear disease (acute and recurrent otitis media and chronic middle-ear effusion), respiratory symptoms (cough, phlegm, wheeze, breathlessness), more severe asthma, and SIDS in children (Figure 7-3).

Data are emerging that other combusted tobacco products expose users to many of the same toxicants as cigarette smoke and likely increase the risk of many of the same diseases, and that smokeless tobacco causes several forms of cancer and oral diseases. Data on novel tobacco products such as electronic nicotine delivery devices, including e-cigarettes, are much more limited, but concerns have been raised about some of the chemicals used to generate the aerosol, exposure to metals leached from the device, the toxicity of certain flavorants when they are inhaled, and exposure to nicotine.

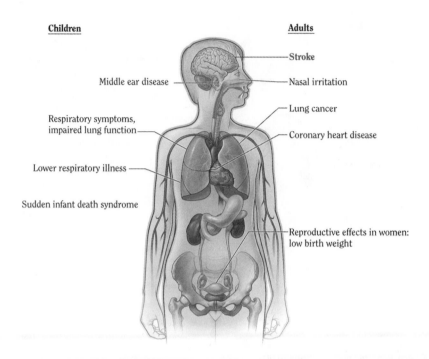

Source: Reprinted from USDHHS (2014).

Figure 7-3. The Health Effect of Passive Smoke on the Human Body

Cigarettes

In 2014, the Surgeon General estimated that cigarette smoking and exposure to secondhand smoke cause more than 480,000 deaths each year (USDHHS 2014)—18% of all deaths in the United States (CDC 2015a). Cigarette smoking is estimated to cause nearly 164,000 cancer deaths each year. Lung cancer is the leading cause of cancer death in the United States, and smoking causes 82% of all lung cancer deaths. Smoking is estimated to cause 27% of all cancer deaths in the United States. Smoking causes more than 100,000 deaths each year from chronic obstructive pulmonary disease in the United States (79% of all chronic obstructive pulmonary disease deaths) and 148,000 deaths from cardiovascular disease and stroke when deaths from both smoking and secondhand smoke are taken into account.

The relative risks for death attributable to diseases caused by smoking and smoking-attributable mortality are shown in Tables 7-1 and 7-2. In addition, the Surgeon General concluded that 5.6 million youths currently aged 0 to

Table 7-1. Relative Risks[a] by Smoking Status and Age Group, Adults Aged 35 Years and Older, United States

Variables	Current Smokers, Years of Age				Former Smokers, Years of Age			
	35–54	55–64	65–74	≥ 75	35–54	55–64	65–74	≥ 75
Men								
Lung cancer	14.3	19.0	28.3	22.5	4.4	4.6	7.8	6.5
Other cancers	1.7	1.9	2.4	2.2	1.4	1.3	1.5	1.5
Coronary heart disease	3.9	3.0	2.8	2.0	1.8	1.5	1.6	1.3
Other heart disease			2.2	1.7			1.3	1.2
Cerebrovascular disease			2.2	1.5			1.2	1.1
Other vascular diseases			7.2	4.9			2.2	1.7
Diabetes mellitus			1.5	1.0			1.5	1.1
Other cardiovascular diseases	2.4	2.5			1.1	1.5		
Influenza, pneumonia, tuberculosis			2.6	1.6			1.6	1.4
Chronic obstructive pulmonary disease			29.7	23.0			8.1	6.6
Influenza, pneumonia, tuberculosis, chronic obstructive pulmonary disease	4.5	15.2			2.2	4.0		
All causes	2.6	3.0	3.0	2.4	1.3	1.5	1.6	1.4
Women								
Lung cancer	13.3	19.0	23.6	23.1	2.6	5.0	6.8	6.4
Other cancers	1.3	2.1	2.1	1.9	1.2	1.3	1.3	1.3
Coronary heart disease	5.0	3.2	3.3	2.2	2.2	1.2	1.6	1.4
Other heart disease			1.8	1.8			1.3	1.3
Cerebrovascular disease			2.3	1.7			1.2	1.1
Other vascular diseases			6.8	5.8			2.3	2.0
Diabetes mellitus			1.5	1.1			1.3	1.1
Other cardiovascular diseases	2.4	2.0			1.0	1.1		
Influenza, pneumonia, tuberculosis			1.8	2.1			1.3	1.2
Chronic obstructive pulmonary disease			38.9	21.0			15.7	7.1
Influenza, pneumonia, tuberculosis, chronic obstructive pulmonary disease	6.4	9.0			1.8	4.8		
All causes	1.8	2.6	2.9	2.5	1.2	1.3	1.5	1.4

Source: Adapted from USDHHS (2014).
Note: For detailed footnotes, see Table 12.3 in USDHHS (2014).
[a]Relative risks rounded to the tenth decimal.

17 years will die prematurely from a smoking-related disease if the rates of youth smoking persist into the future.

Annual smoking-attributable health care expenditures are estimated at $130 billion to $170 billion (with an estimated 60% being paid by public funding such as Medicare, Medicaid, and other federal funding). Thus, 7%

Table 7-2. Annual Deaths and Estimates of Smoking-Attributable Mortality (SAM) for Adults Aged 35 Years and Older, Total and by Gender, United States, 2005–2009

Disease	Men, Attributable Fraction			Women, Attributable Fraction			Total, Attributable Fraction		
	Deaths, No.	SAM	%	Deaths, No.	SAM	%	Deaths, No.	SAM	%
Cancers									
Lung cancer	88,730	74,300	83.74	69,800	56,359	80.74	158,530	130,659	82.42
Other cancers	102,940	26,000	25.26	75,540	10,000	13.24	178,480	36,000	20.17
Total cancers	191,670	100,300	52.33	145,340	63,400	43.62	337,010	163,700	48.50
Cardiovascular and metabolic disease									
Coronary heart disease	218,870	61,800	28.24	193,720	37,500	19.36	412,590	99,300	24.07
Other heart diseases	75,670	13,400	17.71	96,200	12,100	12.58	171,870	25,500	14.84
Cerebrovascular disease	53,610	8,200	15.30	81,300	7,100	8.73	134,920	15,300	11.34
Other vascular disease	14,480	6,000	41.43	15,510	5,500	35.47	29,990	11,500	38.35
Diabetes mellitus	35,200	6,200	17.61	35,600	2,800	7.86	70,810	9,000	12.10
Total cardiovascular and metabolic diseases	397,840	95,600	24.03	422,330	65,000	15.39	820,170	160,600	19.58
Pulmonary disease									
Pneumonia, influenza, tuberculosis	25,300	7,800	30.83	30,290	4,700	15.52	55,590	12,500	22.49
Chronic obstructive pulmonary disease	61,430	50,400	82.04	66,300	50,200	75.71	127,740	100,600	78.76
Total pulmonary diseases	86,730	58,200	67.10	96,590	54,900	56.84	183,320	113,100	61.70
Total cancers, cardiovascular and metabolic diseases, pulmonary diseases	676,240	254,100	37.58	664,260	183,300	27.59	1,340,500	437,400	32.63
Perinatal conditions and sudden infant death syndrome									
Perinatal conditions	5,970	346	5.80	4,620	267	5.78	10,590	613	5.79
Sudden infant death syndrome	1,370	236	17.26	950	164	17.26	2,320	400	17.26
Total perinatal conditions	7,340	582	7.93	5,570	431	7.74	12,900	1,013	7.85

(Continued)

Table 7-2. (Continued)

Disease	Men, Attributable Fraction			Women, Attributable Fraction			Total, Attributable Fraction		
	Deaths, No.	SAM	%	Deaths, No.	SAM	%	Deaths, No.	SAM	%
Residential fires		336			284			620	
Second-hand smoke									
Lung cancer	88,730	4,370	4.93	69,800	2,960	4.24	158,530	7,330	4.63
Coronary heart disease	218,800	19,150	8.75	193,720	14,800	7.64	412,590	33,950	8.23
Total second-hand smoke	307,600	23,530	7.65	263,520	17,760	6.74	571,120	41,280	7.23
Total attributable deaths		278,540			201,770			480,320	

Source: Adapted from USDHHS (2014).

Note: For detailed footnotes, see Table 12.4 in USDHHS (2014).

to 9% of the total U.S. annual spending on health care is attributable to cigarette smoking (USDHHS 2014; CBO 2012). Smoking-attributable productivity losses from premature deaths are estimated to be $150 billion per year (and an additional $6 billion per year from lost productivity because of deaths from secondhand smoke; USDHHS 2014). These productivity costs are underestimated because they do not include lost productivity because of illness, disability, absenteeism, or reduced worker productivity. One study assessed the cost burden (in 2000 dollars) to the smoker, the smoker's family (these costs are generally excluded from cost estimates), and to society, and found that these costs over 60 years were $220,000 for a male smoker and $106,000 for a female smoker, or $40 per pack of cigarettes (Sloan et al. 2004).

Smoking by employees is costly to employers. Additional costs of smokers relative to never smokers include costs related to medical treatment before retirement, illness absences from work, life insurance and disability, housekeeping and maintenance, ventilation, time lost to smoking breaks, fire insurance losses, worker's compensation, and occupational disease compensation. Smokers also may experience lower productivity while at work (Javitz et al. 2006). For example, it is estimated that smokers have 35% more sick days from work. It is estimated that the largest cost driver could be the number of minutes on smoking breaks outside normal breaks because spending five minutes on smoking breaks (in addition to normal break time) reduces employee productivity by 1%. Some studies have suggested that smokers have reduced productivity even while at work, and that cost could be equal to or even larger than the cost of additional time on breaks. Annual medical cost before retirement is estimated to be the next largest cost. Another study estimated that the excess annual cost incurred by private-sector U.S. employers for each employee who smokes, considering excess absenteeism, presenteeism, lost productivity due to smoking breaks, excess health care costs, and pension benefits is $5,816 (Berman et al. 2014).

Tobacco use may also increase the likelihood of poverty. One study estimated that, even after adjusting for a variety of demographic factors, each adult year of smoking was associated with a 4% reduction in net worth. The author concluded that smokers appear to pay for tobacco expenditures out of income that nonsmokers put into savings (Zagorsky 2004). Another U.S. study found that smoking was associated with an increase in food insecurity among low-income families (Armour et al. 2008).

Smokeless Tobacco

Use of smokeless tobacco (defined as any finely cut, ground, powdered, or leaf tobacco that is intended to be placed in the oral cavity) causes addiction; precancerous oral lesions; cancer of the oral cavity, esophagus, and pancreas; and adverse reproductive effects, including low birthweight, preterm birth, and stillbirth. Data are suggestive that some smokeless tobacco products also cause heart disease, stroke, and diabetes (NCI and CDC 2014). On the basis of studies of traditional smokeless tobacco products, the International Agency for Research on Cancer has classified smokeless tobacco as a human carcinogen (IARC 2012). Some studies have also shown a higher risk of hypertension, and lung and cervical cancer, but the data are insufficient to determine whether smokeless tobacco causes these diseases (NCI and CDC 2014).

There is a great diversity of smokeless tobacco products and the level of risk can vary by product characteristics, ingredients, how the products are used, and interaction with other tobacco products (dual or poly-tobacco use). For example, smokeless tobacco products vary in their concentration of nicotine, tobacco-specific nitrosamines, polyaromatic hydrocarbons, toxic metals, and other toxicants. Nitrosamines are formed primarily during tobacco processing, curing, fermentation, and storage. Polyaromatic hydrocarbons are formed during the fire-curing process. A variety of toxic metals have been found in smokeless tobacco products; this is caused by levels of these metals in the soil where the tobacco is grown and from the use of fertilizers. Alkaline agents added to the product increase the absorption of nicotine by the user.

Dual or poly-tobacco use can increase risk because of delayed cessation of cigarette smoking and increased toxicant exposure. Reduced benefit from cessation of cigarette smoking occurs among those who switch to smokeless tobacco rather than quit tobacco use completely. There is also concern that smokeless tobacco use by youths could increase their use of combusted tobacco products. Data to date are mixed, with some studies, but not all, showing that youths who use smokeless tobacco are more likely to smoke cigarettes (NCI and CDC 2014; IARC 2007). However, whether these observations reflect a causal relationship or are merely explained by shared risk factors is unknown.

Higher levels of cotinine (a biomarker of nicotine), nitrosamines, polyaromatic hydrocarbons, and metals have been reported in the serum and urine of smokeless tobacco users, and some data have shown higher levels of certain tobacco-specific nitrosamines in smokeless tobacco users than in cigarette smokers (NCI and CDC 2014; Rostron et al. 2015). The International Agency for Research on Cancer has concluded that smokeless tobacco causes oral, pancreatic, and esophageal cancer (IARC 2012) and it has been estimated that smokeless tobacco–attributable cancers kill more than 2,000 Americans each year (NCI and CDC 2014). Smokeless tobacco contains nicotine, the primary addictive chemical in tobacco products. One study found that 32% of middle- and high-school students who only used smokeless tobacco reported strong cravings for a tobacco product during the past 30 days and 22% reported feeling irritable or restless when not using tobacco (Apelberg et al. 2014).

Cigars

It is estimated that in 2010, regular cigar smoking was responsible for approximately 9,000 premature deaths and almost 140,000 years of potential life lost among adults aged 35 years or older (Nonnemaker et al. 2014). Cigar smoking causes oral, esophageal, laryngeal, and lung cancer (Baker et al. 2000; NCI 1998; Wyss et al. 2013) and may increase the risk of pancreatic, stomach, and bladder cancer (IARC 2004; Shapiro et al. 2000). Regular cigar smokers who inhale, particularly those who smoke several cigars a day, are at increased risk for chronic obstructive pulmonary disease and coronary heart disease (Baker et al. 2000; Jacobs et al. 1999; NCI 1998; Iribarren et al. 1999; Rodriguez et al. 2010). In addition, cigar smokers have a higher risk of fatal and nonfatal stroke than nonsmokers (Katsiki et al. 2013).

A recent systematic review (Chang et al. 2015) found that cigar smoking was associated with increased risk of mortality from all causes, several types of cancers, coronary heart disease, and aortic aneurysm. Mortality risks were greater with increasing number of cigars smoked per day and self-reported level of inhalation. However, any cigar use exposes the mouth and throat to tobacco smoke, and studies have shown that cigar smoking can cause several different types of cancer (oral, esophageal, laryngeal, and stomach cancer) even without inhalation (NCI 1998; Chao et al. 2002). Former cigarette smokers who smoke cigars are more likely to inhale than cigar-only users (USDHHS 2014; NCI 1998), but research also indicates that most cigar smokers do inhale some amount of smoke, even when they do not intend to inhale, and are not aware of doing so (McDonald et al. 2002). In addition, smoking cigars produces secondhand smoke, which causes heart disease and lung cancer in bystanders (Baker et al. 2000; NCI 1998; USDHHS 2006).

Cigar smoke contains many of the same harmful constituents as cigarette smoke and may have equal or higher levels of several harmful compounds (NCI 1998; Chen et al. 2014). An analysis of the 1999–2012 National Health and Nutrition Examination Survey, a nationally representative survey, found that concentrations of a certain nitrosamine, blood cadmium, and lead were higher among cigar smokers compared with nontobacco users and comparable levels were found in daily cigar smokers as in daily cigarette smokers (Chen et al. 2014).

Cigar smoke contains a substantial proportion of its nicotine as un-ionized nicotine, which is easily absorbed through the oral mucosa. Thus, cigar smokers do not need to inhale to ingest significant quantities of nicotine (NCI 1998), and cigars can deliver nicotine concentrations comparable with or higher than those from cigarettes and smokeless tobacco. For example, a cigar can contain as much tobacco as a whole pack of cigarettes, and nicotine yields from smoking a cigar can be up to eight times higher than yields from smoking a cigarette (NCI 1998). Serum cotinine concentrations among cigar smokers have been found to be substantially higher than in non–tobacco users (Chen et al. 2014). Even youth cigar smokers report some measures of addiction. One study found that 6.7% of middle- and high-school students who only smoked cigars reported strong cravings for a tobacco product during the past 30 days, and 7.8% reported sometimes, often, or always feeling irritable or restless when not using tobacco (Apelberg et al. 2014).

Pipes

Pipe smoking causes lip and lung cancer (USDHHS 2004; IARC 2004). Although pipe smoke contains the same toxic chemicals as those found in cigarette smoke, patterns of use can result in lower levels of risk for disease. However, pipe smokers who previously smoked cigarettes are more likely to inhale (USDHHS 2014; Wald and Watt 1997), which increases their risk. Pipe smoking has been linked to orpharyngeal, esophageal, colorectal, pancreas, and laryngeal cancer; cardiovascular disease; cerebrovascular disease; and chronic obstructive pulmonary disease (Henley et al. 2004; USDHHS 1989; IARC 2004; Lange et al. 1992; Rodriguez et al. 2010; Nyboe et al. 1991). Pipe smokers' risk for esophageal cancer is similar to that of cigarette smokers (USDHHS 2004). Pipe smokers have an elevated risk of premature mortality similar to that of cigarette smokers who smoke at comparable consumption levels (Tverdal and Bjartveit 2011). This finding applies to total mortality and mortality for smoking-related diseases (i.e., ischemic heart disease, stroke, cardiovascular disease, and other smoking-related cancers), except for lung cancer for which cigarette smokers had the highest mortality. Even men with the lowest daily consumption of pipe tobacco (fewer than three pipes per day) were found to have significantly higher health risks than never users (Tverdal and Bjartveit 2011). In 1991, it was estimated that pipe smoking kills 1,100 Americans each year (Nelson et al. 1996), but this estimate has not been updated. Pipe tobacco contains nicotine, the primary addictive constituent in tobacco products.

Hookah or Waterpipe

The risks of hookah smoking are less well studied than that of the traditional tobacco products. However, several studies have reported significant nicotine, carbon monoxide, and carcinogen intake during waterpipe use (Schubert et al. 2012; Schubert et al. 2011; Martinasek et al. 2014; Shihadeh and Saleh 2005; Jacob et al. 2011; Jacob et al. 2013). The existence of tobacco-related toxicants, including carcinogens and heavy metals, in waterpipe tobacco smoke may place users at risk for many of the same diseases as cigarette smokers, including lung and esophageal cancer, respiratory illness, cardiovascular disease, and low birthweight (Akl et al. 2010; Rammah et al. 2012; Rammah et al. 2013; WHO 2005; Cobb et al. 2011; Dar et al. 2012; Koul et al. 2011). Concerns have also been raised about the high levels of carbon monoxide produced and the potential for acute carbon monoxide poisoning (WHO 2005). Given that waterpipe tobacco smoking sessions last significantly longer than smoking a cigarette, smoking waterpipe tobacco could potentially be even more dangerous than smoking a cigarette. The WHO Study Group on Tobacco Regulation found that a waterpipe session can be the equivalent of smoking more than 100 cigarettes (WHO 2005).

Waterpipe tobacco contains nicotine, which is the primary addictive chemical in tobacco products. Researchers have observed that waterpipe users are exposed to nicotine in levels that could cause dependence (Cobb et al. 2011; Rastam et al. 2011; Blank et al. 2011). Because waterpipe smoking sessions last longer than smoking a cigarette and there is increased smoke volume, a single session of waterpipe likely exposes users to more nicotine than smoking a cigarette.

Electronic Cigarettes

First introduced in the United States around 2007, electronic cigarettes, or e-cigarettes, are another novel tobacco product whose use is rapidly increasing. Because of the newness of the products, the potential benefits or risks of these products are not yet fully understood. At present, there is significant variability in the concentration of chemicals among products. There is also variability between labeled content and concentration and the actual content and concentration, including nicotine levels (Grana et al. 2014; Davis et al. 2015; Cameron et al. 2014; Etter et al. 2013; Goniewicz et al. 2013; Trehy et al. 2011).

Studies show that e-liquid tobacco products contain nicotine, propylene glycol, glycerin, tobacco-specific nitrosamines, tobacco alkaloids, carbonyls, ethylene glycol, diacetyl, and acetyl propionyl (Etter et al. 2013; Hutzler et al. 2014). Chemicals such as nicotine, carbonyls, tobacco-specific nitrosamines, heavy metals, and volatile organic compounds have also been identified in e-cigarette aerosols (Etter et al. 2013; Goniewicz et al. 2014; Hutzler et al. 2014; Schober et al. 2014; Williams et al. 2013; Schripp et al. 2013). Multiple studies have found much lower levels of carcinogens in e-cigarettes compared to combusted tobacco products (Hecht et al. 2015; Goniewicz et al. 2014), but exposures vary widely across the products, and some chemicals, such as formaldehyde, have been found at levels at, or greater than, that found in cigarettes under certain conditions (Kosmider et al. 2014; Gillman et al. 2015).

Flavored e-cigarettes raise particular concerns because of the potential dangers of these chemical flavorings when inhaled. Chemicals of concern include diacetyl or acetyl propionyl (Farsalinos et al. 2015); diacetyl, 2,3-pentanedione; acetoin (Allen et al. 2016); and aldehydes (Tierney et al. 2015) including cinnamaldehyde (Behar et al. 2014), which pose known inhalation risks (U.S. Department of Labor 2010). Researchers have reported that some e-cigarettes could expose users to levels of respiratory toxicants that exceed recommended workplace limits for breathing these chemicals (Farsalinos et al. 2015). The malfunctioning of certain e-cigarette components (e.g., exploding batteries) are also of concern as are the increasing number of reports of adverse events such as nicotine toxicity and choking hazards.

Some studies have shown that exposure to certain e-cigarettes produces no change in heart rate, complete blood count indices, lung function, cardiac function, or carbon monoxide levels, and that dry cough, dry mouth, and throat irritation decrease with continued use (Vansickel et al. 2010; Callahan-Lyon 2014;

Flouris et al. 2012; Flouris et al. 2013; Farsalinos et al. 2013). Other studies have reported increases in mean heart rate and changes in lung function after exposure to e-cigarette aerosol (Spindle et al. 2015; Chorti et al. 2012).

The long-term health effects of e-cigarettes are unknown, although completely switching from combusted cigarettes to e-cigarettes would likely reduce the risk of tobacco-related disease for individuals unable to quit use of combusted products. However, dual use with combusted products is unlikely to confer a health benefit as duration of use is much more strongly related than intensity of use for lung cancer, heart disease, and chronic obstructive pulmonary disease, and use of e-cigarettes by youths could cause harm (Grana et al. 2013; Tashkin and Murray 2009). Nicotine causes addiction, and some data suggest that nicotine can adversely affect the adolescent brain (USDHHS 2014). Nicotine is also known to cause adverse reproductive outcomes (USDHHS 2012; USDHHS 2014). Although levels of many toxicants are lower than the amounts found in combusted products, some of the chemicals in e-cigarettes have been linked to cancer and other adverse outcomes, so use by youths or former tobacco users should be discouraged. There are anecdotal reports of e-cigarettes helping some cigarette smokers completely switch from cigarettes to e-cigarettes, but data from research are mixed on whether e-cigarettes can help smokers quit, and none have, as yet, been approved as cessation aids (USPSTF 2015).

Pathophysiology

Cardiovascular Disease

It is estimated that cigarette smoking causes more than 99,000 coronary heart disease deaths (24% of the total number) and more than 15,000 stroke deaths (11% of the total number) each year in the United States. Another 34,000 coronary heart disease deaths (8% of the total number) are caused by exposure to secondhand smoke. Secondhand smoke also causes strokes, but there are currently no estimates of the number of deaths. Smoking-induced cardiovascular disease results from a set of interrelated processes: endothelial dysfunction, platelet activation or thrombosis, inflammation, altered lipid metabolism, vasoconstriction causing reduced oxygen and cell nutrient availability, and occlusions and sympathetic nervous system activation causing increased heart rate, increased blood pressure, and increased myocardial contractility that result in increased oxygen and cell nutrient demand. Progress is also being made in understanding the components of cigarette smoke that cause these changes (USDHHS 2010; USDHHS 2014).

The vascular endothelium is critical to normal cardiovascular functioning. Endothelial function requires nitric oxide, and cigarette smoking reduces nitric oxide availability both from exposure to the oxidants and free radicals in cigarette smoke and from free radicals produced by the endothelium itself as a result of smoking-induced enzyme activation within the endothelium. The reactive oxygen species contribute to endothelial dysfunction and they also result in the release of other chemicals, which leads to the expression of pro-inflammatory molecules. These processes result in increased platelet adhesion. Studies have shown that even brief exposure to secondhand smoke results in endothelial damage (USDHHS 2010; USDHHS 2014).

Cigarette smoking promotes thrombosis through multiple mechanisms that increase the number of mature platelets, activate platelets, promote platelet aggregation, increase platelet leukocyte aggregates, increase platelet–fibrinogen binding, increase thrombin and fibrinogen levels, reduce fibrinolysis, and promote the release of clotting factors. The binding of activated platelets to leukocytes causes both inflammatory and prothrombotic effects. Smoking also changes the platelet's membrane structure fluidity and the structure of the fibrin network. Research has also shown that exposure to secondhand smoke is associated with chronic inflammation and that even brief exposure to secondhand tobacco smoke results in a marked activation of platelets (USDHHS 2012; USDHHS 2014; Csordas and Bernhard 2013).

Inflammation plays an important role in the development of atherosclerosis and cardiovascular disease and smoking induces inflammation through multiple pathways. Cigarette smoking causes a chronic inflammatory response as evidenced by increased numbers of leukocytes, fibrinogen, and a variety of inflammatory chemicals. Smoking up-regulates inflammatory genes. Smoking also induces macrophages to release pro-inflammatory agents, reactive oxygen species, and proteolytic enzymes. Macrophage activation also increases the activity of enzymes that degrade collagen and contribute to unstable atherosclerotic plaques (USDHHS 2014).

Cigarette smoke also stimulates the accumulation of cholesterol within macrophages. In addition, nicotine increases heart rate, blood pressure, and the constriction of blood vessels, increasing cardiac demand for oxygen (USDHHS 2014).

Autopsy studies show that smoking in adolescence and young adulthood causes early abdominal aortic atherosclerosis in young adults (USDHHS 2012). Other mechanisms by which smoking might injure the abdominal aorta include chronic inflammation and damage to elastin (USDHHS 2010; USDHHS 2014). The chronic inflammatory state induced by smoking is also thought to be a critical element in the development, progression, and rupture of cerebral aneurysms, a process that results in intracranial hemorrhage (USDHHS 2014).

Cancer

Tobacco smoke contains more than 7,000 chemicals, and at least 70 of these can cause cancer (USDHHS 2010; IARC 2012). These include polycyclic aromatic hydrocarbons, tobacco-specific nitrosamines, aromatic amines, and volatile carcinogens such as formaldehyde, acetaldehyde, 1,3-butadiene, and benzene, as well as various metals (USDHHS 2014). Chemical analysis of the smoke from pipes, cigars, cigarettes, and hookah smoke shows that carcinogens are found in the smoke of all of these tobacco products.

Smokeless tobacco contains more than 4,000 chemicals and more than 30 carcinogens, and levels of tobacco-specific nitrosamines and other carcinogens in smokeless tobacco are often at levels hundreds of times higher than what foods and beverages may legally contain and may also be higher than the amounts found in cigarette smoke (NCI and CDC 2014; Rostron et al. 2015). Tobacco-specific nitrosamines are the most abundant strong carcinogens in smokeless tobacco, two of which are designated as Group 1 human carcinogens (i.e., the agent is definitely carcinogenic to humans) by the International Agency for Research on Cancer (IARC 2012). Smokeless tobacco also contains polonium-210, polynuclear aromatic hydrocarbons, heavy metals, and formaldehyde (NCI and CDC 2014).

More than 50 carcinogens have been identified in secondhand smoke. Secondhand smoke is also classified as a Group 1 carcinogen (USDHHS 2006). Secondhand smoke is qualitatively similar in composition to mainstream smoke, but many carcinogens found in mainstream smoke appear in greater concentration in secondhand smoke. These carcinogens are absorbed by humans at measurable doses. For example, exposure to secondhand smoke causes a significant increase in urinary levels of nitrosamine metabolites. The mechanisms by which secondhand smoke causes lung cancer are thought to be similar to those observed in smokers. The lower relative risk is attributable to the lower carcinogenic dose (USDHHS 2006). Levels of carcinogens are much lower in e-cigarettes compared with conventional cigarettes, but still higher compared with non–tobacco users.

Most constituents of cigarette smoke are metabolized by the body, a process that for these carcinogens, creates reactive compounds that can bind to DNA creating DNA adducts. If the DNA adducts are not fixed by the body's DNA repair enzymes, they can cause miscoding during DNA replication, which can result in a permanent mutation in the DNA sequence. If this mutation occurs in an important section of a cellular oncogene or in a tumor-suppressor gene, the result can be uncontrolled proliferation, further mutations, and cancer. Some constituents of tobacco smoke or their metabolites can also bind directly to cellular receptors, leading to activation of protein kinases, growth receptors, and other pathways that can cause cancer. The inflammation caused by tobacco smoke can promote tumor growth. Cigarette smoke also has co-carcinogens that enhance the smoke's carcinogenic effects. Furthermore, cigarette smoke induces oxidative damage and gene promoter methylation, which also likely contribute to cancer development (USDHHS 2014). Less direct mechanisms of cancer causation are also implicated. For example, smoking may act synergistically with *H. pylori*, a known cause of stomach cancer (IARC 2012).

Specific carcinogens found in tobacco and tobacco smoke have been linked with specific tobacco-related cancers. For example, nitrosamines, polyaromatic hydrocarbons, 1,3-butadiene, and cadmium cause lung cancer, and nitrosamines are implicated in oral cancer. Heterocyclic amines are intestinal carcinogens, furan is a liver carcinogen, aromatic amines are bladder carcinogens, and benzene, 1,3-butadiene, and formaldehyde are known to cause leukemia. Pancreatic cancer can be produced in animals with the tobacco-specific nitrosamine NNN (IARC 2012), nitrosamines have also been found in the cervical mucus (Prokopczyk et al. 1997), and smokers' cervical mucus is mutagenic (IARC 2012). Similarly, the urine of smokers is more mutagenic than the urine of nonsmokers (IARC 2012). Cigarette smoke is the major source of benzene exposure in the United States (Wallace 1996).

Chronic Lung and Other Respiratory Diseases

The pathogenesis of emphysema comprises four interrelated events: (1) chronic exposure to cigarette smoke leads to inflammatory and immune cell recruitment within the terminal airspaces of the lung; (2) these inflammatory cells release proteinases that damage the extracellular matrix of the lung; (3) endothelial cells and other structural cells undergo cell death because of oxidant stress and loss of matrix-cell attachment; and (4) ineffective repair of elastin and other extracellular matrix components result in airspace enlargement. For example, acrolein in cigarette smoke has been shown to exert its toxicity through oxidative damage and chronic inflammation in a feedback loop (Yeager et al. 2016). Eventually the inflammatory process becomes independent of smoking as the matrix fragments themselves can continue to drive the inflammation.

In addition, airway colonization by microorganisms also sustains the inflammation (USDHHS 2014). The airflow obstruction leads to hypoxemia, which is further exacerbated by the inhaled carbon monoxide from cigarette smoke (USDHHS 1984). Strong evidence demonstrates that active smoking across adolescence and young adulthood limits lung growth. Smokers also exhibit a more rapid, dose-related decline in pulmonary function with age than do nonsmokers (USDHHS 1984; USDHHS 2012). Smoking also decreases tracheal mucus velocity, increases mucus secretion, causes chronic airway inflammation and exaggerated airway responsiveness, increases epithelial permeability, and damages parenchymal cells (USDHHS 1990).

The Surgeon General has concluded that there is a causal relationship between active smoking and wheezing severe enough to be diagnosed as asthma in susceptible child and adolescent populations. The Surgeon General has also concluded that smoking causes active primary tuberculosis, recurrent tuberculosis, and other pulmonary infections, including 12,500 deaths (22% of the total number) each year from pneumonia, influenza, and tuberculosis (USDHHS 2014). It is believed that the effects of smoking on the immune system is the reason for the increased risk for these diseases in smokers. However, the specific mechanisms by which cigarette smoking influences the risk of infection and, in the case of TB, reactivation of latent TB infection, are not completely understood (USDHHS 2014).

There are multiple mechanisms by which secondhand smoke causes injury to the respiratory tract. Increased airway wall thickness has been reported in infants exposed to maternal smoking, and secondhand smoke increases bronchial hyperreactivity in children and adults. Altered immune responses may also play a role in secondhand smoke–induced asthma exacerbation and enhanced susceptibility to respiratory infections (USDHHS 2006).

Reproductive Outcomes

Cigarette smoking is estimated to cause more than 1,600 deaths each year from prenatal and perinatal adverse outcomes. Although the mechanisms by which tobacco use causes the known adverse reproductive outcomes is not fully understood, it has been hypothesized that exposure to cigarette smoke results in fetal growth restriction through hypoxia caused by the products of combustion (e.g., carbon monoxide), nicotine-mediated vasoconstriction of uteroplacental vessels, or both. For example, genes that encode enzymes associated with the metabolism of other compounds found in tobacco smoke, such as nitrosamines and polycyclic aromatic hydrocarbons, have been associated with preterm delivery and restricted fetal growth.

Smokeless tobacco use has also been associated with an increase in the risk for being small for gestational age, suggesting that nicotine makes a modest contribution to the effects of tobacco use on fetal growth, but that there is a larger contribution for nicotine combined with the products of combustion in tobacco smoke. Nicotine may also be implicated in stillbirth and perinatal mortality. Maternal use of smokeless tobacco increases the risk of infant apnea to the same extent as maternal smoking. Data suggest that nicotinic acetylcholine receptors in the brainstem control cardiopulmonary integration and arousal in early life. Nicotine also appears to affect adrenal maturation, resulting in a blunted adrenal protective response to hypoxia. An impaired response to hypoxia and impaired arousal may also explain the causal relationship between prenatal and postnatal exposure to tobacco smoke and SIDS (USDHSS 2014).

Possible mechanisms for congenital malformations include maternal smoking interfering with normal organ development in offspring through fetal hypoxia, alterations in essential nutrients, teratogenic effects, and DNA damage. Smoke constituents of concern include carbon monoxide, nicotine, cadmium, and polyaromatic hydrocarbons (USDHHS 2014).

Other Adverse Health Outcomes

Inflammation, oxidative stress, vascular insufficiency, and hypoxia are all potential contributors to smoking-caused age-related macular degeneration (USDHHS 2014). Many aromatic compounds and trace metals in cigarette smoke are capable of damaging lens proteins, but generally cadmium, lead, thiocyanate, and aldehydes are the most frequently linked to lens damage and cataracts (USDHHS 2004).

With regard to periodontal disease, some evidence indicates that smokers may be more likely than nonsmokers to harbor specific periodontal pathogens. There is substantial evidence that smoking affects both localized and systemic components of the immune system, but the link between this effect and periodontal disease has not been established. Research has also suggested that the peripheral vasoconstrictive effect of tobacco smoke and nicotine reduces gingival blood flow and thereby impairs the delivery of oxygen and nutrients to gingival tissue and there is some evidence of reduced blood flow in gingival tissues. Research has also suggested that reduced repair capacity was likely the major mechanism involved in smoking-associated periodontal destruction (USDHHS 2014).

Cigarette smoking is estimated to cause 9,000 deaths (13% of the total number) from diabetes each year (USDHHS 2014). There are multiple mechanisms through which smoking could cause diabetes. First, although smokers tend to be thinner than nonsmokers, many studies have shown that smoking is independently associated with an increased risk of central obesity, and central obesity is a well-established risk factor for insulin resistance and diabetes. Second, smoking increases inflammatory markers, increases oxidative stress, and impairs endothelial function, all mechanisms that are related to the development of insulin resistance and irregularities in glucose metabolism. Third, nicotine has been shown to aggravate insulin resistance, and cigarette smoking has been shown to worsen metabolic control. Finally, neuronal nicotinic acetylcholine receptors are present on pancreatic islet and beta cells and nicotine can reduce the release of insulin from the islet cells (USDHHS 2014).

There are multiple constituents in tobacco smoke that can alter immune function. These include nicotine (which affects cellular immunity either directly through nicotinic cholinergic receptors or indirectly through its effect on the nervous system), acrolein (which has potent suppressive effects on immune cells), and polyaromatic hydrocarbons (which cause both proinflammatory and immunosuppressive effects). Alteration of the immune system, including stimulating autoimmunity, is believed to contribute to why smoking is a causal factor for rheumatoid arthritis (USDHHS 2014).

Although the mechanisms are not fully understood, multiple mechanisms have some data supporting their contribution to smoking-induced erectile dysfunction. These include endothelial dysfunction, reduced endothelial synthesis or neuronal transmission of nitric oxide (the principal mediator of penile erection), oxidative stress, and nicotine-induced vasoconstriction (USDHHS 2014).

Similarly, multiple mechanisms appear to be involved with smoking-attributable hip fractures, including toxic effects of nicotine or cadmium on bone, decreased intestinal calcium absorption, reduced intake and lower levels of vitamin D, altered metabolism of adrenal cortical and gonadal hormones, and reduced bone density because of lower body weight, earlier menopause (from lower levels of estrogen), and the reduced physical activity of smokers (USDHHS 2004).

Nicotine Dependence

In alkaline media, the nicotine molecule is un-ionized and readily absorbed. Thus, inhaled smoke is easily absorbed from the lung, smokeless tobacco's alkaline pH facilitates absorption from the mouth, and nicotine can be absorbed orally from unlit cigars as well as through inhaled smoke. Nicotine distributes rapidly to the brain whether administered orally or by inhalation. For example, when tobacco smoke is inhaled, nicotine is absorbed into the arterial bloodstream and reaches the brain within 10 seconds. Nicotine then crosses the blood–brain barrier and binds to specific receptors in the brain, resulting in the release of neurotransmitters and other chemicals, including acetylcholine, serotonin, dopamine, gamma aminobutyric acid, endogenous opioid peptides, pituitary hormones, and catecholamines (USDHHS 1988).

Nicotine is a psychoactive drug with stimulant and depressive effects. Nicotine's effects depend on the dose, rates of administration and elimination, and tolerance level of the person. Smokers dose themselves throughout the day, maintaining blood levels sufficient for them to avoid withdrawal symptoms. Smokeless tobacco users also maintain sustained levels of blood nicotine. Absorption is slower than with cigarettes, but more prolonged (USDHHS 1988).

Adolescents appear to be particularly vulnerable to the adverse effects of nicotine on the brain. Based on our knowledge of adolescent brain development, results of animal studies, and some data from studies of adolescent and young adult smokers, it is likely that nicotine exposure during adolescence adversely affects cognitive development (USDHHS 2014).

Abstinence regularly produces a withdrawal syndrome that is attenuated by re-administration of nicotine. Among nicotine-dependent tobacco users, withdrawal symptoms (craving for nicotine; irritability, frustration, or anger; anxiety; difficulty concentrating; restlessness; decreased heart rate; increased appetite; and weight gain) begin within 24 hours of cessation and peak within a few days. Acute symptoms may persist for 10 days or more, but cravings for tobacco can persist for years. There is also a behavioral component to nicotine dependence. For regular smokers in particular, smoking has become so intertwined with activities of daily living, resulting in multiple "cues" each day that can trigger cravings and relapse (USDHHS 1988).

Descriptive Epidemiology

High-Risk Populations

Cigarette Smoking

In 2014, an estimated 40 million American adults (16.8%) were current smokers (ever smoked 100 cigarettes and smoked every day or some days at the time of the survey). Smoking prevalence was higher for men (18.8%) than for women (14.8%; Table 7-3). By age, prevalence was highest among those aged 25 to 44 years (20.0%). Smoking prevalence was 9.5% among Asians, 11.2% among Hispanics, 17.5% among African Americans, 18.2% among whites, and 29.2% among American Indians and Alaska Natives. Formal educational attainment is strongly associated with smoking prevalence and cessation rates. In 2014, smoking prevalence was highest among people with a general educational development degree (GED; 43.2%) and those with 9 to 11 years of education (29.5%) and only a high-school diploma (21.7%); and lowest for persons with an undergraduate (7.9%) or graduate (5.4%) degree (CDC 2015b). In 2014, smoking prevalence was higher for persons living below the poverty level (26.3%) than for those living at or above that level (15.2%). In 2014, current smoking was also higher among persons who identified as gay, lesbian, or bisexual (23.9%), compared with those who identified as straight (16.6%; CDC 2015b).

In 2012, the percentage of ever smokers aged 18 years and older who had quit was 55.3% for men and 54.8% for women and 57.1% for whites, 53.6% for Hispanics, 51.8% for Asians, 44.1% for African Americans, and 48.2% for American Indians and Alaska Natives (USDHHS 2014). In 2012, the percentage of ever smokers who had quit was lowest among the group with 9 to 11 years of education (43.5%) and highest among persons with a college degree or greater (73.9%; USDHHS 2014).

In 2014, it was estimated that, on average, every day 2,600 youths aged younger than 18 years smoked their first cigarette (SAMHSA 2014a). Tobacco use generally begins in early adolescence and, among those who had ever

Table 7-3. Percentage of Persons Aged 18 Years and Older Who Were Current Cigarette Smokers, by Sex and Selected Characteristics, National Health Interview Survey, United States, 2014

Characteristics	Men, %	Women, %	Total, %
Race/ethnicity			
White, non-Hispanic	19.3	17.2	18.2
African American, non-Hispanic	22.1	13.7	17.5
Hispanic	14.8	7.6	11.2
American Indian/Alaska Native, non-Hispanic	25.6	32.5	29.2
Asian, non-Hispanic	14.5	5.1	9.5
Education			
0–12 years (no diploma)	26.6	19.5	22.9
≤8 years	16.4	11.3	13.7
9–11 years	33.3	25.9	29.5
12 years (no diploma)	29.8	21.0	25.7
GED	46.6	38.9	43.0
High-school graduate	24.7	18.8	21.7
Some college	19.8	19.6	19.7
Associate degree	21.2	13.7	17.1
Undergraduate degree	9.1	6.9	7.9
Graduate degree	5.8	5.0	5.4
Age group, years			
18–24	18.5	14.8	16.7
25–44	22.9	17.2	20.0
45–64	19.4	16.8	18.0
≥ 65	9.8	7.5	8.5
Poverty status			
At or above	17.5	13.1	15.2
Below	30.4	23.3	26.3
Unknown	14.9	17.7	16.4
Total	18.8	14.8	16.8

Source: Adapted from CDC (2015b).
Note: For detailed footnotes and 95% confidence intervals, see Table, Percentage of adults who were current cigarette smokers, by selected characteristics—National Health Interview Survey, United States, 2005 and 2014, in CDC (2015b).

smoked cigarettes daily, almost 80% first tried a cigarette before age 18 years. Little initiation occurs after age 24 years and essentially none after age 30 years (USDHHS 2014). In 2015, 9.3% of high-school students and 2.3% of middle-school students were current cigarette smokers (had smoked in the past 30 days), corresponding to about 1.6 million adolescents. Among high-school students, the prevalence of cigarette smoking was higher for boys (10.7%) than girls (7.7%) and lower for non-Hispanic black students (5.7%), compared to non-Hispanic white (10.2%) and Hispanic (9.0%) students. Among middle-school students, prevalence of cigarette smoking was comparable between boys (2.3%) and girls (2.2%; Singh et al. 2016).

Use of Other Tobacco Products

In recent years, the marketplace for tobacco products has become increasingly diverse, with the introduction of new tobacco products, such as e-cigarettes, and the re-emergence of traditional products, such as certain types of cigars. The Population Assessment of Tobacco and Health (PATH) Study is a nationally representative longitudinal cohort study of approximately 46,000 Americans that provides a comprehensive assessment of tobacco use in the United States, its determinants, and its impacts. According to the PATH Study, in 2013–2014, the prevalence of current use of any tobacco products among adults aged 18 years and older was 27.6%. After cigarettes, the most commonly reported tobacco products used every day or on some days were cigars including traditional cigars, cigarillos, and filtered cigars (7.8%), followed by e-cigarettes (5.5%), hookah (4.2%), smokeless tobacco (3.4%), and pipe tobacco (1.1%). Whereas the overwhelming majority of adult cigarette smokers are daily smokers, many of the other products are more likely to be used on a nondaily basis (Hyland et al. 2016).

In the PATH Study, the prevalence of current cigar smoking among men (12.8%) is greater than among women (3.3%), as is the prevalence of current smokeless tobacco use (6.7% in men vs. 0.4% in women). The prevalence of current use of e-cigarettes and hookah is more comparable in men and women (e-cigarettes: 6.2% in men vs. 5.0% in women; hookah: 5.0% in men vs. 3.4% in women). For all products other than cigarettes, the prevalence of current use in young adults aged 18 to 24 years is equal to or higher than other age groups. This difference in prevalence by age is particularly pronounced for hookah smoking, with hookah use higher than the use of any other tobacco product, except for cigarette smoking, among 18- to 24-year-olds. A substantial proportion of adult tobacco users report the current use of more than one tobacco product. In 2013–2014, almost 40% of current tobacco users reported using more than one product, with the most common combination being cigarettes and e-cigarettes (Hyland et al. 2016).

In 2014, it was estimated, on average, that almost 2,600 youths aged younger than 18 years smoked their first cigar and 1,300 youths under the age of 18 tried smokeless tobacco for the first time (SAMHSA 2014b). In 2015, 16.0% of high-school students in the United States reported past-30-day e-cigarette use, followed by cigarettes (9.3%), cigars (8.6%), hookah (7.2%), and smokeless tobacco products (6.0%). A similar pattern was observed for middle-school students. Among high-school students, e-cigarettes were the most widely used tobacco product among non-Hispanic white (17.2%) and Hispanic students (16.4%). Among non-Hispanic blacks, however, cigars were the most prevalent product used (12.8%). Among high-school students, boys were more likely than girls to use e-cigarettes, cigars, and smokeless tobacco, whereas current use of hookah was comparable between boys and girls. Overall, in 2015, 25.3% of high-school students (3.8 million) and 7.4% of middle-school students (880,000) reported past-30-day use of any tobacco product and 13.0% of high-school and 3.3% of middle-school students reported past-30-day use of two or more tobacco products* (Singh et al. 2016).

Geographic Distribution

In 2013, adult smoking prevalence varied substantially by state, ranging from 10.3% in Utah to 27.3% in West Virginia. Even greater geographic variation is observed for adult male smokeless tobacco use, with prevalence ranging from 2.5% in New Jersey and the District of Columbia to 18.2% in West Virginia (CDC 2016f). Youth tobacco prevalence data are not available for all states, but in 2013, cigarette smoking prevalence among high-school students ranged from 4.4% in Utah to 19.6% in West Virginia (41 states reporting); current cigar use ranged from 4.1% in Utah to 17.1% in Arkansas (36 states reporting); and current smokeless tobacco use ranged from 2.6% in Utah to 15.9% in West Virginia (38 states reporting; Kann et al. 2014).

Time Trends

Adults

In the early part of the 20th century, the predominant forms of tobacco used by Americans were chewing tobacco, pipes, and cigars (USDHHS 2014). The first half of the 20th century saw a dramatic increase in annual per capita

---

*Tobacco products in this survey included e-cigarettes, hookah, cigarettes, cigars, smokeless tobacco, snus, pipes, bidis, and dissolvable tobacco.

consumption of cigarettes to a peak of 4,345 in 1963, corresponding to more than half a pack a day per person in the United States. Except for an increase from 1971 through 1973, consumption has steadily declined since then (Figure 7-4). Per capita cigarette consumption was 1,232 in 2011, the lowest level in more than 70 years.

Over the same time period, consumption of cigars and loose tobacco has increased, in part because of tax differentials between cigarettes, large cigars, and pipe tobacco (CDC 2012a). Total consumption of cigars increased from 6.2 billion sticks in 2000 to 13.7 billion in 2011, in part because of the rise in smaller little filtered cigars and cigarillos, compared with the historical dominance of large, traditional cigars. Total consumption of loose tobacco (i.e., roll-your-own cigarette tobacco and pipe tobacco) increased from 9 billion cigarette equivalents in 2000 to 20 billion in 2011. As a result, total consumption of combustible tobacco (i.e., cigarettes, cigars, pipe tobacco, and roll-your-own cigarette tobacco) declined over this period, but not at the same rate as the substantial decline observed for cigarettes (CDC 2012a).

In recent years, sales of smokeless tobacco products have increased in the United States. According to an analysis of U.S. convenience store sales data compiled by Nielsen Research Company, unit sales of smokeless tobacco products increased by 56.8% from 2005 to 2011 (Delnevo et al. 2014). Growth in unit sales was driven by moist snuff products, which accounted for more than 90% of the convenience store sales market. Less than 10% of the market was

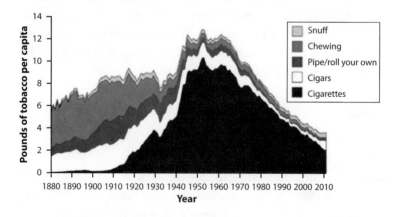

Source: Reprinted from USDHHS (2014).

Figure 7-4. Per Capita Consumption of Different Forms of Tobacco in the United States, 1880–2011

made up of chewing tobacco, snus, dry snuff, and dissolvable tobacco products (Delnevo et al. 2014). In recent years, sales of e-cigarettes have grown dramatically. Between 2012 and 2013, sales of e-cigarettes in traditional U.S. retail channels more than doubled (Giovenco et al. 2015). According to the market research firm, Euromonitor International (2016), in 2015, e-liquids was the fastest-growing individual "vapor product" category, with a 57% value sales increase to reach U.S. $1.0 billion. This contrasted significantly with "vapor products" as a whole, which grew by 29% to reach U.S. $3.5 billion in 2015.

Cigarette smoking prevalence among adults has declined dramatically from 42.4% in 1965 to 16.8% in 2014 (CDC 2016e). Before 1964, the prevalence of smoking among men had already begun to decline, while smoking among women was on the rise (USDHHS 2014). Although men historically had much higher smoking prevalence than women, the gap narrowed over time as more women started smoking and a greater decline in smoking prevalence was observed among men. Since about 1985, declines in smoking prevalence are occurring at a comparable rate for women and men (USDHHS 2014). Although some differences in the rate of smoking prevalence declines have been observed by race/ethnicity, prevalence has nonetheless declined substantially in African Americans, whites, and Hispanics from 1965 to 2011. Smoking prevalence has declined fastest for persons with 16 or more years of education and slowest for persons with 9 to 11 years of education (USDHHS 2014). The prevalence of daily smoking has declined considerably, as well. From 1991 to 2011, the prevalence of daily smoking declined by 7.8 percentage points in men and 6.8 percentage points in women (USDHHS 2014).

According to estimates from the National Health Interview Survey, the prevalence of smokeless tobacco use every day or some days among U.S. adult males decreased from 1987 to 2000, but has increased slightly between 2000 and 2010, particularly among those aged 18 to 24 years (USDHHS 2014). During the same time period, smokeless tobacco use among women has remained extremely low. Similarly, the prevalence of current cigar smoking among women in the United States has remained very low, while the prevalence of adult cigar smoking has remained relatively stable since the late 1990s (USDHHS 2014).

Youths

The prevalence of current smoking (smoking within the past 30 days) among high-school seniors decreased from 37% in 1975 to 29% in 1981, was then relatively stable until 1992, increased to 36% by 1997, and then decreased to 11.4%

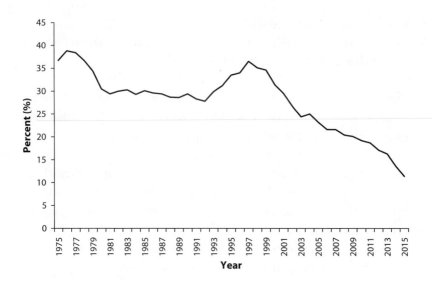

Source: Data from University of Michigan (2015).

Figure 7-5. Trends in Current (Past-30-Day) Cigarette Smoking by High-School Seniors, United States, 1975–2015

in 2015 (Figure 7-5). Similarly, prevalence among 10th graders increased from 21% in 1991 to 30% in 1996 and then decreased to 6% in 2015. The prevalence of smoking among eighth graders increased from 14% in 1991 to 21% in 1996 and then decreased to 4% in 2015. Similar patterns were seen for daily smoking. A larger decline in current smoking prevalence occurred among African American high-school students from 1977 to 1992 (37% to 9%) than among white high-school students (38% to 32%). Smoking prevalence among African American high-school students increased to 15% in 1998 but then decreased to 7% in 2015. Among high-school seniors, smoking prevalence was higher for girls than for boys until 1990; since 1991, it has been somewhat higher for boys than girls (University of Michigan 2015).

Among middle- and high-school students in the United States, overall tobacco use has remained stable over the past several years; however, the types of products used have shifted dramatically (Figure 7-6). For example, from 2011 through 2015 among high-school students, the prevalence (past-30-day use) of cigarette smoking dropped from 15.8% to 9.3%, the prevalence of cigar smoking dropped from 11.6% to 8.6%, and the prevalence of smokeless tobacco use dropped from 7.9% to 6.0%. Conversely, the current use of e-cigarettes rose dramatically, from 1.5% to 16.0% and the current use of hookahs rose from

4.1% to 7.2%. As a result, e-cigarettes are now the most widely used tobacco product among high-school students in the United States. Similar findings were observed among middle-school students (Singh et al. 2016).

Causes of Smoking Initiation

Modifiable Risk Factors

No single factor causes a young person to begin using tobacco. The factors that influence the likelihood that an adolescent or young adult will experiment with tobacco, become an intermittent user, progress to regular use, or become dependent are multifactorial and may operate at different levels of influence. Important factors associated with trial or progression to regular use include demographic characteristics and intrapersonal factors (such as age, gender,

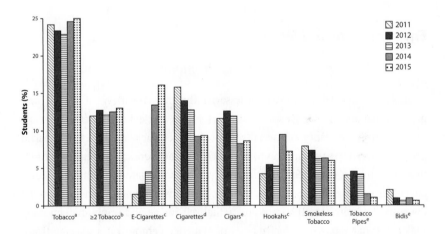

Source: Data from CDC (2016g).
aTobacco is use of cigarettes, cigars, smokeless tobacco, e-cigarettes, hookahs, tobacco pipes, and/or bidis.
b≥2 tobacco is defined as preceding 30-day use of two or more of the following product types: cigarettes, cigars, smokeless tobacco, e-cigarettes, hookahs, tobacco pipes and/or bidis.
cNonlinear increase ($p < 0.05$).
dLinear decrease ($p < 0.05$).
eNonlinear decrease ($p < 0.05$).

Figure 7-6. Percentage of High-School Students Who Used Tobacco in the Preceding 30 Days, by Tobacco Product, National Youth Tobacco Survey, 2011–2015

socioeconomic status [SES], race/ethnicity, negative affect, poor academic achievement, and genetic factors), social or normative influences (such as peer and familial influences and perceived norms related to tobacco use), and cultural or environmental influences (such as the marketing of tobacco products and countermarketing efforts, portrayal of tobacco in the popular culture, accessibility of tobacco products, and policies aimed to reduce access to exposure to tobacco product marketing and secondhand smoke).

It is generally believed that the social and environmental influences are more likely to influence trying and experimenting with tobacco, and intrapersonal factors are more likely to predict frequent use, when development of nicotine dependence plays a larger role (USDHHS 2012). However, it is important to note that there is considerable variation in the trajectories of tobacco initiation and uptake of regular use and the factors that drive the development of tobacco use behavior in youths and young adults (see, for example, Fuemmeler et al. 2013).

Environmental Influences

Tobacco Industry Advertising and Promotion

Youths are exposed to tobacco messages through a variety of media and promotional activities (e.g., sponsorship of events and entertainment, point-of-sale displays, distribution of specialty items, Internet, social media, etc.). Tobacco product advertising uses images to portray the attractiveness and perceived function of smoking (independence, maturity, slimness, glamour, self-confidence, adventure seeking, and youthful activities). Such advertisements capitalize on the disparity between a youth's ideal and actual self-image and imply that smoking may close that gap. An extensive body of evidence demonstrates the significant role that marketing plays on awareness of smoking, brand recognition, attitudes, intentions, and smoking initiation among adolescents (USDHHS 2012).

In 2013, almost $9 billion was spent to market cigarettes in the United States (FTC 2016a) and another $503 million was spent on smokeless tobacco product marketing (FTC 2016b). As increasing restrictions have limited the ability of the tobacco industry to advertise in some traditional channels, the majority of promotional expenditures were spent on efforts to reduce the price of cigarettes, including price discounts, promotions, and coupons. Tobacco industry discounting strategies (e.g., coupons, two-for-one offers) reduce the price of tobacco products and lower prices correlate with increased use by adolescents and young adults. Younger smokers are more likely than older smokers to use price discounts (Pierce et al. 2005; White et al. 2006).

Studies show an association among advertising expenditures and youth brand preference, tobacco marketing exposure and initiation, and favorable beliefs toward smoking in response to marketing exposure (Pechman and Ratneshawr 1994; Pierce et al. 1994; Pierce et al. 1998; Pollay et al. 1996; USDHHS 1994; USDHHS 2012). The Surgeon General, the Institute of Medicine (IOM), the U.S. Food and Drug Administration (FDA), the National Cancer Institute (NCI), and the U.K. Scientific Committee on Tobacco and Health have all concluded that tobacco marketing influences young people to smoke (FDA 1996; Lynch and Bonnie 1994; Scientific Committee on Tobacco and Health 1998; USDHHS 1994; USDHHS 2001; USDHHS 2012; NCI 2008). A systematic review reported in the Cochrane Database of Systematic Reviews evaluated 19 longitudinal studies and concluded that "tobacco advertising and promotion increases the likelihood that adolescents will start to smoke" (Lovato et al. 2011). Teens appear to be three times more sensitive to cigarette advertising than adults (Pollay et al. 1996). One study reported that teens were more likely to be influenced to smoke by tobacco advertising than by peer pressure (Evans et al. 1995).

Data from the National Youth Tobacco Survey has demonstrated continued significant exposure to tobacco marketing among adolescents. From 2000 to 2012, the percentage of middle- and high-school students in the United States exposed to tobacco advertisements through the Internet increased from 22.3% to 43.0%, while the percentage exposed through newspapers or magazines (65.0% to 36.9%) and at retail stores (87.8% to 76.2%) declined over the same period. For all three channels, exposure to tobacco advertising remains above Healthy People 2020 goals (Agaku et al. 2014a). Recent data also demonstrated widespread exposure to marketing of e-cigarettes among adolescents. In 2014, it was estimated that 68.9% of middle- and high-school students (18.3 million) were exposed to e-cigarette advertisements through one of the following sources: retail stores, Internet, TV and movies, and newspaper and magazines (Singh et al. 2016). This widespread exposure to marketing has coincided with e-cigarettes becoming the most widely used tobacco product among middle- and high-school students in the United States.

Several prevention campaigns of the tobacco industry have been shown to increase youth smoking. For example, those exposed to the Philip Morris "Think Don't Smoke" campaign were more likely to be open to the possibility of smoking (Farrelly et al. 2002). Youths exposed to tobacco industry parent-targeted advertisements (such as the Philip Morris "Talk to Your Kids" campaign) had lower perceived harm of smoking, stronger approval of smoking, stronger intentions to smoke in the future, and greater likelihood of having smoked in the past 30 days (Wakefield et al. 2006). Another study showed that tobacco company prevention ads engendered more favorable attitudes toward tobacco companies among adolescents (Henriksen et al. 2006).

Smoking in Entertainment Media

Smoking in the movies has emerged as a tobacco control issue. Several studies have reported that exposure to smoking in the movies increases youth initiation, particularly among adolescents with nonsmoking parents (Dalton et al. 2003; Distefan et al. 2004). A recent meta-analysis found a nearly two-fold increase in the likelihood of smoking onset and current or established smoking among youths and young adults associated with increased exposure to smoking in movies (USDHHS 2012). The Surgeon General's report on preventing tobacco use in youths and young adults concludes that "there is a causal relationship between depictions of smoking in the movies and the initiation of smoking among young people" (USDHHS 2012). Smoking in the United States has declined since the 1950s, and smoking in the movies likewise decreased from 1950 to 1980–1982; however, it rebounded to 1950 levels in 2002 (10.9 incidents per hour; Glantz et al. 2004). From 2002 to 2015, the total number of tobacco incidents in youth-rated movies dropped by approximately half. However, almost 60% of PG-13 movies still showed smoking or other tobacco use (CDC 2016a).

Access to Tobacco Products

Although the majority of adolescent tobacco users report obtaining tobacco products from social sources (Tanski et al. 2016), and retailers are prohibited from selling cigarettes and other tobacco products to minors, tobacco products are still accessible to youths from a variety of sources. According to the 2012 National Youth Tobacco Survey, 20% of 15- to 17-year-old smokers reported buying a pack of cigarettes themselves and about 37% reported having someone else buy a pack of cigarettes for them. Among high-school cigar smokers, 31.4% reported buying it themselves and 25.5% reported asking someone else to buy it for them (IOM 2015). According to the PATH study, the primary retail locations for cigarette, cigarillo, and smokeless tobacco purchases by or for adolescents (ages 15 to 17 years) are gas stations and convenience stores. Conversely, e-cigarettes and hookah are more likely to be purchased in specialty tobacco shops, smoke shops, and hookah bars or cafes (Tanski et al. 2016). Studies have shown that active enforcement of minimum age policies increase retailer compliance and reduce tobacco availability to youths. Although increased compliance is associated with an increase in the use of social sources, evidence suggests that this replacement is incomplete, therefore resulting in an overall reduction in accessibility and use (IOM 2015).

Social and Normative Influences

Youth tobacco use behavior is influenced by societal norms, local community norms, parental and family behavior, and peer behavior. Social norms change over time. Smoking has gone from a common, accepted behavior to a less frequent and increasingly restricted one. However, community norms, such as living in a tobacco-producing state, clearly influence both youth and adult prevalence (CDC 2009). Countermarketing campaigns help change social norms. There is also some evidence that smoke-free laws challenge the perception of smoking as a normal adult behavior (Siegel et al. 2005).

Parental smoking increases the likelihood of children smoking by modeling the behavior and providing easy access to tobacco. Having several close friends who smoke is also associated with smoking among adolescents (USDHHS 1994; USDHHS 2012), likely due both to nonsmokers starting smoking as a result of their friends smoking and the adolescents who smoke starting to associate with other smokers. Youths tend to overestimate the prevalence of smoking among their peers and this overestimation has been shown to be associated with smoking initiation (USDHHS 2012). Religious participation has generally been shown to protect against tobacco use, because of direct religious prohibitions or social influences that tend to promote healthier behaviors (USDHHS 2012).

Similarly, for smokeless tobacco use, perceived approval of use by parents and peers; easy access to the product; use of cigarettes, alcohol, marijuana, or other drugs; engaging in other risky behaviors; living with someone else who uses smokeless tobacco; and having peers who use smokeless tobacco increase the risk of its use by young people (USDHHS 1994). Lower price also increases smokeless tobacco use (Ohsfeldt et al. 1997). Smokeless tobacco use is also more strongly associated with sports, such as baseball. A recent analysis of the National Youth Tobacco Survey found that high-school athletes were almost twice as likely to use smokeless tobacco as non-athletes (Agaku et al. 2015).

Intrapersonal Influences

Individual Psychosocial Factors

Individual risk factors for tobacco use include weaker attachment to parents and family, strong attachment to peers and friends, perception that smoking is more common than is actually true, risk taking and rebelliousness, weaker commitment to school and religion, the belief that smoking can control weight and moods, and having a positive image of smokers (USDHHS 2001). A consistent association has been found between negative affect and adolescent smoking, which may be bidirectional (i.e., negative affect can facilitate continued smoking, and prospective studies have found that smoking during adolescence predicts onset of negative mood and depressive symptoms; USDHHS 2012).

Personal Characteristics

Age, gender, and parental education and income are important predictors of adolescent tobacco use. Although the prevalence of smoking is relatively similar among boys and girls, boys are much more likely to be smokeless tobacco users and cigar smokers (Singh et al. 2016). Racial/ethnic differences have been observed in the types of tobacco products used by adolescents. For example, African-American high-school students are less likely to be cigarette smokers, e-cigarette users, and smokeless tobacco users, compared with White and Hispanic youths, but are more likely to be cigar smokers (Singh et al. 2016). Although the relationships between tobacco use and sexual identity have not been well studied in adolescents, young adult sexual minorities (particularly women) are more likely to report cigarette smoking than straight adults (Johnson et al. 2016).

Tobacco Product Design

Product design features may influence the likelihood that nonusers experiment with and continue to use tobacco products. For example, tobacco products can contain chemicals, such as ammonia, that increase the proportion of free nicotine available, which is more easily absorbed by the body. Filter tip ventilation can also increase free nicotine and reduces the harshness of cigarette smoking (USDHHS 2010). Many tobacco products are available in flavors that appeal to youths and young adults, and the presence of flavors in combusted tobacco products have been shown to mask the harshness and irritation associated with their use. Several recent studies have observed high levels of the use of flavored tobacco products among adolescent tobacco users. For example, in the 2014 National Youth Tobacco Survey, 70% of middle- and high-school students currently using tobacco products reported using flavored products in the past 30 days (Corey et al. 2015). In another national study, almost 80% of past-30-day adolescent tobacco users reported the use of flavored tobacco products. In addition, approximately 80% of adolescents who ever tried a tobacco product reported that the first product they used was flavored (Ambrose et al. 2015).

Nicotine Dependence

Nicotine dependence is the predominant reason for the continuation and maintenance of tobacco use. However, recent research suggests that, for some adolescents, symptoms of nicotine dependence can develop early in the process of smoking initiation and at relatively low levels of use. One tool that has been validated to assess dependence among adolescents is the Hooked on Nicotine Checklist (HONC). In a recent study conducted in a Florida high school, investigators found that 56% of smokeless tobacco users and 57% of smokers that reported smoking fewer than 100 cigarettes in their lifetime, endorsed one or more of the HONC symptoms (DiFranza et al. 2012). A recent national study of middle- and high-school users of cigarettes, cigars, or smokeless tobacco found that more than 40% of past-30-day users reported recent strong cravings to use tobacco (Apelberg et al. 2014). Among the factors that were associated with increased reporting of dependence symptoms were use of more than one tobacco product, greater frequency of use, earlier age at initiation, and being female (Apelberg et al. 2014). Emerging evidence suggests that the adolescent brain may be particularly vulnerable to the addictive properties of nicotine, including through alterations in structure and function that may influence lifelong susceptibility to addiction (USDHHS 2012).

Perceptions of Health Risks and Risk of Dependence

Youths do not fully understand the risks of tobacco use. A 1999 survey of youths aged 14 to 22 years reported that 40% of smokers and 25% of nonsmokers underestimated or did not know the likelihood of smoking-related deaths; more than 40% did not know or underestimated the number of years of life lost to smoking. Young people assume that they will stop before harmful effects occur and do not believe that they personally are at risk from tobacco use (Romer and Jamieson 2001). About one quarter of middle- and high-school students in the United States believe that intermittent smoking causes little or no harm (Amrock and Weitzman 2015). Youths also underestimate the risks of becoming addicted to nicotine and do not expect to continue to smoke (USDHHS 1994). It may be only after the first failed quit attempt that youths realize they are nicotine-dependent and that quitting will not be easy.

Products that are viewed as potentially "safer" can influence youth behavior. For example, youths who smoke low-tar cigarettes reported that they thought these products were safer, less addictive, and easier to quit than regular cigarettes (Kropp and Halpern-Felsher 2004). There has been a rapid increase in e-cigarette use by youths, and although "they come in flavors I like" was the most commonly cited reason for use, the second and third most common reasons were "I use [the product] because they might be less harmful to me than cigarettes" (79%) and "I use [the product] because they might be less harmful to people around me than cigarettes" (78%; Ambrose et al. 2015). The belief that they are not harming themselves and can easily quit when they want could lead to greater youth tobacco use.

Causes of Smoking Continuation

The development of nicotine dependence is the predominant reason for the continued and sustained use of tobacco through adulthood. Societal factors also influence continued tobacco use, including the perception that some tobacco products are safer, tobacco industry advertising and promotion, inadequate understanding of the health risks, social norms around tobacco use, and lower prices for tobacco products. These factors are summarized briefly in the next paragraphs.

Nicotine Dependence

In the United States, the majority of smokers regret ever having started, and report wanting to quit and making at least one quit attempt in the past year; however, the percentage who successfully quit each year is low (Fong et al.

2004; CDC 2011). Nicotine, a psychoactive substance present in all tobacco products, is the primary reason why individuals persist in their use of tobacco (USDHHS 2010). According to the U.S. Surgeon General, the factors that influence developing nicotine dependence include

> (1) the effects of the product itself, including the addictive constituents, their phar-
> macokinetics and pharmacodynamics, and the design of the product that delivers
> the addictive constituents; (2) the response of the host, including genetic suscepti-
> bility and physiological response; and (3) the environmental setting that deter-
> mines the availability of, accessibility to, and norms for use of the product
> (USDHHS 2010).

One measure of nicotine dependence that predicts future cessation is earlier time to first cigarette in the morning (Baker et al. 2007). In the United States, about two thirds of daily smokers report smoking a cigarette within the first 30 minutes of waking (Rodu et al. 2015). The extent of nicotine addiction in users of other tobacco products is influenced, in part, by the amount of nicotine present and bioavailable in different tobacco products and how it is delivered to the body (USDHHS 2010). However, almost 40% of adult tobacco users use more than one type of product (Hyland et al. 2016), which may serve to sustain nicotine exposure and contribute to maintaining tobacco dependence.

Incomplete Understanding of Health Risks

Data from the United States suggest that most smokers are informed to some degree about the major adverse health effects of smoking, such as lung cancer, heart disease, and lung cancer from secondhand smoke (ITC Project 2014). However, other risks are less well understood and misperceptions about nicotine and nicotine-replacement products and misperceptions about the relative safety of what were formerly known as "low-tar" cigarettes are common (Cummings et al. 2004). For example, despite bans on the misleading descriptors such as "light" or "low-tar" cigarettes, many smokers still have misperceptions about these products (Borland et al. 2008; Brown et al. 2012). In addition, nearly all smokers underestimate the severity and the magnitude of the risks from smoking. They also tend to believe that their own health risk is lower than that of other smokers (Weinstein 1998; Arnett 2000; Weinstein 2005). Youths are especially likely to discount information about the risks of tobacco experimentation because they do not fully understand the addictiveness of tobacco products and do not expect to become long-term smokers (Slovic 2000; Weinstein 2005).

Tobacco product changes that infer a reduced risk are appealing to smokers. For example, since the 1970s, after being introduced to the U.S. market, low-tar and low-nicotine cigarettes rapidly increased their market share. Low-tar cigarettes were specifically marketed to such smokers with such tags as "All the fuss about smoking got me thinking I'd either quit or smoke True. I smoke True" (Lorillard 1976), and evidence suggests that the persons most likely to initially use low-tar cigarettes were those most concerned about smoking and most interested in quitting. Product changes that imply a safer way to continue to consume tobacco may provide a rationalization for smokers to postpone quitting. The use of novel tobacco products may also be influenced by harm perceptions. For example, among adult current e-cigarette users in the PATH study, the most widely endorsed reasons for use were that the product may be less harmful to them and those around them than cigarettes (Hyland et al. 2016).

Tobacco Industry Advertising

Pro-tobacco advertising is thought to maintain adult smoking by (1) creating attitudes and images that reinforce the desirability of smoking and that remind smokers of enjoyable occasions associated with smoking, (2) reducing smokers' motivation to quit through attractive imagery and implicit alleviation of fears about the health consequences of smoking, and (3) reminding former smokers of the reasons and situations in which they smoked to encourage them to relapse (USDHHS 1989). According to the NCI, the weight of evidence "demonstrates a causal relationship between tobacco advertising and promotion and increased tobacco use, as manifested by increased smoking initiation and increased per capita tobacco consumption in the population" (NCI 2008). Recent studies have also suggested that marketing and pack displays at the point of sale may influence impulse buys among current smokers, which could impede attempts to quit smoking (Siahpush 2016a; Siahpush 2016b; Carter et al. 2009).

Lower Price

Price is an important driver of tobacco use. Lower prices increase tobacco consumption and higher prices decrease consumption (Chaloupka et al. 2011; Warner et al. 2014). Adolescents, young adults, adults with lower educational attainment or lower SES, African Americans, and Hispanics are more sensitive to price increases (CDC 1998; USDHHS 2000; Farrelly et al. 2001; Thomas et al. 2008). These populations are also more likely to use coupons and other discounts to reduce the price (White et al. 2006), although the use of any price minimization behaviors (e.g., coupons, purchasing generic brands, purchasing in cartons to reduce unit price) is relatively widespread among U.S. smokers (Xu et al. 2013). Engaging in price-minimizing behavior has been found to reduce the likelihood that smokers will quit in the future (Licht et al. 2011). The association between price and demand has also been observed for diverse tobacco products, including novel products, such as e-cigarettes (Huang et al. 2014; NCI and CDC 2014).

Individual Factors

Individual factors influencing continued tobacco use among adults include lower educational attainment and lower SES. Smokers with low SES are less likely to intend to quit, make a quit attempt, and successfully quit (Reid et al. 2010) and the disparity in smoking prevalence by SES has grown over time (Kanjilal et al. 2006). These may be mediated by lower understanding of the health hazards of smoking, less supportive home and work environments for quitting, living in disadvantaged neighborhoods, greater negative affect and greater stress, and lower quitting self-efficacy (i.e., confidence in being able to successfully quit; Sorensen et al. 2002; Businelle et al. 2010).

Interventions

Prevention of Tobacco Use

Comprehensive tobacco prevention programs that may include mass media campaigns; price increases on tobacco products; regulatory initiatives such as those that ban advertising to youths, restrictions on youth access to tobacco, and establishment of smoke-free public and workplace environments; and statewide, community-wide, and school-based programs and policies
are effective in reducing the initiation, prevalence, and intensity of smoking among youths and young adults (USDHHS 2000; USDHHS 2014; CPSTF 2014; IOM 2007). The specific interventions with the strongest evidence of effectiveness to prevent tobacco use initiation are raising the prices of tobacco products, sustained public education media campaigns, and smoke-free policies.

The primary intervention to prevent exposure to secondhand smoke is the implementation of comprehensive smoke-free policies (CPSTF 2014; USDHHS 2006; USDHHS 2014).

Price

There is a robust body of evidence on the effectiveness of price increases on reducing youth initiation (USDHHS 2000; USDHHS 2014; CPSTF 2014; FCTC 2016). Price increases are also one of the most effective interventions to increase cessation. The Surgeon General, an NCI consensus panel, and the Community Preventive Services Task Force (CPSTF) all recommend price increases as a primary strategy to reduce youth and adult tobacco use (NCI 1993; USDHHS 2000; USDHHS 2012; CPSTF 2014; USDHHS 2014). Studies show that a 10% increase in cigarette price will result in a 3% to 5% reduction in overall cigarettes consumed. Increases in cigarette prices decrease the prevalence of smoking and also the average number of cigarettes smoked by smokers.

Youths and young adults are two to three times more responsive than adults to changes in cigarette prices (USDHHS 2012). The CPSTF estimated that a 20% increase in price would be associated with a 14.8% reduction in demand among youths, including a 7.2% reduction in the proportion of young adults who use tobacco, an 8.6% median reduction in initiation among young people, and an 18.6% median increase in cessation among young people. For adults, the CPSTF estimated that a 20% increase in tobacco unit price would be associated with a 7.4% reduction in demand among adults, including a 3.6% reduction in the proportion of adults who use tobacco, and a 6.5% increase in cessation among adults (CPSTF 2014).

Other tobacco products also respond to price interventions (e.g., smokeless tobacco; USDHHS 2000; Ohsfeldt et al. 1997). The estimated tax elasticity of the prevalence of smokeless tobacco use among male high-school students ranged from -0.197 to -0.121, and the estimated tax elasticity of days using smokeless tobacco ranged from -0.085 to -0.044. A study on price and cigar use reported that, after controlling for laws on smoke-free air and on youth access, the price elasticity of the prevalence of cigar smoking among middle- and high-school youths was estimated to be -0.34 (Ringel et al. 2005). However, prices need to be kept aligned among various tobacco products or use can shift to less expensive forms of tobacco (Delnevo et al. 2004; USDHHS 2000; GAO 2012).

Public Education Efforts

Public education media campaigns, when combined with other interventions, are an effective strategy to reduce initiation and prevalence and increase cessation (NCI 2008; USDHHS 2000; USDHHS 2012; USDHHS 2014; CPSTF 2014; CDC 2014). The CPSTF reported that sustained mass-reach health communication interventions decreased tobacco use among adults by 5 percentage points, the prevalence of tobacco use among young people aged 11 to 24 years by 3.4 percentage points, and the initiation of tobacco use among young people aged 11 to 24 years by 6.7 percentage points. These public education campaigns also increased cessation by 3.5 percentage points and increased calls to quitlines by 132% (CPSTF 2014).

Youth-focused campaigns have been developed and evaluated in several states and nationally. It was estimated that 20% of the decline in youth smoking prevalence in the late 1990s was a result of the American Legacy Foundation's "Truth" media campaign (Farrelly et al. 2005a). However, these campaigns need to be sustained. In Minnesota, when a youth-focused media campaign was ended, youth susceptibility to initiate smoking increased from 43% to 53% within six months (CDC 2004a).

Public education campaigns change social norms about tobacco use, increase awareness of the health hazards of smoking and exposure to second-hand smoke, educate about tobacco industry actions, provide motivations for people to quit, inform tobacco users about resources available to help them quit, and support policy efforts.

Studies in a variety of countries have reported that graphic health warnings improve understanding of the health risks of tobacco use, discourage initiation, and prompt interest in trying to quit (Health Canada 2004; Australian Government Department of Health 2009; FCTC 2016; USDHHS 2012). Stronger warning labels in Australia appear to have had a larger effect on quitting behavior than the old labels, and half of Canadian smokers said that warning labels had contributed to their desire to quit or to cut back on their consumption (Kenkel and Chen 2000).

Advertising Bans

Evidence for the effectiveness of advertising bans is mixed. The apparent lack of effect in some studies may be attributable, in part, to these bans being frequently circumvented. For example, after the broadcast ban went into effect in the United States, tobacco advertising shifted to other media—newspapers, magazines, outdoor signs, transit, and point of sale (FTC 2016a). Studies suggest that partial bans are not effective, but that complete bans can decrease consumption and reduce youth tobacco use (FCTC 2016; Saffer and Chaloupka 1999; USDHHS 2012; NCI 2008).

Minors' Access Restrictions

Studies consistently show that enforcement of minors' access provisions decreases retailer sales to minors, but data on the impact on smoking behavior is mixed (Stead and Lancaster 2005). However, because minors do not start buying tobacco products until they are using the products fairly regularly, daily smoking may be a more appropriate outcome measure than initiation or past-30-day use (DiFranza et al. 2009). The CPSTF concluded that minors' access interventions are effective when implemented in conjunction with other community interventions (CPSTF 2014). The IOM reported that increasing the minimum age of legal access to tobacco products, particularly to age 21 or 25, will likely lead to substantial reductions in smoking prevalence and reductions in smoking-related mortality. The report noted that although changes in the minimum age of legal access to tobacco products would directly apply to individuals who are aged 18 years or older, the largest proportionate reduction in the initiation of tobacco use will likely occur among adolescents aged 15 to 17 years (IOM 2015).

Continued enforcement of minors' access provisions is critical to increase retailer compliance (Lynch and Bonnie 1994). An IOM report recommends requiring state licensing of all retail outlets that sell tobacco products, verifying the age of purchasers, banning the use of self-service displays and vending machines, restricting direct access to tobacco products, and selling products only in a face-to-face exchange (IOM 2007).

School-Based Tobacco Prevention Programs

The Surgeon General has concluded that school-based programs with evidence of effectiveness, containing specific components, can produce at least short-term effects, but noted that these programs produce larger and more sustained effects when they are implemented in combination with other initiatives such as mass media public education campaigns, family programs, and state and community programs. Data suggest that the most effective programs are those that are interactive, address social influences, include components on intentions not to use tobacco, use peer leaders, add community components, and include life skills practice. Programs that showed evidence of longer-term effectiveness contained at least 15 sessions including some up to at least ninth grade (USDHHS 2012).

Eliminating Exposure to Secondhand Smoke

In 2006, the Surgeon General concluded that eliminating smoking in indoor spaces fully protects nonsmokers, but that separating smokers from nonsmokers, cleaning the air, and ventilating buildings cannot eliminate exposure to secondhand smoke (USDHHS 2006). The CPSTF has concluded that smoke-free policies reduce exposure to secondhand smoke, reduce the prevalence of tobacco use, increase the number of tobacco users who quit, reduce the initiation of tobacco use among young people, and reduce tobacco-related morbidity and mortality, including acute cardiovascular events (CPSTF 2014).

Studies have shown dramatic declines in respirable particle and carcinogenic particulate polycyclic aromatic hydrocarbon levels after smoking bans were implemented (CDC 2004b; Repace 2004). Other studies have shown improvements in respiratory symptoms, sensory irritation, and lung function in hospitality workers after implementation of smoke-free laws (Eisner et al. 1998; Farrelly et al. 2005b). The CPSTF concluded that smoke-free policies can reduce health care costs substantially and both the CPSTF and the Surgeon General have concluded that these policies do not have an adverse economic impact on businesses, including the hospitality industry (CPSTF 2014; USDHHS 2012).

Screening

One of the most important screening strategies for health care professionals is to ask about a patient's tobacco use. Such information should be ascertained on every visit and documented in the medical record (Fiore et al. 2008). Routine screening for tobacco use is critical for ensuring that all tobacco users receive effective treatment every time they are seen by a health care professional.

Biochemical measures are available to assess whether a person is a smoker or is exposed to secondhand smoke. For example, cotinine (the major metabolite of nicotine) can be measured in blood, urine, and saliva (USDHHS 2006). These measures are generally used in research or surveillance studies but are not recommended for use as part of routine clinical care of tobacco users. Clinicians should be aware that pregnant women may underreport smoking and that the use of multiple choice questions as opposed to a yes-or-no question, can increase disclosure among pregnant women by as much as 40% (Fiore et al. 2008).

Treatment

Interventions proven to increase cessation include increasing the price of tobacco products, sustained public education media campaigns, smoke-free policies (discussed previously), reducing the out-of-pocket costs of treatment, telephone cessation quitlines, mobile phone–based cessation interventions, and health care system changes that ensure that all tobacco users are screened and treated every time they are seen by a health professional (Fiore et al. 2008; CPSTF 2014). There is also a robust evidence base about the specific clinical interventions that increase cessation rates (Fiore et al. 2008; FCTC 2016).

Reducing Out-of-Pocket Costs of Treatment

Although 70% of smokers want to quit (CDC 2011) and more than 50% try to quit each year (Agaku et al. 2014b), only about one third use available effective treatments when trying to quit (CDC 2011). Reducing the barriers to obtaining treatment is critical to increasing the number of smokers who successfully quit. The CPSTF and Public Health Service (PHS) Clinical Practice Guideline both recommend reducing the out-of-pocket costs for effective treatment interventions through comprehensive insurance coverage because such coverage increases use of treatment and the number of successful quitters (Fiore et al. 2008). The CPSTF estimated that the median increase in cessation with coverage was 4.3 percentage points (CPSTF 2014).

Telephone Cessation Quitlines

Telephone cessation quitlines increase quitting success and are recommended by the PHS guideline, the CPSTF, Cochrane Reviews, and the Surgeon General (Fiore et al. 2008; CPSTF 2014; Stead et al. 2013; USDHHS 2014). Telephone quitlines provide practical advice to smokers interested in quitting about how to deal with withdrawal symptoms and the challenges of quitting. Quitlines increase access to treatment because they are free; generally available days, evenings, and weekends; do not require transportation or childcare arrangements; and provide individually tailored help. In addition, the semi-anonymous nature of the phone counseling encourages candid discussion and the use of structured protocols promotes consistent quality control. Some quitlines also provide free nicotine replacement therapy (USDHHS 2014).

Individual Cessation Interventions

The 2008 PHS Clinical Practice Guideline reported the following findings: brief clinician advice to quit is effective (30% increase in cessation rates), and more intensive counseling is even more effective (doubles the cessation rate). Counseling can be delivered as individual, group, or telephone counseling. Medications approved by the FDA increase cessation by twofold to threefold (Fiore et al. 2008). These findings are consistent with other published recommendations. Although there are anecdotal reports about smokers using e-cigarettes to quit smoking, the data are mixed in studies published to date. At this time, no e-cigarette has been approved as an effective cessation aid (USPSTF 2015).

Cessation counseling or coaching provides practical advice about quitting and provides social support to tobacco users as they try to quit. Using counseling and medication together or combining medications results in higher cessation rates (Fiore et al. 2008). A major problem, however, is that physicians are not providing the effective treatments (Jamal et al. 2012), few tobacco users use these effective treatments (CDC 2011), and there is also evidence that tobacco users use fewer doses of the medications and use medication for a shorter period than recommended, which may contribute to lower success rates (Fiore et al. 2008).

As 70% of smokers see a physician and 53% see a dentist each year (Tomar et al. 1996), clinicians have frequent opportunities for treating tobacco users. The PHS Clinical Practice Guideline concluded that effective tobacco use treatments should be offered to every patient who uses tobacco, recommending a brief intervention (three minutes) called the "Five A's" (Fiore et al. 2008):

- Ask every patient at every visit if he or she uses tobacco and document the patient's status in the medical chart (e.g., as a vital sign).
- Advise all tobacco users to quit.
- Assess patients' interest in quitting.
- Assist smokers in quitting by helping them set a quit date, recommending or prescribing FDA-approved medications unless contraindicated,

and providing or referring patients to more intensive individual, group, or telephone counseling.

- Arrange for follow-up (by telephone or by scheduling a return appointment) to assess progress and encourage relapsed smokers to try again.

Patients not yet willing to quit smoking should receive a motivational intervention to promote later quit attempts. These recommendations assume that office systems will be developed to ensure the routine assessment of tobacco use and appropriate treatment (Fiore et al. 2008).

Unfortunately, studies have been mixed for youth cessation interventions (McDonald et al. 2003), although counseling interventions have some evidence of effectiveness (Fiore et al. 2008). Current recommendations are to provide opportunistic advice to quit and offer help to youths interested in quitting. Intensive efforts to recruit adolescents into treatment are not currently recommended, because this effort is difficult and expensive, and attrition is high (Backinger et al. 2003).

Tobacco-use treatment for adults is extremely cost-effective, more so than other commonly covered preventive interventions, such as mammography, treatment for mild-to-moderate hypertension, and treatment for hypercholesterolemia (Cromwell et al. 1997; Cummings et al. 1989; Fiore et al. 2008). An analysis of recommended clinical preventive services that ranked the services based upon disease impact, treatment effectiveness, and cost-effectiveness concluded that treatment of tobacco use among adults ranked first (along with childhood immunizations and aspirin therapy to prevent cardiovascular events in high-risk adults).

Tobacco-use treatment also had the lowest delivery rate among the top-ranked preventive services (Maciosek et al. 2006). One study found that the cost of a moderately priced cessation program (brief clinical interventions, free telephone counseling, and free nicotine replacement therapy) paid for itself within four years because of lower hospital costs among successful quitters compared with continuing smokers (Wagner et al. 1995). Another study of Medicaid recipients found that every $1 in program costs was associated with $3.12 in medical savings (Richard et al. 2012). Provision of preventive services is also associated with increased patient satisfaction (Schauffler and Rodriguez 1994).

Mobile Phone–Based Cessation Interventions

Mobile phone–based cessation interventions use interactive features to deliver evidence-based information, strategies, and behavioral support. Typically, participants receive text messages that support their quit attempt. Content may be adapted for specific populations and messages may be tailored for individuals. These interventions may be automated, and they may include text responses provided on demand to participants encountering urges to smoke. These interventions can also be coordinated with additional interventions, such as Internet-based cessation services or provision of medications (CPSTF 2014).

Examples of Evidence-Based Interventions

State-Based Comprehensive Tobacco Prevention and Control Programs

Comprehensive tobacco control programs are funded as ongoing efforts to implement and coordinate evidence-based population-level interventions to prevent the initiation of tobacco use among youths and young adults, promote quitting among adults and youths, eliminate exposure to secondhand smoke, and identify and eliminate tobacco-related disparities among population groups (CDC 2014a; USDHHS 2014). A comprehensive approach optimizes synergies from applying a mix of educational, clinical, regulatory, economic, and social strategies.

Following the establishment of the first statewide tobacco control programs in Minnesota in 1985 and California in 1989, comprehensive tobacco control programs began to develop during the 1990s. The American Stop Smoking Intervention Study (ASSIST) was established in 17 states in 1991, the Robert Wood Johnson Foundation–funded SmokeLess States coalitions were established in 19 states starting in 1993, CDC funded 32 non-ASSIST states and the District of Columbia through its Initiatives to Mobilize for the Prevention and Control of Tobacco Use program in 1994, and CDC launched the National Tobacco Control Program by providing funding to all 50 states and the District of Columbia, the territories, and selected national networks and tribal support centers in 1999. All 50 states and the District of Columbia currently have state tobacco control programs that are funded through various revenue streams, including tobacco excise tax revenues, tobacco industry settlement payments, state general funds, the federal government, or nonprofit organizations (CDC 2014a; CTFK 2015a).

States that have made larger investments in comprehensive tobacco control programs have seen larger declines in cigarettes sales than the nation as a whole, and the prevalence of smoking among adults and youths has declined faster, as spending for tobacco control programs has increased. In Florida, a comprehensive program reduced the prevalence of smoking among middle- and high-school students. Florida recently reported that its high-school smoking rate fell to 6.9% in 2015, one of the lowest rates ever reported by any state. In the first three years of its youth-directed tobacco control program, Florida reduced high-school and middle-school smoking by almost three percentage points per year and has cut its high-school smoking rate by 75% since 1998 (CTFK 2016a). Similarly, declines in the prevalence of both adult and youth smoking in New York State outpaced declines nationally, resulting in smoking-attributable personal health care expenditures that were $4.1 billion less than they would have been had the prevalence remained unchanged (USDHHS 2014). In addition, the longer the states invest in comprehensive tobacco control programs, the greater and faster the impact. In California, which has the nation's first and longest-running comprehensive state tobacco control program, the prevalence of cigarette smoking among adults declined from 22.7% in 1988 to 11.9% in 2010 (USDHHS 2014).

California has also seen improved health outcomes. Lung cancer incidence has declined three times more rapidly in California than in the rest of the country, and six tobacco-related cancers now have a lower incidence rate in California than in the rest of the United States (lung/bronchus, esophagus, larynx, bladder, kidney, and pancreas; California Department of Health Services 2006). Faster reductions in cardiovascular disease than in the rest of the country have also been reported. It is estimated that the program was associated with 33,000 fewer heart disease deaths from 1989 to 1997 than would have been expected (Fichtenberg and Glantz 2000). California has reported that, for every dollar spent on the program, statewide health care costs are reduced by more than $3.60 (CTFK 2016a).

Similarly, Massachusetts reported that its program paid for itself through declines in smoking among pregnant women (CTFK 2016a). The CDC estimates that the annual cost to implement comprehensive state tobacco control programs ranges from $7.41 to $10.53 per capita for all 50 states and the District of Columbia combined (CDC 2014). Subsequent to the infusion of billions of dollars to states from the Master Settlement Agreement, increases in state funding for tobacco control occurred, though generally not at CDC-recommended levels, and since then state funding for comprehensive tobacco control programs has fallen dramatically despite the fact that research has demonstrated that comprehensive tobacco prevention and control programs decrease consumption (Farrelly et al. 2003), decrease youth smoking prevalence (Tauras et al. 2005), decrease adult smoking prevalence (Pechacek et al. 2008), reduce disease burden, and are cost-effective (CTFK 2016a). One study noted that larger, more established programs may be more efficient, and concluded that if states had begun investing at the CDC-recommended minimum funding levels in 1994, the aggregate sales decline would have doubled by 2000 (Farrelly et al. 2003). Another national analysis reported that had states spent the CDC-recommended minimum levels, youth smoking prevalence would have been between 3% and 14% lower than the observed rate (Tauras et al. 2005).

Evidence-based recommendations have outlined the specific interventions that comprise a comprehensive program. Effective interventions to decrease initiation include raising the price of tobacco products, public education media campaigns combined with other interventions (such as price increases or community interventions), smoke-free policies, and community mobilization around minors' access when combined with other interventions (CPSTF 2014). Effective interventions to reduce exposure to secondhand smoke include smoking bans or restrictions. Effective interventions to increase cessation include raising the price of tobacco products, sustained public education media campaigns (in conjunction with other interventions), telephone quitlines, mobile phone cessation interventions, reduced out-of-pocket costs of treatment (i.e., insurance coverage), and smoke-free policies. Provider reminders alone or in combination with provider training also increase quitting (CPSTF 2014).

It is important that tobacco control efforts encompass all tobacco products, not just cigarettes. Components of a comprehensive approach include (CDC 2014a; USDHHS 2014)

- State and community interventions (policy interventions, coalition building, and community interventions with high-risk populations).
- Mass-reach health communication interventions (youth- and adult-focused campaigns, quitline marketing, and campaigns focused on tobacco-free environments), and restrictions on tobacco industry marketing.
- Cessation interventions (quitline services, mobile phone–based cessation interventions, comprehensive insurance coverage in both public and private sectors, health system transformation to improve screening and treatment of tobacco use).

- Surveillance and evaluation (tobacco use, attributable disease and economic costs, program impact).
- Infrastructure, administration, and management (accountability, monitor grants, and contracts).

Sustaining funding for state tobacco control programs has been a continued challenge. For example, all four of the initial tobacco control programs have sustained cuts. By 2004, the Massachusetts program had been virtually eliminated (a 92% cut) and the California, Arizona, and Oregon programs severely reduced (45%, 37%, and 69%, respectively; CTFK 2006). Florida's campaign was cut 99%, eliminating the effective statewide "Truth" marketing campaign (Schroeder 2004).

In 1998, the Master Settlement Agreement provided $246 billion over 25 years to the states to compensate them for Medicaid and Medicare costs for treating smokers (CTFK 2015a; USDHHS 2014). Although it was expected that states would fund comprehensive tobacco control programs with the proceeds, in most cases, the funds have been used for other purposes, particularly as states experienced budget deficits in the first few years of the 21st century. In 2015, the states provided just 14% of the tobacco prevention funding recommended by CDC. Only one state was funding its tobacco prevention program at the CDC-recommended level and only four other states were funding at even half the CDC's recommended funding level (CTFK 2016b). Total funding for tobacco control programs dropped 27% between 2002 and 2005 and then increased 33% by 2009. However, the funding of $468 million in 2015 is well below the level of funding in 2002, which was 749.7 million (CTFK 2016b). The Robert Wood Johnson Foundation also decreased their investment in tobacco prevention and control and national funding to the Truth Initiative (formerly the American Legacy Foundation) through the Master Settlement Agreement, but Truth funding then increased in 2013.

Federal and State Tobacco Excise Taxes

As of March 2016, the federal cigarette tax was $1.01 per pack (increased from $0.39 in April 2009) and as of January 2016, state excise taxes ranged from $0.17 in Missouri to $4.35 in New York with a median tax of $1.53 per pack (Federation of Tax Administrators 2016).

Taxes on other tobacco products are more variable. As of December 31, 2015, Florida, Pennsylvania, and the District of Columbia did not tax cigars

(CDC 2016b). Cigar tax rates are widely variable and can be levied as percentage of wholesale price (ranging from 6.6% to 95%), percentage of manufacturer price (ranging from 5% to 75%), and tax per 10 cigars (ranging from $0.01 to $2.18) in March 2016 (CTFK 2015b). States tax little cigars in one of three ways: (1) defined and taxed separately as "little cigars," (2) defined as and taxed as "tobacco products," or (3) defined as and taxed as "cigarettes." As of December 2015, only one state did not tax little cigars in any manner. Pennsylvania does not tax pipe tobacco. As of December 31, 2015, three states tax pipe tobacco on a per-ounce basis and the remaining states tax pipe tobacco on a percentage of a specified cost. Three states do not tax roll-your-own tobacco. Four states tax roll-your-own tobacco on a per-ounce basis and the remaining states tax roll-your-own tobacco on a percentage of a specified cost.

Taxes on smokeless tobacco are usually measured in either a dollar amount per ounce or as a percentage of a price (such as the wholesale or manufacturer's price) and the calculations vary by state. There are five types of smokeless tobacco, and the states can tax all of the products equally under a broad definition, or separately, by specific product types. Pennsylvania does not tax any form of smokeless tobacco products (CDC 2016b). As of March 2016, some states and localities were starting to tax e-cigarettes. Some were taxing as a percentage of price (generally percentage of wholesale price, but could be percentage of retail price), with Minnesota being an example with a tax of 95% of wholesale price. Others were taxing by volume (Louisiana, North Carolina, Kansas, and the District of Columbia) or by nicotine level (concentration), as was proposed in Indiana, Montana, New Mexico, and North Carolina, or by unit and by volume (as Chicago did at $0.80/unit + $0.55/mL; Boyle et al. 2016; CTFK 2015b). Except for ad valorum taxes, the effect of taxes attenuates over time (and with inflation), so regular increases are needed.

In addition, parity of taxation across tobacco products reduces switching to cheaper products. Tobacco industry discounting strategies also reduce the impact of tax increases (USDHHS 2014). There is evidence that the tobacco industry uses discounting strategies more heavily in states with more robust tobacco control programs or to specific populations (Loomis et al. 2006; Pierce et al. 2005). Other tobacco control strategies that have an impact on price include restrictions on free samples of tobacco products, restrictions on coupons or discounting, prohibiting the sale of single cigarettes ("loosies"), efforts to combat smuggling, and restrictions on Internet or mail-order sales.

Public Education Campaigns and Restrictions on Tobacco Industry Marketing

Tobacco industry spending on cigarette advertising nearly tripled from 1997 to 2003 (to $15.1 billion), with the proportion used for coupons and discounts increasing from 27% to 87%. Expenditures then decreased to $8 billion in 2010 and then rose to $8.9 billion by 2013 (FTC 2016a). The largest single category of these expenditures continues to be price discounts paid to cigarette retailers or wholesalers to reduce the price of cigarettes to consumers, which accounted for $8.3 billion (93.1% of total advertising and promotional expenditures in 2013). Smokeless tobacco companies spent $503.2 million on advertising and promotion in 2013, up from $282.7 million on advertising in 2005 and price discounts and promotions account for 56.2% of the 2013 advertising budget (FTC 2016b).

Other tobacco company promotional money goes toward supporting cultural and sporting events and minority organizations. The resulting financial dependence may buy silence or active opposition to tobacco control proposals. In 1994, arts organizations in New York that had been recipients of tobacco philanthropy spoke out against an ordinance to ban smoking in public places (Quindlen 1994). The inverse correlation between the percentage of a magazine's health articles that discuss smoking and cigarette advertising revenue as a percentage of the magazine's total advertising revenue suggests that tobacco money also affects editorial decisions (USDHHS 2001; Maroney et al. 2001). Studies have also shown a correlation between tobacco industry donations to politicians and lack of support for tobacco prevention and control legislation (Givel and Glantz 2001).

Efforts have been made to reduce advertising that targets children. The Federal Trade Commission filed suit against R. J. Reynolds in 1997, alleging that the Joe Camel symbol enticed children to smoke. Later that year, the company announced that they were discontinuing Joe Camel in the United States (Ono and Ingersoll 1997). In 2004, R. J. Reynolds settled a lawsuit with 13 states over their "Kool Mixx" marketing campaign, which the states alleged targeted urban minority youths in violation of the Master Settlement Agreement (Maryland Attorney General 2008). In 2006, R. J. Reynolds settled a lawsuit with 38 states over their candy-, fruit-, and alcohol-flavored cigarettes and agreed to restrictions on the marketing of flavored cigarettes (NAAG 2006).

The 1997 MSA imposed some restrictions on cigarette marketing in the United States. There could no longer be (1) brand name sponsorship of concerts, team sporting events, or events with a significant youth audience; (2) sponsorship of events in which paid participants were underage; (3) tobacco brand names in stadiums and arenas; (4) cartoon characters in tobacco advertising, packaging, and promotions; (5) payments to promote tobacco products in entertainment settings, such as movies; (6) sale of merchandise with brand-name tobacco logos; and (7) transit and outdoor advertising (including billboards; USDHHS 2000). The federal Public Health Cigarette Smoking Act of 1969 preempted most state advertising restrictions (The Public Health Cigarette Smoking Act of 1969), but with passage of the Tobacco Control Act, many of the preemptions were lifted (Tobacco Control Act 2009). The law does not allow states to regulate the content of cigarette advertisements or to prescribe health warnings on tobacco products, but does allow states to regulate the time, place, and manner of advertising.

Prohibiting retail products that have tobacco images or brands; eliminating images of tobacco use in television and the movies seen by children; restricting advertising in magazines and other print media with high youth readership; eliminating tobacco company sponsorship of school, cultural, or sporting events (and banning tobacco logos at such events); and eliminating candy cigarettes or shredded bubble gum that is packaged to look like smokeless tobacco are other ways to reduce youth exposure to pro-tobacco messages. For cigarettes and smokeless tobacco products, the Tobacco Control Act of 2009 prohibits brand name sponsorship of athletic, musical, or other social events; teams; and merchandise such as hats and T-shirts with brand names or logos (although corporate names are allowed). Separating Major League Baseball and smokeless tobacco use will also provide better role models for youths. Several Major League teams or cities have banned smokeless tobacco use (Rohan and Goodman 2016), and Minor League Baseball is teaming up with FDA on FDA's adolescent smokeless tobacco prevention campaign (part of FDA's "Real Cost" youth prevention campaign; FDA 2016d).

Stronger health warnings can increase consumer understanding of the health risks of tobacco use. The Tobacco Control Act increased the size of health warnings on smokeless tobacco products to 30% of the two primary surfaces and 20% of the advertising (Tobacco Control Act 2009). The act also required FDA to require graphic health warnings on cigarette packs. The FDA promulgated a regulation that required such warnings, but the tobacco industry sued and the courts ruled that the graphic warnings adopted in FDA's regulation violated the First Amendment. The court of appeals remanded the matter to the agency, and FDA has indicated that the agency will undertake research to support a new rulemaking consistent with the Tobacco Control Act (Almasy 2013).

Sustained countermarketing campaigns are important to counteract the promotion of tobacco products. Effective campaigns for youths include hard-hitting, "edgy" campaigns such as Florida's, and later Legacy's (now the Truth Initiative's), "Truth" campaign (Murphy-Hoefer et al. 2008) and FDA's "The Real Cost" campaign (FDA 2016c). Effective campaigns for adults, such as CDC's "Tips From a Former Smoker" campaign often tell the stories of real people who had been harmed by tobacco use. Public education media campaigns have been shown to be very effective in driving calls to quitlines (CDC 2012b). In fact, limited quitline resources often require states to carefully titrate media buys to control call volume, so that demand does not overwhelm their ability to provide services (CDC 2004c).

Smoke-Free or Tobacco-Free Policies

Although the purpose of smoke-free policies is to reduce secondhand smoke exposure, these policies also reduce consumption, increase quitting, decrease relapse, and reduce initiation (USDHHS 2012; USDHHS 2014; CPSTF 2014). Tobacco-free policies have been implemented in federal facilities (U.S. Department of Health and Human Services and U.S. Department of Defense), by federal law (in indoor facilities that are regularly or routinely used to provide services to children; USDHHS 2006), in transportation venues (airplanes, trains), and in the private sector (hospitals, some hotel chains, private workplaces; ANR 2016). In 2016, the Department of Housing and Urban Development issued a proposed rule that would make indoor areas of public housing smoke-free (DHUD 2016).

As of January 1, 2016, 24 states and two territories had comprehensive indoor smoke-free policies that included all workplaces, restaurants, and bars (ANR 2016). Fifty percent of the U.S. population is covered by these state laws. As of December 31, 2015, 28 states prohibited smoking in bars and 34 states prohibited smoking in restaurants. Thirty-four states had 100% smoke-free indoor air laws in both government and private worksites and four others covered government worksites but not private worksites (CDC 2016c). As of January 1, 2016, there were 4,565 states, commonwealths, territories, and municipalities with laws in effect that restrict where smoking is allowed, including

802 municipalities that had a local law in effect that required workplaces, restaurants, and bars to be 100% smoke-free (ANR 2016). There are 475 cities and counties that restrict e-cigarette use in 100% smoke-free venues. There are also 1,475 colleges and universities with 100% smoke-free campuses. Of these, 1,128 are 100% tobacco-free and 802 prohibit the use of e-cigarettes anywhere on campus. However, as of January 1, 2016, 13 states had legislation that pre-empted localities from enacting laws to restrict smoking in public places that were more stringent than state laws (ANR 2016). In addition to reducing the number and degree of protection afforded by local regulations, preemption prevents the public education that occurs as a result of the debate and community organization around the issue.

Despite substantial progress, 58 million Americans are still exposed to secondhand smoke (CDC 2015c). Homes and workplaces are the primary locations for adult exposure, and homes, schools, and public places are important sources for children (USDHHS 2006). A study examining cotinine levels in a nationally representative survey reported that 12% of nonsmoking adults living in counties with extensive smoke-free laws were exposed to secondhand smoke, compared with 35% in counties with limited coverage and 46% in counties with no law (Pickett et al. 2006).

Improving Public and Private Insurance Coverage of Tobacco-Use Treatment

Insurance coverage for tobacco-use treatment has historically been very poor in both the public and private sectors. However, under the Affordable Care Act, smoking cessation coverage with no co-pays was mandated (with some exceptions; Table 7-4). On May 2, 2014, the federal government provided guidance on this topic. The guidance stated that the departments would consider the relevant health plans to be in compliance with the preventive service requirement for tobacco cessation if they cover, for example, screening for tobacco use; individual, group, and phone counseling (at least 10 minutes per session); all FDA-approved tobacco cessation medications (prescription and over-the-counter) when prescribed by a health care provider; at least two quit attempts per year, four sessions of counseling, and 90 days of medication per quit attempt; no prior authorization requirement for treatment; and no cost-sharing requirement. Although private plans are not allowed to charge co-pays for preventive services, this prohibition does not apply to traditional Medicaid programs.

Table 7-4. Tobacco Cessation Coverage: How Did the ACA Change Requirements for What Plans Should Be Covering to Help Smokers Quit?[a]

Insurance Type	Who?	Required Coverage Before ACA	Required Coverage Now
Medicare	Age 65+ or some disabled individuals	• Four sessions of individual counseling • Four prescription cessation medications • Up to two quit attempts per year	• Four sessions of individual counseling • Four prescription cessation medications • Up to two quit attempts per year • No cost-sharing • Annual prevention visit
Traditional Medicaid	Low-income or disabled individuals, eligibility varies by state	No federal requirements, coverage varied by state	For pregnant women: • Individual, group, and phone counseling • All tobacco cessation medications (prescription and OTC) • No cost-sharing For all Medicaid enrollees: • All tobacco cessation medications (prescription and OTC) • Coverage of counseling varies by state or plan • Cost-sharing varies by state or plan
Medicaid Expansion	Low-income or disabled individuals, up to 138% of Federal Poverty Level in states that expand Medicaid	Not applicable— Medicaid expansion did not exist before ACA	• Tobacco cessation treatment as a preventive service • No cost-sharing • At least one tobacco cessation medication
Individual insurance plans[b]	Individuals not buying insurance through an employer or part of a group, including through state health insurance marketplaces	No tobacco cessation requirements	• Tobacco cessation treatment as a preventive service • No cost-sharing • One to three tobacco cessation medications, depending on the benchmark plan

(Continued)

Table 7-4. (Continued)

Insurance Type	Who?	Required Coverage Before ACA	Required Coverage Now
Small group plans[b]	Individuals buying insurance through their small employer (100 or fewer full-time employees) or another small group, including through state health insurance marketplaces	No tobacco cessation requirements	• Tobacco cessation treatment as a preventive service • No cost-sharing • One to three tobacco cessation medications, depending on the benchmark plan
Employer-provided plans (large group/self-insured)[b]	Employees receiving insurance coverage through their employer	No tobacco cessation requirements	• Tobacco cessation treatment as a preventive service • No cost-sharing medications

Source: Adapted with permission from ALA (2014).

Note: benchmark plan=the plan each state has chosen to set the standard for other plans in the State Health Insurance Marketplace; cost-sharing=money a patient must pay when receiving treatment or filling a prescription, such as copays, deductibles, and coinsurance; OTC medication=over-the-counter medication you can buy without a prescription.

[a]The Patient Protection and Affordable Care Act (ACA) was passed in March 2010, and many of its major provisions have been implemented over the last four years, culminating in new insurance coverage available to many Americans starting January 1, 2014.

[b]Excluding plans that are "grandfathered" (those that were in operation on before March 2010 and have not made significant changes) and do not have to meet ACA requirements.

As of June 2015, nine states had published plans documenting that they covered all evidence-based cessation treatments for all Medicaid patients. However, all nine states have barriers to accessing such treatment, such as co-payments or prior authorization requirements for some treatments (ALA 2014). As of June 2015, 31 states reported that they covered individual counseling for all populations and plans and 10 states covered group counseling for all populations and plans. In addition, 30 states covered all seven FDA-approved cessation medications for all populations and plans. However, as of December 31, 2015, only 9 states provided comprehensive coverage for all participants, and all had barriers to accessing the benefit (CDC 2016d). The most common barriers included prior authorization requirements, limits on duration, annual limits on quit attempts, and required co-payments (CDC 2016d). Medicare Part B covers up to eight face-to-face visits in a 12-month period at no cost as long as it is provided by a qualified doctor or other Medicare-recognized practitioner (CMS 2016).

Restricting Minors' Access

In 1992, Congress enacted the Synar Amendment, requiring every state to have a law prohibiting tobacco sales to minors aged younger than 18 years, to enforce the law, to conduct annual statewide inspections of tobacco outlets to assess the rate of illegal tobacco sales to minors, and to develop a strategy and time frame to reduce the statewide illegal sales rate to 20% or less (SAMHSA 1996). States not meeting the requirement are at risk to lose substance abuse and mental health grant funding. In 2013, all states and the District of Columbia met the overall goal of a 20% violation rate (USDHHS 2014), and the average retailer violation rate decreased from 40% in 1997 to 9.6% in 2013. However, as of December 31, 2015, 22 states had laws that included preemptive minors' access language preventing stronger local legislation (CDC 2015d). Federal law regarding sales to minors for cigarettes, smokeless tobacco, and roll-your-own tobacco products has been in effect and enforced by FDA since 2010 and the final rule asserting jurisdiction over all products meeting the definition of a tobacco product extends this federal minimum age of 18 years to all tobacco products (FDA 2016b). The federal regulation requires retailers to verify a purchaser's age by photographic identification for all purchasers aged younger than 27 years and not to sell to persons aged younger than 18 years. The sales restrictions to minors include Internet sales (FDA 2010). The FDA has educated retailers and issued warning letters, assessed fines, and issued no-tobacco-sales orders to reduce sales to minors (FDA 2016a).

In 2015, the IOM published a report on the impact of raising the minimum age for purchase of tobacco products to ages 19, 21, and 25 years. The committee concluded that increasing the minimum legal age for tobacco products will likely prevent or delay initiation of tobacco use by adolescents and young adults, and that adolescents aged 14 to 17 years would be impacted the most. The committee concluded that there would be a 3% decrease in prevalence of tobacco use among those adults if the minimum age were raised to 19 years, a 12% decrease if it were raised to 21 years, and a 16% decrease if it were raised to 25 years (IOM 2015).

Federal regulation bans sales of cigarettes as single cigarettes ("loosies") or in packs smaller than 20-count packs. Federal regulations also prohibit free samples of cigarettes and "covered" newly deemed tobacco products and allow free samples of smokeless tobacco only in qualified adult-only facilities; prohibit the sale of cigarettes, smokeless tobacco, and "covered" newly deemed tobacco products through vending machines and self-service displays (for cigarettes and smokeless tobacco products), except in facilities where individuals aged younger than 18 years are not present or permitted at any time; prohibit the sale or distribution of brand-identified promotional nontobacco items such as hats and T-shirts (for cigarettes and smokeless tobacco products); and prohibit sponsorship of sporting and other events, teams, and entries in a brand name (for cigarettes and smokeless tobacco products), but permits such sponsorship in a corporate name (FDA 2010).

As commercial sales to minors decrease, "social" sources (other adolescents, parents, and older friends) may become more important. Thus, a comprehensive approach is needed so that individuals, as well as retailers, do not provide tobacco to minors (USDHHS 2000).

State-Based Telephone Cessation Quitlines

In 1992, California became the first state to have a quitline. Other states followed, although funding has been erratic, with some states losing and then regaining financial support. In 2004, the federal government developed a national network of quitlines. This network, supported by NCI, has a single portal number, 1-800-QUIT NOW, that routes callers to their state's quitline. As part of the initiative, CDC provided funding to states to support quitline services. Some quitlines offer free nicotine replacement therapy with the counseling service (USDHHS 2014). However, for most states, funding is not robust enough to allow widespread promotion and the provision of counseling and medication to all tobacco users interested in quitting. It has been estimated that up to 16% of smokers would use a quitline service, but current quitlines have the capacity to only serve 1% of smokers (Fiore et al. 2004; CDC 2014a).

Product Regulation

In 2009, Congress gave FDA the authority to regulate tobacco products. This regulatory authority was immediate for cigarettes, smokeless tobacco, and roll-your-own tobacco, but FDA could expand the authorities to other products. The FDA finalized a rule to assert jurisdiction over all tobacco products in May of 2016 (FDA 2016b). This rule is under legal challenge as of June 2016. For regulated products, the FDA authorities are quite broad and include the following:

1. Certain requirements in the law enable FDA, as the regulatory agency, to obtain information that allows it to better understand the composition, exposure, and harms of tobacco products including:
   a. Registration and listing: Manufacturers must register manufacturing facilities and provide a list of all their regulated products.
   b. Ingredient reporting: Manufacturers must provide a list of ingredients for regulated products.
   c. Reporting of harmful and potential harmful constituents (HPHC): Manufacturers must report levels by brand and sub-brand. The FDA established an initial list of 93 HPHCs but allowed manufacturers to initially report on 20 of them.
   d. Submission of health information: Manufacturers must submit all documents related to health, toxicology, behavioral, and physiologic effects that were developed within six months after enactment of the statute and, upon request, all documents related to research on heath, toxicology, behavior, physiology, and marketing.
2. The law restricts product changes that could affect public health. The law requires manufacturers to inform FDA of any changes to existing products or about any new tobacco products. New products cannot be introduced to market without FDA evaluating the science and determining if they meet the requirements for marketing.

3. The law prohibits false or misleading claims of reduced risk and requires manufacturers to submit data showing that allowing the marketing of a modified-risk tobacco product would (or is expected to) reduce the risk of tobacco-related disease and benefit the population as a whole. The law also prohibits misleading descriptors such as light, low, or mild without FDA authorization.

4. The law authorizes FDA to restrict the marketing and distribution of tobacco products. FDA prohibits
   a. Sales to people aged younger than 18 years and requires proof of age by photo identification for purchasers aged younger than 27 years.
   b. Sales of cigarette packs with fewer than 20 cigarettes.
   c. The distribution of free samples of cigarettes and "covered" newly deemed tobacco products; restricts the distribution of free samples of smokeless tobacco products.
   d. Brand-name sponsorship of athletic, musical, or other social events; teams for cigarettes and smokeless tobacco products.
   e. Hats and T-shirts, etc., with brand names or logos for cigarettes and smokeless tobacco products.
   f. Sales in vending machines except in adult-only facilities; self-service displays for cigarettes and smokeless tobacco products except in adult-only facilities.

5. The law gives FDA the authority to issue product standards that are appropriate for the protection of public health, which could include standards to decrease product appeal, toxicity, or addictiveness. A ban on flavors (except for menthol and tobacco flavors) in cigarettes was implemented directly from the law.

6. Because FDA is a regulatory agency, FDA can require compliance with the law and FDA regulations.
   a. FDA conducts inspections of tobacco retailers to ensure that they are not selling regulated tobacco products to minors or selling products that are not legally on the market, including Internet retailers.
   b. FDA also inspects manufacturing facilities that manufacture, prepare, compound, or process regulated products at least every two years.

7. The FDA can educate the public about the harms of tobacco. For example:
   a. The law increased the size of the health warnings on smokeless tobacco products to 30% of the two principle surfaces and 20% of advertisements and mandated four specific health warnings.

    b. The deeming rule of 2016 required a nicotine warning on roll-your-own tobacco products and "covered" newly deemed tobacco products and an additional five warnings for cigars. The warnings cover 30% of the two principle surfaces of the package and 20% of advertisements.

    c. The law mandates that FDA require graphic health warnings of cigarettes, comprising 50% of the front and back of the pack and 20% of advertisements.

    d. The FDA is required to publish quantities of harmful and potentially harmful constituents by brand and sub-brand in a way that is understandable and not misleading.

    e. The FDA can conduct public education campaigns.

8. The FDA can conduct research on tobacco products, which could include funding scientific studies that expand the science for regulatory action and evaluation.

Although the regulatory authorities are quite broad, there are limitations. For example, in general, FDA's regulatory authorities (through the Center for Tobacco Products) do not extend to setting tax rates for tobacco products; regulating therapeutic products, such as those marketed to treat tobacco dependence; setting clean indoor air policies; regulating tobacco growing; requiring the reduction of nicotine yields to zero; or banning all cigarettes, smokeless tobacco products, little cigars, other cigars, pipe tobacco, or roll-your-own tobacco products (Tobacco Control Act 2009).

Areas of Future Research

Continued research on the effect of various public health actions on reducing tobacco use is important in adapting interventions to maintain and increase effectiveness. Key issues include the following:

- Research on promising public health interventions, particularly research to support regulatory action at the federal, state, and local level.
- Evaluations of state tobacco prevention and control programs to inform best practices.
- Monitoring tobacco industry practices and developing interventions to counteract these practices.
- Understanding the changing patterns of tobacco use (increased use of non-cigarette tobacco products and increase in dual or poly-tobacco product use among both youths and adults).

- Assessing tobacco use and developing effective interventions for reducing tobacco use in disparate populations.
- Research to understand the population health impacts of product changes.
- Improved tobacco-use treatment interventions and finding ways to increase access to treatment.

The reduction in tobacco use in the United States is considered a public health triumph (Eriksen et al. 2007; Figure 7-7) but it is only half achieved. Perhaps most important, large disparities in tobacco use across groups defined by race, ethnicity, educational level, and SES and across regions of the country have emerged over the past 50 years. The diversification of product use and the increasing pattern of dual or poly-tobacco product use among both youths and adults have undermined progress in reducing overall tobacco use. For example, there was no reduction in youth tobacco use from 2011 to 2015 (Singh et al. 2016).

A research agenda that adapts to the changing tobacco control landscape to continually identify the important emerging research needs, leads to improved tobacco control interventions, and determines ways to quickly translate relevant research findings into action are critical. Careful evaluations

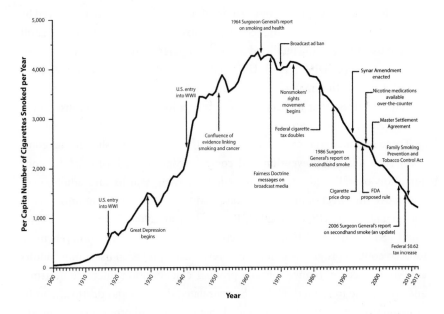

Source: Data from USDHHS (2014) and Warner (1985).

Figure 7-7. Adults Per Capita Cigarette Consumption and Major Smoking and Health Risks, United States, 1900–2012

of specific interventions, timely evaluation of new and innovative strategies, and "macro"-level analyses of the impact of interventions on tobacco use, health outcomes, and health care and productivity costs will be useful to inform future interventions. The United States can learn from the successes of other countries, but many countries, particularly low- and middle-income countries, will need expertise and financial help from the developed world to effectively deal with the emerging epidemic of tobacco use.

Non-use of tobacco is already an accepted norm in many socially defined groups in the United States, and continuing to change the social norms to reduce the acceptability of tobacco use offers great promise (California Department of Health Services 2006). Sustained public education campaigns are a critical element for educating the public, which results in social norm change (Goldman and Glantz 1998). Sustained campaigns at the national or state level are critical to reducing tobacco use, but will need to focus on the diverse products that are popular with youths and adults. For example, tobacco industry promotion of smokeless tobacco and e-cigarettes "for when you can't smoke" could negate the impact of smoke-free policies on increasing cessation.

Prevention programs have demonstrated the ability to delay smoking initiation. However, these programs are most effective when they are reinforced by policy interventions such as higher tobacco taxes, interventions to reduce adult tobacco use, mass media public education campaigns, and supportive community programs (USDHHS 1994; USDHHS 2000; CPSTF 2014; USDHHS 2014; USDHHS 2012) that make smoking unappealing to youths. Communication should also stress that tobacco use results in a loss of control because of the addictiveness of nicotine.

Three national studies and a review by the CPSTF have shown that comprehensive tobacco prevention and control programs reduce cigarette consumption overall and smoking prevalence among youths and adults, over and above the effect of any tax increase that funded the program or occurred concurrently (Farrelly et al. 2003; Pechacek et al. 2008; Tauras et al. 2005). The CPSTF concluded that studies consistently showed that comprehensive tobacco control programs reduce the prevalence of tobacco use among adults and young people, reduce tobacco product consumption, increase quitting, and contribute to reductions in tobacco-related diseases and deaths. In addition, the Community Guide concluded that increases in program funding are associated with increases in program effectiveness (CPSTF 2014). However, with the changing landscape of products being used by youths and adults, tobacco prevention and control programs need to focus on the entire spectrum of popular tobacco products, including cigars, smokeless tobacco, hookah, and e-cigarettes and measure their impact in terms of tobacco use overall, rather than just cigarette smoking.

Finally, FDA's broad regulatory authorities have the potential to greatly reduce the harms from tobacco use, particularly through its use of product standards that can require manufacturers to make changes that could reduce tobacco products' appeal, toxicity, or addictiveness. But even without product standards, FDA's premarket review requirements and enforcement actions are keeping more hazardous products off the market, and the FDA enforcement actions against retailers who sell to minors complement state actions to reduce tobacco use.

The challenge of the 21st century is to accelerate progress so that the morbidity, mortality, and disability caused by any tobacco product no longer occur in the United States or internationally. Although there has been a lot of discussion about the potential role of certain tobacco products, such as e-cigarettes, as reduced risk products that could help smokers who cannot quit transition away from cigarettes, this area is still fundamentally a research question—what is the impact of these products on individual health risk, initiation, cessation, relapse back to tobacco use, dual product use, and net public health impact? And, even if the outcome of that research suggests a net positive impact of these products on public health, a concerted public health effort to implement proven strategies to reduce all forms of tobacco use, particularly by youths, is still a priority.

Full implementation of proven interventions would accelerate the reduction in tobacco use among youths and adults; prevent disease, disability, and death for millions of Americans; increase productivity; and save health care costs. Reducing tobacco use is a shared responsibility of federal, state, and local governments; the public health community; the health care system; the private sector; and individual communities. If each sector did its part to fully implement the proven strategies, one could expect faster progress in reducing tobacco use. As the Surgeon General said in 2000, "The issue is not that we don't know what to do, but the failure to implement what we know works" (USDHHS 2000). A concerted effort is needed, analogous to the efforts to eliminate the morbidity and mortality from polio or smallpox. The leading preventable cause of death in Western societies (and the world) deserves no less.

Acknowledgment

The findings and conclusions in this chapter are those of the authors and do not necessarily represent the official position of the Food and Drug Administration.

Resources

American Cancer Society, http://www.cancer.org

American Heart Association, http://www.heart.org

American Lung Association, http://www.lung.org

Americans for Nonsmokers' Rights, http://www.no-smoke.org

Campaign for Tobacco Free Kids, http://www.tobaccofreekids.org

Centers for Disease Control and Prevention, Office on Smoking and Health, http://www.cdc.gov/tobacco

Food and Drug Administration, Center for Tobacco Products, http://www.fda.gov/tobacco

National Cancer Institute, Cancer Information Service, http://www.cancer.gov/contact/contact-center

National Cancer Institute, Tobacco Control Research Branch, http://www.tobaccocontrol.cancer.gov

Truth Initiative (formerly American Legacy Foundation), http://truthinitiative.org

US Department of Health and Human Services, BeTobaccoFree.gov, http://www.betobaccofree.gov

Suggested Reading

Centers for Disease Control and Prevention. *Best Practices for Comprehensive Tobacco Control Programs—2014*. National Center for Chronic Disease Prevention and Health Promotion, Office on Smoking and Health. 2014. Available at: http://www.cdc.gov/tobacco/stateandcommunity/best_practices/pdfs/2014/comprehensive.pdf.

Community Preventive Services Task Force. Reducing tobacco use and secondhand smoke exposure. 2014. Available at: http://www.thecommunityguide.org/tobacco/index.html.

Fiore MC, Jaen CR, Baker TB, et al. *Treating Tobacco Use and Dependence Clinical Practice Guidelines, 2008 Update*. Rockville, MD: US Department of Health and Human Services, Public Health Service; 2008.

Orleans CT, Slade J, eds. *Nicotine Addiction; Principles and Management.* New York, NY: Oxford University Press; 1993.

US Department of Health and Human Services. *The Health Consequences of Smoking—Nicotine Addiction: A Report of the Surgeon General.* Rockville, MD: Public Health Service, Centers for Disease Control and Prevention, Office on Smoking and Health; 1988.

US Department of Health and Human Services. *The Health Benefits of Smoking Cessation: A Report of the Surgeon General.* Atlanta, GA: US Department of Health and Human Services, Centers for Disease Control and Prevention, Office on Smoking and Health; 1990. DHHS Publication (CDC) 90–8416.

US Department of Health and Human Services. *Reducing Tobacco Use: A Report of the Surgeon General.* Washington, DC: Centers for Disease Control and Prevention, Office on Smoking and Health; 2000.

US Department of Health and Human Services. *The Health Consequences of Smoking: A Report of the Surgeon General.* Atlanta, GA: Centers for Disease Control and Prevention, Office on Smoking and Health; 2004.

US Department of Health and Human Services. *The Health Consequences of Involuntary Exposure to Tobacco Smoke. A Report of the Surgeon General.* Atlanta, GA: Centers for Disease Control and Prevention, Office on Smoking and Health; 2006.

US Department of Health and Human Services. *How Tobacco Smoke Causes Disease— The Biology and Behavioral Basis for Smoking-Attributable Disease. A Report of the Surgeon General.* Atlanta, GA: Centers for Disease Control and Prevention, Office on Smoking and Health; 2010.

US Department of Health and Human Services. *The Health Consequences of Smoking—50 Years of Progress. A Report of the Surgeon General.* Rockville, MD: Centers for Disease Control and Prevention, Office on Smoking and Health; 2014. Available at: http://www.surgeongeneral.gov/library/reports/50-years-of-progress/full-report.pdf.

References

Agaku I, King B, Dube S. Trends in exposure to pro-tobacco advertisements over the Internet, in newspapers/magazines, and at retail stores among US middle and high school students, 2000–2012. *Prev Med.* 2014a;58:45–52.

Agaku IT, King BA, Dube SR; Centers for Disease Control and Prevention. Cigarette smoking among adults—United States, 2005–2012. *MMWR Morb Mortal Wkly Rep.* 2014b;63(2):29–34.

Agaku IT, Singh TS, Everett Jones S, et al. Combustible and smokeless tobacco use among high school athletes—United States, 2001–2013. *MMWR Morb Mortal Wkly Rep*. 2015;64(34):935–939.

Akl EA, Gaddam S, Gunukula SK, Honeine R, Jaoude PA, Irani J. The effects of water-pipe tobacco smoking on health outcomes: a systematic review. *Int J Epidemiol*. 2010;39(3):834–857.

Allen JG, Flanigan SS, LeBlanc M, et al. Flavoring chemicals in e-cigarettes: dia-cetyl,2,3-pentanedione, and acetoin in a sample of 51 products, including fruit-, candy-, and cocktail-flavored e-cigarettes. *Environ Health Perspect*. 2016;124(6):733–739.

Almasy S. FDA changes course on graphic warning labels for cigarettes. CNN. 2013. Available at: http://www.cnn.com/2013/03/19/health/fda-graphic-tobacco-warnings. Accessed April 11, 2016.

Ambrose BK, Day HR, Rostron B, et al. Flavored tobacco product use among US youth aged 12–17 years, 2013–2014. *JAMA*. 2015;314(17):1871–1873.

American Lung Association (ALA). *Helping Smokers Quit: Tobacco Cessation Coverage*. 2014. Available at: http://www.lung.org/our-initiatives/tobacco/cessation-and-prevention/helping-smokers-quit.html. Accessed August 21, 2016.

American Lung Association (ALA). Tobacco cessation coverage: what is required? 2016. Available at: http://www.lung.org/assets/documents/tobacco/helping-smokers-quit-required.pdf. Accessed August 19, 2016.

American Nonsmokers' Rights Foundation (ANR). Smokefree lists, maps, and data. 2016. Available at: http://www.no-smoke.org/goingsmokefree.php?id=519. Accessed March 25, 2016.

Amrock SM, Weitzman M. Adolescents' perceptions of light and intermittent smoking in the United States. *Pediatrics*. 2015;135(2):246–254.

Apelberg BJ, Corey CG, Hoffman AC, et al. Symptoms of tobacco dependence among middle and high school tobacco users: results from the 2012 National Youth Tobacco Survey. *Am J Prev Med*. 2014;47(2 suppl 1):S4–S14.

Armour BS, Pitts MM, Lee CW. Cigarette smoking and food insecurity among low-income families in the United States, 2001. *Am J Health Promot*. 2008;22(6):386–392.

Arnett JJ. Optimistic bias in adolescent and adult smokers and nonsmokers. *Addict Behav*. 2000;25(4):625–632.

Australian Government Department of Health. Evaluation of the effectiveness of the graphic health warnings on tobacco product packaging 2008. 2009. Available at: http://webarchive.nla.gov.au/gov/20140801094931/http://www.health.gov.au/internet/main/

publishing.nsf/Content/phd-tobacco-eval-graphic-health-warnings-exec-sum. Accessed February 24, 2016.

Backinger CL, McDonald P, Ossip-Klein DJ, et al. Improving the future of youth smoking cessation. *Am J Health Behav.* 2003;27(suppl):S170–S184.

Baker F, Ainsworth SR, Dye JT, et al. Health risks associated with cigar smoking. *JAMA.* 2000;284(6):735–740.

Baker TB, Piper ME, McCarthy DE, et al. Time to first cigarette in the morning as an index of ability to quit smoking: implications for nicotine dependence. *Nicotine Tob Res.* 2007;9(suppl 4):S555–S570.

Behar RZ, Davis B, Wang Y, et al. Identification of toxicants in cinnamon-flavored electronic cigarette refill fluids. *Toxicol In Vitro.* 2014;28(2):198–208.

Berman M, Crane R, Seiber E, Munur M. Estimating the cost of a smoking employee. *Tob Control.* 2014;23(5):428–433.

Blank MD, Cobb CO, Kilgalen B, et al. Acute effects of waterpipe tobacco smoking: a double-blind, placebo-control study. *Drug Alcohol Depend.* 2011;116(1–3):102–109.

Borland RR, Fong GT, Yon GG, et al. What happened to smokers' beliefs about light cigarettes when "light/mild" brand descriptors were banned in the U.K.? Findings from the International Tobacco Control (ITC) four country survey. *Tob Control.* 2008;17(4):256–262.

Boyle R, Boon A, Chaloupka FJ, Amato M. How should we tax electronic nicotine delivery systems—analyzing current evidence to inform future policy. Podium presentation at: the 2016 Society for Research on Nicotine and Tobacco 22nd Annual Meeting; March 2–5, 2016; Chicago, IL.

Brown A, McNeill A, Mons U, Guignard R. Do smokers in Europe think all cigarettes are equally harmful? *Eur J Public Health.* 2012;22(suppl 1):35–40.

Businelle MS, Kendzor DE, Reitzel LR, et al. Mechanisms linking socioeconomic status to smoking cessation: a structural equation modeling approach. *Health Psychol.* 2010;29(3):262–273.

California Department of Health Services. California tobacco control update 2006: the social norm change approach. Sacramento, CA: California Department of Health Services, Tobacco Control Section; 2006. Available at: https://www.cdph.ca.gov/programs/tobacco/Documents/Archived%20Files/CTCPUpdate2006.pdf. Accessed April 5, 2016.

Callahan-Lyon P. Electronic cigarettes: human health effects. *Tob Control.* 2014;23(suppl 2):ii36–ii40.

Cameron JM, Howell CN, White JR, et al. Variable and potentially fatal amounts of nicotine in e-cigarette nicotine solutions. *Tob Control.* 2014;23(1):77–78.

Campaign for Tobacco-Free Kids (CTFK). *A Broken Promise to Our Children: The 1998 State Tobacco Settlement Eight Years Later.* Washington, DC: Campaign for Tobacco-Free Kids; 2006.

Campaign for Tobacco-Free Kids (CTFK). *Broken Promises to Our Children: A State-by-State Look at the 1998 State Tobacco Settlement 17 Years Later.* 2015a. Available at: http://www.tobaccofreekids.org/content/what_we_do/state_local_issues/settlement/FY2016/Broken%20Promises%20to%20Our%20Children%2012.7.15.pdf. Accessed April 4, 2016.

Campaign for Tobacco-Free Kids (CTFK). State excise tax rates for non-cigarette tobacco products. 2015b. Available at: http://www.tobaccofreekids.org/research/factsheets/pdf/0169.pdf. Accessed March 20, 2016.

Campaign for Tobacco-Free Kids (CTFK). Comprehensive statewide tobacco prevention programs save money. 2016a. Available at: https://www.tobaccofreekids.org/research/factsheets/pdf/0168.pdf. Accessed April 5, 2016.

Campaign for Tobacco Free Kids (CTFK). Total annual state tobacco prevention spending FY1999–FY2016. 2016b. Available at: http://www.tobaccofreekids.org/content/what_we_do/state_local_issues/settlement/FY2016/4.%20Graph%20-%20Total%20Annual%20State%20Tob%20Prev%20Spending%201999-2016%2012.4.15.pdf. Accessed April 5, 2016.

Carter OB, Mills BW, Donovan RJ. The effect of retail cigarette pack displays on unplanned purchases: results from immediate postpurchase interviews. *Tob Control.* 2009;18(3):218–221.

Centers for Disease Control and Prevention (CDC). Addition of prevalence of cigarette smoking as a nationally notifiable condition—June 1996. *MMWR Morb Mortal Wkly Rep.* 1996;45(25):537.

Centers for Disease Control and Prevention (CDC). Response to increases in cigarette prices by race/ethnicity, income, and age groups—United States, 1976–1993. *MMWR Morb Mortal Wkly Rep.* 1998;47(29):605–609.

Centers for Disease Control and Prevention (CDC). Effect of ending an antitobacco youth campaign on adolescent susceptibility to cigarette smoking—Minnesota, 2002–2003. *MMWR Morb Mortal Wkly Rep.* 2004a;53(14):301–304.

Centers for Disease Control and Prevention (CDC). Indoor air quality in hospitality venues before and after implementation of a clean indoor air law—Western New York, 2003. *MMWR Morb Mortal Wkly Rep.* 2004b;53(44):1038–1041.

Centers for Disease Control and Prevention (CDC). *Telephone Quitlines: A Resource for Development, Implementation, and Evaluation.* 2004c. Available at: http://www.cdc.gov/tobacco/quit_smoking/cessation/quitlines/pdfs/quitlines.pdf. Accessed April 5, 2016.

Centers for Disease Control and Prevention (CDC). State-specific prevalence and trends in adult cigarette smoking—United States, 1998–2007. *MMWR Morb Mortal Wkly Rep.* 2009;58(9):221–226.

Centers for Disease Control and Prevention (CDC). Quitting smoking among adults— United States, 2001–2010. *MMWR Morb Mortal Wkly Rep.* 2011;60(44):1513–1519.

Centers for Disease Control and Prevention (CDC). Consumption of cigarettes and combustible tobacco—United States, 2000–2011. *MMWR Morb Mortal Wkly Rep.* 2012a;61(30):565–569.

Centers for Disease Control and Prevention (CDC). Increases in quitline calls and smoking cessation website visitors during a national tobacco education campaign— March 19–June 10, 2012. *MMWR Morb Mortal Wkly Rep.* 2012b;61(34):667–670.

Centers for Disease Control and Prevention (CDC). *Best Practices for Comprehensive Tobacco Control Programs—2014.* 2014. Available at: http://www.cdc.gov/tobacco/ stateandcommunity/best_practices/pdfs/2014/comprehensive.pdf. Accessed April 5, 2016.

Centers for Disease Control and Prevention (CDC). Deaths and mortality. National Center for Health Statistics. 2015a. Available at: http://www.cdc.gov/nchs/fastats/ deaths.htm. Accessed February 21, 2016.

Centers for Disease Control and Prevention (CDC). Current cigarette smoking among adults—United States, 2005–2014. *Morb Mortal Wkly Rep.* 2015b;64(44):1233–1240.

Centers for Disease Control and Prevention (CDC). Secondhand smoke. CDC Vital Signs. 2015c. Available at: http://www.cdc.gov/vitalsigns/tobacco. Accessed April 5, 2016.

Centers for Disease Control and Prevention (CDC). State system preemption fact sheet. 2015d. Available at: https://chronicdata.cdc.gov/Legislation/STATE-System-Preemption-Fact-Sheet/uu8y-j6ga. Accessed April 4, 2016.

Centers for Disease Control and Prevention (CDC). Smoking in the movies. 2016a. Available at: http://www.cdc.gov/tobacco/data_statistics/fact_sheets/youth_data/movies. Accessed April 20, 2016.

Centers for Disease Control and Prevention (CDC). STATE system excise tax fact sheet. 2016b. Available at: https://chronicdata.cdc.gov/Legislation/STATE-System-Excise-Tax-Fact-Sheet/tsmn-nssw. Accessed April 4, 2016.

Centers for Disease Control and Prevention (CDC). STATE system smokefree indoor air fact sheet. 2016c. Available at: https://chronicdata.cdc.gov/Legislation/STATE-System-Smokefree-Indoor-Air-Fact-Sheet/vgq2-kkcg. Accessed April 4, 2016.

Centers for Disease Control and Prevention (CDC). STATE system Medicaid coverage of tobacco cessation treatments fact sheet. 2016d. Available at: https://chronicdata.cdc.

gov/Cessation-Coverage-/STATE-System-Medicaid-Coverage-of-Tobacco-Cessatio/ ukav-hn33. Accessed April 4, 2016.

Centers for Disease Control and Prevention (CDC). Trends in current cigarette smoking among high school students and adults, United States, 1965–2014. 2016e. Available at: http://www.cdc.gov/tobacco/data_statistics/tables/trends/cig_smoking. Accessed April 18, 2016.

Centers for Disease Control and Prevention (CDC). Chronic disease indicators—online query tool. 2016f. Available at: http://www.cdc.gov/cdi. Accessed March 4, 2016.

Centers for Disease Control and Prevention (CDC). National Youth Tobacco Survey. 2016g. Available at: http://www.cdc.gov/tobacco/data_statistics/surveys/nyts. Accessed August 22, 2016.

Centers for Medicare and Medicaid Services (CMS). Smoking and tobacco use cessation counseling to stop smoking or using tobacco products. 2016. Available at: https://www.medicare.gov/coverage/smoking-and-tobacco-use-cessation.html#1368. Accessed April 11, 2016.

Chaloupka FJ, Straif K, Leon ME. Effectiveness of tax and price policies in tobacco control. *Tob Control.* 2011;20(3):235–238.

Chang CM, Corey CG, Rostron BJ, et al. Systematic review of cigar smoking and all cause and smoking related mortality. *BMC Public Health.* 2015;15:390.

Chao A, Thun MJ, Henley SJ, Jacobs EJ, McCullough ML, Calle EE. Cigarette smoking, use of other tobacco products, and stomach cancer mortality in US adults: the Cancer Prevention Study II. *Int J Cancer.* 2002;101(4):380–389.

Chen J, Kettermann A, Rostron BL, Day HR. Biomarkers of exposure among US cigar smokers: an analysis of 1999–2012 National Health and Nutrition Examination Survey (NHANES) data. *Cancer Epidemiol Biomarkers Prev.* 2014;23(12):2906–3015.

Chorti MK, Poulianti K, Jamurtas A, et al. Effects of active and passive electronic and tobacco cigarette smoking on lung function. *Toxicol Lett.* 2012;21(1S):64.

Cobb CO, Shihadeh A, Weaver MF, Eissenberg T. Waterpipe tobacco smoking and cigarette smoking: a direct comparison of toxicant exposure and subjective effects. *Nicotine Tob Res.* 2011;13(2):78–87.

Community Preventive Services Task Force (CPSTF). Reducing tobacco use and secondhand smoke exposure. 2014. Available at: http://www.thecommunityguide.org/tobacco/index.html. Accessed February 24, 2016.

Congressional Budget Office (CBO). Raising the excise tax on cigarettes: effects on health and the federal budget. 2012. Available at: http://www.cbo.gov/sites/default/files/cbofiles/attachments/06-13-Smoking_Reduction.pdf. Accessed January 26, 2016.

Corey CG, Ambrose BK, Apelberg BJ, King BA. Flavored tobacco product use among middle and high school students—United States, 2014. *MMWR Morb Mortal Wkly Rep*. 2015;64(38):1066–1070.

Cromwell J, Bartosch WJ, Fiore MC, et al. Cost-effectiveness of the clinical practice recommendations in the AHCPR guideline for smoking cessation. *JAMA*. 1997;278(21): 1759–1766.

Csordas A, Bernhard D. The biology behind the atherothrombotic effects of cigarette smoke. *Nat Rev Cardiol*. 2013;10(4):219–230.

Cummings KM, Hyland A, Giovino GA, Hastrup JL, Bauer JE, Bansal MA. Are smokers adequately informed about the health risks of smoking and medicinal nicotine? *Nicotine Tob Res*. 2004;6(suppl 3):S333–S340.

Cummings SR, Rubin SM, Oster G. The cost-effectiveness of counseling smokers to quit. *JAMA*. 1989;261(1):75–79.

Dalton MJ, Sargent J, Beach M, et al. Effect of viewing smoking in movies on adolescent smoking initiation: a Cohort Study. *Lancet*. 2003;362(9380):281–285.

Dar N, Bhat G, Shah I, et al. Hookah smoking, nass chewing, and oesophageal squamous cell carcinoma in Kashmir, India. *Br J Cancer*. 2012;107(9):1618–1623.

Davis B, Dang M, Kim J, et al. Nicotine concentrations in electronic cigarette refill and do-it-yourself liquids. *Nicotine Tob Res*. 2015;17(2):134–141.

Delnevo C, Wackowski O, Giovenco D, et al. Examining market trends in the United States smokeless tobacco use: 2005–2011. *Tob Control*. 2014;23(2):107–112.

Delnevo CD, Hrywna M, Foulds J, Steinberg MB. Cigar use before and after a cigarette excise tax increase in New Jersey. *Addict Behav*. 2004;29(9):1799–1807.

Department of Housing and Urban Development (DHUD). Instituting smoke-free public housing, proposed rule. 2016. Available at: http://portal.hud.gov/hudportal/documents/huddoc?id=smoke-freepublichousing.pdf. Accessed April 5, 2016.

DiFranza JR, Savageau JA, Fletcher KE. Enforcement of underage sales laws as a predictor of daily smoking among adolescents—a national study. *BMC Public Health*. 2009;9:107.

DiFranza JR, Sweet M, Savageau JA, Ursprung WW. The assessment of tobacco dependence in young users of smokeless tobacco. *Tob Control*. 2012;21(5):471–476.

Distefan J, Pierce JP, Gilpin EA. Do favorite movie stars influence adolescent smoking initiation? *Am J Public Health*. 2004;94(7):1239–1244.

Eisner MD, Smith AK, Blanc PD. Bartenders' respiratory health after establishment of smoke-free bars and taverns. *JAMA*. 1998;280(22):1909–1914.

Eriksen MP, Green LW, Husten CG, Pedersen LL, Pechacek TF. Thank you for not smoking: the public health response to tobacco-related mortality in the United States. In: Ward JW, Warren C, eds. *Silent Victories: The History and Practice of Public Health in Twentieth-Century America*. New York, NY: Oxford University Press; 2007.

Etter J, Zather E, Svensson S. Analysis of refill liquids for electronic cigarettes. *Addiction*. 2013;108(9):1671–1679.

Euromonitor International. Vapour devices in the US. 2016. Available at: http://www. euromonitor.com/vapour-products-in-the-us/report. Accessed August 21, 2016.

Evans N, Farkas A, Gilpin E, Berry C, Pierce JP. Influence of tobacco marketing and exposure to smokers on adolescent susceptibility to smoking. *J Natl Cancer Inst*. 1995;87(20):1538–1545.

Family Smoking Prevention and Tobacco Control and Federal Retirement Reform (Tobacco Control Act), Pub L No. 111-31 (2009). Available at: https://www.gpo.gov/fdsys/pkg/PLAW-111publ31/html/PLAW-111publ31.htm. Accessed April 4, 2016.

Farrelly M, Davis KC, Haviland ML, et al. Evidence of a dose–response relationship between "Truth" antismoking ads and youth smoking prevalence. *Am J Public Health*. 2005a;95(3):425–431.

Farrelly M, Pechacek T, Chaloupka F. The impact of tobacco control program expenditures on aggregate cigarette sales: 1981–2000. *J Health Econ*. 2003;22(5):843–859.

Farrelly MC, Bray JW, Pechacek T, Woollery T. Response by adults to increases in cigarette prices by sociodemographic characteristics. *South Econ J*. 2001;68(1):156–165.

Farrelly MC, Healton CG, Davis KC, Messeri P, Hersey JC, Haviland ML. Getting to the truth: evaluating national tobacco countermarketing campaigns. *Am J Public Health*. 2002;92(6):901–907.

Farrelly MC, Nonnemaker JM, Chou R, et al. Changes in hospitality workers' exposure to secondhand smoke following the implementation of New York's smoke-free law. *Tob Control*. 2005b;14(4):236–241.

Farsalinos K, Tsiapras D, Kyrzopoulos S, et al. Immediate effects of electronic cigarette use on coronary circulation and blood carboxyhemoglobin levels: comparison with cigarette smoking. *Eur Heart J*. 2013;34(suppl 1):13.

Farsalinos KE, Kistler KA, Gillman G, Voudris V. Evaluation of electronic cigarette liquids and aerosol for the presence of selected inhalation toxins. *Nicotine Tob Res*. 2015;17(2):168–174.

Federal Trade Commission (FTC). Federal Trade Commission cigarette report for 2013. 2016a. Available at: https://www.ftc.gov/system/files/documents/reports/federal-trade-commission-cigarette-report-2013/2013cigaretterpt.pdf. Accessed April 19, 2016.

Federal Trade Commission (FTC). Federal Trade Commission smokeless tobacco report for 2013. 2016b. Available at: https://www.ftc.gov/reports/federal-trade-commission-smokeless-tobacco-report-2013. Accessed April 19, 2016.

Federation of Tax Administrators. *State Excise Tax Rates on Cigarettes.* 2016. Available at: http://www.taxadmin.org/assets/docs/Research/Rates/cigarette.pdf. Accessed March 10, 2016.

Fichtenberg CM, Glantz SA. Associations of the California tobacco control program with declines in cigarette consumption and mortality from heart disease. *N Engl J Med.* 2000;343(24):1772–1777.

Fiore MC, Coyle RT, Curry SJ, et al. Preventing three million premature deaths and helping five million smokers to quit. A national action plan for tobacco cessation. *Am J Public Health.* 2004;94(2):205–210.

Fiore MC, Jaen CR, Baker TB, et al. *Treating Tobacco Use and Dependence Clinical Practice Guideline, 2008 Update.* US Department of Health and Human Services, Public Health Service. 2008. Available at: http://www.ahrq.gov/sites/default/files/wysiwyg/professionals/clinicians-providers/guidelines-recommendations/tobacco/clinicians/update/treating_tobacco_use08.pdf. Accessed February 24, 2016.

Flouris AD, Chorti MS, Poulianiti KP, et al. Acute impact of active and passive electronic cigarette smoking on serum cotinine and lung function. *Inhal Toxicol.* 2013;5(2):91–101.

Flouris AD, Poulianiti KP, Chorti MS, et al. Acute effects of electronic and tobacco cigarette smoking on complete blood count. *Food Chem Toxicol.* 2012;50(10): 3600–3603.

Fong GT, Hammond D, Laux FL, et al. The near-universal experience of regret among smokers in four countries: findings from the International Tobacco Control Policy Evaluation Survey. *Nicotine Tob Res.* 2004;6(suppl 3):S341–S351.

Food and Drug Administration (FDA). Regulations restricting the sale and distribution of cigarettes and smokeless tobacco products to protect children and adolescents—final rule. *Fed Regist.* 1996;61(41):314–375.

Food and Drug Administration (FDA). Regulations restricting the sale and distribution of cigarettes and smokeless tobacco to protect children and adolescents. *Fed Regist.* 2010;75(53):13225.

Food and Drug Administration (FDA). Compliance, enforcement and training. 2016a. Available at: http://www.fda.gov/TobaccoProducts/GuidanceComplianceRegulatory Information/default.htm. Accessed April 5, 2016.

Food and Drug Administration (FDA). Deeming tobacco products to be subject to the federal Food, Drug, and Cosmetic Act, as amended by the Family Smoking Prevention and Tobacco Control Act; restrictions on the sale and distribution of tobacco products and required warning statements for tobacco products; final rule. *Fed Regist.* 2016b; 81(90):28974–29106.

Food and Drug Administration (FDA). The Real Cost. 2016c. Available at: http://therealcost.betobaccofree.hhs.gov/index.html?utm_source=bing&utm_medium=cpc&utm_campaign=Bully%206%2F15&utm_term=cigarette%20guy&utm_content=Bully%2Creative&gclid=CNiU_p-gt8sCFc5MNwodXXIKQg&gclsrc=ds#Addiction. Accessed March 10, 2016.

Food and Drug Administration (FDA). The Real Cost campaign. 2016d. Available at: http://www.fda.gov/TobaccoProducts/PublicHealthEducation/PublicEducation Campaigns/TheRealCostCampaign. Accessed May 27, 2016.

Framework Convention on Tobacco Control (FCTC). Adopted guidelines. 2016. Available at: http://www.who.int/fctc/treaty_instruments/adopted/en. Accessed February 26, 2016.

Fuemmeler B, Lee C-T, Ranby K, et al. Individual- and community-level correlates of cigarette-smoking trajectories from age 13 to 32 in a US population-based sample. *Drug Alcohol Depend.* 2013;132(1–2):301–308.

Gillman IG, Kistler KA, Stewart EW, Paolantonio AR. Effect of variable power levels on the yield of total aerosol mass and formation of aldehydes in e-cigarette aerosols. *Regul Toxicol Pharmacol.* 2015;75:58–65.

Giovenco D, Hammond D, Corey C, et al. E-cigarette market trends in traditional US retail channels, 2012–13. *Nicotine Tob Res.* 2015;17(10):1279–1283.

Givel MS, Glantz SA. Tobacco lobby political influence on US state legislatures in the 1990s. *Tob Control.* 2001;10(2):124–134.

Glantz SA, Kacirk KA, McCulloch C. Back to the future: smoking in movies in 2002 compared with 1950 levels. *Am J Public Health.* 2004;94(2):261–263.

Goldman LK, Glantz SA. Evaluation of antismoking advertising campaigns. *JAMA.* 1998;279(10):772–777.

Goniewicz ML, Knysak J, Gawron M, et al. Levels of selected carcinogens and toxicants in vapour from electronic cigarettes. *Tob Control.* 2014;23(2):133–139.

Goniewicz ML, Kuma T, Gawron M, et al. Nicotine levels in electronic cigarettes. *Nicotine Tob Res.* 2013;15(1):158–166.

Government Accountability Office (GAO). Large disparities in rates for smoking products trigger significant market shifts to avoid higher taxes. 2012. Available at: http://www.gao.gov/assets/600/590192.pdf. Accessed February 24, 2016.

Grana R, Benowitz N, Glantz SA. e-Cigarettes: a scientific review. *Circulation.* 2014;129(19):1972–1986.

Grana RL, Benowitz N, Glantz SA, Background paper on e-cigarettes (electronic nicotine delivery systems), prepared for World Health Organization Tobacco Control Initiative. 2013. Available at: http://escholarship.org/uc/item/13p2b72n#page-5. Accessed February 20, 2016.

Health Canada. *Building on Success. A Proposal for New Health-Related Information on Tobacco Product Labels: A Consultation Paper.* 2004. Available at: http://www.hc-sc. gc.ca/hc-ps/consult/_2004/advert-publicite/draft-ebauche-eng.php. Accessed August 21, 2016.

Hecht SS, Carmella SG, Kotandeniya D, et al. Evaluation of toxicant and carcinogen metabolites in the urine of e-cigarette users versus cigarette smokers. *Nicotine Tob Res.* 2015;17(6):704–709.

Henley SJ, Thun MJ, Chao A, et al. Association between exclusive pipe smoking and mortality from cancer and other disease. *J Natl Cancer Inst.* 2004;96(11):853–861.

Henriksen L, Dauphinee AL, Wang Y, Fortmann SP. Industry sponsored anti-smoking ads and adolescent reactance: test of a boomerang effect. *Tob Control.* 2006;15(1):13–18.

Huang J, Tauras J, Chaloupka FJ. The impact of price and tobacco control policies on the demand for electronic nicotine delivery systems. *Tob Control.* 2014;23(suppl 3): iii41–iii47.

Hutzler C, Paschke M, Kruschinski S, Henkler F, Hahn J, Luch A. Chemical hazards present in liquids and vapors of electronic cigarettes. *Arch Toxicol.* 2014;88(7): 1295–1308.

Hyland A, Conway K, Borek N, et al. Highlighted findings from wave 1 of the Population Assessment of Tobacco and Health (PATH) Study. Plenary presentation at: the 2016 Society for Research on Nicotine and Tobacco 22nd Annual Meeting; March 2–5, 2016; Chicago, IL.

Institute of Medicine (IOM). *Ending the Tobacco Problem: A Blueprint for the Nation.* Washington, DC: The National Academies Press; 2007.

Institute of Medicine (IOM). *Public Health Implications of Raising the Minimum Age of Legal Access to Tobacco Products.* Washington, DC: The National Academies Press;

2015. Available at: http://www.nap.edu/read/18997/chapter/1#ii. Accessed February 26, 2016.

International Agency for Research on Cancer (IARC). *Smoking and Tobacco Control Monograph no. 9. Tobacco Smoke and Involuntary Smoking. IARC Monographs on the Evaluation of Carcinogenic Risks to Humans.* Vol. 83. 2004. Available at: http://www.ncbi.nlm.nih.gov/books/NBK316407. Accessed February 17, 2016.

International Agency for Research on Cancer (IARC). *Smokeless Tobacco and Some Related Nitrosamines. IARC Monographs on the Evaluation of Carcinogenic Risks to Humans.* Vol. 89. 2007. Available at: http://monographs.iarc.fr/ENG/Monographs/vol89/mono89.pdf. Accessed February 21, 2016.

International Agency for Research on Cancer (IARC). *A Review of Human Carcinogens: Personal Habits and Indoor Combustions. IARC Monographs on the Evaluation of Carcinogenic Risks to Humans.* Vol. 100E. World Health Organization, IARC. 2012. Available at: http://monographs.iarc.fr/ENG/Monographs/vol100E/mono100E.pdf. Accessed February 21, 2016.

Iribarren C, Tekawa I, Sidney S, et al. Effect of cigar smoking on the risk of cardiovascular disease, chronic obstructive pulmonary disease, and cancer in men. *New Engl J Med.* 1999;340(23):1773–1780.

ITC Project. *ITC United States National Report. Findings from the Wave 1 to 8 Surveys (2002–2011).* Waterloo, ON: University of Waterloo; Charleston, SC: Medical University of South Carolina; 2014.

Jacob P, Raddaha AHA, Dempsey D, et al. Nicotine, carbon monoxide, and carcinogen exposure after a single use of a waterpipe. *Cancer Epidemiol Biomarkers Prev.* 2011;20(11):2345–2353.

Jacob P III, Abu Raddaha AH, Dempsey D, et al. Comparison of nicotine and carcinogen exposure with waterpipe and cigarette smoking. *Cancer Epidemiol Biomarkers Prev.* 2013;22(5):765–772.

Jacobs EJ, Thun MJ, Apicella LF. Cigar smoking and death from coronary heart disease in a prospective study. *Arch Intern Med.* 1999;159(20):2413–2418.

Jamal A, Dube SR, Malarcher AM, Shaw L, Engstrom MC; Centers for Disease Control and Prevention. Tobacco use screening and counseling during physician office visits among adults—National Ambulatory Medical Care Survey and National Health Interview Survey, United States, 2005–2009. *MMWR Suppl.* 2012;61(2):38–45.

Javitz HS, Zbikowski SM, Swan GE, Jack LM. Financial burden of tobacco use: an employer's perspective. *Clin Occup Environ Med.* 2006;5(1):9–29.

Johnson SE, Holder-Hayes E, Tessman GK, et al. Tobacco product use among sexual minority adults: findings from the 2012–2013 National Adult Tobacco Survey. *Am J Prev Med.* 2016;50(4):e91–e100.

Kanjilal S, Gregg EW, Cheng YJ, et al. Socioeconomic status and trends in disparities in 4 major risk factors for cardiovascular disease among US adults, 1971–2002. *Arch Intern Med.* 2006;166(21):2348–2355.

Kann L, Kinchen S, Shanklin SL, et al. Youth Risk Behavior Surveillance—United States, 2013. *MMWR Surveill Summ.* 2014;63(4):1–168.

Katsiki N, Papadopoulou SK, Fachantidou AI, Mikhailidis DP. Smoking and vascular risk: are all forms of smoking harmful to all types of vascular disease? *Public Health.* 2013;127(5):435–441.

Kenkel D, Chen L. Consumer information and tobacco use. In: Jha P, Chaloupka F, eds. *Tobacco Control in Developing Countries.* New York, NY: Oxford University Press; 2000.

Kosmider L, Sobczak A, Fik M, et al. Carbonyl compounds in electronic cigarette vapors—effects of nicotine solvent and battery output voltage. *Nicotine Tob Res.* 2014;16(10):1319–1326.

Koul PA, Hajni MR, Sheikh MA, et al. Hookah smoking and lung cancer in the Kashmir valley of the Indian subcontinent. *Asian Pac J Cancer Prev.* 2011;12(2):519–524.

Kropp RY, Halpern-Felsher BL. Adolescents' beliefs about the risks involved in smoking "light" cigarettes. *Pediatrics.* 2004;114(4):445–451.

Lange P, Nyboe J, Appleyard M, Jensen G, Schnohr P. Relationship of the type of tobacco and inhalation pattern to pulmonary and total mortality. *Eur Respir J.* 1992;5(9):1111–1117.

Licht AS, Hyland AJ, O'Connor RJ, et al. How do price minimizing behaviors impact smoking cessation? Findings from the International Tobacco Control (ITC) Four Country Survey. *Int J Environ Res Public Health.* 2011;8(5):1671–1691.

Loomis BR, Farrelly MC, Mann NH. The association of retail promotions for cigarettes with the Master Settlement Agreement, tobacco control programmes and cigarette excise taxes. *Tob Control.* 2006;15(6):458–463.

Lorillard. I smoke True. 1976. Pollay Tobacco Ad Collection. Bates no. true0307. Available at: https://industrydocuments.library.ucsf.edu/tobacco/docs/#id=mmjg0026. Accessed April 29, 2016.

Lovato C, Watts A, Stead L. Impact of tobacco advertising and promotion on increasing adolescent smoking behaviours. *Cochrane Database Syst Rev.* 2011;5(10):CD003439.

Lynch BS, Bonnie RJ. *Growing Up Tobacco Free: Preventing Nicotine Addiction in Children and Youths.* Washington, DC: National Academies Press; 1994.

Maciosek MV, Coffield AB, Edwards NM, Flottemesch TJ, Goodman MJ, Solberg LI. Priorities among effective clinical preventive services: results of a systematic review and analysis. *Am J Prev Med.* 2006;31(1):52–61.

Maroney CL, Sesko A, Whelan EM, Dunston A. Tobacco and women's health: a survey of popular women's magazines: August 1999–August 2000. American Council on Science and Health. 2001. Available at: http://acsh.org/news/2001/08/01/tobacco-and-womens-health-a-survey-of-popular-womens-magazines-august-1999-august-2000. Accessed May 16, 2016.

Martinasek MP, Ward KD, Calvanese AV. Change in carbon monoxide exposure among waterpipe bar patrons. *Nicotine Tob Res.* 2014;16(7):1014–1019.

Maryland Attorney General. Attorney General Gansler commemorates 10th anniversary of historic tobacco settlement: decade of public health gains marked by vigorous enforcement. 2008. Available at: https://www.oag.state.md.us/Press/2008/112008.htm. Accessed August 19, 2016.

McDonald IJ, Bhatia RS, Hollett PD. Deposition of cigar smoke particles in the lung: evaluation with ventilation scan using (99m)Tc-labeled sulfur colloid particles. *J Nuclear Med.* 2002;43(12):1591–1595.

McDonald P, Colwell B, Backinger CL, Husten C, Maule CO. Better practices for youth tobacco cessation: evidence of review panel. *Am J Health Behav.* 2003;27(suppl 2):S144–S158.

Murphy-Hoefer R, Hyland A, Higbee C. Perceived effectiveness of tobacco counter-marketing advertisements among young adults. *Am J Health Behav.* 2008;32(6):725–734.

National Association of Attorneys General (NAAG). Forty-one attorneys general and R.J. Reynolds reach historic settlement to end the sale of flavored. 2006. Available at: http://www.naag.org/naag/media/naag-news/flavored.php. Accessed April 5, 2015.

National Cancer Institute (NCI). *The Impact of Cigarette Excise Taxes on Smoking Among Children and Adults: Summary Report of a National Cancer Institute Expert Panel.* Washington, DC: NCI; 1993.

National Cancer Institute (NCI). *Cigars: Health Effects and Trends.* 1998. Available at: http://cancercontrol.cancer.gov/brp/tcrb/monographs/9/m9_complete.PDF. Accessed February 17, 2016.

National Cancer Institute (NCI). *The Role of the Media in Promoting and Reducing Tobacco Use.* 2008. Available at: http://cancercontrol.cancer.gov/brp/tcrb/monographs/19/m19_complete.pdf. Accessed February 24, 2016.

National Cancer Institute and Centers for Disease Control and Prevention (NCI and CDC). *Smokeless Tobacco and Public Health: A Global Perspective.* 2014. NIH Publication no. 14-7983. Available at: http://cancercontrol.cancer.gov/brp/tcrb/global-perspective/index.html. Accessed February 17, 2016.

Nelson DE, Davis RM, Chrismon JH, et al. Pipe smoking in the United States, 1965–1991: prevalence and attributable mortality. *Prev Med.* 1996;25(2):91–99.

Nonnemaker J, Rostron B, Hall P, MacMonegle A, Apelberg B. Mortality and economic costs from regular cigar use in the United States, 2010. *Am J Public Health.* 2014; 104(9):e86–e91.

Nyboe JG, Jensen G, Appleyard M, et al. Smoking and the risk of first acute myocardial infarction. *Am Heart J.* 1991;122(2):438–447.

Ohsfeldt RL, Boyle RG, Capilouto E. Effects of tobacco excise taxes on the use of smokeless tobacco products in the USA. *Health Econ.* 1997;6(5):525–531.

Ono Y, Ingersoll B. RJR retires Joe Camel, adds sexy smokers. *Wall Street Journal.* July 11, 1997:B1.

Pechacek T, Farrelley M, Thomas K, Nelson D. The impact of tobacco control programs on adult smoking. *Am J Public Health.* 2008;98(2):304–309.

Pechman C, Ratneshawr S. The effects of antismoking and cigarette advertising on young adolescents' perceptions of peers who smoke. *J Consum Res.* 1994;21: 236–251.

Pickett MS, Schober SE, Brody DJ, et al. Smoke–free laws and secondhand smoke exposure in US non-smoking adults, 1999–2000. *Tob Control.* 2006;15(4):302–307.

Pierce JP, Choi WS, Gilpin EA, Farkas AJ, Berr CC. Tobacco industry promotion of cigarettes and adolescent smoking. *JAMA.* 1998;279(7):511–515.

Pierce JP, Gilmer TP, Lee L, Gilpin EA, de Beyer J, Messer K. Tobacco industry price-subsidizing promotions may overcome the downward pressure of higher prices on initiation of regular smoking. *Health Econ.* 2005;14(10):1061–1071.

Pierce JP, Lee L, Gilpin EA. Smoking initiation by adolescent girls, 1944–1988. An association with targeted advertising. *JAMA.* 1994;271(8):608–611.

Pollay R, Siddarth S, Siegel M, et al. The last straw? Cigarette advertising and realized market shares among youths and adults, 1979-1993. *J Mark.* 1996;60:1–16.

Prokopczyk B, Cox JE, Hoffmann D, et al. Identification of tobacco specific carcinogen in the cervical mucus of smokers and nonsmokers. *J Natl Cancer Inst.* 1997;89(12): 868–873.

The Public Health Cigarette Smoking Act of 1969, Pub L 91–222. Available at: https://www.gpo.gov/fdsys/pkg/STATUTE-84/pdf/STATUTE-84-Pg87-2.pdf. Accessed August 21, 2016.

Quindlen A. Quid pro quo. *New York Times.* October 8, 1994. Available at: http://www.nytimes.com/1994/10/08/opinion/public-private-quid-pro-quo.html. Accessed April 5, 2014.

Rammah M, Dandachi F, Salman R, Shihadeh A, El-Sabban M. In vitro cytotoxicity and mutagenicity of mainstream waterpipe smoke and its functional consequences on alveolar type II derived cells. *Toxicol Lett.* 2012;211(3):220–231.

Rammah M, Dandachi F, Salman R, Shihadeh A, El-Sabban M. In vitro effects of waterpipe smoke condensate on endothelial cell function: a potential risk factor for vascular disease. *Toxicol Lett.* 2013;219(2):133–142.

Rastam S, Eissenberg T, Ibrahim I, Ward KD, Khalil R, Maziak W. Comparative analysis of waterpipe and cigarette suppression of abstinence and craving symptoms. *Addict Behav.* 2011;36(5):555–559.

Reid JL, Hammond D, Boudreau C, Fong GT, Siahpush M, ITC Collaboration. Socioeconomic disparities in quit intentions, quit attempts, and smoking abstinence among smokers in four western countries: findings from the International Tobacco Control Four Country Survey. *Nicotine Tob Res.* 2010;12(suppl 1):S20–S33.

Repace J. Respirable particles and carcinogens in the air of Delaware hospitality venues before and after a smoking ban. *J Occup Environ Med.* 2004;46(9):887–905.

Richard P, West K, Ku L. The return on investment of a Medicaid tobacco cessation program in Massachusetts. *PLoS ONE.* 2012;7(1):e29665.

Ringel JS, Wasserman J, Andreyeva T. Effects of public policy on adolescents' cigar use: evidence from the National Youth Tobacco Survey. *Am J Public Health.* 2005; 95(6):995–998.

Rodriguez J, Jiang R, Johnson WC, MacKenzie BA, Smith LJ, Barr RG. The association of pipe and cigar use with cotinine levels, lung function, and airflow obstruction: a cross-sectional study. *Ann Intern Med.* 2010;152(4):201–210.

Rodu B, Plurphanswat N, Fagerstrom K. Time to first use among daily smokers and smokeless tobacco users. *Nicotine Tob Res.* 2015;17(7):882–885.

Rohan T, Goodman JD. Mets and Yankees brace for a future without smokeless tobacco. *New York Times.* March 22, 2016. Available at: http://www.nytimes.com/2016/03/23/sports/the-mets-and-the-yankees-brace-for-a-future-without-smokeless-tobacco.html?emc=edit_tnt_20160322&nlid=68586528&tntemail0=y&_r=0. Accessed April 5, 2016.

Romer D, Jamieson P. Do adolescents appreciate the risks of smoking? Evidence from a National Survey. *J Adolesc Health*. 2001;29(1):12–21.

Rostron BL, Chang CM, van Bemmel DM, Yang X, Blount BC. Nicotine and toxicant exposure among US smokeless tobacco users: results from 1999 to 2012 National Health and Nutrition Examination Survey Data. *Cancer Epidemiol Biomarkers Prev*. 2015;24(12):1–9.

Saffer H, Chaloupka F. Tobacco advertising: economic theory and international evidence. National Bureau of Economic Research. 1999. Available at: http://www.nber.org/papers/w6958.pdf. Accessed April 5, 2015.

Schauffler HH, Rodriguez T. Availability and utilization of health promotion programs and satisfaction with health plan. *Med Care*. 1994;32(12):1182–1196.

Schober W, Szendrei K, Matzen W, et al. Use of electronic cigarettes (e-cigarettes) impairs indoor air quality and increases FeNO levels of e-cigarette consumers. *Int J Hyg Environ Health*. 2014;217(6):628–637.

Schripp T, Markewitz D, Uhde E, et al. Does e-cigarette consumption cause passive vaping? *Indoor Air*. 2013;23(1):25–31.

Schroeder S. Tobacco control in the wake of the 1998 Master Settlement Agreement. *N Eng J Med*. 2004;350(3):293–301.

Schubert J, Hahn J, Dettbarn G, et al. Mainstream smoke of the waterpipe: does this environmental matrix reveal a significant source of toxic compounds? *Toxicol Lett*. 2011;205(3):279–284.

Schubert J, Heinke V, Bewersdorff J, Luch A, Schulz TG. Waterpipe smoking: the role of humectants in the release of toxic carbonyls. *Arch Toxicol*. 2012;86(8):1309–1316.

Scientific Committee on Tobacco and Health. *Report of the Scientific Committee on Tobacco and Health*. London, England: The Stationery Office; 1998.

Shapiro JA, Jacobs EJ, Thun MJ. Cigar smoking in men and risk of death from tobacco-related cancers. *J Natl Cancer Inst*. 2000;92(4):333–337.

Shihadeh A, Saleh R. Polycyclic aromatic hydrocarbons, carbon monoxide, "tar," and nicotine in the mainstream smoke aerosol of the narghile waterpipe. *Food Chem Toxicol*. 2005;43(5):655–661.

Siahpush M, Shaikh RA, Hyland A, et al. Point-of-sale cigarette marketing, urge to buy cigarettes, and impulse purchases of cigarettes: results from a population-based survey. *Nicotine Tob Res*. 2016a;18(5):1357–1362.

Siahpush M, Shaikh RA, Smith D, et al. The association of exposure to point-of-sale tobacco marketing with quit attempt and quit success: results from a prospective study of smokers in the United States. *Int J Environ Res Public Health*. 2016b;6(2):E203.

Siegel M, Albers AB, Cheng DM, Biener L, Rigotti NA. Effect of local restaurant smoking regulations on progression to established smoking among youths. *Tob Control*. 2005; 14(5):300–306.

Singh T, Arrazola RA, Corey CG, et al. Tobacco use among middle and high school students—United States, 2011–2015. *MMWR Morb Mortal Wkly Rep*. 2016;65(14):361–367.

Singh T, Marynak K, Arrazola R, et al. Vital signs: exposure to electronic cigarette advertising among middle school and high school students—United States, 2014. *MMWR Morb Mortal Wkly Rep*. 2016;64(52):1403–1408.

Sloan FA, Ostermann J, Conover C, Taylor DH, Picone G. *The Price of Smoking*. Cambridge, MA: MIT Press; 2004.

Slovic P. What does it mean to know a cumulative risk? Adolescents' perceptions of short-term and long-term consequences of smoking. *J Behav Dec Making*. 2000;13(2):259–266.

Sorensen G, Emmons K, Stoddard AM, Linnan L, Avrunin J. Do social influences contribute to occupational differences in quitting smoking and attitudes toward quitting? *Am J Health Promot*. 2002;16(3):135–141.

Spindle T, Breland A, Karaoghlanian N, et al. Preliminary results of an examination of electronic cigarette use puff topography: the effect of a mouthpiece-based topography measurement device on plasma nicotine and subjective effects. *Nicotine Tob Res*. 2015;17(2):142–149.

Stead LF, Hartmann-Boyce J, Perera R, Lancaster T. Telephone counselling for smoking cessation. *Cochrane Database Syst Rev*. 2013. Available at: http://www.cochrane.org/ CD002850/TOBACCO_is-telephone-counselling-effective-as-part-of-a-programme-help-people-stop-smoking. Accessed February 26, 2016.

Stead LF, Lancaster T. Interventions for preventing tobacco sales to minors. *Cochrane Database Syst Rev*. 2005. Available at: http://www.ncbi.nlm.nih.gov/books/NBK99240/ #ch6.s5. Accessed February 26, 2016.

Substance Abuse and Mental Health Services Administration (SAMHSA). Tobacco regulation for substance abuse prevention and treatment block grants. *Fed Regist*. 1996;61(13):1492–1502.

Substance Abuse and Mental Health Services Administration (SAMHSA). FFY 2013 annual Synar reports: youth tobacco sales. 2014a. Available at: http://store.samhsa.gov/ shin/content//SYNAR-14/SYNAR-14.pdf. Accessed April 6, 2016.

Substance Abuse and Mental Health Services Administration (SAMHSA). Results from the 2014 National Survey on Drug Use and Health: detailed tables. 2014b. Available at: http://www.samhsa.gov/data/sites/default/files/NSDUH-DetTabs2014/NSDUH-DetTabs2014.htm#tab4-10a. Accessed April 18, 2016.

Tanski SE, Emond JA, Stanton CA, et al. Youth access to tobacco products in the United States: findings from wave 1 (2013–14) of the Population Assessment of Tobacco and Health (PATH) Study. Poster presentation at: the 2016 Society for Research on Nicotine and Tobacco 22nd Annual Meeting; March 2–5, 2016; Chicago, IL.

Tashkin DP, Murray RP. Smoking cessation in chronic obstructive pulmonary disease. *Respir Med*. 2009;103(7):963–974.

Tauras JA, Chaloupka F, Farrelly M, et al. State tobacco control spending and youth smoking. *Am J Public Health*. 2005;95(2):338–344.

Thomas S, Fayter D, Misso K, et al. Population tobacco control interventions and their effects on social inequalities in smoking: systematic review. *Tob Control*. 2008; 17(4): 230–237.

Tierney PA, Karpinski CD, Brown JE, Luo W, Pankow JF. Flavour chemicals in electronic cigarette fluids. *Tob Control*. 2015;25(e1):e10–e15.

Tomar SL, Husten CG, Manley WM. Do dentists and physicians advise tobacco users to quit? *J Am Dent Assoc*. 1996;127(2):259–265.

Trehy ML, Ye W, Hadwiger ME, et al. Analysis of electronic cigarette cartridges, refill solutions, and smoke for nicotine and nicotine related impurities. *J Liq Chromatogr Relat Technol*. 2011;34(14):1442–1458.

Tverdal A, Bjartveit K. Health consequences of pipe versus cigarette smoking. *Tob Control*. 2011;20(2):123–130.

University of Michigan. Monitoring the Future. 2015 data from in-school surveys of 8th-, 10th-, and 12th-grade students. 2015. Available at: http://www.monitoringthefuture.org/data/15data.html#2015data-cigs. Accessed April 18, 2016.

US Department of Health and Human Services (USDHHS). *The Health Consequences of Smoking: Chronic Obstructive Lung Disease*. 1984. Available at: http://profiles.nlm.nih.gov/NN/B/C/C/S. Accessed February 22, 2016.

US Department of Health and Human Services (USDHHS). *The Health Consequences of Smoking—Nicotine Addiction: A Report of the Surgeon General*. 1988. DHHS Publication (CDC) 88-8406. Available at: http://profiles.nlm.nih.gov/NN/B/B/Z/D. Accessed February 22, 2016.

US Department of Health and Human Services (USDHHS). *Reducing the Health Consequences of Smoking: 25 Years of Progress: A Report of the Surgeon General.* Atlanta, GA: Centers for Disease Control and Prevention, Office on Smoking and Health; 1989.

US Department of Health and Human Services (USDHHS). *The Health Benefits of Smoking Cessation: A Report of the Surgeon General.* 1990. DHHS Publication (CDC) 90–8416. Available at: http://profiles.nlm.nih.gov/NN/B/B/C/T. Accessed February 22, 2016.

US Department of Health and Human Services (USDHHS). *Preventing Tobacco Use Among Young People: A Report of the Surgeon General.* Atlanta, GA: Centers for Disease Control and Prevention, National Center for Chronic Disease Prevention and Health Promotion, Office on Smoking and Health; 1994.

US Department of Health and Human Services (USDHHS). *Reducing Tobacco Use: A Report of the Surgeon General.* 2000. Available at: http://www.cdc.gov/tobacco/data_statistics/sgr/2000/complete_report/pdfs/fullreport.pdf. Accessed February 24, 2016.

US Department of Health and Human Services (USDHHS). *Women and Smoking: A Report of the Surgeon General.* 2001. Available at: http://www.ncbi.nlm.nih.gov/books/NBK44303. Accessed April 5, 2016.

US Department of Health and Human Services (USDHHS). *The Health Consequences of Smoking: A Report of the Surgeon General.* 2004. Available at: http://www.cdc.gov/tobacco/data_statistics/sgr/2004/complete_report/index.htm. Accessed February 17, 2016.

US Department of Health and Human Services (USDHHS). *The Health Consequences of Involuntary Exposure to Tobacco Smoke. A Report of the Surgeon General.* 2006. Available at: http://www.cdc.gov/tobacco/data_statistics/sgr/2006/index.htm. Accessed February 17, 2016.

US Department of Health and Human Services (USDHHS). *How Tobacco Smoke Causes Disease—The Biology and Behavioral Basis for Smoking-Attributable Disease. A Report of the Surgeon General.* Atlanta, GA: Centers for Disease Control and Prevention, Office on Smoking and Health; 2010.

US Department of Health and Human Services (USDHHS). *Preventing Tobacco Use Among Youth and Young Adults: A Report of the Surgeon General, 2012.* 2012. Available at: http://www.ncbi.nlm.nih.gov/books/NBK99237. Accessed February 21, 2016.

US Department of Health and Human Services (USDHHS). *The Health Consequences of Smoking—50 Years of Progress. A Report of the Surgeon General.* 2014. Available at: http://www.surgeongeneral.gov/library/reports/50-years-of-progress/full-report.pdf. Accessed February 17, 2016.

US Department of Labor. Occupational exposure to flavoring substances: health effects and hazard control. SHIB 10-14-2010. 2010. Available at: https://www.osha.gov/dts/shib/shib10142010.html. Accessed February 20, 2016.

US Preventive Services Task Force (USPSTF). Tobacco smoking cessation in adults, including pregnant women: behavioral and pharmacotherapy interventions. 2015. Available at: http://www.uspreventiveservicestaskforce.org/Page/Document/Update-SummaryFinal/tobacco-use-in-adults-and-pregnant-women-counseling-and-interventions1. Accessed February 26, 2016.

Vansickel AR, Cobb CO, Weaver MF, et al. A clinical laboratory model for evaluating the acute effects of electronic cigarettes: nicotine delivery profile and cardiovascular and subjective effects. *Cancer Epidemiol Biomarkers Prev.* 2010;19(8):1945–1953.

Wagner EH, Curry SJ, Grothaus L, et al. The impact of smoking and quitting on health care use. *Arch Intern Med.* 1995;155(16):1789–1795.

Wakefield M, Terry-McElrath Y, Emery S, et al. Effect of televised, tobacco company–funded smoking prevention advertising on youth smoking-related beliefs, intentions, and behavior. *Am J Public Health.* 2006;95(12):2154–2160.

Wald NJ, Watt HC. Prospective study of effect of switching from cigarettes to pipes or cigars on mortality from three smoking related diseases. *Brit Med J.* 1997;314(7098):1860–1863.

Wallace L. Environmental exposure to benzene: an update. *Environ Health Perspect.* 1996;104(suppl 6):1129–1136.

Warner KE. Cigarette advertising and media coverage of smoking and health. *N Engl J Med.* 1985;312(6):384–388.

Warner KE, Sexton DW, Gillespie BW, Levy DT, Chaloupka FJ. Impact of tobacco control on adult per capita cigarette consumption in the United States. *Am J Public Health.* 2014;104(1):83–89.

Weinstein ND. Accuracy of smokers' risk perceptions. *Ann Behav Med.* 1998;20(2):135–140.

Weinstein ND. Smokers' unrealistic optimism about their risk. *Tob Control.* 2005;14(1):55–59.

White VM, White MM, Freeman K, Gilpin EA, Pierce JP. Cigarette promotional offers: who takes advantage? *Am J Prev Med.* 2006;30(3):225–231.

Williams M, Villarreal A, Bozhilov K, Lin S, Talbot P. Metal and silicate particles including nanoparticles are present in electronic cigarette cartomizer fluid and aerosol. *PLOS One.* 2013;8(3):1–11.

World Health Organization (WHO). WHO Framework Convention on Tobacco Control. 2003. Available at: http://www.who.int/tobacco/framework/WHO_FCTC_english.pdf. Accessed May 16, 2016.

World Health Organization Study Group on Tobacco Product Regulation (WHO). Waterpipe tobacco smoking: health effects, research needs, and recommended actions by regulators. WHO Tobacco Free Initiative. 2005. Available at: http://www.who.int/tobacco/global_interaction/tobreg/Waterpipe%20recommendation_Final.pdf. Accessed February 20, 2016.

Wyss A, Hashibe M, Chuang SC. Cigarette, cigar, and pipe smoking and the risk of head and neck cancers: pooled analysis in the International Head and Neck Cancer Epidemiology Consortium. *Am J Epidemiol*. 2013;178(5):679–690.

Xu X, Pesko MF, Tynan MA, Gerzoff RB, Malarcher AM, Pechacek TF. Cigarette price-minimization strategies by US smokers. *Am J Prev Med*. 2013;44(5):472–476.

Yeager RP, Kushman M, Chemerynski S, et al. Proposed mode of action for acrolein respiratory toxicity associated with inhaled tobacco smoke. *Toxicol Sci*. 2016;151(2):347–364.

Zagorsky JL. The wealth effects of smoking. *Tob Control*. 2004;13(4):370–374.

8

DIET AND NUTRITION

Cassandra Greenwood, BS, Rachel Sippy, MPH,
Bethany Weinert, MD, MPH, and Alexandra Adams, MD, PhD

Introduction

Healthy eating habits are necessary for health and survival, yet we eat for more than sustenance. Foods are deeply connected to our cultures, memories, lifestyles, and emotions. Every sector of society influences food and beverage choices (USDHHS and USDA 2015). Families, schools, and employers create social norms through policies and environments that can either facilitate or hinder healthy eating behaviors. Conversely, the food and beverage industry drives choice and consumption through marketing, portion sizes, food ingredients, disclosure of nutritional information, location of grocery stores, offerings in restaurants, and pricing (Cannuscio et al. 2014; Ferguson et al. 2012; USDHHS and USDA 2015). Similarly, the entertainment and sports industries have an impact on product placement, promotion, and availability of healthy foods at sport, movie, and other entertainment venues.

Health care providers and insurers also influence patient behavior through standards, practices, and incentives. Federal, state, and local governments set priorities for prevention, provide incentives and funding for nutrition assistance programs, and stimulate efforts in planning, land use, and transportation. For example, the Patient Protection and Affordable Care Act, commonly referred to as ACA, was signed into law in 2010. Under Section 2705, employers are allowed to promote wellness programs. For example, they may reimburse part or all of a fitness center membership, provide a reward to employees for attending periodic public health education seminars, and make available diagnostic testing that rewards for participation, not outcomes (Patient Protection and Affordable Care Act 2010).

Poor nutrition has many consequences. It is linked to most major chronic diseases, including obesity, type 2 diabetes, cardiovascular disease (CVD),

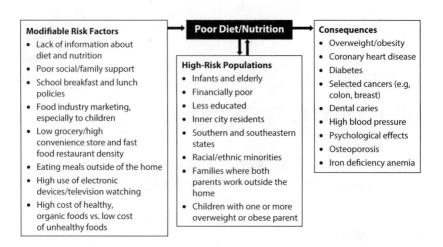

Source: Adapted from Malas et al. (2010).

Figure 8-1. Poor Diet and Nutrition: Causes, Consequences, and High-Risk Groups

hypertension, poor oral health, osteoporosis, iron deficiency anemia, and many cancers (USDHHS and USDA 2015; GBD 2013 Risk Factors Collaborators 2015; WHO 2015). As nutrition is one of the major modifiable risk factors for chronic disease, it could have a significant impact on global chronic disease burden (WHO 2015).

Public health nutrition must take a population-based approach to simultaneously address food security, health promotion, and disease prevention. The challenge for public health is to provide leadership across the public, nonprofit, and business sectors that will result in norms and environments where the healthiest food choices are also the most affordable and readily accessible to all segments of society, as well as to partner with these sectors to enact change. The purpose of this chapter is to describe and discuss the downstream consequences of poor nutrition, the upstream modifiable risk factors that cause poor nutrition, the high-risk populations for poor nutrition, and the associated conditions and diseases related to poor nutrition (Figure 8-1).

Significance

As noted in Figure 8-1, the consequences of poor nutrition are numerable and severe. Some nutrition-related factors, such as high blood pressure, high cholesterol, low fruit and vegetable intake, high body mass index (BMI), and alcohol consumption are leading contributors to chronic disease in developed countries (WHO 2013; Liu 2013). Poor nutrition accounts for 11.3 million deaths and 241.4 million disability-adjusted life years (DALYs) annually, while malnutrition is responsible for another 1.7 million deaths and 176.9 million DALYs (GBD 2013 Risk Factors Collaborators 2015). However, a lack of access to proper nutrition and food insecurity are prevalent for many in the United States. More than 49 million people experienced food insecurity more than once in 2008 and more than 23 million Americans live in food deserts—areas that are more than one mile away from a supermarket (Nord et al. 2009; USDA 2009).

Noncommunicable diseases such as diabetes, cancer, and CVDs kill more than 38 million people worldwide each year (WHO 2015). In the United States, about half of all adults have one or more noncommunicable disease, accounting for 86% of all health care spending in 2010 (Gerteis et al. 2014). The *Dietary Guidelines for Americans*, as outlined in Table 8-1, provides dietary

Table 8-1. Dietary Guidelines for Americans

1. Eat a variety of highly nutritious foods and beverages within the basic food groups.
2. Eat two cups of fruit and two and a half cups of vegetables per day, selecting from all five vegetable groups (dark green, orange, legumes, starchy vegetables, and other vegetables).
3. Eat three or more ounce equivalents of whole grain foods per day, with at least half of all daily grain intake being from whole grains.
4. Eat a variety of protein foods, including seafood, lean meats and poultry, eggs, legumes (beans and peas), seeds, and soy products.
5. Drink up to three cups per day of fat-free or low-fat milk or equivalent milk products, such as low-fat cheese or yogurt.
6. Consume less than 10% of calories from saturated fatty acids by replacing them with monounsaturated and polyunsaturated fatty acids and consume less than 300 milligrams per day of dietary cholesterol.
7. Your total fat consumption should be between 25% and 30% of your total calories, and the majority of your daily fats should come from polyunsaturated or monounsaturated sources such as fish, nuts, and vegetable oils.
8. Eat foods that are high in fiber.
9. Consume less than 10% of calories per day from added sugars.
10. Reduce daily sodium intake to less than 2,300 milligrams and further reduce intake to 1,500 milligrams among persons who are aged 51 years and older and those of any age who are African American or have hypertension, diabetes, or chronic kidney disease.
11. If alcohol is consumed, it should be consumed in moderation—up to one drink per day for women and up to two drinks per day for men—and only by adults of legal drinking age.

Source: Compiled from USDA (2005); USDHHS and USDA (2010); and USDHHS and USDA (2015).

recommendations throughout the lifecycle for proper health and a decreased risk of chronic disease (USDHHS and USDA 2015). However, all available data show that we are falling far short of domestic and worldwide nutrition targets (USDHHS and USDA 2010; WHO 2013). The majority of Americans consume more than the recommended amounts of solid fat and added sugars, refined grains, sodium, and saturated fat, while eating less fruits and vegetables, whole grains, and dairy products than recommended (USDA and USDHHS 2010).

Pathophysiology

Studies have shown that good nutrition can be preventive against certain diseases and lowers risks for adverse health outcomes, whereas poor nutrition—whether an excess or insufficient amount of calories and nutrients—is a risk factor for many diseases. Given the amount and complexity of dietary research, only some of the most important relationships will be described in the next paragraphs to illustrate ways that nutrition affects chronic disease biology.

Fruits and Vegetables

An adequate intake of fruits and vegetables has long been associated with a lower risk of many chronic diseases, including some cancers, type 2 diabetes, CVD, and obesity (CDC 2013; Liu 2013; Appleton et al. 2016). The protection appears to come from a variety of nutrients found in fruits and vegetables, including dietary fiber, vitamin C, vitamin E, folic acid, potassium, selenium, and phytochemicals such as terpenes, carotenoids, lycopene, isothiocyanates, dithiolthiones, and flavonoids (Liu 2013).

One mechanism for the association between fruits and vegetables and reduced risk of CVD may be through antioxidants such as vitamin C, beta-carotene, and flavonoids. They may act by reducing oxidized cholesterol levels in the body, thereby protecting arteries from damage by slowing or inhibiting the development of atherosclerotic plaques made up of low-density lipoprotein (LDL) particles (Willcox et al. 2008). However, as of yet, studies lack sufficient and conclusive evidence that antioxidants prevent or reduce risk of CVD, especially in supplemental forms (Sesso et al. 2008; NIH 2013). Higher consumption of antioxidants such as vitamins E and C has also been associated with lower total and LDL cholesterol (IOM 2000). A second protective mechanism for CVD may be through a reduction of serum cholesterol caused by soluble fiber found in fruits and vegetables. Studies have found a reduction in both coronary events and coronary deaths for each incremental increase in fiber consumption (Pereira et al. 2004; Theuwissen and Mensink 2008).

Natural substances in fruits and vegetables may also be responsible for a decreased risk of some cancers. Antioxidants are theorized to protect cell membranes and DNA from oxidative damage (Wolfe et al. 2008; World Cancer Research Fund and American Institute for Cancer Research 2007). As yet, however, the lack of high-quality studies exploring the role of antioxidants has provided inconclusive evidence of their effect on long-term disease prevention (NIH 2013). In addition, phytochemicals such as isothiocyanates, dithiolthiones, and indoles appear to induce enzymatic detoxification systems and block tumor production or growth. Isoflavones, found in soybeans and other legumes, may keep endogenous estrogens from binding to cell receptors, which may reduce the risk of associated cancers. Phenolic acids found in fruits may inhibit activity of other receptors necessary for cancer development (Zamora-Ros et al. 2013; Lim et al. 2016; Dikmen et al. 2011).

Fruits and vegetables are thought to influence body weight through a variety of mechanisms. Their high content of water and fiber and low fat content result in low energy density. Such foods have been associated with greater post-meal satiety. Nevertheless, studies examining an association between increased fruit and vegetable consumption and weight control are inconsistent (Järvi et al. 2016; Kaiser et al. 2014; Mytton et al. 2014; Bertioa et al. 2015). This may be attributable at least in part to the inherent complexity, multiple contributing factors, and long-term nature of dietary research.

Dietary Fiber

For hundreds of years, people have been consuming dietary fiber for its accompanying health benefits (Fuller et al. 2016). Many studies have shown an association between higher consumption of dietary fiber and reduced incidence of coronary heart disease and some cancers. Several potential mechanisms for this association have been proposed. Insoluble dietary fiber is found in grains, fruits, vegetables, and nuts. It speeds transit time and increases stool bulk, thereby decreasing exposure to and concentration of carcinogens in the gut (Aune et al. 2011). It also binds bile acids that can potentially act as promoters of carcinogenesis. Production of short-chain fatty acids, such as butyrate, occurs as dietary fiber is fermented in the colon. These short-chain fatty acids may protect against cancer by promoting differentiation, inducing apoptosis, or inhibiting secondary bile acid production (Bultman 2014; Cho et al. 2014). Many case–control studies have demonstrated a somewhat lower risk of cancer with high consumption of dietary fiber, yet large prospective studies have been largely inconsistent (Aune et al. 2011; Huang et al. 2015; Park et al. 2005).

In terms of CVD, soluble fiber (β-glucan), found in the endosperm cell walls of oats, has been shown to lower blood cholesterol levels, likely by binding bile acids, thereby preventing reabsorption (Fuller et al. 2016; Othman et al. 2011). Furthermore, dietary fiber appears to be inversely associated with blood insulin levels, which may have benefits for the prevention of insulin resistance and type 2 diabetes (Yu et al. 2014).

Dietary Fat and Red Meat

Different types of fats affect our bodies in different ways. Trans fats and saturated fats can have adverse effects on health, whereas others, such as monounsaturated fats, have significant benefits. For example, women who consumed the lowest proportions of saturated fatty acids and trans fatty acids had reduced risk of coronary heart disease, CVD, and stroke. Two large prospective cohort studies found that replacing just 5% of energy intake of saturated fats with equal amounts from polyunsaturated fats, monounsaturated fats, or whole grain carbohydrate sources, was associated with a 25%, 15%, and 9% lower risk of coronary heart disease, respectively (Li et al. 2015). Other studies find that a reduced intake of saturated fatty acids and cholesterol can reduce total cholesterol and LDL, leading to lower rates of atherosclerosis, ischemic stroke, and myocardial infarction (Chang et al. 2014; Seo et al. 2005). Replacing saturated fatty acids with polyunsaturated or monounsaturated fatty acids also results in decreased LDL cholesterol (Baum et al. 2012).

Other fats are beneficial to a healthy diet, particularly omega-3 fatty acids and monounsaturated oils. Several studies show an inverse relationship between intake of omega-3 fatty acids and cancer. Omega-3 fatty acids are present in fish oils and in some vegetables. One hypothesis is that omega-3 fatty acids alter the immune response to cancer cells and influence transcription factor activity and gene expression (Larsson et al. 2004). Another hypothesis is that omega-3 fatty acids reduce circulating markers of inflammation, thus potentially protecting against heart disease, atherosclerosis, rheumatoid arthritis, and psychiatric disease (Yan et al. 2013; Calder 2015; Lee et al. 2006).

Although some epidemiological studies have supported this hypothesis, clinical trials are not definitive. In some studies, monounsaturated oils, such as olive oil, have also shown a protective effect on health, particularly heart disease (Guasch-Ferré et al. 2014).

Red meat can result in both positive health benefits and negative health outcomes. In moderation, red meat is a rich source of iron, folate, zinc, selenium, vitamins A and B12, and protein (Ekmekcioglu et al. 2016). Diets in developing countries or lower-income communities are predominantly composed of cereal and legume-based foods with low bioavailable iron. In addition, the folate in red meat is of higher bioavailability than that provided in plant-based sources, which may explain the greater prevalence of iron deficiency anemia in populations that do not consume adequate amounts of red meat (Ekmekcioglu et al. 2016; Moshe et al. 2013).

However, high intake of red meat has been associated with some cancers, principally colorectal cancer (Cross et al. 2010; Demeyer et al. 2015). The possible mechanisms include the polycyclic hydrocarbons and mutagenic amines that can be generated by cooking at high temperatures; the nitrites and other similar compounds found in salted, smoked, and processed meats that can be converted to toxic N-nitroso compounds within the colonic wall; and the high level of iron, which can lead to the formation of mutagenic free radicals in the gut wall (Cross et al. 2010; Demeyer et al. 2015). The World Health Organization recently classified processed meat as carcinogenic to humans, and red meat was classified as probably carcinogenic to humans (Bouvard et al. 2015).

Dairy Products and Milk

Dairy intake offers many benefits to a balanced diet. Dairy products are rich sources of protein, calcium, potassium, vitamin B12, riboflavin, magnesium, phosphorous, and, when fortified, vitamin D (Heaney 2013). However, consumption can be precluded in many populations by lactose or milk protein intolerance. It is estimated that 80 million Americans have lactose intolerance or lactose malabsorption (Levitt et al. 2013).

Daily consumption of low-fat milk products has been shown to be protective against some chronic diseases, including osteoporosis, CVD, and colon cancer (USDHHS and USDA 2010; World Cancer Research Fund and American Institute for Cancer Research 2007). Milk contains beneficial fatty acids, vitamins, minerals, and bioactive compounds that positively affect overall nutrition (Heaney 2013; Dugan and Fernandez 2014). Calcium in dairy products directly inhibits lipid accumulation in cells and increases fecal excretion of lipids (Bendsen et al. 2008). In addition, calcium from food, but not supplements, preserves thermogenesis during calorie restriction (Zemel 2004).

Despite the benefits of milk intake on nutrition, whole and 2% milk products contain a considerable amount of saturated fat and extra calories. The *Dietary Guidelines for Americans* recommends that all adults consume up to three servings of low-fat or nonfat milk, or equivalent milk products such as low-fat yogurt, each day (USDHHS and USDA 2010). Although overall consumption of milk has decreased progressively since 1970, low-fat and nonfat milk intake has increased and whole-fat milk consumption has decreased drastically (Stewart et al. 2013).

Sugar-Sweetened Beverages

Soda, energy drinks, and sports drinks account for the highest amount of added sugar consumption in the United States, easily outnumbering the consumption percentages of added sugar from desserts, candy, and ready-to-eat cereals (Malik and Hu 2015). Sugar-sweetened beverages include soft drinks; fruit drinks; sweetened waters, teas, and coffees; and energy drinks that are sweetened by high-fructose corn syrup or sucrose but excludes naturally occurring sugars and artificial sweeteners (Malik and Hu 2015; Le Bodo et al. 2015). Overconsumption of energy-dense, nutrient-poor beverages has been associated with obesity, dental caries, diabetes, and cardiovascular risks (Malik et al. 2010; Malik and Hu 2015; Zheng et al. 2015). The low-cost, convenience, variety of options, lack of satiety, and aggressive and widespread marketing campaigns all contribute to the high intake of sugar-sweetened beverages (Drewnowski and Bellisle 2007; Le Bodo et al. 2015).

Descriptive Epidemiology

High-Risk Populations

The U.S. population is at high risk of developing diet-related chronic disease. Our energy-dense diet includes saturated fats, red meat, and sugars and few vegetables, fruits, and whole grains. Surveillance of nutritional intake is difficult, especially within current public health and health care infrastructure, and relies on national surveys or epidemiological studies, such as the National

Health and Nutrition Examination Survey (NHANES) and the Behavioral Risk Factor Surveillance System (BRFSS; Bauer et al. 2014). These efforts reveal disparities in dietary quality among demographic groups.

Sex

Dietary quality varies by sex; this difference only begins in adulthood. Women have better healthy eating habits (Hiza et al. 2013) and a better-quality diet (Ervin 2011; Rehm et al. 2015), consuming more fruits and vegetables (Grimm et al. 2012; Hiza et al. 2013). Older men and women had no significant difference in healthy eating indices (Hiza et al. 2013). Younger women have more disordered eating behaviors compared to men (Lundahl et al. 2015), and women prefer to use diet modification for weight reduction, whereas men focus on physical activity (Grebitus et al. 2015). Women are also better than men at using portion-control strategies (Spence et al. 2015).

Age and Life Course

In children and adolescents, taste preferences, family support for healthy foods, and food availability are strongly correlated with a healthy, balanced diet (Neumark-Sztainer et al. 2003; Shepherd et al. 2006). Youths gravitate toward heavily marketed, energy-dense foods unless parents model healthy eating and set limits (Gidding et al. 2006). Poor dietary habits established at an early age are often carried into adulthood and can be difficult to change (Guo et al. 2002).

Aging involves many psychosocial, economic, and physiological changes. Metabolism slows, nutritional requirements change, and the pleasure of eating may wane (de Graaf et al. 1994; Bernstein and Munoz 2012; Wolfe et al. 2015). Data from NHANES and BRFSS suggest that older adults have the best healthy eating indices compared to younger groups (Grimm et al. 2012; Hiza et al. 2013); this indication may reflect survival bias, as those with a better diet may be better able to survive to older ages. Despite this finding, many older adults struggle to meet dietary recommendations because of factors such as disability, caregiver limitations, or living arrangements (Bernstein and Munoz 2012).

Race and Ethnicity

While the percentage of individuals meeting dietary guidelines within any racial/ethnic group is poor (Kirkpatrick et al. 2012), the data on which group is most likely to meet recommended dietary guidelines are complex. Among older adults, there are very few differences in diet between racial groups (Hiza et al. 2013). Hispanic children and adults are most likely to meet healthy food guidelines (Hiza et al. 2013; Kirkpatrick et al. 2012). Non-Hispanic blacks are least likely to achieve healthy diets, compared to other groups (Ervin 2011; Kirkpatrick et al. 2012; Hiza et al. 2013; Rehm et al. 2015). This effect is seen starting in childhood (Hiza et al. 2013). Asian Americans have been documented to consume more fruits and vegetables in general than other populations, and Asian American children also frequently consume milk, meat, unenriched white rice, and high-fat and high-sugar items (Satia 2009; Diep et al. 2015). Studies have found that low percentages of American Indians meet the recommended number of fruits and vegetables per day from the USDA (Basiotis et al. 1999; Berg et al. 2012). These differences are largely attributable to a variety of interlinked sociocultural, environmental, and psychobiological factors (Zhang and Wang 2012).

Income

As the affluence of a community decreases, access to healthy food also decreases (Morland et al. 2002). In a given week, about 20% of low-income households do not purchase fruits and vegetables, twice the rate for higher-income homes (Blisard et al. 2004). Energy-dense diets with poor nutritional value are more likely to be consumed by persons of lower economic means, whereas whole grains, lean meats, fish, low-fat milk products, and fresh fruits and vegetables are more likely to be consumed by those with greater means (Darmon and Drewnowski 2008; Doubeni et al. 2012; Grimm et al. 2012; Kirkpatrick et al. 2012). Conversely, children in low-income groups tend to have better fruit and vegetable scores than their high-income peers; this is thought to reflect participation in food benefit programs (Hiza et al. 2013) and the efforts of food-insecure adults to mitigate dietary insufficiency in their children (Dinour et al. 2007; Kant and Graubard 2007).

The relationship between income and diet quality holds along a gradient of income levels, indicating a positive relationship between low income and poor nutrition (Darmon and Drewnowski 2008; Hiza et al. 2013). Research suggests that this effect can be mitigated by nutrition education (Middaugh et al. 2012), as cost is only one component of the decision to consume healthy foods (Williams et al. 2010).

Education

Education and income are highly interrelated, and both have been shown to strongly correlate with nutrition and chronic disease, although nutritional education may be more important than income for fruit and vegetable consumption (Mullie et al. 2009; Wenrich et al. 2010; Middaugh et al. 2012). Higher consumption of fruits, vegetables, and foods with vitamins A and C, calcium, and potassium have been associated with higher levels of education (Kant and Graubard 2007; Ervin 2011; Hiza et al. 2013). Maternal education is positively related to the nutritional content of home meals, with college-educated primary food providers spending the most per capita for fruits and vegetables (Blisard et al. 2004).

Food Insecurity

Food insecurity is a growing area of research in nutrition. It describes limited or unstable access to healthy foods and can have major impacts on physical and mental health (Dinour et al. 2007). Purchasing power is a new term related to having money to purchase food (Escaron et al. 2013). Although closely linked to socioeconomic status, it also incorporates the safety, quality, and adequacy of available foods, cyclical patterns of economic and food benefit resources, and food behavior coping mechanisms (Dinour et al. 2007; Leung et al. 2014). Food insecurity has been linked to poor diet (Leung et al. 2014), obesity, and hunger, although these relationships are complex (Dinour et al. 2007), and may be modified by participation in food benefit programs (Larson and Story 2011). Highly palatable but nutritionally poor foods may be consumed more by the food-insecure as a coping mechanism (Leung et al. 2014). Food insecure households are more likely to be headed by blacks, Hispanics, or single parents, and prevalence varies from 2.9% to 22.0%, depending on the state (Coleman-Jensen et al. 2015). The highest rates of food insecurity, up to 75%, have been noted in rural American Indian populations (Pardilla et al. 2014; Gordon and Oddo 2012).

Genetics and Microbiome

There is mounting evidence of the importance of genetic factors and the microbiome as determinants, mediators, or modifiers of healthy diets and disease outcomes. Genetics have an impact on food metabolism or weight gain, which in turn affect health outcomes (Bordoni and Capozzi 2014;

Qi et al. 2014; Nettleton et al. 2015). Genetics are also associated with food choice and eating behaviors (Bordoni and Capozzi 2014; Qi et al. 2014; Hughes and Frazier-Wood 2016).

The microbiome—the community of microorganisms that inhabit the human body—serves an important role in human health. Long-term diet is believed to have the greatest influence on gut microbiome diversity (Xu and Knight 2015). Given the association between the microbiome and obesity, diabetes, and other nutrition-related diseases, there is increasing research into the relationship between diet and microbiome, and how they influence each other (Xu and Knight 2015; Vipperla and O'Keefe 2016). There is ongoing research on genetics, epigenetics, "microbiome health," and modification as a method of disease reduction (Hughes and Frazier-Wood 2016; Vipperla and O'Keefe 2016). Once the complexities of the genetics–diet–microbiome–disease relationship are better understood, genetics may become a tool for nutritional advice and the microbiome may become a modifiable risk factor.

Geographic Distribution

Within the United States, there are important and long-standing regional differences in food consumption patterns. Fish is consumed more frequently in coastal areas. Fruit and vegetable consumption is lower, and saturated fat consumption higher, in regions that also have high rates of obesity such as the South and lower Midwest. Sometimes described as the "stroke belt," many Southern states maintain diets high in added fats, fried foods, processed meats, and sugary drinks (Judd et al. 2014). Southern and Midwestern states have the lowest proportion of adults consuming two or more fruits each day, and Midwestern states and U.S. territories had the lowest proportion of adults consuming three or more vegetables each day (Grimm et al. 2012).

Local food availability also affects disease rates. People who live more than a mile away from a supermarket are 25% less likely to eat a healthy diet compared with those with a supermarket nearby (Moore et al. 2008). In many inner-city neighborhoods, full-spectrum supermarkets offering a variety of fresh produce and other foods have relocated to more affluent neighborhoods, causing a reduction in healthy dietary options within those communities (Moore et al. 2008). Rural communities are also at high risk of poor diet and nutritional health problems (Befort et al. 2012; Lutfiyya et al. 2012; O'Connor and Wellenius 2012), and likewise struggle with access to fresh food (Calancie et al. 2015).

Climate change is affecting, and will continue to affect, the growing season for plants. The United States' average length of growing season has increased by nearly two weeks since the 20th century (USEPA 2016). However, many countries will be negatively impacted with decreases in growing season length and water shortages (Mora et al. 2015).

Industrial Development and Immigration

Diets in Western, developed countries contain many animal products and saturated fat, with many readily available, energy-dense foods. Observational studies of populations that migrate from countries with low rates of chronic disease show that disease patterns of the acculturating migrants shift toward those of the new environment (Delavari et al. 2013), even though many migrants arrive practicing healthier behaviors than people in the United States (Perez-Escamilla 2011). As an immigrant spends more time in the United States, he or she adapts a poorer diet (Perez-Escamilla 2011), and is more likely to become overweight or obese (Tovar et al. 2012). Thus, in transitional groups, it is important to preserve healthy diets and prevent the uptake of highly advertised, inexpensive, low-nutrient foods, especially by children.

Time Trends

Since NHANES was first administered in 1971, there have been many changes in food consumption. The quantity of food and beverages consumed, the fraction of meals eaten outside the home, portion sizes, and energy density have increased significantly. Energy intake has increased by 196 kcal per day for men and 283 kcal per day for women (Wright et al. 2004; Kant and Graubard 2006). The percentage of men and women with an ideal, healthy diet increased over 1999 to 2008, but remains below 1.4% (Huffman et al. 2012). Between 1994 and 2005, the frequency of fruit and vegetable consumption had declined, with only 25% of adults eating the recommended minimum of five daily servings (Casagrande et al. 2007; Blanck et al. 2008). This trend continued from 2000 to 2009, with decreasing proportions of people report eating two or more fruits per day (Foltz et al. 2010).

Portion sizes have increased both inside and outside the home, and portions for snacks, soft drinks, and fruit drinks have grown markedly (Nielsen 2003; English et al. 2015). Fewer people in the United States report eating all three meals, and more report snacking as a significant source of their daily caloric intake (Kant and Graubard 2015). Projections of healthy diet scores for 2020 are below those targeted by the American Heart Association's 2020 Strategic Impact Goals (Huffman et al. 2012).

Between 1965 and 2002, calories per capita from beverages increased from 12% to 21% of daily caloric intake (Duffey and Popkin 2007). In 2002, 30% of Americans were drinking 25% or more of their daily calories, with higher intakes coming from alcohol, soda, fruit drinks, and other sweetened beverages. Since 2000, intake of high-caloric beverages has declined, with increased purchasing of low-caloric or no-sweetener beverages (Popkin and Nielsen 2003).

Causes

Modifiable Risk Factors

Like any complex human behavior, diet choice is determined by multiple factors working independently and concurrently. Factors that promote healthy eating include time, location, psychology, social relationships, culture, and environment (Swinburn et al. 1999). These risk factors can be related to personal or individual preferences, sociocultural factors, built environment, or macro environment. Understanding these factors can help in the design of innovative interventions (Story et al. 2008).

Because these interacting factors work on multiple levels, an ecological approach is the most inclusive model by which to address both barriers to and

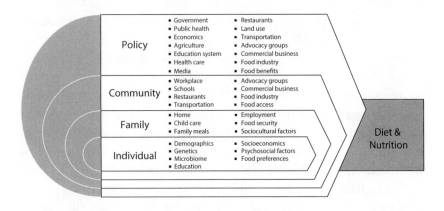

Source: Based on IOM 2007.

Figure 8-2. Social Ecological Approach to Diet and Nutrition

opportunities for healthy eating (IOM 2005; IOM 2007; Story et al. 2008). Such a model (Figure 8-2; IOM 2007) can help to assess forces, direct efforts, and interactions within and among individuals; families, peers, and social groups; institutions and communities; businesses, nonprofits, and government programs; and larger forces of society and culture. As research expands and interventions become more creative, this ecological approach will help organize interventions at local, regional, state, and national levels.

Individual-Level Factors

Self-efficacy, strong social support, and knowledge of nutritional benefits are strong predictors of fruit and vegetable intake (Shaikh et al. 2008). Other potential predictors include perceived barriers, strength of intention, attitudes and beliefs, and autonomous motivation to consume a healthy diet. Susceptibility to portion size effects also varies by individual (English et al. 2015). Emotional state and stress are important determinants of diet and eating patterns (Tate et al. 2015). The ability of a given individual to handle stress affects whether he or she will consume unhealthy foods under stress (i.e., emotion-driven eating; Tate et al. 2015). Individuals recognize that "food cravings" influence their diet and can identify particular triggers for cravings; despite the connection of cravings to obesity and unhealthy food consumption, many individuals do not see these cravings and their subsequent indulgence as problematic (Malika et al. 2015). The nature and demands of individual lifestyle can affect one's ability to eat a healthy diet (Jilcott et al. 2011); food "convenience" ranks highly among the factors influencing purchases (Kirkpatrick 2012).

Personal preference for certain qualities of foods, including taste, texture, and appearance, can vary considerably from person to person. Preference can override nutritional knowledge and drive resistance to the adoption of a healthy diet. In the absence of economic barriers and poor availability, personal preference is the best predictor of food choice (Clark 1998; Eertmans et al. 2001; Rozin 2001). There is ample evidence that marketing and nutrition education with taste testing of new foods, as well as introduction of healthy foods early in life, can alter population taste preferences.

Family and Social Environment

Families provide considerable influence on dietary habits, through learned behavior, parent or peer modeling, household food purchasing, and regularity of family meals (Gillman et al. 2000; van der Horst et al. 2006; Cruwys et al. 2015). Beliefs regarding what or how much is eaten are influenced by those with whom we eat and the social acceptableness of eating patterns (i.e., perceived norms; Cruwys et al. 2015; Sawka et al. 2015). Family meals are important to healthy eating. As more families have multiple members working long hours outside the home, the number of family meals can become limited and replaced by unhealthy snacking, missed meals, or fast food. Adolescents in particular resort to low-cost, energy-dense foods when there is little parental oversight (Grimm et al. 2004); child and adolescent eating patterns are particularly influenced by peers in the absence of parents (Sawka et al. 2015). Strong parental modeling and enforcement of home rules for healthy eating are promising strategies to improve nutrition (Story et al. 2008).

Community Environments

It is easier for an individual to make healthy dietary choices when supported by a physical environment with access to affordable, varied, nutritious foods (USDHHS 2000). Food cost is considered second only to taste in its effect on dietary choice (Glanz et al. 1998). Costs are influenced by supply-and-demand factors including consumer demand, season, government subsidies and regulations, food advertising, and geographic distribution of food production, supermarkets, restaurants, and other food outlets. Food prices have a more significant effect on the food choices of individuals at lower socioeconomic strata than individuals at higher socioeconomic levels (Beydoun and Wang 2008). Although there is a perception of less-healthy foods being cheaper than healthy foods, a relationship between the healthiness of food and its cost is likely false (Davis and Carlson 2015).

The built environment strongly affects access to healthy food options (Glanz and Yaroch 2004; Penney et al. 2015). Access to large supermarkets or a mix of markets with a variety of competitively priced, nutritious foods has been associated with better dietary practices (Larson et al. 2009; Penney et al. 2015). As the number of supermarkets in a community increases, fruit and vegetable consumption proportionally increases (Morland et al. 2002), though the mechanisms by which increased supermarket access affect diet are unclear (Cummins et al. 2014; Dubowitz et al. 2015; Penney et al. 2015). Areas of lower socioeconomic status, minority communities, and rural areas have few options for food purchasing and increasingly rely on fast food and convenience stores (Pothukuchi 2005; Powell et al. 2007; Dubowitz et al. 2015). In such areas, shopping may be limited to convenience stores tending to stock foods high in fat, salt, and sugar with little produce, whole grains, or lean meat (Glanz et al. 2005; Larson et al. 2009). This has been a major contributor to growing health disparities for low-income, minority communities.

People in the United States are eating a greater proportion of meals and snacks away from home (Kant and Graubard 2004). Between 1977 and 2006, the reported percentage of daily energy obtained via meals outside the home increased from 23.4 to 33.9% (Poti and Popkin 2011). Food consumed outside the home has low nutrition and is served in portions far above recommended amounts (Guthrie et al. 2002; Poti and Popkin 2011; Batada et al. 2012; Urban et al. 2016); the public is largely unaware of this problem (Briefel and Johnson 2004; Burton et al. 2006; Sinclair et al. 2014). However, restaurants may be willing to improve their menu and portion sizes if approached (Crixell et al. 2014).

The schools' environment influences dietary behavior at formative ages; children may consume two meals and several snacks each day at school. Most food at school is provided through the U.S. Department of Agriculture (USDA), which must meet federal standards. Child nutrition programs, like the School Breakfast Program and National School Lunch Program, were upgraded to align with public health recommendations in 2009, with the assistance of the Institute of Medicine (IOM 2010). Pressure from Congress, the Institute of Medicine, some states, and school boards to regulate all foods and beverages sold at schools (USGAO 2005) led to the Healthy, Hunger-Free Kids Act of 2010 and the "Smart Snacks in School" guidelines, which took effect in 2014 (USDA 2015b). No research has yet been published on the health impacts of these changes. The Child and Adult Care Food Program also provides nutritious meals and snacks to child and adult care institutions and family or group day care homes—more than 3.3 million children and 120,000 chronically impaired disabled adults receive food from this program each day (USDA 2015).

As children transition to adulthood, they move from school to work environments. Workplace modifications can have real impacts on dietary habits (Matson-Koffman et al. 2005; Strickland et al. 2015), particularly for low-income workers (Special Committee on Health, Productivity, and Disability Management 2009). Most programs have used behavior interventions or improved access to information, but others secured positive changes following alterations in both access and availability to healthy food (Anderson et al. 2009). Workplaces may improve diets by increasing access to healthy foods onsite, making it easier for employees to bring meals from home, implementing workplace health programs, or modifying schedules (Strickland et al. 2015). Improving workplace social networks and social norms also resulted in significant improvements to dietary choices (Sorensen et al. 2007).

Outer Spheres of Influence

On the broadest level, economics, mass media, and public policy modulate the complexities of food choice. Food companies are the second-largest advertiser on television, spending billions of dollars and competing vigorously to entice consumers to select their products (Lake and Townshend 2006; Kraak and Story 2015). In the United States, more than 80% of the $30 billion spent annually on food advertising is for sugar-laden, convenience, or fast foods (Harrison and Marske 2005). Children exposed to advertisements for unhealthy foods consume more food as a result (Boyland et al. 2016). There is evidence that advertising for healthy foods and diets could be used to improve dietary behaviors (Kraak and Story 2015), though effects may vary across demographic groups (Forwood et al. 2015).

Modifications to existing policy or introduction of new policy can also greatly affect access to healthy foods. These changes may include food or menu nutritional labeling practices, food labeling policy, food quality regulation, restrictions against using food benefits to purchase unhealthy foods, encouragement of using food benefits to purchase healthy foods, simplification of benefits, modification of benefit cycles, nutrition education, and improving built food environments (Dinour et al. 2007; Kirkpatrick 2012). Modification of the Supplemental Nutrition Assistance Program (SNAP; formerly the Food Stamp Program) in 2008 and the Special Supplemental Nutrition Program for Women, Infants, and Children (WIC) program in 2009 aimed to promote healthy food choices (Larson and Story 2011); changes to WIC have been shown to improve healthy food access and intake (Schultz et al. 2015). When nutrition labeling is added to a menu, it can help people make better eating choices, but only if contextual or interpretive information is also provided (Sinclair et al. 2014). Simplifying the use of SNAP at farmer's markets increased utilization by 38% each month (Kirkpatrick 2012). Nutrition education such as MyPlate helps to teach proper serving sizes and portion control (Fisher et al. 2015). Additional research is needed to determine which policies are most cost-effective and appropriate in a given population.

Population-Attributable Risk

Of the top-10 highest risks contributing to mortality in the United States, three are dietary and two are directly affected by diet (GBD 2013 Risk Factors Collaborators et al. 2015). Estimating the population-attributable risk (PAR) attributable to diet is difficult. Poor nutrition is associated with many chronic diseases throughout the life course. Estimates for PAR may determine specific components of food or broad dietary measures associated with all-cause mortality or specific diseases. High trans fatty acid consumption is estimated to contribute to 7% of all mortalities (Kiage et al. 2013). Consumption of charbroiled or smoked meats is one source of polyaromatic hydrocarbon exposure, which is attributed to 1.3% to 2.8% of all cases of kidney stones (Shiue 2016). An examination of sugar-sweetened beverages found them to be linked to 2.2% of all deaths (Singh et al. 2015), and the fraction of type 2 diabetes cases attributed to sugar-sweetened, artificially sweetened, and fruit juice beverages is 8.7% (Imamura et al. 2015). Having an American Heart Association healthy diet score of two or less (on a scale of zero to five) is attributed to 1.8% of all deaths, 13.2% of CVD deaths, and 20.6% of ischemic heart disease deaths (Yang et al. 2012). Another study estimated 12% of all deaths as attributable to not following dietary guidelines (Kant et al. 2009). Because of potential biases, these may be underestimates (Greenberg et al. 2007)

Evidence-Based Interventions

Prevention

Since 1980, the U.S. Department of Health and Human Services (USDHHS) and the USDA have updated the *Dietary Guidelines for Americans (Dietary Guidelines)* in line with new public health science on a five-year basis. The *Dietary Guidelines* are targeted to meet the dietary needs of Americans aged two years and older (USDHHS and USDA 2015). The *Dietary Guidelines* focus on healthy eating patterns rather than individual nutrients and food groups, making healthy shifts rather than large dietary changes, and utilizing the social–ecological model to address all layers of influence that shape an individual's eating patterns. The new *Dietary Guidelines* are (1) follow a healthy eating pattern across the lifespan; (2) focus on variety, nutrient density, and amount; (3) limit calories from added sugars and saturated fats and reduce sodium intake; (4) shift to healthier food and beverage choices; and (5) support healthy eating patterns for all. The nutrition recommendations are summarized in Table 8-1.

The *Dietary Guidelines* emphasize eating a balanced diet with the majority of food coming from fruits, vegetables, whole grains, legumes, and low-fat or fat-free milk or milk equivalent. They encourage limiting saturated fats, trans fats, added sugars, salt, and alcohol. Weight maintenance, regular physical activity, and attention to food safety are also stressed. Recommendations for special population groups such as children and adolescents, pregnant and breastfeeding women, and older adults are added when applicable.

The *Dietary Guidelines* form the basis of MyPlate, an interactive food guide developed by the USDA. It was introduced in 2011 to replace MyPyramid (USDA 2011). MyPlate is intended as a graphic display to help all Americans know what to eat. MyPlate is USDA's interactive food guide. At the website (https://www.supertracker.usda.gov), people can enter their age, sex, weight, height, and level of physical activity to calculate personalized diet and exercise

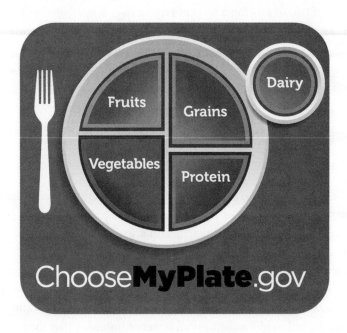

Source: Reprinted from USDA (2011).
Note: For more information about MyPlate, see https://www.choosemyplate.gov and http://www.hsph. harvard.edu/nutritionsource/.
Figure 8-3. MyPlate

recommendations based on the *Dietary Guidelines*. The output details the grains, vegetables, fruits, milk, meat and beans, oils, discretionary calories, and physical activity the individual needs on a daily basis. A pictorial representation of MyPlate is shown in Figure 8-3.

Federal food and nutrition education programs such as WIC, child nutrition programs, and SNAP use the *Dietary Guidelines* as the foundation for their programs. Other target audiences include policymakers, health care providers, nutritionists, nutrition educators, and the food industry.

The *Dietary Guidelines* have been modified over time to reflect the most current evidence including systematic reviews and food pattern modeling. For example, the recommended healthy U.S.-style eating pattern incorporates evidence from the long-term trial, Dietary Approaches to Stop Hypertension (DASH). The DASH eating plan showed reductions in blood pressure, LDL-cholesterol, and CVD events and mortality (Appel et al. 1997; Obarzanek et al. 2001; Salehi-Abargouei et al. 2013). The DASH diet is low in saturated fat, added sugars, and sodium, and it promotes fruits, vegetables, whole grains, fish, poultry, low-fat dairy, and nuts. On the basis of evidence evaluated by the Dietary Guidelines Advisory Committee, the *Dietary Guidelines* now also include the healthy Mediterranean-style eating pattern and the healthy vegetarian eating pattern as healthy options. The Mediterranean eating pattern emphasizes more seafood and fruits and less dairy than the healthy U.S.-style eating pattern, and the vegetarian eating pattern includes more soy, nuts, seeds, legumes, and whole grains and does not include meat, poultry, or seafood (DGAC 2015).

Screening

Public health practitioners can find nutrition surveillance data in the national surveys that together make up the National Nutrition Monitoring System surveys (IOM 2007). Cross-sectional and longitudinal surveys include measures of diet; physical activity; biological measures such as weight, anemia, CVD risk factors, and diabetes; school food; school health policies and programs; and youth media. Surveys with state-specific data include the BRFSS, Pediatric Nutrition Surveillance, the Youth Risk Factor Behavioral Surveillance System, School Health Policies and Practices Study, and the National Survey of Children's Health. Similarly, state-specific data about participation in USDA nutrition assistance programs that are available annually can be calculated at the county level (FRAC 2015; CFPA 2015). A growing number of states, counties, and cities are conducting their own surveys and developing new approaches, such as Geographic Information Systems, to map and evaluate factors contributing to dietary, physical activity, and obesity risks. An emerging approach is the use of the electronic health record to monitor health and its association with location (Guilbert et al. 2012).

Food disappearance data provide information about quantities of foods and nutrients in retail food distribution each year. The data are calculated by adding all foods produced in the United States, inventories from the previous year, and imported food, then subtracting year-end inventories, exported foods, and foodstuffs used for nonfood purposes. The final result is the quantity and nutrient value of food available for human consumption. Because the data are for foods available for purchase but not necessarily eaten, they overestimate food actually consumed. However, because the USDA Economic Research Service has been tracking data on agricultural commodities since 1909, the statistics allow analysis of trends in food availability.

U.S. food consumption data are collected through the national food survey, What We Eat in America, which involves obtaining two 24-hour dietary recalls for each participant in NHANES. Its inaugural year was 2002, when two formerly separate surveys from two federal agencies combined their efforts. The former surveys were NHANES and USDA's Continuing Survey of Food Intakes by Individuals. Before 2002, data were collected for each survey in discrete intervals with no surveillance in off-years. Now, fewer individuals are sampled, but surveillance is continuous. Data available include types and amounts of foods consumed as well as information on the food nutrients and energy.

Treatment

Several instruments have been developed to assess overall dietary quality. Short-term recall and diet record methods have traditionally been unrepresentative of dietary intake, time-intensive, and costly (Willett 2013). Thus, although the 24-hour dietary recall is the gold standard in research, it is costly, time-consuming, and difficult to administer. Therefore, epidemiologists have sought other means of measuring food intake. Food frequency questionnaires (FFQs) are the most popular form of assessing dietary quality in public health practice (see examples at http://epi.grants.cancer.gov/diet/screeners). The basic food frequency questionnaire consists of two parts: a food list and a section to mark the frequency of intake. The underlying principle behind the FFQ is that dietary intake over long periods, such as weeks or months, is more important than

Table 8-2. Healthy Eating Index 2010 Components and Scoring System

HEI-2010 Component	Maximum	Standard for Maximum Score	Standard for Minimum Score of Zero
▲ Adequacy (higher score indicates higher consumption)			
Total fruit	5	≥0.8 cup equiv./1,000 kcal	No fruit
Whole fruit	5	≥0.4 cup equiv./1,000 kcal	No whole fruit
Total vegetables	5	≥1.1 cup equiv./1,000 kcal	No vegetables
Greens and beans	5	≥0.2 cup equiv./1,000 kcal	No dark-green vegetables, beans, or peas
Whole grains	10	≥1.5 ounce equiv./1,000 kcal	No whole grains
Dairy	10	≥1.3 cup equiv./1,000 kcal	No dairy
Total protein foods	5	≥2.5 ounce equiv./1,000 kcal	No protein foods
Seafood and plant proteins	5	≥0.8 ounce equiv./1,000 kcal	No seafood or plant proteins
Fatty acids	10	(PUFAs+MUFAs)/SFAs>2.5	(PUFAs+MUFAs)/SFAs<.2
▼ Moderation (higher score indicates lower consumption)			
Refined grains	10	≤1.8 ounce equiv./1,000 kcal	≥4.3 ounce equiv./1,000 kcal
Sodium	10	≤1.1 gram/1,000 kcal	≥2.0 grams/1,000 kcal
Empty calories	20	≤19% of energy	≥50% of energy

Source: Reprinted from The Center for Nutrition Policy and Promotion (2013).
Note: HEI=Healthy Eating Index; MUFA=monounsaturated fatty acid; PUFA=polyunsaturated fatty acid; SFA=saturated fatty acid.

sampling data from a few specific days (Willett 2013). Although sampling data on specific days may be more exact, the crude data collected over longer periods are more essential to assessing dietary quality. In addition, individuals can often easily recall the routine consumption frequency of certain foods, as opposed to specific meals eaten in the past (Willett 2013).

Many other dietary instruments have been designed for the purpose of assessing the quantity and quality of dietary intake. These include such instruments as food frequency screeners, 3-day recalls, food diaries, food records, and other variations of the aforementioned instruments.

One such instrument, the Healthy Eating Index, is depicted in Table 8-2. Developed by the USDA, the Healthy Eating Index assesses 12 aspects of dietary consumption (Table 8-2) and provides a validated tool for public health practitioners to track population characteristics and help modulate interventions (Guenther et al. 2014). Such tools have helped reveal associations between population characteristics and nutrition.

Examples of Evidence-Based Interventions

Economic concerns and a growing awareness of the role of social determinants are accelerating the pressure to use social marketing, environmental change, and policy as affordable and effective large-scale approaches for populations. They are seen as powerful complements to traditional educational and community organizing techniques (Story et al. 2008; Mozaffarian et al. 2012).

Large-Scale Initiatives

Historically, the drive to use large-scale approaches for healthy nutrition promotion started with the National Cancer Institute–Kellogg's Campaign in the early 1980s. The then-controversial partnership between government and industry used a marketing approach that included mass media advertising, information on cereal boxes, in-store merchandising, and other commercial techniques to reach the general adult market and health professionals. The campaign increased consumer awareness of diet–cancer relationships and extended beyond the Kellogg's brand to a wide range of bran products (Levy and Stokes 1987).

The largest and longest-running partnership for nutrition and chronic disease prevention is the National 5 a Day Program, now renamed Fruits & Veggies—More Matters. The program was originally created by the California Department of Health Services in 1988 (Foerster et al. 1995). In 1991, the National Cancer Institute and the Produce for Better Health Foundation entered into a partnership based on California's 5 a Day—for Better Health! Campaign (Foerster et al. 1995). The National 5 a Day Program used a social marketing approach to focus on specific market segments with a carefully designed communications campaign delivered in multiple channels (Heimendinger and Chapelsky 1996).

To assess the effectiveness of the National 5 a Day Program, an external evaluation and two large national randomized phone-based surveys were conducted (Stables et al. 2002). The external evaluation concluded that the low-cost effort should be continued and expanded, and the phone surveys found significant increases in fruit and vegetable consumption, a higher percentage of individuals reporting that they ate at least five servings of fruit and vegetables a day, and a greater number meeting the then-current *Dietary Guidelines* (23% in 1991 to 26% in 1997). In addition, awareness of the 5 a Day message increased (7% to 19%), correlating again with greater fruit and vegetable consumption.

In March 2007, the 5 a Day message was transitioned to Fruits & Veggies—More Matters in accord with the near-doubling of recommended levels of fruits and vegetables in the 2005 *Dietary Guidelines*. Governmental leadership as the national health authority shifted to the Centers for Disease Control and Prevention (CDC), and the Produce for Better Health Foundation continued to provide a single point of contact for the estimated 1,000 fruit and vegetable industry licensees. Leadership expanded to include other members of the National Fruit and Vegetable Alliance steering committee, namely the USDA, the National Cancer Institute, the California Department of Public Health, the National Council of Fruit and Vegetable Nutrition Coordinators, the National Alliance for Nutrition and Activity, the American Cancer Society, the American Diabetes Association, the Produce Marketing Association, the United Fresh Produce Association, the Canned Food Alliance, the Frozen Food Institute, and the American Heart Association. As with 5 a Day, state agencies are licensed by CDC, or the Produce for Better Health Foundation, to serve as health authorities, implement interventions, and ensure conformity among public and nonprofit partners. Campaign awareness increased from 12% in 2007 to 18% in 2010 after the message re-branding to Fruits & Veggies—More Matters (Pivonka et al. 2011).

An example of another successful large-scale campaign is the 1% or Less Campaign. The 1% or Less Campaign sought to shift consumption from whole milk, 2% milk, or high-fat milk products to 1%, skim milk, or low-fat milk products—thereby increasing consumption of milk with 1% fat or less and reducing saturated fat intake (Maddock et al. 2007; Reger et al. 2000; Reger et al. 1998). It showed dramatic short-term sales increases by using paid advertising and public relations, with and without community-level programming, with the combination of both approaches being more effective, reaching more people, and therefore being more cost-effective than community programming alone (Reger et al. 1999; Booth-Butterfield and Reger 2004). Similar effects on high-fat milk intake have been reported in ethnically diverse communities, which were sustained far beyond the conclusion of the intervention (Maddock et al. 2007).

Site-Based Interventions

Worksites

The rising cost of health care benefits, together with lost work productivity attributable to obesity and other chronic diseases, is driving employer and policy interest in worksite modifications and programs that can reach employed adults in venues where they spend more than half their waking hours. A 2009 systematic review illustrated the promise of worksite interventions (Anderson et al. 2009). The review showed that, among 47 studies exploring worksite nutrition and physical activity programs, there were modest improvements in employee weight status at 6 to 12 months of follow-up. Another review of worksite nutrition interventions found a small but positive effect on diet (Ni Mhurchu et al. 2010).

A subsequent 2011 meta-analysis of 22 studies provided further evidence that workplace interventions are effective at reducing employee bodyweight, especially when an environmental component is added (Verweij et al. 2011). Examples of environmental interventions included worksite prompts, point-of-choice messages, healthy options on cafeteria menus and in vending machines, employee recognition programs, management training, and health objectives as management goals (Goetzel et al. 2009). Additional examples and resources for environmental interventions are available at the CDC Healthier Worksite Initiative website, including lactation support for breastfeeding mothers and healthier foods at meetings (https://www.cdc.gov/workplacehealthpromotion). Other reviews of worksite interventions found more modest effects on nutrition, however (Maes et al. 2012; Geaney et al. 2013).

Schools

Schools offer a venue to reach virtually all children and youths through education, skill-building, environmental change, and social support. Most large interventions in schools have shown a positive effect on both dietary attitudes and the consumption of a healthy diet (Thomson and Ravia 2011; Evans et al. 2012a; Wang et al. 2015).

Farm-to-school and school garden programs have been shown to improve fruit and vegetable consumption for children (CDC 2011; Dietz 2009, Langellotto and Gupta 2012; Mozaffarian et al. 2012). Several Wisconsin elementary schools participated in a farm-to-school program through

AmeriCorps and showed improvements in availability of fruits and vegetables at school lunch, increased student knowledge and willingness to try fruits and vegetables, and increased consumption for students with the lowest fruit and vegetable intake at baseline (Bontrager Yoder et al. 2014). A program for sixth-grade students in the San Francisco school district provided weekly garden-based learning as a part of the science curriculum for four months and found that participating students had an increased willingness to taste vegetables and greater variety of vegetables eaten when compared to controls (Ratcliffe et al. 2011).

There is also evidence that multicomponent obesity prevention programs at schools can improve student nutrition and weight (Van Cauwenberghe et al. 2010; Nixon et al. 2012). The Switch program in 10 elementary schools in Minnesota and Iowa was designed to increase fruit and vegetable consumption, increase physical activity, and reduce screen time in third through fifth graders (Gentile et al. 2009). The program used a social–ecological framework including family-, school-, and community-level components. Parents were given monthly packets of behavior-change tools, teachers integrated core concepts into their existing curriculum, and the community participated in advertising and other media emphasizing key health messages. The program was successful in increasing parent- and child-reported fruit and vegetable consumption (Gentile et al. 2009). Other programs utilizing both school- and community-level interventions have demonstrated positive outcomes including Shape Up Somerville (Economos et al. 2013) and the CATCH trial—Coordinated Approach to Child Health—(Hoelscher et al. 2010). State and local health departments have used similar models of community–school partnerships (Cousins et al. 2011). However, a multisector approach was recently used in the Identification and prevention of Dietary- and lifestyle-induced health EFfects In Children and infantS (IDEFICS) study with 8 countries in Europe and did not result in significant change (Baranowski and Lytle 2015).

Preschool Interventions

Changes targeting early childhood will reach a large number of children as early care and education providers, especially child care centers, reach large numbers of children for prolonged periods of time each day. More than 50% of children aged five years or younger with a mother working full-time spend more than 35 hours per week in child care (Capizzano and Main 2005). In addition, providers have existing infrastructure for meeting the nutritional and activity needs of children, which may be enhanced to more effectively improve nutrition. Licensing and accreditation standards that shape the early care and education setting offer additional points for intervention. Implementing wellness policies and training caregivers in best practices for nutrition can promote healthy weight and good nutrition for young children in child care settings (Lyn et al. 2015). These factors make interventions focused on the early care and education setting particularly strategic (Nader et al. 2012; Larson et al. 2011). Emerging evidence that attendance in child care may be associated with childhood obesity suggests that intervention in this setting may not only be opportune, but also critical (Larson et al. 2011; Benjamin Neelon et al. 2015).

Faith-Based Organizations

Comprehensive interventions supported by respected spiritual leaders and using approaches such as peer support, motivational interviewing, community coalitions, health fairs, grocery store promotions, cooking classes, healthy options at church meals, and printed materials as part of established religious infrastructures have been shown to be effective (Lancaster et al. 2014). Participants reported that some of the more influential dietary interventions included serving vegetables or fruits in church and verbal or printed messages from spiritual leaders (Lancaster et al. 2014). Fit Body and Soul, a faith-based diabetes prevention program, demonstrated improvements in participants' weight status after 12 program sessions; 48% of participants lost at least 5% of baseline body weight (Dodani and Fields 2010). Another faith-based diabetes prevention program utilizing community health advisors saw no difference between the intervention group and controls, however (Faridi et al. 2010).

Interventions Focusing on Specific Populations

Emerging Community Approaches

Increasing access to a diverse array of nutritious foods is needed to ensure population improvements in nutrition, particularly in low-income communities (IOM and National Research Council 2009). Increasingly, advocates, public health departments, and occasionally urban planning committees are working to bring full-service supermarkets into low-income communities, increase healthy foods stocked by small food stores, support community gardens, start farmers' markets, expand community-supported agriculture, organize farm-to-institution networks, and stimulate other direct-marketing opportunities for locally grown foods (IOM and National Research Council 2009; Khan et al. 2009, Litt et al. 2011; Girard et al. 2012, Evans et al. 2012b; Quandt et al. 2013). The availability of a mix of nutritious foods requires not only expanding product offerings at grocery and convenience stores but also working with food preparers, restaurants, and fast-food entities to replace unhealthy meal choices with more nutritious options. Food policy councils in cities, counties, and states have emerged as a cross-cutting political response to bring diverse stakeholders together (Wisconsin Department of Health Services and Division of Public Health 2012).

The Federal Safety Net

The USDA's 15 nutrition assistance programs are designed to work together to provide healthy food to all schoolchildren and a nutrition safety net for America's low-income families. These programs serve one in four Americans over the course of a year with a budget exceeding $100 billion dollars (Oliveira 2016).

The 40-year-old WIC program starts at the beginning of life by providing high-risk pregnant and breastfeeding women with incomes less than 185% Federal Poverty Level (FPL) and their children up to age five years with nutrition education, links to health care, and grocery store vouchers for specific foods that are rich in nutrients needed for pregnancy, growth, and development. In 2015, federal funding totaled about $6 billion and reached eight million women and children in an average month (Oliveira 2016). As a discretionary program, WIC's funding level must be re-appropriated by Congress each year. In most states, the department of public health administers the federal program and provides WIC services through a network of local public and nonprofit agencies.

In 2009, the WIC food package was updated to also provide, among other things, fresh fruits and vegetables, whole grains, and low-fat milk products. A review of the literature indicates that these changes have led to increased consumption of whole grains among WIC recipients; decreased the purchasing of juice, whole milk, and white bread; and improved access to healthier foods at WIC vendors (Schultz et al. 2015). However, fruit and vegetable consumption increased only minimally, and there were mixed results for breast-feeding rates (Schultz et al. 2015).

The National School Lunch Program is USDA's largest program for America's schoolchildren. In most states, it is administered through the state education agency to local education agencies such as school districts, and the great majority of public schools participate to serve about 30 million students every school day with federal funds totaling approximately 13 billion dollars (Oliveira 2016). The School Lunch Program subsidizes but does not fully pay the school's cost of free, reduced-price, and full-priced lunches. The amount of federal subsidy is based on the students' family income, where the divisions are as follows: less than 130% FPL (free), 130% to 185% FPL (reduced-price), or greater than 185% FPL (full-priced). Some states and localities augment the federal reimbursements, while most schools make up the difference by charging students for reduced-price and full-priced meals. The percentage of free, reduced-price lunch enrollment is a criterion of child and community poverty used in many community, state, and national statistics.

In a 2009 study of almost 400 public schools participating in the National School Lunch Program, most of the *Dietary Guidelines* recommendations were not being met (Crepinsek et al. 2009). Although schools met standards for protein, minerals, and vitamins, lunches exceeded saturated fat and sodium standards and were deficient in fiber (Crepinsek et al. 2009). Then, the 2010 Healthy Hunger-Free Kids Act was passed, taking effect in 2012–2013. The act required the National School Lunch Program to meet nutrition standards set by the *Dietary Guidelines* (Johnson et al. 2016). The changes required an increase in the availability of whole grains, fruits, and vegetables; an increase in the portion sizes for fruits and vegetables; calorie limits by age; and a decrease in the amount of sodium in school lunches (Schwartz et al. 2015). Several studies have shown that improving school lunch nutrition standards increased students' healthy food choices without increasing food waste (Johnson et al. 2016; Schwartz et al. 2015; Cohen et al. 2014).

Formerly known as food stamps, SNAP is an entitlement program considered the centerpiece of the U.S. food security safety net. It uses Electronic Benefit Transfer cards rather than vouchers to provide households with gross incomes less than 130% FPL with a monthly cash allotment for food. The value of the food benefit is based on the cost of USDA's Thrifty Food Plan. All foods, except hot, ready-to-eat items, qualify. Even liquor and convenience stores may be certified by the USDA if the food they carry meets minimum federal requirements. Complex means testing to determine eligibility typically is administered through state and local social services departments. It includes household income, the number of qualifying household members, specific types of expenses, documentation of U.S. citizenship or residency, and regular recertification.

In 2015, SNAP served more than 45 million persons per month, and it provided $126.83 per month per person for food (Oliveira 2016). Increasingly, this program serves working poor, elderly, and newly unemployed families, and yet only an estimated 85% of eligible Americans participated in 2013 (Eslami 2015). Although SNAP addresses food insecurity, recent studies suggest that participants have lower-quality diets and higher rates of obesity than those with the same income who do not participate (Leung et al. 2013; Hilmers et al. 2014). There is public support for SNAP policy changes, however, such as restricting the purchase of sugar-sweetened beverages and incentivizing the purchase of healthier foods (Long et al. 2014).

The obesity prevention and nutrition education side of SNAP (SNAP-Ed) is reimbursed as an optional administrative activity that requires detailed documentation of in-kind state share funds from nonfederal sources. Budgets and activities require annual federal approval of a SNAP-Ed state plan. Although the amount per state depends on the matching funds a state can identify, all states now offer some SNAP-Ed. In 2016, states qualified for $408 million in matching federal reimbursement (Ward 2015). In the United States, SNAP-Ed and WIC are the two largest sources of nutrition education funding. One study of SNAP-Ed programming in California found that it was associated with increased fruit and vegetable consumption in adults and children and decreased fast food consumption in adults (Molitor et al. 2015). Another study of six different SNAP-Ed programs had mixed results, however (Williams et al. 2015).

Additional federal nutrition assistance programs at USDA include the School Breakfast Program, the Child and Adult Care Food Programs, Summer Food Service Program, and Afterschool Snacks. They are updated by Congress approximately every five years through the Child Nutrition and WIC reauthorization. About every five years, SNAP and other, more agriculturally based programs, such as the Fresh Fruit and Vegetable Snack Program, the WIC Farmer's Market Nutrition Program, the Senior Farmer's Market Nutrition Program, and some commodity and emergency food programs, are reauthorized in a statute commonly known as the Farm Bill.

Eliminating Racial Disparities

Programming aimed at ethnic minority groups has lagged even though these groups bear a disproportionate burden of chronic disease, much of it attributable to poor nutrition (IOM and National Research Council 2009; Stuart-Shor et al. 2012, Nierkens et al. 2013). A review of 17 interventions focusing on ethnic minorities for tobacco cessation, physical activity, and diet found that cultural adaptations had significant effects on outcomes for five studies, and many other studies showed a positive trend. The study concluded that effective interventions incorporated a "package" of multiple cultural adaptations, used interventions of greater intensity, and emphasized family values. Some successful cultural adaptations included materials written or spoken in preferred languages and tailored to the local community, community health workers (CHWs) and case managers trained in cultural sensitivity, and family education sessions (Nierkens et al. 2013).

One randomized controlled trial included in the review targeted Hispanic individuals with newly diagnosed type 2 diabetes and analyzed the effectiveness of a CHW program, *Amigos en Salud* (Babamoto et al. 2009). Participants were randomized to the CHW program, case management, or standard provider care in three Los Angeles clinics. The CHWs were bilingual and Hispanic, had personal experience with diabetes, and received formal training. The CHWs provided culturally appropriate, individualized education sessions as well as regular telephone follow-up. The program was based on the Transtheoretical, or Stages of Change, Model. Participants randomized to the CHW program had greater improvements in health status, diabetes medication adherence, and nutrition including fruit and vegetable consumption ($p < .05$; Babamoto et al. 2009).

Community-based participatory research methods have been utilized in many successful behavioral interventions in ethnic minority groups. The WORD (Wholeness, Oneness, Righteousness, Deliverance), a faith-based diabetes prevention program focusing on a rural African-American community, successfully used community-based participatory research to improve weight status for participants (Kim et al. 2008). The WORD was a cultural adaptation of the Diabetes Prevention Program, which was a major clinical trial aimed at discovering whether either diet and exercise or the drug metformin could delay or prevent the onset of type 2 diabetes (Diabetes Prevention Program 2006). Trained community members led weekly group sessions that emphasized physical activity, nutrition, and the connection between faith and health. After the eight-week initial intervention, there was a statistically significant average weight loss of 3.00 pounds (±0.87; Kim et al. 2008). The WORD has now been translated into a randomized controlled trial design for sustained weight loss over 18 months and will expand to include 30 churches (Yeary et al. 2015).

Policy Approaches

Although federal policies focus most directly on nutrition for women, children, and those with lesser means, the effects of poor nutrition on health have far reaching effects on nearly everyone. Policies that shape the supply, production, distribution, and promotion of food can have significant clout in shaping population dietary behavior (Hood et al. 2012).

Agriculture Policy

Food and agricultural policy helps determine which crops farmers will produce and the prices they will get, thereby influencing the food products that retailers, food services, and restaurants offer the public. Federal agriculture policy has supported particular crop production through funding for research, enhancement of infrastructure, and subsidies (Franck et al. 2013). In particular, long-standing policies have promoted the production of grains, corn, and soybeans (Franck et al. 2013).

Such crops can be converted to energy-dense food products laden with either simple sugars or saturated fats. Individuals often make choices about nutrition by their pocketbooks and not health benefits (Franck et al. 2013). Current food and agricultural policy is seen as artificially lowering the costs of nutritionally deficient food products, making them more attractive to price-conscious processors of food and consumers. However, some economic models have predicted that eliminating these subsidies would have minimal impact on caloric consumption and obesity rates (Franck et al. 2013).

Approximately every five years, there is the opportunity to change federal agricultural policy through the Farm Bill. The Farm Bill governs several domestic food policies, including SNAP, the Emergency Food Assistance Program, Child Nutrition Reauthorization Act, and the Commodity Food Assistance Program. A much more diverse set of stakeholders became engaged in the 2008 Farm Bill, many of whom sought better alignment of agriculture policy with public health policies in nutrition, conservation, sustainable local food systems, climate change, the preservation of agricultural land, and economic development. The latest Farm Bill (2014) maintained previous SNAP eligibility requirements, included additional funding to support healthy food purchases such as fruits and vegetables, and increased support for The Emergency Food Assistance Program (USDA 2014a).

Nutrition Right-to-Know

Consumption of food from restaurants continues to grow; currently, almost half of all food dollars are spent on "away-from-home" foods (VanEpps et al. 2016). Until recently, there have been no federal requirements for restaurants or volume food packaging used by commercial or school food services to carry Nutrition Fact labels. As a part of the Affordable Care Act, however, chain restaurants and vending machines with 20 or more locations will soon have to disclose nutrition information, with requirements anticipated to take effect in December 2016 (VanEpps et al. 2016). Unwilling to wait, in 2008, New York City became the first city to require restaurants to post the calorie content of their menu. California became the first state to do so. Early results from studies of restaurant menu labeling are mixed, but suggest that nutrition labeling may lead to healthier purchases in certain situations. For example, higher-income individuals are more likely to use nutrition labels in purchasing decisions (VanEpps et al. 2016).

School Wellness Policies

Policy within the public school system has also received rigorous review and criticism. In 2006, Congress mandated that schools develop wellness policies to improve the physical activity and nutrition of children. The Healthy, Hunger-Free Kids Act of 2010 updated the National School Lunch Program nutrition standards. The Institute of Medicine made clear recommendations for federally funded school meal programs as well as the sale of competitive foods in schools, such as foods and beverages sold from vending machines (IOM 2012). Although there was no call for dismissal of private food vendors, the report urged that healthy food choices be used as an adjunct to federal meal programs. The Healthy, Hunger-Free Kids Act of 2010 has required that competitive foods also meet USDA nutrition standards in schools served by federal meal programs. Early results suggest that such regulations of competitive foods may decrease consumption of unhealthy foods and reduce student weight gain if applied comprehensively (Taber et al. 2012; Chriqui et al. 2014).

Advertising to Children

The significant and detrimental effect that food marketing can have on dietary choice, particularly in children, has been refuted by advertisers and food producers. However, in 2006, an expert committee found a clear connection between advertising, adverse dietary choices, and overall declining childhood nutrition, concluding that television advertising has significant influence on the food preferences, purchase requests, and dietary choices of children (IOM 2012). The committee made strong recommendations for a more balanced approach to food marketing, including more emphasis on promoting fruits and vegetables.

The Federal Trade Commission, the USDHHS, and the American Academy of Pediatrics have echoed these recommendations and issued similar statements (Story et al. 2008). The Federal Communications Commission has created a task force to address the effects of mass media on childhood nutrition and obesity (Miller 2007). In December 2006, several of the top food producers and marketers in the United States developed the Children's Food and Beverage Advertising Initiative to include more advertising for healthier foods, better dietary practices, and improved physical activity (Story et al. 2008). An early assessment of the initiative suggests that more work needs to be done (Powell et al. 2013). Food marketing expenditures declined; however, there was also a shift in spending toward unprotected markets such as newer online media, product placements, athletic sponsorships, and advertisements directed at older children (Powell et al. 2013).

Areas of Future Research

In the past decade, there has been a change in large food manufacturers and some fast food restaurants to remove artificial food coloring, artificial flavoring, trans fats, and preservatives from their products. Some of these companies also pledged to remove high-fructose corn syrup. At the same time, there has been an increase in the number of farmers' markets across the United States. In 1994 there were fewer than 2,000 farmers' markets, but by 2014 there were more than 8,000 (USDA 2014b). Besides supporting the local economy, it increases availability of locally grown produce, organic products, and other homemade food items that lack artificial ingredients. This shift might represent the public's increased awareness and subsequent demand for healthier, fresher food (USDA 2014b).

Likewise, food gardening is increasing in popularity in the United States. A report from the National Gardening Association found that 35% of all households in America, or 42 million households, are growing food at home or in a community garden—a 17% increase from 2008 to 2013 (National Gardening Association 2014). Community gardens offer community members the opportunity to participate in the maintenance of a garden in exchange for fresh and affordable produce. They, too, are showing growths in numbers; community garden participation in the United States doubled since 2008 to 4 million households participating (National Gardening Association 2014). In low-income communities with limited access to fresh produce, community gardens are especially promising to improve access to healthy foods. Much is still to be learned, but the literature suggests room for cautious optimism. Still, studies are needed to determine the long-term impact on eating habits from the increases in farmers' markets, community gardens, and food gardening.

This chapter has introduced issues and trends in public health nutrition. It has illustrated that, although vast areas of intervention research and theory should be explored, there are many proven effective solutions in the public health literature, and broad-based solutions are percolating within communities. The disparities in nutrition between socioeconomic, racial, and geographic divides that lead to chronic disease are being exposed, and concern about vulnerable groups who live in environments that promote poor nutrition, especially low-income families, children, and the elderly, is creating urgency. Understanding the gaps and interconnections in policy and environmental information, built environment, community intervention, and surveillance systems increases clarity about opportunities for change. As the burden of poor nutrition grows, so has the willingness to find solutions. These solutions have been increasingly brokered by broad-based partnerships, multilevel interventions, public policy, and collaborative efforts among health care, mass media, communities, and the producers of food.

Intervention resources and research for dietary change are needed in proportion to the magnitude of the problem. Much is to be learned through experience operating and evaluating programs, and much will be gained by adopting common, preferably validated, measures of environmental influence (Glanz et al. 2005). The focus must be on advancing research and interventions in parallel that focus on the many environmental and individual factors that affect food choice (Story et al. 2008). For public health applications, priorities include delineating the elements of sector- and population-specific interventions, understanding marketplace factors such as economic incentives and disincentives, sponsoring effective mass communications, and understanding

how organizations on the national, state, regional, and local levels can complement and gain synergy from each others' efforts.

From a systems perspective, the Institute of Medicine released a report
that examines factors related to childhood overweight and obesity. The report
focused on preventing obesity in children aged five years or younger (IOM
2011). The resulting policy recommendations are to focus on these areas:

- Assess, monitor, and track growth from birth to age five.
- Increase physical activity in young children.
- Decrease sedentary behavior in young children.
- Help adults increase physical activity and decrease sedentary behavior in
  young children.
- Promote the consumption of a variety of nutritious foods, and encourage
  and support breast-feeding during infancy.
- Create a healthful eating environment that is responsive to children's
  hunger and fullness cues.
- Ensure access to affordable healthy foods for all children.
- Help adults increase children's healthy eating.
- Limit young children's screen time and exposure to food and beverage
  marketing.
- Use social marketing to provide consistent information and strategies
  for the prevention of childhood obesity in infancy and early childhood.
- Promote age-appropriate sleep durations among children.

Given the scope of the food system, it is not surprising that large-scale, comprehensive initiatives that require a mix of professional disciplines and stakeholders
are needed to increase access to healthy food, collaborate with other stakeholders,
generate resources, and deliver communication programs. Specialists needed at
the table include those in the fields of public health nutrition, health education,
marketing, epidemiology, mass communications and public relations, health
care providers and insurers, policy, community organizing, schools, business,
design and creative arts, culinary arts and retail merchandising, public health
law, resource development, applied research, evaluation, and administration.
Although some of the specialties may be available through public–private partnerships, public health agencies need dedicated resources for these functions. The
challenges in nutrition are large, but the growing interest and innovation is equally
large. As public health interventions become more multifaceted, wider-reaching,
and creative, the prospect of a healthier global diet grows more promising.

Resources

American Dietetic Association, http://www.eatright.org

Association of State Public Health Nutritionists, http://www.asphn.org

Center for Food Safety and Applied Nutrition, Food and Drug Administration, http://www.fda.gov/AboutFDA/CentersOffices/OfficeofFoods/CFSAN

Center for Nutrition Policy and Promotion, U.S. Department of Agriculture, http://www.cnpp.usda.gov

Department of Nutrition for Health and Development, World Health Organization, http://www.who.int/nmh/about/nhd/en

Division of Nutrition, Physical Activity, and Obesity, Centers for Disease Control and Prevention, http://www.cdc.gov/nccdphp/dnpao/index.html

Feeding America, http://www.feedingamerica.org

Food and Nutrition Service, U.S. Department of Agriculture, http://www.fns.usda.gov

Food Research and Action Center, http://frac.org

Let's Move!, http://www.letsmove.gov

National Gardening Association, http://www.garden.org

School Nutrition Association, http://www.schoolnutrition.org

Supplemental Nutrition Assistance Program—Nutrition Education (SNAP-Ed), https://snaped.fns.usda.gov

Suggested Reading

Institute of Medicine. *Early Childhood Obesity Prevention Policies.* 2011. Available at: http://www.nationalacademies.org/hmd/~/media/Files/Report%20Files/2011/Early-Childhood-Obesity-Prevention-Policies/Young%20Child%20Obesity%202011%20Recommendations.pdf.

Institute of Medicine. *Accelerating Progress in Obesity Prevention: Solving the Weight of the Nation.* Washington, DC: The National Academies Press; 2012.

Nord M, Andrews M, Carlson S. Household food security in the United States, 2008. 2009. Economic Research Report no. 83. Available at: http://www.ers.usda.gov/media/184956/err83_1_.pdf.

US Department of Agriculture. Access to affordable and nutritious food measuring and understanding food deserts and their consequences: report to Congress. 2009. Available at: http://www.ers.usda.gov/media/242675/ap036_1_.pdf.

US Department of Agriculture, US Department of Health and Human Services. *Dietary Guidelines for Americans, 2010.* 7th ed. Washington, DC: US Government Printing Office; 2010.

US Department of Health and Human Services and US Department of Agriculture. *Dietary Guidelines for Americans, 2015-2020.* 8th ed. Washington, DC: US Government Printing Office; 2015.

References

Anderson LM, Quinn TA, Glanz K, et al. The effectiveness of worksite nutrition and physical activity interventions for controlling employee overweight and obesity: a systematic review. *Am J Prev Med.* 2009;37(4):340–357.

Appel LJ, Moore TJ, Obarzanek E, et al. A clinical trial of the effects of dietary patterns on blood pressure: DASH Collaborative Research Group. *N Engl J Med.* 1997;336(16): 1117–1124.

Appleton KM, Hemingway A, Saulais L, et al. Increasing vegetable intakes: rationale and systematic review of published interventions. *Eur J Nutr.* 2016;55(3):869–896.

Aune D, Chan DS, Lau R, et al. Dietary fibre, whole grains, and risk of colorectal cancer: systematic review and dose-response meta-analysis of prospective studies. *BMJ.* 2011;343:d6617.

Babamoto KS, Sey KA, Camilleri AJ, Karlan VJ, Catalasan J, Morisky DE. Improving diabetes care and health measures among Hispanics using community health workers: results from a randomized controlled trial. *Health Educ Behav.* 2009;36(1):113–126.

Baranowski T, Lytle L. Should the IDEFICS outcomes have been expected? *Obes Rev.* 2015;16(suppl 2):162–172.

Bastiotis P, Lino M, Anand R. The diet quality of American Indians: Evidence from the continuing survey of food intakes by individuals. *Fam Econ Nutr Rev.* 1999;12(2):44–46.

Batada A, Bruening M, Marchlewicz EH, Story M, Wootan MG. Poor nutrition on the menu: children's meals at America's top chain restaurants. *Child Obes.* 2012;8(3):251–254.

Bauer UE, Briss PA, Goodman RA, Bowman BA. Prevention of chronic disease in the 21st century: elimination of the leading preventable causes of premature death and disability in the USA. *Lancet.* 2014;384(9937):45–52.

Baum SJ, Kris-Etherton PM, Willett WC, et al. Fatty acids in cardiovascular health and disease: a comprehensive update. *J Clin Lipidol.* 2012;6(3):216–234.

Befort CA, Nazir N, Perri MG. Prevalence of obesity among adults from rural and urban areas of the United States: findings from NHANES (2005–2008). *J Rural Health.* 2012;28(4):392–397.

Bendsen NT, Hother AL, Jensen SK, Lorenzen JK, Astrup A. Effect of dairy calcium on fecal fat excretion: a randomized crossover trial. *Int J Obes (Lond).* 2008;32(12):1816–1824.

Benjamin Neelon SE, Andersen CS, Morgen CS, et al. Early child care and obesity at 12 months of age in the Danish National Birth Cohort. *Int J Obes.* 2015;39(1):33–38.

Berg CJ, Daley CM, Nazir N, et al. Physical activity and fruit and vegetable intake among American Indians. *J Community Health.* 2012;37(1):65–71.

Bernstein M, Munoz N; Academy of Nutrition and Dietetics. Position of the Academy of Nutrition and Dietetics: food and nutrition for older adults: promoting health and wellness. *J Acad Nutr Diet.* 2012;112(8):1255–1277.

Bertioa ML, Mukamal KJ, Cahill LE, et al. Changes in intake of fruits and vegetables and weight change in United States men and women followed for up to 24 years: analysis from three prospective cohort studies. *PLoS Med.* 2015;12(9):e1001878.

Beydoun MA, Wang Y. How do socio-economic status, perceived economic barriers and nutritional benefits affect quality of dietary intake among US adults? *Eur J Clin Nutr.* 2008;62(3):303–313.

Blanck HM, Gillespie C, Kimmons JE, Seymour JD, Serdula MK. Trends in fruit and vegetable consumption among US men and women, 1994–2005. *Prev Chronic Dis.* 2008;5(2):A35.

Blisard N, Stewart H, Joliffe D. *Low-Income Households' Expenditures on Fruits and Vegetables.* Washington, DC: US Department of Agriculture; 2004. Agricultural Economic Report no. 833.

Bontrager Yoder AB, Liebhart JL, McCarty DJ, et al. Farm to elementary school programming increases access to fruits and vegetables and increases their consumption among those with low intake. *J Nutr Educ Behav.* 2014;46(3):341–349.

Booth-Butterfield S, Reger B. The message changes belief and the rest is theory: the 1% or less milk campaign and reasoned action. *Prev Med.* 2004;39(3):581–588.

Bordoni A, Capozzi F. Foodomics for healthy nutrition. *Curr Opin Clin Nutr Metab Care.* 2014;17(5):418–424.

Bouvard V, Loomis D, Guyton KZ, et al. Carcinogenicity of consumption of red and processed meat. *Lancet Oncol.* 2015;16(16):1599–1600.

Boyland EJ, Nolan S, Kelly B, et al. Advertising as a cue to consume: a systematic review and meta-analysis of the effects of acute exposure to unhealthy food and nonalcoholic beverage advertising on intake in children and adults. *Am J Clin Nutr.* 2016;103(2):519–533.

Briefel RR, Johnson CL. Secular trends in dietary intake in the United States. *Annu Rev Nutr.* 2004;24:401–431.

Bultman SJ. Molecular pathways: gene–environment interactions regulating dietary fiber induction of proliferation and apoptosis via butyrate for cancer prevention. *Clin Cancer Res.* 2014;20(4):799–803.

Burton S, Creyer EH, Kees J, Huggins K. Attacking the obesity epidemic: the potential health benefits of providing nutrition information in restaurants. *Am J Public Health.* 2006;96(9):1669–1675.

Calancie L, Leeman J, Jilcott Pitts SB, et al. Nutrition-related policy and environmental strategies to prevent obesity in rural communities: a systematic review of the literature, 2002–2013. *Prev Chronic Dis.* 2015;12:E57.

Calder PC. Marine omega-3 fatty acids and inflammatory processes: effects, mechanisms and clinical relevance. *Biochim Biophys Acta.* 2015;1851(4):469–484.

California Food Policy Advocates (CFPA). 2015. Available at: http://cfpa.net. Accessed March 9, 2016.

Cannuscio CC, Hillier A, Karpyn A, Glanz K. The social dynamics of healthy food shopping and store choice in an urban environment. *Soc Sci Med.* 2014;122:13–20.

Capizzano JA, Main R. Many young children spend long hours in child care. Vol. 22. Washington, DC: Urban Institute, Center on Labor, Human Services, and Population; 2005.

Casagrande SS, Wang Y, Anderson C, Gary TL. Have Americans increased their fruit and vegetable intake? The trends between 1988 and 2002. *Am J Prev Med.* 2007;32(4): 257–263.

Center for Nutrition Policy and Promotion, US Department of Agriculture. Fact sheet no. 2. 2013. Available at: http://www.cnpp.usda.gov. Accessed August 15, 2016.

Centers for Disease Control and Prevention (CDC). *Strategies to Prevent Obesity and Other Chronic Diseases: The CDC Guide to Strategies to Increase the Consumption of Fruits and Vegetables.* Atlanta, GA: US Department of Health and Human Services; 2011.

Centers for Disease Control and Prevention (CDC). State indicator report on fruits and vegetables, 2013. Atlanta, GA: US Department of Health and Human Services; 2013.

Chang CL, Torrejon C, Jung UJ, Graf K, Deckelbaum RJ. Incremental replacement of saturated fats by n-3 fatty acids in high-fat, high-cholesterol diets reduces elevated plasma lipid levels and arterial lipoprotein lipase, macrophages and atherosclerosis in LDLR-/- mice. *Atherosclerosis*. 2014;234(2):401–409.

Cho Y, Turner ND, Davidson LA, Chapkin RS, Carroll RJ, Lupton JR. Colon cancer cell apoptosis is induced by combined exposure to the n-3 fatty acid docosahexaenoic acid and butyrate through promoter methylation. *Exp Biol Med (Maywood)*. 2014;239(3):302–310.

Chriqui JF, Pickel M, Story M. Influence of school competitive food and beverage policies on obesity, consumption, and availability: a systematic review. *JAMA Pediatr*. 2014;168(3):279–286.

Clark JE. Taste and flavour: their importance in food choice and acceptance. *Proc Nutr Soc*. 1998;57(4):639–643.

Cohen JWF, Richardson S, Parker E, Catalano PJ, Rimm EB. Impact of the new US Department of Agriculture school meal standards on food selection, consumption, and waste. *Am J Prev Med*. 2014;46(4):388–394.

Coleman-Jensen A, Rabbitt MP, Gregory C, Singh A. Household food security in the United States in 2014. Washington, DC: Economic Research Service, US Department of Agriculture; 2015. ERR-194.

Cousins JM, Langer SM, Rhew LK, Thomas C. The role of state health departments in supporting community-based obesity prevention. *Prev Chronic Dis*. 2011;8(4):A87.

Crepinsek MK, Gordon AR, McKinney PM, Condon EM, Wilson A. Meals suffered and served in US public schools: do they meet nutrient standards? *J Am Diet Assoc*. 2009;109(2 suppl):S31–S43.

Crixell SH, Friedman B, Fisher DT, Biediger-Friedman L. Improving children's menus in community restaurants: best food for families, infants, and toddlers (Best Food FITS) intervention, South Central Texas, 2010–2014. *Prev Chronic Dis*. 2014;11:E223.

Cross AJ, Ferrucci LM, Risch A, et al. A large prospective study of meat consumption and colorectal cancer risk: an investigation of potential mechanisms underlying this association. *Cancer Res*. 2010;70(6):2406–2414.

Cruwys T, Bevelander KE, Hermans RC. Social modeling of eating: a review of when and why social influence affects food intake and choice. *Appetite*. 2015;86:3–18.

Cummins S, Flint E, Matthews SA. New neighborhood grocery store increased awareness of food access but did not alter dietary habits or obesity. *Health Aff (Millwood)*. 2014;33(2):283–291.

Darmon N, Drewnowski A. Does social class predict diet quality? *Am J Clin Nutr.* 2008;87(5):1107–1117.

Davis GC, Carslon A. The inverse relationship between food price and energy density: is it spurious? *Public Health Nutr.* 2015;18(6):1091–1097.

de Graaf C, Polet P, van Staveren WA. Sensory perception and pleasantness of food flavors in elderly subjects. *J Gerontol.* 1994;49(3):93–99.

Delavari M, Sonderlund AL, Swinburn B, Mellor D, Renzaho A. Acculturation and obesity among migrant populations in high income countries—a systematic review. *BMC Public Health.* 2013;13:458.

Demeyer D, Mertens B, De Smet S, Ulens M. Mechanisms linking colorectal cancer to the consumption of (processed) red meat: a review. *Crit Rev Food Sci Nutr.* 2015; epub ahead of print May 15, 2015.

Diabetes Prevention Program. 2006. Available at: http://www.diabetesprevention.pitt.edu/index.php/for-the-public/diabetes-prevention-program-dpp. Accessed August 12, 2016.

Diep CS, Foster MJ, McKyer EL, Goodson P, Guidry JJ, Liew J. What are Asian-American youth consuming? A systematic literature review. *J Immigr Minor Health.* 2015;17(2): 591–604.

Dietary Guidelines Advisory Committee (DGAC). *Scientific Report of the 2015 Dietary Guidelines Advisory Committee, Advisory Report to the Secretary of Health and Human Services and the Secretary of Agriculture.* 2015. Available at: http://health.gov/dietaryguidelines/2015-scientific-report/PDFs/Scientific-Report-of-the-2015-Dietary-Guidelines-Advisory-Committee.pdf. Accessed February 10, 2016.

Dietz WH. CDC congressional testimony: benefits of farm-to-school projects, healthy eating and physical activity for school children. Centers for Disease Control and Prevention. 2009. Available at: http://www.cdc.gov/washington/testimony/2009/t20090515.htm. Accessed May 7, 2016.

Dikmen M, Ozturk N, Ozturk Y. The antioxidant potency of *Punica granatum L.* fruit peel reduces cell proliferation and induces apoptosis on breast cancer. *J Med Food.* 2011;14(12):1638–1646.

Dinour LM, Bergen D, Yeh MC. The food insecurity–obesity paradox: a review of the literature and the role food stamps may play. *J Am Diet Assoc.* 2007;107(11):1952–1961.

Dodani S, Fields JZ. Implementation of the Fit Body and Soul, a church-based life style program for diabetes prevention in high-risk African Americans: a feasibility study. *Diabetes Educ.* 2010;36(3):465–472.

Doubeni CA, Schootman M, Major JM, et al. Health status, neighborhood socioeconomic context, and premature mortality in the United States: the National Institutes of Health–AARP Diet and Health Study. *Am J Public Health*. 2012;102(4):680–688.

Drewnowski A, Bellisle F. Liquid calories, sugar, and body weight. *Am J Clin Nutr*. 2007;85(3):651–661.

Dubowitz T, Ghosh-Dastidar M, Cohen DA, et al. Diet and perceptions change with supermarket introduction in a food desert, but not because of supermarket use. *Health Aff (Millwood)*. 2015;34(11):1858–1868.

Duffey KJ, Popkin BM. Shifts in patterns and consumption of beverages between 1965 and 2002. *Obesity*. 2007;15(11):2739–2747.

Dugan CE, Fernandez ML. Effects of dairy on metabolic syndrome parameters: a review. *Yale J Biol Med*. 2014;87(2):135–147.

Economos CD, Hyatt RR, Must A, et al. Shape Up Somerville two-year results: a community-based environmental change intervention sustains weight reduction in children. *Prev Med*. 2013;57(4):322–327.

Eertmans A, Baeyens F, Van de Bergh O. Food likes and their relative importance in human eating behavior: review and preliminary suggestions for health promotion. *Health Educ Res*. 2001;16(4):443–456.

Ekmekcioglu C, Wallne P, Kundi M, Weisz U, Haas W, Hutter HP. Red meat, diseases and healthy alternatives: a critical review. *Crit Rev Food Sci Nutr*. 2016; epub ahead of print April 29, 2016.

English L, Lasschuijt M, Keller KL. Mechanisms of the portion size effect. What is known and where do we go from here? *Appetite*. 2015;88:39–49.

Ervin RB. Healthy Eating Index—2005 total and component scores for adults aged 20 and over: National Health and Nutrition Examination Survey, 2003–2004. *Natl Health Stat Report*. 2011;(44):1–9.

Escaron AL, Meinen AM, Nitzke SA, Martinez-Donate AP. Supermarket and grocery store-based interventions to promote healthful food choices and eating practices: a systematic review. *Prev Chronic Dis*. 2013;10:E50.

Eslami E. *Trends in Supplemental Nutrition Assistance Program Participation Rates: Fiscal Year 2010 to Fiscal Year 2013*. US Department of Agriculture. 2015. Available at: http://www.fns.usda.gov/sites/default/files/ops/Trends2010-2013.pdf. Accessed March 22, 2016.

Evans AE, Jennings R, Smiley AW, et al. Introduction of farm stands in low-income communities increases fruit and vegetable among community residents. *Health Place*. 2012a;18(5):1137–1143.

Evans CE, Christian MS, Cleghorn CL, Greenwood DC, Cade JE. Systematic review and meta-analysis of school-based interventions to improve daily fruit and vegetable intake in children aged 5 to 12 y. *Am J Clin Nutr.* 2012b;96(4):889–901.

Faridi Z, Shuval K, Njike VY, et al. Partners Reducing Effects of Diabetes (PREDICT): a diabetes prevention physical activity and dietary intervention through African-American churches. *Health Educ Res.* 2010;25(2):306–315.

Ferguson CJ, Muñoz ME, Medrano MR. Advertising influences on young children's food choices and parental influence. *J Pediatr.* 2012;130(3):452–455.

Fisher JO, Goran MI, Rowe S, Hetherington MM. Forefronts in portion size. An overview and synthesis of a roundtable discussion. *Appetite.* 2015;88:1–4.

Foerster SB, Kizer KW, Disogra LK, Bal DG, Krieg BF, Bunch KL. California's 5 a Day—for Better Health! campaign: an innovative population-based effort to effect large-scale dietary change. *Am J Prev Med.* 1995;11(2):124–131.

Foltz JL, Grimm KA, Blanck HM, Scanlon KS, Moore LV, Grummer-Strawn LM. *State-Specific Trends in Fruit and Vegetable Consumption Among Adults—United States, 2000–2009.* Vol. 59. Washington, DC: US Department of Health and Human Services; 2010:1125–1130.

Food Research and Action Center (FRAC). 2015. Available at: http://www.frac.org. Accessed March 9, 2016.

Forwood SE, Ahern AL, Hollands GJ, Ng YL, Marteau TM. Priming healthy eating. You can't prime all the people all of the time. *Appetite.* 2015;89:93–102.

Franck C, Grandi SM, Eisenberg MJ. Agricultural subsidies and the American obesity epidemic. *Am J Prev Med.* 2013;45(3):327–333.

Fuller S, Beck E, Salman H, Tapsell L. New horizons for the study of dietary fiber and health: a review. *Plant Foods Hum Nutr.* 2016;71(1):1–12.

Global Burden of Disease (GBD) Study 2013 Risk Factor Collaborators, Forouzanfar MH, Alexander L, et al. Global, regional, and national comparative risk assessment of 79 behavioural, environmental and occupational, and metabolic risks or clusters of risks in 188 countries, 1990–2013: a systematic analysis for the Global Burden of Disease Study 2013. *Lancet.* 2015;386(10010):2287–2323.

Geaney F, Kelly C, Greiner BA, Harrington JM, Perry IJ, Beirne P. The effectiveness of workplace dietary modification interventions: a systematic review. *Prev Med.* 2013;57(5):438–447.

Gentile DA, Welk G, Eisenmann JC, et al. Evaluation of a multiple ecological level child obesity prevention program: switch what you do, view, and chew. *BMC Med.* 2009;7:49.

Gerteis J, Izrael D, Deitz D, et al. *Multiple Chronic Conditions Chartbook.* Rockville, MD: Agency for Healthcare Research and Quality; 2014. AHRQ Publications no. Q14-0038.

Gidding SS, Dennison BA, Birch LL, et al. Dietary recommendations for children and adolescents: a guide for practitioners. *Pediatrics.* 2006;117(2):544–559.

Gillman MW, Rifas-Shiman SL, Frazier AL, et al. Family dinner and diet quality among older children and adolescents. *Arch Fam Med.* 2000;9(3):235–240.

Girard AW, Self JL, McAuliffe C, Olude O. The effects of household food production strategies on the health and nutrition outcomes of women and young children: a systematic review. *Paediatr Perinat Epidemiol.* 2012;26(1):205–222.

Glanz K, Basil M, Maibach E, Goldberg J, Snyder D. Why Americans eat what they do: taste, nutrition, cost, convenience, and weight control concerns as influences on food consumption. *J Am Diet Assoc.* 1998;98(10):1118–1126.

Glanz K, Sallis J, Saelens B, Frank L. Healthy nutrition environments: concepts and measures. *Am J Health Promot.* 2005;19(5):330–333.

Glanz K, Yaroch AL. Strategies for increasing fruit and vegetable intake in grocery stores and communities: policy, pricing, and environmental change. *Prev Med.* 2004;39(2 suppl): S75–S80.

Goetzel RZ, Baker KM, Short ME, et al. First-year results of an obesity prevention program at The Dow Chemical Company. *J Occup Environ Med.* 2009;51(2):125–138.

Gordon A, Oddo V. Addressing child hunger and obesity in Indian Country: report to Congress. Mathmematica Policy Research. 2012. Available at: http://www.fns.usda.gov/sites/default/files/IndianCountry.pdf. Accessed August 12, 2016.

Grebitus C, Hartmann M, Reynolds N. Global obesity study on drivers for weight reduction strategies. *Obes Facts.* 2015;8(1):77–86.

Greenberg JA, Fontaine K, Allison DB. Putative biases in estimating mortality attributable to obesity in the US population. *Int J Obes (Lond).* 2007;31(9):1449–1455.

Grimm GC, Harnack L, Story M. Factors associated with soft drink consumption in school-aged children. *J Am Diet Assoc.* 2004;104(8):1244–1249.

Grimm KA, Foltz JL, Blanck HM, Scanlon KS. Household income disparities in fruit and vegetable consumption by state and territory: results of the 2009 Behavioral Risk Factor Surveillance System. *J Acad Nutr Diet.* 2012;112(12):2014–2021.

Guasch-Ferré M, Hu FB, Martínez-González MA, et al. Olive oil intake and risk of cardiovascular disease and mortality in the PREDIMED Study. *BMC Med.* 2014;12:78.

Guenther PM, Kirkpatrick SI, Reedy J, et al. The Healthy Eating Index-2010 is a valid and reliable measure of diet quality according to the 2010 Dietary Guidelines for Americans. *J Nutr.* 2014;144(3):399–407.

Guilbert TW, Arndt B, Temte J, et al. The theory and application of UW eHealth-PHINEX, a clinical electronic health record–public health information exchange. *WMJ.* 2012;111(3):124–133.

Guo SS, Wu W, Chumlea WC, Roche AF. Predicting overweight and obesity in adulthood from body mass index values in childhood and adolescence. *Am J Clin Nutr.* 2002; 76(3):653–658.

Guthrie JF, Lin BH, Frazao E. Role of food prepared away from home in the American diet, 1977–78 versus 1994–96: changes and consequences. *J Nutr Educ Behav.* 2002;34(3): 140–150.

Harrison K, Marske AL. Nutritional content of foods advertised during the television programs children watch most. *Am J Public Health.* 2005;2005(9):1568–1574.

Heaney RP. Dairy intake, dietary adequacy, and lactose intolerance. *Adv Nutr.* 2013;4(2):151–156.

Heimendinger J, Chapelsky D. The National 5 a Day for Better Health program. *Adv Exp Med Biol.* 1996;401:199–206.

Hilmers A, Chenb T, Dave JM, Thompson D, Cullen KW. Supplemental Nutrition Assistance Program participation did not help low income Hispanic women in Texas meet the dietary guidelines. *Prev Med.* 2014;62:44–48.

Hiza HA, Casavale KO, Guenther PM, Davis CA. Diet quality of Americans differs by age, sex, race/ethnicity, income, and education level. *J Acad Nutr Diet.* 2013;113(2):297–306.

Hoelscher DM, Springer AE, Ranjit N, et al. Reductions in child obesity among disadvantaged school children with community involvement: the Travis County CATCH trial. *Obesity.* 2010;18(suppl 1):S36–S44.

Hood C, Martinez-Donate A, Meinen A. Promoting healthy food consumption: a review of state-level policies to improve access to fruits and vegetables. *WMJ.* 2012; 111(6):283–288.

Huang T, Xu M, Lee A, Cho S, Qi L. Consumption of whole grains and cereal fiber and total and cause-specific mortality: prospective analysis of 367,442 individuals. *BMC Med.* 2015;13:85.

Huffman MD, Capewell S, Ning H, Shay CM, Ford ES, Lloyd-Jones DM. Cardiovascular health behavior and health factor changes (1988–2008) and projections to

2020: results from the National Health and Nutrition Examination Surveys. *Circulation*. 2012;125(21):2595–2602.

Hughes SO, Frazier-Wood AC. Satiety and the self-regulation of food take in children: a potential role for gene–environment interplay. *Curr Obes Rep*. 2016;5(1):81–87.

Imamura F, O'Connor L, Ye Z, et al. Consumption of sugar sweetened beverages, artificially sweetened beverages, and fruit juice and incidence of type 2 diabetes: systematic review, meta-analysis, and estimation of population attributable fraction. *BMJ*. 2015;351: h3576.

Institute of Medicine, Food and Nutrition Board. *Dietary Reference Intakes: Vitamin C, Vitamin E, Selenium, and Carotenoids*. Washington, DC: National Academy Press, 2000.

Institute of Medicine (IOM). *Preventing Childhood Obesity: Health in the Balance*. Committee on Prevention of Obesity in Children and Youth. Washington, DC: The National Academies Press; 2005.

Institute of Medicine (IOM). *Progress in Preventing Childhood Obesity: How Do We Measure Up?* Committee on Preventing Childhood Obesity. Washington, DC: The National Academies Press; 2007.

Institute of Medicine (IOM). *School Meals: Building Blocks for Healthy Children*. Washington, DC: The National Academies Press; 2010.

Institute of Medicine (IOM). Early childhood obesity prevention policies. Report. Washington, DC: The National Academies Press; 2011.

Institute of Medicine (IOM). *Accelerating Progress in Obesity Prevention: Solving the Weight of the Nation*. Washington, DC: The National Academies Press; 2012.

Institute of Medicine (IOM), National Research Council. *Local Government Actions to Prevent Childhood Obesity*. Washington, DC: The National Academies Press; 2009.

Järvi A, Karlström B, Vessby B, Becker W. Increased intake of fruits and vegetables in overweight subjects: effects on body weight, body composition, metabolic risk factors and dietary intake. *Br J Nutr*. 2016;115(10):1760–1768.

Jilcott SB, Moore JB, Wall-Bassett ED, Liu H, Saelens BE. Association between travel times and food procurement practices among female Supplemental Nutrition Assistance Program participants in eastern North Carolina. *J Nutr Educ Behav*. 2011;43(5): 385–389.

Johnson DB, Podrabsky M, Rocha A, Otten JJ. Effect of the Healthy Hunger-Free Kids Act on the nutritional quality of meals selected by students and school lunch participation rates. *JAMA Pediatr*. 2016;170(1):e153918.

Judd SE, Letter AJ, Shikany JM, Roth DL, Newby PK. Dietary patterns derived using exploratory and confirmatory factor analysis are stable and generalizable across race, region, and gender subgroups in the REGARDS study. *Front Nutr.* 2014;1:29.

Kaiser KA, Brown AW, Bohan Brown MM, Shikany JM, Mattes RD, Allison DB. Increased fruit and vegetable intake has no discernible effect on weight loss: a systematic review and meta-analysis. *Am J Clin Nutr.* 2014;100(2):567–576.

Kant AK, Graubard BI. Eating out in America, 1987–2000: trends and nutritional correlates. *Prev Med.* 2004;38(2):243–249.

Kant AK, Graubard BI. Secular trends in patterns of self-reported food consumption of adult Americans: NHANES 1971–1975 to NHANES 1999–2002. *Am J Clin Nutr.* 2006;84(5):1215–1223.

Kant AK, Graubard BI. Secular trends in the association of socio-economic position with self-reported dietary attributes and biomarkers in the US population: National Health and Nutrition Examination Survey (NHANES) 1971–1975 to NHANES 1999–2002. *Public Health Nutr.* 2007;10(2):158–167.

Kant AK, Graubard BI. 40-year trends in meal and snack eating behaviors of American adults. *J Acad Nutr Diet.* 2015;115(1):50–63.

Kant AK, Leitzmann MF, Park Y, Hollenbeck A, Schatzkin A. Patterns of recommended dietary behaviors predict subsequent risk of mortality in a large cohort of men and women in the United States. *J Nutr.* 2009;139(7):1374–1380.

Khan LK, Sobush K, Keener D, et al. Recommended community strategies and measurements to prevent obesity in the United States. *MMWR Recomm Rep.* 2009;58(RR–7): 1–26.

Kiage JN, Merrill PD, Robinson CJ, et al. Intake of trans fat and all-cause mortality in the Reasons for Geographical and Racial Differences in Stroke (REGARDS) cohort. *Am J Clin Nutr.* 2013;97(5):1121–1128.

Kim KH, Linnan L, Campbell MK, Brooks C, Koenig HG, Wiesen C. The WORD (wholeness, oneness, righteousness, deliverance): a faith-based weight-loss program utilizing a community-based participatory research approach. *Health Educ Behav.* 2008; 35(5):634–650.

Kirkpatrick SI. Understanding and addressing barriers to healthy eating among low-income Americans. *J Acad Nutr Diet.* 2012;112(5):617–620.

Kirkpatrick SI, Dodd KW, Reedy J, Krebs-Smith SM. Income and race/ethnicity are associated with adherence to food-based dietary guidance among US adults and children. *J Acad Nutr Diet.* 2012;112(5):624–635.e6.

Kraak VI, Story M. Influence of food companies' brand mascots and entertainment companies' cartoon media characters on children's diet and health: a systematic review and research needs. *Obes Rev.* 2015;16(2):107–126.

Lake A, Townshend T. Obesogenic environments: exploring the built and food environments. *J R Soc Promot Health.* 2006;126(6):261–267.

Lancaster KJ, Carter-Edwards L, Grilo S, Shen C, Schoenthaler AM. Obesity interventions in African American faith-based organizations: a systematic review. *Obes Rev.* 2014;15(suppl 4):159–176.

Langellotto GA, Gupta A. Gardening increases vegetable consumption in school-aged children: a meta-analytical synthesis. *HortTechnology.* 2012;22(4):430–445.

Larson N, Ward DS, Neelon SB, Story M. What role can child-care settings play in obesity prevention? A review of the evidence and call for research efforts. *J Am Diet Assoc.* 2011;111(9):1343–1362.

Larson NI, Story MT. Food insecurity and weight status among US children and families: a review of the literature. *Am J Prev Med.* 2011;40(2):166–173.

Larson NI, Story MT, Nelson MC. Neighborhood environments—disparities in access to healthy foods in the US. *Am J Prev Med.* 2009;36(1):74–81.

Larsson SC, Kumlin M, Ingelman-Sundberg M, Wolk A. Dietary long-chain N-3 fatty acids for the prevention of cancer: a review of potential mechanisms. *Am J Clin Nutr.* 2004;79(6):935–945.

Le Bodo Y, Paquette MC, Vallières M, Alméras N. Is sugar the new tobacco? Insights from laboratory studies, consumer surveys and public health. *Curr Obes Rep.* 2015;4(1): 111–121.

Lee S, Gura KM, Kim S, Arsenault DA, Bistrian BR, Puder M. Current clinical applications of omega-6 and omega-3 fatty acids. *Nutr Clin Pract.* 2006;4(4):323–341.

Leung CW, Blumenthal SJ, Hoffnagle EE, et al. Associations of food stamp participation with dietary quality and obesity in children. *Pediatrics.* 2013;131(3):463–472.

Leung CW, Epel ES, Ritchie LD, Crawford PB, Laraia BA. Food insecurity is inversely associated with diet quality of lower-income adults. *J Acad Nutr Diet.* 2014;114(12): 1943–1953.e2.

Levitt M, Wilt T, Shaukat A. Clinical implications of lactose malabsorption versus lactose intolerance. *J Clin Gastroenterol.* 2013;47(6):471–480.

Levy AS, Stokes RC. Effects of a health promotion advertising campaign on sales of ready-to-eat cereals. *Public Health Rep.* 1987;102(4):398–403.

Li Y, Hruby A, Bernstein AM, et al. Saturated fats compared with unsaturated fats and sources of carbohydrates in relation to risk of coronary heart disease: a prospective cohort study. *J Am Coll Cardiol.* 2015;66(14):1538–1548.

Lim S, Han SH, Kim J, Lee HJ, Lee JG, Lee EJ. Inhibition of hardy kiwifruit (*Actinidia aruguta*) ripening by 1-methylcyclopropene during cold storage and anticancer properties of the fruit extract. *Food Chem.* 2016;190:150–157.

Litt JS, Soobader MJ, Turbin MS, Hale JW, Buchenau M, Marshall JA. The influence of social involvement, neighborhood aesthetics, and community garden participation on fruit and vegetable consumption. *Am J Public Health.* 2011;101(8):1466–1473.

Liu RH. Health-promoting components of fruits and vegetables in the diet. *Adv Nutr.* 2013;4(3):384S–392S.

Long MW, Leung CW, Cheung LWY, Blumenthal SJ, Willett WC. Public support for policies to improve the nutritional impact of the Supplemental Nutritional Assistance Program (SNAP). *Public Health Nutr.* 2014;17(1):219–224.

Lundahl A, Wahlstrom LC, Christ CC, Stoltenberg SF. Gender differences in the relationship between impulsivity and disordered eating behaviors and attitudes. *Eat Behav.* 2015;18:120–124.

Lutfiyya MN, Chang LF, Lipsky MS. A cross-sectional study of US rural adults' consumption of fruits and vegetables: do they consume at least five servings daily? *BMC Public Health.* 2012;12:280.

Lyn R, Maalouf J, Evers S, Davis J, Griffin M. Nutrition and physical activity in child care centers: the impact of a wellness policy initiative on environment and policy assessment and observation outcomes, 2011. *Curr Obes Rep.* 2015;4(2):191–197.

Maddock J, Maglione C, Barnett JD, Cabot C, Jackson S, Reger-Nash B. Statewide implementation of the 1% or less campaign. *Health Educ Behav.* 2007;34(6):953–963.

Maes L, Van Cauwenberghe E, Van Lippevelde W, et al. Effectiveness of workplace interventions in Europe promoting healthy eating: a systematic review. *Eur J Public Health.* 2012;22(5):677–682.

Malas N, Tharp KM, Foerster SB. Diet and nutrition. In: Remington PL, Brownson RC, Wegner MV, ed. *Chronic Disease Epidemiology and Control.* 3rd ed. Washington, DC: American Public Health Association; 2010:160.

Malik VS, Hu FB. Fructose and cardiometabolic health: what the evidence from sugar-sweetened beverages tells us. *J Am Coll Cardiol.* 2015;66(10):1615–1624.

Malik VS, Popkin BM, Bray GA, Després JP, Hu FB. Sugar-sweetened beverages, obesity, type 2 diabetes mellitus, and cardiovascular disease risk. *Circulation.* 2010;121:1356–1364.

Malika NM, Hayman LW Jr, Miller AL, Lee HJ, Lumeng JC. Low-income women's conceptualizations of food craving and food addiction. *Eat Behav.* 2015;18:25–29.

Matson-Koffman DM, Brownstein JN, Neiner JA, Greaney ML. A site-specific literature review of policy and environmental interventions that promote physical activity and nutrition for cardiovascular health: what works? *Am J Health Promot.* 2005;19(3): 167–193.

Middaugh AL, Fisk PS, Brunt A, Rhee YS. Few associations between income and fruit and vegetable consumption. *J Nutr Educ Behav.* 2012;44(3):196–203.

Miller P. Statement of Patti Miller, Vice President, Children Now FCC Task Force on Media and Childhood Obesity. 2007. Available at: http://www.fcc.gov/obesity/march07meeting/Miller.pdf. Accessed March 23, 2016.

Molitor F, Sugerman S, Yu H, et al. Reach of Supplemental Nutrition Assistance Program-Education (SNAP-Ed) interventions and nutrition and physical activity-related outcomes, California, 2011–2012. *Prev Chronic Dis.* 2015;12:E22.

Moore LV, Diez Roux AV, Nettleton JA, Jacobs DR. Associations of the local food environment and diet quality—a comparison of assessments based on surveys and geographic information systems. *Am J Epidemiol.* 2008;167(8):917–924.

Mora C, Caldwell IR, Caldwell JM, Fisher MR, Genco BM, Running SW. Suitable days for plant growth disappear under projected climate change: potential human and biotic vulnerability. *PLoS Biol.* 2015;13(6):e1002167.

Morland K, Wing S, Diez Roux A. The contextual effect of the local food environment on residents' diets: the atherosclerosis risk in communities study. *Am J Public Health.* 2002;92(11):1761–1767.

Moshe F, Amitai Y, Korchia G, et al. Anemia and iron deficiency in children: association with red meat and poultry consumption. *J Pediatr Gastroenterol Nutr.* 2013;57(6): 722–727.

Mozaffarian D, Afshin A, Benowitz NL, et al. Population approaches to improve diet, physical activity, and smoking habits: a scientific statement from the American Heart Association. *Circulation.* 2012;126(12):1514–1563.

Mullie P, Guelinckx I, Clarys P, Degrave E, Hulens M, Vansant G. Cultural, socioeconomic and nutritional determinants of functional food consumption patterns. *Eur J Clin Nutr.* 2009;63(11):1290–1296.

Mytton OT, Nnoaham K, Eyles H, Scarborough P, Ni Mhurchu C. Systematic review and meta-analysis of the effect of increased vegetable and fruit consumption on body weight and energy intake. *BMC Public Health.* 2014;14:886.

Nader PR, Huang TTK, Gahagan S, Kumanyika S, Hammond RA, Christoffel KK. Next steps in obesity prevention: altering early life systems to support healthy parents, infants, and toddlers. *Child Obes.* 2012;8(3):195–204.

National Gardening Association. *Garden to Table: A 5-Year Look at Food Gardening in America.* National Gardening Association. 2014. Available at: http://garden.org/learn/articles/view/3819. Accessed August 12, 2016.

National Institutes of Health (NIH). Antioxidants: in depth. 2013. Available at: https://nccih.nih.gov/health/antioxidants/introduction.htm. Accessed March 25, 2016.

Nettleton JA, Follis JL, Ngwa JS, et al. Gene × dietary pattern interactions in obesity: analysis of up to 68317 adults of European ancestry. *Hum Mol Genet.* 2015;24(16): 4728–4738.

Neumark-Sztainer D, Wal M, Perry C, Story M. Correlates of fruit and vegetable intake among adolescents. Findings from Project EAT. *Prev Med.* 2003;37(3):198–208.

Ni Mhurchu C, Aston LM, Jebb SA. Effects of worksite health promotion interventions on employee diets: a systematic review. *BMC Public Health.* 2010;10:62.

Nielsen SJ, Popkin BM. Patterns and trends in food portion sizes. *JAMA.* 2003;289(4): 450–453.

Nierkens V, Hartman MA, Nicolaou M, et al. Effectiveness of cultural adaptations of interventions aimed at smoking cessation, diet, and/or physical activity in ethnic minorities. A systematic review. *PLoS One.* 2013;8(10):e73373.

Nixon CA, Moore HJ, Douthwaite W, et al. Identifying effective behavioural models and behaviour change strategies underpinning preschool and school-based obesity prevention interventions aimed at 4-6-year-olds: a systematic review. *Obes Rev.* 2012; 13(suppl 1):106–117.

Nord M, Andrews M, Carlson S. Household food security in the United States, 2008. US Department of Agriculture. 2009. Economic Research Report no. 83. Available at http://www.ers.usda.gov/media/184956/err83_1_.pdf. Accessed August 12, 2016.

Obarzanek E, Sacks FM, Vollmer WM, et al. Effects on blood lipids of a blood-pressure-lowering diet: the dietary approaches to stop hypertension (DASH) trial. *Am J Clin Nutr.* 2001;74(1):80–89.

O'Connor A, Wellenius G. Rural–urban disparities in the prevalence of diabetes and coronary heart disease. *Public Health.* 2012;126(10):813–820.

Oliveira V. *The Food Assistance Landscape: FY 2015 Annual Report, EIB-150.* US Department of Agriculture. 2016. Available at: http://www.ers.usda.gov/media/2031346/eib150.pdf. Accessed March 22, 2016.

Othman RA, Moghadasian MH, Jones PJ. Cholesterol-lowering effects of oat β-glucan. *Nutr Rev.* 2011;69(6):299–309.

Park Y, Hunter DJ, Spiegelman D, et al. Dietary fiber intake and risk of colorectal cancer: a pooled analysis of prospective cohort studies. *JAMA.* 2005;294(22):2849–2857.

Patient Protection and Affordable Care Act, 42 USC § 2705 (2010).

Pardilla M, Prasad D, Suratkar S, Gittelsohn J. High levels of household food insecurity on the Navajo Nation. *Public Health Nutr.* 2014;14(1):58–65.

Penney TL, Brown HE, Maguire ER, Kuhn I, Monsivais P. Local food environment interventions to improve healthy food choice in adults: a systematic review and realist synthesis protocol. *BMJ Open.* 2015;5(4):e007161.

Pereira MA, O.'Reilly E, Augustsson K, et al. Dietary fiber and risk of coronary heart disease: a pooled analysis of cohort studies. *Arch Intern Med.* 2004:164:370–376.

Perez-Escamilla R. Acculturation, nutrition, and health disparities in Latinos. *Am J Clin Nutr.* 2011;93(5):1163S–1167S.

Pivonka E, Seymour J, McKenna J, Baxter SD, Williams S. Development of the behaviorally focused Fruits & Veggies—More Matters public health initiative. *J Am Diet Assoc.* 2011;111(10):1570–1577.

Popkin BM, Nielsen SJ. The sweetening of the world's diet. *Obes Res.* 2003;11(11):1325–1332.

Pothukuchi K. Attracting supermarkets to inner-city neighborhoods: economic development outside the box. *Econ Dev Q.* 2005:19:232–244.

Poti JM, Popkin BM. Trends in energy intake among US children by eating location and food source, 1977–2006. *J Am Diet Assoc.* 2011;111(8):1156–1164.

Powell LM, Harris JL, Fox T. Food marketing expenditures aimed at youth: putting the numbers in context. *Am J Prev Med.* 2013;45(4):453–461.

Powell LM, Slater S, Mirtcheva D, Bao Y, Chaloupka FJ. Food store availability and neighborhood characteristics in the United States. *Prev Med.* 2007;44(1):189–195.

Qi Q, Kilpelainen TO, Downer MK, et al. FTO genetic variants, dietary intake and body mass index: insights from 177,330 individuals. *Hum Mol Genet.* 2014;23(25):6961–6972.

Quandt SA, Dupuis J, Fish C, D'Agostino RB II. Feasibility of using a community supported agriculture program to improve fruit and vegetable inventories and consumption in an underresourced urban community. *Prev Chronic Dis.* 2013;10:E136.

Ratcliffe MM, Merrigan KA, Rogers BL, Goldberg JP. The effects of school garden experiences on middle school–aged students' knowledge, attitudes, and behaviors associated with vegetable consumption. *Health Promot Pract.* 2011;12(1):36–43.

Reger B, Wootan M, Booth-Butterfield S. Using mass media to promote healthy eating: a community-based demonstration project. *Prev Med.* 1999;29(5):414–421.

Reger B, Wootan MG, Booth-Butterfield S. A comparison of different approaches to promote community-wide dietary change. *Am J Prev Med.* 2000;18(4):271–275.

Reger B, Wootan MG, Booth-Butterfield S, Smith H. 1% or Less: a community based nutrition campaign. *Public Health Rep.* 1998;113(5):410–419.

Rehm CD, Monsivais P, Drewnowski A. Relation between diet cost and Healthy Eating Index 2010 scores among adults in the United States 2007–2010. *Prev Med.* 2015;73:70–75.

Rozin P. Food preference. In: Smelser NJ, Baltes PB, eds. *International Encyclopedia of the Social and Behavioral Sciences.* Oxford, England: Elsevier; 2001:5719–5722.

Salehi-Abargouei A, Maghsoudi Z, Shirani F, Azadbakht L. Effects of Dietary Approaches to Stop Hypertension (DASH)–style diet on fatal or nonfatal cardiovascular diseases—incidence: a systematic review and meta-analysis on observational prospective studies. *Nutrition.* 2013;29(4):611–618.

Satia JA. Diet-related disparities: understanding the problem and accelerating solutions. *J Am Diet Assoc.* 2009;109(4):610–615.

Sawka KJ, McCormack GR, Nettel-Aguirre A, Swanson K. Associations between aspects of friendship networks and dietary behavior in youth: findings from a systematized review. *Eat Behav.* 2015;18:7–15.

Schultz DJ, Byker Shanks C, Houghtaling B. The impact of the 2009 Special Supplemental Nutrition Program for Women, Infants, and Children food package revisions on participants: a systematic review. *J Acad Nutr Diet.* 2015;115(11):1832–1846.

Schwartz MB, Henderson KE, Read M, Danna N, Ickovics JR. New school meal regulations increase fruit consumption and do not increase total plate waste. *Child Obes.* 2015;11(3):242–247.

Seo T, Qi K, Chang C, et al. Saturated fat-rich diet enhances selective uptake of LDL cholesteryl esters in the arterial wall. *J Clin Invest.* 2005;115(8):2214–2222.

Sesso HD, Buring JE, Christen WG, et al. Vitamins E and C in the prevention of cardiovascular disease in men: the Physicians' Health Study II randomized trial. *JAMA.* 2008;300(18):2123–2133.

Shaikh RA, Yaroch A, Nebeling L, Yeh MC, Resnicow K. Psychosocial predictors of fruit and vegetable consumption in adults. *Am J Prev Med.* 2008;34(6):535–543.

Shepherd J, Harden A, Rees R, et al. Young people and healthy eating: a systematic review of research on barriers and facilitators. *Health Educ Res.* 2006;21(2):239–257.

Shiue I. Urinary polyaromatic hydrocarbons are associated with adult celiac disease and kidney stones: USA NHANES, 2011–2012. *Environ Sci Pollut Res Int.* 2016;23(4):3971–3977.

Sinclair SE, Cooper M, Mansfield ED. The influence of menu labeling on calories selected or consumed: a systematic review and meta-analysis. *J Acad Nutr Diet.* 2014;114(9):1375–1388.e15.

Singh GM, Micha R, Khatibzadeh S, et al. Estimated global, regional, and national disease burdens related to sugar-sweetened beverage consumption in 2010. *Circulation.* 2015;132(8):639–666.

Sorensen G, Stoddard AM, Dubowitz T, et al. The influence of social context on changes in fruit and vegetable consumption: results of the healthy directions studies. *Am J Pub Health.* 2007;97(7):1216–1227.

Special Committee on Health, Productivity, and Disability Management. Healthy workforce/healthy economy: the role of health, productivity, and disability management in addressing the nation's health care crisis: why an emphasis on the health of the workforce is vital to the health of the economy. *J Occup Environ Med.* 2009;51(1):114–119.

Spence M, Lahteenmaki L, Stefan V, Livingstone MBE, Gibney ER, Dean M. Quantifying consumer portion control practices. A cross-sectional study. *Appetite.* 2015;92:240–246.

Stables GJ, Subar AF, Patterson BH, et al. Changes in vegetable and fruit consumption and awareness among US adults: results of the 1991 and 1997 5 a Day for Better Health program surveys. *J Am Diet Assoc.* 2002;102(6):809–817.

Stewart H, Dong D, Carlson A. Why are Americans consuming less fluid milk? A look at generational differences in intake frequency. Washington, DC: US Department of Agriculture, Economic Research Service; 2013. ERR-149.

Story M, Kaphingst KM, Robinson-O'Brien R, Glanz K. Creating healthy food and eating environments: policy and environmental approaches. *Annu Rev Public Health.* 2008;29:253–272.

Strickland JR, Pizzorno G, Kinghorn AM, Evanoff BA. Worksite influences on obesogenic behaviors in low-wage workers in St Louis, Missouri, 2013–2014. *Prev Chronic Dis.* 2015;12:E66.

Stuart-Shor EM, Berra KA, Kamau MW, Kumanyika SK. Behavioral strategies for cardiovascular risk reduction in diverse and underserved racial/ethnic groups. *Circulation.* 2012;125(1):171–184.

Swinburn B, Egger G, Raza F. Dissecting obesogenic environments: the development and application of a framework for identifying and prioritizing environmental interventions for obesity. *Prev Med.* 1999;6(pt 1):563–570.

Taber DR, Chriqui JF, Perna FM, Powell LM, Chaloupka FJ. Weight status among adolescents in states that govern competitive food nutrition content. *Pediatrics*. 2012;130(3): 437–444.

Tate EB, Spruijt-Metz D, Pickering TA, Pentz MA. Two facets of stress and indirect effects on child diet through emotion-driven eating. *Eat Behav*. 2015;18:84–90.

Theuwissen E, Mensink RP. Water-soluble dietary fibers and cardiovascular disease. *Physiol Behav*. 2008;94(2):258–292.

Thomson CA, Ravia J. A systematic review of behavioral interventions to promote intake of fruit and vegetables. *J Am Diet Assoc*. 2011;111(10):1523–1535.

Tovar A, Hennessy E, Pirie A, et al. Feeding styles and child weight status among recent immigrant mother–child dyads. *Int J Behav Nutr Phys Act*. 2012;9:62.

Urban LE, Weber JL, Heyman MB, et al. Energy contents of frequently ordered restaurant meals and comparison with human energy requirements and US Department of Agriculture database information: a multisite randomized study. *J Acad Nutr Diet*. 2016; 116(4):590–598e6.

US Department of Agriculture (USDA). *Dietary Guidelines for Americans 2005 Executive Summary*. Available at: https://health.gov/dietaryguidelines/dga2005/document/html/executivesummary.htm. Accessed August 15, 2015.

US Department of Agriculture (USDA). Access to affordable and nutritious food measuring and understanding food deserts and their consequences: report to Congress. 2009. Available at: http://www.ers.usda.gov/media/242675/ap036_1_.pdf. Accessed August 12, 2016.

US Department of Agriculture (USDA). A brief history of USDA food guides. 2011. Available at: http://www.choosemyplate.gov/sites/default/files/printablematerials/ABriefHistoryOfUSDAFoodGuides.pdf. Accessed March 7, 2016.

US Department of Agriculture (USDA). 2014 Farm Bill highlights. 2014a. Available at: https://www.usda.gov/documents/usda-2014-farm-bill-highlights.pdf. Accessed March 15, 2016.

US Department of Agriculture (USDA), Economic Research Service. Number of US farmers' markets continues to rise. 2014b. Available at: http://www.ers.usda.gov/data-products/chart-gallery/detail.aspx?chartId=48561&ref=collection&embed=True. Accessed August 12, 2016.

US Department of Agriculture (USDA) Food and Nutrition Service. Child and Adult Care Food Program (CACFP). 2015a. Available at: http://www.fns.usda.gov/cacfp/child-and-adult-care-food-program. Accessed August 12, 2016.

US Department of Agriculture. Tools for schools: focusing on smart snacks. Healthier school day 2015. 2015b. Available at: http://www.fns.usda.gov/healthierschoolday/tools-schools-focusing-smart-snacks. Accessed March 31, 2016.

US Department of Health and Human Services (USDHHS) and US Department of Agriculture (USDA). *Dietary Guidelines for Americans, 2010*. 7th ed. Washington, DC: US Government Printing Office; 2010.

US Department of Health and Human Services (USDHHS) and US Department of Agriculture (USDA). *2015–2020 Dietary Guidelines for Americans*. 8th ed. 2015. Available at: http://health.gov/dietaryguidelines/2015/guidelines. Accessed February 9, 2016.

US Department of Health and Human Services (USDHHS). *Healthy People 2010*. Vol. 2. Conference ed. Washington, DC: US Department of Health and Human Services; 2000.

US Environmental Protection Agency (USEPA). *Climate Change Indicators in the United States: Length of Growing Season*. 2016. Available at: http://www.epa.gov/climatechange/indicators. Accessed May 17, 2016.

US Government Accountability Office. School meal programs: competitive foods are widely available and generate substantial revenues for schools. Washington, DC: US Government Accountability Office; 2005. Report GA0-05-563.

Van Cauwenberghe E, Maes L, Spittaels H, et al. Effectiveness of school-based interventions in Europe to promote healthy nutrition in children and adolescents: systematic review of published and "grey" literature. *Br J Nutr*. 2010;103(3):781–797.

van der Horst K, Oenema A, Ferreira I, et al. A systematic review of environmental correlates of obesity-related dietary behaviors in youth. *Health Educ Res*. 2006;22(2):203–226.

VanEpps EM, Roberto CA, Park S, Economos CD, Bleich SN. Restaurant menu labeling policy: review of evidence and controversies. *Curr Obes Rep*. 2016; 5(1):72–80.

Verweij LM, Coffeng J, van Mechelen W, Proper KI. Meta-analyses of workplace physical activity and dietary behaviour interventions on weight outcomes. *Obes Rev*. 2011;12(6):406–429.

Vipperla K, O'Keefe SJ. Diet, microbiota, and dysbiosis: a "recipe" for colorectal cancer. *Food Funct*. 2016;7(4):1731–1740.

Wang Y, Cai L, Wu Y, et al. What childhood obesity prevention programmes work? A systematic review and meta-analysis. *Obes Rev*. 2015;16(7):547–565.

Ward R. Supplemental Nutrition Assistance Program Education (SNAP-Ed) FY 2016 allocation. 2015. Available at: https://snaped.fns.usda.gov/snap/Guidance/FY2016FinalStateSNAP-EdAllocations.pdf. Accessed March 22, 2016.

Wenrich TR, Brown JL, Miller-Day M, Kelley KJ, Lengerich EJ. Family members' influence on family meal vegetable choices. *J Nutr Educ Behav.* 2010;42(4):225–234.

Willcox BJ, Curb JD, Rodriquez BL. Antioxidants in cardiovascular health and disease: key lessons from epidemiologic studies. *Am J Cardiol.* 2008;101(10A):75D–86D.

Willett WC. *Nutritional Epidemiology.* 3rd ed. New York, NY: Oxford University Press; 2013.

Williams L, Ball K, Crawford D. Why do some socioeconomically disadvantaged women eat better than others? An investigation of the personal, social and environmental correlates of fruit and vegetable consumption. *Appetite.* 2010;55(3):441–446.

Williams PA, Cates SC, Blitstein JL, et al. Evaluating the impact of six Supplemental Nutrition Assistance Program education interventions on children's at-home diets. *Health Educ Behav.* 2015;42(3):329–338.

Wisconsin Department of Health Services, Division of Public Health, Nutrition, Physical Activity, and Obesity Program. *Got Access? A Guide for Improving Fruit and Vegetable Access in Wisconsin Communities.* Madison, WI: Wisconsin Department of Health Services; 2012.

Wolfe KL, Kang X, He X, Dong M, Zhang Q, Liu RH. Cellular antioxidant activity of common fruits. *J Agric Food Chem.* 2008;56(18):8418–8426.

Wolfe RR. Update on protein intake: importance of milk proteins for health status of the elderly. *Nutr Rev.* 2015;73(suppl 1):41–47.

World Cancer Research Fund, American Institute for Cancer Research. *Food, Nutrition, Physical Activity, and the Prevention of Cancer: A Global Perspective.* Washington, DC: American Institute for Cancer Research; 2007.

World Health Organization (WHO). *Global Action Plan for the Prevention and Control of Noncommunicable Diseases 2013–2020.* Geneva, Switzerland: WHO; 2013.

World Health Organization (WHO). *Noncommunicable Diseases.* Geneva, Switzerland: WHO; 2015.

Wright JD, Kennedy-Stephenson J, Wang CY, McDowell MA, Johnson CL. Trends in intake of energy and macronutrients—United States, 1971–2000. *MMWR Weekly.* 2004; 53(4):80–82.

Xu Z, Knight R. Dietary effects on human gut microbiome diversity. *Br J Nutr.* 2015;113(suppl):S1–S5.

Yan Y, Jiang W, Spinetti T, et al. Omega-3 fatty acids prevent inflammation and metabolic disorder through inhibition of NLRP3 inflammasome activation. *Immunity.* 2013;38(6):1154–1163.

Yang Q, Cogswell ME, Flanders WD, et al. Trends in cardiovascular health metrics and associations with all-cause and CVD mortality among US adults. *JAMA*. 2012;307(12): 1273–1283.

Yeary KH, Cornell CE, Prewitt E, et al. The WORD (Wholeness, Oneness, Righteousness, Deliverance): design of a randomized controlled trial testing the effectiveness of an evidence-based weight loss and maintenance intervention translated for a faith-based, rural, African American population using a community-based participatory approach. *Contemp Clin Trials*. 2015;40:63–73.

Yu K, Ke MY, Li WH, Zhang SQ, Fang XC. The impact of soluble dietary fibre on gastric emptying, postprandial blood glucose and insulin in patients with type 2 diabetes. *Asia Pac J Clin Nutr*. 2014;23(2):210–218.

Zamora-Ros R, Rothwell JA, Scalbert A, et al. Dietary intakes and food sources of phenolic acids in the European Prospective Investigation Into Cancer and Nutrition (EPIC) study. *Br J Nutr*. 2013;110(8):1500–1511.

Zemel MB. Role of calcium and dairy products in energy partitioning and weight management. *Am J Clin Nutr*. 2004;79(5):907S–912S.

Zhang Q, Wang Y. Socioeconomic and racial/ethnic disparity in Americans' adherence to federal dietary recommendations. *J Acad Nutr Diet*. 2012;112(5):614–616.

Zheng M, Rangan A, Allman-Farinelli M, Rohde JF, Olsen NJ, Heitman BL. Replacing sugary drinks with milk is inversely associated with weight gain among young obesity-predisposed children. *Br J Nutr*. 2015;114(9):1448–1455.

9

PHYSICAL ACTIVITY

Barbara E. Ainsworth, PhD, MPH, FACSM, and
Caroline A. Macera, PhD, FACSM

Introduction

The importance of being physically active has been repeatedly shown in countless studies of various populations. Physically active people have longer life expectancy and are less likely to be diagnosed with chronic diseases such as diabetes, heart disease, and some cancers. In 1996, the first Report of the Surgeon General on Physical Activity and Health summarized the many health benefits associated with physical activity and suggested that the minimum level required to achieve health benefits was a daily expenditure of 150 kilocalories in moderate or vigorous activities (USDHHS 1996). This recommendation is consistent with a 1995 consensus statement issued by the Centers for Disease Control and Prevention (CDC) and American College of Sports Medicine recommending that every adult should accumulate at least 30 minutes of moderate activity most days of the week (Pate et al. 1995).

An update to these guidelines was published in 2008 as the U.S. Physical Activity Guidelines that incorporated a combination of 150 minutes per week of moderate-intensity or 75 minutes per week of vigorous-intensity physical activity (USDHHS 2008). In this update, accumulating the equivalent amount of either moderate or vigorous activity was acceptable. Also, these guidelines highlighted the importance of minimizing sitting, referred to as "sedentary" time, regardless of the type and amount of physical activity obtained during the rest of the day. The causes of not meeting federal guidelines for physical activity or for engaging in sedentary time, health consequences, and populations at high risk are summarized in Figure 9-1 and described in detail in this chapter.

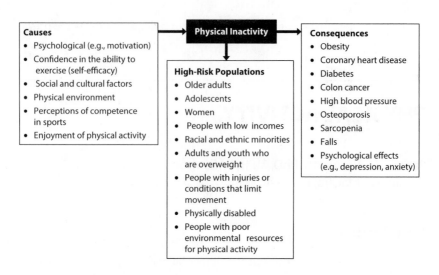

Source: Adapted from Ainsworth and Macera (2010).

Figure 9-1. Physical Inactivity: Causes, Consequences, and High-Risk Groups

Significance

The consequences of physical inactivity are observed among many dimensions of health including physical, physiological, psychological, and societal. Regular physical activity performed at the level recommended by the 2008 guidelines reduces the risks of dying prematurely and developing coronary heart disease, type 2 diabetes, breast cancer, and colon cancer. Regular activity also reduces blood pressure among people with hypertension, promotes psychological well-being, and builds and maintains healthy bones, muscles, and joints so that older adults can avoid falls and maintain functional independence (USDHHS 2008).

A landmark study published in the *Lancet* in 2012 estimated that 10.8% of U.S. deaths were attributed to physical inactivity (Lee et al. 2012). Furthermore, it is estimated that if adults were active at the recommended levels, 6.2% of coronary heart disease, 8.3% of type 2 diabetes, 12.4% of breast cancer, and 12.0% of colon cancer cases could be avoided (Lee et al. 2012). One reason for the major impact that physical inactivity has on morbidity and mortality is its prevalence. Worldwide, it is estimated that 31.1% of adults are not physically active at recommended levels. The levels of inactivity range from 17.0% in Southeast Asia to about 43% in the Mediterranean and in the Americas

(Hallal et al. 2014). These levels are important for global health, as the prevalence of physical inactivity is nearly 40% among people who develop chronic diseases and die prematurely (Lee et al. 2012).

The major economic impact of physical inactivity is felt through medical expenditures and loss of income and productivity associated with disease and disability. A study published in 2015 estimated that medical expenditures for inactive adults were $1,313 higher per year than for active adults. This represents a 26.6% difference in medical costs between inactive and active adults and is estimated to cost an additional $117 billion dollars after accounting for the effects of overweight and obesity on medical expenditures (Carlson et al. 2015).

The low prevalence of physical activity is a significant public health problem that affects various populations, multidimensional in its scope, and interdependent on other factors that may compound its effects. Actions are needed at the personal, social, economic, scientific, legal, and policy levels to reduce the prevalence of physical inactivity in the United States.

Pathophysiology

Several terms, shown in Table 9-1, are used to characterize human movement. *Physical activity* refers to any bodily movement produced by the contraction of skeletal muscle that increases energy expenditure above a basal level (Caspersen 1989). This is contrasted with the term *exercise*, which is planned, structured, and repetitive in the sense that the improvement or maintenance of one or more of the components of physical fitness is the objective (USDHHS 2008; Caspersen 1989). *Physical fitness* is a set of attributes that allows individuals to carry out daily tasks with vigor and alertness, without undue fatigue and with ample energy to enjoy leisure-time pursuits and meet unforeseen emergencies (USDHHS 1996). Components of health-related fitness include cardiorespiratory, muscular, metabolic, morphological, and motor (Bouchard et al. 1994). The terms *frequency, duration,* and *intensity* of an activity are used to measure the *activity dose* or the threshold level of physical activity associated with health benefits (USDHHS 2008).

Another term that is often used concerning physical activity is *leisure*, as in leisure-time physical activity (also called recreational physical activity). This term refers to physical activities performed by a person that are not required as essential activities of daily living and are performed at the discretion of the

Table 9-1. Definitions Used to Characterize Physical Activity

Term	Definition
Physical activity (PA)	Bodily movement that is produced by the contraction of skeletal muscle and that substantially increases energy expenditure (Caspersen 1989). • Occupational • Non-occupational (leisure, family, transportation, household, other activities)
Exercise	Planned, structured, and repetitive bodily movement done to improve or maintain one or more components of physical fitness (Caspersen 1989).
Physical fitness	The ability to perform physical activity (Caspersen 1989). The ability to carry out daily tasks with vigor and alertness, without undue fatigue, and with ample energy to enjoy leisure-time pursuits and to meet unforeseen emergencies (Garber et al. 2011). The ability to perform moderate-to-vigorous levels of physical activity without undue fatigue and the capability of maintaining such ability throughout life (Bouchard et al. 1994). Components of health-related fitness (Bouchard et al. 1994). • Submaximal exercise capacity, maximal aerobic power, heart and lung functions, blood pressure. • Muscular: power, strength, endurance. • Metabolic: glucose tolerance, insulin sensitivity, lipid and lipoprotein metabolism, substrate oxidation characteristics. • Morphological: body mass for height, body composition, subcutaneous fat distribution, abdominal visceral fat, bone density, flexibility. • Motor: agility, balance, coordination, speed of movement, reaction time.
Frequency	The times an activity is performed in a selected period (e.g., 1 week; Ainsworth et al. 2011; Bouchard et al. 1994).
Duration	The minutes or hours one engages in physical activity (Ainsworth et al. 2011; Bouchard et al. 1994).
Intensity	The energy cost of performing an activity (Ainsworth et al. 2011; Bouchard et al. 1994). • METs: The activity metabolic cost divided by the resting metabolic rate. • MET-min: The activity MET level × min of participation. • MET-hours: The activity MET level × hours of participation. • Kilocalories: MET-hours × (body weight in kilograms). • Inactivity (sedentary): 1 to 1.4 METs. • Light intensity: Physical activities from 1.5 to 2.9 METs. • Moderate intensity: Physical activities from 3 to 5.9 METs. • Vigorous intensity: Physical activities ≥ 6 METs.
Activity dose	A threshold for physical activity associated with health benefits. It is generally expressed in terms of energy expenditure, frequency, intensity, or duration (Ainsworth et al. 2000; Bouchard et al. 1994).
Leisure	Activities done in a setting that include the elements of free choice, freedom from constraints, intrinsic motivation, enjoyment, relaxation, personal involvement, and self-expression (Henderson et al. 1996).

(Continued)

Term	Definition
Occupation PA	Activities done during paid employment.
Transportation PA	Physical activity performed when traveling to a destination.
Household PA	Activities performed for the care and maintenance of the home.
Family PA	Activities performed in the care for others.

person (USDHHS 2008). Leisure-time physical activities also apply to activities that include the elements of free choice, freedom from constraints, intrinsic motivation, enjoyment, relaxation, personal involvement, and self-expression (Henderson et al. 1996). Other domains for physical activity include *occupation, transportation, household,* and *family care* physical activity. Incorporating physical activity into all domains should be encouraged, as small amounts of activity accumulated throughout the day can have a positive impact for weight control (Donnelly et al. 2009). However, leisure-time physical activity is a behavior that should be encouraged, as these activities are likely to become habits that endure throughout life.

Physical activity affects all body systems associated with energy production, metabolism, and bodily movement. Table 9-2 shows the acute and chronic changes in body systems and associated disease risks following moderate amounts of physical activity. Acute changes refer to the immediate adaptations in body systems during a physical activity period. Chronic changes refer to long-term adaptations in body systems resulting from regular participation over time (USDHHS 2008). The time required for physical activity participation to produce chronic changes in the body may range from one week (in the neuromuscular system) to several years (some metabolic hormones and enzymes).

Regular physical activity reduces risk factors for coronary heart disease by raising high-density lipoprotein cholesterol, lowering triglycerides, lowering resting and exercise blood pressures, and increasing blood clot dissolving mechanisms. Among people with coronary heart disease, regular physical activity can reduce the threshold for angina pectoris during physical activity and reduce the risks for sudden death. Regular physical activity is inversely associated with obesity and glucose–insulin intolerance and is positively associated with immune function, muscular strength, mobility, psychological well-being, and increased bone mass. Through modifications of these intermediate factors, regular physical activity can reduce

Table 9-2. Acute and Chronic Changes Associated with Disease Risk Following Moderate Amounts of Physical Activity

System	Acute Changes	Chronic Changes
Cardiovascular	Heart rate	CHD risk
	Resting heart rate	Stroke risk
	Stroke volume	CHD rehabilitation
	Maximal stroke volume	Symptoms of claudication
	Cardiac output	
	Maximal cardiac output	
	Systolic blood pressure	
	Hemoglobin	
	Blood volume	
	Blood pressure in hypertensives	
	Blood clot lysis	
	Thrombosis	
Pulmonary	Breath rate and depth	Pulmonary rehabilitation
	Breath rate for submax-activity	
	Oxygen diffusion	
	Dilatation of airways	
Neuromuscular	Rate of nerve impulses	Size of motor nerves
	Mobility	Size of muscle fibers
	Oxygen utilization	Strength
	Mitochondria	Aerobic capacity
	Anaerobic enzymes	Functional independence
	Aerobic enzymes	Fat and carbohydrate utilization
		Muscle flexibility
Skeletal	Bone mass and density	Osteoporosis bone loss
	Tendon and ligament strength	Risk of joint injury
Endocrine	Release of hormones from pituitary (most), adrenal,	Sensitivity of muscles to insulin
	thyroid, parathyroid, kidney, ovaries, testes,	Diabetes
	pancreas (glucagon and insulin), endorphins	Psychological well-being
	Release of glucose during activity	
	Adrenaline release during rest	
Metabolic	Body fat stores	Obesity
	Muscle mass	Cancer
	Ratio of lipid:carbohydrate oxidation	
	HDL-cholesterol	
	Triglycerides	
Immune	Resistance to illness	Cancer
	Leukocyte distribution	Acute illness
	Lymphocyte proliferation	Atherosclerosis and CH
	Innate immunity	
	Humoral immunity	
	Cytokines and cytotoxicity	

Source: Compiled from Bouchard et al. (1994) and Bouchard et al. (2012).
Note: CHD=coronary heart disease; HDL=high-density lipoprotein.

the risks for diabetes mellitus, depression, injuries, osteoporosis, and some forms of cancer associated with immune deficiencies and excess body fat (USDHHS 2008).

The disease risk–reducing and health-enhancing effects of regular, moderate physical activity involve the integration of many body systems. Adaptations to body systems are specific to the imposed demands of the physical activity stress (deVries and Housh 1994). This is called the SAID principle (Specific Adaptations to Imposed Demands). Types of physical activities that impose the greatest stress on most systems simultaneously are aerobic (moderate or vigorous intensity), weight bearing, and resistance activities. These activities include brisk walking, gardening, home repair, most sports and conditioning activities, manual labor occupations, and vigorous house cleaning (Ainsworth et al. 2011).

Bouchard et al. (1994) describe the relationships among habitual physical activity, health-related fitness, and health status. Health-related fitness refers to changes in morphological, muscular, motor, cardiorespiratory, and metabolic systems attributable to regular physical activity. Components in the health-related fitness model are modified by levels of physical activity, health status, heredity, and other factors, such as lifestyle behaviors, personal attributes, and physical and social environments. Regular physical activity can provide a direct effect on health-related fitness, as observed in Table 9-2, or may indirectly modify health-related fitness levels through other changes in health status.

Descriptive Epidemiology

Using a surveillance system can help to monitor the "distribution" of physical activity among the general population and to develop and evaluate interventions. Although these systems rely on self-report rather than objectively measured data and may overestimate actual physical activity, they are the best measures available for surveillance. Not only do self-report measures provide information on types of activity, but they also form the basis for research identifying the long-term health effects of physical activity and have been used to develop physical activity guidelines (Haskell 2012). Although the national surveys already in place provide a framework from which to collect data, physical activity surveillance systems must be updated regularly to ensure that prevalence data on activity patterns and trends are meaningful and complete.

Previous surveillance systems focused on sports and conditioning activities, but many have been updated to provide more information on occupation, transportation, sex-specific, and ethnic-specific physical activities. Such activities may include walking, lifting, and carrying activities during work; walking and cycling to and from work; family care and household activities; and activities relating to religious and cultural traditions.

Currently, surveillance systems commonly assess whether people are meeting the 2008 federal Physical Activity Guidelines, which would include obtaining 150 minutes per week of moderate or vigorous activity in leisure time, occupational time, or for transportation. Examples of moderate-intensity activities include brisk walking, bicycling, vacuuming, gardening, or anything else that causes small increases in breathing or heart rate. Examples of vigorous-intensity activities include running, aerobics, heavy yard work, or anything else that causes large increases in breathing or heart rate. This can be accomplished through lifestyle activities (i.e., household, transportation, occupational, or leisure-time activities). To meet the federal Physical Activity Guidelines, a person should accumulate 150 minutes a week of moderate-intensity aerobic physical activity or 75 minutes a week of vigorous-intensity activity or an equivalent combination of moderate- and vigorous-intensity activity. The guidelines also highlighted the importance of not being sedentary (USDHHS 2008).

Five major population-based surveys measure non-occupational physical activity among the U.S. population. The National Health Interview Survey (NHIS) is a household interview conducted by the National Center for Health Statistics on a representative sample of noninstitutionalized adults aged 18 years and older (NCHS 2016a). Questions on physical activity were included in 1985, 1990, 1991, and 1995. In 1997, the physical activity questions were modified and they have been included every year since. These questions include the frequency, self-assessed intensity, and duration of leisure-time physical activity.

The National Health and Nutrition Examination Survey (NHANES) program began in the early 1960s and refers to a group of studies designed to assess the health and nutritional status of adults and children in the United States. Each survey has focused on different population groups or health topics. Since 1999, the survey has included questions on physical activity with both subjective and objective measurements. This survey covers leisure-time physical activity as well as physical activity obtained through occupation and transportation (NCHS 2016b).

The Behavioral Risk Factor Surveillance System (BRFSS) is a telephone-administered survey conducted monthly by participating states in collaboration with the CDC (CDC 2016a). National estimates are developed from state-specific data. The BRFSS included physical activity items from 1986 through 1992 and in even years from 1994 to 2000 and every odd year from 2001. Questions include the type, frequency, and duration of leisure-time physical activity during the past month. Intensity measures were estimated depending on the type of activity and the age of the respondent. In 2001, modifications to the questions focused on measuring lifestyle activities rather than specific sports. The intensity of the activities (e.g., housework, yard work, walking) was self-assessed as "moderate intensity" if it required an increase in heart rate or breathing, or "vigorous intensity" if it required a large increase in heart rate or breathing. In addition to these questions, there has been one question assessing participation in any leisure-time physical activity (yes or no) that has been asked each year since 1984.

In 2002, the BRFSS initiated the Selected Metropolitan/Micropolitan Area Risk Trends (SMART) project to analyze BRFSS data of 170 selected metropolitan and micropolitan statistical areas with 500 or more respondents. These data can be used to identify emerging health problems, establish and track health objectives, and develop and evaluate public health policies and programs within targeted areas of the United States (CDC 2014).

For adolescents, the Youth Risk Behavior Surveillance System (YRBSS) is a self-administered survey distributed at selected schools (9th through 12th grade). Starting in 1991, the survey included questions about moderate and vigorous physical activities done in the past seven days as well as participation in school-based physical education programs (CDC 2015). The question that assessed vigorous physical activity asked how many days in the past seven days did they exercise or take part in sports that made them sweat or breathe hard. The question to assess moderate physical activity asked how many days in the past seven days did they ride a bicycle or walk for 30 minutes at a time.

Other surveys are conducted as needed; for example, the Youth Media Campaign Longitudinal Survey (YMCLS) was conducted in 2002 to assess the effectiveness of the Youth Media Campaign in increasing levels of physical activity among children and adolescents (CDC 2003). The YMCLS is a national random-digit-dialed telephone survey of children aged 9 to 13 years and their parents. Participation in organized and free-time physical activity was assessed for the seven days preceding the survey. Parents were asked about their perceptions of five potential barriers to the children's participation in physical activity.

For transportation activities, the National Household Travel Survey (NHTS 2016; formerly known as the Nationwide Personal Transportation Survey and the American Travel Survey) assesses commuting activity. This survey is conducted every 5 years. Because transportation activities are not comprehensively measured in other types of surveys, this information on active transportation augments the overall physical activity data. According to the latest report (Whitfield et al. 2015), less than 4% of those surveyed used active transportation regularly for commuting, whereas about 11% to 19% reported active transportation on a 1-day assessment. Among the findings of this report is that active transportation was more common among men, younger respondents, and minority racial/ethnic groups as well as in urban areas. However, active transportation was most common among both the least and most educated groups. This survey helps us understand how active transportation fits into the larger picture of total physical activity.

High-Risk Populations

Results from these surveys consistently report that the prevalence of meeting the Physical Activity Guidelines (based only on leisure-time activity) decreases with age and is lower among women and ethnic minorities compared with men and white populations (CDC 2016a; NCHS 2016a; USDHHS 1996). In Table 9-3, the prevalence of meeting Physical Activity Guidelines is shown for adult men and women by age. About 53% of men and 46% of women aged 18 years and older participated in recommended levels of moderate or vigorous activity in 2014 (NCHS 2015). Among men, the prevalence of physical activity is highest among those between the ages of 18 and 24 years (59%) and lowest among those aged 75 years and older (28%). Similarly, among women, the prevalence of physical activity is highest among those aged 18 to 24 years (54%) and lowest among those aged 75 years and older (46%). Hispanic (41%) and non-Hispanic black (44%) adults were less likely to meet the Physical Activity Guidelines (based on leisure-time activity) compared with non-Hispanic white adults (53%).

Although most of the national physical activity surveys focus on adults, physical inactivity among adolescents is of increasing concern. According to the 2008 guidelines, children and adolescents should have 60 minutes (1 hour) or more of physical activity daily. This hour should consist of primarily of aerobic activity, but should also include some muscle-strengthening and bone-strengthening activities throughout the week.

Table 9-3. Percentage of Adults Aged 18 Years and Older Who Met the 2008 Federal Physical Activity Guidelines for Aerobic Activity through Leisure-Time Aerobic Activity by Age Group and Sex: United States, 2014

Age, Years	Overall, % (95% CI)	Men, % (95% CI)	Women, % (95% CI)
18–24	59.4 (56.4, 62.4)	64.9 (61.3, 68.6)	53.8 (49.4, 58.1)
25–64	50.8 (40.7, 52.0)	53 (51.5, 54.5)	48.8 (47.4, 50.1)
65–74	42.4 (40.3, 44.4)	45.6 (42.8, 48.4)	39.6 (37.0, 42.1)
75 and older	28.1 (26.1, 30.1)	35.2 (31.7, 38.7)	23.1 (20.8, 25.5)
Total	49.2 (48.2, 50.2)	52.6 (51.3, 53.9)	46.1 (44.9, 47.3)

Source: Adapted from NCHS (2015).
Note: CI=confidence interval. Meeting guidelines is defined as engaging in moderate or vigorous leisure-time physical activities for 150 or more minutes per week. These estimates reflect leisure-time activity only, although the 2008 guidelines include all activity, so the actual percentages meeting the guidelines may be underestimated.

The YRBSS provides timely information on the aerobic activity levels of adolescents in grades 9 through 12. The guidelines suggest that adolescents should get at least one hour of physical activity on all seven days a week, but the 2013 YRBSS data found that only 58% of boys and 37% of girls in grades 9 through 12 met this guideline at least five days in the past week (CDC 2015). Additional YRBSS data suggest that about one third of youths in grades 9 through 12 watch television three or more hours per school day and 40% played video games or were using the computer outside of school work three or more hours per school day. According to NHANES data, only about 25% of youths aged 12 to 15 years met the daily physical activity guideline in 2012 (Fakhouri et al. 2014).

Although the detail necessary to assess adherence to these guidelines is not readily available, data from the 2005 YRBSS indicate that more than 90% of children in grades 9 through 12 participated in moderate or vigorous physical activity at least once during the past seven days. Data from the 2002 YMCLS indicate that about 39% of children aged 9 to 13 years participate in organized physical activity, and 77% participate in free-time physical activity. Parents perceive expense to be a major barrier to their child's participation in physical activity (overall 47% report expense as a barrier), and lack of neighborhood safety was cited as a barrier for 16% of parents. These percentages significantly varied by education, race/ethnicity, and parental income (CDC 2003). In spite of the differences in data collection samples and techniques, it is clear that many adolescents are at risk to become inactive adults.

Data from national surveys also identify those who are at high risk for not achieving sufficient levels of physical activity. These include the physically disabled (CDC 2007a; USDHHS 1996) people with injuries (Carlson et al. 2006) or conditions that limit movement (Shih et al. 2006; Butler and Evenson 2014), older adults (Sapkota et al. 2005; USDHHS 1996; Macera et al. 2015), adults who are overweight (CDC 2007b), women (CDC 2007b; Eyler et al. 2003; USDHHS 1996), ethnic minorities (CDC 2004; CDC 2007b), and people with low incomes or educational levels (Eyler et al. 2003; CDC 2007b).

Geographic Distribution

Geographic variations in the prevalence of adults meeting recommended levels of physical activity in non-occupational settings were found with data from the 2001 BRFSS (Reis et al. 2004). The prevalence was highest in the West (49%) and lowest in the South (43%). However, the area of the country may not be as important as the differences found in degree of urbanization (metro, large urban, small urban, and rural). In general, the highest prevalence of non-occupational physical activity was found in large urban areas and the lowest prevalence was found in rural areas. However, further analysis of the data indicated that, even among urbanization levels, people living in the Midwest or the South were less active than people living in the West (Reis et al. 2004). There is some evidence that the pattern of physical activity may explain some difference in urban and rural activity levels. According to subjective and objective data from NHANES, rural respondents were found to be more active overall but less active in objectively measured bouts of 10 minutes or more (Fan et al. 2014).

Another indication that geography may influence physical activity comes from studies relating characteristics of the physical environment (so-called built environment) to physical activity levels of the residents (Committee on Physical Activity, Health, Transportation, and Land Use 2005). The built environment—the physical form of communities—includes land use patterns (i.e., the location of activities across space), large- and small-scale built and natural features (e.g., architectural details, quality of landscaping), and the transportation system (i.e., the facilities and services that link one location to another).

A number of studies have shown that leisure walking and other leisure-time activities are positively associated with access to attractive open spaces and trails (Addy et al. 2004; Giles-Corti and Donovan 2003), availability of sidewalks, and satisfaction with the neighborhood environment (Ball et al. 2001; De Bourdeaudhuij et al. 2003); perceived personal safety (Giles-Corti et al. 2005; Wilson et al. 2004; Zwald et al. 2014); and access to shopping malls for walking (Addy et al. 2004). Walking for transportation is higher in urban areas with street connectivity (Cevero and Duncan 2003; Giles-Corti et al. 2005; Zwald et al. 2014), in places where pedestrians are safe from traffic, and where one lives in a close proximity to destinations for shopping and work (Giles-Corti et al. 2005). Readers are directed to Saelens et al. (2003), Owen et al. (2004), and Duncan et al. (2005) for excellent reviews of this topic.

Time Trends

As shown in Figure 9-2, the prevalence of meeting Physical Activity Guidelines during leisure time increased slightly for adults during the past decade but overall is still below 50% (NCHS 2015). For adolescents overall, one study found that the number of physically active days per week has increased slightly over the nine-year period from 2001 to 2010, and the hours per day of watching TV or playing video games have decreased slightly (Iannotti and Wang 2013). However, nationally representative longitudinal data from the YMCLS conducted from 2002 to 2006 found that the prevalence of meeting guidelines declines as children age and also has declined over time (Wall et al. 2011).

Causes

Modifiable Risk Factors

Identifying factors associated with a physically active lifestyle (also called determinants of physical activity) is important for the development of effective interventions. Although much work remains to be done, several investigators have suggested that correlates of physical activity behaviors involve individual (i.e., demographic, psychological, and biological), interpersonal (i.e., social support, cultural norms and practices), environmental (i.e., social, built, and natural environment), regional or national policy factors (i.e., transport systems, urban planning and architecture, parks and recreation, organized sports, national physical activity plans, advocacy organizations, and the corporate sector), and global efforts (i.e., economic development, media, product markets, urbanization, advocacy efforts, and social and cultural norms;

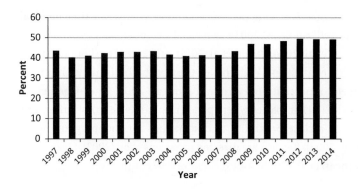

Source: Adapted from NCHS 2015.
Note: Meeting guidelines is defined as engaging in moderate or vigorous leisure-time physical activities for 150 or more minutes per week. These estimates reflect leisure-time activity only, although the 2008 guidelines include all activity, so the actual percentages meeting the guidelines may be underestimated.

Figure 9-2. Percentage of Adults Aged 18 Years and Older Who Met the 2008 Federal Physical Activity Guidelines for Aerobic Activity through Leisure-Time Aerobic Activity, United States, 1997–2014

Bauman et al. 2012). Self-efficacy (confidence in one's ability to be physically active) is strongly related to physical activity participation. As for adults, correlates of physical activity behavior among youths and adolescents are not well identified but include confidence in one's ability to engage in exercise, perceptions of competence in sports, and enjoyment of physical activity (Heitzler et al. 2006; Van Der Horst et al. 2007).

Common barriers to physical activity are lack of time, motivation, social support, facilities, and knowledge of ways to become more physically active (CDC 2004). Certain lifestyle characteristics may promote physical inactivity. These include commuting long distances to work (Zlot et al. 2006), sedentary jobs (Kruger et al. 2006b), watching television (Koezuka et al. 2006), and using computers during leisure time (Zlot et al. 2006). However, more research is needed to understand lifestyle behaviors associated with physically inactive lifestyles.

Among women, fear of assault, cultural expectations, and obligations to family care are also cited as common barriers to being physically active. Women who work full-time and have home and family responsibilities report less physical activity than working women without family care responsibilities. Among minority women, additional barriers may include differences in native languages, acculturation issues, and economic status (CDC 2004; Eyler et al. 2002).

Living in rural areas is associated with lower levels of leisure-time physical activity compared with living in urban areas (Parks et al. 2003; Reis et al. 2004; Wilcox et al. 2000). This may be attributable to differences in activity patterns that focus on activity patterns not captured on sport and recreation–focused questionnaires (e.g., house, yard, and farm work; animal care) or not having environmental supports for leisure-time activity such as sidewalks, parks, and stores near one's home for walking for transportation. More studies are needed to understand physical activity patterns of rural dwellers.

For some individuals, other health conditions may contribute to physical inactivity. Overweight status, chronic and infectious disease, injury, and physical disability may increase the energy cost of physical activity. The conditions may also prohibit one from being physically active. Often, inactivity because of existing health conditions or inaccessible facilities may create a positive feedback response by which the condition may worsen with decreased physical activity.

Population-Attributable Risk

The proportion of physical inactivity attributable to the factors just described has not been estimated. Estimates could be made with more information about relative risks and the prevalence of exposure. For example, if 25% of adults live in communities without sidewalks and persons who live in a neighborhood without a sidewalk are twice as likely to be physically inactive, then about 20% of physical inactivity would be attributable to living in a neighborhood without sidewalks. See Chapter 2 for more information about population-attributable risk.

Evidence-Based Interventions

Prevention

As with any public health problem, prevention works best when operating at many levels: personal, medical, work site, school, and community. To guide prevention efforts and to measure the improvement in the risk profiles of the U.S. population, the government routinely develops national health objectives. The most recent document, *Healthy People 2020*, was published in 2010 and lists 1,200 objectives in 42 focus areas (ODPHP 2016). These objectives provide baseline prevalence data and set 10-year targets for each objective.

Developing and modifying objectives for the next decade is an ongoing process. More information and opportunities for input are available at http://www.healthypeople.gov.

Strategies for improving physical activity among adults and children are summarized by U.S. Preventive Services Task Force (USPSTF 2014) recommendations for clinical and community practice. *The Guide to Clinical Preventive Services* provides updated counseling information for clinicians. This guide contains recommendations for prevention based on a review of evidence-based interventions to prevent 88 different illnesses and conditions. In the 2014 edition, physical activity is recommended as a multicomponent intervention that targets patient conditions such as overweight and obesity, preventing falls in older adults, and type 2 diabetes. The guide notes that linking primary care patients to community-based physical activity programs provides the best setting to enhance primary care clinician counseling.

Released in 2001 and updated annually, *The Guide to Community Preventive Services* (USPSTF 2015) provides evidence-based recommendations for programs and policies designed to promote population health in community settings. Containing intervention approaches for 22 behaviors and conditions, the guide is designed for use by public health professionals, legislators, policymakers, community-based organizations, providers of health care services, researchers, and employers and other purchasers of health care services to promote public health. Recommended intervention approaches have "sufficient evidence" demonstrating effectiveness of the interventions in research studies. Intervention approaches with insufficient evidence are those that need more research showing consistent and desired results.

Recommended intervention approaches for physical activity are grouped into three areas: informational approaches, behavioral and social approaches, and environmental and policy approaches. A list of the types of recommended approaches and those with insufficient evidence for physical activity are highlighted in Table 9-4.

Environmental and Policy Approaches

Understanding and modifying physical activity patterns is the first step in changing this behavior. Two public health approaches to increasing physical activity rely on environmental and policy strategies. Changes in public policy to promote physical activity often arise from grass roots community

Table 9-4. Guide to Community Preventive Services Task Force Findings for Physical Activity Intervention

Approaches	Recommended Methods	Methods with Insufficient Evidence
Behavioral and social	Individually adapted health behavior change programs	Family-based social support
	Social support interventions in community settings	College-based physical education and health education
	Enhanced school-based physical education	
Campaigns and informational	Community-wide campaigns	Stand-alone mass media campaigns
		Classroom-based health education focused on providing information
Environmental and policy	Community-scale urban design and land-use policies	Transportation and travel policies and practices
	Creation of or enhanced access to places for physical activity combined with information outreach activities	
	Street-scale urban design and land-use policies	
	Point-of-decision prompts to encourage use of stairs	

Source: Adapted from USPSTF (2015).

organizations designed to affect change at local, state, and national levels. However, in recent years, there have been increased coordinated efforts among public health, education, and advocacy groups to change policies for programs and facilities that promote regular physical activity in children and adults.

Policy changes can be focused on removing environmental barriers for bicyclists and pedestrians, de-emphasizing automation, building more accessible facilities to enhance movement, requiring school physical education, redirecting the use of state or federal funds to support physical activity initiatives, or subsidizing parks and recreational facilities to provide physical activity programs for people of all ages (Schmid et al. 2006a; Schmid et al. 2006b). An example of an environmental policy is to require architects to design buildings with open, well-lit, safe, and accessible stairways placed in visible locations, such as in the lobby of buildings. This provides an alternative to elevators and escalators.

Other environmental interventions with policy implications can be developed at community levels, within work sites, at schools, and in recreation centers (Heath et al. 2012). For example, community developers and city councils could be encouraged to install bicycle trails, walking trails, and sidewalks in new housing developments. Employers could provide safe and convenient exercise facilities as well as flexible work schedules to promote increased activity during the workday. Other examples of environmental opportunities for promoting physical activity include building bicycling paths and sidewalks along busy streets and providing access to shopping malls and schools as safe, heated, or air-conditioned walking and exercise spaces.

In the past 15 years, numerous state legislation and statutes have been introduced to state legislatures to increase access to and programs for physical activity (National Conference on State Legislators 2016). In a review of the state legislation and statutes database for physical activity provided by the National Conference on State Legislators, nearly every state has introduced legislation to mandate state and local school boards to require school physical education with a focus on activities that can be practiced throughout life.

Similarly, legislation has been introduced in selected states to increase access to open space for recreation, ensure bicycle and pedestrian safety, assess fitness and fatness in school-age children, and to appropriate funding from various sources, such as deposits made on recyclable soda cans, for physical activity programs. Given the public health impact of physical inactivity in terms of personal health, the economy, and societal integration, policy and environmental approaches provide an effective way to increase opportunities for physical activity for people of all ages.

Examples of Evidence-Based Interventions

Many programs conducted over the past decade provide insight as to strategies for behavior change through individual, group, site-based (e.g., schools, worksites, churches, and communities), environmental, and policy interventions and initiatives (see Resources). Within a social–ecological model whereby activities are targeted at the individual, interpersonal, social and cultural, community, and policy levels, various theories of behavior change allow interventions to target groups with messages appropriate to their readiness to modify their behaviors. The Stages of Change Model, also called the Transtheoretical Model, describes five stages to behavior change: (1) precontemplation: one is not thinking about behavior change; (2) contemplation: one is thinking about changing a behavior but has not done anything about it; (3) action: one has adopted a new behavior for less than six months; (4) maintenance: one has practiced a new behavior for longer than six months; and (5) relapse: one has stopped the new behavior but plans to resume the behavior change (Marcus and Simkin 1994). The Stages of Change approach has been used to promote physical activity in individual and physician-based interventions.

The *Guide to Community Preventive Services* endorses three types of physical activity interventions: behavioral and social approaches, campaigns and informational approaches, and environmental and policy approaches. Behavioral and social interventions are designed to increase physical activity by using individually adapted health behavior change programs tailored to meet an individual's interests, readiness for change, and preferences for physical activities. Social support interventions in community settings are designed to change physical activity behaviors through building, strengthening, and maintaining social networks (e.g., walking groups). Enhanced school-based physical education involves curricular changes designed to increase moderate- and vigorous-intensity physical activity in youths and adolescents.

These interventions are grounded in behavioral theories (e.g., social–ecological theory, social support theory) and are designed to increase physical activity, reduce sedentary behaviors, or both. An example of a classic behavioral intervention is Project Active (Dunn et al. 1997), designed to compare a lifestyle (home-based) exercise intervention with a structured, traditional (a health club) exercise intervention. Project Active showed the value of lifestyle physical activity interventions in behavior change. The lifestyle exercise intervention consisted of advising each participant to accumulate at least 30 minutes of moderate-intensity physical activity on most days of the week, in a way unique to each participant's lifestyle. The lifestyle participants also received information and skills needed to increase their self-efficacy for physical activity. The traditional exercise intervention offered structured exercise programs in a health club setting. Both activity programs received motivational messages targeted to participants on the basis of their level of readiness to change their physical activity behaviors.

After the six-month intervention period, both groups had similar reductions in cardiovascular disease risk factors such as total cholesterol, the ratio of total to high-density lipoprotein cholesterol, diastolic blood pressure, and percentage of body fat. At 24 months after the start of the study, declines in aerobic fitness, physical activity, and cardiovascular risk factors occurred in both groups; however, the lifestyle group showed smaller declines.

This suggested that lifestyle and structured physical activity programs are equally effective in maintaining positive changes in aerobic fitness, physical activity, and cardiovascular risk factors (Dunn et al. 1999). As an example of a research-to-practice translation, Project Active has been disseminated as a program for use in classrooms and community settings under the name Active Living Every Day (Blair et al. 2011).

Campaigns and informational approaches aim to increase physical activity through highly visible, broad-based, multicomponent strategies that involve many community sectors. An example of a community-wide campaign is Sumter (South Carolina) County Active Lifestyles (SCAL 2015). The SCAL campaign was developed to promote health and quality of life by advocating a community environment that supports physically active lifestyles and includes partners from the community, organizations, government, and local agencies. Operating with a multilevel framework, SCAL engages in activities designed to increase physical activity opportunities among individuals, social networks, and community organizations. It also seeks to improve environmental supports for physical activity and to advocate policies to enhance active lifestyles.

As noted earlier, environmental and policy approaches often include transdisciplinary partnerships among physical activity, public health, transportation, nonprofit, safety, government, and educational organizations as an effective approach to promoting physical activity in settings that involve multiple disciplines (National Center for Safe Routes to School 2016; Schilling et al. 2009; Sallis et al. 2006; Zimmerman et al. 2016). For example, in 2006, the U.S. Department of Transportation formed the National Safe Routes to School Task Force to develop strategies to assist communities in enabling and encouraging children to walk and bicycle safely to school in each state. The task force includes leaders in health, transportation, education, government, and nonprofit organizations (National Center for Safe Routes to School 2016).

An outgrowth of the Safe Routes to School initiatives are Walking School Bus programs defined as groups of children who walk to school with one or more adults. In a study of improving safety while walking to school, 1,252 fourth-grade children from underserved schools in Houston, Texas, participated in a Walking School Bus with adult volunteers. After five weeks, children who participated in the program were more likely to cross the streets in safe locations than students not participating in the program (Mendoza et al. 2012).

Other examples of public health approaches to promoting physical activity include several national and state campaigns as outlined in the next paragraphs.

U.S. National Physical Activity Plan

The National Physical Activity Plan is a comprehensive set of policies, programs, and initiatives that aim to increase physical activity in all segments of the American population (US National Physical Activity Plan 2016). As a private–public sector collaborative, the plan focuses on various societal sectors to promote physical activity, including business and industry; education; health care; mass media; parks, recreation, fitness, and sports; public health; transportation, land use, and community design; and volunteer and non-profit agencies. Each sector comprises strategies that aim to increase physical activity.

Examples in the health care sector are strategies to make physical activity a patient "vital sign" and that all health care providers assess and discuss physical activity with their patients. An initiative that addresses this strategy is Exercise Is Medicine (EIM; Exercise Is Medicine 2016), a global initiative of the American College of Sports Medicine designed to encourage primary care physicians and other health care providers to include physical activity assessment and recommendations during each office visit. Launched in 2007, EIM provides resources for physical activity vital sign assessment, prescription, counseling, and referral schemes in health care settings.

The ability to incorporate physical activity as a vital sign was demonstrated by Southern California Kaiser Permanente in a study that measured physical activity levels in 1,537,799 patients. Among members completing the questionnaire at a clinic visit, 36% were classified as completely inactive (0 minutes of physical activity per week), 33.3% were insufficiently active (more than 0 but less than 150 minutes per week), and 30.4% met the 2008 Physical Activity Guidelines (150 or more minutes per week; Rohm-Young et al. 2014). The effectiveness of provider-based physical activity promotion in primary care was reviewed in a meta-analysis of 13 randomized controlled trials. Patients receiving physical activity promotion efforts in primary care settings showed a 25% (range 11% to 38%) increase in physical activity after 12 months compared with those not receiving the physical activity efforts (Orrow et al. 2012). Because few physicians have specific training in physical activity promotion and counseling skills, an additional strategy in the health care sector is to include physical activity education in the training of all health care professionals.

Other important sectors for physical activity intervention programs are work sites, schools, and community settings. Work site physical activity promotion can operate at many levels (Proper et al. 2003). Some companies are large enough to provide exercise facilities including showers and changing rooms. Other companies can support physical activity by allowing time off during the day for regular exercise. Still other companies may incorporate physical activity education into their health promotion program along with smoking cessation and nutritional education. Providing a supportive work site environment will help employees to recognize the importance of physical activity and to participate in social interaction as well as physical activity. Work site physical activity may be especially important for adults with family responsibilities that constrain physical activity at home.

In 2011, Evenson and Satinsky (2014) conducted an evaluation of the National Physical Activity Plan to describe the initial accomplishments of the sector teams, and to determine how the sectors operated and achieved cross-sector collaboration, as well as positive experiences and challenges. Using an in-person, Internet-based reporting system, sector leaders provided input about the strengths and limitations of their initial accomplishments. Overall, the sector leaders valued the opportunity to lead the National Physical Activity Plan efforts and identified effective experiences in collaborations with others across sectors. They felt that the sector organization was efficient to accomplish work processes and that working with community members within the sectors was positive. As with many volunteer organizations, efforts were limited by a lack of funding and time and the need for marketing and promotion to bring awareness of sector initiatives. Additional organizational support was needed to increase effectiveness between National Physical Activity Plan Coordinating Committee and the sector members.

National Coalition for Promoting Physical Activity

The National Coalition for Promoting Physical Activity (NCPPA 2016) coordinates the efforts of sports medicine, public health, and corporate agencies to increase physical activity in the United States. The goal of the coalition is to unite the strengths of public, private, and industry efforts into a collaborative partnership to inspire Americans to lead physically active lifestyles to enhance their health and quality of life. The National Coalition for Promoting Physical Activity is open to nonprofit organizations that are membership-based and have identified physical activity and health as a primary mission.

President's Council on Fitness, Sports, and Nutrition

The President's Council on Fitness, Sports, and Nutrition (PCFSN 2016) was established in 1956 to promote physical activity, fitness, and sports for all Americans. Modified in 2008 to include nutrition, its mission is to engage, educate, and empower all Americans to adopt a healthy lifestyle that includes regular physical activity and good nutrition. Members of the council are national leaders in physical activity, fitness, sport, and nutrition who support community, state, and national organizations to promote active lifestyles. Types of activities supported include holding physical activity and fitness programs, promoting healthy eating initiatives, campaigns, and publishing reports to translate research into practice. In addition, the President's Council on Fitness, Sports, and Nutrition provides grass roots support to educators, parents, physicians and health professionals, youth sport coaches and recreation workers, employers, public officials, and community leaders interested in promoting physical activity, fitness, sport, and nutrition.

State Governor's Council on Physical Fitness

State governors' councils on physical fitness are extension of the President's Council on Fitness, Sports and Nutrition (PCFSN 2016) at the state and community levels. The chairs of governors' councils are generally employed by the state health department or the governor's office. Council members are state leaders in physical activity and are appointed to the council by the governor. Physical activity and fitness promotion efforts vary by state. However, they generally include regular meetings of the council, newsletters, awareness campaigns, conferences, and participation on policy decisions.

National Physical Activity Society

Launched in 2006, the National Physical Activity Society (NPAS 2016) (initially named the National Society of Physical Activity Practitioners in Public Health) was developed to provide strategies for communities to promote physical activity among their residents. Strategies focus on policy (Kimber et al. 2009), systems, and environmental approaches to provide resources and directions for practitioners' work on agendas for physical activity, cultivating allies, and raising the public health priority of physical activity. Resources for practitioners include webinars, fact sheets, presentations, small-town success stories, and an annual conference. In collaboration with the American College of Sports Medicine, the National Physical Activity Society supports the Physical Activity in Public Health Specialist Certification (ACSM 2016).

State Health Department Physical Activity Initiatives and Campaigns

Under the leadership of state and local health departments, physical activity initiatives and campaigns are designed to promote physical activity. Examples of initiatives are walking and bicycling events, work site challenges, and physical activity marketing efforts.

Areas of Future Research

The health effects of physical activity have been studied for nearly a half century. In the 1980s and 1990s, the emphasis shifted from performance and cardiorespiratory fitness benefits of exercise to understanding the myriad health benefits that we now know accompany even small increases in moderate activity. In the 2000s and beyond, focus has expanded to measuring and improving physical activity globally, understanding how environmental and policy factors can increase opportunities for people to be physically active, and reducing sedentary behaviors. Consensus conferences have been held to set a research agenda for physical activity, fitness, and health (Bouchard et al. 1994), and recommendations have been written for health-enhancing physical activity for people of all ages (WHO 2010; Physical Activity Guidelines Advisory Committee 2008; Haskell et al. 2007; Nelson et al. 2007; Pate et al. 1995; Sallis and Patrick 1994; USDHHS 1996). Foundations, such as the Robert Wood Johnson Foundation, are supporting research and practice efforts to modify the environment, understand how policies can promote physical activity, and increase physical activity in older adults (Sallis et al. 2002), and the National Institutes of Health has sponsored research grants to advance the assessment of physical activity (USDHHS 2015). Nevertheless, gaps still remain in understanding how to measure physical activity, to translate research to public health practice, and to promote physical activity in underserved sectors of the population. The future directions for research are outlined next.

Measurement of Physical Activity

In the past 25 years, there has been considerable progress in the assessment of physical activity by using questionnaires and objective measures in the field (Strath et al. 2013). Most questionnaires now address moderate and vigorous physical activity on the basis of the recommendations to accumulate at least 150 minutes per week of moderate activity, or to perform 75 minutes per week of vigorous activity (USDHHS 2008). Popular types of physical activity behaviors have also been measured, such as walking for transportation (Ham et al. 2005) and walking a dog (Ham and Epping 2006).

However, it is difficult to assess these behaviors by self-report with sufficient accuracy needed to track long-term trends or measure the success of intervention studies. Low-cost and nonobtrusive uses of integrated technology, such as pedometers, accelerometers, heart rate monitors, and electronic diaries, which identify the amount and type of activities that are performed, are needed for use in physical activity surveillance and intervention study settings (USDHHS 2015). Furthermore, these instruments need to be evaluated and used in diverse groups, including ethnic minorities, older adults, and children.

Adolescent Physical Activity

Adoption of guidelines to promote physical activity in schools (CDC 2016b) and out of school settings (Sallis and Patrick 1994; USDHHS 2008) provides a framework to address the decline in physical activity among adolescents. Despite recent research designed to test interventions to prevent declines in physical activity among adolescent girls (e.g., Stevens et al. 2005), additional research and demonstration projects are needed to identify effective strategies to encourage youths, especially girls and young women, to remain active during adolescence and to balance activity levels with adequate nutrition needed for growth and development.

Environmental and Policy Changes

There is increased awareness and action related to the importance of public policy change to increase physical activity at the population level. In 2004, the CDC and Prevention Research Centers (PRC 2010) established the Physical Activity Policy Research Network to identify existing physical activity policies and determinants of the policies, to describe the process of implementing policies, and to determine the outcomes of physical activity policies. Projects are designed to understand policies related to active transport and national and state physical activity plans (Eyler et al. 2013); explore policy changes in the development of community trails for walking or bicycling; and to determine a policy and environmental research agenda (Brownson et al. 2008).

Nevertheless, continued efforts are needed by community leaders, coalitions, legislators, public health experts, educators, and community residents to effect environmental and policy changes that promote physical activity among people of all ages (Bauman et al. 2006; Schmid et al. 2006a; McKinnon et al. 2011; Heath et al. 2012). These efforts may take the form of working with neighborhood coalitions to adopt residential policies conducive to being physically active, writing letters to the editor of local newspapers, writing position statements for local agencies, and lobbying legislators and city planners to pass laws to require environmental changes that promote physical activity. Additional funding is needed for research into the effectiveness of environmental and policy changes in decreasing the prevalence of physical inactivity, especially in minority and disadvantaged community settings.

Community Physical Activity Promotion

In 1994, King presented an enduring framework for community and public health approaches to promote physical activity (King 1994). Nearly 20 years after the publication of her article, physical activity is regarded as an important behavior for community health promotion (Lamarre and Pratt 2006). There have been systematic reviews of evidence-based interventions to increase physical activity, efforts to increase physical activity nationally (Dietz 2006), development of Pan-American partnerships to increase physical activity in Latin America (Gámez et al. 2006; Schmid et al. 2006b), and collaborative initiatives have been implemented to increase physical activity globally (Pratt et al. 2012; Bull et al. 2010; Kohl et al. 2012; Hallal et al. 2014). Guidelines also have been written on how to evaluate community-based physical activity programs (Martin and Heath 2006). In 2009, a national plan for promoting physical activity was introduced to provide the framework to support a broad and comprehensive national effort to increase physical activity throughout the population.

Despite these activities, continued innovative efforts are still needed to apply evidence-based approaches to increase physical activity in all sectors of the population (Bailey et al. 2013), especially in older adults (de Souto Barreto et al. 2016; Bauman et al. 2016), children and adolescents (USDHHS 2008; Lipnowski et al. 2012), individuals with chronic diseases (Brown et al. 2006; Imperatore et al. 2006), and overweight individuals (Kruger et al. 2006a). Continued attention is needed to address physical activity disparities in underserved communities (Whitt-Glover et al. 2009).

More recent approaches to promoting physical activity involve the use of technology. In 2013, experts in behavior change convened to discuss emerging trends in the use of technology in personal assessment and intervention efforts (King et al. 2015). Two levels were studied—individual and community. Mobile devices used to assess behavior at the individual level include smart phones; motion sensors that monitor physiologic, behavioral, social, and environmental influences on behavior change (e.g., accelerometers, heart-rate monitors, skin conductance and temperature sensors); personal digital assistants to monitor behavior in "real time"; portable global positioning systems that map location and distance traveled (e.g., Personal Activity Location Measurement System); and cameras worn on the body that capture physical activity behaviors (e.g., SenseCam).

Technology also has become popular in behavioral interventions to measure changes in clinical interventions (e.g., Quantified-Self mobile apps). Technologies available at the community level aggregate data across people and larger-scale contexts. Resources include web-based tools and Geographic Information Systems, which are used to assess supports for physical activity in community settings (e.g., Walk-score, Google Earth, Google Streetview). Aggregated, de-identified data collected from mobile devices can monitor personal information for many persons simultaneously to detect collective person–environment interactions in community contexts (e.g., crowd-sourcing, social network–based surveillance), and group observational recording devices can be used to determine the use of community resources (e.g., System for Observing Play and Recreation in Communities).

Innovative technologies have been used in community interventions including visualization media that can construct virtual communities supportive of physical activity and "stealth" interventions that modify sedentary activities to encourage physical activity (e.g., BingoWalk). Although technology is changing the ways individuals and interventions monitor and assess behavior change, challenges exist with matching advances in technology with the needs for assessment and intervention goals, the costs of technology, bridging the digital divide across demographic sectors, and identifying sustainable ways to provide digital and information technology in low-income and under-developed countries (Pratt et al. 2012).

Older Adults

In 2014, 76 million older adults aged 50 to 68 years represented close to one quarter of the U.S. population of 314 million (Pollard and Scommegna 2014). These "baby boomers" are the largest cohort of adults approaching retirement age ever in the United States, with nearly 8,000 adults turning 60 years old every day. By 2030, more than 20% of the U.S. population are projected to be aged 65 years and older, compared with 13% in 2010 (Colby and Ortman 2014). There is an urgent need to understand more about the "efficacy" (i.e., does it work in controlled research settings?) and "effectiveness" (i.e., does it work in real-world settings?) of community-wide physical activity programs designed to maintain physical function and to prevent physiological decline and disability in this aging cohort (Prohaska et al. 2006). Evidence-based physical activity programs designed for younger adults and for older adults in clinical research settings need to be translated for use in older adults in community-wide settings.

An example of such a program is Active for Life—Increasing Physical Activity Levels in Adults Age 50 and Older. Supported by the Robert Wood Johnson Foundation, Active for Life is designed to test the community translation of two empirically validated physical activity interventions (Active Choices and Active Living Every Day) created for midlife and older adults. A total of 5,891 adults aged 50 years and older from nine community-based programs in the United States completed the program. Following program participation, increases in moderate-to-vigorous physical activity and total physical activity, increases in satisfaction with body appearance and function, and decreases in body mass index provided evidence for the program's success (Wilcox et al. 2008). Similar programs are needed for use in community settings to maintain healthy and active lifestyles among adults as they age.

Resources

Guidelines

2008 Physical Activity Guidelines for Americans, https://www.health.gov/paguidelines

The Guide to Clinical Preventive Services, http://www.USPreventiveServicesTaskForce.org

The Guide to Community Preventive Services, http://www.thecommunityguide.org

Healthy People 2020, https://www.healthypeople.gov

Surveillance

Behavioral Risk Factor Surveillance System, http://www.cdc.gov/brfss

National Health Interview Survey, http://www.cdc.gov/nchs/nhis.htm

World Health Organization Global Physical Activity Surveillance, http://www.who.int/chp/steps/GPAQ/en

Youth Media Campaign Longitudinal Survey, http://www.cdc.gov/mmwr/preview/mmwrhtml/mm5233a1.htm

Youth Risk Behavior Survey, http://www.cdc.gov/HealthyYouth/yrbs

Organizations and Agencies

American Cancer Society, http://www.cancer.org

American College of Sports Medicine, http://www.acsm.org

American Heart Association, http://www.aha.orgCenters for Disease Control and Prevention, National Center for Chronic Disease Prevention and Health Promotion, Division of Nutrition and Physical Activity, http://www.cdc.gov

International Society for Physical Activity and Health, http://www.ispah.org

National Association for Health and Fitness: A Network of State and Governor's Councils, http://www.physicalfitness.org

National Center for Bicycling and Walking, http://www.bikewalk.org

National Center on Physical Activity and Disability, http://www.ncpad.org

National Coalition for Promoting Physical Activity, http://www.ncppa.org

National Physical Activity Plan, http://www.physicalactivityplan.org/index.html

National Physical Activity Society, http://physicalactivitysociety.org

National Recreation and Parks Association, http://www.nrpa.org

President's Council for Fitness, Sport and Nutrition, http://www.fitness.gov

Robert Wood Johnson Foundation, http://www.rwjf.org

Society of Health and Physical Educators (SHAPE America), http://www.shapeamerica.org

World Health Organization Physical Activity, http://www.who.int/topics/physical_activity/en

YMCA of the USA, http://www.ymca.net

Policy

National Center for Safe Routes to School, http://www.saferoutesinfo.org

Prevention Research Centers Physical Activity Policy Network, http://prcstl.wustl.edu/Pages/default.aspx

University of South Carolina Prevention Research Center, http://prevention.sph.sc.edu

U.S. Department of Transportation, https://www.transportation.gov/mission/health/physical-activity-transportation

World Health Organization Physical Activity Policy, http://www.euro.who.int/en/health-topics/disease-prevention/physical-activity/policy

Environment

Active Living Research, http://activelivingresearch.org

Association of State and Territorial Health Officials, http://www.astho.org

International Physical Activity and the Environment Network, http://www.ipenproject.org

U.S. Environmental Protection Agency, https://www.epa.gov/aging/index.htm

Suggested Reading

The Global Physical Activity Observatory. 2016. Available at: http://www.globalphysicalactivityobservatory.com. Accessed April 30, 2016.

US Department of Health and Human Services. *Physical Activity and Health: A Report of the Surgeon General.* 1996. Available at: http://www.cdc.gov/nccdphp/sgr/contents.htm. Accessed April 11, 2016.

US Department of Health and Human Services. *2008 Physical Activity Guidelines for Americans.* 2008. Available at: http://www.health.gov/paguidelines. Accessed April 11, 2016.

References

Addy CL, Wilson DK, Kirtland KA, Ainsworth BE, Sharpe P, Kimsey D. Associations of perceived social and physical environmental supports with physical activity and walking behavior. *Aust J Polit Hist.* 2004;94(3):440–443.

Ainsworth BE, Haskell WL, Hermann SD, et al. Compendium of physical activities: a second update of codes and MET values. *Med Sci Sports Exerc.* 2011;43(8):1575–1581.

Ainsworth BE, Macera CA. Physical activity. In: Remington PL, Brownson RC, Wegner MV, ed. *Chronic Disease Epidemiology and Control.* 3rd ed. Washington, DC: American Public Health Association; 2010:200.

American College of Sports Medicine (ACSM). Physical Activity in Public Health Specialist Certification. 2016. Available at: http://certification.acsm.org/acsm-physical-activity-in-public-health-specialist. Accessed April 14, 2016.

Bailey R, Hillman C, Arent S, Petitpas A. Physical activity: an underestimated investment in human capital? *J Phys Act Health.* 2013;10(3):289–308.

Ball K, Bauman A, Leslie E, Owen N. Perceived environmental aesthetics and convenience and company are associated with walking for exercise among Australian adults. *Prev Med.* 2001;33(5):434–440.

Bauman A, Merom D, Bull FC, Buchner DM, Fiatarone Singh MA. Updating the evidence for physical activity: summative reviews of the epidemiological evidence, prevalence, and interventions to promote "active aging." *Gerontologist.* 2016;56(suppl 2): S268–S280.

Bauman A, Reis J, Sallis JF, et al. Correlates of physical activity: why are some people physically active and others not? *Lancet.* 2012;380(9838):258–271.

Bauman AE, Nelson DE, Pratt M, Matsudo V, Schoeppe S. Dissemination of physical activity evidence, programs, policies, and surveillance in the international public health arena. *Am J Prev Med.* 2006;31(4 suppl):S57–S65.

Blair SN, Dunn AL, Marcus BH, Carpenter RA, Jaret P. *Active Living Every Day.* 2nd ed. Champaign, IL: Human Kinetics; 2011.

Bouchard C, Blair SN, Haskell WL, eds. *Physical Activity and Health.* Champaign, IL: Human Kinetics Publishers; 2012.

Bouchard C, Shephard RJ, Stephens T. *Physical Activity, Fitness, and Health: International Proceedings and Consensus Statement.* Champaign, IL: Human Kinetics; 1994.

Brown DW, Brown DR, Heath GW, et al. Relationships between engaging in recommended levels of physical activity and health-related quality of life among hypertensive adults. *J Phys Act Health.* 2006;3(4):137–147.

Brownson RC, Kelly CM, Eyler AA, et al. Environmental and policy approaches for promoting physical activity in the United States: a research agenda. *J Phys Act Health.* 2008;5(4):488–503.

Bull FC, Gauvin L, Bauman A, Shilton T, Kohl HW III, Salmon A. The Toronto charter for physical activity: a global call for action. *J Phys Act Health.* 2010;7(4):421–422.

Butler EN, Evenson KR. Prevalence of physical activity and sedentary behavior among stroke survivors in the United States. *Top Stroke Rehabil.* 2014;21(3):246–255.

Carlson SA, Fulton JE, Pratt M, Yang Z, Adams K. Inadequate physical activity and health care expenditures in the United States. *Prog Cardiovasc Dis.* 2015;57(4):315–323.

Carlson SA, Hootman JM, Powell KS, et al. Self-reported injury and physical activity levels: United States 2000 to 2002. *Ann Epidemiol.* 2006;16(9):712–719.

Caspersen CJ. Physical activity epidemiology: concepts, methods, and applications to exercise science. *Exerc Sport Sci Rev.* 1989;17:423–473.

Centers for Disease Control and Prevention (CDC). Physical activity levels among children Aged 9–13 years—United States, 2002. Youth Media Campaign Longitudinal Survey. Methods and Statistical Reports. 2003. Available at: http://www.cdc.gov/mmwr/preview/mmwrhtml/mm5233a1.htm. Accessed April 11, 2016.

Centers for Disease Control and Prevention (CDC). REACH 2010 surveillance for health status in minority communities—United States, 2001–2002. *MMWR Surveill Summ.* 2004;53(6):1–36.

Centers for Disease Control and Prevention (CDC). Physical activity among adults with a disability—United States. *MMWR Morb Mortal Wkly Rep.* 2007a;56(39):1021–1024.

Centers for Disease Control and Prevention (CDC). Prevalence of regular physical activity among adults—United States, 2001 and 2005. *MMWR Morb Mortal Wkly Rep.* 2007b;56(46):1209–1212.

Centers for Disease Control and Prevention (CDC). SMART: Selected Metropolitan / Micropolitan Area Risk Trends. 2014. Available at: http://www.cdc.gov/brfss/smart/smart_data.htm. Accessed April 11, 2016.

Centers for Disease Control and Prevention (CDC). Youth Risk Behavior Surveillance System. Methods and Statistical Reports. 2015. Available at: http://www.cdc.gov/HealthyYouth/yrbs. Accessed April 11, 2016.

Centers for Disease Control and Prevention (CDC). Behavioral Risk Factor Surveillance System. Methods and Statistical Reports. 2016a. Available at: http://www.cdc.gov/brfss. Accessed April 11, 2016.

Centers for Disease Control and Prevention (CDC). School health guidelines. 2016b. Available at: https://www.cdc.gov/healthyschools/npao/strategies.htm. Accessed August 14, 2016.

Cevero R, Duncan M. Walking, bicycling, and urban landscapes: evidence from the San Francisco Bay area. *Aust J Polit Hist.* 2003;93(9):1478–1483.

Colby SL, Ortman JM. The baby boom cohort in the United States: 2012 to 2060. Washington, DC: US Department of Commerce, Economics and Statistics Administration, US Census Bureau; 2014.

Committee on Physical Activity, Health, Transportation, and Land Use. Does the built environment influence physical activity? Examining the Evidence. Washington, DC: Transportation Research Board; 2005.

De Bourdeaudhuij I, Sallis JF, Saelens BE. Environmental correlates of physical activity in a sample of Belgian adults. *Am J Health Promot*. 2003;18(1):83–92.

de Souto Barreto P, Morley JE, Chodzko-Zajko WH, et al. Recommendations on physical activity and exercise for older adults living in long-term care facilities: a taskforce report. *J Am Med Dir Assoc*. 2016;17(5):381–392.

deVries HA, Housh TJ. *Physiology of Exercise*. 5th ed. Dubuque, IA: Brown and Benchmark Publishers; 1994.

Dietz WH. Canada on the move: a novel effort to increase physical activity among Canadians. *Can J Public Health*. 2006;97(suppl 1):S3–S4.

Donnelly JE, Blair SN, Jakicic JM, et al. American College of Sports Medicine Position Stand. Appropriate physical activity intervention strategies for weight loss and prevention of weight regain for adults. *Med Sci Sports Exerc*. 2009;41(2):459–471.

Duncan MJ, Spence JC, Mummery WK. Perceived environment and physical activity: a meta-analysis of selected environmental characteristics. *Int J Behav Nutr Phys Act*. 2005;2:11.

Dunn AL, Marcus BH, Kampert JB, et al. Reduction in cardiovascular disease risk factors: 6-month results from Project Active. *Prev Med*. 1997;26(6):883–892.

Dunn AL, Marcus BH, Kampert JB, et al. Comparison of lifestyle and structured interventions to increase physical activity and cardiorespiratory fitness—a randomized trial. *JAMA*. 1999;281(4):327–334.

Evenson KR, Santinsky SB. Sector activities and lessons learned around initial implementation of the United States National Physical Activity Plan. *J Phys Act Health*. 2014;11(6):1120–1128.

Eyler AA, Brownson RC, Schmid TL. Making strides toward active living: the policy perspective. *J Public Health Manag Pract*. 2013;19(3 suppl 1):S5–S7.

Eyler AA, Matson-Koffman D, Vest JR, et al. Environmental, policy, and cultural factors related to physical activity in a diverse sample of women: the Women's Cardiovascular Health Network Project—summary and discussion. *Women Health*. 2002;36(2):123–134.

Eyler AA, Matson-Koffman D, Young DR, et al. Quantitative study of correlates of physical activity in women from diverse racial/ethnic groups: the Women's Cardiovascular Health Network Project—summary and conclusions. *Am J Prev Med.* 2003;25(3 suppl 1):93–103.

Exercise Is Medicine. 2016. Available at: http://www.exerciseismedicine.org. Accessed April 14, 2016.

Fakhouri THI, Hughes JP, Burt VL, Song MK, Fulton JE, Ogden CL. Physical activity in US youth aged 12–15 years, 2012. National Center for Health Statistics. 2014. NCHS Data Brief, no. 141. Available at: http://www.cdc.gov/nchs/data/databriefs/db141.pdf. Accessed April 10, 2016.

Fan JX, Wen M, Kowaleski-Jones L. Rural–urban differences in objective and subjective measures of physical activity: findings from the National Health and Nutrition Examination Survey (NHANES) 2003–2006. *Prev Chronic Dis.* 2014;11:E141.

Gámez R, Parra D, Pratt M, Schmid T. *Muévete Bogotá*: promoting physical activity with a network of partner companies. *Promot Educ.* 2006;13(2):138–143.

Garber CE, Blissmer B, Deschenes MR, et al. Quantity and quality of exercise for developing and maintaining cardiorespiratory, musculoskeletal, and neuromotor fitness in apparently healthy adults: guidance for prescribing exercise. *Med Sci Sports Exerc.* 2011;43(7):1334–1359.

Giles-Corti B, Donovan RJ. Relative influences of individual, social environmental, and physical environmental correlates of walking. *Aust J Polit Hist.* 2003;93(9):1583–1589.

Giles-Corti B, Timperio A, Bull F, Pikora T. Understanding physical activity environmental correlates: increased specificity for ecological models. *Exerc Sport Sci Rev.* 2005;33(4):175–181.

Hallal PC, Martins RC, Ramírez A. Physical activity observatory: promoting physical activity worldwide. *Lancet.* 2014;384(9942):471–472.

Ham SA, Epping J. Dog walking and physical activity in the United States. *Prev Chronic Dis.* 2006;3(2):A47.

Ham SA, Macera CA, Lindley C. Trends in walking for transportation in the United States, 1995 and 2001. *Prev Chronic Dis.* 2005;2(4):A14.

Haskell WL. Physical activity by self-report: a brief history and future issues. *J Phys Act Health.* 2012;9(suppl 1):S5–S10.

Haskell WL, Lee I-M, Pate RR, et al. Physical activity and public health: updated recommendation for adults from the American College of Sports Medicine and the American Heart Association. *Med Sci Sports Exerc.* 2007;39(8):1423–1434.

Heath GW, Parra DC, Sarmiento OL, et al. Evidence-based intervention in physical activity: lessons from around the world. *Lancet.* 2012;380(9838):272–281.

Heitzler CD, Martin SL, Duke J, Huhman M. Correlates of physical activity in a national sample of children aged 9–13 years. *Prev Med.* 2006;42(4):254–260.

Henderson KA, Bialeschki MD, Shaw SM, Freysinger VJ. *Both Gains and Gaps: Feminist Perspectives on Women's Leisure.* State College, PA: Venture; 1996.

Imperatore G, Cheng YJ, Williams DE, Fulton JE, Gregg EW. Physical activity, cardiovascular fitness, and insulin sensitivity among US adolescents: the National Health and Nutrition Examination Survey, 1999–2002. *Diabetes Care.* 2006;29(7):1567–1572.

Iannotti R, Wang J. Trends in physical activity, sedentary behavior, diet, and BMI among US adolescents, 2001–2009. *Pediatrics.* 2013;132(4):606–614.

Kimber C, Abercrombie E, Epping JN, Mordecal L, Newkirk J II, Ray M. Elevating physical activity as a public health priority: creation of the National Society of Physical Activity Practitioners in Public Health. *J Phys Act Health.* 2009;6(6):677–681.

King AC. Community and public health approaches to the promotion of physical activity. *Med Sci Sports Exerc.* 1994;26(11):1405–1412.

King AC, Glanz K, Patrick K. Technologies to measure and modify physical activity and eating environments. *Am J Prev Med.* 2015;48(5):630–638.

Koezuka N, Ko M, Allison KR, et al. The relationship between sedentary activities and physical inactivity among adolescents: results from the Canadian Community Health Survey. *J Adolesc Health.* 2006;39(4):515–522.

Kohl HW III, Craig CL, Lambert EV, et al. The pandemic of physical inactivity: global action for public health. *Lancet.* 2012;380(9838):294–305.

Kruger J, Blanck HM, Gillespie C. Dietary and physical activity behaviors among adults successful at weight loss maintenance. *Int J Behav Nutr Phys Act.* 2006a;3:17.

Kruger J, Yore MM, Ainsworth BE, Macera CA. Is participation in occupational physical activity associated with lifestyle physical activity levels? *J Occup Environ Med.* 2006b;48(11):1143–1148.

Lamarre MC, Pratt M. Physical activity and health promotion. *Promot Educ.* 2006; 13(2):88–89,145–146,152–153.

Lee I-M, Shiroma EJ, Lobelo F, Puska P, Blair SN, Katzmarzyk PT. Effect of physical inactivity on major non-communicable diseases worldwide: an analysis of burden of diseases and life expectancy. *Lancet.* 2012;380(9838):219–229.

Lipnowski S, LeBlanc CM; Canadian Paediatric Society Healthy Active Living and Sport Medicine Committee. Healthy active living: physical activity guidelines for children and adolescents. *Paediatr Child Health*. 2012;17(2):209–210.

Macera CA, Cavanaugh A, Bellettiere J. State of the art review: physical activity and older adults. *Am J Lifestyle Med*. 2015; epub ahead of print February 18, 2015.

Marcus BH, Simkin LR. The Transtheoretical Model: applications to exercise behavior. *Med Sci Sports Exerc*. 1994;26(11):1400–1404.

Martin SL, Heath GW. A six-step model for evaluation of community-based physical activity programs. *Prev Chronic Dis*. 2006;3(1):A24.

McKinnon RA, Bowles HR, Trowbridge MJ. Engaging physical activity policymakers. *J Phys Act Health*. 2011;8(suppl 1):S145–S147.

Mendoza JA, Watson K, Chen T, et al. Impact of a pilot Walking School Bus intervention on children's pedestrian safety behaviors: a pilot study. *Health Place*. 2012;18(1):24–30.

National Center for Health Statistics (NCHS). Early release from the 2015 National Health Interview Study. 2015. Available at: http://www.cdc.gov/nchs/data/nhis/earlyrelease/earlyrelease201506_07.pdf. Accessed April 1, 2016.

National Center for Health Statistics (NCHS). National Health Interview Survey. Methods and Statistical Reports. 2016a. Available at: http://www.cdc.gov/nchs/nhis.htm. Accessed April 22, 2016.

National Center for Health Statistics (NCHS). National Health and Nutrition Examination Survey. 2016b. Available at: http://www.cdc.gov/nchs/nhanes.htm. Accessed April 8, 2016.

National Center for Safe Routes to School. 2016. Available at: http://www.saferoutesinfo.org. Accessed April 11, 2016.

National Coalition for Promoting Physical Activity (NCPPA). 2016. Available at: http://www.ncppa.org. Accessed April 14, 2016.

National Conference on State Legislators. Legislation and statute database. 2016. Available at: http://www.ncsl.org/?tabid=17173. Accessed April 13, 2016.

National Household Travel Survey (NHTS). 2016. Available at: http://nhts.ornl.gov. Accessed April 16, 2016.

National Physical Activity Society (NPAS). 2016. Available at: http://physicalactivitysociety.org. Accessed August 10, 2016.

Nelson ME, Rejeski WJ, Blair SN, et al. Physical activity and public health in older adults: recommendation from the American College of Sports Medicine and the American Heart Association. *Med Sci Sports Exerc*. 2007;39(8):1435–1445.

Office of Disease Prevention and Health Promotion (ODPHP). *Healthy People 2020.* 2016. Available at: https://www.healthypeople.gov. Accessed April 13, 2016.

Orrow G, Kinmonth A-L, Sanderson S, Sutton S. Effectiveness of physical activity promotion based in primary care: systematic review and meta-analysis of randomized controlled trials. *BMJ.* 2012;344:e1389.

Owen N, Humpel N, Leslie E, Bauman A, Sallis JF. Understanding environmental influences on walking: review and research agenda. *Am J Prev Med.* 2004;27(1):67–76.

Parks SE, Housemann RA, Brownson RC. Differential correlates of physical activity in urban and rural adults of various socioeconomic backgrounds in the United States. *J Epidemiol Community Health.* 2003;57(1):29–35.

Pate RR, Pratt M, Blair SN, et al. Physical activity and public health: a recommendation from the Centers for Disease Control and Prevention and the American College of Sports Medicine. *JAMA.* 1995;273(5):402–407.

Physical Activity Guidelines Advisory Committee. *Physical Activity Guidelines Advisory Committee Report, 2008.* Washington, DC: US Department of Health and Human Services; 2008.

Pollard K, Scommegna P. Just how many baby boomers are there? Available at: http://www.prb.org/Publications/Articles/2002/JustHowManyBabyBoomersAreThere.aspx. Accessed August 14, 2016.

Pratt M, Sarmiento OL, Montes F, et al. The implications of megatrends in information and communication technology and transportation for changes in global physical activity. *Lancet.* 2012;380(9838):282–293.

President's Council on Fitness, Sports & Nutrition (PCFSN). 2016. Available at: http://www.fitness.gov. Accessed April 14, 2016.

Prevention Research Centers (PRC). Physical Activity Policy Research Network. 2010. Available at: http://paprn.wustl.edu/Pages/Homepage.aspx. Accessed August 14, 2016.

Prohaska T, Belansky E, Belza B, et al. Physical activity, public health, and aging: critical issues and research priorities. *J Gerontol B Psychol Sci Soc Sci.* 2006;61(5): S267–S273.

Proper KI, Koning M, van der Beek A, et al. The effectiveness of worksite physical activity programs on physical activity, physical fitness, and health. *Clin J Sport Med.* 2003;13(2):106–117.

Reis JP, Bowles HR, Ainsworth BE, Dubose KD, Smith S, Laditka JN. Nonoccupational physical activity by degree of urbanization and US geographic region. *Med Sci Sports Exerc.* 2004;36(12):2093–2098.

Rohm-Young D, Coleman KJ, Ngor E, Reynolds K, Sidell M, Sallis RE. Associations between physical activity and cardiometabolic risk factors assessed in a southern California health care system, 2010–2012. *Prev Chronic Dis.* 2014;11:1–8.

Saelens BE, Sallis JF, Frank LD. Environmental correlates of walking and cycling: findings from the transportation, urban design, and planning literatures. *Ann Behav Med.* 2003;25(2):80–91.

Sallis JF, Cervero RB, Ascher W, et al. An ecological approach to creating active living communities. *Annu Rev Public Health.* 2006;27:297–322.

Sallis JF, Kraft K, Linton LS. How the environment shapes physical activity: a transdisciplinary research agenda. *Am J Prev Med.* 2002;22(3):208.

Sallis JF, Patrick K. Physical activity guidelines for adolescents: consensus statement. *Pediatr Exerc Sci.* 1994;6:302–314.

Sapkota S, Bowles HR, Ham SA, Kohl HW III. Adult participation in recommended levels of physical activity—United States, 2001 and 2003. *MMWR Morb Mortal Wkly Rep.* 2005;54:1208–1212.

Schilling JM, Giles-Corti B, Sallis JF. Connecting active living research and public policy: transdisciplinary research and policy interventions to increase physical activity. *J Public Health Policy.* 2009;30(suppl 1):S1–S15.

Schmid TL, Librett J, Neiman A, Pratt M, Salmon A. A framework for evaluating community-based physical activity promotion programs in Latin America. *Promot Educ.* 2006a;13(2):112–118.

Schmid TL, Pratt M, Witmer L. A framework for physical activity policy research. *J Phys Act Health.* 2006b;3:S20–S29.

Shih M, Hootman JM, Kruger J, Helmick CG. Physical activity in men and women with arthritis: National Health Interview Survey, 2002. *Am J Prev Med.* 2006;30(5):385–393.

Stevens J, Murray DM, Catellier DJ, et al. Design of the Trial of Activity in Adolescent Girls (TAAG). *Contemp Clin Trials.* 2005;26(2):223–233.

Strath SJ, Kaminsky LA, Ainsworth BE, et al. Guide to the assessment of physical activity: clinical and research applications. A scientific statement from the American Heart Association. *Circulation.* 2013;128(20):2259–2279.

Sumter County Active Lifestyles (SCAL). 2015. Available at: http://www.sumtercounty activelifestyles.org/about.php. Accessed April 14, 2016.

US Department of Health and Human Services (USDHHS). Improving diet and physical activity assessment. 2015. Available at: http://grants.nih.gov/grants/guide/pa-files/PAR-15-171.html. Accessed April 16, 2016.

US Department of Health and Human Services (USDHHS). *Physical Activity and Health: A Report of the Surgeon General.* Atlanta, GA: Centers for Disease Control and Prevention, National Center for Chronic Disease Prevention and Health Promotion; 1996.

US Department of Health and Human Services (USDHHS). *Physical Activity Guidelines for Americans.* 2008. Available at http://health.gov/paguidelines. Accessed April 1, 2016.

US National Physical Activity Plan. 2016. Available at: http://www.physicalactivityplan.org. Accessed April 30, 2016.

US Preventive Services Task Force (USPSTF). *The Guide to Clinical Preventive Services 2014.* 2014. Available at: http://www.uspreventiveservicestaskforce.org. Accessed April 13, 2016.

US Preventive Services Task Force (USPSTF). *The Guide to Community Preventive Services.* 2015. Available at: http://www.thecommunityguide.org. Accessed April 11, 2016.

Van Der Horst K, Paw MJ, Twisk JW, Van Mechelin W. A brief review on correlates of physical activity and sedentariness in youth. *Med Sci Sports Exerc.* 2007;39(8):1241–1250.

Wall MI, Carlson SA, Stein AD, Lee SM, Fulton JE. Trends by age in youth physical activity: Youth Media Campaign Longitudinal Survey. *Med Sci Sports Exerc.* 2011;43(11):2140–2147.

Whitfield GP, Paul P, Wendel AM. Active transportation surveillance, United States 1999–2012. *MMWR Surveill Summ.* 2015;64(7):1–20.

Whitt-Glover MC, Taylor WC, Floyd MF, Yore MM, Yancey AK, Matthews CE. Disparities in physical activity and sedentary behaviors among US children and adolescents: prevalence, correlates, and intervention implications. *J Public Health Policy.* 2009;30(suppl 1):S309–S334.

Wilcox S, Castro C, King AC, Housemann R, Brownson RC. Determinants of leisure time physical activity in rural compared with urban older and ethnically diverse women in the United States. *J Epidemiol Community Health.* 2000;54(9):667–672.

Wilcox S, Dowda M, Leviton LC, et al. Active for Life: final results from the translation of two physical activity programs. *Am J Prev Med.* 2008;35(4):340–351.

Wilson DK, Kirtland K, Ainsworth BE, Addy CL. Socioeconomic status and perceptions of access and safety for physical activity. *Ann Behav Med*. 2004;28(1):20–28.

World Health Organization. *WHO Global Recommendations on Physical Activity for Health*. 2010. Available at: http://apps.who.int/iris/bitstream/10665/44399/1/9789241599979_eng.pdf. Accessed April 16, 2016.

Zimmerman S, Lieberman M, Kramer K, Sadler B. At the intersection of active transportation and equity. 2016. Available at: http://www.saferoutespartnership.org. Accessed April 14, 2016.

Zlot A, Librett J, Buchner D, Schmidt T. Environmental, transportation, social, and time barriers to physical activity. *J Phys Act Health*. 2006;1:15–21.

Zwald ML, Hipp JA, Corseuil MW, Dodson EA. Correlates of walking for transportation and use of public transportation among adults in St Louis, Missouri, 2012. *Prev Chronic Dis*. 2014;11:E112.

10

ALCOHOL USE

Karly Christensen, BS, Matthew Thomas, MD,
Jordan Mills, DO, PhD, Brienna Deyo, MPH,
Brittany Hayes, MA, and Randall Brown, MD, PhD, FASAM

Introduction

Consumption of alcohol has been a part of numerous societies going as far back as 6000 B.C. (LMU 2016). Ancient texts from Persia, Egypt, Babylon, and China as well as Biblical writers have documented that people have been aware of alcohol's beneficial and harmful effects for nearly as long as people have been drinking (Rubin and Thomas 1992). Like tobacco use, alcohol use has complex physiological, behavioral, social, and political interrelationships. Unlike tobacco use, however, alcohol use is generally not considered to be as harmful. Rather, alcohol consumption needs to be viewed on a continuum from abstinence to low-risk use to risky use, problem drinking, alcohol misuse, alcohol use disorder, and other consequences (Saitz 2005).

The relationship between alcohol consumption and alcohol use disorder is a complicated one. Clearly, a lifetime nondrinker cannot develop an alcohol use disorder. The more one drinks, the more likely one is to suffer negative consequences from one's drinking. The relationship between the amount and duration of alcohol consumption, and the risk of developing an alcohol use disorder is not a linear one. In fact, the vast majority of heavy drinkers do not meet criteria for a use disorder (NIAAA 2008b). Genetics, co-occurring conditions, and a whole host of other factors make some people more sensitive to the effects of alcohol than others. Drinking patterns and the settings in which drinking occurs are also important. The causes, consequences, and groups at high risk for alcohol misuse and for alcohol use disorder are summarized in Figure 10-1.

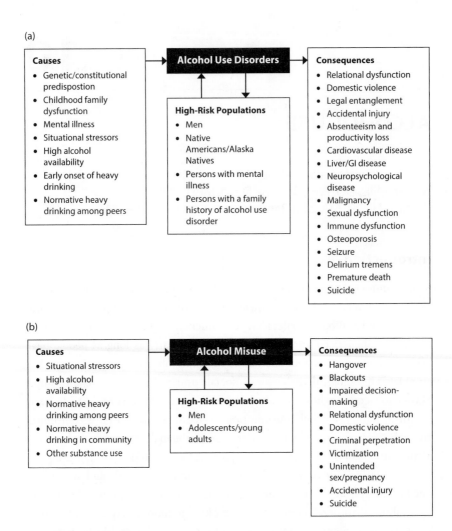

Figure 10-1. Alcohol (a) Use Disorders and (b) Misuse: Causes, Consequences, and High-Risk Groups

For those who choose to consume alcohol, the 2015 Dietary Guidelines for Americans recommend up to one drink a day for women and up to two drinks a day for men (USDHHS and USDA 2015). A drink is defined as 12 ounces of regular beer, 5 ounces of wine, or 1.5 ounces of 80-proof distilled spirits (USDHHS and USDA 2015). Drinking becomes problematic when it causes or elevates the risk for alcohol-related problems or complicates the management of other health problems.

Significance

Alcohol consumption is a part of contemporary life for many. As a result, although most people drink moderately and without ill effect, alcohol use disorders and related consequences are major health problems in the United States. In 2014, 16.3 million Americans aged 18 years and older met the criteria for alcohol use disorders (NIAAA 2016). The Centers for Disease Control and Prevention ranks alcohol as the third leading cause of preventable death in the United States (Mokdad et al. 2004). Alcohol is a contributing cause of more than 200 health conditions (Rehm et al. 2010). Worldwide, alcohol causes 3.3 million deaths (5.9% of total) and a loss of 58.3 million (4% of total) disability-adjusted life years each year (WHO 2014). The presence of an alcohol use disorder increases the relative risk of mortality 3.5 times for men and 4.6 times for women (Roerecke and Rehm 2013).

In economic terms, alcohol-related costs are estimated to have been $250 billion in 2010, the most recent year for which such estimates are available (Sacks et al. 2015). Of these costs, more than 72% are in the form of indirect costs, such as productivity losses attributable to premature mortality, excess morbidity, and crime attributed to alcohol, and only 11% are for medical treatment of alcohol use disorders (Sacks et al. 2015). Alcohol use disorders also contribute to other health problems and thereby increase the use of health care services. More than 30% of patients in short-stay general hospitals have a history of risky or problem alcohol use, regardless of their admitting diagnosis. Beyond its impact on health and economic productivity, alcohol misuse exacts an enormous toll in terms of human suffering. Failed marriages, anguished families, stalled careers, criminal records, and the pain of having loved ones killed or disabled in alcohol-related traffic crashes attest to its destructive power.

Although moderate alcohol use has been accepted in the United States for a long time, its objective physical health benefits have begun to be quantified only in the past 30 years. A substantial body of literature now exists describing the protective effects of low-level alcohol consumption against coronary heart disease (Rimm and Moats 2007).

The caloric density of alcohol (7 kcal/gram) is closer to dietary fat (9 kcal/gram) than carbohydrates (4 kcal/gram) or protein (4 kcal/gram), giving rise to public health concerns that regular alcohol use could increase overall caloric intake, contributing to obesity. Results of prospective studies suggest that light to moderate alcohol use does not increase the risk for obesity, whereas heavy drinking is more consistently associated with weight gain (Traversy and Chaput 2015).

The public has also become increasingly aware of alcohol's general risks, as well as benefits: *Healthy People 2020*, the comprehensive, nationwide health promotion and disease prevention agenda for the second decade of the 21st century, has chosen substance abuse as one of 12 leading health indicators—the major public health concerns in the United States (USDHHS and ODPHP 2014). The overarching goal of the substance abuse chapter is to reduce substance abuse to protect the health, safety, and quality of life for all, especially children. Traffic statistics, news reports, and public health initiatives, however, do not necessarily delineate the health risks and benefits of alcohol consumption for a given individual. The physical and mental health effects of alcohol use may range from beneficial to harmful. Other consequences, such as divorce or loss of a job, are not health-related per se, although they may negatively affect health indirectly through loss of income and concomitant access to health care.

Negative health consequences are of three broad types: (1) the acute consequences of ingesting large doses of alcohol in a short period of time, such as alcohol-related motor vehicle crash injuries and alcohol poisoning; (2) chronic disease consequences, such as alcoholic liver disease and alcoholic cardiomyopathy; and (3) the primary chronic disease of alcohol use disorder. Individuals who suffer from alcohol use disorder often experience other chronic and acute health effects as well. However, an individual need not suffer from alcohol use disorder to suffer negative health consequences of alcohol consumption. For example, motor vehicle accidents and other accidental trauma may occur because of a single episode of binge drinking.

Efforts to develop reliable and effective classification systems and well-founded diagnostic procedures have led to many modifications of the terms used to describe these disorders. The *Diagnostic and Statistical Manual of Mental Disorders, 5th Edition* (*DSM-5*; APA 2013) defines the concept of "alcohol use disorder" in place of the previous terms of "alcohol abuse" and "alcohol dependence" (Table 10-1). Though not strictly accurate clinically, the terms "alcohol use disorder," "alcohol abuse," and "alcoholism" continue to be widely used both among health professionals and the general public, and, to some extent, there is some shared understanding as to their meaning. The National Council on Alcoholism and Drug Dependency and the American Society of Addiction Medicine formulated the following definition:

> Alcoholism is a primary chronic disease with genetic, psychosocial, and environmental factors influencing its development and manifestations. The disease is often progressive and fatal. It is characterized by impaired control over drinking,

preoccupation with the drug alcohol, use of alcohol despite adverse consequences, and distortions of thinking, most notably denial. Each of these symptoms may be continuous or periodic (Morse and Flavin 1992).

Pathophysiology

In keeping with the chronic disease epidemiology orientation of this book, this chapter focuses primarily on the chronic disease of alcohol dependence and the chronic disease consequences of alcohol consumption. However, the negative health consequences of acute excess alcohol consumption are serious and all too common. Alcohol-related traffic crashes, the largest single alcohol-related cause of death (CDC 2004a), represent a public health problem of major significance. Some of the most effective alcohol policy measures relate to drinking and driving; therefore, binge drinking and acute consequences are covered as well.

Alcohol affects every organ of the body, manifesting in a wide array of pathology. Most critical to heavy consumption are the effects of alcohol on

Table 10-1. Terms and Definitions

Term	Clinical Diagnosis	Definition
Alcohol misuse	Not a clinical diagnosis	Alcohol use that presents significant risk of or results in alcohol-attributable consequences.
At-risk alcohol use	Not a clinical diagnosis	A pattern of alcohol use in terms of quantity and frequency that falls outside recommended limits.
Harmful alcohol use	Not a clinical diagnosis	Alcohol use resulting in negative consequences (may or may not meet criteria for alcohol use disorder).
Alcohol use disorder	DSM-5	A pattern of maladaptive use resulting in multiple consequences (such as episodes of withdrawal or exhibiting dysfunction in usual life roles) repetitively over a 12-month time course.
Alcohol abuse	DSM-IV	A pattern of maladaptive use resulting in repetitive consequences in one or more of four areas (such as legal consequences or use in hazardous circumstances) over a 12-month time course.
Alcohol dependence	DSM-IV	A pattern of maladaptive use resulting in repetitive consequences in three or more of seven areas (such as episodes of withdrawal or exhibiting dysfunction in usual life roles) over a 12-month time course.

Source: Compiled from APA (1994) and APA (2013).
Note: DSM-IV=Diagnostic and Statistical Manual of Mental Disorders, Fourth Edition; DSM-5=Diagnostic and Statistical Manual of Mental Disorders, Fifth Edition.

the brain itself. It has been known for millennia that alcohol ingestion creates a pleasurable state of mind. After extremely heavy drinking, it leads to confusion, incoordination, sedation, and coma. The brain adapts to long-term daily exposure to alcohol and eventually functions more normally in its presence, which is known as tolerance. When alcohol is then withdrawn suddenly, this adapted state becomes imbalanced, and tremors, hallucinations, and convulsions may ensue, thus demonstrating physical dependence and withdrawal.

With repeated drinking, susceptible individuals develop an imbalance with regard to the balance of the central nervous system neurotransmitters gamma-aminobutyric acid, an inhibitory neurotransmitter, and glutamate, an excitatory neurotransmitter. After years of heavy use of alcohol, the individual may suffer nutritional deficiency, repeated episodes of trauma, liver failure, and lesions of the brain attributable to the toxic effects of alcohol and its breakdown products. In some, these accumulated insults result in social deterioration, inability to walk, and severely disabling disorders of memory and cognition and, with continued drinking, culminate in death (Dupuy and Chanraud 2016; Costin and Miles 2014).

Problem alcohol use can lead to a variety of chronic health disorders. Liver disease (such as hepatic steatosis, cirrhosis, and fulminant liver failure), the most prominent of these disorders, is the leading cause of death in chronic heavy drinkers (Dufour 2007). Not only is all-cause mortality elevated in these individuals, but these deaths also occur at younger ages (Taylor et al. 1983). Heavy alcohol consumption is one of the two leading causes of acute pancreatitis (gallstones being the other; Dufour and Adamson 2003). Approximately three quarters of the patients with chronic pancreatitis have a history of heavy alcohol consumption (Dufour and Adamson 2003). Chronic alcohol consumption may also lead to chronic, irreversible conditions in other organ systems such as dilated cardiomyopathy, cardiac arrhythmia, hypertension, and stroke. Heavy alcohol use is associated with increased risk of cancer of the oral cavity, nasopharynx, larynx, esophagus, and liver (Corrao et al. 2004; Thakker 1998). For breast cancer in women, the risk rises relatively slowly but steadily with increasing alcohol consumption (Thakker 1998).

Reproductive disorders in both men and women are associated with alcohol consumption. Alcohol-related testicular atrophy may contribute significantly to sexual problems in men (Van Thiel et al. 1975; Anderson et al. 1983). In women, alcohol misuse can lead to anovulation, amenorrhea, and late menopause (Mendelson and Mello 1988; Taneri et al. 2016), and fetal alcohol spectrum disorders in a developing fetus. Alcohol use during pregnancy is the leading preventable cause of birth defects as well as intellectual and neuro-developmental disabilities (Williams and Smith 2015). Pregnant women with underlying alcohol use disorder are particularly vulnerable and may also be susceptible to nutritional deficiencies, which can compound risk to the developing fetus. Folate is of particular concern given the strong relationship between folate deficiency and the development of neural tube and congenital heart defects (Huhta and Linask 2015).

One area of harm reduction for heavy alcohol use is fortification of flour with thiamine to reduce Wernicke–Korsakoff syndrome. Wernicke–Korsakoff syndrome is a form of brain damage from a reduction of energy production in the brain by a deficiency of thiamine (vitamin B1), an important enzyme that helps in the production of this energy. This often goes missed in those with chronic alcoholism and can be missed in as many as 80% of cases of those with alcohol use disorder. It is characterized by encephalopathy, ataxia, and visual symptoms, and, although Wernicke's encephalopathy is reversible by replacement of thiamine in high doses, if not treated soon enough, it can become irreversible and then it is termed Korsakoff's syndrome, which is characterized by memory problems.

Descriptive Epidemiology

In 2010, the United States spent $249 billion on problems associated with excessive alcohol consumption, with 77% of those costs attributed to binge drinking. The costs are estimated as workplace productivity lost, criminal justice costs, health care, and motor vehicle crashes (CDC 2016a).

The physical effects of alcohol consumption vary greatly between individual people, but blood alcohol concentration (BAC) can be used as an indicator for level of impairment caused by alcohol (Table 10-2). Research suggests that men who drink more than four standard drinks per day (or more than 14 per week) and women who drink more than three per day (or more than seven per week) are at increased risk for alcohol-related problems (NIAAA 2005a).

Beer, wine, and other alcoholic beverages differ greatly in the amounts of alcohol they contain per ounce. In fact, the alcohol concentration in the same brand of beer may vary slightly between different states. To be able to compare the amounts of alcohol consumed across a variety of alcoholic beverages, drinks are sometimes expressed in terms of the amount of ethanol (the type of alcohol in alcoholic beverages) they contain. This type of calculation results in

Table 10-2. Effects of Blood Alcohol Concentration

Blood Alcohol Concentration	Typical Effects	Predictable Effects on Driving
0.02%	• Some loss of judgment • Relaxation • Slight body warmth • Altered mood	• Decline in visual functions (rapid tracking of a moving target) • Decline in ability to perform two tasks at the same time (divided attention)
0.05%	• Exaggerated behavior • May have loss of small-muscle control (e.g., focusing your eyes) • Impaired judgment • Usually good feeling • Lowered alertness • Release of inhibition	• Reduced coordination • Reduced ability to track moving objects • Difficulty steering • Reduced response to emergency driving situations
0.08%	• Muscle coordination becomes poor (e.g., balance, speech, vision, reaction time, and hearing) • Harder to detect danger • Judgment, self-control, reasoning, and memory are impaired	• Impaired concentration • Short-term memory loss • Impaired speed control • Reduced information-processing capability (e.g., signal detection, visual search) • Impaired perception
0.10%	• Clear deterioration of reaction time and control • Slurred speech, poor coordination, and slowed thinking	• Reduced ability to maintain lane position and brake appropriately
0.15%	• Far less muscle control than normal • Vomiting may occur (unless this level is reached slowly or a person has developed a tolerance for alcohol) • Major loss of balance	• Substantial impairment in vehicle control, attention to driving task, and in necessary visual and auditory information processing

Source: Reprinted from CDC (2016c).

an apparent per capita alcohol consumption in gallons of ethanol. In 2014, 2.32 gallons of all alcoholic beverages (wine, beer, and spirits) were consumed in the United States, per capita. This estimate includes all individuals aged 14 years and older (Haughwout et al. 2016). Although 14 years is well below the legal drinking age, people aged 14 years and older were included in this calculation because survey data suggest that many young people begin consuming alcohol around this age. Although quite robust, apparent per capita alcohol consumption is a crude measure because it assumes that everyone drinks. Clearly, this is not the case.

Data from national surveys provide data on drinking prevalence, drinking patterns, and problems. Two large national surveys, the National Survey on Drug Use and Health and the National Epidemiologic Survey on Alcohol and Related Conditions, are key sources of information on alcohol use and misuse in the United States. Although both are national population surveys, prevalence estimates for some of the alcohol use outcomes do differ somewhat between the surveys. Research suggests that a number of methodological differences are likely to account for these variations (Grucza et al. 2007). Nevertheless, taken together, these two surveys provide a valuable picture of alcohol use and misuse in this country.

The National Survey on Drug Use and Health is a large annual survey sponsored by the Substance Abuse and Mental Health Services Administration and is one of the primary federal sources of information on the use of illicit drugs, alcohol, and tobacco in the civilian, noninstitutionalized population of the United States aged 12 years and older. This ongoing household survey began in 1971, and was called the National Household Survey on Drug Abuse before 2002. In recent years, this survey has employed a state-based design with an independent, multistage area probability sample within each state and the District of Columbia. The national target sample size is approximately 67,500 persons each year (Hedden et al. 2015). In this survey, the following definitions are used:

- Current drinking: At least one drink in the 30 days before the survey.
- Binge drinking: Five or more drinks on the same occasion on at least 1 day in the past 30 days.
- Heavy drinking: Five or more drinks on the same occasion on each of 5 or more days in the past 30 days.

According to the 2014 survey, slightly more than half of Americans aged 12 years or older (approximately 139.7 million people) reported being current drinkers, 23% (60.9 billion) reported binge drinking, and 6.2% (16.3 million) reported heavy drinking. In 2014, 17 million persons aged 12 years or older were classified with alcohol use disorder (6.4%; Hedden et al. 2015). Table 10-3 illustrates heavy drinking over five years by age, sex, and race/ethnicity.

The National Epidemiologic Survey on Alcohol and Related Conditions is a large, nationwide household survey of the civilian, noninstitutionalized population of the United States, designed and conducted by the National Institute on Alcohol Abuse and Alcoholism of the National Institutes of Health. This longitudinal survey follows the same respondents over a period of years, as opposed to surveying different people each year. Wave 1 of this survey was

Table 10-3. Percentage of Past Monthly Heavy Alcohol Use by Age, Sex, and Race/Ethnicity, 2010–2014

Variable		2010[a]	2011[b]	2012[b]	2013[c]	2014[c]
Total		6.7	6.2	6.5	6.3	6.2
Age, years	12–17	1.7	1.5	1.3	1.2	1
	18–25	13.6	12.1	12.7	11.3	10.8
	26 and older	6.1	5.7	6.1	6.1	6
Sex	Male	10.1	9.4	9.9	9.5	9.3
	Female	3.4	3.2	3.4	3.3	3.2
Race/ethnicity	White, non-Hispanic	7.7	7.1	7.6	7.3	7.1
	Black/African American, non-Hispanic	4.5	4	4.5	4.5	4.5
	American Indian/Alaska Native, non-Hispanic	6.9	11.6	8.5	5.8	9.2
	Native Hawaiian/Pacific Islander, non-Hispanic	[d]	10.5	4.8	5.8	9.2
	Asian, non-Hispanic	2.4	1.6	1.7	2	2
	Two or more races	5.8	5.1	6.8	7.5	5.8
	Hispanic or Latino	5.1	5	5.1	4.8	5.1

Source: Data from SAMHSA (2016b).
Note: Heavy use of alcohol was defined as drinking five or more drinks on the same occasion (i.e., at the same time or within a couple of hours of each other) on each of five or more days in the past 30 days. Heavy alcohol users also were defined as binge users of alcohol.
[a]National Survey on Drug Use and Health 2009–2010.
[b]National Survey on Drug Use and Health 2011–2012.
[c]National Survey on Drug Use and Health 2013–2014.
[d]Low precision; no estimate reported.

conducted from 2001 to 2002 and consisted of 43,093 respondent interviews of people aged 18 years and older (NIAAA 2006a). Wave 2 was conducted from 2004 to 2005, and consisted of 34,653 of the original respondents (NIAAA 2010). Categories of drinkers in this survey include

- Lifetime abstainers: Those respondents who never had one or more drinks in their life.
- Former drinkers: Those who had at least one drink in their life but not in the past year.
- Current drinkers: Those who had at least one drink of any type of alcohol in the year before the survey (NIAAA 2006a)

By comparing the different waves in this survey, changes in drinking habits over time can be examined. During wave 1, approximately 65% of the respondents were current drinkers, 17% were former drinkers, and the remaining 17% were lifetime abstainers. By wave 2, 88% of the wave 1 current drinkers were still current drinkers, 73% of the wave 1 former drinkers had continued to abstain, and 75% of the wave 1 lifetime abstainers were still lifetime abstainers. From consumption-specific data collected in this survey, it is possible to calculate estimates of total ethanol consumption during the past year by summing beverage-specific volumes across the four individual beverage types. Dividing this annual total by 365 yields the average daily volume of ethanol intake, the key statistic used for "drinking level" classification. Drinkers are categorized as follows:

- Light: No more than 0.257 ounce of ethanol per day (i.e., three or fewer drinks per week).
- Moderate: More than 0.257 ounce and up to 1.2 ounces of ethanol per day (i.e., three to 14 drinks per week) for men and up to 0.6 ounce (i.e., three to seven drinks per week) for women.
- Heavier: More than 1.2 ounces of ethanol (i.e., more than two drinks) per day for men and more than 0.6 ounce (i.e., more than one drink) per day for women (NIAAA 2006a).

Data from this longitudinal survey can also indicate the progression of alcohol-related health problems. In wave 1, 83% of adults aged 18 years and older reported ever drinking alcohol, and 65% reported drinking in the past year. However, only a fraction of this group drank sufficient quantities of alcohol to suffer serious health consequences. In wave 1, 13% of current drinkers also had an alcohol use disorder. By wave 2, three years later, 9% of the original current, non–alcohol use disorder drinkers had developed their first incidence of alcohol use disorder. In addition, of those within wave 1 who were identified to be heavier drinkers, by wave 2, 21% had developed alcohol use disorder, 11% had become nicotine dependent, 7% had developed a mood disorder, and another 7% had developed an anxiety disorder.

Adolescents

Alcohol continues to be the most widely used substance of misuse among America's youths, with a higher percentage of those aged 12 to 20 years reporting the use of alcohol in the previous 30 days (22.7%) than tobacco (16.9%) or any illicit drugs (13.6%; SAMHSA 2015). In 2015, 35% of 12th graders, 22% of 10th graders, and 35% of 8th graders reported consuming alcohol within the previous 30 days (Johnston et al. 2016). Roughly one in five people between the ages of 12 to 20 years had consumed alcohol in the previous month, and about one in seven of those individuals between the ages of 12 and 20 years were considered binge drinkers (SAMHSA 2015). Although drinking alcohol before the legal age of 21 years is still prevalent, there has been a decline in the 12- to 20-year-old population from 28.8% in 2002 to 22.7% in 2013 (SAMHSA 2015).

More than 18.6% of individuals begin consuming alcohol before the age of 13 years (CDC 2014). In 2015, the observed prevalence of alcohol consumption among eighth graders was 5% (Johnston et al. 2016). Those who consume alcohol at an early age are also at an increased risk for developing an alcohol use disorder later in life. Largely because of the illegal nature of drinking alcohol before the age of 21 years, young people often attempt to conceal their consumption, which may increase the likelihood of risky behaviors, social problems, and physical problems such as alcohol poisoning. The desire to avoid detection has likely contributed to an increase in the popularity among young people of methods for achieving intoxication without consuming alcoholic beverages that are intended for consumption. For example, the ingestion of alcohol-based hand sanitizer has become an increasingly popular and potentially dangerous practice among American adolescents, as the number of reports to the National Poison Data System continues to rise (Gormley et al. 2012).

Older Americans

The rates of alcohol consumption among adults aged 65 years or older are lower in current drinking, binge drinking, and heavy drinking than in all other adult age groups (SAMHSA 2013b). However, among older individuals who drink, the proportion of heavy drinkers is nearly as high as that in the group aged 16 to 17 years (SAMHSA 2013b). In 2001–2002, among those aged 65 years and older, the 12-month prevalence estimates for *Diagnostic and Statistical Manual of Mental Disorders, Fourth Edition (DSM-IV)*–defined alcohol abuse were 2.4% for men and 0.38% for women. The 12-month prevalence estimates for *DSM-IV* alcohol dependence were 0.39% for men and 0.13% for women (APA 1994; NIAAA 2006a). One reason for the lower prevalence among older individuals may be underreporting. Instruments for detecting use disorders were largely designed and validated in younger samples.

For example, a retired widower who is no longer driving will report no alcohol-related marital or job problems or arrests for drunk driving, regardless of how much alcohol he consumes.

Among clinical populations, estimates of alcohol misuse and alcohol use disorder are substantially higher because problem drinkers of all ages are more likely to present to health care settings. Although rates of alcohol use disorder are lowest in older Americans (>65 years of age), nearly 50% of nursing home residents have some type of alcohol-related problem (NCADD 2015). Many older individuals with an alcohol use disorder developed it earlier in their lives. However, the risk for new cases continues through the later years, even as overall prevalence declines. Late-onset heavy drinking may begin in response to stressful life experiences such as bereavement, declining health, economic changes, or retirement (Dufour 2006). Sensitivity to the physical effects of alcohol increases with age, because of a decrease in total body water and reductions in gastric enzymatic (alcohol dehydrogenase) activity. A 2008 study found that 40% of older adults (aged >65 years) consume alcohol in the United States. Older adults are at an increased risk of experiencing problems from consuming alcohol, especially individuals who take certain medications, have health problems, or drink heavily (NIAAA 2008a). In addition, aging can lower an individual's tolerance for alcohol, which puts some older adults at a higher risk for falls, unintentional injuries, and car crashes (NIAAA 2008a).

Sex

Men are more likely than women to drink alcohol excessively. In fact, men are twice as likely to have engaged in binge drinking in the previous 30 days compared to women. It is estimated that roughly 4.5% of men and 2.5% of women met the criteria for alcohol dependence in 2011 (CDC 2016b). In general men have higher drinking rates than women. However, among the heaviest drinkers, female drinkers equal or surpass male drinkers in the number of problems that result from their drinking (NIDA 2015).

Women are more susceptible to the effects of alcohol primarily because women, pound for pound have lower total body water content than men of comparable size. A woman will achieve a higher concentration of alcohol in her blood than a man after consuming an equivalent amount of alcohol (NIDA 2015). Women are also more likely to develop alcohol use disorders earlier than men. In addition, women are more likely to experience reproductive issues attributable to drinking (IAS 2013). Finally, there is the issue of ethanol metabolism and sex differences in the activity of an alcohol metabolizing enzyme found in the stomach—gastric alcohol dehydrogenase. After a person consumes alcohol, some of it is oxidized in the stomach by alcohol dehydrogenase. The capacity for this form of metabolism is lower in women and may contribute to higher blood alcohol levels than those seen in men at similar levels of acute consumption (Cederbaum 2012).

Race/Ethnicity

Differences in alcohol consumption and problems with and across racial/ethnic minorities have become increasingly important as the proportion of racial/ethnic minorities in the population of the United States has increased. Past studies of what is now referred to as alcohol use disorder and adverse consequences of drinking among racial and ethnic minorities have been criticized for assuming that a given group is homogeneous. Intra-ethnic variations, such as self- assessment of ethnic identification, culture retention, incorporation of mainstream culture, and whether individuals are foreign- or native-born, are important to consider when one is examining alcohol-related questions.

In the 2013 National Survey on Drug Use and Health, 57.7% of whites reported current use of alcohol, which is more than any other racial/ethnic group. Asians reported the lowest rate of current use (34.5%). The rate of binge or heavy drinking was lowest among Asians at 12.4% and highest among Native Hawaiians or other Pacific Islanders at 24.7%. Among youths aged 12 to 17 years, reported current alcohol use was highest among whites (12.9%) and lowest among Asians (8%; SAMHSA 2013a).

Although women are overall less likely to drink than men, the distributions of drinking status and drinking levels are similar for men and women across races/ethnicities. More than half of Asian/Native Hawaiian/Pacific Islander women and about a third of African-American and Hispanic women report being lifetime abstainers. Although men of some racial/ethnic groups are less likely to be drinkers, among those who are, the proportions drinking at the various levels are more similar. Asian/Native Hawaiian/Pacific Islander men who drink are most likely to be light drinkers and least likely to be moderate or heavier drinkers. They are also much less likely to meet criteria for an alcohol use disorder. American Indian/Alaska Native men are slightly more likely to report heavier drinking and somewhat more likely to meet criteria for an alcohol use disorder. Patterns of heavy drinking by race/ethnicity are distributed similarly for both women and men (Table 10-3). Compared with women as a whole, a slightly lower proportion of Asian/Native Hawaiian/Pacific Islander women meet criteria for an alcohol use disorder and nearly double the proportion of Native American/Alaska Native women meet criteria for an alcohol use disorder (NIAAA 2006a).

Hispanic Americans are one of the fastest growing ethnic groups in the United States, accounting for roughly 17% of the national population. However, Hispanics are not a homogeneous population. Nearly 64% of Hispanics in the United States trace their origins to Mexico, and the rest to many other countries (US Census Bureau 2014). Hispanics have higher rates of abstinence from alcohol than non-Hispanic whites. However, the Hispanic individuals who choose to consume alcohol are more likely to drink alcohol in higher volumes than non-Hispanic whites. Hispanic women traditionally do not drink outside of the family; however, because of acculturation, this does not tend to apply to young Hispanic women in the United States. Acculturation is the process of adapting to a new culture; this not only includes the language but also the norms, behaviors, and beliefs (NIAAA 2015c).

The national origin among Hispanics is another factor that has an impact on the trends in alcohol consumption. Among Hispanic men, those from Puerto Rico on average have more drinks per week (16.9 drinks) than those of any other national origin. Men from Mexico rank second in drinks per week (15.9 drinks). Men from Central or South America drink more per week than men from Cuba (8.9 vs. 4 drinks). Women from Puerto Rico consume significantly more alcohol per week (9.5 drinks) than women from Mexico (3.0 drinks; NIAAA 2015a).

Native Americans are particularly likely to suffer some of the potential adverse effects of heavy alcohol use, particularly hepatic cirrhosis, although there are indications of improvement. The age-adjusted chronic liver disease and cirrhosis death rate (72.4 deaths per 100,000) for American Indians and Alaska Natives (AI/AN) for years 1979 to 1981 has decreased to 43.1 for years 2007 to 2009. However, though significantly reduced, the 2007 to 2009 rate still represented a rate 4.7 times higher than the general population rate of 9.2 for 2008 (IHS 2015). The age-specific alcohol-related death rate for AI/AN men was higher for all age groups in comparison with AI/AN women. However, rates among AI/AN women were much higher than for women of all races in the U.S. population (IHS 2015). In 2013, chronic liver disease and cirrhosis accounted for 5.5% of all AI/AN deaths, compared to 1.4% in the white population (NCHS 2014).

College Drinking

Consumption of alcohol on college campuses is considered a social norm. Roughly four out of five college students consume alcohol, and about half of those students binge drink. Of those students who consume alcohol, about 20% meet the criteria for alcohol use disorder (NIAAA 2015b). Men on average binge drink more often than women; however, the gender gap has been narrowing since 1993 (White et al. 2013). College students who misuse alcohol more frequently experience sexual assault, engage in risky sexual behaviors, experience academic consequences, and suffer unintentional injuries (NIAAA 2015b).

On average, one in four women are sexually assaulted on college campuses every year, and 50% of reported sexual assaults involve alcohol use (Abbey 2002). Though much less likely than for women, men also experience sexual assault on college campuses. Approximately 1 in 16 men have reported sexual assault while in college (NSVRC 2015). Not all sexual assaults take place in the presence of heavy alcohol consumption, but the high frequency of the two conditions co-occurring suggest that alcohol does play a role in some sexual assaults (Abbey 2011).

Alcohol is also likely to affect academics, particularly for heavy drinkers. There is an inverse relationship between alcohol consumption level and college academic performance. One out of four students who drink reports missing class, doing poorly in exams, and falling behind in class. Of those students who drink, the binge drinkers are six times more likely to do poorly on exams or projects than non–binge drinkers (NIAAA 2015b).

Social Stigma

Both the social consequences and the health impacts of alcohol consumption vary significantly among socioeconomic classes, sexes, levels of education, and racial/ethnic groups. Different levels of alcohol consumption are socially acceptable among different groups of people and in different circumstances. For example, alcohol consumption is often highly stigmatizing for people who are unstably housed; however, it is socially expected among some groups of university undergraduates. Even binge use and intoxication are frequently viewed as normative behavior for the latter, whereas greater degrees of stigma are frequently attached to such behavior for the former group.

Social situations for different groups of people can intersect to increase the social and health consequences of alcohol consumption. In 2016, Bellis found that individuals of lower socioeconomic status were more likely to smoke tobacco, binge drink, and drink spirits, beer, or cider when compared to individuals of higher socioeconomic status. The lifestyle factors associated with socioeconomic status combined to increase the risk of developing alcohol-related health problems including fatty liver disease (Bellis et al. 2016). A higher prevalence of very excessive drinking has been reported among men with lower levels of educational attainment (Van Oers et al. 1999).

Genetic and Constitutional Factors

Extensive evidence points toward a significant contribution of genetics to the development of alcohol use disorder. Twin studies indicative of significantly increased risk for identical twins (as opposed to fraternal twins or other siblings) are an example of one such type of evidence (Kendler et al. 1997; Prescott et al. 1999). Approximately 50% of the vulnerabilities leading to alcohol use disorder can be explained by genetic factors (Schuckit 2009; McGue 1999). The risk for the male and female children of those with alcohol use disorder is similar, indicating that the increased prevalence of alcohol use disorder among men is more likely attributable to cultural than to genetic factors (Eng et al. 2005). It appears that genetic influence upon important intermediate factors may be primary drivers of the process leading to alcohol use disorder. Primary examples of these intermediate factors include low level of response to alcohol (or high constitutional tolerance), personality characteristics (such as impulsivity or novelty seeking), a flushing response to alcohol, and psychological factors and mental illness (Schuckit 2009).

Geographic Distribution

As mentioned earlier, apparent per capita consumption calculations are based on the total population of a given state or region. Such data underestimate average consumption for the actual number of individuals who drink alcohol because the percentage of people who abstain varies considerably from state to state. Starting in 1999, national surveys were expanded to produce state-level estimates. The samples in each state are selected to represent proportionately the geography and demography of that state. The samples are interviewed with audio computer-assisted self-interviewing for more sensitive populations, to facilitate confidentiality, and in-person interviews are used with the less sensitive populations (SAMHSA 2016a).

The National Survey on Drug Use and Health reports state estimates for 23 measures of substance use or mental health problems including several measures of alcohol use and alcohol use disorder. In 2013 to 2014, the rate of past-month alcohol use in states among all persons aged 12 years or older ranged from a low of 31.9% in Utah to a high of 68.0% in the District of Columbia (Table 10-4). Figure 10-2 presents the geographic distribution of current drinking by state. The highest rates of past-month alcohol use occurred in the group aged 18 to 25 years, with the District of Columbia having the highest rate (73.9%) for this age group and Utah having the lowest rate (36.6%) from 2013 to 2014 (SAMHSA 2016b).

The Behavioral Risk Factor Surveillance System conducted by individual states and coordinated by the Centers for Disease Control and Prevention (CDC) is the world's largest ongoing telephone health survey system, tracking health conditions and risk behaviors in the United States yearly since 1984. Currently, data are collected monthly in all 50 states, the District of Columbia, Puerto Rico, the U.S. Virgin Islands, and Guam. State prevalence data are available for the following three alcohol consumption variables: (1) adults (aged 18 years and older) who had at least one drink of alcohol within the past 30 days, (2) heavy drinkers (adult men who have more than two drinks per day and adult women who have more than one drink per day), and (3) binge drinkers (men who had five or more drinks on one occasion and women who had four or more drinks on one occasion, in the past 30 days). The magnitude and distribution of these state-specific prevalence rates for past-month alcohol consumption by state are roughly similar to those in national surveys. The CDC website (http://www.cdc.gov/brfss) provides a number of features especially useful to public health professionals including interactive databases such as the State Prevalence Data Charts and Maps, which make it possible to view specific alcohol variables by state and map them. The Web Enabled Analysis Tool permits researchers to create cross-tabulation reports and perform logistic analysis of these data.

Table 10-4. Alcohol Use and Binge Alcohol Use in Past Month and Alcohol Misuse in Past Year by Age Group and State: Percentages, Annual Averages

| | Age Group, Years | | | | | | | | | | | |
| | 12+ | | | 12 to 17 | | | 18 to 25 | | | 26+ | | |
State	Past Month Use	Past Month Binge	Past Year AUD	Past Month Use	Past Month Binge	Past Year AUD	Past Month Use	Past Month Binge	Past Year AUD	Past Month Use	Past Month Binge	Past Year AUD
National total	52	23	6.5	52	6.2	2.8	60	38	13	56	22	5.9
Alabama	45	22	5.8	10	6.0	2.8	51	33	11	48	22	5.3
Alaska	54	23	6.7	9.0	5.0	2.1	56	39	13	59	22	6.2
Arizona	52	23	7.6	12	6.4	3.4	58	37	13	56	23	7.2
Arkansas	42	21	5.2	9.9	5.9	2.6	55	37	10	44	20	4.7
California	51	22	6.6	12	6.4	2.7	58	37	13	54	22	6.0
Colorado	62	26	7.5	14	6.9	3.4	67	41	14	66	25	6.9
Connecticut	60	24	6.8	13	6.3	2.7	66	42	14	65	23	6.1
Delaware	57	23	6.2	11	5.6	2.5	63	41	14	61	22	5.3
District of Columbia	68	34	10	13	6.0	2.5	74	49	15	71	33	9.2
Florida	53	21	6.0	12	5.6	2.8	58	34	11	57	21	5.6
Georgia	49	21	6.2	11	5.4	2.3	54	32	12	53	21	5.7
Hawaii	50	24	6.8	11	5.9	2.5	59	42	13	52	24	6.3
Idaho	47	20	6.7	11	6.1	3.5	50.	33	12	52	20	6.1
Illinois	56	26	6.2	11	5.5	2.3	61	41	14	60	26	5.5
Indiana	51	22	6.7	11	6.3	3.0	62	39	13	54	21	6.0
Iowa	56	25	6.2	11	6.4	2.6	69	47	14	59	24	5.3
Kansas	54	24	7.4	11.2	6.5	2.8	61	40	14	58	21	6.8
Kentucky	42	20	5.5	9.0	5.1	2.4	55	34	12	44	19	4.8
Louisiana	49	24	6.0	12	6.8	2.6	56	34	10	53	24	5.7

(Continued)

Table 10-4. (Continued)

State	Age Group, Years 12+ Past Month Use	12+ Past Month Binge	12+ Past Year AUD	12 to 17 Past Month Use	12 to 17 Past Month Binge	12 to 17 Past Year AUD	18 to 25 Past Month Use	18 to 25 Past Month Binge	18 to 25 Past Month AUD	26+ Past Month Use	26+ Past Month Binge	26+ Past Year AUD
Maine	59	23	5.7	12	6.8	2.7	66	43	13	63	22	4.9
Maryland	58	23	6.7	12	6.2	2.9	63	35	12	63	22	6.3
Massachusetts	62	24	6.7	13	7.0	3.0	70	44	14	66	23	5.7
Michigan	54	25	6.1	12	6.1	2.4	63	42	13	58	24	5.4
Minnesota	59	24	6.3	11	5.1	2.4	65	42	13	64	23	5.6
Mississippi	42	20	5.8	9.8	4.9	2.3	53	31	10	44	20	5.5
Missouri	51	25	6.4	11	6.7	2.7	6	41	13	54	25	5.7
Montana	58	24	7.6	11	6.5	3.5	65	43	16	63	23	6.8
Nebraska	57	24	7.5	10	6.3	2.8	65	43	16	62	23	6.6
Nevada	55	24	6.8	14	6.6	3.1	58	37	12	59	24	6.3
New Hampshire	64	25	7.6	64	7.4	3.6	71	46	17	69	23	6.5
New Jersey	57	23	6.5	14	8.0	3.3	61	38	12	61	22	6.0
New Mexico	48	24	6.9	9.7	6.1	2.6	56	37	13	52	24	6.4
New York	56	24	6.6	13	6.7	2.7	61	38	12	60	23	6.1
North Carolina	47	20	6.1	10	5.6	2.5	55	33	12	50	20	5.6
North Dakota	59	28	7.7	11	7.0	3.5	70	49	15	62	26	6.7
Ohio	54	25	6.7	11	6.3	2.7	62	41	13	58	25	61
Oklahoma	49	24	6.4	11	6.0	2.1	59	37	11	52	24	6.0
Oregon	57	22	7.0	13	7.4	3.4	63	40	13	61	21	6.3
Pennsylvania	57	24	6.6	13	6.8	2.7	64	43	14	61	23	5.9
Rhode Island	58	25	7.7	13	5.8	2.9	65	43	16	61	24	6.6

(Continued)

Table 10-4. (Continued)

| | Age Group, Years | | | | | | | | | | | |
| | 12+ | | | 12 to 17 | | | 18 to 25 | | | 26+ | | |
State	Past Month Use	Past Month Binge	Past Year AUD	Past Month Use	Past Month Binge	Past Year AUD	Past Month Use	Past Month Binge	Past Year AUD	Past Month Use	Past Month Binge	Past Year AUD
South Carolina	48	22	5.9	9.6	5.4	2.6	58	36	11	51	21	5.5
South Dakota	55	26	7.6	9.3	6.4	3.0	64	45	15	59	25	6.8
Tennessee	43	18	5.4	9.4	5.23	2.5	53	31	11	45	17	4.7
Texas	47	22	6.5	11	5.8	2.8	56	34	12	51	22	6.1
Utah	32	16	5.4	6.8	5.2	2.5	37	26	11	35	15	4.6
Vermont	61	23	7.2	14	7.4	3.6	71	47	15	64	21	6.2
Virginia	53	23	7.1	11	5.7	2.8	62	41	15	56	22	6.2
Washington	54	20	6.7	10	5.7	2.9	59	36	13	58	20	6.0
West Virginia	39	19	6.3	9.7	6.3	3.4	53	37	12	39	18	5.8
Wisconsin	63	30	7.8	14	7.1	3.9	69	50	16	67	29	6.8
Wyoming	62	25	7.5	11	7.4	3.5	63	43	14	59	24	6.9

Source: Data from SAMHSA (2016b).

Note: AUD=alcohol use disorder. Estimates are based on a survey-weighted hierarchical Bayes estimation approach. Binge alcohol use is defined as drinking five or more drinks on the same occasion (i.e., at the same time or within a couple of hours of each other) on at least 1 day in the past 30 days; dependence and abuse are based on Diagnostic and Statistical Manual of Mental Disorders, Fourth Edition, definitions.

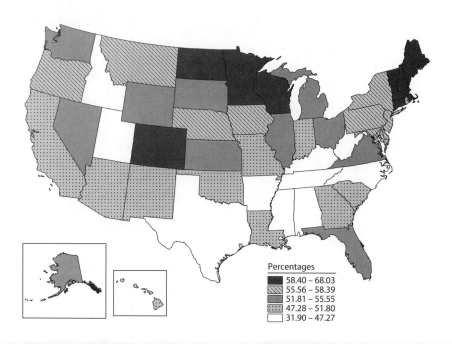

Source: Reprinted from SAMHSA (2014).

Figure 10-2. Alcohol Use in the Past Month among Individuals Aged 12 Years or Older, by State: Percentages, Annual Averages Based on 2013 and 2014 National Survey on Drug Use and Health

According to National Survey on Drug Use and Health, binge alcohol use is defined as drinking five or more drinks on the same occasion for men, and four or more drinks on the same occasion for women on at least 1 day in the 30 days before the survey. Nationally, 22.9% of all persons aged 12 years or older reported binge alcohol use in 2013 to 2014 (Table 10-4). For that same period, the past-month rate of binge use ranged from 15.9% in Utah to 34.0% in the District of Columbia (SAMHSA 2016b). In addition, 7.7% of the population aged 12 years or older met criteria for alcohol use disorder in the past year with the rate among those aged 18 to 25 years being highest (12.6%). New Hampshire had the highest rate (17.2%) and Louisiana had the lowest rate (10.1%) of alcohol use disorder (SAMHSA 2016b).

Another useful resource for information on alcohol consumption in the United States is Chronic Disease Indicators, a collaborative effort of the Council of State and Territorial Epidemiologists, the National Association of Chronic Disease Directors, and the National Center for Chronic Disease

Prevention and Health Promotion at the CDC, which allows public health officials in states and territories to uniformly define, collect, and report chronic disease data that are important to public health practice (Pelletier et al. 2005; CDC 2004b). This cross-cutting set of 90 indicators is divided into seven categories, one of which is tobacco and alcohol use. Included in this category are the following alcohol items:

- Alcohol use among youths.
- Binge drinking among youths.
- Binge drinking among adults aged 18 years and older.
- Binge drinking among women of childbearing age.
- Heavy drinking among adult women aged 18 years and older.
- Heavy drinking among adult men aged 18 years and older.
- Mortality from chronic liver disease.

Data for the indicators are derived from nine sources. The CDC website (http://www.cdc.gov/nccdphp/cdi) is interactive and allows comparisons among states on the different categories of indicators. The website also serves as a gateway with hyperlinks to additional information and survey information.

Time Trends

Beginning in 1934, following Prohibition, per capita alcohol consumption generally increased (excluding fluctuations during and immediately following World War II), reaching a peak of 2.76 gallons of ethanol in 1980 and 1981, and declining during the remainder of the 1980s. After a slight increase in 1990, per capita alcohol consumption decreased slightly from 1991 to 1998. From 1999 to 2005, per capital alcohol consumption has gradually increased reaching 2.24 gallons of ethanol in 2005 (Lakins et al. 2007). Alcohol consumption has continued to increase from 2.24 gallons in 2005 to 2.34 gallons in 2015 (Haughwout et al. 2015).

Beer consumption has remained relatively stable over the past 40 years, peaking in 1981 and gradually decreasing since that time (Lakins et al. 2007). In 2005, beer comprised approximately 53% of the per capita alcohol consumption from all alcoholic beverages combined. Wine consumption increased throughout the 1980s, peaked in 1986, and then decreased until 1996. Since then, wine consumption has gradually increased reaching 1.36 gallons of ethanol per capita in 2005, the same level as in 1988. In 2005, wine represented about 16% of the per capita alcohol consumption from all alcoholic beverages (Lakins et al. 2007). According to the National Institute on Alcohol Abuse and Alcoholism, per capita consumption of ethanol from all alcoholic beverages combined in 2014 was 2.32 gallons, representing a 0.4% decrease from 2.33 gallons in 2013 (Haughwout et al. 2016). In addition, the overall per capita consumption of alcohol by census region between 2013 and 2014 revealed a decrease of 0.4% in the Northeast and West, no change in the Midwest, and 0.9% decrease in the South (Haughwout et al. 2016; Figure 10-3).

Long-term time trends in the prevalence of alcohol use disorder in the United States are difficult to assess. Since the 1971, large-scale U.S. and international surveys have produced a range of rates of the prevalence of current and lifetime of what is now known as alcohol use disorder utilizing a range of diagnostic criteria (*DSM-III, DSM-IIIR, DSM-IV, DSM-5*). Given the range of rates over time, location, and diagnostic criteria, it is very difficult to differentiate true time trends from methodological variations.

The National Longitudinal Alcohol Epidemiologic Survey, the National Epidemiologic Survey on Alcohol and Related Conditions, and the National Survey on Drug Use and Health are three large national surveys that serve as

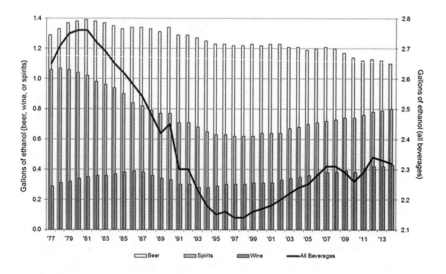

Source: Reprinted from Haughwout (2016).

Figure 10-3. Gallons of Beer, Spirits, Wine, and All Beverages, 1977 to 2014

the main sources of data on alcohol use in the United States. The Longitudinal Alcohol Epidemiologic Survey was conducted during 1991 and 1992, and the first wave of the National Epidemiologic Survey on Alcohol and Related Conditions was conducted during 2001 and 2002. Because of the timing of the surveys, it is possible to present accurate trends in the prevalence of alcohol use disorder across these years. During the 10 years between these surveys, the prevalence of alcohol use disorders in the general population declined from 4.4% to 3.8%. Notably, the prevalence of alcohol use disorders decreased among men while remaining stable among women, decreased among whites and Hispanics, and increased among young black and Hispanic men and young Asian women (NIAAA 2006a; NIAAA 2006b; Grant et al. 2004). In 2014, the National Survey on Drug Use and Health found the prevalence of alcohol use disorder among people aged 12 years or older to be 6.4% (Hedden et al. 2015). All three surveys used *DSM-IV* diagnostic criteria (Grant et al. 2015).

With the Alcohol Related Disease Impact System, recently revised by the CDC, it is now possible to calculate the alcohol-attributable deaths in the United States or in individual states over time. These estimates are obtained by multiplying the number of deaths from a particular alcohol-related condition by its alcohol-attributable fraction. Certain conditions (e.g., alcoholic cirrhosis of the liver) are, by definition, 100% alcohol-attributable. For the majority of the chronic conditions profiled in this system, alcohol-attributable fractions are obtained by using relative risk estimates from meta-analyses and prevalence data on alcohol use from the state-based telephone surveys. For all ages, between 2006 and 2010, there were an estimated 87,798 alcohol-attributable deaths from both acute and chronic causes, including 62,104 male and 25,693 female deaths (CDC 2013).

In 1999, the National Center for Health Statistics reported 19,469 "alcohol-induced" deaths (Kung et al. 2008). The category "alcohol-induced" includes not only deaths from dependent and nondependent use of alcohol, but also accidental poisoning by alcohol, alcoholic polyneuropathy, alcoholic liver disease, and others. Alcohol-induced causes exclude accidents, homicides, and other causes that could be indirectly related to alcohol use. Among these exclusions are alcohol-related motor vehicle crashes—a significant cause of death. In 2013, 31% of total traffic fatalities can be attributed to a driver with a BAC of 0.08% or higher, which amounts to 10,076 deaths in that year alone (NHTSA 2014). From 1999 to 2013, there has been a decrease in the number of deaths attributable to alcohol-related motor vehicle crashes. However, despite this decline, drinking and driving still accounted for roughly 30% of all driving fatalities in 2013 (NHTSA 2014).

Causes

Modifiable Risk Factors

Aspects of culture and environment are potentially points of intervention for the reduction of alcohol-related harms. The influence of alcohol advertising on young people is a subject of much debate. Recent reviews of the literature indicate that, although many ecological studies suggested little effect, longitudinal studies enrolling individual subjects show clear links between advertising and behavior (Hastings et al. 2005; Anderson et al. 2009). Although ecological designs complicate causal attribution, their results potentially imply that access to alcohol, and local and peer drinking norms, also may be significant contributors to the development of problem alcohol use. Studies of alcohol outlet density indicate a greater prevalence of use disorders in neighborhoods with increased alcohol availability (Campbell et al. 2009; Pearson et al. 2014; Murphy et al. 2014; Paschall et al. 2012). These and related data have been deemed compelling enough by the Task Force on Community Preventive Services to prompt their formal recommendation of limiting outlet density as an intervention to reduce alcohol-related harms (TFCPS 2009).

Age of onset of drinking is a modifiable risk factor in that early onset of drinking poses an increased risk for lifetime alcohol-related problems. Almost half (46%) of individuals who develop symptoms of *DSM-IV*–defined alcohol dependence had started drinking before the age of 16 years (Hingson et al. 2006). Parent and other adult alcohol use appears to influence the likelihood of heavy drinking in adolescence (Paschall et al. 2012; Haugland et al. 2013; Mares et al. 2013), and as a result, an adolescent's choice between drinking and non-drinking peer groups can be correlated with home drinking environment (Wang et al. 2015).

Young adolescents with higher communal goals appear to be at greater risk in an alcohol-using peer group. For those with lower goals in terms of wide social acceptance, the perception of acceptability of alcohol use appears to be associated with acceptance into a group of peers prone to experience social anxiety, circumvention, or shyness, which they may choose to manage with alcohol (Meisel and Colder 2015).

Population-Attributable Risk

Estimates of relative risk of adverse health outcomes by degrees of alcohol misuse are available. For example, estimates of fatal motor vehicle crash by BAC have been produced (Zador et al. 2000). Examining relative risk across six age and sex groups, at a BAC of 0.035%, the relative risk ranged from 2.6 to 4.6; at a BAC of 0.065%, from 5.8 to 17.3; at a BAC of 0.09%, from 11.4 to 52; at a BAC of 1.125%, from 29.3 to 240.9; and at a BAC of 0.220%, from 382 to 15,560. Compared with other drivers, drivers aged 16 to 20 years had an increased relative risk of fatal crashes with no alcohol involvement. Among these young drivers, relative risk increased substantially even at BACs less than 0.02%. The relative risk curve increased fastest with increasing BAC among male drivers aged 16 to 20 years (Zador et al. 2000).

Attributable risk estimates for hypertension associated with heavy drinking in the United States have been published (NIAAA 2010). Just over 10% of the population that had met criteria for being heavier drinkers (an average of more than one drink per day for women and two drinks per day for men) three years before they were hypertensive. Breast cancer risk is also increased with heavier drinking, increasing risk up to 6.1% in white women who drink two or more drinks daily (Clarke et al. 2006).

Psychosocial and environmental risk factors for alcohol use among the general population are shown in Table 10-5. Most studies of these risk factors focus on particular alcohol-related outcomes such as violence or traffic fatalities.

Prevention and Control

Prevention

Prevention measures aim to reduce negative alcohol-related consequences through multiple strategies employed at the individual and community level. Such measures include policies regulating alcohol-related behavior on the one hand and community and educational interventions seeking to influence drinking behavior on the other. Most programs are focused on immediate goals, such as decreasing binge drinking among youths or preventing driving after drinking. If successful, however, these programs could also affect longer-term health consequences such as problem alcohol use, liver disease, alcohol use disorder, and mortality. Research has demonstrated that rates of alcohol

Table 10-5. Environmental Risk Factors for Increased Alcohol Consumption

Factor	Examples
Home drinking environment	• Parent use of alcohol
	• Family traditions
Local policies regulating alcohol behavior	• Open intoxicants laws
	• Drunk-driving penalties
Level of enforcement of local police regulating alcohol behavior	• Level of police presence at events
	• Drunk-driving checkpoints
Community or cultural drinking norms or customs	• Drinking at sporting events
	• Drinking at family meals
Price of alcohol in retail settings	• Sales
	• Discount liquor outlets
Outlet density of retail outlets that sell alcohol	• How far apart the stores are
Happy hours and bar or restaurant drink specials	• Buckets of beer
	• Boots of beer
Outlet density of bars and restaurants	• How far apart the bars or restaurants are
Advertising	• Sales advertised in newspapers
	• Drink specials advertised on sandwich boards

Source: Based on Fone et al. (2003).

consumption, intoxication, and driving after drinking rates are sensitive to the price of alcoholic beverages. Underage individuals and young adults are particularly affected by the cost of alcohol. Studies show that increases in price significantly reduce the number of drinks consumed by this population. Happy hours, drinking contests, "all-you-can-drink" specials, and other promotions encourage overconsumption by reducing prices, a potent incentive to drinking large amounts of alcohol in short time periods. As of January 1, 2015, 16 states had ordinances either prohibiting or restricting "happy hour" types of promotions. In states where these ordinances are not in place, communities may pass local ordinances prohibiting or restricting these practices (APIS 2015), but almost no literature exists on enforcement and adjudication of these laws.

Nearly every state prohibits sales and service of alcohol to obviously intoxicated people (NHTSA 2005). Again, little research is available to determine how these laws are enforced, the extent to which they are complied with, and the impact enforcement and compliance might have on public health outcomes (NHTSA 2005). Multiple examples of prevention efforts are included later in this chapter in the section Examples of Public Health Interventions.

Screening

Preventive health services include early intervention programs that focus on identifying people who are drinking in unhealthy ways or are beginning to experience adverse consequences of their alcohol use. Screening all patients for alcohol problems, particularly in primary health care settings, is a medical necessity. The U.S. Preventive Services Task Force recommends routine screening of adults for alcohol misuse in the primary care setting as well as brief counseling interventions for individuals with alcohol misuse (USPSTF 2004). Such brief counseling has been shown to reduce alcohol consumption and alcohol-related harms (USPSTF 2004).

Structured interviews and self-report instruments are useful for screening. Both are rapid, inexpensive, noninvasive, and relatively accurate tools. A number of screening instruments are available. A specific screening instrument should be selected on the basis of staff experience and training, available testing time, and characteristics of the patient population.

The CAGE questionnaire derives its name from a mnemonic for attempts to cut down on drinking, annoyance with criticisms about drinking, guilt about drinking, and using alcohol as an eye-opener (APA 2002). The responses to each question are scored with a 1 or a 0, the higher the score, the more clinically significant the response becomes (APA 2002). CAGE is an internationally used assessment instrument for identifying alcoholism. It is particularly popular with primary care providers. CAGE has been translated into several languages. The CAGE questions can be used in the clinical setting with informal phrasing. It has been demonstrated that they are most effective when used as part of a general health history and should not be preceded by questions about how much or how frequently the patient drinks (Steinweg and Worth 1993). It is popular for screening in the primary care setting because it is short, simple, easy to remember, and has been proven effective for detecting a range of alcohol problems (NIAAA 2005b). The CAGE questionnaire can be self-administered or asked by a clinician; it poses four overt yes–no questions. Because it takes less than a minute to administer, the CAGE can be woven into a standard, brief clinical history.

A major limitation of the CAGE, however, is that it does not address current consumption levels or consequences. The Alcohol Use Disorders Identification Test (Table 10-6) is a 10-question instrument that includes questions about the current quantity and frequency of alcohol use, as well as current binge drinking, symptoms of alcohol use disorder, and alcohol-related problems (Bohn et al. 1995). The Alcohol Use Disorders Identification Tool, which was developed by the World Health Organization, takes about five minutes to complete, has been tested internationally in primary care settings, and found to be highly valid and reliable (NIAAA 2005a; Babor et al. 2001). It is especially useful in screening women and minorities. It also shows promise in screening adolescents and young adults. Even more efficient, the first three questions of the Alcohol Use Disorders Identification Tool have been validated as an initial screen and termed the AUDIT-C.

The National Institute on Alcohol Abuse and Alcoholism, with guidance from physicians, nurses, advanced practice nurses, physician assistants, and clinical researchers, has produced an updated edition of *Helping Patients Who Drink Too Much: A Clinician's Guide* (NIAAA 2005a). This guide is intended for primary care and mental health clinicians and features guidelines on screening and brief intervention. The guide is available in English and Spanish and comes with a variety of supporting materials including downloadable versions of the Alcohol Use Disorders Identification Tool in both English and Spanish, preformatted progress notes and templates, training materials, and patient education materials. The guide and related materials are available at https://www.niaaa.nih.gov/guide.

Clinical laboratory tests can be used in conjunction with self-report instruments to enhance objectivity. Several clinical laboratory tests are available to assist in the detection of alcohol use, misuse, and its consequences, such as alcoholic hepatitis, anemia, and thrombocytopenia. Serum concentrations of the transaminase enzymes produced by the liver are frequently used in the medical setting. These include alanine aminotransferase, aspartate aminotransferase, and gamma-glutamyl transpeptidase. Elevations of these enzymes are sensitive for alcohol-related liver injury, but not particularly specific, because all types of liver damage and a wide variety of diseases can cause elevated serum activity of these enzymes. Results may be more discriminating when interpreted in conjunction with routine hematological tests, such as mean corpuscular volume and red cell distribution width. Both mean corpuscular volume, an index of red blood cell volume, and red cell distribution width, an index of variability of red blood cell size, are standard components of routine complete blood count tests and both increase with excessive alcohol intake over time because of the adverse nutritional and bone marrow–toxic effects of regular heavy alcohol consumption.

Table 10-6. Alcohol Use Disorder Identification Test (AUDIT)

Question	0	1	2	3	4
1. How often do you have a drink containing alcohol?[a]	Never	Monthly or less	Two to four times a month	Two to three times a week	Four or more times a week
2. How many drinks containing alcohol do you have on a typical day when you are drinking?[a]	One or two	Three or four	Five or six	Seven to nine	Ten or more
3. How often do you have five or more drinks on one occasion?[a]	Never	Less than monthly	Monthly	Weekly	Daily or almost daily
4. How often during the last year have you found that you were not able to stop drinking once you had started?	Never	Less than monthly	Monthly	Weekly	Daily or almost daily
5. How often during the last year have you failed to do what was normally expected of you because of drinking?	Never	Less than monthly	Monthly	Weekly	Daily or almost daily
6. How often during the last year have you needed a first drink in the morning to get yourself going after a heavy drinking session?	Never	Less than monthly	Monthly	Weekly	Daily or almost daily
7. How often during the last year have you had a feeling of guilt or remorse after drinking?	Never	Less than monthly	Monthly	Weekly	Daily or almost daily
8. How often during the last year have you been unable to remember what happened the night before because of your drinking?	Never	Less than monthly	Monthly	Weekly	Daily or almost daily
9. Have you or someone else been injured because of your drinking?	No		Yes, but not in the last year		Yes, during the last year
10. Has a relative, friend, doctor, or other health care worker been concerned about your drinking or suggested you cut down?	No		Yes, but not in the last year		Yes, during the last year

TOTAL AUDIT SCORE:

AUDIT scores between 8 and 15 are most appropriate for simple advice focused on the reduction of hazardous drinking. Scores between 16 and 19 suggest brief counseling and continued monitoring. Scores > 20 warrant further diagnostic evaluation for alcohol use disorder.

Source: Based on AUDIT-C, which is available for use in the public domain at http://www.integration.samhsa.gov/images/res/tool_auditc.pdf.

Note: To reflect drink serving sizes in the United States (14 grams of pure alcohol), the number of drinks in question three was changed from six to five. The first 3 questions of the AUDIT comprise the AUDIT-C, a 3-item alcohol screen scored on a scale of 0 to 12. A positive score for identifying alcohol misuse or active alcohol use disorders is ≥ 4 in men and ≥ 3 in women.

[a]

In recent years, carbohydrate-deficient transferrin has emerged as a bio-marker of sustained heavy alcohol consumption. Compared to BAC, which is reflective of recent drinking only (within the past 12 hours), elevated blood carbohydrate-deficient transferrin reflects sustained heavy alcohol use (more than five drinks per day for at least two weeks; Maenhout et al. 2012). However, recent evidence suggests that carbohydrate-deficient transferrin may have limited sensitivity in obese individuals, women, and those with liver disease (Fagan et al. 2014). Some studies have examined the usefulness of combining the carbohydrate-deficient transferrin and gamma-glutamyl transpeptidase tests, finding that, at least in men, using both tests is more precise than using either marker alone (Hietala et al. 2006). Alcohol metabolites can be detected in urine to provide additional objective information regarding recent alcohol use. There are numerous assays in development to quantify each of the differ-ent metabolites, including ethyl sulfate, phosphatidylethanol, fatty acid ethyl esters, and ethyl glucuronide. Ethyl glucuronide is used most often in the med-ical setting because this metabolite may be detectable for up to 80 hours after a single episode of drinking.

Treatment

Unlike traditional specialty treatments that are designed for people who have alcohol use disorder, brief interventions (short one-on-one counseling sessions) are very effective for people who drink in ways that are harmful or abusive. Brief interventions generally aim to moderate a person's drinking to sensible levels and to eliminate harmful drinking practices including binge drinking (NIAAA 2005c). Brief interventions differ from most other treatments for alcohol problems because they are generally restricted to four or fewer sessions; are usually performed in a treatment setting not specific for alcohol use disorder, typically a primary care context; and are commonly performed by personnel who have not specialized in addiction treatment. Brief interventions are inex-pensive, can readily be incorporated into many settings, and are reasonably effective. Brief interventions in no way preclude subsequent application of more intensive intervention. People who do not respond well can be referred for further treatment.

Despite evidence that brief interventions are useful and effective in the primary care setting, they are not yet a routine practice. One survey of pri-mary care physicians found that, although most (88%) reported asking their patients about alcohol use, only 13% used standard screening instruments. A survey of primary care patients revealed that more than half said that their physician did nothing about their substance abuse and nearly as many said their physician never diagnosed their condition (NIAAA 2005c). New technology such as computerized interventions may offer an effective alternate means of implementing brief interventions, particularly in settings in which time constraints or lack of resources or training in intervention techniques are factors (NIAAA 2005c).

Alcohol use disorder is a complex disorder, not a single straightforward entity. Clinicians and researchers have long recognized the heterogeneity of individuals with alcohol use disorder. To improve clinical management and to understand the complexity of genetic and environmental influences on the disorder, efforts have been made to develop alcohol use disorder subtypes (Moss et al. 2010). Researchers with NIAAA, who recently analyzed the large national sample of individuals with alcohol dependence, but now known as alcohol use disorder, available in national surveys, reported five distinct subtypes of the disease: young adult, young antisocial, functional, intermediate familial, and chronic severe subtype (Moss et al. 2010). Because these data are derived from the general population rather than from individuals with alcohol use disorder in treatment, they provide a broader and more accurate picture of the true heterogeneity of alcohol use disorder in the general population (Moss et al. 2010).

A number of treatments is available within the specialist treatment system. In many cases, the beginning phase is detoxification, the set of interventions aimed at managing acute intoxication and alcohol withdrawal. Abstinence from alcohol may lead to the alcohol withdrawal syndrome, the cluster of symptoms observed in people who stop drinking alcohol following continuous heavy consumption. Milder manifestations of alcohol withdrawal include tremulousness, seizures, and hallucinations, typically occurring within 6 to 48 hours after the last drink. Much more serious is delirium tremens, which includes profound confusion, hallucinations, and severe autonomic nervous system overactivity, typically beginning 48 to 96 hours after the last drink (Table 10-7).

Many withdrawal symptoms appear to result in part from overactivity of the sympathetic nervous system. As such, the preferred medications are benzodiazepines, which help to dampen the racing sympathetic nervous system while also preventing seizures. There is also some support for a role for anticonvulsant medications in this setting (Hammond et al. 2015). Ongoing research indicates that repeated, untreated alcohol withdrawal episodes may increase the risk of

Table 10-7. Alcohol Withdrawal Signs and Physical Symptoms

Level	Onset[a]	Symptoms	Physical Signs
Mild	Early	• Anxiety • Sleep disturbances • Vivid dreams • Anorexia • Nausea • Headache	• Tachycardia (fast heart rate) • Hypertension (elevated blood pressure) • Hyperactive reflexes • Sweating • Hyperthermia • Tremor
Mild–moderate	Early	Perceptual disturbances, including • Visual (e.g., shadows) • Auditory (e.g., "buzzing or clicking") • Tactile (e.g., "pins and needles")	Hallucinations • Visual (e.g., seeing people or animals) • Auditory (e.g., hearing noncommanding voices) • Formication (e.g., feeling of bugs crawling on them)
Seizures	Within 8 to 24 hours	Risk is increased with • History of any type of seizure • Concomitant use of benzodiazepines before withdrawal	Kindling effect (the more times someone experiences withdrawal, the more likely they are to have seizures)
Delirium tremens	Within 72 to 96 hours	Confusion and disorientation (e.g., a person may think the hospital is his or her home and that the hospital staff are people they actually know as acquaintances)	• Tachycardia • Tremor • Diaphoresis (sweating) • Fever • Sometimes severe agitation • Sometimes low-level psychomotor activity

[a] The timing of onset may vary and progression of symptoms and signs is not always linear from mild to moderate to seizures to delirium tremens; they may go directly to any stage mentioned in the table.

seizures and other complications during detoxification (NIAAA 1997). Third-party payers sometimes prefer to manage payment for detoxification separately from the longer term, definitive, behavioral treatment for alcohol use disorder. This unbundling of services may result in fragmentation of care. In addition, reimbursement for detoxification may not cover counseling, leading to frequent inadequate treatment (SAMHSA 1997).

No single definition of treatment exists and no standard terminology describes the different dimensions and elements of treatment. Describing a facility as providing inpatient care or ambulatory services characterizes only one aspect of treatment: the setting. The continuum of treatment settings, from most to least intensive, includes inpatient hospitalization, residential treatment, intensive outpatient treatment, and outpatient treatment. All specialized alcohol treatment programs have three broad goals: (1) reducing alcohol misuse or achieving an alcohol-free life, (2) maximizing multiple aspects of life functioning, and (3) preventing or reducing the frequency and severity of relapse. Within each treatment approach, a variety of treatment services are provided to achieve specific goals (SAMHSA 1997). The emphasis may change, from pharmacological intervention to treat withdrawal to behavioral therapy, mutual-help support, and relapse prevention efforts during the initial care and stabilization phase, and continued Alcoholics Anonymous participation after discharge from formal treatment. The principal elements of most treatment programs include (Table 10-8).

- Pharmacotherapies that discourage alcohol use, suppress withdrawal symptoms, block or diminish cravings, or treat coexisting psychiatric problems.
- Psychosocial or psychological interventions that modify destructive interpersonal feelings, attitudes, and behaviors through individual, group, marital, or family therapy.

Examples of Public Health Interventions

Multiple successful prevention and intervention strategies that could serve as effective components of a public health effort are outlined here. Examples of policy measures relating to alcohol include regulation of the price of beverages, a minimum legal drinking age of 21 years, 0.08% BAC limits for drivers aged 21 years and older, zero-tolerance laws (laws that make it illegal for drivers younger than age 21 years to drive after drinking alcohol, typically setting the BAC at 0.00% to 0.02%), administrative license revocation laws, server liability, warning labels, and limitations on numbers, types, hours of operation, and locations of outlets that sell alcoholic beverages.

Underage youths obtain alcohol from friends, coworkers, parents, siblings, and strangers. Policies that address youth social access to alcohol include beer keg registration, alcohol use restrictions on public property, alcohol restrictions at community events, and social host liability. Underage youths also obtain alcohol from licensed alcohol establishments such as bars, convenience stores, liquor stores, grocery stores, and restaurants. Policies that address reducing

Table 10-8. U.S. Food and Drug Administration–Approved Medications for Abstinence in Alcohol Use Disorder

Medication, Generic (Brand Name)	Method of Action	Contraindications, Cautions, Adverse Events
disulfiram (Antabuse)	Causes aversive symptoms after ingestion of alcohol.	• Drowsiness • Fatigue • Visual symptoms • Liver damage
naltrexone (Revia [oral]; Vivitrol [injectable])	Decreases the rewards or reinforcing effects of alcohol.	• Cannot be using any opioid pain medications • Cannot be used in people with liver disease • Can cause GI upset upon starting it
acamprosate (Campral)	Acts on same neuroreceptors that alcohol does (GABA).	• Patients must be abstinent from alcohol and receive psychosocial treatment • Mild GI upset and itchiness • Rarely worsening depression and suicide completion

Source: Compiled from Jonas et al. (2014); Myrick et al. (2009); Ries et al. (2014).
Note: GABA=gamma-aminobutyric acid; GI=gastrointestinal.

commercial access include compliance checks, administrative penalties, responsible beverage service training, checking age identification, regulations or bans on home delivery of alcohol, minimum age of seller requirements, and alcohol warning posters. Restrictions on alcohol advertising and on alcohol sponsorship can be instituted through local ordinances or state laws, or can be implemented voluntarily by a business, event, or organization (Toomey and Wagenaar 2002).

Maintaining the minimum legal drinking age at 21 years and zero tolerance laws continue to be effective in reducing the proportion of fatal crashes involving young drivers under the influence of alcohol (Voas et al. 2003). As of March, 2016, all states and the District of Columbia had enacted laws making it illegal to operate a motor vehicle with a BAC of 0.08% or greater for motor vehicle drivers aged 21 years and older to further reduce alcohol-related traffic crashes (GHSA 2016). A recent meta-analysis of 0.08% BAC laws in 19 jurisdictions showed a statistically significant decline of 14.8% in the rate of drinking drivers in fatal crashes after the 0.08% law was introduced. The reductions were greater in states that also had an administrative license suspension or revocation law and implemented frequent sobriety checkpoints (Tippetts et al. 2005). Extensive information on other alcohol policies can be found at the Alcohol Policy Information System at http://www.alcoholpolicy.niaaa.nih.gov.

The Task Force on Community Preventive Services produces *The Community Guide*, which provides evidence-based recommendations for programs and policies to promote population health. Interventions directed to the general population recommended in *The Community Guide* include outlet density and zoning restrictions. Interventions directed to underage drinkers include enhanced enforcement of laws prohibiting the sale of alcohol to minors (CPSTF 2016).

Many successful community interventions have been implemented. One example is the Communities Mobilizing for Change on Alcohol, a community organizing program designed to reduce teen (13–20 years of age) access to alcohol by changing community policies and practices. This program seeks both to limit youth access to alcohol and to communicate a clear message to the community that underage drinking is inappropriate and unacceptable. The program involves community members in seeking and achieving changes in local public policies and the practices of community institutions that can affect youth access to alcohol. The interventions are based on established research that has demonstrated the importance of the social and policy environment in facilitating or impeding drinking among youths.

The Communities Mobilizing for Change on Alcohol was first implemented and evaluated in a fully randomized 5-year trial across 15 U.S. communities. Since that initial trial in the early 1990s, numerous communities in the United States, Sweden, and other countries have implemented interventions based closely on this model (Wagenaar et al. 2000a; Wagenaar et al. 2000b). Materials, training, and resources are available (see http://nrepp.samhsa.gov).

Education of primary health care providers is an evolving public health intervention. Tobacco, alcohol, and other drug use must become a standard part of every medical history. Health care providers for population subgroups at high risk should be made more aware of the need for routine use of alcohol misuse screening and intervention. Hospitalized trauma patients represent one such population. The American Medical Association and the American Society of Addiction Medicine recommend that BACs be ascertained in all such patients and, when positive, that individuals be evaluated and treated for their alcohol problems as well as the traumatic injury.

Public health officials strengthen and magnify their impact in addressing alcohol problems when they work in collaboration with other health care professionals, designated public officials, and community groups dedicated to the prevention and treatment of alcohol use disorder. All too often, public health practitioners in chronic disease control and alcohol and drug use disorder professionals are located in different state or local agencies and may not even know each other. Appropriate communication and care coordination in primary care and public health settings (and, hence, reduction of alcohol-related harms) is complicated by federal (Confidentiality of Alcohol and Drug Abuse Patient Records 1987) and state statutes, which limit such communication and these practices. Tension between patient confidentiality and improving population health are factors that contribute to the fragmentation in the communication.

Areas of Future Research and Demonstration

Research on alcohol risk and use disorder vulnerabilities (genetic and environmental) continues to flourish. The neural basis of alcohol use disorder is also being clarified, thanks in part to advanced imaging techniques, such as functional magnetic resonance imaging. Research showing that drinking is influenced by multiple neurotransmitter systems, neuromodulators, hormones, and intracellular networks points to a number of potential target sites for pharmacotherapy. Treatment research continues to seek effective pharmacotherapies and behavioral interventions, and to develop more effective means of their dissemination and implementation in general medical settings, such as primary care and emergency departments.

Progress in the genetics of alcoholism has been explosive, and may serve as a guide in the future to which individuals might benefit most from which categories of pharmacotherapy. As genes are identified and their functions explicated, not only will we be in a better position to identify individuals at increased genetic risk, but we will also be in a better position to clarify environmental factors that further increase risk or that confer protection. Important advances are being made in our understanding of individual vulnerabilities to alcohol-related complications. We are also gaining a much clearer understanding of alcohol's protective effects against coronary artery disease. Results of this research will more fully inform public health policymakers and practitioners. Issues under investigation of particular interest to public health professionals include

- Neurobiological mechanisms explaining the heritability of and vulnerability to alcohol use disorders.
- Potential for mobile technology–based interventions to support behavior change and recovery.
- The differential impact that alcohol use disorders have upon minority groups in terms of morbidity and mortality.

- The gene–environment interplay explaining age of first drink, age of first intoxication, age of onset of regular drinking, and contribution to the development of alcohol use disorder.
- New pharmacotherapies to assist in recovery from alcohol use disorders.
- Neural mechanisms of addiction and recovery.
- Developmental science related to brain reward circuits and the risk for adolescent heavy drinking, related complications, and progression to alcohol use disorder.
- Constitutional vulnerabilities to the development of alcohol-related liver disease.
- Development and optimization of brief cognitive interventions to prevent progression of alcohol misuse to more severely disordered drinking.
- Development of valid electronic alcohol risk screening modalities.
- Development of further primary care–based interventions for alcohol use disorders.
- Elucidating the impact of heavy alcohol consumption on the immune system.
- Developing models to facilitate recovery in the setting of alcohol use disorders and comorbid psychiatric conditions, such as posttraumatic stress disorder, bipolar spectrum disorders, and in the setting of sexual victimization and domestic violence.
- Clarification of neighborhood factors contributing to unhealthy alcohol consumption patterns.
- Wearable, noninvasive technologies for alcohol monitoring.
- Clarification of mechanisms of and vulnerability to fetal alcohol spectrum disorders.

Resources

Recent Surveillance Reports

Chen CM, Yi H. *Trends in Alcohol-Related Morbidity Among Community Hospital Discharges, United States, 2000–2012.* Bethesda, MD: National Institute on Alcohol Abuse and Alcoholism, National Institutes of Health; 2014. Surveillance Report no. 99. Available at: http://pubs.niaaa.nih.gov/publications/surveillance.htm.

Chen CM, Yi H, Faden VB. *Trends in Underage Drinking in the United States, 1991–2013.* Bethesda, MD: National Institute on Alcohol Abuse and Alcoholism, National Institutes of Health; 2015. Surveillance Report no. 101. Available at: http://pubs.niaaa.nih.gov/publications/surveillance.htm.

Haughwout SP, Lavalle RA, Castle IP. *Apparent Per Capita Alcohol Consumption: National, State, and Regional Trends, 1977–2014.* Bethesda, MD: National Institute on Alcohol Abuse and Alcoholism, National Institutes of Health; 2016. Surveillance Report no. 104. Available at: http://pubs.niaaa.nih.gov/publications/surveillance.htm.

Useful Websites

National Institute on Alcohol Abuse and Alcoholism (NIAAA), National Institutes of Health, http://www.niaaa.nih.gov

NIAAA-sponsored websites (accessible through the NIAAA website or at the following URLs):

- The Coolspot, http://www.thecoolspot.gov
- National Epidemiologic Survey on Alcohol and Related Conditions, https://www.niaaa.nih.gov/research/nesarc-iii
- College Drinking Prevention, http://www.collegedrinkingprevention.gov
- Alcohol Policy Information System, http://www.alcoholpolicy.niaaa.nih.gov

Substance Abuse and Mental Health Services Administration (SAMHSA), http://www.samhsa.gov

Links to resources on the SAMHSA website:

- Preventing and reducing underage drinking, http://www.samhsa.gov/underage-drinking
- Statistics, reports, and data from all of the SAMHSA major national databases, including National Survey on Drug Use and Health, https://nsduhweb.rti.org/respweb/homepage.cfm
- National Registry of Evidence-Based Programs and Practices, http://www.nrepp.samhsa.gov
- Screening, Brief Intervention, Referral, and Treatment, http://www.samhsa.gov/sbirt
- SAMHSA's Substance Abuse Treatment Facility Locator, https://findtreatment.samhsa.gov

The referral helpline run by SAMHSA's Center for Substance Abuse Treatment: 1-800-662-HELP.

Centers for Disease Control and Prevention, http://www.cdc.gov

- Chronic Disease Indicators, http://www.cdc.gov/nccdphp/cdi
- Behavioral Risk Factor Surveillance System, http://www.cdc.gov/brfss
- National Center for Health Statistics, http://www.cdc.gov/nchs; the NCHS homepage provides a link to an alphabetical list of topics including "alcohol use" (http://

www.cdc.gov/nchs/fastats/alcohol.htm), which provides information on the prevalence of alcohol use, alcohol-induced mortality, and other alcohol information.

Other Resources

American Society of Addiction Medicine, http://www.asam.org

National Association of State Alcohol and Drug Abuse Directors, http://www.nasadad.org

National Council on Alcoholism and Drug Dependence, http://www.ncadd.org

Suggested Reading

Recent issues of *NIAAA Alcohol Alerts* (a twice yearly bulletin that summarizes key findings in an important area of alcohol research). Available at: http://www.arcr.niaaa.nih.gov/arcr/alert.htm

- No. 88: eHealth Technology and What It Means for the Alcohol Field
- No. 87: Measuring the Burden of Alcohol
- No. 86: Epigenetics—A New Frontier for Alcohol Research
- No. 85: The Link between Stress and Alcohol
- No. 84: The Genetics of Alcoholism

Helping Patients Who Drink Too Much: A Clinician's Guide (2005), http://www.niaaa.nih.gov/guide (Continuing Medical Education credits available for physicians)

References

Abbey A. Alcohol-related sexual assault: a common problem among college students. *J Stud Alcohol Suppl.* 2002;(suppl 14):118–128.

Abbey A. Alcohol's role in sexual violence perpetration: theoretical explanations, existing evidence, and future direction. *Drug Alcohol Rev.* 2011;30(5):481–489.

Alcohol Policy Information System (APIS). Alcohol beverages pricing: drink specials. 2015. Available at: http://alcoholpolicy.niaaa.nih.gov/alcohol_beverages_pricing_drink_specials.html. Accessed May 18, 2016.

American Psychiatric Association (APA). *Diagnostic and Statistical Manual of Mental Disorders, Fourth Edition.* Washington, DC: American Psychiatric Association; 1994.

American Psychiatric Association (APA). CAGE Questionnaire. National Institutes of Health. 2002. Available at: http://pubs.niaaa.nih.gov/publications/inscage.htm. Accessed May 18, 2016.

American Psychiatric Association (APA). *Diagnostic and Statistical Manual of Mental Disorders, Fifth Edition.* Arlington, VA: American Psychiatric Publishing; 2013.

Anderson P, de Bruijn A, Angus K, Gordon R, Hastings G. Impact of alcohol advertising and media exposure on adolescent alcohol use: a systematic review of longitudinal studies. *Alcohol Alcohol.* 2009;44(3):229–243.

Anderson RA, Willis BR, Oswald C, Zaneveld LJD. Male reproductive tract sensitivity to ethanol: a critical overview. *Pharmacol Biochem Behav.* 1983;18(suppl 1): 305–310.

Babor TF, Higgins-Biddle J, Saunders J, Monteiro M. *AUDIT: The Alcohol Use Disorders Identification Test Guidelines for Use in Primary Care.* 2nd ed. Geneva, Switzerland: World Health Organization; 2001.

Bellis M, Hughes K, Nicholls J, Sharon S, Gilmore I, Jones L. The alcohol harm paradox: using a national survey to explore how alcohol may disproportionally impact health in deprived individuals. *BMC Public Health.* 2016;16:111.

Bohn MJ, Babor TF, Kranzler HR. The Alcohol Use Disorders Identification Test (AUDIT): validation of a screening instrument for use in medical settings. *J Stud Alcohol.* 1995;56(4):423–432.

Campbell CA, Hahn RA, Elder R, et al. The effectiveness of limiting alcohol outlet density as a means of reducing excessive alcohol consumption and alcohol-related harms. *Am J Prev Med.* 2009;37(6):556–569.

Cederbaum AI. Alcohol metabolism. *Clin Liver Dis.* 2012;16(4):667–685.

Centers for Disease Control and Prevention. Alcohol-attributable deaths and years of potential life lost—United States, 2001. *MMWR Morb Mortal Wkly Rep.* 2004a;53(37): 866–870.

Centers for Disease Control and Prevention (CDC). Indicators for chronic disease surveillance. *MMWR Recomm Rep.* 2004b;53(RR–11):1–6.

Centers for Disease Control and Prevention (CDC). *Alcohol and Public Health: Alcohol Related Disease Impact (ARDI).* 2013. Available at: http://nccd.cdc.gov/DPH_ARDI/Default/Report.aspx?T=AAM&P=f6d7eda7-036e-4553-9968-9b17ffad620e&R=d7a9b303-48e9-4440-bf47-070a4827e1fd&M=AD96A9C1-285A-44D2-B76D-BA2AE037F-C56&F=&D=. Accessed May 18, 2016.

Centers for Disease Control and Prevention (CDC). Youth Risk Behavior Surveillance—United States, 2013. *MMWR Suppl.* 2014;64(4):1–168.

Centers for Disease Control and Prevention (CDC). Excessive drinking is draining the U.S. economy. National Center for Chronic Disease Prevention and Health Promotion,

Division of Population Health. 2016a. Available at: http://www.cdc.gov/features/cost-sofdrinking. Accessed May 12, 2016.

Centers for Disease Control and Prevention (CDC). Excessive alcohol use and risks to men's health. 2016b. Available at: http://www.cdc.gov/alcohol/fact-sheets/mens-health.htm. Accessed May 12, 2016.

Centers for Disease Control and Prevention (CDC). Impaired driving: get the facts. 2016c. Available at: http://www.cdc.gov/motorvehiclesafety/impaired_driving/impaired-drv_factsheet.html. Accessed May 19, 2016.

Clarke CA, Purdie DM, Glaser SL. Population attributable risk of breast cancer in white women associated with immediately modifiable risk factors. *BMC Cancer.* 2006;6:170.

Community Preventive Services Task Force (CPSTF). The Community Guide. 2016. Available at: http://www.thecommunityguide.org. Accessed August 12, 2016.

Confidentiality of Alcohol and Drug Abuse Patient Records, 52 *Federal Register* 21809 (1987). Available at: http://www.ecfr.gov/cgi-bin/text-idx?rgn=div5;node=42%3A1.0.1.1.2. Accessed May 19, 2016.

Corrao G, Bagnardi V, Zambon A, La Vecchia C. A meta-analysis of alcohol consumption and the risk of 15 diseases. *Prev Med.* 2004;38(5):613–619.

Costin BN, Miles MF. Molecular and neurologic responses to chronic alcohol use. *Handb Clin Neurol.* 2014;125:157–171.

Dufour MC. Alcohol use and abuse. In: Pathy MSJ, Sinclair AJ, Morley JE, eds. *Principles and Practice of Geriatric Medicine.* Vol. 1. 4th ed. Chichester, England: Wiley and Sons; 2006: 157–168.

Dufour MC. Alcoholic liver disease. In: Talley NJ, Locke GR III, Saito YA, eds. *GI Epidemiology.* Malden, MA: Blackwell; 2007:231–237.

Dufour MC, Adamson MD. The epidemiology of alcohol-induced pancreatitis. *Pancreas.* 2003;27(4):286–290.

Dupuy M, Chanraud, S. Imaging the addicted brain: alcohol. *Int Rev Neurobiol.* 2016;129:1–31.

Eng MY, Schuckit MA, Smith TL. The level of response to alcohol in daughters of alcoholics and controls. *Drug Alcohol Depend.* 2005;79(1):83–93.

Ewing JA. Detecting alcoholism: the CAGE Questionnaire. *JAMA.* 1984;252(13):1905–1907.

Fagan KJ, Irvine KM, McWhinney BC, et al. Diagnostic sensitivity of carbohydrate deficient transferrin in heavy drinkers. *BMC Gastroenterol.* 2014;14:97.

Fone D, Farewell D, White J, Lyons R, Dunstan F. Socioeconomic patterning of excessive alcohol consumption and binge drinking: a cross sectional study of multilevel associations with neighborhood deprivation. *BMJ Open.* 2003;3(4):e002337.

Gormley NJ, Bronstein AC, Rasimas JJ, et al. The rising incidence of intentional ingestion of ethanol-containing hand sanitizers. *Crit Care Med.* 2012;40(1):290–294.

Governors Highway Safety Association (GHSA). Drunk driving laws. 2016. Available at: http://www.ghsa.org/html/stateinfo/laws/impaired_laws.html. Accessed May 19, 2016.

Grant B, Goldstein R, Saha T, et al. Epidemiology of DSM-5 alcohol use disorder: results from the National Epidemiologic Survey on Alcohol and Related Conditions III. *JAMA Psychiatry.* 2015;72(8):757–766.

Grant BF, Stinson FS, Dawson DA, et al. Prevalence and co-occurrence of substance use disorders and independent mood and anxiety disorders: results from the National Epidemiologic Survey on Alcohol and Related Conditions. *Arch Gen Psychiatry.* 2004;61(8):807–816.

Grucza RA, Abbacchi AM, Przybeck TR, Gfroerer JC. Discrepancies in estimates of prevalence and correlates of substance use and disorders between two national surveys. *Addiction.* 2007;102(4):623–629.

Hammond CJ, Niciu MJ, Drew S, Arias AJ. Anticonvulsants for the treatment of alcohol withdrawal syndrome and alcohol use disorders. *CNS Drugs.* 2015;29(4):293–311.

Hastings G, Anderson S, Cooke E, Gordon R. Alcohol marketing and young people's drinking: a review of the research. *J Public Health Policy.* 2005;26:296–311.

Haughwout S, LaVallee R, Castle I-J. Apparent per capita alcohol consumption: national, state, and regional trends, 1977–2013. National Institutes of Health. 2015. Available at: http://pubs.niaaa.nih.gov/publications/surveillance102/CONS13.pdf. Accessed May 18, 2016.

Haughwout SP, Lavelle RA, Castle I-JP. Apparent per capita consumption: national, state, and regional trends: 1977–2014. National Institute on Alcohol Abuse and Alcoholism. 2016. Available at: http://pubs.niaaa.nih.gov/publications/surveillance104/CONS14.htm. Accessed May 18, 2016.

Haugland SH, Holmen TL, Ravndal E, Bratberg GH. Parental alcohol misuse and hazardous drinking among offspring in a general teenage population: gender-specific findings from the Young-HUNT 3 study. *BMC Public Health.* 2013;13:1140.

Hedden SL, Kennet J, Lipari R, et al. Behavioral health trends in the United States: results from the 2014 National Survey on Drug Use and Health. Substance Abuse and Mental Health Services Administration. 2015. Available at: http://www.samhsa.gov/data/sites/default/files/NSDUH-FRR1-2014/NSDUH-FRR1-2014.htm. Accessed May 12, 2016.

Hietala J, Koivisto H, Anttila P, Niemela O. Comparison of the combined marker GGT–CDT and the conventional laboratory markers of alcohol abuse in heavy drinkers, moderate drinkers and abstainers. *Alcohol Alcohol.* 2006;41(5):528–533.

Hingson R, Heeren T, Winter M. Age at drinking onset and alcohol dependence: age at onset, duration, and severity. *Arch Pediatr Adolesc Med.* 2006;160(7):739–746.

Huhta J, Linask K. When should we prescribe high-dose folic acid to prevent congenital heart defects? *Curr Opin Cardiol.* 2015;30(1):125–131.

Indian Health Services (IHS). *Trends in Indian Health: 2014 Edition.* US Department of Health and Human Services. 2015. Available at: https://www.ihs.gov/dps/includes/themes/newihstheme/display_objects/documents/Trends2014Book508.pdf. Accessed May 16, 2016.

Institute of Alcohol Studies (IAS). Women and alcohol factsheet. London, UK: Alcohol Health Alliance; 2013. Available at: http://www.ias.org.uk/uploads/pdf/Factsheets/Women%20and%20alcohol%20factsheet%20May%202013.pdf.

Johnston L, O'Malley P, Miech R, Jerald B, Schulenberg J. *Monitoring the Future: National Survey Results on Drug Use, 1975–2015: Overview, Key Findings on Adolescent Drug Use.* University of Michigan Institute for Social Research and National Institute on Drug Abuse, National Institutes of Health. 2016. Available at: http://www.monitoringthefuture.org/pubs/monographs/mtf-overview2015.pdf. Accessed May 12, 2016.

Jonas DE, Amick HR, Feltner C, et al. *Pharmacotherapy for Adults With Alcohol-Use Disorders in Outpatient Settings.* Agency for Healthcare Research and Quality. 2014. Available at: http://www.ncbi.nlm.nih.gov/books/NBK208590. Accessed April 7, 2016.

Kendler KS, Prescott CA, Neale MC, Pedersen NL. Temperance board registration for alcohol abuse in a national sample of Swedish male twins, born 1902 to 1949. *Arch Gen Psychiatry.* 1997;54(2):178–184.

Kung HC, Hoyert DL, Xu JQ, Murphy SL. Deaths: final data for 2005. *Natl Vital Stat Rep.* 2008:56(10):1–120.

Lakins NE, Williams GD, Yi H. *Apparent Per Capita Alcohol Consumption: National, State, and Regional Trends, 1977–2005.* National Institute on Alcohol Abuse and Alcoholism, Alcohol Epidemiologic Data System. 2007. Surveillance Report no. 82. Available at: http://pubs.niaaa.nih.gov/publications/surveillance82/CONS05.pdf. Accessed August 12, 2016.

Loyola Marymount University (LMU). *History of Alcohol Use.* Heads Up. 2016. Available at: http://academics.lmu.edu/headsup/forstudents/historyofalcoholuse. Accessed May 11, 2016.

Maenhout TM, De Buyzere ML, Delanghe JR. Non-oxidative ethanol metabolites as a measure of alcohol intake. *Clin Chim Acta.* 2012;415:322–329.

Mares SH, Lichtwarck-Aschoff A, Engels RC. Intergenerational transmission of drinking motives and how they relate to young adults' alcohol use. *Alcohol Alcohol.* 2013;48(4): 445–451.

McGue M. The behavioral genetics of alcoholism. *Curr Dir Psychol Sci.* 1999;8(4):109–115.

Meisel SN, Colder CR. Social goals and grade as moderators of social normative influences on adolescent alcohol use. *Alcohol Clin Exp Res.* 2015;39(12):2455–2462.

Mendelson JH, Mello NK. Chronic alcohol effects on anterior pituitary and ovarian hormones in healthy women. *J Pharmacol Exp Ther.* 1988;245(2):407–412.

Mokdad AH, Marks JS, Stroup DF, Gerberding JL. Actual causes of death in the United States, 2000. *JAMA.* 2004;291(10):1238–1245.

Morse RM, Flavin DK. The definition of alcoholism. *JAMA.* 1992;268(8):1012–1014.

Moss HB, Chen CM, Yi H-Y. Prospective follow-up of empirically derived alcohol dependence subtypes in wave 2 of the National Epidemiologic Survey on Alcohol and Related Conditions (NESARC): recovery status, alcohol use disorders and diagnostic criteria, alcohol consumption behavior, health status, and treatment seeking. *Alcohol Clin Exp Res.* 2010;34(6):1073–1083.

Murphy A, Roberts B, Ploubidis GB, Stickley A, McKee M. Using multi-level data to estimate the effect of an "alcogenic" environment on hazardous alcohol consumption in the former Soviet Union. *Health Place.* 2014;27:205–211.

Myrick H, Malcolm R, Randall PK, et al. A double-blind trial of gabapentin versus lorazepam in the treatment of alcohol withdrawal. *Alcohol Clin Exp Res.* 2009;33(9):1582–1588.

National Center for Health Statistics (NCHS). Deaths, percent of total deaths, and death rates for the 15 leading causes of death in 5-year age groups, by race and sex: United States, 2013. Centers for Disease Control and Prevention. 2014. Available at: http://www.cdc.gov/nchs/data/dvs/lcwk1_2013.pdf. Accessed May 16, 2016.

National Council on Alcoholism and Drug Dependence (NCADD). Alcohol, drug dependence and seniors. 2015. Available at: https://www.ncadd.org/about-addiction/seniors/alcohol-drug-dependence-and-seniors. Accessed May 12, 2016.

National Highway Traffic Safety Administration (NHTSA). Research report: Preventing over- consumption of alcohol—sales to the intoxicated and "happy hour" (drink special) laws. Washington, DC: National Highway Traffic Safety Administration; 2005. DOT HS 809 878.

National Highway Traffic Safety Administration (NHTSA). Alcohol-impaired driving. US Department of Transportation. 2014. Available at: http://www-nrd.nhtsa.dot.gov/Pubs/812102.pdf. Accessed May 18, 2016.

National Institute on Alcohol Abuse and Alcoholism (NIAAA). Treatment of alcoholism and related problems. *Ninth Special Report to Congress on Alcohol and Health.* Bethesda, MD: National Institute on Alcohol Abuse and Alcoholism; 1997. NIH Publication 97-4017.

National Institute on Alcohol Abuse and Alcoholism (NIAAA). Helping patients who drink too much: a clinician's guide. National Institutes of Health. 2005a. Available at: http://pubs.niaaa.nih.gov/publications/Practitioner/CliniciansGuide2005/guide.pdf.

National Institute on Alcohol Abuse and Alcoholism (NIAAA). Screening for alcohol use and alcohol-related problems. Alcohol Alert. 2005b:65. Available at: http://pubs. niaaa.nih.gov/publications/aa65/AA65.htm. Accessed August 14, 2016.

National Institute on Alcohol Abuse and Alcoholism (NIAAA). Brief interventions. Alcohol Alert. 2005c:66. Available at: http://pubs.niaaa.nih.gov/publications/AA66/ AA66.htm. Accessed August 14, 2016.

National Institute on Alcohol Abuse and Alcoholism (NIAAA). National Epidemiologic Survey on Alcohol and Related Conditions. National Institutes of Health. 2006a. Available at: http://pubs.niaaa.nih.gov/publications/AA70/AA70.htm. Accessed May 18, 2016.

National Institute on Alcohol Abuse and Alcoholism (NIAAA). Alcohol use and alcohol use disorders in the United States: main findings from the 2001–2002 National Epidemiologic Survey on Alcohol and Related Conditions (NESARC). National Institutes of Health. 2006b. Available from: http://pubs.niaaa.nih.gov/publications/NESARC_ DRM/NESARCDRM.htm. Accessed May 12, 2016.

National Institute on Alcohol Abuse and Alcoholism (NIAAA). Older adults. National Institutes of Health. 2008a. Available at: http://www.niaaa.nih.gov/alcohol-health/ special-populations-co-occurring-disorders/older-adults. Accessed May 12, 2016.

National Institute on Alcohol Abuse and Alcoholism (NIAAA). *Alcohol and Other Drugs.* 2008b. Available at: http://pubs.niaaa.nih.gov/publications/AA76/AA76.htm. Accessed May 11, 2016.

National Institute on Alcohol Abuse and Alcoholism (NIAAA). Alcohol use and alcohol use disorders in the United States, a 3-year follow up: main findings from the 2004–2005 wave 2 National Epidemiologic Survey on Alcohol and Related Conditions (NESARC). National Institutes of Health. 2010. Available at: http://pubs.niaaa.nih.gov/ publications/NESARC_DRM2/NESARC2DRM.htm. Accessed May 12, 2016.

National Institute on Alcohol Abuse and Alcoholism (NIAAA). Alcohol use disorder: a comparison between *DSM–IV* and *DSM–5.* National Institutes of Health. 2015a. Available at: http://pubs.niaaa.nih.gov/publications/dsmfactsheet/dsmfact.htm. Accessed May 18, 2016.

National Institute on Alcohol Abuse and Alcoholism (NIAAA). College drinking. National Institutes of Health. 2015b. Available at: http://pubs.niaaa.nih.gov/publications/CollegeFactSheet/CollegeFact.htm. Accessed May 16, 2016.

National Institute on Alcohol Abuse and Alcoholism (NIAAA). Alcohol and the Hispanic community. National Institutes of Health. 2015c. Available at: http://pubs.niaaa.nih.gov/publications/HispanicFact/HispanicFact.htm. Accessed May 16, 2016.

National Institute on Alcohol Abuse and Alcoholism (NIAAA). Alcohol facts and statistics. National Institutes of Health. 2016. Available at: http://www.niaaa.nih.gov/alcohol-health/overview-alcohol-consumption/alcohol-facts-and-statistics. Accessed May 12, 2016.

National Institute on Drug Abuse (NIDA). Sex and gender differences in substance use. National Institutes of Health. 2015. Available at: https://www.drugabuse.gov/publications/research-reports/substance-use-in-women/sex-gender-differences-in-substance-use. Accessed August 14, 2016.

National Sexual Violence Resource Center (NSVRC). Statistics about sexual violence. 2015. Available at: http://www.nsvrc.org/sites/default/files/publications_nsvrc_factsheet_media-packet_statistics-about-sexual-violence_0.pdf. Accessed May 18, 2016.

Paschall MJ, Grube JW, Thomas S, Cannon C, Treffers R. Relationships between local enforcement, alcohol availability, drinking norms, and adolescent alcohol use in 50 California cities. *J Stud Alcohol Drugs*. 2012;73(4):657–665.

Pearson AL, Bowie C, Thornton LE. Is access to alcohol associated with alcohol/substance abuse among people diagnosed with anxiety/mood disorder? *Public Health*. 2014;128(11):968–976.

Pelletier AR, Siegel PZ, Baptiste MS, Maylahn C. Revisions to chronic disease surveillance indicators, United States, 2004. *Prev Chronic Dis*. 2005;2(3):A15.

Prescott CA, Aggen SH, Kendler KS. Sex differences in the sources of genetic liability to alcohol abuse and dependence in a population-based sample of U.S. twins. *Alcohol Clin Exp Res*. 1999;23(7):1136–1144.

Rehm J, Baliunas D, Borges GL, et al. The relation between different dimensions of alcohol consumption and burden of disease: an overview. *Addiction*. 2010;105(5):817–843.

Ries RK, Fiellin DA, Miller SC, Saitz R. *ASAM Principles of Addiction Medicine*. 5th ed. Philadelphia, PA: Lippincott Williams and Wilkins; 2014.

Rimm EB, Moats C. Alcohol and coronary heart disease: drinking patterns and mediators of effect. *Ann Epidemiol*. 2007;17:S3–S7.

Roerecke M, Rehm J. Alcohol use disorders and mortality: a systematic review and meta-analysis. *Addiction*. 2013;108(9):1562–1578.

Rubin E, Thomas AP. Effects of alcohol on the heart and cardiovascular system. In: Mendelson JH, Mello NK, eds. *Medical Diagnosis and Treatment of Alcoholism*. New York, NY: McGraw-Hill; 1992:263–287.

Sacks JJ, Gonzales KR, Bouchery EE, Tomedi LE, Brewer RD. 2010 national and state costs of excessive alcohol consumption. *Am J Prev Med*. 2015;49(5):e73–e79.

Saitz R. Unhealthy alcohol use. *N Engl J Med*. 2005;352:596–607.

Schuckit MA. An overview of genetic influences in alcoholism. *J Subst Abuse Treat*. 2009;36(1):S5–S14.

Steinweg DL, Worth H. Alcoholism: the keys to the CAGE. *Am J Med*. 1993;94(5):520–523.

Substance Abuse and Mental Health Services Administration (SAMHSA). *TIP 24: A Guide to Substance Abuse Services for Primary Care Clinicians*. Rockville, MD: Center for Substance Abuse Treatment; 1997. DHHS Publication no. (SMA) 97-3139.

Substance Abuse and Mental Health Services Administration (SAMHSA). *Results From the 2013 National Survey on Drug Use and Health: Mental Health Findings*. US Department of Health and Human Services. 2013a. Available at: http://www.samhsa.gov/data/sites/default/files/NSDUHmhfr2013/NSDUHmhfr2013.pdf. Accessed May 11, 2016.

Substance Abuse and Mental Health Services Administration (SAMHSA). *Results From the 2013 National Survey on Drug Use and Health: Summary of National Findings*. Center for Behavioral Health Statistics and Quality, US Department of Health and Human Services. 2013b. Available at: http://www.samhsa.gov/data/sites/default/files/NSDUHresultsPDFWHTML2013/Web/NSDUHresults2013.htm. Accessed May 12, 2016.

Substance Abuse and Mental Health Services Administration (SAMHSA). *2013–2014 National Survey on Drugs and Health National Maps of Prevalence Estimates, by State*. 2014. Available at: http://www.samhsa.gov/data/sites/default/files/NSDUHsaeMaps2014/NSDUHsaeMaps2014.pdf.

Substance Abuse and Mental Health Services Administration (SAMHSA). Underage drinking declined between 2002 and 2013. US Department of Health and Human Services. 2015. Available at: http://www.samhsa.gov/data/sites/default/files/report_1978/Spotlight-1978.pdf. Accessed August 16, 2016.

Substance Abuse and Mental Health Services Administration (SAMHSA). About population data/NSDUH. US Department of Health and Human Services. 2016a. Available at: http://www.samhsa.gov/data/population-data-nsduh/about. Accessed May 18, 2016.

Substance Abuse and Mental Health Services Administration (SAMHSA). National Survey on Drug Use and Health. US Department of Health and Human Services. 2016b. Available at: https://nsduhweb.rti.org/respweb/homepage.cfm. Accessed August 14, 2016.

The Task Force on Community Preventive Services (TFCPS). Recommendations for reducing excessive alcohol consumption and alcohol-related harms by limiting alcohol outlet density. *Am J Prev Med*. 2009;37(6):570–571.

Taneri PE, Kiefte-de Jong JC, Bramer WM, Daan NM, Franco OH, Muka T. Association of alcohol consumption with the onset of natural menopause: a systematic review and meta-analysis. *Hum Reprod Update*. 2016;22(4):516–528.

Taylor JR, Combs-Orme T, Taylor DA. Alcohol and mortality: diagnostic considerations. *J Stud Alcohol*. 1983;44(1):17–25.

Thakker KD. An overview of health risks and benefits of alcohol consumption. *Alcohol Clin Exp Res*. 1998;22(suppl 7):285S–298S.

Tippetts AS, Voas RB, Fell JC, Nichols JL. A meta-analysis of .08 BAC laws in 19 jurisdictions in the United States. *Accid Anal Prev*. 2005;37(1):149–161.

Toomey TL, Wagenaar AC. Environmental policies to reduce college drinking: options and research findings. *J Stud Alcohol*. 2002;(suppl 14):193–205.

Traversy G, Chaput J-P. Alcohol consumption and obesity: an update. *Curr Obes Rep*. 2015;4(1):122–130.

US Census Bureau. ACS demographic and housing estimates: 2010–2014 American Community Survey 5-year estimates. DP05. 2014. Available at: http://factfinder.census.gov/faces/tableservices/jsf/pages/productview.xhtml?src=CF. Accessed May 16, 2016.

US Department of Health and Human Services, Office of Disease Prevention and Health Promotion (USDHHS and ODPHP). *Healthy People 2020*. 2014. Available at: https://www.healthypeople.gov. Accessed May 11, 2016.

US Department of Health and Human Services, US Department of Agriculture (USDHHS and USDA). Appendix 9. Alcohol. In: *2015-2020 Dietary Guidelines for Americans*. 8th ed. 2015. Available at: http://health.gov/dietaryguidelines/2015/guidelines. Accessed May 11, 2016.

US Preventive Services Task Force (USPSTF). Screening and behavioral counseling interventions in primary care to reduce alcohol misuse: recommendation statement. *Ann Intern Med*. 2004;140(7):554–556.

Van Oers J, Bongers I, Van de Goor L, Garretsen H. Alcohol consumption, alcohol-related problems, problem drinking, and socioeconomic status. *Alcohol Alcohol.* 1999;34(1):78–88.

Van Thiel DH, Gavaler JS, Lester R, Goodman MD. Alcohol-induced testicular atrophy. An experimental model for hypogonadism occurring in chronic alcoholic men. *Gastroenterology.* 1975;69(2):326–332.

Voas RB, Tippetts AS, Fell JC. Assessing the effectiveness of minimum legal drinking age and zero tolerance laws in the United States. *Accid Anal Prev.* 2003;35(4):579–587.

Wagenaar AC, Murray DM, Toomey TL. Communities Mobilizing for Change on Alcohol (CMCA): effects of a randomized trial on arrests and traffic crashes. *Addiction.* 2000a;95(2):209–217.

Wagenaar AC, Murray DM, Gehan JP, et al. Communities Mobilizing for Change on Alcohol: outcomes from a randomized community trial. *J Stud Alcohol.* 2000b;61(1): 85–94.

Wang C, Hipp JR, Butts CT, Jose R, Lakon CM. Alcohol use among adolescent youth: the role of friendship networks and family factors in multiple school studies. *PLoS One.* 2015;10(3):e0119965.

White A, Hingson R; National Institute on Alcohol Abuse and Alcoholism. The burden of alcohol use: excessive alcohol consumption and related consequences among college students. *Alcohol Res.* 2013;35(2):201–218.

Williams JF, Smith VC; The Committee on Substance Abuse. Fetal alcohol spectrum disorders. *Pediatrics.* 2015;136(5):e1395–e1406.

World Health Organization (WHO). *Global Status Report on Alcohol and Health, 2014.* 2014. Available at: http://www.who.int/substance_abuse/publications/global_alcohol_report/en. Accessed May 11, 2016.

Zador PL, Krawchuk SA, Voas RB. Alcohol-related relative risk of driver involvement in fatal crashes in relation to driver age and sex: an update using 1996 data. Washington, DC: National Highway Traffic Safety Administration; 2000. DOT HS 809 050.

PART III. MIDSTREAM CHRONIC CONDITIONS

11

OBESITY

Deborah A. Galuska, PhD, MPH, and Heidi M. Blanck, PhD, CAPT USPHS

Introduction

Obesity is complex, common, and costly condition that results in poorer health and quality of life. However, it has the potential to be prevented and managed. This chapter examines the epidemiology of obesity, its health and economic consequences, and the evidence for prevention and treatment strategies.

Obesity is defined as the accumulation of excess fat. In clinical and public health settings, it is most often assessed by the body mass index (BMI), a measure of weight that accounts for height and is estimated as weight in kilograms divided by height in meters squared (kg/m^2). Although BMI does not directly measure the amount of fat, it is easily assessed in clinic and large population settings, and correlates reasonably well with more direct measures of body fat assessed through techniques such as skinfold thickness or dual x-ray absorptiometry (CDC 2012). For adults, an absolute value of BMI—a BMI greater than or equal to 30—is used to define obesity. The obese category can be subdivided into three classes: class 1 is BMI 30.0 to 34.9; class 2 is BMI 35.0 to 39.9; and class 3 (also called extreme obesity) is BMI greater than or equal to 40 (NIH 1998).

For children and adolescents aged 2 to 19 years, because of their growth patterns, the classification of weight status is relative; BMI is compared to age- and sex-specific percentiles on the Centers for Disease Control and Prevention (CDC) growth charts and obesity is defined as a BMI greater than or equal to the 95th percentile for age and sex (CDC 2015a).

Significance

The burden of obesity and its sequelae in the United States is significant (Figure 11-1). In 2011 to 2014, more than a third of adults (36.5%) and one sixth

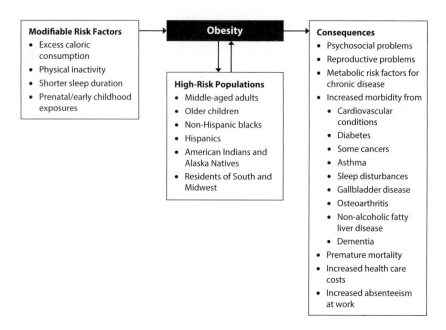

Figure 11-1. Obesity: Causes, Consequences, and High-Risk Groups

of children and adolescents aged 2 to 19 years (17.0%) in the United States had obesity (Ogden et al. 2015). Obesity is associated with an increased risk of a multitude of deleterious health outcomes that can be grouped into five major categories: (1) psychosocial, (2) reproductive, (3) metabolic risk factors for chronic disease, (4) morbidity, and (5) mortality. The relationship of these outcomes with obesity has been extensively reviewed for both adults and children and is summarized in the next paragraphs.

Psychosocial

Obesity may affect how people feel about themselves as well as how others in society feel about them. In general, obesity is associated with individual feelings of lower self-esteem for both adults and children (Sikorski et al. 2015). In addition, individuals with obesity may be perceived negatively by others and be the target of discrimination in a variety of settings (Puhl and Brownell 2001; Puhl and Heuer 2009); the strongest evidence supports prejudice or discrimination in the employment settings. Obesity also may be correlated with lower levels of socioeconomic achievement, in particular for women

(Puhl et al. 2005; Puhl and Heuer 2009). Furthermore, obesity affects mental health as it is associated with an increased risk of depression (Luppino et al. 2010).

Reproductive

Among women, obesity can negatively affect menstrual function and fertility (NIH 1998; Sarwer et al. 2006). Women with obesity experience complications both during pregnancy including hypertension or pre-eclampsia (Marchi et al. 2015) and gestational diabetes (Sarwer et al. 2006; Chu et al. 2007a; Marchi et al. 2015), as well as complications during labor and delivery (Marchi et al. 2015) including an increased risk of cesarean delivery (Sarwer et al. 2006; Chu et al. 2007c; Marchi et al. 2015). Maternal obesity is also associated with increased adverse effects for the child including high birthweight (Marchi et al. 2015), stillbirths (Chu et al. 2007b; Marchi et al. 2015), fetal death (Marchi et al. 2015), and a range of congenital anomalies (Marchi et al. 2015; Stothard et al. 2009).

Metabolic Risk Factors for Chronic Disease

The positive association between excess weight and risk factors for chronic disease, in particular cardiovascular disease (CVD) and type 2 diabetes, has been documented for both adults (NIH 2013) and children (Reilly et al. 2003; Güngör 2014). These risk factors include elevated blood pressure, dyslipidemias, and insulin resistance. Obesity is also associated with higher levels of inflammatory markers such as C-reactive protein (Bastien et al. 2014; Iyengar et al. 2015). These chronic disease risk factors are more likely to cluster in overweight and obese persons than in normal-weight persons (Camhi and Katzmarzyk 2011; Wildman et al. 2008). Childhood adiposity is associated with adult adiposity (Simmonds et al. 2016), and through this mechanism may also influence the risk of obesity-related conditions in adulthood.

Morbidity

Obesity is associated with greater morbidity from a number of chronic conditions including some of the leading causes of death. Among adults, obesity or higher weight status increases the risk of cardiovascular conditions such as coronary heart disease (Bogers et al. 2007; NIH 2013), ischemic and hemorrhagic stroke (NIH 2013; Strazzullo et al. 2010), type 2 diabetes (NIH 2013; Vazquenz et al. 2007), and some cancers including colorectal, endometrial, postmenopausal breast, pancreatic, esophageal, liver, thyroid, and kidney cancer (Wang et al. 2016; World Cancer Research Fund 2007). In addition to being related to these leading causes of death, obesity is also associated with other health conditions that affect quality of life. These include asthma (Beuther and Sutherland 2007), sleep disturbances (Schwartz et al. 2008), gallbladder disease (Aune et al. 2015), osteoarthritis (Bliddal et al. 2014), and nonalcoholic fatty liver disease (Angulo 2007). Table 11-1 documents the relative risks for the association of obesity with select outcomes.

Table 11-1. Relative Risks for the Association Between Body Mass Index (BMI) and Select Health Outcomes as Estimated by Meta-analyses

Health Outcome (Source)	Adjusted Relative Risk[a]	Comparison
Cancer		
Breast, postmenopausal (Wang et al. 2016)	1.11	Per 5 kg/m² increase
Endometrial (Bergström et al. 2001)	2.52	BMI≥30 vs. BMI 20.0–24.0
Colorectal, male (Wang et al. 2016)	1.13	Per 5 kg/m² increase
Colorectal, female	1.06	
Esophagus/gastric, male (Wang et al. 2016)	1.11	Per 5 kg/m² increase
Esophagus/gastric, female	1.07	
Kidney, male (Wang et al. 2016)	1.18	Per 5 kg/m² increase
Kidney, female	1.21	
Liver, male (Wang et al. 2016)	1.21	Per 5 kg/m² increase
Liver, female	1.20	
Pancreas, male (Wang et al. 2016)	1.10	Per 5 kg/m² increase
Pancreas, female	1.08	
Thyroid, male (Wang et al. 2016)	1.16	Per 5 kg/m² increase
Thyroid, female	1.09[b]	
Coronary heart disease, unadjusted for blood pressure and cholesterol levels (Bogers et al. 2007)	1.81	BMI≥30 vs. BMI 18.5–24.0
Coronary heart disease, adjusted for blood pressure and cholesterol levels	1.49	BMI≥30 vs. BMI 18.5–24.0
Diabetes (Vazquenz et al. 2007)	1.87	Standard deviation of BMI (4.3 units)
Stroke, ischemic (Strazzullo et al. 2010)	1.64	Obese vs. normal weight[c]

[a]Variables adjusted for vary by study.
[b]Not statistically significant.
[c]Definition of obesity and normal weight varied by study within the meta-analysis.

Obesity also affects cognitive health. Obesity during midlife appears to be associated with a small but increased risk of dementia; however, obesity in late life is associated with a lower risk (Pedditizi et al. 2016).

Children also experience morbidities associated with their weight, many of them similar to those experienced by adults. These include respiratory problems such as asthma and sleep apnea, orthopedic problems such as Blount's disease (a growth disorder of the tibia that causes the bowing of legs) and slipped capital femoral epiphysis (a separation of the ball of the hip joint from the thigh bone), and gastrointestinal problems such a gallbladder disease (Güngör 2014). Severe obesity in childhood is a risk factor for type 2 diabetes in childhood (Weiss et al. 2005). Childhood obesity is also associated with increased risk of cardiometabolic morbidity in adulthood (Reilly and Kelly 2011).

Mortality

Among adults, meta-analyses conclude that obesity or high weight status is associated with greater all-cause mortality (Berrington de Gonzalez et al. 2010; Flegal et al. 2013; McGee and the Diverse Populations Collaboration 2005; Whitlock et al. 2009) and a number of cause-specific mortalities including CVD (Berrington de Gonzalez et al. 2010; McGee and the Diverse Populations Collaboration 2005) and some cancers (Berrington de Gonzalez et al. 2010; Whitlock et al. 2009). However, one meta-analysis did not find a significant association between obesity and cancer in men (McGee and the Diverse Populations Collaboration 2005). One meta-analysis estimated that, compared to persons with a BMI of 18.5 to 25.0, those with a BMI of 30 (obese) or higher had a relative risk of 1.22 for all-cause mortality, 1.48 for CVD, and 1.07 for cancer (McGee and the Diverse Populations Collaboration 2005). The association between obesity and mortality may weaken with age; a study using National Health and Nutrition Examination Survey data found no association among adults aged 70 years and older (Flegal et al. 2005). Among children, overweight or obesity is associated with increased overall mortality (Reilly and Kelly 2011) in adulthood. Whether this association is independent of adult obesity is unclear.

Economic

Obesity-related health conditions pose economic costs for society. For example, a recent meta-analysis reported that medical costs associated with obesity accounted for approximately $150 billion in 2014 U.S. dollars (Kim and Basu 2016). One study in this meta-analysis estimated that the total medical costs were about 9.1% of total annual medical spending (Finkelstein et al. 2009). Because the more serious consequences of weight appear in adulthood, the costs of obesity for children are smaller but not insignificant. One study found that elevated BMI (obesity or overweight) was associated with an additional $14.1 billion annual costs related to outpatient visits, prescription drugs, and emergency room visits for children aged 6 to 19 years (Trasande and Chatterjee 2009). In addition, childhood obesity, if maintained, can have significant life-time medical costs in the range of $12,660 to $19,630 excess costs (Finkelstein et al. 2014). In addition to increased medical costs, obesity is also associated with increased costs in the workplace related to increased absenteeism and presenteeism (Finkelstein et al. 2010).

Pathophysiology

Obesity affects multiple physiologic processes and organs and has an impact on disease through these pathways. Three more established biological mechanisms are briefly described here. However, as more research is conducted, new pathways and a better understanding of the complex interrelationships between pathways will continue to emerge.

Biomechanical changes caused by large body mass are one mechanism that links obesity with disease. For example, increased cardiac burden as a result of size is thought to cause adverse changes to the heart muscle and the efficiency of the heart's function and contribute to heart failure (Bastien et al. 2014). Stress on load-bearing joints as well as gait abnormalities caused by insufficient muscle mass to support excess weight are hypothesized to contribute to joint degeneration and osteoarthritis (Vincent et al. 2012). Obesity may contribute to sleep apnea through the narrowing of the upper airway caused by fat deposited there or by the association of obesity with reduced lung volume (Schwartz et al. 2008).

Metabolic changes associated with adipose tissue are a second mechanism that links obesity with health outcomes. For example, increased total and free circulating estrogen levels caused by the conversion of androgens to estrogens in adipose tissue is hypothesized as one link between obesity and some reproductive cancers in women (Iyengar et al. 2015). Obesity might also exert its effect on multiple diseases including CVD, cancers, and diabetes, through its association with increased circulation of free fatty acids and their deleterious effect on lipoprotein metabolism and insulin resistance (Bastien et al. 2014; Iyengar et al. 2015; Tchernof and Despres 2013).

The association of obesity with a chronic low level of inflammation is another biologic mechanism that links obesity with health. Pro-inflammatory factors produced by adipose tissue are hypothesized to adversely affect many obesity-related diseases through mechanisms such as their effect on insulin resistance (Bastien et al. 2014), direct tissue damage (Iyengar et al. 2015; Vincent et al. 2012), their interaction with other biological process such as estrogen biosynthesis at a local level (Iyengar et al. 2015), or their effect on the response of the neuromuscular system (Schwartz et al. 2008).

Obesity might also exert its effect on health outcomes through non-biological mechanisms. For example, the visibility of obesity and the associated negative experiences persons with obesity have is one mechanism that potentially links obesity with depression and lower socioeconomic achievement (Puhl and Heuer 2009). Embarrassment or negative experiences in the medical care setting might also negatively affect whether persons with obesity seek medical care (Puhl and Heuer 2009).

In addition, both children and adults with obesity report an overall lower quality of life than those of normal weight. This appears to be mediated through both the social and medical consequences of obesity (Doll et al. 2000; Schwimmer et al. 2003).

Descriptive Epidemiology

High-Risk Populations

Data from the National Health and Nutrition Examination Surveys provide evidence that obesity differentially affects certain demographic subgroups of the population characterized by sex, race/ethnicity, age (Ogden et al. 2015), and socioeconomic status (May et al. 2013a; Ogden et al. 2010). Among adults in 2011 to 2014, the prevalence of obesity was higher among women (38.3%) than men (34.3%). Racial/ethnic differences vary by sex (Figure 11-2). Among men, the prevalence of obesity was approximately the same for Hispanics (39.0%) and non-Hispanic blacks (37.5%), slightly lower for non-Hispanic whites (33.6%), and lowest for non-Hispanic Asians (11.2%). In contrast, among women, non-Hispanic blacks (56.9%) had the highest prevalence followed by Hispanics (45.7%), non-Hispanic whites (35.5%), and non-Hispanic Asians (11.9%).

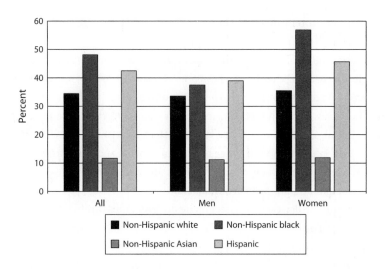

Source: Adapted from Ogden et al. (2015).

Note: Estimates are age-adjusted by the direct method to the U.S. Census population with the age groups 20 to 39 years, 40 to 59 years, and 60 years and older. Obesity is defined as body mass index greater than or equal to 30.

Figure 11-2. Prevalence of Obesity Among Adults Aged 20 Years and Older, by Sex and Race and Hispanic Origin, 2011–2014

For both men and women, obesity was highest among those aged 40 to 59 years, and lowest among those aged 20 to 39 years. In 2007 to 2010, for both men and women, those who were college graduates had the lowest prevalence of obesity (May et al. 2013a). The association of income with obesity is complex. In 2005 to 2008, household income poverty threshold was inversely associated with obesity in non-Hispanic white women and positively associated with obesity in Mexican-American men and non-Hispanic black men. No significant associations were observed for other demographic subgroups (Ogden et al. 2010). Based on self-reported data, American Indians and Alaska Natives have about a 50% higher crude prevalence of obesity compared to non-Hispanic whites (Cobb et al. 2014).

Among children and adolescents aged 2 to 19 years in 2011 to 2014, the prevalence of obesity was similar for boys (16.9%) and girls (17.1%; Ogden et al. 2015). Among boys (Figure 11-3), Hispanics (22.4%) had the highest prevalence of obesity followed by non-Hispanic blacks (18.4%); both of these prevalences were higher than those for non-Hispanic whites (14.3%) and non-Hispanic

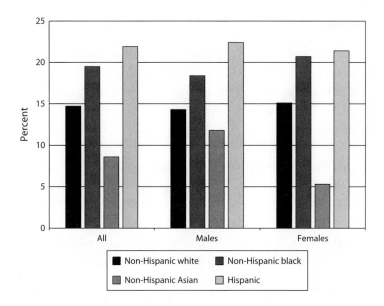

Source: Adapted from Ogden et al. (2015).

Note: Obesity defined as body mass index greater than or equal to 95th percentile on Centers for Disease Control and Prevention growth charts.

Figure 11-3. Prevalence of Obesity Among Youths Aged 2 to 19 Years, by Sex and Race and Hispanic Origin, 2011–2014

Asians (11.8%). Among girls (Figure 11-3), Hispanics (21.4%) and non-Hispanic blacks (20.7%) had a similar prevalence of obesity with a slightly lower prevalence for non-Hispanic whites (15.1%) and substantially lower prevalence for non-Hispanic Asians (5.3%). The prevalence in children aged 2 to 5 years (8.9%) was approximately half that of those aged 6 to 11 years (17.5%) and 12 to 19 years (20.5%), a pattern consistent for boys and girls.

Geographic Distribution

In 2015, the state-specific prevalence of adult obesity based on self-report ranged from 20.2% in Colorado to 36.2% in Louisiana (CDC 2016). In general, the prevalence of obesity was lowest among states in the West and Northeast, and highest among states in the Midwest and South. Similar geographic patterns are observed for the prevalence of obesity based on self-report among adolescents (Kann et al. 2016).

Time Trends

During the 1980s and 1990s, the prevalence of obesity more than doubled for both adults and children (Fryar et al. 2014; Ogden et al. 2002). Between 1999–2000 and 2013–2014, the prevalence of obesity continued to increase for adults (30.5% to 37.7%) and youths aged 2 to 19 years (13.9% to 17.2%). However, despite the overall increase during this period, in more recent years, the trends for youths were stable and may even be improving; between 2003–2004 and 2013–2014, youth prevalence did not change significantly overall (Ogden et al. 2015) and may have declined for children aged two to five years (Ogden et al. 2016). Other studies support this trend in children. For example, in the past decade, declines in childhood obesity have been observed in low-income children aged two to four years (May et al. 2013b), and schoolchildren in New York City (Berger et al. 2011) and Philadelphia (Robbins et al. 2012).

Causes

Conceptually, excessive weight gain is ultimately caused by an imbalance between energy intake and energy expenditure. However a complex interplay of multiple factors at the individual (e.g., genetics, knowledge, attitudes, health status) and population level (e.g., environments and policies that support diet and physical activity) can affect energy intake, metabolism, and expenditure. A more complete description of this interplay is beyond the scope of this chapter but can be found in more comprehensive reviews (IOM 2005; USDHHS 2010). Key modifiable risk factors at the individual level are described in the next paragraphs.

Modifiable Risk Factors

Diet, particularly as it relates to the overconsumption of calories, is one modifiable risk factor for obesity. Calories are obtained from four dietary sources: carbohydrates, proteins, fats, and alcohol. In general, the energy density of fats (9 kcal/g) and alcohol (7 kcal/g) are approximately twice that of carbohydrates (4 kcal/g) and proteins (4 kcal/g; National Research Council 1989). As such, one strategy promoted to prevent weight gain is reducing the consumption of high-calorie–low-nutrient foods or increasing the consumption of lower-calorie nutrient-dense foods. An evidence review conducted for the 2015–2020 Dietary Guidelines for Americans concluded that there was moderate evidence that dietary patterns that are "higher in vegetables, fruits, and whole grains; include seafood and legumes; are moderate in dairy products (particularly low and non-fat dairy) and alcohol; lower in meats (including red and processed meats), and low in sugar-sweetened foods and beverages, and refined grains are associated with favorable outcomes related to healthy body weight (including lower BMI, waist circumference, or percent body fat) or risk of obesity." (DGAC 2015).

Whether the consumption of specific foods or types of foods leads to weight gain is not clear, however, in part because foods and food groups are not eaten in isolation of each other. A recent review of reviews found evidence, albeit inconsistent, for an inverse relation between overweight or obesity and increased consumption of fruits and vegetables, increased consumption of nuts and seeds, and increased consumption of whole grains (Fardet and Boire 2014). The review found the most consistent evidence, however, existed for a positive relationship between increased sugar-sweetened beverage consumption and weight. This association is found for both children and adults and across multiple study designs (Malik et al. 2013). Sugar-sweetened beverages, in addition to their contribution to caloric intake, are also hypothesized to contribute to weight gain because calories consumed in this liquid form may not be as satiating and may only partially be compensated for in later meals during the day (Malik and Hu 2015).

Interventions to alter caloric intake are challenging because of the complex relationships between an individual's physiological triggers and responses to hunger, satiety, and food intake; their beliefs and attitudes about food; their environmental exposure to certain foods and marketing of foods; and characteristics of food such as satiety and palatability (Blundell and Stubbs 2007; IOM 2005).

Another modifiable risk factor for obesity is low physical activity. Total daily energy expenditure consists of three components: basal and resting metabolic expenditure, the thermic effect of eating, and physical activity (Bouchard and Shepard 1994; USDHHS 1996). Because physical activity appears to be the most modifiable component of energy expenditure, it is the target of interventions to alter energy expenditure. Among adults, epidemiologic studies have demonstrated an inverse relationship between physical activity and obesity in cross-sectional studies and a relationship between increases in physical activity and less weight gain in longitudinal studies (PAGAC 2008). Similar findings have been observed for children (PAGAC 2008; Strong et al. 2005).

In addition to the direct effects of energy intake via diet and energy expenditure through physical activity, other modifiable risk factors for weight gain have been proposed. Sedentary behaviors may be a risk factor independent of lower physical activity. One sedentary behavior that has received attention is television viewing among children. Hypothesized mechanisms for the influence of television viewing on adiposity include the replacement of more intense physical activities, poor dietary patterns while watching television, and the influence of television commercials on the foods consumed in the house (Woodward-Lopez et al. 2006). A 2004 synthesis of the observational and experimental evidence for the relationship between television viewing and adiposity in children found a significant, albeit small, association between increased television viewing and obesity (Marshall et al. 2004). However, a more recent meta-analysis of interventions to reduce screen time in children did not find reductions in BMI among children (Wahi et al. 2011).

Another modifiable risk factor for obesity is sleep quality; shorter sleep duration has been associated with higher weight status in both children (Patel and Hu 2008; Ruan et al. 2015) and adults (Patel and Hu 2008). Proposed mechanisms for this association include the potential influence of less sleep on fatigue, which might reduce physical activity behaviors; on increased waking time and, thus, increased opportunities to eat; or on physiological processes that might increase hunger and calorie intake or slow energy expenditure through thermoregulation (Patel and Hu 2008; Ruan et al. 2015).

Prenatal or early childhood exposures are also modifiable risk factors for childhood obesity. For example, excessive weight gain during pregnancy is associated with higher weight during childhood (Lau et al. 2014; Mamum et al. 2014). Other hypothesized maternal risk factors associated with childhood obesity include gestational diabetes, tobacco use during pregnancy, and pre-pregnancy weight status (Woo Baidal et al. 2015). In early childhood, longer breastfeeding has been associated with lower childhood weight status in some but not all systematic reviews and meta-analyses (Woo and Martin 2015). Whether this association is causal is still unclear.

An emerging area of modifiable risk factors is the role of the gut microbiome. The gut microbiome appears to be different for those with obesity and those without. One proposed mechanism linking the microbiome with weight gain is the relative efficiency of different microbes in breaking down dietary polysaccharides, providing additional energy to humans. The composition of the diet and its interaction with host's genetic factors is one factor thought to influence the types of microbes that exist in the gut (Patterson et al. 2016).

Another emerging area is the role of certain environmental chemicals on obesity. These chemicals are thought to disrupt the endocrine system and potentially change metabolic set points and metabolism (Heindel et al. 2015).

Population-Attributable Risk

The relative contribution of modifiable risk factors to causing obesity is not clear. The state of science in obesity research precludes the estimation of population-attributable risk for most proposed risk factors for obesity because either the assumptions of the population-attributable risk cannot be met or the estimates needed for the calculation are not available. This is particularly true for dietary risk factors. The limitations in the literature include (1) the lack of consensus on the causal link between many hypothesized risk factors and obesity, (2) the limited number of longitudinal studies that have addressed the incidence of obesity (as compared to weight change), (3) the difficulty in establishing an independent effect of different dietary behaviors that are often highly correlated, and (4) difficulty in disentangling caloric intake from caloric expenditure, which are interdependent in weight control.

Evidence-Based Interventions

Prevention

Obesity prevention focuses on limiting unhealthy weight gain. For children, this is the prevention of weight gain beyond that needed for growth and development, and for adults, this is the prevention of weight gain among those of normal weight as well as the prevention of further weight gain among those with overweight or obesity. Although individuals can undertake actions to prevent weight gain, this section will focus on population-based strategies. In their 2012 report on "Accelerating Progress in Childhood Obesity," the Institute of Medicine stated that the goal of population obesity prevention was to "create, through directed societal change, an environmental–behavioral synergy to foster the achievement and maintenance of healthy weight among individuals and the population at large" (IOM 2012). These population-level strategies can be done at the level of behavioral settings, sectors, or social norms and values (IOM 2005). In addition to population strategies that specifically address the social and physical environments for diet and physical activity, actions that alter the overall conditions or the context in which people live, often called the social determinants of health (CDC 2015b), also have the potential to affect obesity. Examples include adequate income that allows purchase of healthy foods or safe communities that allow people to be active outdoors.

Over the past several decades, numerous expert bodies have made recommendations related to population strategies for obesity prevention (CDC 2011; IOM 2009; IOM 2011; IOM 2012; Khan et al. 2009; TFCPS 2009; USDHHS 2010; White House Task Force on Childhood Obesity 2010). These are described in more detail in the next paragraphs. However, two common themes occur across these recommendations: (1) a focus on both diet and physical activity and (2) the promotion of a multilevel approach that both helps individuals learn how to make healthier choices and provides supportive environments for making these choices.

Obesity prevention efforts have been directly targeted to four key population settings; a brief description of current evidence and recommendations for these settings is provided.

Early Care and Education and Schools

Interventions for obesity prevention in early care and education settings as well as schools are promoted because of the large amount of time children spend in these settings exposed to opportunities to eat and be active, the potential for promoting life habits, the potential to engage and influence parents as decision-makers and role models, and the potential to influence the adults employed in these settings. Numerous expert bodies including CDC (CDC 2011; Khan et al. 2009), the Institute of Medicine (IOM 2011; IOM 2012), the U.S. Surgeon General (USDHHS 2010), and the White House Task Force on Childhood Obesity (White House Task Force on Childhood Obesity 2010) have recommended the implementation of obesity prevention strategies for schools or early care and education settings.

Much of the evidence on the effectiveness of these interventions exists for those done at the facility or organizational level. Systematic reviews of facility-level interventions document limited to moderate evidence that interventions conducted in the child care setting can have a positive impact on weight status (DGAC 2015; Sisson et al. 2016; Wang et al. 2015) or behaviors related to weight status such as diet, physical activity, or television viewing (Sisson et al. 2016). Compared to early care and education settings, more studies have been done in schools. In general, systematic reviews of these studies have found moderate to strong evidence that school-based interventions can improve weight status (Langford et al. 2014; Wang et al. 2015; Waters et al. 2011), particularly for multicomponent interventions or those for younger children (Waters et al. 2011).

In addition to facility-level interventions done in a limited number of facilities, federal, state, and local policies have the potential to have an impact on the practices, curriculum, and teacher training at large numbers of facilities. For example, at the federal level, the Healthy, Hunger Free Kids Act of 2010 set new nutritional standards for foods served and sold in schools as a condition of receiving federal funding (USDA 2013). At the state level, licensing standards govern the practices of child care facilities. The National Resource Center for Health and Safety in Child Care and Early Education has identified 47 licensing standards components considered to be high impact for obesity prevention (NRC 2014). Examples include having a written nutrition plan or limiting screen time.

Worksites

Both the amount of time adults spend in the work environment as well as the direct and indirect costs of poor health to employers are the impetus for worksite interventions. Intervening in the worksite to prevent or control obesity has been recommended by the Community Preventive Services Task Force (TFCPS 2009) and the Institute of Medicine (IOM 2012). Systematic reviews had found limited to strong evidence (Anderson et al. 2009; Gudzune et al. 2013; Verweij et al. 2011) for a positive effect on weight status; across all reviews, the most promising interventions appear to include both diet and physical activity and target both the individual at work as well as the worksite environment.

Community-Level Interventions

Expert recommendations about what communities or local government can do to prevent obesity have focused primarily on what should be done in different community-based settings. In addition to those for child care, schools, and worksites, recommendations exist related to healthy food retail and community design to support physical activity, as well as zoning and incentive policies to support physical activity and to address access to healthy and less healthy foods (IOM 2009; IOM 2012; Khan et al. 2009). The evidence that multicomponent interventions implemented across community settings prevent weight gain is limited but evolving. One systematic review that examined community-based childhood obesity interventions concluded that the community interventions that combined diet and physical activity and included schools as one place for intervention were most promising (Bleich et al. 2013). Community-level interventions focusing on weight gain prevention in adults are rare. However, a number of community interventions carried out during the 1970s and 1980s designed to address CVD risk factors, but not weight specifically, demonstrated minimal impact on weight (WHO 1999).

Screening

Clinical screening for obesity is recommended for both adults and children. For adults, the U.S. Preventive Services Task Force (USPSTF) recommends that all patients be screened for obesity and that those with a BMI of 30 kg/m^2 or higher be offered intensive, multicomponent behavioral interventions; the BMI is the recommended screening tool (Moyer 2012). High-intensity interventions are defined as 12 to 26 sessions in year. The multiple components include "behavioral management activities such as setting weight loss goals, improving diet or nutrition and physical activity, addressing barriers to change, self-monitoring, and strategizing how to maintain lifestyle changes" (Moyer 2012).

For children and adolescents aged 6 to 18 years, the USPSTF also recommends screening for obesity and the offering of or referral for intensive counseling and behavioral interventions (USPSTF 2010). As in adults, the screening tool is the BMI. Effective interventions are moderate to high intensity, defined as greater than 25 hours of child or family contact over a 6-month period, and address diet and physical activity as well as behavioral management strategies. Similar to the USPSTF, a 2007 expert committee recommended yearly assessment of weight and height; those children with age- and sex-specific BMI over the 85th percentile are to be followed up with a more comprehensive clinical assessment that includes measurement of pulse, blood pressure, and fasting lipids as well as family history (Barlow 2007). In addition, on the basis of the level of BMI, these children should also receive interventions of varying intensities.

For children, whether to screen in the school setting has also been debated (IOM 2005; Nihiser et al. 2007; Westwood et al. 2007). As of 2012, 25 states had legislation that required schools to monitor BMI (Ruggieri and Bass 2015). A recent review of issues related to screening programs identified concerns about confidentiality, the need for additional resources, and parental issues such as failure to follow up with a health care provider (Ruggieri and Bass 2015). However, benefits for the programs may include providing parents accurate information about their child's weight that can be used to take further action, and using data in the aggregate for surveillance and for justification of school-based interventions.

Treatment

Among adults, weight loss in the range of 5% to 10% of the baseline weight appears to have a positive impact on health (NIH 2013). A review of clinical trials documented an association between weight loss and positive changes in blood pressure, lipid profiles, and blood glucose (NIH 2013). Weight loss also appears to improve function in persons suffering from osteoarthritis (Bliddal et al. 2014). Among high-risk individuals, weight loss also reduces the risk of type 2 diabetes (NIH 2013). For example, the U.S. Diabetes Prevention Program intervention found a lifestyle intervention that recommended a 5% to 7% weight loss and 150 minutes of physical activity per week resulted in a reduced incidence of type 2 diabetes in individuals with prediabetes (Knowler et al. 2002). Whether weight loss affects cardiovascular risk factors among children is less clear. One systematic review found limited evidence for changes in insulin resistance, but not other risk factors with behavioral interventions (Whitlock et al. 2010).

For adults and children alike, a variety of approaches can be used to facilitate weight loss. These include dietary modification, physical activity, behavioral modification, pharmacotherapy, and surgery. The effectiveness and appropriateness of each modality have been extensively reviewed and they are summarized here.

Dietary Modification

A primary goal of dietary modification for weight loss is to reduce energy intake. For adults, on the basis of evidence from randomized controlled weight-loss trials, calorie reductions in the range of 500 to 750 calories per day or total caloric intake of 1,200 to 1,500 calories per day for women and 1,500 to 1,800 calories per day for men facilitate weight losses in the range of one to two pounds per week (NIH 2013). A variety of dietary approaches can lead to caloric reduction and subsequent weight loss. One review found that when caloric reduction is achieved, comparable weight losses over 6 to 12 months are observed for diets that are lower versus higher fat, protein, carbohydrate, or glycemic load; calorie-restricted dietary patterns (e.g., Mediterranean-style) versus energy-restricted, lower fat only; or use meal replacements versus conventional foods (NIH 2013).

Current recommendations for weight loss among children focus on changing dietary patterns to be healthier over the reduction of a specific number of calories (Barlow 2007). However, as in adults, current evidence is not sufficient to recommend a particular macronutrient composition of diets (Hoelscher et al. 2013).

Physical Activity

Because it increases energy expenditure, physical activity has a role in weight loss. The use of physical activity as the sole weight-loss strategy in volumes realistic for most people can result in only modest weight loss for both adults (Donnelly et al. 2009; NIH 1998; PAGAC 2008; Shaw et al. 2006) and children (Kelley et al. 2014). As such, most current recommendations for weight loss include physical activity as an adjunct to diet and calorie reduction (Barlow 2007; Jensen et al. 2014). For adults, physical activity combined with diet improves weight loss more than diet or physical activity alone (NIH 1998; Shaw et al. 2006).

The amount of physical activity needed for weight loss is unclear and, in part, depends on whether and to what extent calories are also being reduced. Current recommendations conclude that adults who are overweight or have obesity initially should aim for 150 minutes per week of moderate-intensity physical activity (Donnelly et al. 2009), and children should aim for one hour or more of daily physical activity (Barlow 2007). However, more may be needed (PAGAC 2008). Even in the absence of weight loss, physical activity appears to improve the risk profile of persons with excess weight (PAGAC 2008; Shaw et al. 2006).

Behavioral Therapies

Weight loss appears to be enhanced when persons develop strategies to address the day-to-day challenges of changing their diet or physical activity habits (NIH 2013; Whitlock et al. 2010) and, thus, inclusion of these strategies is a recommended component of weight-loss therapies for both adults (Jensen et al. 2014; Moyer 2012) and children (USPSTF 2010). Examples of these strategies include tracking of weight, the amount of food consumed, and frequency of physical activity; limiting one's exposure to calorie-dense foods or situations in which they are served; setting realistic and specific goals; and problem-solving (NIH 2013; Moyer 2012).

Pharmacological and Surgical Therapies

Pharmacological and surgical therapies can be used to facilitate weight loss in select individuals. A limited number of drugs are approved by the U.S. Food and Drug Administration for the long-term treatment of obesity including orlistat, lorcaserin, and phentermine plus topiramate–extended release. Orlistat acts by blocking the digestion and absorption of fat by inhibiting gastric lipases (Atkinson 2005) whereas the other two drugs act as appetite suppressants (Yanovski and Yanovski 2014). A recent review concluded that, when combined with lifestyle interventions, use of these drugs results in an average of 3% (orlistat and lorcaserin) to 9% (top-dose phentermine plus topiramate–extended release) additional one-year weight loss relative to placebo (Yanovski and Yanovski 2014). In addition to the drugs previously mentioned, two more recently approved are liraglutide injections and bupropion plus naltrexone. In general, for adults, drugs are recommended as an adjunct to behavioral therapies and for potential use in those who have obesity (BMI≥30) or those with a BMI of 27 or higher with obesity-related comorbidities (Apovian et al. 2015).

The purpose of surgical interventions is to reduce caloric intake by changing the structure of the gastrointestinal tract. This can be done in two ways: changes that limit the intake of food (restrictive) and changes that limit the absorption of nutrients (malabsorptive; DeMaria 2007). Procedures include gastric stapling, adjustable gastric banding, proximal Roux-en-Y gastric bypass, and biliopancreatic diversion. These surgeries result in substantial weight loss (NIH 2013; Paulus et al. 2015) and are associated with a reduction in multiple morbidities in the short term in adolescents (Paulus et al. 2015) and a reduction in comorbidities, particularly related to diabetes, two to three years after the surgery for adults (NIH 2013), with some evidence of longer-term impacts on morbidities and all-cause mortality (Sjöström et al. 2013). However, these procedures are associated with medical complications (DeMaria 2007; Inge 2016) and require a major lifestyle change related to food consumption. For both adults and adolescents, surgical interventions are recommended only for select persons with severe obesity who have been unsuccessful in using less-invasive methods of weight loss (Jensen et al. 2014; Pratt et al. 2009).

Weight-Loss Maintenance

Once weight is lost, an important next step is the long-term maintenance of the loss. However, this is a struggle for many (Douketis et al. 2005; Weiss et al. 2007). Evidence of what strategies help people remain successful comes from clinical trials (NIH 2013; Soleymani et al. 2016); strategies reported from participants in the National Weight Loss Registry, a registry of persons who persons who have lost at least 30 pounds and kept it off for a year (Wing and Phelan 2005); and other observational studies (Donnelly et al. 2009; PAGAC 2008). Similar to the strategies for weight loss, success in weight-loss maintenance appears to be related to continued attention to comprehensive lifestyle modification (NIH 2013; Soleymani et al. 2016). Strategies that may contribute to success include high levels of physical activity in the range of 200 to 360 minutes per week (Donnelly et al. 2009; PAGAC 2008; Wing and Phelan 2005); diet strategies such as planning of meals, continued use of low-calorie or low-fat diets, eating breakfast, or following consistent diet patterns (Soleymani et al. 2016; Wing and Phelan 2005); and behavioral modification techniques such as self-monitoring of caloric intake, physical activity, and weight (Soleymani et al. 2016; Wing and Phelan 2005). Among those who lost weight through formal weight-loss programs, continued provision of a comprehensive program also improved success (NIH 2013; Soleymani et al. 2016).

Examples of Evidence-Based Interventions

As described previously, a number of evidence-based intervention strategies can be used to address weight or obesity at the individual or population level. Four illustrative examples are described here.

At the individual level, one intervention strategy is to work directly with individuals to help them lose weight. Evidence suggests that high-intensity, face-to-face interventions that include prescriptions for moderately reduced-calorie diet and increased physical activity and the use of behavioral strategies to facilitate adherence to these recommendations are effective in achieving this goal (NIH 2013). Examples of this type of intervention include those designed for the Diabetes Prevention Program (Knowler et al. 2002) or the Trials of Hypertension Prevention, Phase II study (Stevens et al. 2001).

At the population level, obesity-related behaviors such as diet or physical activity can be addressed without a specific aim to reduce weight. For example, to increase physical activity, the *Community Guide to Preventive Services* has recommended population-level interventions such as community-wide campaigns, social support programs, interventions to improve access to places for physical activity combined with information outreach, and street-scale or community-scale urban design and land-use policies (GCPS 2013; Heath et al. 2006; Kahn et al. 2002).

Several examples of population-level, place-based interventions exist. An example of a multilevel intervention addressing both diet and physical activity in a single setting is the Nutrition and Physical Activity Self-Assessment for Child Care intervention. This intervention, which targets the child care setting, has as a goal to improve their nutrition and physical activity environments. This is done through staff education as well as by working with staff to assess and change their child care environments and policies as they relate to nutrition and physical activity. A recent study found that the intervention, when delivered by a trained health professional, was associated with improvements in the quality and quantity of nutrition and physical activity policies at the center level as well as a small but significant relative change in BMI z-scores for children when compared with control centers (Alkon et al. 2014).

An example of a population strategy that used a multicomponent approach across multiple settings instead of a single setting was Shape Up Somerville. This intervention, whose goal was to prevent weight gain in young children, was implemented across the school, home, and community settings in Somerville, Massachusetts. It included information interventions such as curriculum changes and education of parents through newsletters and parent nutrition forums as well as interventions designed to change policy and environments such as school wellness policy development, walk-to-school programs, school food service changes, and designation of restaurants with healthier options. The project found a small but significant decline in BMI z-score for children in the intervention community as compared to the control communities in both the first and second year of the intervention (Economos et al. 2007; Economos et al. 2013).

Areas of Future Research

Given the magnitude of the obesity problem, progress in addressing obesity could be enhanced by additional research on the topics of prevention and treatment strategies at the individual and population level, disparities, translation, and information to inform decision-makers. At the individual level, research that further characterizes the complex interactions between behaviors and physiological processes that contribute either to causing obesity or the health effects of obesity will help the development of more targeted interventions. One promising area might include the role of the microbiome in obesity as well as how the microbiome might be changed by diet or clinical interventions. Another topic for research at the individual level that merits further attention is weight loss and treatment. These efforts could include understanding the unique barriers to diet and physical activity among those with morbid obesity as well as understanding how to best clinically manage their obesity-related comorbidities. Among adults and children who successfully lose weight, the health impact of this loss could be enhanced by better identifying the strategies to maintain this weight loss in the long term. Another important question is whether clinical weight-loss interventions could be enhanced by clinical decision supports generated through electronic medical records or by linkages to supports and services within the community.

More information is also needed on effective population prevention strategies across all settings. One topic for further development is identifying the necessary or most effective components of multicomponent or multilevel interventions and whether these components differ depending on the characteristics of the population served in the setting. Another important topic to examine is how federal or state policies might enhance or deter community- or facility-level interventions that alter nutrition and physical activity best practices.

Translational research is another need. Research that examines how to facilitate the wide-scale implementation of interventions determined to be effective in research settings would help practitioners in various settings identify the best ways to adopt, adapt, and maintain use of effective interventions over time. This research could include the development of metrics to assess intervention fidelity and dosage. Another type of translational research could identify effective communication and social marketing strategies for translating scientific information about physical activity, diet, and obesity to the lay public with a particular emphasis on how new communication technologies could be used.

Another area that merits further development is research that addresses the disparities in obesity levels, particularly for African-American and Hispanic populations. Researchers could work with affected groups and community coalitions to better characterize the cultural, behavioral, and environmental barriers to diet and physical activity, and to develop and evaluate interventions to address these barriers. Another topic for disparities research is to examine whether population-level policy and environmental interventions have equal uptake and effectiveness in different subgroups in the population or whether these types of interventions might increase instead of decrease disparities attributable to factors such as social conditions or differences in nutrition and health literacy.

Finally, policymakers and decision-makers would benefit from research that better informs their decision-making. This research could include studies that document natural experiments in policy implementation; evaluate the cost and cost-effectiveness of various options to address the problem of obesity; examine potential co-benefits of health interventions, and examine public perception and support for various intervention options. Additional work in the development of models that compare the relative cost and impact of different intervention options such as those developed for the Childhood Obesity Intervention Cost-Effectiveness Study (CHOICES) (Gortmaker et al. 2015) or that estimate the long-term impacts of interventions on overall health and the economy would also benefit policymakers.

Acknowledgment

The findings and conclusions in this chapter are those of the authors and do not necessarily represent the official position of the Centers for Disease Control and Prevention.

Resources

Centers for Disease Control and Prevention

- Overweight and obesity, http://www.cdc.gov/obesity/index.html
- Healthy Schools, http://www.cdc.gov/healthyschools/obesity/facts.htm
- National Center for Health Statistics, http://www.cdc.gov/nchs/index.htm

National Academies of Sciences, Engineering, and Medicine

- National Academies Press, Institute of Medicine reports, http://www.nap.edu

National Institutes of Health

- Weight-Control Information Network, http://www.niddk.nih.gov/health-information/health-communication-programs/win/Pages/default.aspx

Robert Wood Johnson Foundation

- Childhood obesity, http://www.rwjf.org/en/our-focus-areas/topics/childhood-obesity.html

References

Alkon A, Crowley AA, Neelon SE, et al. Nutrition and physical activity randomized control trial in child care centers improves knowledge, policies, and children's body mass index. *BMC Public Health*. 2014;14:215.

Anderson LM, Quinn TA, Glanz K, et al. The effectiveness of worksite nutrition and physical activity interventions for controlling employee overweight and obesity: a systematic review. *Am J Prev Med*. 2009;37(4):340–357.

Angulo P. Obesity and nonalcoholic fatty liver disease. *Nutr Rev*. 2007;65(6 pt 2):S57–S63.

Apovian CM, Aronne LJ, Bessesen DH, et al. Pharmacological management of obesity: an Endocrine Society clinical practice guideline. *J Clin Endocrinol Metab*. 2015;100(2): 342–362.

Atkinson RL. Management of obesity: pharmacotherapy. In: Kopelman PG, Caterson ID, Dietz WH, eds. *Clinical Obesity in Adults and Children*, 2nd ed. Malden, MA: Blackwell; 2005:380–393.

Aune D, Norat T, Vatten LJ. Body mass index, abdominal fatness and the risk of gallbladder disease. *Eur J Epidemiol*. 2015;30(9):1009–1019.

Barlow SE, Expert Committee. Expert Committee recommendations regarding the prevention, assessment, and treatment of child and adolescent overweight and obesity: summary report. *Pediatrics*. 2007;120(suppl 4):S164–S192.

Bastien M, Poirier P, Lemieux I, Depres JP. Overview of epidemiology and contribution of obesity to cardiovascular disease. *Prog Cardiovasc Dis*. 2014;6(4):369–381.

Berger M, Konty K, Day S, et al. Obesity in K–8 students—New York City, 2006–07 to 2010–11 school years. *MMWR Morb Mortal Wkly Rep*. 2011;60(49):1673–1678.

Bergström A, Pisani P, Tenet V, Wolk A, Adami HO. Overweight as an avoidable cause of cancer in Europe. *Int J Cancer*. 2001;91(3):421–430.

Berrington de Gonzalez A, Hartge P, Cerhan J, et al. Body-mass index and mortality among 1.46 million white adults. *N Engl J Med*. 2010;363(23):2211–2219.

Beuther DA, Sutherland ER. Overweight, obesity, and incident asthma: a meta-analysis of prospective epidemiologic studies. *Am J Respir Crit Care Med*. 2007;175(7):661–666.

Bleich SN, Segal J, Wu Y, Wilson R, Wang Y. Systematic review of community-based childhood obesity prevention studies. *Pediatrics*. 2013;132(1):e201–e210.

Bliddal H, Leeds AR, Christensen R. Osteoarthritis, obesity and weight loss: evidence, hypothesis and horizons—a scoping review. *Obes Rev*. 2014;15(7):578–586.

Blundell JE, Stubbs RJ. Diet composition and the control of food intake in humans. In: Bray GA, Bouchard C, eds. *Handbook of Obesity*. New York, NY: Informa Healthcare; 2007:427–460.

Bogers RP, Bemelmans WJ, Hoogenveen RT, et al. Association of overweight with increased risk of coronary heart disease partly independent of blood pressure and cholesterol levels. *Arch Intern Med*. 2007;167(16):1720–1728.

Bouchard C, Shepard RJ. Physical activity, fitness, and health: the model and key concepts. In: Bouchard C, Shepard RJ, Stephens T, eds. *Physical Activity, Fitness, and Health: International Proceedings and Consensus Statement*. Champaign, IL: Human Kinetics Publishers; 1994:77–88.

Camhi SM, Katzmarzyk PT. Prevalence of cardiovascular risk factor clustering and body mass index in adolescents. *J Pediatr*. 2011;159(2):303–307.

Centers for Disease Control and Prevention (CDC). School health guidelines to promote healthy eating and physical activity. *MMWR Recomm Rep*. 2011;60(RR–5):1–76.

Centers for Disease Control and Prevention (CDC). Overweight and obesity: defining adult overweight and obesity. 2012. Available at: http://www.cdc.gov/obesity/adult/defining.html. Accessed April 16, 2016.

Centers for Disease Control and Prevention (CDC). Overweight and obesity: defining childhood obesity. 2015a. Available at: http://www.cdc.gov/obesity/childhood/defining.html. Accessed April 16, 2016.

Centers for Disease Control and Prevention (CDC). Social determinants of health: know what affects health. 2015b. Available at: http://www.cdc.gov/socialdeterminants. Accessed April 16, 2016.

Centers for Disease Control and Prevention (CDC). Overweight and obesity: obesity prevalence maps. 2016. Available at: http://www.cdc.gov/obesity/data/prevalence-maps.html. Accessed September 20, 2016.

Chu SY, Callaghan WM, Kim SY, et al. Maternal obesity and risk of gestational diabetes mellitus. *Diabetes Care*. 2007a;30(8):2070–2076.

Chu SY, Kim SY, Lau J, et al. Maternal obesity and risk of stillbirth: a meta-analysis. *Am J Obstet Gynecol*. 2007b;197(3):223–228.

Chu SY, Kim SY, Schmid CH, et al. Maternal obesity and risk of cesarean delivery: a meta-analysis. *Obes Rev*. 2007c;8(5):385–394.

Cobb N, Epsey D, King J. Health behaviors and risk factors among American Indians and Alaska Natives, 2000–2010. *Am J Public Health*. 2014;104(suppl 3):S481–S489.

DeMaria EJ. Bariatric surgery for morbid obesity. *New Engl J Med.* 2007;356(21):2176–2183.

Dietary Guidelines Advisory Committee (DGAC). *Scientific Report of the 2015 Dietary Guidelines Advisory Committee: Advisory Report to the Secretary of Health and Human Services and the Secretary of Agriculture, 2015.* Washington, DC: US Department of Agriculture and US Department of Health and Human Services; 2015.

Doll HA, Petersen SEK, Stewart-Brown SL. Obesity and physical and emotional well-being: associations between body mass index, chronic illness, and the physical and mental components of the SF-36 questionnaire. *Obes Res.* 2000;8(2):160–170.

Donnelly JE, Blair SN, Jakicic JM, et al. American College of Sports Medicine Position Stand. Appropriate physical activity intervention strategies for weight loss and prevention of weight regain for adults. *Med Sci Sports Exerc.* 2009;41(2):459–471.

Douketis JD, Macie C, Thabane L, Williamson DF. Systematic review of long-term weight loss studies in obese adults: clinical significance and applicability to clinical practice. *Int J Obes.* 2005;29(10):1153–1167.

Economos CD, Hyatt RR, Goldberg JP, et al. A community intervention reduces BMI z-score in children: Shape Up Somerville first year results. *Obesity.* 2007;15(5):1325–1336.

Economos CD, Hyatt RR, Must A, et al. Shape up Somerville two-year results: a community-based environmental change intervention sustains weight reduction in children. *Prev Med.* 2013;57(4):322–327.

Fardet A, Boirie Y. Associations between food and beverage groups and major diet-related chronic diseases: an exhaustive review of pooled/meta-analyses and systematic reviews. *Nutr Rev.* 2014;72(12):741–762.

Finkelstein EA, DiBonaventura MD, Burgess SM, Hale BC. The costs of obesity in the workplace. *J Occup Environ Med.* 2010;52(19):971–976.

Finkelstein EA, Graham WC, Malhotra R. Lifetime direct medical costs of childhood obesity. *Pediatrics.* 2014;133(5):854–862.

Finkelstein EA, Trogdon JG, Cohen JW, Dietz W. Annual medical spending attributable to obesity: payers and service-specific estimates. *Health Aff (Millwood).* 2009;8(5):w822–w831.

Flegal KM, Graubard BI, Williamson DF, Gail MH. Excess deaths associated with underweight, overweight, and obesity. *JAMA.* 2005;293(15):1861–1867.

Flegal KM, Kit BK, Orpana H, Graubard BI. Association of all-cause mortality with overweight and obesity using standard body mass index categories: a systematic review and meta-analysis. *JAMA.* 2013;309(1):71–82.

Fryar CD, Carroll MD, Ogden CL. *Prevalence of Overweight, Obesity, and Extreme Obesity Among Adults: United States, 1960–1962 Through 2011–2012.* NCHS Health E-Stat.

Hyattsville, MD: National Center for Health Statistics, US Department of Health and Human Services; 2014.

Gortmaker SL, Long MW, Resch SC, et al. Cost effectiveness of childhood obesity interventions: evidence and methods for CHOICES. *Am J Prev Med.* 2015;49(1):102–111.

Gudzune K, Hutfless S, Maruthur N, Wilson R, Segal J. Strategies to prevent weight gain in workplace and college settings: a systematic review. *Prev Med.* 2013;57(4):268–277.

Guide to Community Preventive Services (GCPS). Increasing physical activity. 2013. Available at: http://www.thecommunityguide.org/pa/index.html. Accessed May 30, 2016.

Güngör NK. Overweight and obesity in children and adolescents. *J Clin Res Pediatr Endocrinol.* 2014;6(3):129–143.

Heath GW, Brownson RC, Kruger J, et al. The effectiveness of urban design and land use and transport policies and practices to increase physical activity: a systematic review. *J Phys Act Health.* 2006;3(suppl 1):S55–S76.

Heindel JJ, Newbold R, Schug TT. Endocrine disruptors and obesity. *Nat Rev Endocrinol.* 2015;11(11):653–661.

Hoelscher DM, Kirk S, Ritchie L, Cunningham-Sabo L. Position of the Academy of Nutrition and Dietetics: interventions for the prevention and treatment of pediatric overweight and obesity. *J Acad Nutr Diet.* 2013;113(10):1375–1394.

Inge TH, Courcoulas A, Jenkins TM, et al. Weight loss and health status after bariatric surgery in adolescents. *New Engl J Med.* 2016;374(2):113–123.

Institute of Medicine (IOM). *Preventing Childhood Obesity: Health in the Balance.* Koplan JP, Liverman CT, Kraack VI, eds. Washington, DC: National Academies Press; 2005.

Institute of Medicine (IOM). *Local Government Actions to Prevent Childhood Obesity.* Washington, DC: The National Academies Press; 2009.

Institute of Medicine (IOM). *Early Childhood Obesity Prevention Policies.* Washington, DC: National Academies Press; 2011.

Institute of Medicine (IOM). *Accelerating Progress in Obesity Prevention: Solving the Weight of the Nation.* Washington, DC: National Academies Press; 2012.

Iyengar NM, Hudis CA, Dannenberg AJ. Obesity and cancer: local and systematic mechanisms. *Annu Rev Med.* 2015;66:297–309.

Jensen MD, Ryan DH, Apovian CM, et al. 2013 AHA/ACC/TOS Guideline for the Management of Overweight and Obesity in Adults: a report of the American College of Cardiology/American Heart Association Task Force on Practice Guidelines and the Obesity Society. *Circulation.* 2014;129(25 suppl 2):S102–S138.

Kahn EB, Ramsey LT, Brownson RC, et al. The effectiveness of interventions to increase physical activity: a systematic review. *Am J Prev Med.* 2002;22(suppl 4):73–107.

Kann L, McManus T, Harris WA, et al. Youth Risk Behavior Surveillance—United States, 2015. *MMWR Surveill Summ.* 2016;65(6):1–174.

Kelley GA, Kelley KS, Pate RR. Effects of exercise on BMI *z*-score in overweight and obese children and adolescents: a systematic review with meta-analysis. *BMC Pediatr.* 2014;14:225.

Khan LK, Sobush K, Keener D, et al. Recommended community strategies and measurements to prevent obesity in the United States. *MMWR Recomm Rep.* 2009;58(RR-7):1–26.

Kim DD, Basu A. Estimating the medical care costs of obesity in the United States: systematic review, meta-analysis, and empirical analysis. *Value Health.* 2016;19(5);602–613.

Knowler WC, Barrett-Connor E, Fowler SE, et al. Reduction in the incidence of type 2 diabetes with lifestyle intervention or metformin. *N Engl J Med.* 2002;346(6):393–403.

Langford R, Bonell CP, Jones HE, et al. The WHO health promoting school framework for improving the health and well-being of students and their academic achievement. *Cochrane Database Syst Rev.* 2014;(4):CD008958.

Lau EY, Liu J, Archer E, McDonald SM, Liu J. Maternal weight gain in pregnancy and risk of obesity among offspring: a systematic review. *J Obes.* 2014;2014:524939.

Luppino FA, de Wit LM, Bouvy PF, et al. Overweight, obesity, and depression: a systematic review and meta-analysis of longitudinal studies. *Arch Gen Psychiatry.* 2010;67(3):220–229.

Malik VS, Hu FB. Fructose and cardiometabolic health. What the evidence from sugar-sweetened beverages tells us. *J Am Coll Cardiol.* 2015;66(14):1615–1624.

Malik VS, Pan A, Willett WC, Hu FB. Sugar-sweetened beverages and weight gain in children and adults: a systematic review and meta-analysis. *Am J Clin Nutr.* 2013;98(4):1084–1102.

Mamum AA, Mannan M, Doi SA. Gestational weight gain in relation to offspring obesity over the life course: a systematic review and bias-adjusted meta-analysis. *Obes Rev.* 2014;15(4):338–347.

Marchi J, Berg M, Dencker A, Olander EK, Begley C. Risks associated with obesity in pregnancy, for the mother and baby: a systematic review of reviews. *Obes Rev.* 2015;16(8):621–638.

Marshall SJ, Biddle SJH, Gorely T, Cameron N, Murdey I. Relationships between media use, body fatness and physical activity in children and youth: a meta-analysis. *Int J Obes.* 2004;28(10):1238–1246.

May AL, Freedman D, Sherry B, Blanck HM. Obesity—United States, 1999–2010. *MMWR Suppl.* 2013a;62(3):120–128.

May AL, Pan L, Sherry B, et al. Vital signs: obesity among low-income, preschool-aged children—United States, 2008–2011. *MMWR Morb Mortal Wkly Rep.* 2013b;62(31):629–634.

McGee DL, the Diverse Populations Collaboration. Body mass index and mortality: a meta-analysis based on person-level data from twenty-six observational studies. *Ann Epidemiol.* 2005;15(2):87–97.

Moyer VA; US Preventive Services Task Force. Screening for and management of obesity in adults: US Preventive Services Task Force recommendation statement. *Ann Intern Med.* 2012;157(5):373–378.

National Institutes of Health (NIH). *Clinical Guidelines on the Identification, Evaluation, and Treatment of Overweight and Obesity in Adults: The Evidence Report.* Bethesda, MD: US Department of Health and Human Services, NIH; 1998.

National Institutes of Health (NIH). *Managing Overweight and Obesity in Adults: Systematic Evidence Review From the Obesity Expert Panel, 2013.* Rockville, MD: US Department of Health and Human Services, NIH; 2013.

National Research Council. Committee on Diet and Health. Calories: total macronutrient intake, energy expenditure, and net energy stores. In: *Diet and Health: Implications for Reducing Chronic Disease Risk.* Washington, DC: National Academies Press; 1989:139–158.

National Resource Center for Health and Safety in Child Care and Early Education. *Achieving a State of Healthy Weight: 2014 Update.* Aurora, CO: University of Colorado Denver; 2014.

Nihiser AJ, Lee SM, Wechsler H, et al. Body mass index measurement in schools. *J Sch Health.* 2007;77(10):651–671.

Ogden CL, Carroll MD, Fryar CD, Flegal KM. *Prevalence of Obesity Among Adults and Youth: United States, 2011–2014.* NCHS Data Brief no. 219:1–8. Hyattsville, MD: US Department of Health and Human Services, National Center for Health Statistics; 2015.

Ogden CL, Carroll MD, Lawman HG, et al. Trends in obesity prevalence among children and adolescents in the United States, 1988–1994 through 2013–2014. *JAMA.* 2016; 315(21):2292–2299.

Ogden CL, Flegal KM, Carroll MD, Johnson CL. Prevalence and trends in overweight among US children and adolescents, 1999–2000. *JAMA.* 2002;288(14):1728–1732.

Ogden CL, Lamb MM, Carroll MD, Flegal KM. *Obesity and Socioeconomic Status in Adults: United States, 2005–2008.* Hyattsville, MD: National Center for Health Statistics, US Department of Health and Human Services; 2010. NCHS Data Brief no. 50:1–7.

Patel SR, Hu FB. Short sleep duration and weight gain: a systematic review. *Obesity.* 2008;16(3):643–653.

Patterson E, Ryan PM, Cryan JF, et al. Gut microbiota, obesity and diabetes. *Postgrad Med J.* 2016;92(1087):1–15.

Paulus GF, de Vaan LE, Verdam FJ, Bouvy ND, Ambergen TA, van Heurn LW. Bariatric surgery in morbidly obese adolescents: a systematic review and meta-analysis. *Obes Surg.* 2015;25(5):860–878.

Pedditizi E, Peters R, Beckett N. The risk of overweight/obesity in mid-life and late life for the development of dementia: a systematic review and meta-analysis of longitudinal studies. *Age Aging.* 2016;45(1):14–21.

Physical Activity Guidelines Advisory Committee (PAGAC). *Physical Activity Guidelines Advisory Committee Report, 2008.* Washington, DC: US Department of Health and Human Services; 2008.

Pratt JS, Lenders CM, Dionne EA, et al. Best practice updates for pediatric/adolescent weight loss surgery. *Obesity (Silver Spring).* 2009;17(5):901–910.

Puhl R, Brownell KD. Bias, discrimination, and obesity. *Obes Res.* 2001;9(12):788–805.

Puhl RM, Henderson KE, Brownell KD. Social consequence of obesity. In: Kopelman PG, Caterson ID, Dietz WH, eds. *Clinical Obesity in Adults and Children*, 2nd ed. Malden, MA: Blackwell; 2005:29–45.

Puhl RM, Heuer CA. The stigma of obesity: a review and update. *Obesity (Silver Spring).* 2009;17(5):941–964.

Reilly JJ, Kelly J. Long-term impact of overweight and obesity in childhood and adolescence on morbidity and premature mortality in adulthood: systematic review. *Int J Obes.* 2011;35(7):891–898.

Reilly JJ, Methven E, McDowell ZC, et al. Health consequences of obesity. *Arch Dis Child.* 2003;88(9):748–752.

Robbins JM, Mallya G, Polansky M, Schwarz DF. Prevalence, disparities, and trends in obesity and severe obesity among students in the Philadelphia, Pennsylvania, School District, 2006–2010. *Prev Chronic Dis.* 2012;9:E145.

Ruan H, Xun P, Cai W, He K, Tang Q. Habitual sleep duration and risk of childhood obesity: systematic review and dose-response meta-analysis of prospective cohort studies. *Sci Rep.* 2015;5:16160.

Ruggieri DG, Bass SB. A comprehensive review of school-based body mass index screening programs and their implications for school health: do the controversies accurately reflect the research? *J Sch Health.* 2015;85(1):61–72.

Sarwer DB, Allison KC, Gibbons LM, Tuttman Markowitz J, Nelson DB. Pregnancy and obesity: a review and agenda for future research. *J Women's Health*. 2006;15(6):720–733.

Schwartz AR, Patil SP, Laffan AM, Polotsky V, Schneider H, Smith PL. Obesity and obstructive sleep apnea: pathogenic mechanisms and therapeutic approaches. *Proc Am Thorac Soc*. 2008;5(2):185–192.

Schwimmer JB, Burwinkle TM, Varni JW. Health-related quality of life of severely obese children and adolescents. *JAMA*. 2003;289(14):1813–1819.

Shaw K, Gennat H, O'Rourke P, Del Mar C. Exercise for overweight or obesity. *Cochrane Database Syst Rev*. 2006;(4):CD003817.

Sikorski C, Luppa M, Luck T, Riedel-Heller SG. Weight stigma "gets under the skin"— evidence for an adapted psychological medication framework: a systematic review. *Obesity (Silver Spring)*. 2015;23(2):266–276.

Simmonds M, LLewellyn A, Owen CG, Woolacott N. Predicting adult obesity from childhood obesity: a systematic review and meta-analysis. *Obesity Rev*. 2016;17(2):95–107.

Sisson SB, Krampe M, Anundson K, Castles S. Obesity prevention and obesogenic behavior interventions in child care: a systematic review. *Prev Med*. 2016;87:57–69.

Sjöström L. Review of the key results from the Swedish Obese Subjects (SOS) trial—a prospective controlled intervention study of bariatric surgery. *J Intern Med*. 2013;273(3):219–234.

Soleymani T, Daniel S, Garvey WT. Weight maintenance: challenges, tools and strategies for primary care physicians. *Obes Rev*. 2016;17(1):81–93.

Stevens VJ, Obarzanek E, Cook NR, et al. Long-term weight loss and changes in blood pressure: results of the trials of hypertension prevention, phase II. *Ann Intern Med*. 2001;134(1):1–11.

Stothard KJ, Tennant PW, Bell R, Rankin J. Maternal overweight and obesity and the risk of congenital anomalies: a systematic review and meta-analysis. *JAMA*. 2009;301(6):636–650.

Strazzullo P, D'Elia L, Cairella G, et al. Excess body weight and incidence stroke: meta-analysis of prospective studies with 2 million participants. *Stroke*. 2010;41(5): e418–e426.

Strong WB, Malina RM, Blimkie CJ, et al. Evidence-based physical activity for school-age youth. *J Pediatrics*. 2005;146(6):732–737.

Task Force on Community Preventive Services (TFCPS). A recommendation to improve employee weight status through worksite health promotion programs that target nutrition, physical activity, or both. *Am J Prev Med*. 2009;37(4):358–359.

Tchernof A, Despres JP. Pathophysiology of human visceral obesity: an update. *Physiol Rev.* 2013;93(1):359–404.

Trasande L, Chatterjee S. The impact of obesity on health service utilization and costs in childhood. *Obesity.* 2009;17(9):1749–1754.

US Department of Agriculture (USDA). National School Lunch Program and School Breakfast Program: nutrition standards for all foods sold in school as required by the Healthy, Hunger-Free Kids Act of 2010. Fed Regist. 2013;78(125):39068–39120.

US Department of Health and Human Services (USDHHS). *Physical Activity and Health: A Report of the Surgeon General.* Atlanta, GA: Centers for Disease Control and Prevention, National Center for Chronic Disease Prevention and Health Promotion; 1996.

US Department of Health and Human Services (USDHHS). *The Surgeon General's Vision for a Healthy and Fit Nation.* Rockville, MD: USDHHS, Office of the Surgeon General; 2010.

US Preventive Services Task Force (USPSTF). Screening for obesity in children and adolescents: US Preventive Services Task Force recommendation statement. *Pediatrics.* 2010;125(2):361–367.

Vazquenz G, Duval S, Jacobs DR Jr, Silventoinen K. Comparison of body mass index, waist circumference, and waist/hip ratio in predicting incident diabetes: a meta-analysis. *Epidemiol Rev.* 2007;29:115–128.

Verweij LM, Coffeng J, van Mechelen W, Proper KI. Meta-analyses of workplace physical and dietary behavior interventions on weight control outcomes. *Obes Rev.* 2011;12(6):406–429.

Vincent HK, Heywood K, Connelly J, Hurley RW. Obesity and weight loss in the treatment and prevention of osteoarthritis. *PM R.* 2012;4(5 suppl):S49–S67.

Wahi G, Parkin PC, Beyene J, Uleryk EM, Birken CS. Effectiveness of interventions aimed at reducing screen time in children: a systematic review and meta-analysis of randomized controlled trials. *Arch Pediatr Adolesc Med.* 2011;165(11):979–986.

Wang J, Yang DL, Chen ZZ, Gou BF. Associations of body mass index with cancer incidence among populations, genders, and menopausal status: a systematic review and meta-analysis. *Cancer Epidemiol.* 2016;42:1–8.

Wang Y, Cai L, Wu Y, et al. What childhood obesity prevention programmes work? A systematic review and meta-analysis. *Obes Rev.* 2015;16(7):547–565.

Waters E, de Silva-Sanigorski A, Hall BJ, et al. Interventions for preventing obesity in children. *Cochrane Database Syst Rev.* 2011;(12):CD001871.

Weiss EC, Galuska DA, Khan LK, Gillespie C, Serdula MK. Weight regain in US adults who experienced substantial weight loss, 1999–2002. *Am J Prev Med.* 2007;33(1):34–40.

Weiss R, Taksali SE, Tamorlane WV, et al. Predictors of changes in glucose tolerance in obese youth. *Diabetes Care.* 2005;28(4):902–909.

Westwood M, Fayter D, Hartley S, et al. Childhood obesity: should primary school children be routinely screened? A systematic review and discussion of the evidence. *Arch Dis Child.* 2007;92(5):416–422.

White House Task Force on Childhood Obesity. *Solving the Problem of Childhood Obesity Within a Generation: Report to the President.* 2010. Available at: http://www.letsmove. gov/sites/letsmove.gov/files/TaskForce_on_Childhood_Obesity_May2010_FullReport. pdf. Accessed April 16, 2016.

Whitlock EP, O'Connor EA, Williams SB, Beil TL, Lutz KW. Effectiveness of weight management interventions in children: a targeted systematic review for the USPSTF. *Pediatrics.* 2010;125(2):e396–e418.

Whitlock G, Lewington S, Sherliker P, et al. Body-mass index and cause-specific mortality in 900,000 adults: collaborative analyses of 57 prospective studies. *Lancet.* 2009;373(9669):1083–1096.

Wildman RP, Muntner P, Reynolds K, et al. The obese without cardiovascular risk factor clustering and the normal weight with cardiometabolic risk factor clustering: prevalence and correlates of 2 phenotypes among the US population (NHANES 1999–2004). *Arch Intern Med.* 2008;168(15):1617–1624.

Wing RR, Phelan S. Long-term weight loss maintenance. *Am J Clin Nutr.* 2005;82 (1 suppl):222S–225S.

Woo Baidal JA, Locks LM, Cheng ER, Blake-Lamb TL, Perkins ME, Taveras EM. Risk factors for childhood obesity in the first 1,000 days. *Am J Prev Med.* 2016;50(6):761–779.

Woo JG, Martin LJ. Does breastfeeding protect against childhood obesity? Moving beyond observational evidence. *Curr Obes Rep.* 2015;4(2):207–216.

Woodward-Lopez G, Ritchie LD, Gerstein DE, Crawford PB. *Obesity: Dietary and Developmental Influences.* Boca Raton, FL: CRC Press; 2006.

World Cancer Research Fund, American Institute for Cancer Research. *Food, Nutrition, Physical Activity, and the Prevention of Cancer: A Global Perspective.* Washington, DC: American Institute for Cancer Research; 2007.

World Health Organization (WHO). *Obesity: Preventing and Managing the Global Epidemic.* Geneva, Switzerland: WHO; 1999.

Yanovski SZ, Yanovski JA. Long-term drug treatment for obesity. *JAMA.* 2014;311(1): 74–86.

12

DIABETES

Donald B. Bishop, PhD, Patrick J. O'Connor, MD, MA, MPH,
Renée S.M. Kidney, PhD, MPH, and Debra Haire-Joshu, PhD

Introduction

Diabetes mellitus designates a group of diseases characterized by myriad metabolic abnormalities including abnormal metabolism of glucose. Type 1 diabetes, which comprises 5% to 10% of all diabetes cases, is caused by immune-mediated β-cell destruction, which leads to absolute insulin deficiency and a need for insulin treatment over time (CDC 2014). Type 2 diabetes, which accounts for 90% to 95% of all diagnosed cases of diabetes (CDC 2014) is caused by resistance to insulin and is more common in the elderly and in persons who are overweight (Halban et al. 2014; Samuel et al. 2010; Taylor 2013).

In 2012, approximately 29.1 million people in the United States had diabetes of any type. More than a quarter of these, 8.1 million, are undiagnosed (CDC 2014), in part because type 2 diabetes symptoms develop gradually and it can take several years before severe symptoms occur.

The prevalence of diagnosed diabetes has risen dramatically since the 1950s, with the rate accelerating in the mid-1990s to the 2000s. The National Health Interview Survey shows that only 0.9% of the U.S. population had diabetes in 1958, 2.0% in 1973, 2.6% in 1988, and 4.9% in 2003, and it finally rose to 7.2% in 2013 (DDT 2014). These changes largely mirror increases in the rate of obesity during the 1980s, 1990s, and 2000s, but other factors, including better care for people with diabetes leading to increased lifespan, an aging population, and a population that is growing more diverse, with people from racial and ethnic backgrounds that tend to have higher risks of diabetes, have also contributed (Geiss et al. 2014). Models have been developed to forecast what diabetes prevalence will look like in the future. The expectation that incidence rates will continue to rise with obesity must shape those public health actions we can take now to forestall and ultimately reject that outcome. Using 2010 data as a baseline, with an estimated 14% of adults with prevalent diabetes (diagnosed and undiagnosed), models suggest prevalence will rise. A low-incidence future scenario would predict 24.7% or one in four adults will have diabetes and a higher-incidence scenario, one keeping track with rates observed in the 2000s, predicts that 32.8% or one in three adults will have diabetes in 2050 (Boyle et al. 2010).

Significance

Mortality

Often, the significance of a disease is summed up by talking about mortality related to the disease. Because most people with diabetes do not die as a direct result of it, tracking deaths attributable to diabetes as the primary cause is only telling a fraction of the diabetes story. Diabetes has been ranked among the leading causes of death in the United States since 1932 (Harris 1993), but recently dropped from sixth to seventh (Heron 2015). Listed as the main cause of death on 69,071 certificates in 2010, diabetes was named a main or contributing case in 234,051 death certificates and this number is still only capturing 35% to 40% of the true number of deaths (approximately 600,000) related to diabetes (Heron 2015; McEwen et al. 2006). However, mortality data do provide insight into disparities. In 2012, 2.9% of all deaths were attributed to diabetes as a main cause (rate 23.9 per 100,000 deaths). By race/ethnicity, diabetes ranked the seventh leading cause of death (2.7% of all deaths) for whites, but ranked fourth for blacks (4.4% of deaths), fourth for American Indians/Alaska Natives (6.0% of deaths), and fifth for Asians or Pacific Islanders (3.8% of deaths). The pattern holds when one compares non-Hispanic whites (seventh leading cause; 2.5% of deaths) to Hispanics (fourth leading cause, 5.0% of deaths; Heron 2015).

Mortality for people with diabetes has not followed a simple trajectory, but is currently declining. Between 1970 and 2000, the age-adjusted all-cause mortality rate for men declined from 42.6 of 1,000 to 24.4 of 1,000, similar to trends for the general population. The trend was the opposite for women, with increasing mortality leading to similar rates for men and women by the turn of the century (Gregg et al. 2007a; Gregg et al. 2007b). Rates for both men and women then began a 23% decline through 2006 (Gregg et al. 2012).

High mortality rates for people with diabetes are driven by the burden of multiple complications and comorbid conditions, especially cardiovascular disease (CVD). A pooled analysis of cohort studies compared all-cause mortality rates for people who did not have diabetes, stroke, or myocardial infarction (MI) at the start of the study. Mortality rates for a 60-year-old without any cardiometabolic conditions were 6.8 per 1,000 person-years. For those with diabetes, the mortality rate was 15.6 per 1,000 person years. Adding MI or stroke increased rates to approximately 32.0 per 1,000 person years, and both conditions increased mortality to 59.5 per 1,000 person years. Life expectancy was reduced by 12 years for people with diabetes and one condition and 15 years for those with both conditions (Di Angelantonio et al. 2015). The effect of diabetes on mortality and life expectancy also varies with age. A registry study showed that younger people with diabetes were more likely to die of any cause or CVD as compared to age-matched individuals without diabetes; for CVD-related deaths adjusted hazard ratios were 2.86, 1.93, 1.35, and 0.98 for adults with diabetes who were aged younger than 55 years, 55 to 64 years, 65 to 74 years, and 75 years or older, respectively (Tancredi et al. 2015).

Morbidity

Over the course of the disease, diabetes leads to a variety of disabling and life-threatening complications. For people with diabetes aged older than 65 years, heart disease and stroke were noted on 68% and 16% of their death certificates, respectively; 67% have controlled or uncontrolled high blood pressure (BP); and 28% aged 40 years or older have diabetic retinopathy, the leading cause of blindness. Diabetes is the leading cause of kidney failure, accounting for 44% of new cases. Between 60% and 70% of people with diabetes have mild to severe forms of nervous system failure and 30% aged older than 40 years have impaired sensation in their feet. Diabetic neuropathy is a major contributing cause of lower-extremity amputations with more than 60% of nontraumatic lower-limb amputations occurring in people with diabetes (CDC 2011). The 2010 age-standardized rate for diabetes complications among U.S. adults with diabetes per 1,000 persons is acute MI: 4.5; stroke: 5.3; amputation: 2.8; and end-stage renal disease: 2.0 events. The incidence of blindness is 3.0 to 3.4 events per 1,000 person years, and the risk of amputation is 1.3 to 2.6 events per 1,000 person years, much lower than the incidence of major cardiovascular events (Hippisley-Cox and Coupland 2015). Almost one third of people with diabetes have periodontal disease, and, in general, people with diabetes are more susceptible to severe complications during pregnancy, are vulnerable to life-threatening events such as diabetic ketoacidosis, and are more susceptible to other illnesses and often have a worse prognosis (CDC 2011).

Lower Extremity Amputations

Between 1988 and 2009, the number of diabetes-related nontraumatic lower extremity amputations declined from an age-adjusted 7.3 per 1,000 to 3.2 per 1,000 (Table 12-1). For adults with diabetes, rates increased in the early 1990s and declined between 1997 and 2008 by 8.6% each year, with much of the decline occurring in the population aged 75 years and older. Despite these improvements, the rate among people aged 40 years and older with diabetes is still higher than for adults aged 40 years and older without diabetes (3.9 vs. 0.5 hospitalizations per 1,000 people). Men and blacks have higher rates of hospitalization for nontraumatic lower extremity amputations than women and whites, respectively. The authors posit that higher rates among blacks may be

Table 12-1. Age-Adjusted Hospital Discharge Rates for First-Listed Complications per 1,000 Population with Diabetes, United States, 1988–2009

Complications	Hospital Discharge Rate, per 1,000[a]		
	1988	1998	2009
Diabetes, any-listed	379.4 (450.8)	292.4 (396.2)	223.7 (267.0)
Diabetes	113.3 (73.6)	69.6 (48.9)	13.4 (19.9)
Major CVD	72.3 (142.8)	64.3 (127.8)	43.7 (81.1)[b]
Ischemic heart disease	34.5 (63.6)	25.2 (48.5)	14.7 (26.9)[b]
Heart failure	18.9 (30.4)	19.2 (31.3)	13.4 (19.9)[b]
Stroke	12.5 (18.6)	11.9 (17.7)	7.3 (10.8)[b]
Diabetic ketoacidosis	35.7 (12.6)	25.4 (9.0)	22.0 (7.1)
Lower extremity conditions[c]	19.0 (28.0)	16.9 (23.5)	14.9 (15.7)
Lower extremity amputation	7.3 (8.9)	7.0 (8.2)	3.2 (3.3)

Source: Adapted from CDC (2012).
Note: CVD = cardiovascular disease.
[a]Crude rates are in parentheses.
[b]Data are for 2006.
[c]Lower extremity conditions combines peripheral arterial disease, ulcer/inflammation/infection, and neuropathy.

attributable to higher rates of peripheral artery disease and peripheral neuropathy (Li et al. 2012).

End-Stage Renal Disease

End-stage renal disease, or kidney failure, requiring dialysis or kidney transplant, is a complication strongly linked with diabetes. The U.S. Renal Data System reports that of the 661,648 prevalent U.S. cases in 2013, 39% were attributed to diabetes as a primary cause. About 13% of diabetes-related cases were attributable to type 1 diabetes, and 55.3% occurred among adults aged 22 to 64 years, even though rates increase with age. Prevalence rates have increased over time as a result of better disease management. Age-, sex-, and race/ethnicity-adjusted rates were 1.9 per 1,000 population per year in 2013, with the rate per diabetic population nearly five times higher at 10.8 per 1,000 population per year, with higher rates for blacks or African Americans (21.0) and Hispanics (14.8) compared to whites (8.7). The rate of incident cases has declined since the early 2000s to 0.15 per 1,000 population per year (USRDS 2015).

Disability

Largely because of long-term complications, disability affects 20% to 50% of the diabetic population. A greater percentage of people with diabetes experience physical limitations versus people without diabetes (66% vs. 29%; Ryerson et al. 2003). Mobility disabilities among adults with diabetes increase with age, affecting 59.1%, 68.1%, and 78.7% of those aged 45 to 64 years, 65 to 74 years, and 75 years and older, respectively (Caspersen et al. 2012). A recent meta-analysis demonstrated that people with diabetes had approximately 1.7 times the odds of having a physical limitation—mobility disability, limitations in instrumental activities of daily living (activities including preparing meals or doing housework), or limitations in activities of daily living such as eating or dressing—compared to those without diabetes (Ryerson et al. 2003; Wong et al. 2013). Visual disabilities affect approximately 20% of adults with diabetes aged older than 45 years (Caspersen et al. 2012) and depression can compound disability as shown in data from the 1999 National Health Interview Survey. Functional disability was reported for 51% of people with diabetes, 78% of adults with diabetes and depression, and 24% of adults with neither diabetes nor depression (Egede 2004). Although many different conditions can lead to disability, we will highlight two: arthritis and dementia, because of their high prevalence and potential to influence our aging population.

In national surveys 48.1% (9.6 million) adults with diabetes also report having arthritis. Adults with diabetes are 1.4 times more likely to report having arthritis and 55.0% of them report that their arthritis limited daily activities. Age-adjusted rates of arthritis are highest among non-Hispanic whites and African Americans. Women were more likely to experience arthritis with age-adjusted prevalence of 37.6% (95% confidence interval [CI]=35.7, 39.4) versus 27.8% (95% CI=26.0, 29.5%) for men (Cheng et al. 2012). Arthritis can limit quality of life and prevent people from engaging in physical activity that can aid diabetes management. After correcting for age, only 27.6% of adults with diabetes and arthritis met recommended physical activity levels; 35.1% reported no physical activity. Arthritis rates increased with increasing body mass index (BMI), with age-adjusted rates of 21.7%, 25.7%, and 38.7% for normal, overweight, and obese adults with diabetes, respectively.

A 2013 meta-analysis suggested that 8% of the population-attributable risk for Alzheimer's disease, one specific type of dementia, might be attributed to diabetes (Vagelatos and Eslick 2013). The relationships between diabetes and dementia are complex and still being worked out as exemplified in the following studies. A Canadian medical records study assessed incident diabetes among older adults (interquartile range for age: 69–78 years) and followed them for dementia onset. Individuals with diabetes had 16% higher rates of dementia. Rates were slightly higher for men and individuals in the lowest income category. Risk of dementia was greatest for adults with vascular problems: cerebrovascular disease (hazard ratio [HR]=2.03), peripheral vascular disease (HR=1.47), and chronic kidney disease (HR=1.44). Medications modified risk, with statins causing a reduction (HR=0.78).

Associations between hypoglycemia and dementia may not indicate a causal relationship, but might be a marker for cognitive status (e.g., poor cognition leads to failure to eat, or taking too much medication leads to hypoglycemia; Haroon et al. 2015). A systematic review of diabetes and Alzheimer's disease reported a pooled adjusted risk ratio of 1.57 (95% CI=1.41, 1.75) and strong interactions with smoking and hypertension. Overall, studies examining the effect of Apo-ε4 genotype on risk found a positive association, and significant heterogeneity was found. Pathology findings suggest that cerebrovascular pathology plays a role in Alzheimer's development (Vagelatos and Eslick 2013).

Mental Health

Mental health and diabetes are strongly intertwined, and efforts to address diabetes increasingly focus on addressing both conditions. People with type 2 diabetes are more likely to experience major depressive disorder over their lifetime than people without type 2 diabetes (Penckofer et al. 2014). Approximately one in four people with type 2 diabetes have clinically significant depression (Semenkovich et al. 2015); evidence suggests that diabetes can lead to depression and that people with depression are more likely to develop diabetes (Snoek et al. 2015; Tabak et al. 2014). Diabetes is also common among people with schizophrenia and psychoses. A literature review showed the median diabetes prevalence among people with schizophrenia across studies was 15% and that people with psychoses were twice as likely to have diabetes compared to people with other mental illnesses, and two to five times as likely as the general population (Ward and Druss 2015).

Increased risk may be inherent with schizophrenia and other psychoses, but some medications used to manage serious mental illness also contribute to increased risk (Ward and Druiss 2015). Whether use of antidepressive medications increases diabetes risk is an unresolved question, but medication use is associated with greater odds of having diabetes. Long-term outcomes for individuals with depression and schizophrenia are often poorer. Individuals with comorbid diabetes and psychoses are treated less frequently than others with diabetes, quality of care is lower, and outcomes including hospitalizations and mortality are more common (Ward and Druss 2015). Depressive symptoms can contribute to poorer self-care and worsening diabetes (Snoek et al. 2015). Occurring with depression or independently, diabetes distress is an emotional response toward negative stressors having to do with having diabetes. Severity of diabetes distress is correlated with treatment burden and can influence self-care behaviors and health of people with diabetes.

Economic Costs

Diabetes has a negative economic impact for individuals and is an exceptionally costly disease from the societal point of view. The estimated direct medical costs of diabetes in 2012 were $176 billion, an increase of 48% over the 2007 estimate. An estimated 23% of U.S. health care expenditures were for care of the 8% of people with diabetes. Costs often focus on older adults for whom diabetes is more common, but people aged younger than 65 years accounted for 40% of total health care expenditures, despite the fact that their average per capita health care expenditures are half those of adults aged 65 years and older. Accounting for differences in age and sex, medical expenditures were 2.3 times greater for people with diabetes ($13,741 vs. $5,853; ADA 2013). Indirect costs are difficult to accurately estimate, but a conservative estimate put the annual cost of absences, reduced performance or attendance at work, reduced labor force participation, and mortality related to diabetes at $68.6 billion in 2012 (ADA 2013).

Excess medical spending for people with diabetes increased from $2,588 per person in the late 1980s to $5,378 per person in 2011. Prescription medications accounted for 55% of the increase, whereas costs of inpatient visits, outpatient visits, and emergency department or other spending contributed 24%, 15%, and 6%, respectively (Zhuo et al. 2015a). The increased spending on prescriptions is attributable to increased use (Schmittdiel et al. 2014; Zhuo et al. 2015b) and increased cost for medications (Zhuo et al. 2015b). Rates of hospitalization and emergency department use have decreased, but the visits themselves are costlier (Zhuo et al. 2015b).

Pathophysiology

Type 1 diabetes is a disorder characterized by an inability to produce insulin because of autoimmune destruction of the β cells in the pancreas. It is a disease that most often starts in childhood but can also occur in adults of any age. Classic symptoms include polydipsia, polyphagia, and polyuria alongside overt hyperglycemia and an immediate need for exogenous insulin replacement (Atkinson 2012). The manifestation of type 1 diabetes is preceded by the development of autoantibodies, marking the loss of immunological tolerance to β cells. Once two or more diabetes-related autoantibodies are present, the progression to type 1 diabetes is 75% over 10 years and all but certain in 20 years (Ziegler et al. 2013).

The etiology and pathophysiology of type 2 diabetes is complex. In general, people with type 2 diabetes have insulin resistance, which means they cannot make efficient use of insulin in the muscle or liver, despite sufficient insulin production early in the course of the disease. Obesity and hyperinsulinemia are characteristic of this early phase, and obesity accentuates the insulin resistance (Samuel et al. 2010; Taylor 2013). Over time, the pancreas fails to produce enough insulin to compensate adequately for the insulin resistance and hyperglycemia begins (Halban et al. 2014). Type 2 diabetes is a progressive disease, and response to treatment varies over time. Clinical application of advances in genetics have been slow in coming, and currently the mechanism of action that accounts for high remission rates of type 2 diabetes after bariatric surgery are incompletely understood.

Occurrence of gestational diabetes mellitus (GDM) is associated with increased risk of subsequent type 2 diabetes. Between 20% and 60% of women who had GDM will progress to diabetes within 5 to 10 years (Tabak et al. 2012). Risk factors for GDM include older maternal age, family history of type 2 diabetes, GDM in a previous pregnancy, and adiposity, with step-wise increases in risk among overweight, obese, and morbidly obese women (Zhang and Ning 2011).

A recent study (Bardenheier et al. 2015b) examined GDM prevalence trends by age, state, and region for 19 states and by race/ethnicity for 12 states. Between 2000 and 2010, the age-standardized prevalence of GDM increased from 3.71 to 5.77 per 100 deliveries (relative increase 56%). In the 12 states reporting race and ethnicity, the relative increase was highest for Hispanics (66%). Gestational diabetes can result in significant adverse outcomes for the fetus, which are only partially preventable through appropriate screening and intervention (Landon et al. 2009). Current controversy about the best way to diagnosis GDM has led to divergent recent estimates of its prevalence in pregnancy (Metzger et al. 2010; Ryan 2011).

Prediabetes, or blood glucose levels that are higher than normal, but not high enough to be considered diabetes, is defined by a fasting plasma glucose (FPG) of 100 to 125 milligrams per deciliter (mg/dL), or an glycated hemoglobin test (HbA1c) of 5.7% to 6.4%, in the absence of overt diabetes. Impaired glucose tolerance (IGT) is defined as a two-hour plasma glucose level between 140 and 199 mg/dL on a 75-gram oral glucose tolerance test (ADA 2016b). Both are associated with insulin resistance and β-cell dysfunction, abnormalities that begin before glucose changes are detected (Tabak et al. 2012). Prediabetes is a strong risk factor for the future development of diabetes and is also associated with early nephropathy, small-fiber neuropathy, diabetic retinopathy, and increased risk of macrovascular disease (Tabak et al. 2012). Prevalence of prediabetes was an estimated 38% (95% CI=34.7, 41.3) of U.S. adults in 2011 to 2012. Prediabetes rates increase with age and are 28.2%, 44.9%, and 49.5% in U.S. adults who are aged 20 to 44 years, 45 to 64 years, and 65 years or older, respectively (Menke et al. 2015).

Prediabetes progresses to overt diabetes at rates depending on demographic and clinical factors. Meta-analyses suggest that about 5% to 10% of people with prediabetes develop diabetes each year; however, risk is not equal across all people with prediabetes. Rates were higher for people with both impaired fasting glucose (IFG) and IGT, who experienced a 15% to 19% annual incidence of diabetes compared to 4% to 6% and 6% to 9% for isolated IGT and isolated IFG, respectively (Tabak et al. 2012). Among Dutch adults aged 45 years or older, risk of progression from prediabetes to diabetes was 74% (95% CI=67.6, 80.5) over the person's lifetime, with risk increasing with increasing BMI (Ligthart et al. 2016). The most recent data available did not find statistically significant differences in prediabetes prevalence by gender or by race/ethnicity (Menke et al. 2015).

Diabetes complications may be classified as macrovascular or microvascular complications. Macrovascular complications include accelerated atherosclerosis resulting in MI, stroke, or peripheral vascular disease. Up to 50% of adults with diabetes will ultimately die of macrovascular events or their sequellae, and a study of the Danish National Diabetes Cohort demonstrated that there were more than 45 macrovascular deaths for every one renal death from 1995 to 2008 (Hansen et al. 2012). Drivers of excess macrovascular complications in diabetes include high BP, high low-density lipoprotein cholesterol, low high-density lipoprotein cholesterol, smoking, increased fibrinogen levels, and plasminogen activator inhibitor levels, which increase the tendency of the blood to clot, and many other factors. Microvascular complications include disorders of the eye, kidney, and foot, which increase risk of blindness, renal failure, and amputation.

The age-adjusted relative risk in 2010 for certain major complications based on the presence or absence of diabetes was as follows: acute MI, 1.8 (95% CI=1.3, 2.3); stroke, 1.5 (95% CI=1.1, 2.0); lower extremity amputation, 10.5 (95% CI=6.0, 15.0), and end-stage renal disease, 6.1 (95% CI=5.7, 6.3; Gregg et al. 2014b). This compares well to 1990 when relative risks for these same complications were calculated at 3.8 (95% CI=3.3, 4.2); 3.1 (95% CI=2.7, 3.5); 18.8 (95% CI=15.1, 22.6); and 13.7 (95% CI=12.6, 14.9), respectively (Gregg et al. 2014b). Hospital discharge rates for most macrovascular and microvascular complications have dropped substantially in recent decades (see Table 12-1).

Effective multifactorial therapy can substantially reduce complications and mortality in type 1 diabetes (Nathan et al. 2009) and type 2 diabetes

(Gaede et al. 2008). In the aggregate, these data suggest that adequate BP, lipid, glucose, and tobacco control, plus appropriate aspirin use, are important, and that glucose-control goals should be individualized for type 2 diabetes, including less intensive glycemic goals for patients with severe or frequent hypoglycemia (Ismail-Beigi et al. 2010). Large randomized trials in type 2 diabetes found that near-normal glycemic control achieved through pharmacological means over a 3.5- to 5-year period reduced nonfatal cardiovascular events 10% to 15%, but failed to reduce mortality (Patel et al. 2008). Of particular concern is a large North American randomized trial that showed more intensive glucose control using then-current glucose-lowering medications was associated with a 22% increased risk of death (Gerstein et al. 2008; Zoungas et al. 2014).

Although many patients fail to reach HbA1c, BP, or low-density lipoprotein cholesterol goals, there has been impressive progress in diabetes care in the past 10 years, and the median HbA1c level nationally is now approximately 7% (Ali et al. 2013). With respect to the cost-effectiveness of diabetes treatment, a Centers for Disease Control and Prevention (CDC) analysis reported in 2002 that the cost per quality-adjusted life year (QALY) of life saved by aggressive HbA1c control was $41,384, but increased with age at diagnosis and ranged from about $9,600 for patients aged 25 to 34 years to $2.1 million for patients aged 85 to 94 years. By comparison, the cost-effectiveness ratio for intensive hypertension control was $1,959 per QALY (cost-saving), and low-density lipoprotein cholesterol control with statins is close to cost-saving if a generic statin is used (CDC Diabetes Cost-Effectiveness Group 2002).

Descriptive Epidemiology

High-Risk Populations

Not everyone is equally likely to develop diabetes or to experience comorbidities associated with the disease. Risk factors for developing type 2 diabetes are well-defined and form the basis of recommendations for diabetes and prediabetes screening (ADA 2016b; Siu 2015). They include older age, high-risk race/ethnicity, family history of diabetes, overweight and obese BMI, low levels of physical activity, cardiovascular risk factors, and antecedent diagnoses of prediabetes or gestational diabetes (ADA 2016b; Siu 2015). The impact of other risk factors such as low income or educational status may be independent, or may be mediated through higher rates of smoking or biological risk factors.

Age

The strongest risk factor for diabetes is aging, reflecting in part the changes in insulin sensitivity and other physiological processes that accompany aging. Unadjusted diabetes prevalence estimates for 2012 showed increases with age: 4.1%, 16.2%, and 25.9% for adults aged 20 to 44 years, 45 to 64 years, and 65 years and older, respectively (CDC 2014). Diabetes incidence rates were 3.6, 12.0, and 11.5 new cases per 1,000 people for adults aged 20 to 44 years, 45 to 64 years, and 65 years and older, respectively, in 2012. Absolute rates of hospitalization and mortality increase with age independent of diabetes status, so comparisons to non-diabetic populations are needed to assess the relative risk of hospitalization or mortality attributable to diabetes. Diabetes results in proportionally more mortality at younger ages versus older ages (e.g., 50 vs. 70 years; Hansen et al. 2012; Tancredi et al. 2015).

Race and Ethnicity

The prevalence of diagnosed diabetes varies widely in the United States by race and ethnicity, ranging from 7.6% for whites to 15.9% for American Indians/Alaska Natives (Selvin et al. 2014). Increased prevalence and incidence of type 2 diabetes in populations of color are reflected across all age ranges and are consistent both for diagnosed and undiagnosed diabetes (The et al. 2013; Becerra and Becerra 2015; Hamman et al. 2014). People of color also have lower rates of achieving recommended diabetes care goals (AHRQ 2015), higher hospitalizations rates for diabetes-related comorbidities, and higher mortality rates.

Family History

Family history of diabetes is a strong risk factor for diabetes. Diabetes prevalence was 30% for persons with high familial risk, 14.8% for moderate risk, and 5.9% for average risk, corresponding with adjusted diabetes rates that were 2.4 and 5.8 times greater for people with moderate and high familial risk, respectively (Valdez et al. 2007). Pointing toward a role for environmental factors as well as genetic factors driving familial risk is the observation that risk is also shared among spouses; a recent study showed that spousal diabetes associated with an odds ratio (OR) of 2.32 (95% CI = 1.87, 3.98) for diabetes or prediabetes after adjustment for BMI (Leong et al. 2014). Although shared environmental and genetic characteristics contribute to the predictive power of family history, recent work suggests that many of the factors explaining the association may be unknown (Scott et al. 2013).

Income

Low income is consistently associated with increased diabetes risk and with poorer clinical outcomes. In the United States in 2010, the age-standardized prevalence of diagnosed diabetes was 10.6% for poor, 9.6% for near-poor, 7.6% for middle-income, and 6.4% for high-income adults (Beckles and Chou 2013). Similar trends are observed for low education and other indicators of low socioeconomic position (Beckles and Chou 2013). Longitudinal studies support the association between low income and diabetes incidence, and suggest that this is more consistent for women than for men (Demakakos et al. 2012; Insaf et al. 2014; Maty et al. 2005; Robbins et al. 2005; Smith et al. 2011). In some studies, lower income during childhood and adulthood both exert independent effects on risk (Demakakos et al. 2012; Insaf et al. 2014; Maty et al. 2005; Smith et al. 2011; Stringhini et al. 2013).

Diabetes may affect the ability of some people to work and earn income. In the United States, people with diabetes are 40% more likely to leave the workforce early (Rumball-Smith et al. 2014) and more likely to stop working because of poor health or to work under disability status (Tunceli et al. 2005). Community income is also related to diabetes outcomes; 2012 rates of hospital admission rates for uncontrolled diabetes without complications were 40 per 100,000 adult population in areas with median incomes in the lowest quartile, as compared to 20, 10, and slightly less than 10 for the second, third, and fourth quartiles of median income (AHRQ 2015). This association may reflect correlation between individual and community-level income.

Obesity

Overweight and obesity are key drivers of diabetes risk and the global diabetes epidemic (Hu 2011) and are potentially modifiable risk factors (see Chapter 11).

Geographic Distribution

In the United States, diabetes prevalence varies significantly by region. The Northeast has the lowest age-adjusted prevalence at 6.3%, followed by the West (7.3%), Midwest (7.9%), and South (8.8%). Prevalence is significantly higher in all three regions as compared to the Northeast (Beckles et al. 2013).

Recently, scientists at the CDC proposed the existence of a diabetes belt, similar to the stroke belt in which states have high age-adjusted stroke mortality (Barker et al. 2011). The diabetes belt of 644 counties in the southern United States includes all of Mississippi; most of Alabama, Tennessee, and West Virginia; large portions of Louisiana, Kentucky, Georgia, and South Carolina; and parts of Arkansas, Texas, Virginia, and North Carolina. In 2007 to 2008, the prevalence of diabetes in these counties was 11.7% compared with 8.5% for the rest of the country. Diabetes risk factors that are more common in these counties include more non-Hispanic African Americans (23.8% vs. 8.6%), higher rates of obesity (32.9% vs. 26.1%), and fewer people with a college degree (24.1% vs. 34.3%). Models suggest that 30% of the excess risk for people living in the diabetes belt is attributed to modifiable risk factors (Barker et al. 2011).

Diabetes prevalence is also higher in U.S. counties with the lowest median incomes. Factors correlated with lower incomes that may explain some of the relationship includes a high degree of food insecurity and increased sedentariness. In the United States, 43% of individuals with incomes below the poverty line are considered food-insecure and many impoverished areas lack access to fresh food. Higher levels of violence may increase sedentary behavior and limit outdoor physical activity, and economically deprived communities may lack geographic access to parks and economic access to exercise facilities (Levine 2011).

Spatial correlation for diabetes-associated behaviors or outcomes has also been reported. Margolis et al. (2011) demonstrated that the incidence of lower-extremity limb amputation among Medicare beneficiaries is clustered by hospital referral region and appears unrelated to the cost of care for either lower extremity limb amputation or diabetes. Lower extremity limb amputations appeared to be less common in hospital referral regions with lower diabetes prevalence but more common in hospital referral regions with generally lower socioeconomic status, a higher percentage of African Americans, higher prevalence of diabetic foot ulcer, and higher rate of mortality among those with diabetic foot ulcer, but these differences could not fully explain the effect of location (Margolis et al. 2011).

Although these spatial patterns are important to understand, it is also important to develop models that explore the contribution of risk factors at both the individual and community levels. For example, in the Boston Area Community Health (BACH) study, nonrandom spatial patterning of type 2 diabetes prevalence was observed in Boston neighborhoods in addition to higher diabetes rates for black and Hispanic residents compared to their white counterparts. Individual demographics explained 22% of the neighborhood-to-neighborhood variation in type 2 diabetes incidence. Neither the racial disparities nor much of the neighborhood variation was explained by census-tract level measures of poverty or other neighborhood characteristics (Piccolo et al. 2015).

In contrast, the Multi-ethnic Study of Atherosclerosis (MESA) utilized a model that did not focus on racial disparities and used both Geographic Information Systems data and individual-level assessments of nearness of healthy food and other neighborhood characteristics to describe neighborhoods and observe neighborhood effects on type 2 diabetes incidence. In adjusted models, living in a neighborhood with greater physical activity options was associated with lower diabetes incidence as was having greater exposure to healthy food. The results were observed for self-reported metrics of neighborhood food and physical activity environment from community members and not Geographic Information Systems measures, suggesting that the metrics capture different information (Christine et al. 2015).

Time Trends

This chapter opened by describing the dramatic increase in diabetes, mostly driven by type 2 diabetes, since the 1950s. This is still the main story and public health challenge for diabetes. We addressed the causes: improved care for people with diabetes, which increases lifespan; demographic changes, including our aging population and our increasingly diverse population; and rising obesity. Obesity is a reflection of our modern lifestyles characterized by overnutrition and low levels of physical activity (Hu 2011). Diabetes prevalence increased between 1998 and 2012 for all ages, men and women, all races/ethnicities, all levels of educational attainment, and across income levels. When stratified by BMI, the proportion of adults with diabetes only increased for those with a BMI of 30 or greater (18.0% in 1988–1994 vs. 20.1 in 2011–2012; Menke et al. 2015). In recent years, increased diabetes screening and more inclusive diagnostic criteria for diabetes may have contributed to increased estimates of diabetes prevalence. The rate of undiagnosed diabetes declined from 40.3% in 1988 through 1994 to 31.0% in 2011 through 2012, but the decline was limited to adults aged 45 to 64 years and those aged 65 years and older (Menke et al. 2015).

Recent national surveillance data suggest that national diabetes prevalence plateaued in the late 2000s, ending a decades-long rise. Incidence peaked around 2008 and has since decreased (Geiss et al. 2014). The same pattern was also observed among a large group of patients enrolled in managed care organizations, the Surveillance, Prevention, and Management of Diabetes Mellitus (SUPREME-DM) study (Nichols et al. 2015). These changes may be related to the national obesity rate plateauing between 2003 to 2004 and 2011 to 2012 (Geiss et al. 2014) Widespread recent use of HbA1c as a diagnostic test may also decrease the number of diabetes cases detected (Geiss et al. 2014; Nichols et al. 2015). Although diabetes incidence appears to have declined overall, it was still increasing as of 2012 for non-Hispanic Black and Hispanic adults, and especially among adults aged 20 to 44 years and adults who completed less than a high-school education (Geiss et al. 2014).

Diabetes in Pregnancy

Diabetes in pregnancy, whether pre-existing diabetes or new-onset GDM, is on the rise. An analysis of hospitalization data from 19 states showed overall age-standardized rates of pre-gestational diabetes (diabetes diagnosed before pregnancy) increased across all ages and race/ethnicity groups between 2000 and 2010 from 0.65 per 100 deliveries to 0.89 per 100 deliveries. The largest changes were observed in many Western states (Bardenheier et al. 2015a). This statistic coupled with national data showing that adults aged 20 to 44 years are the least likely age group to have blood sugar levels in control and that this group has not shown improvements in blood sugar control over time (Ali et al. 2013) paints a disturbing picture. Uncontrolled diabetes in pregnancy is associated with severe outcomes, including birth defects. For example, pregnancies complicated by pre-gestational diabetes have 3.8 times the odds of having congenital heart defects (Simeone et al. 2015). Improving glycemic control among these women could prevent about 2,700 cases of congenital heart defects annually (Simeone et al. 2015).

Age-adjusted rates of GDM rose between 2000 and 2010 from 3.71 to 5.77 per 100 deliveries between 2000 and 2010 in the 19 states with available data. The greatest increases were observed in the Midwest and West, increasing 69% and 64%, respectively. Gestational diabetes increased for all ages, including female adolescents and women aged 15 to 19 years and 20 to 24 years, who experienced increases of around 50% to 60%. Not all of the increase in GDM was attributable to older average maternal ages at delivery. Rates increased for all race/ethnicity groups by 4.1% from 2000 to 2010. The challenges associated with GDM pregnancies also increased: the proportion with pre-eclampsia increased from 9.8% to 11.0% and the proportion complicated by pre-pregnancy hypertension rose (Bardenheier et al. 2015b).

Diabetes among Children and Youth

Diabetes among children and youth has grown more common in the United States during the past decade according to the SEARCH for Diabetes in Youth Study (SEARCH). Between 2001 and 2009, the prevalence of any form of diabetes increased from 1.8 to 2.2 per 1,000 youth, meaning that approximately 192,000 children or youth have diabetes in the United States. Both type 1 and type 2 diabetes increased: 21.1% (95% CI=15.6, 27.0) for type 1 to a rate of 1.93 per 1,000 for children and youth of all ages and 30.5% (95% CI=17.3, 45.1%) for type 2 to a rate of 0.46 per 1,000 youth aged 10 to 19 years (Dabelea et al. 2014).

Similarly, incidence also increased between 2001 and 2009, with an estimated 18,400 U.S. children diagnosed with type 1 and 5,000 with type 2 diabetes every year, up from 15,000 and 3,700, respectively. Type 1 incidence increased for all age groups except those aged zero to four years. Increases in type 1 diabetes were especially notable among non-Hispanic whites aged five years and older (Hamman et al. 2014). Minority youth aged 10 to 19 years were more likely to be diagnosed with type 2 diabetes than their non-Hispanic white counterparts. Incidence rates were 1.20 per 1,000 among American Indian youth, 1.06 per 1,000 for Black youth, 0.79 per 1,000 for Hispanic youth, and 0.17 per 1,000 for white youth (Dabelea et al. 2014). Among American Indian/Alaska Natives aged 15 to 19 years who were diagnosed with diabetes, 80% of diabetes diagnoses were type 2 diabetes compared to 35% of new diagnoses among Hispanic youth and 5.5% among non-Hispanic white youth (Pettitt et al. 2014).

Because the causes of type 1 diabetes are not well-understood, reasons behind the increase are unclear. However, increases have been reported around the world (citations within Hamman et al. 2014). Type 2 diabetes among youth represents a different phenomenon. Several decades ago, type 2 diabetes among youth was not reported. The increasing rates of type 2 diabetes among youth mirror increases among adults. Youth who are Hispanic or non-white are more likely to be affected, just as minority adults are. Income and socioeconomic status factors also contribute as they do in adults; in the SEARCH study 60% to 70% of youth with diabetes, especially those with type 2 diabetes, came from low-resourced homes. In addition, disparities in diabetes care such as BP checks, HbA1c testing, and eye examinations, as well as increased complication rates, are evident among minority youth (Hamman et al. 2014), raising concerns about the future health of these individuals. A recent report showed that individuals diagnosed with type 2 diabetes during youth or early adulthood (ages 15 to 30 years) have higher standardized mortality ratios than adults diagnosed between the ages of 40 and 50 years (Al-Saeed et al. 2016).

Estimates of Prevalence Versus Lifetime Risk for Diabetes

Increasing prevalence of diabetes is often the soundbite that we hear. In fact, we closed the introduction of this chapter with these numbers: increasing diabetes incidence could result in as many as one in three adults having diabetes in 2050 (Boyle et al. 2010). It only tells part of the story; examining lifetime risk is also important as it quantifies at the individual level the number of lives touched by this condition. For individuals aged 20 years in 2010, the estimated risk of developing diabetes during their lifetime is 40.2% for men and 39.3% for women, compared with 20.4% and 26.7%, for men and women who were aged 20 years in the late 1980s (Gregg et al. 2014a). Diagnosis of diabetes at a young age, 20 years, is expected to decrease life expectancy by six to seven years for both men and women, a smaller reduction in life expectancy than before. The reduction in life expectancy decreases with increasing age at diabetes diagnosis. However, because more people are living with diabetes, the total number of years spent living with diabetes has increased by 156% for men and 70% for women overall (Gregg et al. 2014a).

Causes

Modifiable Risk Factors

Previous sections described known risk factors for type 2 diabetes and how both type 1 and type 2 diabetes are distributed spatially, which may be correlated with these risk factors. In this section, we focus attention on known risk factors for type 2 diabetes that are modifiable at individual, community, and societal levels through individual behavior change, changing societal norms, and establishing and enforcing policies that promote healthy behaviors. Table 12-2 highlights some examples that fall into three broad

Table 12-2 Risk Factors for Diabetes with Relative Risk

Risk Factor	Unit of Comparison	Relative Risk for Diabetes	Source
Obesity and metabolic syndrome	Metabolically unhealthy obese	8.9	Bell et al. 2014
	Metabolically healthy obese	4.0	
Women with gestational diabetes (GDM)	GDM status	7.4	Bellamy et al. 2009
Dietary glycemic load (GL)	100-g increment of GL per day	1.5	Livesey et al. 2013
Smoking	Heavy (≥ 20 cigarettes/day)	1.6	Willi et al. 2007
	Light (< 20 cigarettes/day)	1.3	
Low birthweight and later lifestyle	Per kg lower birthweight	1.5	Li et al. 2015b
	Per unhealthy lifestyle factor	2.1	
	Per birthweight and lifestyle factor	2.9	
Fasting insulin when young	3–6-year-olds 1-SD increase fasting insulin	2.0	Sabin et al. 2015
Higher body mass index (BMI) when young	9–18-year-olds with 1-SD increase BMI	1.5	
Sleep (quality and quantity)	Difficulty maintaining sleep	1.8	Cappuccio et al. 2010
	Difficulty initiating sleep	1.6	
	Long duration (> 8–9 hours/night)	1.5	
	Short duration (< 5–6 hours/night)	1.3	
High systolic blood pressure (SBP)	20 mm Hg higher per unit SBP	1.6	Emdin et al. 2015
High diastolic blood pressure (DBP)	10 mm Hg higher per unit DBP	1.5	
Low socioeconomic position	Low education or income	1.4	Agardh et al. 2011
Television	Two hours of TV per day	1.2	Grontved et al. 2011
Depression	Use of antidepressants	1.3	Pan et al. 2010

categories: overweight and obesity, lifestyle factors, and socioeconomic position and the factors that travel with it.

Addressing obesity across the lifespan and not just in adulthood is needed. People who are overweight are more likely to develop diabetes (Bell et al. 2014) and that risk appears to be established early, as lower birthweight (Li et al. 2015b) and higher BMIs in childhood predict diabetes status (Sabin et al. 2015). Many lifestyle factors contribute to obesity. Diets including greater consumption of sugar-sweetened beverages (Hu 2011) or higher sugar content in one's overall diet are associated with diabetes risk (Livesey et al. 2013). Smoking also increases diabetes risk in a dose-dependent manner (Willi et al. 2007). Lower levels of physical activity are associated with higher diabetes rates (Hu 2011); unsurprisingly, sedentary behaviors such as TV watching are associated with diabetes (Grontved and Hu 2011). Duration and quality of sleep influences metabolic pathways; too much or too little sleep is associated with increased diabetes risk (Cappuccio et al. 2010). Finally, socioeconomic position linked to income, educational attainment, and health literacy predicts risk (Agardh et al. 2011) and vice versa. Socioeconomic position also influences the ability to engage in physical activity and consume healthier foods and can, in turn, increase diabetes risk or the development of complications.

There is strong evidence that influencing risk factors can reduce diabetes risk in populations of individuals at increased risk of developing diabetes: people with prediabetes and women with a history of GDM (7.4-fold increased risk; Bellamy et al. 2009). Healthier diets and increasing physical activity to 150 minutes per week can lead to a 58% reduction in diabetes risk over three years among adults with prediabetes. Treatment with metformin, which improves insulin action in the liver to reduce glucose formation, also reduces risk, by about 31% overall (Knowler et al. 2002), with most of the effect concentrated among people with a very high risk of developing diabetes (Sussman et al. 2015).

Population-Attributable Risk

Population-attributable risk aims to assess the degree to which each risk factor contributes to overall diabetes risk in the population. Estimates of population-attributable risk for diabetes are largely dependent upon the population being examined and how the question is framed or, in other words, what variables are included in the model. An examination of predominantly white, educated, female health care providers in the Nurses' Health Study found that 91% of the population-attributable risk could be explained by elevated BMI, poor diet, lack of exercise, smoking, and abstinence from alcohol (Hu et al. 2001). The effects of heavy drinking were not considered in the Nurses' Health Study. See Crandall et al. (2009) and Liang and Chikritzhs (2014) for discussions on the relationship between alcohol and diabetes.

A subsequent analysis with the Nurses' Health Study and the Health Professionals Follow-up Study also included non-adult risk factors and found different estimates of population-attributable risk; 22% of the risk was attributable to birthweight, 59% to adult lifestyle characteristics (dietary pattern, physical activity, smoking status, and alcohol consumption), and 18% to the interaction between birthweight and adult lifestyle. Among men and women with normal birthweights, 57% of diabetes cases could have been prevented if people had consumed better diets, had more physical activity, did not smoke, and had moderate alcohol consumption. The estimate increased to the original 91% with the inclusion of healthy BMI (< 25), but few individuals were in this grouping and the population-attributable risk was higher for women than men (94% vs. 81%; Li et al. 2015b).

Results from the Multiethnic Cohort Study suggest that most (83%) type 2 diabetes cases in women could be prevented if all modifiable risk factors were eliminated. Although BMI was a major component of risk, the population-attributable risk varied by ethnic group: 50% of cases could be prevented among men if BMI was less than 25 kg/m^2; however, this varied by ethnic group, with 38% of the population-attributable risk attributable to BMI in Japanese-American men, 60% among Native Hawaiian men, and 65% among white men (Steinbrecher et al. 2011).

The importance of lifestyle factors on risk of GDM is also evident. Using information from the Nurses' Health Study to inform national estimates, approximately 33% of risk is attributed to obesity, 11% to not adhering to a healthy diet, 11% to not exercising regularly, and 6% to smoking (Zhang et al. 2014). Analyses using birth records come to similar conclusions, with about 40% of GDM cases attributed to obesity, with rates that vary by race/ethnicity: approximately 15% for Asian/Pacific Islanders, 40% for non-Hispanic whites, 50% for blacks, and a little less than 60% for American Indians/Alaska Natives (Kim et al. 2012; Kim et al. 2013).

Because diabetes is a known cardiovascular risk factor, the population-attributable risk due to diabetes for CVD should be examined. Known

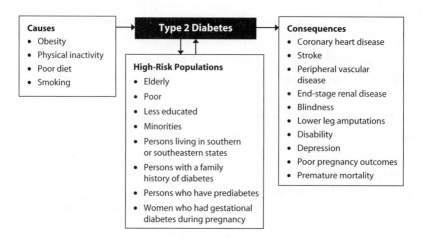

Source: Adapted from Bishop et al. (2010).

Figure 12-1. Type 2 Diabetes: Causes, Consequences, and High-Risk Groups

cardiovascular risk factors contributed to 68% and 51% of the population-attributable risk for women and men, respectively. Diabetes has a larger population-attributable risk for U.S. women compared to men (21% vs. 14%). Population-attributable risk was greater for blacks (28%) compared to whites (13%) in the 1990s, reflecting increasing population-attributable risk for blacks between the 1980s and 1990s (Cheng et al. 2014). The causes, consequences, and high-risk groups for type 2 diabetes are summarized in Figure 12-1.

Interventions

Prevention

Type 1 Diabetes

Although there is still no durable cure for type 1 diabetes, much progress has been made in identifying the causes of the disease, its pathogenesis, and risk factors. The capacity to assess risk and predict disease development has further enabled the identification and recruitment of high-risk infants into large-scale investigations that are bringing us closer to learning how to prevent type 1 diabetes. Most of these studies have been conducted on recent-onset type 1 diabetes by attempting to interrupt the progression of the disease to preserve remaining β-cell function and potentially reduce the severity of the disease and prevent further deterioration (Skyler 2013; i.e., tertiary prevention). Recent and current investigations can be divided into (1) primary prevention: before the development of autoimmunity; (2) secondary prevention: once autoanti-bodies are present; and (3) tertiary: after recent onset of the disease and early enough in the process that there are still β cells to be preserved (Wherrett 2014). Results to date for tertiary prevention have not shown lasting benefit or resolution of type 1 diabetes, but hope remains that ultimately long-term remission can be achieved through immunotherapy treatment started early in the disease process (Chatenoud et al. 2012).

Many of the current and most recent studies are focused on primary or secondary prevention in young infants who have been identified as at high risk of developing type 1 diabetes. To prevent the development of type 1 diabetes, primary prevention studies attempt to avoid or alter exposure to identified environmental triggers before the development of autoimmunity and the destruction of β cells can occur (Wherrett 2014). All such studies have been on infants and young children at high risk for type 1 diabetes, meaning a first-degree relative with type 1 diabetes and the presence of high-risk human leukocyte antigen (HLA) genes in the child (Simmons and Michels 2014). Because the population for these studies is so young, they must be conducted with minimal risk and have been limited to dietary interventions.

The primary prevention dietary intervention studies include exposure to infant formulas free of cow's milk and bovine insulin, infant formula supplemented with omega-3 fatty acid docosahexaenoic acid, delayed exposure to gluten-containing foods, and vitamin D supplementation (Skyler 2013; Wu et al. 2013), on the theory that exposure to complex dietary proteins may increase risk of β-cell autoimmunity in children at genetic risk for type 1 diabetes (Akerblom et al. 2005).

Cow's milk formula containing bovine insulin is known to induce autoimmune responses to insulin and observational studies have suggested that delayed introduction of gluten-containing foods or cereals into the diet might help prevent the development of islet autoimmunity in children (Ziegler et al. 2003). Diets high in omega-3 fatty acids have been linked retrospectively to lower risk of islet autoimmunity and diabetes in children (Norris et al. 2007). A meta-analysis of four case–control studies and one cohort study found that the risk of type 1 diabetes was reduced 29% in infants who were supplemented with vitamin D compared to those infants not supplemented (pooled OR=0.71; 95% CI=0.60, 0.84; Zipitis and Akobeng 2008). And yet, when these apparent dietary factors have been tested in medical trials, a cause–effect relationship with type 1 diabetes has not yet been demonstrated (Skyler 2015).

Secondary prevention studies targeting children and adults with diabetes auto-antibodies already present have tested the effects of nicotinamide, insulin injections, oral insulin, nasal insulin, glutamic acid decarboxylase, and cyclosporine. Despite a growing number of large studies, to date there are no trials that have successfully delayed or prevented type 1 diabetes (Skyler 2013; Skyler 2015).

Type 2 Diabetes

The prevention or delayed onset of type 2 diabetes has been clearly demonstrated in numerous large clinical trials published since 1997 including three successful interventions: the Chinese Da Qing Study, Finnish Diabetes Prevention Study, and US Diabetes Prevention Program (Knowler et al. 2002; Pan et al. 1997; Tuomilehto et al. 2001). These studies clearly show that both lifestyle and pharmacological interventions prevent or delay the onset of type 2 diabetes in high-risk, prediabetes (IGT or IFG) populations. In these trials, the development of diabetes was reduced 25% to 60% at follow-up, with the largest reductions accomplished most often through lifestyle interventions that supported weight loss and increased physical activity (Knowler et al. 2009).

In the Da Qing IGT and Diabetes Study in China, 110,000 people were screened for IGT and type 2 diabetes. Of these, 577 were identified as having IGT, then randomly assigned into four groups: control, diet only, exercise only, and diet plus exercise. At six-year follow-up, the diet, exercise, and diet-plus-exercise intervention groups displayed 31%, 46%, and 42% reductions in diabetes incidence compared with controls (Pan et al. 1997). At 20-year follow-up, the cumulative diabetes prevalence was 80% in the combined lifestyle intervention groups versus 93% in the control group, with the intervention groups averaging 3.6 fewer years with diabetes (Li et al. 2008). At the 23-year follow-up, the incidence of CVD mortality, all-cause mortality, and occurrence of diabetes was 11.9%, 28.1%, and 72.6% in the combined lifestyle intervention groups and 19.6%, 38.4%, and 89.9% in the control group, respectively (Li et al. 2014).

In the Finnish Diabetes Prevention study (Tuomilehto et al. 2001), 522 overweight subjects with IGT were randomly assigned into a lifestyle intervention or control group. The treatment goal was to reduce weight by 5%, perform moderate-to-vigorous exercise at least 30 minutes a day, limit total and saturated fat, and increase consumption of fiber. After three years of follow-up, the incidence of type 2 diabetes was reduced by 58% in the intervention group. Follow-up conducted three years after the intervention ended (median follow-up: seven years) demonstrated long-term effects: the absolute difference in diabetes risk between intervention and control remained at about 15% with a 43% reduction in relative risk (Lindstrom et al. 2006). Thirteen years after baseline, the relative risk reduction was 38%. Most who had maintained lifestyle goals at the conclusion of the intervention remained diabetes-free after 13 years, with diabetes incidence 32% lower in the intervention group than controls in 2009 (Lindstrom et al. 2013).

The Diabetes Prevention Program (DPP) Research Group, conducted in the United States, randomly assigned 3,234 adults with IGT and a BMI greater than 24 kg/m² to placebo, metformin (850 mg twice daily), or a lifestyle modification program. The two major goals of the DPP lifestyle intervention were a minimum of 7% weight loss or weight maintenance and a minimum of 150 minutes per week of physical activity (Knowler et al. 2002). The DPP included (1) individual case managers or "lifestyle coaches"; (2) frequent contact; (3) a structured, 16-session core curriculum including behavioral self-management strategies; (4) supervised physical activity; (5) a maintenance intervention; (6) a "toolbox" of adherence strategies; (7) tailoring of materials and strategies to address ethnic diversity; and (8) an extensive network of training, feedback, and clinical support to reach these goals (Sanders Thompson et al. 2015; Tabak et al. 2015). The average follow-up was 2.8 years with respective incidence rates for diabetes in the placebo, metformin, and lifestyle groups of 11.0, 7.8, and 4.8 per 100 person-years. This represents a 58% and 31% risk reduction in the lifestyle and metformin groups compared with the placebo. The effect of the lifestyle intervention was associated with reduced risk for all age and racial/ethnic groups and in both sexes, but was especially effective in the older age group (60–85 years), whereas metformin was less effective than in younger adults.

The DPP Outcomes Study was a long-term follow-up (2002–2014) of the DPP (1996–2001) participants (Knowler et al. 2009) investigating whether the delay in the development of diabetes was sustained for up to 12 additional years beyond the three-year average treatment in the DPP. Participants in lifestyle and metformin groups were encouraged to continue the interventions and all participants were offered a group lifestyle intervention. At the 10-year follow-up, average of diabetes incidence was reduced by 34% in those initially randomized to lifestyle change and by 18% in those initially randomized to metformin compared with placebo (Knowler et al. 2009). Among women without a history of GDM, lifestyle but not metformin reduced progression to diabetes (Aroda et al. 2015). At the 15-year follow-up, incidence was 27%

lower for the lifestyle group and 18% lower for metformin versus placebo. The DPP participants in both the lifestyle change and metformin groups also had lower use of antidiabetic medications compared to participants originally assigned to placebo. Aggregate microvascular outcome between the treatment groups and the placebo found no overall difference; however, those who did not develop diabetes compared to those who did had a 28% lower prevalence of microvascular complications (DPPRG 2015).

Lifestyle or metformin interventions of the DPP were cost-effective (Herman et al. 2013). The DPP Outcomes Study revealed that the cumulative QALYs accrued over 10 years were greater for lifestyle (6.89) than metformin (6.79) or placebo (6.74; DPPRG 2012a). Further analyses revealed lifestyle cost of $12,878 per QALY, whereas metformin had slightly lower costs and nearly the same QALYs as placebo. Lifestyle proved to be cost-effective whereas metformin was marginally cost-saving compared with placebo (DPPRG 2012a).

Several pharmacological agents, including metformin, α-glucosidase inhibitors, orlistat, and thiazolidinedione, have shown various levels of success in decreasing incident diabetes. Of these, metformin has the strongest evidence base and demonstrated long-term safety as a pharmacological therapy for diabetes prevention (DPPRG 2012b; Hostalek et al. 2015). Other drugs used in pharmacological interventions are more costly, have potentially dangerous side effects, are generally less effective than lifestyle interventions, and are less likely than diet and physical activity to be of general benefit to the human body for diseases other than diabetes (Srinivasan and Florez 2015).

On the basis of the evidence, the American Diabetes Association (ADA) developed a position statement that recommends that patients with prediabetes be referred to an intensive diet and physical activity behavioral counseling program based on the DPP, which targets a loss of 7% of body weight and increases moderate-intensity physical activity to at least 150 minutes per week (ADA 2016a). The use of metformin is recommended for those with IFG or IGT if they have any of the following characteristics: aged younger than 60 years, BMI greater than or equal to 35 kg/m^2, and previous GDM. Because of costs and potential side effects, further consideration is needed for the use of other drugs in individuals with IFG or IGT. Metformin use rates in prediabetes are now less than 4%, and lifestyle interventions are used in a minority of prediabetes patients. Increased use of both of these proven interventions is likely the optimal way forward (Sussman et al. 2015).

Prevention of Type 2 Diabetes in Youth

The strong evidence that type 2 diabetes can be delayed or prevented by life-style modification or pharmacology in adults has yet to be extensively replicated among youth or young adults (Balk et al. 2015). The positive recommendation from the Community Preventive Services Task Force (Pronk and Remington 2015) for combined diet and physical activity promotion programs for preventing diabetes in adults and adolescents was based on an evidence review that was only able to include two studies focused on adolescents, and the 39 included studies on adults had an age range of 43 to 65 years (Balk et al. 2015), missing a young adult population at growing risk. Fortunately, since that review, two new studies (Hannon et al. 2015; Hingle et al. 2015) have appeared in the literature, both of which, in partnership with the YMCA, are adapting the YDPP to make this group-based version of the DPP suitable for families, with one focusing on families in which the mother has had GDM or prediabetes (Hannon et al. 2015). There is also a recently reported feasibility study of a technology-based lifestyle coaching program focused on diet and physical activity that incorporates use of a handheld device and digital platforms for young adults with prediabetes aged 18 to 29 years (Cha et al. 2014).

In the Type 2 Diabetes in Adolescents and Youth (TODAY) Study, 699 youth aged 10 to 17 years within two years since diagnosis of diabetes were enrolled into one of three treatment arms: metformin, metformin plus intensive lifestyle modification, or metformin plus rosiglitazone (Zeitler et al. 2012). The objective of the study was to maintain glycemic control, but the rate of failure for the three arms was 52%, 39%, and 47%, respectively, with an average progression to failure of 3.86 years (Tryggestad and Willi 2015). Notably, intensive lifestyle modification combined with metformin added little or nothing to metformin alone. By comparison, the A Diabetes Outcome Progression Trial (ADOPT) study in adults using metformin and rosiglitazone individually experienced failure rates of only 21% and 15% over a five-year period (Kahn et al. 2006). In the TODAY study, youth experienced complications and comorbidities similar to adults but on a much accelerated timeline (Tryggestad and Willi 2015), underscoring the need to aggressively pursue measures to prevent obesity in children through diet and physical activity at a point at which such measures can be most effective.

Several lifestyle change studies conducted with children in school settings have attempted to reduce or prevent the onset of obesity in high-risk youth, through physical activity or dietary interventions. Reviews and meta-analyses

of school-based and clinic-based interventions have identified the longer duration of an intervention and the inclusion of a strong parental component as
being critical to achieving successful lifestyle change and weight loss outcomes
(Amini et al. 2015; Gonzalez-Suarez et al. 2009; Kelishadi and Azizi-Soleiman
2014; Nixon et al. 2012).

The National Institute of Diabetes and Digestive and Kidney Diseases and
the ADA sponsored a collaborative diabetes-specific research initiative called
Studies to Treat or Prevent Pediatric Type 2 Diabetes (Baranowski et al. 2006;
Hartstein et al. 2008). This collaboration launched the HEALTHY Study in 2006,
a 2.5-year study to examine the effects of a multicomponent, school-based program addressing risk factors for diabetes among children whose race or ethnic
group and socioeconomic status placed them at high risk for obesity and type 2
diabetes. A total of 4,603 students from 42 schools participated and underwent
measurements of BMI, waist circumference, and fasting glucose and insulin levels at the beginning of sixth grade and the end of eighth grade (Hirst et al. 2009).
Findings revealed no significant differences in the primary outcome of overweight and obesity. Although the intervention did not have an impact on obesity
or overweight prevalence across groups, the intervention did result in significantly greater reductions in various indexes of adiposity, which may reduce risk
of childhood-onset type 2 diabetes (Foster et al. 2010; Marcus et al. 2013).

Prevention of type 2 diabetes in youth necessarily includes the early detection
of prediabetes followed by clinic- and family-based interventions that typically
include nutrition education, physical activity, behavioral modification, and, in
some cases, use of metformin or other pharmacologic interventions (Hingle
et al. 2015; Niemeier et al. 2012). There is a growing awareness that communication about health through intrafamilial sharing of diabetes risk and the sense
of ethnic identity, can provide a strong incentive for organizing effective, culturally sensitive prevention efforts in those communities most victimized by widespread diabetes (Bascones-Martinez et al. 2011; Brezo et al. 2006; Burnet et al.
2011; Chambers et al. 2015; Reinschmidt et al. 2010; Teufel-Shone et al. 2005).

Screening

Prediabetes and Diabetes

The benefits of primary prevention of diabetes are firmly established, because
preventing or delaying the onset of diabetes appears to substantially reduce
long-term complications of diabetes. An estimated 86 million American adults

are now classified as having prediabetes (CDC 2014) and most do not know they have it (Geiss et al. 2010), pointing to the need for improved identification.

The U.S. Preventive Services Task Force currently recommends screening for abnormal blood glucose and diabetes in those aged 40 to 70 years who also have BMI of 25 or greater (Siu 2015). The ADA suggests much broader, less evidence-based screening of (1) all those aged 45 years and older, (2) those aged 19 to 45 years with a BMI of 25 or greater (BMI≥23 in Asian Americans) who have one or more additional risk factors for diabetes, and (3) adolescents who are overweight or obese and have two or more risk factors for diabetes. The ADA list of risk factors for diabetes includes physical inactivity, first-degree relative with diabetes, high-risk race or ethnicity, history of gestational diabetes or a baby weighing greater than 9 pounds, polycystic ovary syndrome, previous diagnosis of prediabetes, hypertension, high-density lipoprotein cholesterol less than 35 mg/dL (0.90 mmol/L) or triglycerides greater than 250 mg/dL (2.82 mmol/L), history of CVD, or acanthosis nigricans (dark patches of skin with thick, velvety texture that most often appear on armpits, groin, and neck; ADA 2016b). Both groups recommend that candidates who screen normal be re-screened in 3 years.

Population screening specifically for type 1 diabetes is not generally recommended for asymptomatic low-risk individuals because of the absence of approved therapeutic interventions (ADA 2016b). The ADA indicates that physicians should consider referring relatives of those with type 1 diabetes for antibody testing for risk assessment in the setting of a clinical research study (ADA 2016b). It is important to recall that any patient presenting with symptoms suggestive of diabetes, such as need to urinate frequently, increased thirst and fluid intake, increased appetite, fatigue, blurry vision, or recurrent infections be evaluated for diabetes independent of screening criteria (O'Connor et al. 2006).

In the absence of diabetes, a diagnosis of prediabetes is established by (1) an HbA1c between 5.7% and 6.4% inclusive, (2) a fasting plasma glucose of 100 to 125 mg/dL inclusive, or (3) an 75-gram oral glucose tolerance test with the two-hour glucose of 140 to 200 mg/dL (11.1 mmol/L). Diagnosis of diabetes can be established by (1) an HbA1c of 6.5% or greater, confirmed by a second test in this list, (2) a fasting plasma glucose greater than 126 mg/dL (7.0 mmol/L) confirmed on repeat testing a different day or by a different test on this list, (3) an oral glucose tolerance test with the two-hour glucose greater than 200 mg/dL (11.1 mmol/L), or (4) a random plasma glucose greater than 200 mg/dL in a patient with typical symptoms (ADA 2016b).

Gestational Diabetes

Early diagnosis and aggressive treatment of GDM has been shown to reduce fetal morbidity and mortality (Horvath et al. 2010). Therefore, the National Institutes of Health (Vandorsten et al. 2013) and the American College of Obstetrics and Gynecology (Committee on Practice Bulletins—Obstetrics 2013) recommend that high-risk pregnant women be screened for GDM between the 24th and 28th weeks of pregnancy with a 50-gram (g) nonfasting one-hour oral glucose tolerance test. When the screening test is positive (one-hour plasma glucose greater than or equal to 140 mg/dL [7.8 mmol/L] or greater than or equal to 135 mg/dL in high-risk populations), a three-hour 100-g oral glucose tolerance test is subsequently administered. A diagnosis of GDM is confirmed when any two glucose values equal or exceed these limits: fasting, 105 mg/dL; one hour, 190 mg/dL; two hours, 165 mg/dL; three hours, 145 mg/dL (ADA 2016b).

An alternative strategy to screen for GDM has been suggested by The International Association of Diabetes and Pregnancy Study Group (Metzger et al. 2010). Experts are divided on the benefits of the two screening strategies, the alternative strategy would roughly triple the incidence of GDM and has not been endorsed by most expert groups because it may medicalize pregnancy for millions of women, provides only marginal additional benefits to the baby, requires a fasting test for all women, and increases costs (Metzger et al. 2010).

Treatment

Diabetes mellitus is a chronic illness that requires lifelong care. Effective treatment is ideally provided by a health care team that includes a physician, a diabetes educator, a dietitian, and others. Yet, the majority of all diabetes care is necessarily self-care (Nuovo et al. 2007). Therefore, treatment should include not only thorough initial evaluation, establishment of treatment goals, development of a management plan, cardiovascular risk factor reduction, and recognition of and care for complications, but also patient education in self-management and ongoing support. Standards of medical care patient education criteria have been published by various entities (ADA 2016c).

Type 1 Diabetes

The Diabetes Control and Complications Trial, the longest prospective study for type 1 diabetes, showed that adequate blood glucose control (HbA1c 7%

vs. 9%) slows or prevents development of major microvascular and macrovascular diabetes complications (Nathan et al. 2009). Patients with type 1 diabetes need insulin injections to survive; multiple daily insulin injections or use of an insulin infusion pump are usually required. Nutritional and caloric intake must be synchronized with insulin administration, with adjustments for varying levels of physical activity (ADA 2016c). The use of continuous glucose monitoring and more sophisticated insulin pumps is revolutionizing treatment of type 1 diabetes in the United States (Bergenstal et al. 2013). Maintaining a physically active lifestyle confers additional benefits and should be an important goal of treatment (Guelfi et al. 2007; Rachmiel et al. 2007). Development of increasingly effective islet cell transplantation techniques and other novel therapies have raised hopes that a durable cure for type 1 diabetes may emerge in coming years (Bruni et al. 2014).

Type 2 Diabetes

The cornerstones of type 2 diabetes care are adequate BP, lipid, glucose, tobacco, and weight management, caloric restriction, and physical activity (ADA 2016c). Nearly all type 2 diabetes patients eventually require pharmacotherapy for adequate management of BP, lipids, and glucose. Early use of metformin for glucose control and statins for lipid management are currently recommended. About 70% of type 2 diabetes patients have elevated BP, and many require treatment with two or more BP-lowering medications to achieve adequate BP control. Thus, it is not surprising that the average person newly diagnosed with diabetes is taking six medications, which increases to eight medications one year after diabetes diagnosis (Schmittdiel et al. 2014). This high treatment burden is one reason for high rates of medication nonadherence, and efforts to provide "minimally disruptive health care" for those with diabetes and related chronic diseases may be considered (Montori 2016; Montori and Rodriguez-Gutierrez 2016). From both the public health and clinical point of view, effective management of BP, lipids, tobacco use, and appropriate aspirin use are often as important if not more important than aggressive glucose control in type 2 diabetes (Gaede et al. 2008; Patel et al. 2008).

A wide range of pharmacological agents are available to help achieve glucose goals in type 2 diabetes. Initial treatment with metformin is widely recommended because metformin reduces cardiovascular mortality (Holman 2013; Holman et al. 2008), causes little hypoglycemia or weight gain, has favorable lipid effects, and has a proven safety record (Inzucchi et al. 2015).

Metformin cannot be used in those with uncompensated congestive heart failure or advanced chronic kidney disease. Other agents used to control glucose in type 2 diabetes include insulins, sulfonylureas, α-glucosidase inhibitors, thiazolidinedione, incretin agonists, dipeptidyl peptidase-4 inhibitors, sodium-glucose co-transporter-2 inhibitors, and others (Nathan 2015).

Short-term studies of cardiovascular safety over two to five years suggest that several agents increase congestive heart failure hospitalizations, whereas others may reduce cardiovascular and overall mortality (Inzucchi et al. 2015; Zinman et al. 2016; Zinman et al. 2015). However, more studies are needed to confirm these initial findings. A detailed discussion of pharmacotherapy for management of glucose, BP, and lipids is beyond the scope of this chapter, but may be found in standard medical reference books or online. In addition, it is worth noting that bariatric surgery offers some patients with type 2 diabetes an opportunity to achieve at least a temporary remission of the diabetic state, with commensurate reductions in risk of subsequent microvascular and macrovascular complications. The benefits and risks of bariatric surgery vary greatly across different groups of type 2 diabetes patients, especially by age and duration of diabetes (Schauer et al. 2015).

Diabetes treatment requires the active involvement of the patient. Patient readiness to change predicts improved diabetes care (O'Connor et al. 2004) and lower levels of health literacy are associated with poorer diabetes outcomes (Laramee et al. 2007; Schillinger et al. 2006; Schillinger et al. 2002). There is a growing body of well-conducted randomized studies on diabetes patient education and diabetes self-management interventions that show small but important benefits to many patients; benefits are realized across varied delivery settings and populations (Lepard et al. 2015; Ricci-Cabello et al. 2014; Sherifali et al. 2015) and through the Internet and interactive technology (Pereira et al. 2015; Wood et al. 2015).

An intervention recommended by the national Task Force on Community Preventive Services—diabetes self-management education—teaches people to manage their own diabetes with the goal of optimizing metabolic control, prevention or early detection of acute and chronic complications, and optimizing quality of life at an acceptable cost both for the patient and the health care system (Siminerio 2006; Task Force on Community Preventive Services 2002). Self-monitoring of blood glucose levels is important in insulin-treated patients and in patients prone to hypoglycemia without symptoms. In other patients, self-monitoring of blood glucose has not been shown to improve outcomes.

However, it often provides important information during episodes of acute illnesses, and can be used by patients to assess the impact of eating, physical activity, and stress on glucose levels (Malanda et al. 2012).

Continuing care is crucial in the management of diabetes, and frequent evaluation and adjustment in therapy may be required. Care can be effectively delivered through primary care, subspecialty care, or disease management models of care (Glasgow 2003; Wagner et al. 2001). Essential components of diabetes management on a population basis include identification of individuals or populations with diabetes, use of guidelines or performance standards to manage those identified, information systems to track and monitor interventions and patient- or population-based outcomes, and measurement and management of patient and population outcomes (Task Force on Community Preventive Services 2002).

Despite impressive improvement in diabetes care over the past decade, there is a persistent gap between recommended and actual levels of diabetes control. Analysis of data from national surveys conducted between 1999 and 2010 showed that people with self-reported diabetes have made significant improvement in meeting their treatment goals. Unfortunately 33% to 49% had still not met their targets for glycemic control, BP, or lipid cholesterol. Only 14% had met targets for all three and avoiding tobacco (Ali et al. 2013). Factors that contribute to this gap include lack of health insurance, low health literacy, patient nonadherence to lifestyle or pharmacologic therapy, failure of providers to intensify lifestyle or pharmacological therapy in a timely and persistent way until recommended goals of therapy are achieved, and inability to address external influences on outcomes within the patient's environment that are beyond the influence of the treatment setting.

Translating Diabetes Evidence-Based Research into Public Health Practice

Discrepancies exist between evidence-based, efficacious interventions, like those deployed in the DPP trial, and what is feasible for implementation in real-world settings. The approach taken in the large clinical trials (Chiasson et al. 2002; Knowler et al. 2009; Li et al. 2015a; Lindstrom et al. 2013) to prevent or delay diabetes onset have been resource-intense (e.g., one-on-one interventions like in the DPP trial [Herman et al. 2013]) and focused on adults at greatest risk of developing diabetes (Albright and Gregg 2013). Whether or not clinic-based interventions will reach populations in greatest need is unclear, especially because those at greatest risk for developing diabetes often have fewer resources and poorer access to health care.

Moving diabetes prevention from research to implementation, a process that requires both cultural adaptation and feasibility, has been a focus of implementation research in recent years. Numerous practical clinical trials tested the translation of the DPP into real world settings, often adapting delivery to include more cost-effective, group-based or technology approaches (Tabak et al. 2015). These studies have varied by at-risk population enrolled (e.g., overweight individuals, prediabetes, and type of diabetes) and setting (e.g., churches [Dodani and Fields 2010; Faridi et al. 2010], worksites [Miller et al. 2015; Weinhold et al. 2015], and home-based settings [Haire-Joshu et al. 2008]) with varying but generally positive behavior change results.

Tabak and colleagues (2015) reviewed 44 articles published between 2004 and 2013 on adaptations of the original DPP curriculum. Of 44 studies reviewed, eight took place in churches, 18 in medical settings, and 10 in community centers. Eight targeted specific population groups and 15 made cultural adaptations to the DPP. Lay health workers were used in 18 of the studies but health care settings typically relied on medical staff whose ethnicity matched the target population for program delivery. Five of the studies that made cultural adaptations used the community-based participatory research framework. Most studies (58%) used a pre–post design without a control group but there were also nine randomized controlled trials. Studies that adapted program content to meet the needs of a specific cultural group (e.g., including culturally appropriate recipes or encouraging participation in local or traditional physical activities) found that matching the facilitator to the participants aided the process and that adaptations increased the relevance of the program for participants. Because of the heterogeneity of the programs, the degree to which modifications in the original evidence-based programs might have altered impact could not be assessed. A relatively common adaptation was to reduce the number of sessions from 16 to 12. Most of the studies failed to report on such important implementation outcomes as cost. Both cost and sustainability data are essential to the future expansion of the DPP group-based model into more communities and settings.

One promising intervention for broad population impact is the YMCA model for the Diabetes Prevention Program (YDPP). Low-income, overweight participants (n=509) were recruited to the YDPP trial. When compared to standard care, YDPP participants achieved a 2.3 kg weight loss after one year; there was a dose–response relationship with a 5.3 kg weight loss for those attending nine or more sessions. The YMCA model showed the promise of DPP dissemination and success in achieving a meaningful weight loss at 12 months among low-income adults (Ackermann et al. 2015).

An article published in February 2016 described a 12-month randomized trial to test whether a widely available commercial weight-management program (Weight Watchers) might provide an additional alternative for individuals with prediabetes (Marrero et al. 2016). The commercial program has a core curriculum that is evidence-based and includes the same behavioral change topics as the DPP: self-monitoring of weight, intake, and activity; dietary modification; physical activity; stimulus control; and relapse prevention. A difference from YDPP and other DPP adaptations was that the weight-loss program used a "loop" model in which sessions were repeated frequently and at multiple times and locations, allowing the participant more flexibility by not having to commit to 16 sequentially scheduled weekly sessions as in the YDPP. At the 6- and 12-month follow-ups, the intervention group lost significantly more weight than controls and had significantly greater improvements in HbA1c and high-density lipoprotein cholesterol levels. The investigators felt that this was a viable alternative to the YDPP in part because it would be cost-competitive and the "loop" model provided much more flexibility. In addition, it is a commercial program that is much more widely available than the YDPP.

In a review on the prevention of type 2 diabetes, it was noted that roughly half of the risk for type 2 diabetes can be attributed to environmental exposure and that overweight is clearly the most critical risk factor and should be the primary target, especially in the young (Hussain et al. 2007). The authors suggested, on the basis of their review, that the first objective should be to target people with IGT with increased physical activity and altered diet and, second, to introduce population-based measures that would encourage increased physical activity and decreased consumption of energy-dense foods in the community. Population-based approaches to prevent diabetes to date have been mostly synonymous with population-based approaches to preventing obesity (Baranowski et al. 2006; Jenum et al. 2006; Marcus et al. 2013; see Chapter 11).

Upstream population-based measures, by definition, involve policy and environmental changes such as increased physical activity opportunities built into the school day and urban planning concepts such as "complete streets," which make possible and encourage alternative forms of transportation such as walking and biking. Although such upstream interventions appear to have great potential for ending the obesity and diabetes epidemics, rigorous scientific studies to demonstrate their worth are exceedingly difficult to conduct. The breadth, scale, and complexity of population-based interventions are not well-suited to assessment through the parameters of a clinical trial. This is because policies or interventions put in place in one community setting will probably need to be adapted in another community because of structural and cultural differences. Even if the policy or program is close to identical, it may be received very differently in each setting because of the differences between communities that may either support or hinder the change. There is, however, a rapidly developing science for measuring cultural adaptation and implementation of programs such as the group-based DPPs and other "natural experiments" (Gregg et al. 2013) to better measure, evaluate, and understand the cultural adaptation, translation, and implementation that has taken place and their effect on the fidelity of the intervention in achieving the intended outcomes (Chou 2015; Tabak et al. 2015; Venditti and Kramer 2013).

Another means of disseminating DPP-like interventions to a wider public is through use of the Internet. One recent study tested the feasibility and effectiveness of a web-based lifestyle intervention based on the DPP for women with recent gestational diabetes (Nicklas et al. 2014) called *Balance after Baby*, delivered over the first postpartum year, and found that women in the intervention group lost a mean of 2.8 kg at 12 months compared to the controls who gained 4.0 kg ($p=.035$). In another program called *Prevent*, an online social network translation of the DPP lifestyle intervention, participants achieved a 5.4% weight loss at 16 weeks and 4.8% at one year compared to baseline with an HbA1c reduction of 0.37% (Sepah et al. 2014).

Examples of Evidence-Based Interventions

The systems that have an impact on diabetes in the United States are vast, and include myriad organizations and other stakeholders. In this section, we will largely focus on diabetes within the governmental public health system.

The National Diabetes Prevention Program

In 2010 Congress authorized the CDC to establish and lead the national DPP through passage of the Diabetes Prevention Act of 2009, which amended the

Public Health Service Act to direct the Secretary of Health and Human Services to act through the CDC to establish a national diabetes prevention program targeted at persons at high risk for diabetes. The CDC national DPP facilitates the dissemination of the adapted group-based low-cost DPP lifestyle change program so that quality programs are available to at-risk populations with pre-diabetes throughout the country. To achieve this end, CDC relies on its many partnerships with state health departments, community-based organizations, health insurers, employers, health care systems, academia, and other government agencies.

The CDC national DPP has four core elements:

1. Training of a workforce that can implement the program cost-effectively.
2. A recognition program to ensure quality, lead to reimbursement, and allow CDC to develop a program registry.
3. Intervention sites to build infrastructure and provide the program.
4. Health marketing to support program uptake by increasing referrals through the health care system and the private sector for use of the prevention program. (Albright et al. 2013)

The CDC established the Diabetes Training and Technical Assistance Center at Emory University to provide comprehensive training services across the country for lifestyle coaches, and established the Diabetes Prevention Recognition Program to

1. Ensure the quality, consistency, and broad dissemination of lifestyle change for people at high risk for type 2 diabetes.
2. Develop and maintain a registry of organizations able to deliver an effective lifestyle program.
3. Provide technical assistance to organizations that have applied for recognition to help these organizations achieve the necessary standard and subsequently maintain that standard.

Although the need for standards is clear, strict adherence can hamper the ability of states and local communities to adapt the DPP to their population. The United Health Group and the YMCA were the first organizations to formally partner with the CDC in the national DPP under the Diabetes Prevention and Control Alliance.

A critical element to wider dissemination of the DPP model is reimbursement. Some states such as Minnesota allow for payment through Medicaid to community health workers to lead the 16-session class. Very recently (March 2016) the DPP received a critical boost when the Secretary of Health and Human Services announced that the independent Office of the Actuary in the Centers for Medicare and Medicaid Services (CMS) certified that expansion of the DPP would reduce net Medicare spending and improve quality of patient care without limiting coverage or benefits. It was the first time a preventive service model from the CMS Innovation Center has become eligible for expansion into the Medicare program. In making this determination, the Department of Health and Human Services relied on an evaluation of the YDPP (CMS 2016; Hinnant et al. 2016).

Albright and Gregg (2013) provide a discussion of the merits of taking a "high-risk" versus "population-wide" public health approach to diabetes, suggesting that both approaches are necessary when those with prediabetes or diabetes are close to half the adult population. They suggest the need for a multi-tiered approach that links type and intensity of intervention to appropriate level of risk and describe a four-tiered model for prediabetes. The first tier, with the highest level of risk of developing diabetes, are those with HbA1c greater than or equal to 5.7% but less than 6.5% with FPG greater than 110 and 10-year diabetes risk of 30% to 40%. The second tier are those with FPG greater or equal to 100 mg/dL and less than 126 mg/dL and a 20% to 30% 10-year risk of diabetes. It is the people in these first two tiers who are prioritized for structured lifestyle change programs and observation. The third tier consists of those at moderate 10-year risk for diabetes of between 10% and 20% and two or more risk factors who should receive brief education or counseling. The fourth tier with the lowest risk, a 0% to 10% 10-year risk for diabetes and no more than one risk factor, are targeted by whole-population strategies alone, including such changes as alterations in the built environment or higher taxes on unhealthy food items.

The CDC's focus in the past several years with the advent of the DPP has moved decidedly toward high-risk prevention, although there are still many others who champion a population-based approach that includes an environment conducive to healthy diets and increased physical activity. Resources are scarce at all levels of government, but the DPP model has the advantage of being effective and relatively low-cost. With a growing opportunity for reimbursement through Medicaid and Medicare and the extension of the DPP model more broadly in both the public and private sector, the future appears hopeful.

Areas of Future Research

Prevention

It is clear that in the face of the diabetes and obesity epidemics, primary prevention of diabetes through weight management, increased levels of physical activity, and healthier diet, is a critical public health and clinical research priority. There is strong evidence that lifestyle interventions and metformin use delay progression to diabetes in high-risk adults, but most of these individuals have still not been exposed to these effective interventions (Knowler et al. 2009; Lindstrom et al. 2013; Schmittdiel et al. 2013; Schmittdiel et al. 2015). Cost-effectiveness of both metformin and lifestyle interventions in prediabetes patients appears to be good, and metformin use may be cost-saving (Herman et al. 2013).

For lifestyle interventions that prevent diabetes to be effectively adopted and widely disseminated, several research needs should be addressed as summarized by Samuel-Hodge et al. (2006) and Siminerio (2008). These include

1. Determine the necessary intensity, frequency, and duration of physical activity.
2. Better elucidate healthy or preventive dietary components and amounts.
3. Investigate effectiveness of lifestyle interventions for obese adults with normal glucose tolerance or prediabetes.
4. Examine potential effectiveness of lifestyle interventions conducted in diverse community settings that rely on "nonselective" community recruitment (e.g., the YDPP).
5. Quantify the role of physical activity independent of weight loss.
6. Explore effectiveness of lifestyle weight loss interventions in combination with public health (physical and social environment) or pharmacological interventions.
7. Identify maximally effective lifestyle behavior change maintenance strategies.
8. Track long-term outcomes of lifestyle interventions on diabetes complications.
9. Strengthen population-based lifestyle intervention study designs to include careful measurement of both processes and outcomes and the assessment of community and environmental indicators of risks and outcome (Siminerio 2008).

Additional questions include (Ackermann 2015)

1. What is the most effective way to identify individuals at high risk for prediabetes?
2. What changes in the health system and policy are needed to support and sustain lifestyle intervention?
3. What roles, responsibilities, and resources are most suitably placed in the hands of the physician, the health care system, or public health in a manner that will ensure effective collaboration?

The contribution of a recognitions program for DPP and other providers and the impact of publicly reported provider performance measurement on delivery of preventive services and diabetes care deserve more attention. It would be unfortunate if community-based organizations that may excel in reaching high-risk populations would be discouraged from engaging those most in need because of concern about not achieving recognition standards or performance goals that may be more difficult to achieve in certain subgroups of patients or certain community settings.

Treatment

The benefits of BP, lipid, glucose, and tobacco management are apparent, but less than 20% of those with diabetes meet currently recommended goals in all these domains. Efforts to improve the delivery of coordinated and effective health care using a team model are an ongoing research and policy challenge. The care of minority patients with diabetes is on average even worse, and focused efforts to reduce health disparities by race, ethnicity, and socioeconomic position are especially needed. In the face of increasing pharmaceutical costs, efforts to develop more cost-effective approaches to diabetes care are needed. Development and deployment of more effective diabetes education and self-care models is urgently needed (Sperl-Hillen et al. 2011), as is development of more effective provider education (Sperl-Hillen et al. 2014).

Clinical decision support systems to support team models of diabetes care and provide personalized and prioritized evidence-based recommendations to individual patients need further development (Bright et al. 2012; O'Connor et al. 2011). Shared decision-making (Legare et al. 2014) and patient-centered care (Dwamena et al. 2012) are other important research areas. Public health or population-based diabetes registries have been implemented in New York City and in many large health care delivery systems. In some of these care systems, there have been dramatic improvements in diabetes care since 1994. The use of electronic medical record system–derived registries that monitor HbA1c, BP, low-density lipoprotein cholesterol, total cholesterol, and reversible cardiovascular risk and treatment patterns have revolutionized chronic disease surveillance and will likely lead to new approaches to diabetes management on a population basis in the near future (Desai et al. 2015; Vazquez-Benitez et al. 2015).

Team care models in primary care medical homes and other care settings often include pharmacists and expanded-role nurses and educators, and have shown promise as a way to improve care for diabetes and other chronic diseases. Further work to understand the potential impact of primary care medical homes, shared care between primary care providers and subspecialists, and social media approaches that may augment existing models of diabetes care and education is needed.

Efforts to identify biomarkers that can help predict risk of certain complications and differential response to various classes of drugs have been discussed for decades, but few such markers are currently available for use in clinical practice. Eventually, such markers may make it possible to more effectively tailor primary and secondary diabetes prevention strategies to individuals.

Cost-Effectiveness and Policy Studies

Various prediction models are available to examine the cost utility of specific diabetes prevention and care strategies (Bannister et al. 2014; Herman et al. 2013). The cost-effectiveness of diabetes treatment strategies necessarily change over time with changes in pharmaceutical costs and standards of care. A CDC study in 2002 on cost-effectiveness of type 2 diabetes treatments suggested that the mean cost of adding one QALY through intensive glucose control was approximately $41,000, but ranged from $9,614 per QALY when diabetes was diagnosed at ages 25 to 34 years to $2.1 million per QALY when diabetes was diagnosed at ages 80 to 94 years. This analysis also indicated that efforts to control BP and lipids may be cost saving for many patients, from the payer perspective (CDC Diabetes Cost-Effectiveness Group 2002). Updated cost-effectiveness analyses that model the use of new classes of medications and evolving guidelines are very much needed.

The cost-effectiveness of behavioral interventions (e.g., diet plus exercise) for patients with type 2 diabetes is well-established, with data from the DPP demonstrating the cost-effectiveness of lifestyle change (nutrition and physical activity) and metformin intervention for prediabetes (Herman et al. 2013). Recent data summarized by the National Institutes of Health quantify the impact of lifestyle risk factors and the expected benefits of their successful modification on cardiovascular risk. These data can be used to model the cost utility of nutrition and physical activity interventions (Eckel et al. 2014). Perhaps the strongest case can be made for primary prevention to lower incidence of type 2 diabetes through more physical activity, dietary change, weight management, use of metformin, and reduced smoking.

The influence of the social and physical environment and socioeconomic status on diabetes onset and progression of type 2 diabetes are becoming increasingly well documented and understood (Agardh et al. 2011; Auchincloss et al. 2009; Christine et al. 2015; Gaskin et al. 2014; Walker et al. 2014; Zuijdwijk et al. 2013) and make plain the need for a public health response capable of addressing the underlying issues in the social (stress, overwork, fragmented social systems) and physical (barriers to healthy eating and activity) environment in a multitude of cultures and settings. There is a great need for research on diabetes that is informed by the social and cultural context in which it occurs, including examination of family and friendship ties, community norms, the structure of community services, and health policy.

Goodman et al. (2006) argue that such prevention efforts need to focus more on the social, cultural, community, and environmental factors that contribute to health disparities than on behavioral modification strategies. Their recommended approach to a comprehensive community effort includes (1) facilitating a meaningful and central role for the community, (2) giving primary attention to participatory processes before best practices, (3) emphasizing cultural relevance in intervention design sensitive to the cultural and racial or ethnic makeup of the community, and (4) incorporating a social-ecology approach that is holistic and addresses larger environmental influences and not individual behavior change alone. At the clinic level, their concerns are mirrored in the Reach, Effectiveness, Adoption, Implementation, and Maintenance framework, proposed by Glasgow (2003) that emphasizes the importance of developing evidence-based interventions that balance effectiveness with generalizability (i.e., adoptability and effectiveness across many diverse settings). An excellent example of this approach and methodology is a school-based physical activity intervention to prevent diabetes in the Hualapai Indian community in Arizona (Teufel-Shone et al. 2014).

Successful efforts to blunt the diabetes epidemic will require close collaboration among the health care, business, and public health sectors of our society within a framework of strong government and community partnership. Upstream public policy interventions that involve government actions directed at entire populations or communities that alter tax structures, reinforce health promotion, and increase access to healthy food and physical activity opportunities within neighborhoods and communities are foundational to any comprehensive strategy of diabetes treatment and prevention. Such strategies are also among the most difficult to initiate and maintain for a sufficiently long period to permit adequate policy-relevant analysis of impact and cost-effectiveness.

Resources

American Association of Diabetes Educators, http://www.diabeteseducator.org

American Diabetes Association, http://www.diabetes.org

Diabetes. Guide to Community Preventive Services, Centers for Disease Control and Prevention (CDC), http://www.thecommunityguide.org/diabetes

Diabetes centers:

Diabetes Research Centers, https://diabetescenters.org

Centers for Diabetes Translation Research, http://www.diabetes-translation.org

The National Institute of Diabetes and Digestive and Kidney Diseases (NIDDK), http://www.niddk.nih.gov/research-funding/research-programs/Pages/diabetes-centers.aspx

Diabetes Prevention Program Outcomes Study, https://dppos.bsc.gwu.edu

Diabetes Public Health Resource, National Center for Chronic Disease Prevention and Health Promotion, Centers for Disease Control and Prevention, http://cdc.gov/diabetes/home/index.html

- National Diabetes Prevention Program, http://www.cdc.gov/diabetes/prevention/index.html
- Native Diabetes Wellness Program, http://www.cdc.gov/diabetes/ndwp/index.html
- National Diabetes Education Program, http://www.cdc.gov/diabetes/ndep/index.html (joint program of CDC and NIDDK)
- Prevent Diabetes STAT: Screen/Test/Act Today, http://ama-assn.org/sub/prevent-diabetes-stat (joint program of CDC and the American Medical Association)

- Diabetes data and statistics, http://www.cdc.gov/diabetes/data/index.html
- CDC-supported programs and initiatives, www.cdc.gov/diabetes/programs Juvenile Diabetes Research Foundation International, http://www.jdrf.org

National Diabetes Information Clearinghouse: Directory of Diabetes Organizations, http://www.niddk.nih.gov/health-information/health-topics/Diabetes/Documents/Directory_Diabetes_Orgs_508.pdf

Suggested Reading

American Diabetes Association. Clinical Practice Recommendations 2016. *Diabetes Care.* 2016:38(suppl 1). Available at: http://care.diabetesjournals.org/content/38/Supplement_1.

Centers for Disease Control and Prevention. *Effective Public Health Strategies to Prevent and Control Diabetes: A Compendium.* US Department of Health and Human Services. 2013. Available at: https://stacks.cdc.gov/view/cdc/23434.

Centers for Disease Control and Prevention. *National Diabetes Statistics Report: Estimates of Diabetes and Its Burden in the United States, 2014* [in English and Spanish]. US Department of Health and Human Services. 2014. Available at: http://www.cdc.gov/diabetes/data/statistics/2014statisticsreport.html.

Centers for Disease Control and Prevention. *Diabetes Report Card.* US Department of Health and Human Services, Centers for Disease Control and Prevention. 2015. Available at http://www.cdc.gov/diabetes/library/reports/congress.html.

Institute for Clinical Systems Improvement. *Diabetes Mellitus in Adults, Type 2; Diagnosis and Management.* Updated July 2014. Available at: https://www.icsi.org/guidelines__more/catalog_guidelines_and_more/catalog_guidelines/catalog_endocrine_guidelines/diabetes.

Narayan KMV, Williams D, Gregg EW, Cowie CC. *Diabetes Public Health: From Data to Policy.* New York, NY: Oxford University Press, 2011.

Partnership for Prevention. *Diabetes Self-Management Education (DSME): Establishing a Community-Based DSME Program for Adults With Type 2 Diabetes to Improve Glycemic control—An Action Guide. The Community Health Promotion Handbook: Action Guides to Improve Community Health.* Washington, DC: Partnership for Prevention; 2008. Available at: http://www.prevent.org/actionguides.

University of Chicago. *The Effectiveness of Diabetes Prevention Programs in Community Settings.* New York State Health Foundation. 2015. Available at: http://nyshealthfoundation.org/uploads/resources/report-diabetes-prevention-in-community-settings.pdf.

References

Ackermann RT. Diabetes prevention at the tipping point: aligning clinical and public health recommendations. *Ann Intern Med.* 2015;163(6):475–476.

Ackermann RT, Liss DT, Finch EA, et al. A randomized comparative effectiveness trial for preventing type 2 diabetes. *Am J Public Health.* 2015;105(11):2328–2334.

Agardh E, Allebeck P, Hallqvist J, Moradi T, Sidorchuk A. Type 2 diabetes incidence and socio-economic position: a systematic review and meta-analysis. *Int J Epidemiol.* 2011;40(3):804–818.

Agency for Healthcare Research and Quality (AHRQ). *2014 National Healthcare Quality and Disparities Report—Chartbook on Effective Treatment.* Rockville, MD: AHRQ; 2015.

Akerblom HK, Virtanen SM, Ilonen J, et al. Dietary manipulation of beta cell autoimmunity in infants at increased risk of type 1 diabetes: a pilot study. *Diabetologia.* 2005;48(5):829–837.

Al-Saeed AH, Constantino MI, Molyneaux L, et al. An inverse relationship between age of type 2 diabetes onset and complication risk and mortality: the impact of youth-onset type 2 diabetes. *Diabetes Care.* 2016;39(5):823–829.

Albright AL, Gregg EW. Preventing type 2 diabetes in communities across the U.S.: the national Diabetes Prevention Program. *Am J Prev Med.* 2013;44(suppl 4):S346–S351.

Ali MK, Bullard KM, Gregg EW. Achievement of goals in U.S. diabetes care, 1999–2010. *N Engl J Med.* 2013;369(3):287–288.

American Diabetes Association (ADA). Economic costs of diabetes in the U.S. in 2012. *Diabetes Care.* 2013;36(4):1033–1046.

American Diabetes Association (ADA). Prevention or delay of type 2 diabetes. Sec. 4. In: Standards of Medical Care in Diabetes—2016. *Diabetes Care.* 2016a;39(suppl 1): S36–S38.

American Diabetes Association (ADA). Classification and diagnosis of diabetes. Sec. 2. In: Standards of Medical Care in Diabetes—2016. *Diabetes Care.* 2016b;39(suppl 1): S13–S22.

American Diabetes Association (ADA). Standards of Medical Care in Diabetes—2016, abridged for primary care providers. *Clin Diabetes.* 2016c;34(1):3–21.

Amini M, Djazayery A, Majdzadeh R, Taghdisi MH, Jazayeri S. Effect of school-based interventions to control childhood obesity: a review of reviews. *Int J Prev Med.* 2015; 6:68.

Aroda VR, Christophi CA, Edelstein SL, et al. The effect of lifestyle intervention and metformin on preventing or delaying diabetes among women with and without gestational diabetes: the Diabetes Prevention Program outcomes study 10-year follow-up. *J Clin Endocrinol Metab.* 2015;100(4):1646–1653.

Atkinson MA. The pathogenesis and natural history of type 1 diabetes. *Cold Spring Harb Perspect Med.* 2012;2(11):a007641.

Auchincloss AH, Diez Roux AV, Mujahid MS, Shen M, Bertoni AG, Carnethon MR. Neighborhood resources for physical activity and healthy foods and incidence of type 2 diabetes mellitus: the multi-ethnic study of atherosclerosis. *Arch Intern Med.* 2009;169(18):1698–1704.

Balk EM, Earley A, Raman G, Avendano EA, Pittas AG, Remington PL. Combined diet and physical activity promotion programs to prevent type 2 diabetes among persons at increased risk: a systematic review for the Community Preventive Services Task Force. *Ann Intern Med.* 2015;163(6):437–451.

Bannister CA, Poole CD, Jenkins-Jones S, et al. External validation of the UKPDS risk engine in incident type 2 diabetes: a need for new type 2 diabetes-specific risk equations. *Diabetes Care.* 2014;37(2):537–545.

Baranowski T, Cooper DM, Harrell J, et al. Presence of diabetes risk factors in a large U.S. eighth-grade cohort. *Diabetes Care.* 2006;29(2):212–217.

Bardenheier BH, Imperatore G, Devlin HM, Kim SY, Cho P, Geiss LS. Trends in pre-pregnancy diabetes among deliveries in 19 U.S. states, 2000–2010. *Am J Prev Med.* 2015a;48(2):154–161.

Bardenheier BH, Imperatore G, Gilboa SM, et al. Trends in gestational diabetes among hospital deliveries in 19 U.S. States, 2000–2010. *Am J Prevent Med.* 2015b;49(1):12–19.

Barker LE, Kirtland KA, Gregg EW, Geiss LS, Thompson TJ. Geographic distribution of diagnosed diabetes in the U.S.: a diabetes belt. *Am J Prev Med.* 2011;40(4):434–439.

Bascones-Martinez A, Matesanz-Perez P, Escribano-Bermejo M, Gonzalez-Moles MA, Bascones-Ilundain J, Meurman JH. Periodontal disease and diabetes—review of the literature. *Med Oral Patol Oral Cir Bucal.* 2011;16(6):e722–e729.

Becerra MB, Becerra BJ. Disparities in age at diabetes diagnosis among Asian Americans: implications for early preventive measures. *Prev Chronic Dis.* 2015;12:E146.

Beckles G, Chou C. Diabetes—United States, 2006 and 2010. *MMWR Suppl.* 2013;62(3):99–104.

Bell JA, Kivimaki M, Hamer M. Metabolically healthy obesity and risk of incident type 2 diabetes: a meta-analysis of prospective cohort studies. *Obes Rev.* 2014;15(6):504–515.

Bellamy L, Casas JP, Hingorani AD, Williams D. Type 2 diabetes mellitus after gestational diabetes: a systematic review and meta-analysis. *Lancet*. 2009;373(9677):1773–1779.

Bergenstal RM, Klonoff DC, Garg SK, et al. Threshold-based insulin-pump interruption for reduction of hypoglycemia. *N Engl J Med*. 2013;369(3):224–232.

Bishop DB, O'Connor PJ, Desai J. Diabetes. In: Remington PL, Brownson RC, Wegner MV, ed. *Chronic Disease Epidemiology and Control*. 3rd ed. Washington, DC: American Public Health Association; 2010:304.

Boyle J, Thompson T, Gregg E, Barker L, Wiliamson D. Projection of the year 2050 burden of diabetes in the US adult population: dynamic modeling of incidence, mortality, and prediabetes prevalence. *Popul Health Metr*. 2010;8:29.

Brezo J, Royal C, Ampy F, Headings V. Ethnic identity and type 2 diabetes health attitudes in Americans of African ancestry. *Ethn Dis*. 2006;16(3):624–632.

Bright TJ, Wong A, Dhurjati R, et al. Effect of clinical decision-support systems: a systematic review. *Ann Intern Med*. 2012;157(1):29–43.

Bruni A, Gala-Lopez B, Pepper AR, Abualhassan NS, Shapiro AJ. Islet cell transplantation for the treatment of type 1 diabetes: recent advances and future challenges. *Diabetes Metab Syndr Obes*. 2014;7:211–223.

Burnet DL, Plaut AJ, Wolf SA, et al. Reach-out: a family-based diabetes prevention program for African American youth. *J Natl Med Assoc*. 2011;103(3):269–277.

Cappuccio FP, D'Elia L, Strazzullo P, Miller MA. Quantity and quality of sleep and incidence of type 2 diabetes: a systematic review and meta-analysis. *Diabetes Care*. 2010;33(2):414–420.

Caspersen CJ, Thomas GD, Boseman LA, Beckles GLA, Albright AL. Aging, diabetes, and the public health system in the United States. *Am J Public Health*. 2012;102(8):1482–1497.

Centers for Disease Control and Prevention (CDC). National diabetes fact sheet: national estimates and general information on diabetes and prediabetes in the United States, 2011. Atlanta, GA: US Department of Health and Human Services, CDC; 2011.

Centers for Disease Control and Prevention (CDC), Division of Diabetes Translation. Hospitalization. 2012. Available at: http://www.cdc.gov/diabetes/statistics/hospitalization_national.htm. Accessed August 23, 2016.

Centers for Disease Control and Prevention (CDC). *National Diabetes Statistics Report: Estimates of Diabetes and Its Burden in the United States, 2014*. Atlanta, GA: US Department of Health and Human Services, CDC; 2014.

Centers for Disease Control and Prevention (CDC) Diabetes Cost-Effectiveness Group. Cost-effectiveness of intensive glycemic control, intensified hypertension control, and serum cholesterol level reduction for type 2 diabetes. *JAMA*. 2002;287(19): 2542–2551.

Centers for Medicare and Medicaid Services (CMS), Office of the Actuary. Certification of Medicare Diabetes Prevention Program. 2016. Available at: https://www.cms. gov/Research-Statistics-Data-and-Systems/Research/ActuarialStudies/Downloads/ Diabetes-Prevention-Certification-2016-03-14.pdf. Accessed May 1, 2016.

Cha E, Kim KH, Umpierrez G, et al. A feasibility study to develop a diabetes prevention program for young adults with prediabetes by using digital platforms and a handheld device. *Diabetes Educ*. 2014;40(5):626–637.

Chambers RA, Rosenstock S, Neault N, et al. A home-visiting diabetes prevention and management program for American Indian youth: the Together on Diabetes Trial. *Diabetes Educ*. 2015;41(6):729–747.

Chatenoud L, Warncke K, Ziegler AG. Clinical immunologic interventions for the treatment of type 1 diabetes. *Cold Spring Harb Perspect Med*. 2012;2(8):a007716.

Cheng S, Claggett B, Correia AW, et al. Temporal trends in the population attributable risk for cardiovascular disease: the Atherosclerosis Risk in Communities Study. *Circulation*. 2014;130(10):820–828.

Cheng YJ, Imperatore G, Caspersen CJ, Gregg EW, Albright AL, Helmick CG. Prevalence of diagnosed arthritis and arthritis-attributable activity limitation among adults with and without diagnosed diabetes: United States, 2008–2010. *Diabetes Care*. 2012; 35(8):1686–1691.

Chiasson JL, Josse RG, Gomis R, Hanefeld M, Karasik A, Laakso M. Acarbose for prevention of type 2 diabetes mellitus: the STOP-NIDDM randomised trial. *Lancet*. 2002;359(9323):2072–2077.

Chou CH, Burnet DL, Meltzer DO, Huang ES; University of Chicago. *The Effectiveness of Diabetes Prevention Programs in Community Settings*. New York, NY: New York State Health Foundation; 2015.

Christine PJ, Auchincloss AH, Bertoni AG, et al. Longitudinal associations between neighborhood physical and social environments and incident type 2 diabetes mellitus: the Multi-ethnic Study of Atherosclerosis (MESA). *JAMA Intern Med*. 2015;175(8):1311–1320.

Committee on Practice Bulletins—Obstetrics. Practice Bulletin No. 137: gestational diabetes mellitus. *Obstet Gynecol*. 2013;122(2 pt 1):406–416.

Crandall JP, Polsky S, Howard AA, et al. Alcohol consumption and diabetes risk in the diabetes prevention program. *Am J Clin Nutr*. 2009;90(3):595–601.

Dabelea D, Mayer-Davis EJ, Saydah S, et al. Prevalence of type 1 and type 2 diabetes among children and adolescents from 2001 to 2009. *JAMA*. 2014;311(17):1778–1786.

Demakakos P, Marmot M, Steptoe A. Socioeconomic position and the incidence of type 2 diabetes: the ELSA study. *Eur J Epidemiol*. 2012;27(5):367–378.

Desai JR, Vazquez-Benitez G, Xu Z, et al. Who must we target now to minimize future cardiovascular events and total mortality? Lessons from the Surveillance, Prevention and Management of Diabetes Mellitus (SUPREME-DM) cohort study. *Circ Cardiovasc Qual Outcomes*. 2015;8(5):508–516.

Diabetes Prevention Program Research Group (DPPRG). The 10-year cost-effectiveness of lifestyle intervention or metformin for diabetes prevention: an intent-to-treat analysis of the DPP/DPPOS. *Diabetes Care*. 2012a;35(4):723–730.

Diabetes Prevention Program Research Group (DPPRG). Long-term safety, tolerability, and weight loss associated with metformin in the Diabetes Prevention Program outcomes study. *Diabetes Care*. 2012b;35(4):731–737.

Diabetes Prevention Program Research Group (DPPRG). Long-term effects of lifestyle intervention or metformin on diabetes development and microvascular complications over 15-year follow-up: the diabetes prevention program outcomes study. *Lancet Diabetes Endocrinol*. 2015;3(11):866–875.

Di Angelantonio E, Kaptoge S, Wormser D, et al. Association of cardiometabolic multimorbidity with mortality. *JAMA*. 2015;314(1):52–60.

Division of Diabetes Translation (DDT). *Long-Term Trends in Diabetes*. Atlanta, GA: Centers for Disease Control and Prevention; 2014.

Dodani S, Fields JZ. Implementation of the Fit Body and Soul, a church-based life style program for diabetes prevention in high-risk African Americans: a feasibility study. *Diabetes Educ*. 2010;36(3):465–472.

Dwamena F, Holmes-Rovner M, Gaulden CM, et al. Interventions for providers to promote a patient-centered approach in clinical consultations. *Cochrane Database Syst Rev*. 2012;(12):CD003267.

Eckel RH, Jakicic JM, Ard JD, et al. 2013 AHA/ACC guideline on lifestyle management to reduce cardiovascular risk: a report of the American College of Cardiology/American Heart Association Task Force on Practice Guidelines. *Circulation*. 2014;129(25 suppl 2): S76–S99.

Egede LE. Diabetes, major depression, and functional disability among U.S. adults. *Diabetes Care*. 2004;27(2):421–428.

Emdin CA, Anderson SG, Woodward M, Rahimi K. Usual blood pressure and risk of new-onset diabetes: evidence from 4.1 million adults and a meta-analysis of prospective studies. *J Am Coll Cardiol.* 2015;66(14):1552–1562.

Faridi Z, Shuval K, Njike VY, et al. Partners Reducing Effects of Diabetes (PREDICT): a diabetes prevention physical activity and dietary intervention through African-American churches. *Health Educ Res.* 2010;25(2):306–315.

Foster GD, Linder B, Baranowski T, et al. A school-based intervention for diabetes risk reduction. *N Engl J Med.* 2010;363(5):443–453.

Gaede P, Lund-Andersen H, Parving HH, Pedersen O. Effect of a multifactorial intervention on mortality in type 2 diabetes. *N Engl J Med.* 2008;358(6):580–591.

Gaskin DJ, Thorpe RJ II, McGinty EE, et al. Disparities in diabetes: the nexus of race, poverty, and place. *Am J Public Health.* 2014;104(11):2147–2155.

Geiss L, James C, Gregg E, Albright A, Williamson D, Cowie C. Diabetes risk reduction behaviors among U.S. adults with prediabetes. *Am J Prev Med.* 2010;38(4):403–409.

Geiss LS, Wang J, Cheng YJ, et al. Prevalence and incidence trends for diagnosed diabetes among adults aged 20 to 79 years, United States, 1980–2012. *JAMA.* 2014;312(12):1218–1226.

Gerstein HC, Miller ME, Byington RP, et al. Effects of intensive glucose lowering in type 2 diabetes. *N Engl J Med.* 2008;358(24):2545–2559.

Glasgow RE. Translating research to practice: lessons learned, areas for improvement, and future directions. *Diabetes Care.* 2003;26(8):2451–2456.

Gonzalez-Suarez C, Worley A, Grimmer-Somers K, Dones V. School-based interventions on childhood obesity: a meta-analysis. *Am J Prev Med.* 2009;37(5):418–427.

Goodman RM, Yoo S, Jack L II. Applying comprehensive community-based approaches in diabetes prevention: rationale, principles, and models. *J Public Health Manag Pract.* 2006;12(6):545–555.

Gregg EW, Ali MK, Moore BA, et al. The importance of natural experiments in diabetes prevention and control and the need for better health policy research. *Prevent Chronic Dis.* 2013;10:E14.

Gregg EW, Cheng YJ, Narayan KM, Thompson TJ, Williamson DF. The relative contributions of different levels of overweight and obesity to the increased prevalence of diabetes in the United States: 1976–2004. *Prev Med.* 2007a;45(5):348–352.

Gregg EW, Cheng YJ, Saydah S, et al. Trends in death rates among U.S. adults with and without diabetes between 1997 and 2006: findings from the National Health Interview Survey. *Diabetes Care*. 2012;35(6):1252–1257.

Gregg EW, Gu Q, Cheng YJ, Narayan KM, Cowie CC. Mortality trends in men and women with diabetes, 1971 to 2000. *Ann Intern Med*. 2007b;147(3):149–155.

Gregg EW, Li Y, Wang J, et al. Changes in diabetes-related complications in the United States, 1990-2010. *N Engl J Med*. 2014b;370(16):1514–1523.

Gregg EW, Zhou X, Cheng Y, Albright A, Venkat Narayan K, Thompson T. Trends in lifetime risk and years of life lost due to diabetes in the USA, 1985–2011: a modelling study. *Lancet Diabetes Endocrinol*. 2014a;2(11):867–874.

Grontved A, Hu FB. Television viewing and risk of type 2 diabetes, cardiovascular disease, and all-cause mortality: a meta-analysis. *JAMA*. 2011;305(23):2448–2455.

Guelfi KJ, Jones TW, Fournier PA. New insights into managing the risk of hypoglycaemia associated with intermittent high-intensity exercise in individuals with type 1 diabetes mellitus: implications for existing guidelines. *Sports Med*. 2007;37(11):937–946.

Haire-Joshu D, Elliott MB, Caito NM, et al. High 5 for Kids: the impact of a home visiting program on fruit and vegetable intake of parents and their preschool children. *Prev Med*. 2008;47(1):77–82.

Halban PA, Polonsky KS, Bowden DW, et al. Beta-cell failure in type 2 diabetes: postulated mechanisms and prospects for prevention and treatment. *J Clin Endocrinol Metab*. 2014;99(6):1983–1992.

Hamman R, Bell R, Dabelea D, et al. The SEARCH for diabetes in youth study: rationale, findings, and future directions. *Diabetes Care*. 2014;37(12):3336–3344.

Hannon TS, Carroll AE, Palmer KN, Saha C, Childers WK, Marrero DG. Rationale and design of a comparative effectiveness trial to prevent type 2 diabetes in mothers and children: the ENCOURAGE healthy families study. *Contemp Clin Trials*. 2015;40:105–111.

Hansen MB, Jensen ML, Carstensen B. Causes of death among diabetic patients in Denmark. *Diabetologia*. 2012;55(2):294–302.

Haroon NN, Austin PC, Shah BR, Wu J, Gill SS, Booth GL. Risk of dementia in seniors with newly diagnosed diabetes: a population-based study. *Diabetes Care*. 2015;38(10):1868–1875.

Harris MI. Undiagnosed NIDDM: clinical and public health issues. *Diabetes Care*. 1993;16(4):642–652.

Hartstein J, Cullen KW, Reynolds KD, Harrell J, Resnicow K, Kennel P. Impact of portion-size control for school a la carte items: changes in kilocalories and macronutrients purchased by middle school students. *J Am Diet Assoc.* 2008;108(1):140–144.

Herman WH, Edelstein SL, Ratner RE, et al. Effectiveness and cost-effectiveness of diabetes prevention among adherent participants. *Am J Manag Care.* 2013;19(3):194–202.

Heron M. *Deaths: Leading Causes for 2012.* Atlanta, GA: Centers for Disease Control and Prevention, National Center for Health Statistics, National Vital Statistics System; 2015.

Hingle MD, Turner T, Kutob R, et al. The EPIC kids study: a randomized family-focused YMCA-based intervention to prevent type 2 diabetes in at-risk youth. *BMC Public Health.* 2015;15(1):1253.

Hinnant L, Razi S, Lewis R, et al. Evaluation of the Health Care Innovation Awards: Community Resource Planning, Prevention, and Monitoring, Annual Report 2015. Awardee-Level Findings:

YMCA of the USA. RTI International. 2016. Available at: https://innovation.cms.gov/Files/reports/hcia-ymcadpp-evalrpt.pdf. Accessed May 1, 2016.

Hippisley-Cox J, Coupland C. Development and validation of risk prediction equations to estimate future risk of blindness and lower limb amputation in patients with diabetes: cohort study. *BMJ.* 2015;351:h5441.

Hirst K, Baranowski T, DeBar L, et al. HEALTHY study rationale, design and methods: moderating risk of type 2 diabetes in multi-ethnic middle school students. *Int J Obes (Lond).* 2009;33(suppl 4):S4–S20.

Holman RR. Type 2 diabetes mellitus in 2012: optimal management of T2DM remains elusive. *Nat Rev Endocrinol.* 2013;9(2):67–68.

Holman RR, Paul SK, Bethel MA, Matthews DR, Neil HA. 10-year follow-up of intensive glucose control in type 2 diabetes. *N Engl J Med.* 2008;359(15):1577–1589.

Horvath K, Koch K, Jeitler K, et al. Effects of treatment in women with gestational diabetes mellitus: systematic review and meta-analysis. *BMJ.* 2010;340:c1395.

Hostalek U, Gwilt M, Hildemann S. Therapeutic use of metformin in prediabetes and diabetes prevention. *Drugs.* 2015;75(10):1071–1094.

Hu FB. Globalization of diabetes: the role of diet, lifestyle, and genes. *Diabetes Care.* 2011;34(6):1249–1257.

Hu FB, Manson JE, Stampfer MJ, et al. Diet, lifestyle, and the risk of type 2 diabetes mellitus in women. *N Engl J Med.* 2001;345(11):790–797.

Hussain A, Claussen B, Ramachandran A, Williams R. Prevention of type 2 diabetes: a review. *Diabetes Res Clin Prac.* 2007;76(3):317–326.

Insaf TZ, Strogatz DS, Yucel RM, Chasan-Taber L, Shaw BA. Associations between race, lifecourse socioeconomic position and prevalence of diabetes among US women and men: results from a population-based panel study. *J Epidemiol Community Health.* 2014;68(4):318–325.

Inzucchi SE, Bergenstal RM, Buse JB, et al. Management of hyperglycemia in type 2 diabetes, 2015: a patient-centered approach: update to a position statement of the American Diabetes Association and the European Association for the Study of Diabetes. *Diabetes Care.* 2015;38(1):140–149.

Ismail-Beigi F, Craven T, Banerji MA, et al. Effect of intensive treatment of hyperglycaemia on microvascular outcomes in type 2 diabetes: an analysis of the ACCORD randomised trial. *Lancet.* 2010;376(9739):419–430.

Jenum AK, Anderssen SA, Birkeland KI, et al. Promoting physical activity in a low-income multiethnic district: effects of a community intervention study to reduce risk factors for type 2 diabetes and cardiovascular disease: a community intervention reducing inactivity. *Diabetes Care.* 2006;29(7):1605–1612.

Kahn SE, Haffner SM, Heise MA, et al. Glycemic durability of rosiglitazone, metformin, or glyburide monotherapy. *N Engl J Med.* 2006;355(23):2427–2443.

Kelishadi R, Azizi-Soleiman F. Controlling childhood obesity: a systematic review on strategies and challenges. *J Res Med Sci.* 2014;19(10):993–1008.

Kim SY, England L, Sappenfield W, et al. Racial/ethnic differences in the percentage of gestational diabetes mellitus cases attributable to overweight and obesity, Florida, 2004–2007. *Prev Chronic Dis.* 2012;9:E88.

Kim SY, Sappenfield W, Sharma AJ, et al. Racial/ethnic differences in the prevalence of gestational diabetes mellitus and maternal overweight and obesity, by nativity, Florida, 2004–2007. *Obesity (Silver Spring).* 2013;21(1):E33–E40.

Knowler WC, Barrett-Connor E, Fowler SE, et al. Reduction in the incidence of type 2 diabetes with lifestyle intervention or metformin. *N Engl J Med.* 2002;346(6): 393–403.

Knowler WC, Fowler SE, Hamman RF, et al. 10-year follow-up of diabetes incidence and weight loss in the Diabetes Prevention Program Outcomes Study. *Lancet.* 2009; 374(9702):1677–1686.

Landon MB, Spong CY, Thom E, et al. A multicenter, randomized trial of treatment for mild gestational diabetes. *N Engl J Med.* 2009;361(14):1339–1348.

Laramee AS, Morris N, Littenberg B. Relationship of literacy and heart failure in adults with diabetes. *BMC Health Serv Res.* 2007;7:98.

Légaré F, Stacey D, Turcotte S, et al. Interventions for improving the adoption of shared decision making by healthcare professionals. *Cochrane Database Syst Rev.* 2014;(9): CD006732.

Leong A, Rahme E, Dasgupta K. Spousal diabetes as a diabetes risk factor: a systematic review and meta-analysis. *BMC Med.* 2014;12:12.

Lepard MG, Joseph AL, Agne AA, Cherrington AL. Diabetes self-management interventions for adults with type 2 diabetes living in rural areas: a systematic literature review. *Curr Diab Rep.* 2015;15(6):608.

Levine JA. Poverty and obesity in the U.S. *Diabetes.* 2011;60(11):2667–2668.

Li Y, Burrows NR, Gregg EW, Albright A, Geiss LS. Declining rates of hospitalization for nontraumatic lower-extremity amputation in the diabetic population aged 40 years or older: U.S., 1988–2008. *Diabetes Care.* 2012;35(2):273–277.

Li Y, Ley SH, Tobias DK, et al. Birth weight and later life adherence to unhealthy lifestyles in predicting type 2 diabetes: prospective cohort study. *BMJ.* 2015b;351: h3672.

Li R, Qu S, Zhang P, et al. Economic evaluation of combined diet and physical activity promotion programs to prevent type 2 diabetes among persons at increased risk: a systematic review for the Community Preventive Services Task Force. *Ann Intern Med.* 2015a;163(6):452–460.

Li G, Zhang P, Wang J, et al. The long-term effect of lifestyle interventions to prevent diabetes in the China Da Qing diabetes prevention study: a 20-year follow-up study. *Lancet.* 2008;371(9626):1783–1789.

Li G, Zhang P, Wang J, et al. Cardiovascular mortality, all-cause mortality, and diabetes incidence after lifestyle intervention for people with impaired glucose tolerance in the Da Qing Diabetes Prevention Study: a 23-year follow-up study. *Lancet Diabetes Endocrinol.* 2014;2(6):474–480.

Liang W, Chikritzhs T. Alcohol consumption during adolescence and risk of diabetes in young adulthood. *Biomed Res Int.* 2014;2014:795741.

Ligthart S, van Herpt T, Lenning M, et al. Lifetime risk of developing impaired glucose metabolism and eventual progression from prediabetes to type 2 diabetes: a prospective cohort study. *Lancet Diabetes Endocrinol.* 2016;4(1):44–51.

Lindstrom J, Ilanne-Parikka P, Peltonen M, et al. Sustained reduction in the incidence of type 2 diabetes by lifestyle intervention: follow-up of the Finnish Diabetes Prevention Study. *Lancet.* 2006;368(9548):1673–1679.

Lindstrom J, Peltonen M, Eriksson JG, et al. Improved lifestyle and decreased diabetes risk over 13 years: long-term follow-up of the randomised Finnish Diabetes Prevention Study (DPS). *Diabetologia*. 2013;56(2):284–293.

Livesey G, Taylor R, Livesey H, Liu S. Is there a dose–response relation of dietary glycemic load to risk of type 2 diabetes? Meta-analysis of prospective cohort studies. *Am J Clin Nutr*. 2013;97(3):584–596.

Malanda UL, Welschen LM, Riphagen II, Dekker JM, Nijpels G, Bot SD. Self-monitoring of blood glucose in patients with type 2 diabetes mellitus who are not using insulin. *Cochrane Database Syst Rev*. 2012;(1):CD005060.

Marcus MD, Hirst K, Kaufman F, Foster GD, Baranowski T. Lessons learned from the HEALTHY primary prevention trial of risk factors for type 2 diabetes in middle school youth. *Curr Diab Rep*. 2013;13(1):63–71.

Margolis DJ, Hoffstad O, Nafash J, et al. Location, location, location: geographic clustering of lower-extremity amputation among Medicare beneficiaries with diabetes. *Diabetes Care*. 2011;34(11):2363–2367.

Marrero DG, Palmer KN, Phillips EO, Miller-Kovach K, Foster GD, Saha CK. Comparison of commercial and self-initiated weight loss programs in people with prediabetes: a randomized control trial. *Am J Public Health*. 2016;106(5):949–956.

Maty SC, Everson-Rose SA, Haan MN, Raghunathan TE, Kaplan GA. Education, income, occupation, and the 34-year incidence (1965–99) of type 2 diabetes in the Alameda County Study. *Int J Epidemiol*. 2005;34(6):1274–1281.

McEwen LN, Kim C, Haan M, et al. Diabetes reporting as a cause of death: results from the Translating Research Into Action for Diabetes (TRIAD) study. *Diabetes Care*. 2006;29(2):247–253.

Menke A, Casagrande S, Geiss L, Cowie CC. Prevalence of and trends in diabetes among adults in the United States, 1988–2012. *JAMA*. 2015;314(10):1021–1029.

Metzger BE, Gabbe SG, Persson B, et al. International association of diabetes and pregnancy study groups recommendations on the diagnosis and classification of hyperglycemia in pregnancy. *Diabetes Care*. 2010;33(3):676–682.

Miller CK, Nagaraja HN, Weinhold KR. Early weight-loss success identifies nonresponders after a lifestyle intervention in a worksite diabetes prevention trial. *J Acad Nutr Diet*. 2015;115(9):1464–1471.

Montori VM. Selecting the right drug treatment for adults with type 2 diabetes. *BMJ*. 2016;352:i1663.

Montori VM, Rodriguez-Gutierrez R. The triumph of innovation and the hard work of caring for patients with diabetes. *Ann Intern Med.* 2016;164(2):127–128.

Nathan DM. Diabetes: advances in diagnosis and treatment. *JAMA.* 2015;314(10):1052–1062.

Nathan DM, Zinman B, Cleary PA, et al. Modern-day clinical course of type 1 diabetes mellitus after 30 years' duration: the diabetes control and complications trial/epidemiology of diabetes interventions and complications and Pittsburgh epidemiology of diabetes complications experience (1983–2005). *Arch Intern Med.* 2009;169(14):1307–1316.

Nichols GA, Schroeder EB, Karter AJ, et al. Trends in diabetes incidence among 7 million insured adults, 2006–2011: the SUPREME-DM project. *Am J Epidemiol.* 2015;181(1):32–39.

Nicklas JM, Zera CA, England LJ, et al. A web-based lifestyle intervention for women with recent gestational diabetes mellitus: a randomized controlled trial. *Obstet Gynecol.* 2014;124(3):563–570.

Niemeier BS, Hektner JM, Enger KB. Parent participation in weight-related health interventions for children and adolescents: a systematic review and meta-analysis. *Prev Med.* 2012;55(1):3–13.

Nixon CA, Moore HJ, Douthwaite W, et al. Identifying effective behavioural models and behaviour change strategies underpinning preschool- and school-based obesity prevention interventions aimed at 4–6-year-olds: a systematic review. *Obes Rev.* 2012;13(suppl 1):106–117.

Norris JM, Yin X, Lamb MM, et al. Omega-3 polyunsaturated fatty acid intake and islet autoimmunity in children at increased risk for type 1 diabetes. *JAMA.* 2007;298(12):1420–1428.

Nuovo J, Balsbaugh T, Barton S, et al. Interventions to support diabetes self-management: the key role of the patient in diabetes care. *Curr Diabetes Rev.* 2007;3(4):226–228.

O'Connor PJ, Asche SE, Crain AL, et al. Is patient readiness to change a predictor of improved glycemic control? *Diabetes Care.* 2004;27(10):2325–2329.

O'Connor PJ, Gregg E, Rush WA, Cherney LM, Stiffman MN, Engelgau MM. Diabetes: how are we diagnosing and initially managing it? *Ann Fam Med.* 2006;4(1):15–22.

O'Connor PJ, Sperl-Hillen JM, Rush WA, et al. Impact of electronic health record clinical decision support on diabetes care: a randomized trial. *Ann Fam Med.* 2011;9(1):12–21.

Pan A, Lucas M, Sun Q, et al. Bidirectional association between depression and type 2 diabetes mellitus in women. *Arch Intern Med.* 2010;170(21):1884–1891.

Pan XR, Li GW, Hu YH, et al. Effects of diet and exercise in preventing NIDDM in people with impaired glucose tolerance. The Da Qing IGT and Diabetes Study. *Diabetes Care*. 1997;20(4):537–544.

Patel A, MacMahon S, Chalmers J, et al. Intensive blood glucose control and vascular outcomes in patients with type 2 diabetes. *N Engl J Med*. 2008;358(24):2560–2572.

Penckofer S, Doyle T, Byrn M, Lustman PJ. State of the science: depression and type 2 diabetes. *West J Nurs Res*. 2014;36(9):1158–1182.

Pereira K, Phillips B, Johnson C, Vorderstrasse A. Internet delivered diabetes self-management education: a review. *Diabetes Technol Ther*. 2015;17(1):55–63.

Pettitt DJ, Talton J, Dabelea D, et al. Prevalence of diabetes in U.S. youth in 2009: the SEARCH for Diabetes in Youth study. *Diabetes Care*. 2014;37(2):402–408.

Piccolo RS, Duncan DT, Pearce N, McKinlay JB. The role of neighborhood characteristics in racial/ethnic disparities in type 2 diabetes: results from the Boston Area Community Health (BACH) Survey. *Soc Sci Med*. 2015;130:79–90.

Pronk NP, Remington PL. Combined diet and physical activity promotion programs for prevention of diabetes: Community Preventive Services Task Force recommendation statement. *Ann Intern Med*. 2015;163(6):465–468.

Rachmiel M, Buccino J, Daneman D. Exercise and type 1 diabetes mellitus in youth; review and recommendations. *Pediatr Endocrinol Rev*. 2007;5(2):656–665.

Reinschmidt KM, Teufel-Shone NI, Bradford G, et al. Taking a broad approach to public health program adaptation: adapting a family-based diabetes education program. *J Prim Prev*. 2010;31(1–2):69–83.

Ricci-Cabello I, Ruiz-Perez I, Rojas-Garcia A, Pastor G, Rodriguez-Barranco M, Goncalves DC. Characteristics and effectiveness of diabetes self-management educational programs targeted to racial/ethnic minority groups: a systematic review, meta-analysis and meta-regression. *BMC Endocr Disord*. 2014;14:60.

Robbins JM, Vaccarino V, Zhang H, Kasl SV. Socioeconomic status and diagnosed diabetes incidence. *Diabetes Res Clin Pract*. 2005;68(3):230–236.

Rumball-Smith J, Barthold D, Nandi A, Heymann J. Diabetes associated with early labor-force exit: a comparison of sixteen high-income countries. *Health Aff (Millwood)*. 2014;33(1):110–115.

Ryan EA. Diagnosing gestational diabetes. *Diabetologia*. 2011;54(3):480–486.

Ryerson B, Tierney EF, Thompson TJ, et al. Excess physical limitations among adults with diabetes in the U.S. population, 1997–1999. *Diabetes Care*. 2003;26(1):206–210.

Sabin MA, Magnussen CG, Juonala M, et al. Insulin and BMI as predictors of adult type 2 diabetes mellitus. *Pediatrics*. 2015;135(1):e144–e151.

Samuel VT, Petersen KF, Shulman GI. Lipid-induced insulin resistance: unravelling the mechanism. *Lancet*. 2010;375(9733):2267–2277.

Samuel-Hodge CD, Hill-Briggs F, Gary TL. Lifestyle intervention for prevention and treatment of type 2 diabetes. *Nurs Clin North Am*. 2006;41(4):567–588,vii.

Sanders Thompson VL, Johnson-Jennings M, Bauman AA, Proctor E. Use of culturally focused theoretical frameworks for adapting diabetes prevention programs: a qualitative review. *Prev Chronic Dis*. 2015;12:E60.

Schauer DP, Arterburn DE, Livingston EH, et al. Impact of bariatric surgery on life expectancy in severely obese patients with diabetes: a decision analysis. *Ann Surg*. 2015;261(5):914–919.

Schillinger D, Barton LR, Karter AJ, Wang F, Adler N. Does literacy mediate the relationship between education and health outcomes? A study of a low-income population with diabetes. *Public Health Rep*. 2006;121(3):245–254.

Schillinger D, Grumbach K, Piette J, et al. Association of health literacy with diabetes outcomes. *JAMA*. 2002;288(4):475–482.

Schmittdiel JA, Brown SD, Neugebauer R, et al. Health-plan and employer-based wellness programs to reduce diabetes risk: The Kaiser Permanente Northern California NEXT-D Study. *Prev Chronic Dis*. 2013;10:E15.

Schmittdiel JA, Desai J, Schroeder EB, et al. Methods for engaging stakeholders in comparative effectiveness research: a patient-centered approach to improving diabetes care. *Healthc (Amst)*. 2015;3(2):80–88.

Schmittdiel JA, Raebel MA, Dyer W, et al. Prescription medication burden in patients with newly-diagnosed diabetes: A SUrveillance, PREvention, and ManagEment of Diabetes Mellitus (SUPREME-DM) Study. *J Am Pharm Assoc*. 2014;54(4):374–382.

Scott RA, Langenberg C, Sharp SJ, et al. The link between family history and risk of type 2 diabetes is not explained by anthropometric, lifestyle or genetic risk factors: the EPIC-InterAct study. *Diabetologia*. 2013;56(1):60–69.

Selvin E, Parrinello C, Sacks D, Coresh J. Trends in prevalence and control of diabetes in the United States, 1988–1994 and 1999–2010. *Ann Intern Med*. 2014;160:517–525.

Semenkovich K, Brown ME, Svrakic DM, Lustman PJ. Depression in type 2 diabetes mellitus: prevalence, impact, and treatment. *Drugs*. 2015;75(6):577–587.

Sepah SC, Jiang L, Peters AL. Translating the Diabetes Prevention Program into an online social network: validation against CDC standards. *Diabetes Educ*. 2014;40(4):435–443.

Sherifali D, Bai JW, Kenny M, Warren R, Ali MU. Diabetes self-management programmes in older adults: a systematic review and meta-analysis. *Diabet Med.* 2015; 32(11):1404–1414.

Simeone RM, Devine OJ, Marcinkevage JA, et al. Diabetes and congenital heart defects: a systematic review, meta-analysis, and modeling project. *Am J Prev Med.* 2015;48(2):195–204.

Siminerio LM. Implementing diabetes self-management training programs: breaking through the barriers in primary care. *Endocr Pract.* 2006;12(suppl 1):124–130.

Siminerio LM. Approaches to help people with diabetes overcome barriers for improved health outcomes. *Diabetes Educ.* 2008;34(suppl 1):18s–24s.

Simmons K, Michels AW. Lessons from type 1 diabetes for understanding natural history and prevention of autoimmune disease. *Rheum Dis Clin North Am.* 2014;40(4):797–811.

Siu AL. Screening for abnormal blood glucose and type 2 diabetes mellitus: U.S. Preventive Services Task Force recommendation statement. *Ann Intern Med.* 2015;163(11):861–868.

Skyler JS. Primary and secondary prevention of type 1 diabetes. *Diabet Med.* 2013;30(2): 161–169.

Skyler JS. Prevention and reversal of type 1 diabetes—past challenges and future opportunities. *Diabetes Care.* 2015;38(6):997–1007.

Smith BT, Lynch JW, Fox CS, et al. Life-course socioeconomic position and type 2 diabetes mellitus: The Framingham Offspring Study. *Am J Epidemiol.* 2011;173(4):438–447.

Snoek FJ, Bremmer MA, Hermanns N. Constructs of depression and distress in diabetes: time for an appraisal. *Lancet Diabetes Endocrinol.* 2015;3(6):450–460.

Sperl-Hillen J, Beaton S, Fernandes O, et al. Comparative effectiveness of patient education methods for type 2 diabetes: a randomized controlled trial. *Arch Intern Med.* 2011;171(22):2001–2010.

Sperl-Hillen J, O'Connor PJ, Ekstrom HL, et al. Educating resident physicians using virtual case-based simulation improves diabetes management: a randomized controlled trial. *Acad Med.* 2014;89(12):1664–1673.

Srinivasan S, Florez JC. Therapeutic challenges in diabetes prevention: we have not found the "exercise pill." *Clin Pharmacol Ther.* 2015;98(2):162–169.

Steinbrecher A, Morimoto Y, Heak S, et al. The preventable proportion of type 2 diabetes by ethnicity: the multiethnic cohort. *Ann Epidemiol.* 2011;21(7):526–535.

Stringhini S, Batty GD, Bovet P, et al. Association of lifecourse socioeconomic status with chronic inflammation and type 2 diabetes risk: the Whitehall II prospective cohort study. *PLoS Med.* 2013;10(7):e1001479.

Sussman JB, Kent DM, Nelson JP, Hayward RA. Improving diabetes prevention with benefit based tailored treatment: risk based reanalysis of diabetes prevention program. *BMJ*. 2015;350:h454.

Tabak AG, Akbaraly TN, Batty GD, Kivimaki M. Depression and type 2 diabetes: a causal association? *Lancet Diabetes Endocrinol*. 2014;2(3):236–245.

Tabak AG, Herder C, Rathmann W, Brunner E, Kivimaki M. Prediabetes: a high-risk state for diabetes development. *Lancet*. 2012;379(9833):2279–2290.

Tabak RG, Sinclair KA, Baumann AA, et al. A review of Diabetes Prevention Program translations: use of cultural adaptation and implementation research. *Transl Behav Med*. 2015;5(4):401–414.

Tancredi M, Rosengren A, Svensson AM, et al. Excess mortality among persons with type 2 diabetes. *N Engl J Med*. 2015;373(18):1720–1732.

Task Force on Community Preventive Services. Recommendations for healthcare system and self-management education interventions to reduce morbidity and mortality from diabetes. *Am J Prev Med*. 2002;22(suppl 4):10–14.

Taylor R. Type 2 diabetes: etiology and reversibility. *Diabetes Care*. 2013;36(4):1047–1055.

Teufel-Shone NI, Drummond R, Rawiel U. Developing and adapting a family-based diabetes program at the U.S.–Mexico border. *Prev Chronic Dis*. 2005;2(1):A20.

Teufel-Shone NI, Gamber M, Watahomigie H, Siyuja TJ Jr, Crozier L, Irwin SL. Using a participatory research approach in a school-based physical activity intervention to prevent diabetes in the Hualapai Indian community, Arizona, 2002–2006. *Prev Chronic Dis*. 2014;11:E166.

The NS, Richardson A, Gordon-Larsen P. Timing and duration of obesity in relation to diabetes: findings from an ethnically diverse, nationally representative sample. *Diabetes Care*. 2013;36:865–872.

Tryggestad JB, Willi SM. Complications and comorbidities of T2DM in adolescents: findings from the TODAY clinical trial. *J Diabetes Complications*. 2015;29(2):307–312.

Tunceli K, Bradley CJ, Nerenz D, Williams LK, Pladevall M, Elston Lafata J. The impact of diabetes on employment and work productivity. *Diabetes Care*. 2005;28(11):2662–2667.

Tuomilehto J, Lindstrom J, Eriksson JG, et al. Prevention of type 2 diabetes mellitus by changes in lifestyle among subjects with impaired glucose tolerance. *N Engl J Med*. 2001;344(18):1343–1350.

US Renal Data System (USRDS), National Institute of Diabetes and Digestive and Kidney Diseases. *2015 USRDS Annual Data Report: Epidemiology of Kidney Disease in the United States*. Bethesda, MD: National Institutes of Health; 2015.

Vagelatos NT, Eslick GD. Type 2 diabetes as a risk factor for Alzheimer's disease: the confounders, interactions, and neuropathology associated with this relationship. *Epidemiol Rev.* 2013;35:152–160.

Valdez R, Yoon PW, Liu T, Khoury MJ. Family history and prevalence of diabetes in the U.S. population: the 6-year results from the National Health and Nutrition Examination Survey (1999–2004). *Diabetes Care.* 2007;30(10):2517–2522.

Vandorsten JP, Dodson WC, Espeland MA, et al. NIH Consensus Development Conference: Diagnosing Gestational Diabetes Mellitus. *NIH Consens State Sci Statements.* 2013;29(1):1–31.

Vazquez-Benitez G, Desai JR, Xu S, et al. Preventable major cardiovascular events associated with uncontrolled glucose, blood pressure, and lipids and active smoking in adults with diabetes with and without cardiovascular disease: a contemporary analysis. *Diabetes Care.* 2015;38(5):905–912.

Venditti EM, Kramer MK. Diabetes prevention program community outreach: perspectives on lifestyle training and translation. *Am J Prev Med.* 2013;44(suppl 4):S339–S345.

Wagner EH, Glasgow RE, Davis C, et al. Quality improvement in chronic illness care: a collaborative approach. *Jt Comm J Qual Improv.* 2001;27(2):63–80.

Walker RJ, Smalls BL, Campbell JA, Strom Williams JL, Egede LE. Impact of social determinants of health on outcomes for type 2 diabetes: a systematic review. *Endocrine.* 2014;47(1):29–48.

Ward M, Druss B. The epidemiology of diabetes in psychotic disorders. *Lancet Psychiatry.* 2015;2(5):431–451.

Weinhold KR, Miller CK, Marrero DG, Nagaraja HN, Focht BC, Gascon GM. A randomized controlled trial translating the Diabetes Prevention Program to a university worksite, Ohio, 2012–2014. *Prev Chronic Dis.* 2015;12:E210.

Wherrett DK. Trials in the prevention of type 1 diabetes: current and future. *Can J Diabetes.* 2014;38(4):279–284.

Willi C, Bodenmann P, Ghali WA, Faris PD, Cornuz J. Active smoking and the risk of type 2 diabetes: a systematic review and meta-analysis. *JAMA.* 2007;298(22):2654–2664.

Wong E, Backholer K, Gearon E, et al. Diabetes and risk of physical disability in adults: a systematic review and meta-analysis. *Lancet Diabetes Endocrinol.* 2013;1(2):106–114.

Wood FG, Alley E, Baer S, Johnson R. Interactive multimedia tailored to improve diabetes self-management. *Nurs Clin North Am.* 2015;50(3):565–576.

Wu YL, Ding YP, Gao J, Tanaka Y, Zhang W. Risk factors and primary prevention trials for type 1 diabetes. *Int J Biol Sci.* 2013;9(7):666–679.

Zeitler P, Hirst K, Pyle L, et al. A clinical trial to maintain glycemic control in youth with type 2 diabetes. *N Engl J Med*. 2012;366(24):2247–2256.

Zhang C, Ning Y. Effect of dietary and lifestyle factors on the risk of gestational diabetes: review of epidemiologic evidence. *Am J Clin Nutr*. 2011;94(suppl 6):1975s–1979s.

Zhang C, Tobias DK, Chavarro JE, et al. Adherence to healthy lifestyle and risk of gestational diabetes mellitus: prospective cohort study. *BMJ*. 2014;349:g5450.

Zhuo X, Zhang P, Kahn HS, Bardenheier BH, Li R, Gregg EW. Change in medical spending attributable to diabetes: national data from 1987 to 2011. *Diabetes Care*. 2015a;38(4):581–587.

Ziegler AG, Rewers M, Simell O, et al. Seroconversion to multiple islet autoantibodies and risk of progression to diabetes in children. *JAMA*. 2013;309(23):2473–2479.

Ziegler AG, Schmid S, Huber D, Hummel M, Bonifacio E. Early infant feeding and risk of developing type 1 diabetes-associated autoantibodies. *JAMA*. 2003;290(13):1721–1728.

Zinman B, Lachin JM, Inzucchi SE. Empagliflozin, cardiovascular outcomes, and mortality in type 2 diabetes. *N Engl J Med*. 2016;374(11):1094.

Zinman B, Wanner C, Lachin JM, et al. Empagliflozin, cardiovascular outcomes, and mortality in type 2 diabetes. *N Engl J Med*. 2015;373(22):2117–2128.

Zipitis CS, Akobeng AK. Vitamin D supplementation in early childhood and risk of type 1 diabetes: a systematic review and meta-analysis. *Arch Dis Child*. 2008;93(6):512–517.

Zoungas S, Chalmers J, Neal B, et al. Follow-up of blood-pressure lowering and glucose control in type 2 diabetes. *N Engl J Med*. 2014;371(15):1392–1406.

Zuijdwijk CS, Cuerden M, Mahmud FH. Social determinants of health on glycemic control in pediatric type 1 diabetes. *J Pediatr*. 2013;162(4):730–735.

13

HIGH BLOOD PRESSURE

Leonelo E. Bautista, MD, DrPH, MPH

Introduction

Arterial blood pressure is the force the circulating blood exerts on the walls of the larger, low-resistance arteries of the vascular system. High blood pressure (also called hypertension) is asymptomatic, because blood pressure cannot be perceived. However, high blood pressure has a large impact on morbidity and mortality in almost all populations because of its high prevalence and strong association with the incidence of cardiovascular and renal disease (Figure 13-1). Fortunately, hypertension is fairly easy to diagnose and blood pressure control results in significant health benefits.

The precise blood pressure levels defining high blood pressure are those above which blood pressure–lowering interventions have been shown to significantly reduce the risk of stroke and coronary heart disease (Evans and Rose 1971; Zanchetti and Mancia 2012). Accordingly, the definition of high blood pressure has changed over time as new knowledge on the consequences of hypertension and on the benefits of blood pressure lowering has accumulated. Although arbitrary, the definition of hypertension is very useful for clinicians making treatment decisions, for epidemiologic surveillance, and for public health policy formulation.

Pathophysiology

Mean arterial pressure is the product of cardiac output, the volume of blood pumped by the heart by unit of time, and systemic vascular resistance, the force that small peripheral arteries oppose to the circulation of the blood. The mechanisms that cause essential hypertension are not completely understood. However, it is well recognized that the kidney, the sympathetic nervous system,

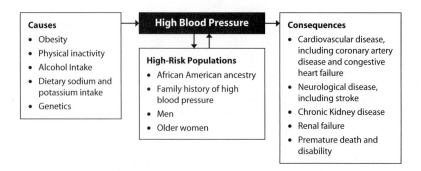

Source: Reprinted from Bautista (2010).

Figure 13-1. High Blood Pressure: Causes, Consequences, and High-Risk Groups

and the renin–angiotensin system play central roles in blood pressure regulation. Under normal conditions, the human body maintains a precise balance between the intake and output of fluids and electrolytes. If this balance is compromised, the volume of body fluids could expand or contract to a point at which the circulatory system would fail. The long-term regulation of body fluids volume depends greatly on the ability of the kidneys to excrete and reabsorb sodium chloride. When the extracellular concentration of sodium increases, the blood volume increases, leading to an increase in cardiac output and blood pressure. In response to the increase in blood pressure, the kidney increases sodium excretion, leading to lower blood volume, reduced cardiac output, and normal blood pressure. Conversely, when blood pressure falls below normal, the kidney retains water and sodium as a way to increase blood volume and cardiac output and re-establish normal blood pressure.

All forms of essential hypertension are characterized by impaired pressure natriuresis, a condition in which a blood pressure higher than normal is required to stimulate the kidney to excrete sodium as a way to maintain normal body fluid volumes. Impaired pressure natriuresis could be caused by intrarenal or extrarenal factors. A reduced glomerular filtration rate or an increased tubular reabsorption of sodium are intrarenal mechanisms that may lead to hypertension. When the intrinsic balance between glomerular filtration rate and tubular reabsorption is altered, blood pressure increases as a way to increase natriuresis and preserve normal body fluid volume.

Increased activity of the sympathetic nervous system is an extrarenal mechanism often associated with the pathogenesis of hypertension. In fact, increased sympathetic activity has been proposed as a mechanism for obesity and stress-related hypertension. Activation of the sympathetic nervous system can cause short-term increases in blood pressure by increasing heart rate, heart contractility, and cardiac output, and by increasing vasoconstriction and systemic vascular resistance. More importantly, activation of renal sympathetic activity increases sodium retention, impairs pressure natriuresis, and could lead to hypertension.

Disorders that induce arterial vasoconstriction or sodium retention can also play a role in the pathogenesis of hypertension. For example, an increased activity of the renin–angiotensin system results in high levels of angiotensin II, a powerful vasoconstrictor that helps to maintain blood pressure in situations in which blood volume or cardiac contractility are low. High levels of angiotensin II increase vasoconstriction and systemic vascular resistance and also impair pressure natriuresis. Thus, high angiotensin II could lead to chronic hypertension because higher levels of blood pressure are needed to preserve normal sodium excretion and body fluid volume. Finally, vasodilating (e.g., nitric oxide) and vasoconstricting (e.g., endothelin-1) factors produced by the vascular endothelium in response to mechanical and biochemical agonists participate in blood pressure control, but their role on the pathogenesis of hypertension has yet to be fully elucidated.

Measurement of Blood Pressure and Diagnosis of High Blood Pressure

Owing to blood pressure's intrinsic variability, the diagnosis of high blood pressure has traditionally been based on the average of at least two blood pressure measurements made on at least two sequential clinic visits, using a mercury sphygmomanometer and the auscultatory method (Chobanian et al. 2003). Though the auscultatory method using a mercury sphygmomanometer remains the gold standard for blood pressure measurement, its accuracy is compromised by the common use of suboptimal measurement procedures (Burgess et al. 2011; Villegas et al. 1995). Also, environmental concerns have led to a worldwide ban on the use of mercury devices in the clinical setting (Jones et al. 2003; Asayama et al. 2016; Environmental Working Group 2000). As a result, in developed countries, the mercury sphygmomanometer and the auscultatory method have been progressively phased out and replaced by automatic oscillometric devices for blood pressure measurement in clinical practice. A clear-cut advantage of oscillometric devices is the potential to obtain multiple measurements while reducing the observer bias resulting from misidentification of Korotkoff sounds and terminal digit preference (Reid et al. 2005; Tobe and Izzo 2016; Myers et al. 2009).

In spite of their widespread use, significant concerns remain regarding the use of oscillometric devices. Knowledge on the risk associated with high blood pressure and on the benefits of blood pressure reduction through treatment has been mostly based on auscultatory measurements using mercury sphygmomanometers (Grim and Grim 2016; Tobe and Izzo 2016) and it is still unclear how this knowledge translates to oscillometric measures. Also, the accuracy of validated oscillometric devices in clinical practice is uncertain (Wan et al. 2010), particularly in elderly patients and patients with arrhythmias or very high or very low blood pressure (Jones et al. 2003; Landgraf et al. 2010; Stergiou et al. 2009a; Stergiou et al. 2012; Ga 2001; Stergiou et al. 2009b).

Ambulatory blood pressure monitoring was originally used for research, but is now proposed as a way to improve the diagnosis of high blood pressure (Ritchie et al. 2011; Gorostidi et al. 2015; Krakoff 2015; O'Brien et al. 2013; O'Brien 2003) by screening out and avoiding treatment in patients whose blood pressure is high in a medical setting but normal in an ambulatory setting, a phenomenon called white coat hypertension (Pickering 1996; Pickering and White 2008). This phenomenon has been detected in 20% to 40% of all hypertensive patients (Thomas et al. 2016; Gorostidi et al. 2015; Pickering et al. 1988). However, if multiple blood pressure measures are taken in at least two clinic visits, following standard protocols (Chobanian et al. 2003), the prevalence of white coat hypertension in individuals without a previous diagnosis of hypertension is closer to 9% (Shimbo et al. 2009; Fogari et al. 1996; Ogedegbe et al. 2008; Stergiou et al. 2000; Stergiou et al. 2005).

Another main argument for the use of ambulatory blood pressure monitoring is that it is a better predictor of cardiovascular morbidity and mortality than clinic blood pressure (O'Brien 2003; Krakoff 2015). This is just a consequence of ambulatory blood pressure being an average of a larger number of measurements than clinic blood pressure, and it has not been replicated in studies with repeated clinic measures (Mancia et al. 2006; Sega et al. 2005; Woodiwiss et al. 2009).

There are also concerns regarding the reproducibility of ambulatory blood pressure monitoring (Keren et al. 2015; van der Steen et al. 1999; Palatini et al. 1994) and the use of cutpoints to define high blood pressure (O'Brien et al. 2013) that are mostly supported by consensus agreement and differ from cutpoints derived from outcome studies (de la Sierra 2013; Redon and Lurbe 2014; Kikuya et al. 2007; Ohkubo et al. 1998). However, the main hurdle for the replacement of clinic blood pressure by ambulatory blood pressure is that most of our knowledge on the impact of blood pressure on cardiovascular risk, risk stratification, and blood pressure management has been guided by clinic blood pressure, and it is uncertain whether ambulatory blood pressure–guided diagnosis and treatment would lead to improved prevention of cardiovascular complications to a degree that justifies its added complexity and costs (Mancia and Verdecchia 2015; de la Sierra 2013; Redon and Lurbe 2014; Grim and Grim 2016).

Home blood pressure monitoring, which was originally developed as a product for consumers without the endorsement of any scientific society, is now proposed as a way to improve blood pressure control in treated patients (Yarows and Staessen 2002). The use of this approach and ambulatory blood pressure monitoring to diagnose high blood pressure has been recently endorsed in several (Daskalopoulou et al. 2015; Task Force for the Management of Arterial Hypertension of the ESH and ESC 2013; Krause et al. 2011; Shimamoto et al. 2014; Piper et al. 2015; Siu 2015), but not all, international high blood pressure management guidelines (Table 13-1; Chobanian et al. 2003; Weber et al. 2014; Campbell et al. 2014).

Regardless of the measuring approach and diagnostic procedures, standard guidelines must be followed to obtain accurate and reliable clinic and ambulatory blood pressure measurements (Pickering et al. 2005; Parati et al. 2008; Parati et al. 2014). For more than three decades, individuals aged 18 years and older who are not acutely ill and have systolic blood pressure 140 millimeters of mercury (mm Hg) or higher or diastolic blood pressure 90 mm Hg or higher have been diagnosed as hypertensive, because they have an important increase in cardiovascular risk and they benefit from additional examinations or blood pressure–lowering interventions (JNC 1977). This definition of hypertension is employed throughout this chapter.

However, current guidelines vary significantly in terms of the approach and cutpoints used for diagnosing high blood pressure (Table 13-1). Guidelines currently used in the United States (shown under JNC 7 in Table 13-1) include normal blood pressure (systolic blood pressure < 120 mm Hg and diastolic blood pressure < 80 mm Hg), prehypertension (systolic blood pressure 120–139 mm Hg or diastolic blood pressure 80–89 mm Hg), stage 1 hypertension (systolic

Table 13-1. Blood Pressure (Systolic/Diastolic, mm Hg) Staging According to International Guidelines for the Evaluation and Treatment of High Blood Pressure among Adults

Stage	JNC 7[a] (2003)	CHEP[b] (2015) Office BP	ABPM	ESH/ESC/JHS[c] (2013/2014) Office BP	ABPM	UK-NICE[d] (2011) Office BP and ABPM
Optimal				<120/80		
Normal	<120/80			120–129/ 80–84		
High normal		130–139/ 85–89		130–139/ 85–89		
Prehyper- tension	120–139/ 80–89					
Hypertension			Daytime[e]		Daytime[e]	Daytime
Stage 1 (mild)	140–159/ 90–99[f]	140–159/ 90–99 ≥135/85[g]	≥135/≥85	140–159/ 90–99	≥135/≥85	≥140/90 and ≥135/85 <160/100 and <150/90
					Night time ≥120/≥70	
			24-hour ≥130/≥80		24-hour ≥130/≥80	
Stage 2 (moderate)	≥160/≥100			160–179/ 100–109		≥150/95 and ≥160/100
Stage 3 (severe)			≥180/≥110	≥180/110		

Note: ABPM=ambulatory blood pressure monitoring; BP=blood pressure.

[a]JNC 7=Joint National Committee on Prevention, Detection, Evaluation, and Treatment of High Blood Pressure (Chobanian et al. 2003). A more recent guideline (JNC 8) was published in 2014, but made no changes to blood pressure staging (James et al. 2014).

[b]CHEP=*Canadian* Hypertension Education Program (Daskalopoulou et al. 2015). Oscillometric devices preferred over auscultation. There is no rest period needed before measurement.

[c]ESH=*European* Society of Hypertension; ESC=European Society of Cardiology; JSH=Japanese Society of Hypertension (Task Force for the Management of Arterial Hypertension of the ESH and ESC 2013; Shimamoto et al. 2014).

[d]NICE=*National* Institute for Health and Care Excellence (United Kingdom). Clinical guideline (National Clinical Guideline Centre 2011).

[e]Same cutpoints are used for home blood pressure monitoring.

[f]This cutpoint is also recommended by the American Society of Hypertension and the International Society of Hypertension (Weber et al. 2014).

[g]Hypertension defined as ≥135/85 when using oscillometric automated devices.

blood pressure 140–159 or diastolic blood pressure 90–99 mm Hg), and stage 2 hypertension (systolic blood pressure ≥ 160 mm Hg or diastolic blood pressure ≥ 100 mm Hg; Chobanian et al. 2003). The term "prehypertension" was introduced a few years ago to emphasize the need for preventive interventions, because individuals with blood pressures in the prehypertensive range have been found to be three to seven times more likely to become hypertensive and two times more likely to develop cardiovascular diseases (Vasan et al. 2001a; Vasan et al. 2001b), and can benefit from non-pharmacologic interventions aimed to reduce blood pressure (He et al. 2000; Sacks et al. 2001; Whelton et al. 2002b).

Significance

The Worldwide Impact of High Blood Pressure

High blood pressure (hypertension) imposes an extraordinary health burden in almost all populations because of its high prevalence and the large increase in the risk of cardiovascular and renal disease among individuals with this condition.

Estimates of the prevalence of high blood pressure come mostly from epidemiologic studies in which cases are defined by using the average of multiple blood pressure readings taken in a single evaluation, instead of multiple sequential clinic visits. However, most prospective studies linking blood pressure and cardiovascular risk have relied on this epidemiologic definition of high blood pressure (Kannel et al. 1971; MacMahon 2000). It is estimated that, in 2008, 40% of adults aged 25 years and older in the world were hypertensive (Chow et al. 2013; WHO 2011). Also, from 1980 to 2008, the number of individuals with high blood pressure increased by 62%, from 600 million to almost 1 billion because of population growth and aging (Danaei et al. 2012). By 2025, 1.56 billion individuals in the world will have hypertension (Kearney et al. 2005).

According to a worldwide study, high blood pressure is the leading single contributor to the global burden of disease (WHO 2009; Lim et al. 2010). About 9.4 million deaths per year (13% of all deaths in the world) are caused by high blood pressure, which is responsible for at least 45% of deaths attributed to ischemic heart disease, and 51% of deaths attributed to stroke (WHO 2009). In 2010, the number of disability-adjusted life years (DALYs) attributed to high blood pressure was 173.6 million (7.0% of the total), considerably larger than that for smoking (136.9 million), alcohol intake (120.6 million), obesity (93.6 million), high fasting plasma glucose (89.0 million), and high total cholesterol (40.9 million; Lim et al. 2010).

Global age-standardized systolic blood pressure decreased at a rate of 1 mm Hg per decade from 1980 to 2008 (Danaei et al. 2012). However, although in high-income countries there was a strong decline of 7.3 mm Hg during the period, in low-income countries there was an increase of 3.3 mm Hg, with little change in middle-income countries (Danaei et al. 2012; Anand and Yusuf 2011). In 2008, approximately 40% of adults aged 25 years and older in the world were hypertensive, 46% in the African Region (the highest) and 35% in the Americas (the lowest; Chow et al. 2013; WHO 2011). Overall, the prevalence of hypertension in high-income countries (35%) is lower than that in low- and middle-income countries (40%; Chow et al. 2013; WHO 2011; WHO 2013). As a result of the absolute increase in the number of individuals in the world with systolic blood pressure in the range from greater than 110 to 115 mm Hg, high blood pressure moved up from being the fourth-ranked risk factor for burden of disease in 1990 to the leading risk factor in 2010 (Lim et al. 2010).

The effect of blood pressure on cardiovascular mortality has been estimated in a meta-analysis of cohort studies in more than 1 million adults (Lewington et al. 2002). In this study, an increase of 20 mm Hg in systolic blood pressure increased the coronary heart disease death rate by 50% in those aged 80 to 89 years, 70% in those aged 70 to 79 years, 90% in those aged 60 to 69 years, and 100% in those aged 50 to 59 years and 40 to 49 years. Corresponding changes for an increase of 10 mm Hg in diastolic blood pressure were 40%, 60%, 80%, 90%, and 110%. For the same age groups and systolic blood pressure difference, the risk of stroke mortality increased by 50%, 100%, 130%, 160%, and 180%, respectively. Corresponding changes associated with diastolic blood pressure were 60%, 110%, 150%, 190%, and 190%. These results show that the relative effect of high blood pressure on cardiovascular mortality is higher in younger individuals. However, the absolute differences in mortality are larger in older individuals, because cardiovascular disease mortality increases with age. The relative increase in mortality associated with an absolute difference in blood pressure was the same at all levels of blood pressure down to at least 115 mm Hg of systolic blood pressure and 75 mm Hg of diastolic blood pressure (Lewington et al. 2002).

Descriptive Epidemiology (United States)

Blood Pressure Patterns by Gender, Age, and Race

Average blood pressure and prevalence of high blood pressure depend strongly on age, gender, and race/ethnicity. Average blood pressure increases with age in most populations, except isolated populations with low sodium intake (Bazzano et al. 2007; Whelton 1994; Wolf-Maier et al. 2003). Age-related changes in blood pressure are mostly explained by the loss of elasticity of the aorta and other large arteries (arterial stiffness) that occurs normally with aging. Age- and gender-related changes in blood pressure are illustrated here with data from the National Health and Nutrition Examination Survey (NHANES) in the United States (National Center for Health Statistics 1996; National Center for Health Statistics 2006).

Systolic blood pressure increases with age in both men and women, from about 110 mm Hg in women at age 20 to about 160 mm Hg at age 80; and from about 120 mm Hg in men at age 20 to about 150 mm Hg at age 80. As a consequence, systolic blood pressure is higher in young men than in young women, but becomes higher in women than in men around age 50 for whites and Hispanics and around age 40 for African Americans (Figure 13-2). Gender- and age-specific average systolic blood pressure tends to be higher among African Americans than in other racial/ethnic groups.

Average diastolic blood pressure increases with age until about age 50 and remains constant or decreases thereafter (Figure 13-3). Among whites and Hispanics, diastolic blood pressure peaks and then levels off at around age 40 in men and age 50 in women. Corresponding changes occur around age 50 and 60 years among African Americans. Diastolic blood pressure is slightly and consistently higher among men than in women of the same age and race/ethnicity.

Estimates of the prevalence of high blood pressure in the United States are based on data from NHANES 2011–2014 (Table 13-2). The overall prevalence of high blood pressure in U.S. adults aged 20 years and older was 27.3%, but ranged from about 4% in those aged 20 to 29 years to 80% in those aged 80 to 89 years. Similar to average systolic blood pressure, the prevalence of high blood pressure is higher in young men than in young women, but higher in older women than in older men (Table 13-2; Figure 13-4). This pattern is consistent in all race/ethnicity groups, but the age at which high blood pressure prevalence becomes higher in women than in men is about 30 years in African Americans and 50 years in other race/ethnicity groups.

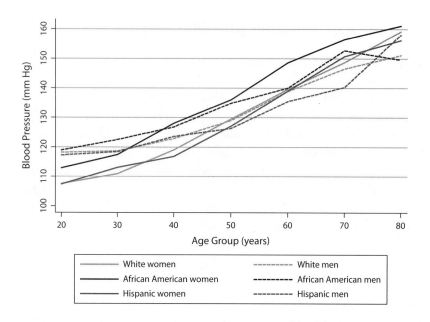

Source: Data from National Health and Nutrition Examination Survey 1999-2004 (CDC 1999-2000; CDC 2001-2002; CDC 2003-2004).

Figure 13-2. Average Systolic Blood Pressure by Age, Gender, and Race

Data on the incidence of high blood pressure are limited because they require active follow-up of populations with frequent blood pressure measurements for long periods of time. The incidence of hypertension in a community-based sample of mostly white individuals aged 35 to 79 years from Western New York was 21.9% in six years (Stranges and Donahue 2015). The risk of developing high blood pressure among Framingham Heart Study participants free of the condition at age 55 or 65 years was about 90% in their median residual lifetime expectancy (20 years for 65-year-olds and 25 years for 55-year-olds; Vasan et al. 2002).

In addition to age, the incidence of high blood pressure depends greatly on starting blood pressure values. Individuals with systolic blood pressure less than 140 mm Hg and diastolic blood pressure 85 to 89 mm Hg are two to three times more likely to develop high blood pressure than those with similar systolic blood pressure and diastolic blood pressure less than 85 mm Hg (Leitschuh et al. 1991). Among Framingham Heart Study participants with optimum (systolic < 120 mm Hg/diastolic < 80 mm Hg), normal (systolic < 130/diastolic < 85 mm Hg), or high-normal (systolic 130–139 mm Hg/diastolic 85–89 mm Hg)

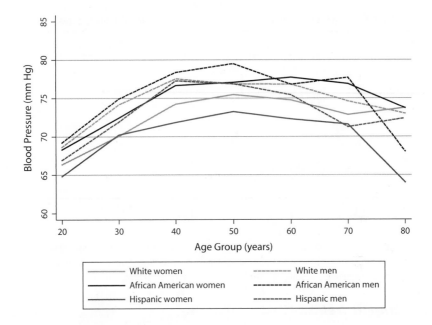

Source: Data from National Health and Nutrition Examination Survey 1999–2004 (CDC 1999–2000; CDC 2001–2002; CDC 2003–2004).

Figure 13-3. Average Diastolic Blood Pressure by Age, Gender, and Race

blood pressure according to Joint National Committee on Prevention, Detection, Evaluation, and Treatment of High Blood Pressure (JNC) 6 (JNC 6 1997), the four-year risk of high blood pressure was 5.1%, 18.1%, and 39.4% in individuals aged 35 to 64 years and 18.5%, 29.0%, and 52.5% in individuals aged 65 to 94 years, respectively (Vasan et al. 2001b).

Race/ethnicity also has a large impact in high blood pressure incidence. In the Atherosclerosis Risk in Communities (ARIC) cohort (n = 15,972) the 6-year risks of high blood pressure in men and women were 27% and 30% among African Americans, and 17% and 16% among whites, respectively (Fuchs et al. 2001).

In 2013, the death rate attributable to hypertension in the United States was 19.9 per 100,000 (Mozaffarian et al. 2016). From 1994 to 2004, the age-adjusted death rate for hypertension increased 2.5% per year (Rosamond et al. 2007), but from 2003 to 2013 the increase slowed down to 0.8% per year (Mozaffarian et al. 2016). The estimated total cost of hypertension for 2011 to 2012 was $48.6 billion (Mozaffarian et al. 2016).

Table 13-2. Prevalence of Hypertension (%) by Gender and Age in the United States

Age	Women	Men	All
20–29	2.7	5.2	4.0
30–39	11.6	15.2	3.4
40–49	23.1	25.2	24.2
50–59	39.2	46.1	42.6
60–69	58.2	57.0	57.6
70–79	71.7	69.1	70.6
80–89	83.5	74.1	79.9
All	27.6	27.0	27.3

Source: National Health and Nutrition Examination Survey, 2011–2014 (CDC 2011–2012; CDC 2013–2014).

Note: Hypertension was defined as systolic blood pressure greater than or equal to 140 mm Hg or diastolic blood pressure greater than or equal to 90 mm Hg or self-reported history of a diagnosis of hypertension plus current use of antihypertensive medication. Pregnant women were excluded.

Geographic Trends

The prevalence of high blood pressure is higher in states and communities with a higher proportion of African Americans, such as the South and Southeastern United States (Hajjar and Kotchen 2003b; Olives et al. 2013). However, there is also evidence that African Americans and whites living or born in Southern states are at higher risk of developing high blood pressure (Kershaw et al. 2010; Kiefe et al. 1997).

Time Trends

Overall, the age-adjusted average systolic and diastolic blood pressure in the U.S. population aged 18 to 74 years decreased from 131 to 119 mm Hg and from 83 to 73 mm Hg, respectively, from 1971 to 1991 (Burt et al. 1995). Correspondingly, the age-adjusted prevalence of high blood pressure declined by 16%, from 36.3% to 20.4%. This decline was observed across all age, gender, and racial/ethnic groups, with the exception of African American men aged 50 years and older, who experienced a small increase (Burt et al. 1995). During this period, the distribution of both systolic and diastolic blood pressure in the whole U.S. population shifted downward, suggesting population-wide behavioral and environmental influences on blood pressure, and not only a reduction in average blood pressure among treated hypertensive patients (Goff et al. 2001). Moreover, there is evidence that the age-related increase in both systolic

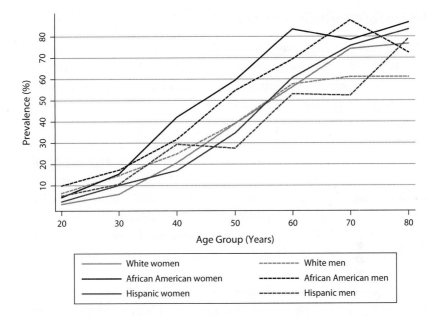

Source: Data from National Health and Nutrition Examination Survey 1999-2004 (CDC 1999-2000; CDC 2001-2002; CDC 2003-2004).

Figure 13-4. Prevalence of Hypertension by Age, Gender, and Race

and diastolic blood pressure is slower in more recent birth cohorts than in earlier birth cohorts (Goff et al. 2001).

The downward trend in the prevalence of high blood pressure in the United States reversed during 1998 to 2000. During that period, the age-adjusted prevalence increased from 25.0% to 28.7% (Hajjar and Kotchen 2003a). Larger increases occurred among persons aged 60 years and older (7.5%) and in women (5.6% compared to 2.2% in men), particularly those of African American race/ethnicity (7.2%). An increase in average body mass index (BMI) observed during the same period was responsible for more than 50% of the increase in prevalence, independently of age, gender, and race/ethnicity (Hajjar and Kotchen 2003a). More recent data indicate that the prevalence of high blood pressure has stabilized or may be decreasing (Whelton 2015; Yoon et al. 2015). Comparable prevalence estimates from recent waves of NHANES were 24.1% in 1988 to 1994, 30.2% in 1999 to 2002, 32.1% in 2003 to 2006, and 32.2% in 2009 to 2012, with a 2% absolute decrease in age-adjusted prevalence for the last period (Whelton 2015; NCHS 2015).

Impact on Morbidity and Mortality

Relative risk and population-attributable risk for various outcome diseases associated with hypertension are shown in Table 13-3. Among middle-class whites participating in the Framingham study, those with high blood pressure were about two times more likely to develop coronary heart disease (Kannel 1996). However, in a more recent cohort study including a large sample of African Americans, high blood pressure was a stronger predictor of coronary heart disease in African-American women than in other race–sex groups, with a relative risk of 4.8, compared to 2.0 in African-American men, 2.1 in white women, and 1.6 in white men (Jones et al. 2002). Limited data from cohort studies suggest that high blood pressure doubles the risk of coronary heart disease in Hispanics (pooled relative risk: 1.9; D'Agostino et al. 2001; Otiniano et al. 2005; Wei et al. 1996) but no gender-specific estimates have been reported in this ethnic group.

High blood pressure is the strongest independent risk factor for stroke. Estimates of the relative risk of stroke associated with high blood pressure have been remarkably consistent in different cohort studies (Li et al. 2005; Ohira et al. 2006; Qureshi et al. 2002). In these cohorts, the incidence of stroke was on average 2.2 times higher in hypertensive compared to normotensive

Table 13-3. Relative Risk and Population-Attributable Risk for Diseases Associated with Hypertension in Men (M) and Women (W) by Race/Ethnicity, United States, 2011–2014

		Population-Attributable Risk, %[b]							
		White		African American		Hispanic		All	
Disease	Relative Risk[a]	M	W	M	W	M	W	M	W
Coronary heart disease	2.2	18.5	28.7	29.8	63.1	22.9	23.7	19.6	42.6
Stroke	2.2	31.2	30.5	33.8	35.1	27.7	28.6	30.7	30.6
Congestive heart failure	1.8	23.2	22.7	25.4	26.5	20.4	21.1	22.8	22.7
Chronic kidney disease	1.7	20.9	20.4	22.9	24.0	18.3	19.0	20.6	20.5

[a]Relative risks were calculated by the author by pooling the estimates from the references cited in the text (for coronary heart disease the relative risks were 1.66 in men and in women).

[b]Population attributable risks were calculated by the author by using Levin's formula (Szklo and Nieto 2007). Estimates of the prevalence of hypertension used in the calculations correspond to 2011–2014 (see Table 13-2).

participants. The relative effect of high blood pressure on stroke does not seem to depend on race or gender (Kittner et al. 1990; Lawes et al. 2004; MacMahon et al. 1990).

High blood pressure is also a major risk factor for the development of congestive heart failure, with hypertensive subjects developing this condition 1.8 times more frequently than normotensive subjects (Levy et al. 1996; McNeill et al. 2006; Williams et al. 2002). Although the increase in risk is similar in men and women (Kannel et al. 1994), it is currently uncertain whether the effect of high blood pressure on the risk of congestive heart failure depends on race.

High blood pressure can also lead to the development of chronic kidney disease (see Chapter 22), a progressive loss of renal function, and to end-stage renal disease, an advanced stage of chronic kidney disease requiring dialysis or renal transplant as a form of renal replacement therapy (Levey et al. 2003). The average relative risk from three prospective cohort studies of high blood pressure and risk of chronic kidney disease (glomerular filtration rate <60 mL/min per 1.73 m^2) was 1.72 (95% confidence interval = 1.49, 1.97; Fox et al. 2004; Kurella et al. 2005; Yamagata et al. 2007). End-stage renal disease incidence also increases progressively with higher levels of blood pressure. Pooled estimates from three large cohort studies show that the relative risk of end-stage renal disease associated with high–normal blood pressure, stage 1, stage 2, stage 3, and stage 4 hypertension as compared to optimal blood pressure (JNC 5 and 6 stages; JNC 6 1997; JNC 5 1993) were 1.5, 2.0, 2.8, 4.8, and 7.0, respectively (Haroun et al. 2003; Williams et al. 2002; Klag et al. 1997). The strength of the association between blood pressure and chronic kidney disease is similar in men and women (Haroun et al. 2003) and in African Americans and whites (Klag et al. 1997).

A considerable fraction of all new cases of cardiovascular disease in the United States is attributable to high blood pressure. About 20% of all cases of coronary heart disease in men and almost 43% in women are attributable to high blood pressure (Table 13-3). It is unknown whether a similar gender disparity also occurs in Hispanics. The larger absolute impact among women is attributable to both a larger relative risk and higher prevalence of high blood pressure in women than in men. Almost 30% of all cases of coronary heart disease in white women are associated with high blood pressure, compared to 63% in African American women. Approximately 30% of all strokes, 22% of all cases of congestive heart failure, and 20% of all cases of chronic kidney disease are attributable to high blood pressure. Overall, about one out of every four cases of cardiovascular diseases in the United States could be theoretically prevented by eliminating high blood pressure.

The population-attributable risks presented in Table 13-3 likely underestimate the impact of elevated blood pressure, because they do not take into account that the risk of developing cardiovascular disease increases even with blood pressure levels within the "normal range." Indeed, individuals with systolic blood pressure between 130 and 139 mm Hg and diastolic blood pressure between 85 and 89 mm Hg are 2.5 and 1.6 times more likely to develop cardiovascular disease, respectively, than those with systolic blood pressure less than 120 mm Hg and diastolic blood pressure less than 80 mm Hg (Vasan et al. 2001a). In the ARIC study, the risk of ischemic stroke increased about 50% for each increase of 19 mm Hg in systolic blood pressure (Ohira et al. 2006). Also, in the Framingham cohort, an increase of 20 mm Hg in systolic blood pressure or 10 mm Hg in diastolic blood pressure was associated with corresponding increases of 56% and 24%, respectively, in the incidence of congestive heart failure (Haider et al. 2003). Finally, an increase of 16 mm Hg in systolic blood pressure or 10 mm Hg in diastolic blood pressure resulted in a similar increase of 76% in the risk of end-stage renal disease (Klag et al. 1996).

The effect of high blood pressure on cardiovascular complications varies by racial/ethnic group and by age. In middle-aged Europeans and Americans, coronary heart disease is the main complication of high blood pressure, whereas stroke is more important among Asians and older individuals (Staessen et al. 2003). African Americans tend to have higher prevalence of high blood pressure and higher rates of high blood pressure–related complications than other racial groups. The relative effect of blood pressure is larger in younger persons, but the absolute effect is larger in older individuals.

The impact of blood pressure on disease incidence also depends on the type of blood pressure. In those aged younger than 50 years, diastolic blood pressure is the strongest predictor of coronary heart disease. From ages 50 to 59 years, systolic blood pressure, diastolic blood pressure, and their difference (pulse pressure) are equally predictive of coronary heart disease. For those aged 60 years and older, pulse pressure becomes a better predictor than systolic blood pressure, and higher levels of diastolic blood pressure are associated with lower risk of coronary heart disease (Franklin et al. 2001). Moreover, systolic blood pressure seems to be a better predictor of stroke incidence than diastolic blood pressure and pulse pressure (Bowman et al. 2006; Inoue et al. 2006; Kannel et al. 1981; Nielsen et al. 1997; Psaty et al. 2001). Systolic blood pressure and pulse pressure also confer a greater risk of congestive heart disease than diastolic blood pressure (Chae et al. 1999; Haider et al. 2003; Vaccarino et al. 2000). Although all blood pressure measurements are directly associated with increased risk of chronic kidney disease, results from a large observational study and from several clinical trials suggest that systolic blood pressure is a stronger predictor of chronic kidney disease than diastolic blood pressure and pulse pressure (Klag et al. 1996; Mentari and Rahman 2004).

Causes

Various genetic and environmental factors promote the development and persistence of high blood pressure (Figure 13-1). Non-modifiable risk factors for high blood pressure include age, gender, and genetic susceptibility. Known modifiable risk factors include high dietary intake of sodium and low dietary intake of potassium, alcohol intake, obesity, and low levels of physical activity. Other potential risk factors have been identified, but it is still uncertain whether they have an independent effect on blood pressure levels. These include low birthweight; socioeconomic status; insulin resistance; dietary intake of fat, protein, calcium, and fiber; mild chronic inflammation; and psychological and emotional stress.

Genetic Factors

Blood pressure level aggregates in families, partly as a result of shared genetic predisposition. In fact, about 40% of the variability in blood pressure is explained by genetic factors (Harrap et al. 2000), and the risk of developing high blood pressure in persons aged younger than 50 years doubles for each first-degree relative with a history of high blood pressure (Hopkins and Hunt 2003). However, identifying genetic causes has been particularly difficult, because blood pressure is regulated by multiple mechanisms involving multiple nonallelic genes with small additive effects. The altered mechanism cannot be identified in 90% of the cases, because high blood pressure looks the same in all individuals. This compromises our ability to identify gene variants (alleles) or combinations of variants (haplotypes) associated with the development of high blood pressure.

Obesity

Excessive accumulation of body fat commonly leads to higher blood pressure. This effect could be mediated by overactivation of the sympathetic nervous system and the renin–angiotensin system, and by alterations in endothelial and renal function. The prevalence of high blood pressure in U.S. adults (NHANES 2011–2014) increases progressively with BMI (weight in kilograms/[height in meters]^2 [kg/m^2]), from 13.3% in those with normal BMI (<25 kg/m^2) to 29.0% in those with overweight (BMI≥25 and <30 kg/m^2) and 41.6% in those with obesity (BMI≥30 kg/m^2). Combining data from two large cohort studies, Field et al. (2001) showed that the risk of high blood pressure increased 2.1, 2.7, 2.4, and 3.9 times in overweight women, obese women, overweight men, and obese men, respectively, compared to those with normal BMI. About 46% of all new cases of hypertension in men and women in the United States could be attributable to overweight, and 38% of the cases in women and 45% of the cases in men could be attributed to obesity. Overall, 46% of all new cases of high blood pressure are attributable to overweight and obesity combined (Table 13-4). Multiple randomized controlled trials of non-pharmacological weight reduction interventions have corroborated the effect of obesity on blood pressure (see Lifestyle Modifications section; Neter et al. 2003).

Salt Intake

A high dietary intake of salt (sodium chloride) is associated with the development of high blood pressure. A high intake of salt over prolonged periods of time compromises the kidney's capacity to excrete sodium, leading to a persistent increase in blood volume and blood pressure. The International Study of Salt and Blood Pressure (INTERSALT), a standardized epidemiologic study of more than 10,000 persons from 32 countries, showed that an increase of 100 millimoles (mmol) per day of urinary sodium (an additional intake of approximately five grams of salt) increased systolic blood pressure by 3 to 6 mm Hg and diastolic blood pressure by 0 to 3 mm Hg (Stamler 1997). In a more recent study of more than 23,000 individuals, systolic and diastolic blood pressures were 7.2 and 3.0 mm Hg higher, respectively, in those with a daily salt intake 12.6 grams or more per day compared to 4.6 grams or less day (Khaw et al. 2004). Accordingly, the risk of having a systolic blood pressure equal to or greater than 160 mm Hg was about 2.5 times higher in those in the highest compared to the lowest salt intake group. In fact, the population-attributable risk of high blood pressure for a salt intake of more than 4.6 grams per day is about 30% in the United States (Table 13-4). The relationship between salt intake and blood pressure has been confirmed in multiple randomized controlled trials of sodium intake reduction (Cutler et al. 1997; He and MacGregor 2004; Sacks et al. 2001).

Table 13-4. Relative Risk and Population-Attributable Risk for Risk Factors for
Hypertension, United States, 1999–2003

Risk Factor	Relative Risk[a]	Population-Attributable Risk, %
Overweight and obesity	2.5	46.0
Salt intake (> 4.6 g/day)	1.5[b]	30.4
Alcohol intake in men[c]	1.2	15.5
Alcohol intake in women[c]	1.5	5.0
Low physical activity[d]	1.7	16.6

[a]Relative risks were calculated by pooling the estimates mentioned in the text and prevalence of risk factors came from the National Health and Nutrition Examination Survey 1999–2004 (CDC 1999–2000; CDC 2001–2002; CDC 2003–2004).

[b]This is a conservative estimate based on the report of Khaw et al. 2004.

[c]Exposure corresponds to one or more drinks per day in men and four or more drinks per day in women.

[d]Exposure corresponds to less than three hours per week of moderate or vigorous physical activity.

Potassium Intake

Increased dietary intake of potassium has been associated with lower blood pressure (Dyer et al. 1994). Administration of dietary potassium increases renal sodium and chloride excretion, reduces blood volume, and decreases blood pressure (Gallen et al. 1998). In INTERSALT, an increase of 30 mmol per day in urinary potassium excretion was associated with an independently significant reduction of 2.0 mm Hg in systolic and 1.1 mm Hg in diastolic blood pressure (Dyer et al. 1994). However, large epidemiologic studies using dietary records have failed to show an independent association between potassium intake and self-reported incidence of high blood pressure (Ascherio et al. 1992; Ascherio et al. 1996). This is probably explained by inaccuracy in the measurement of dietary potassium intake. On the contrary, randomized clinical trials have confirmed that potassium supplementation is associated with significant reductions in systolic and diastolic blood pressure (Whelton et al. 1997).

Alcohol Intake

There is ample evidence linking alcohol intake and high blood pressure. Although the biological mechanisms of the long-term effect of alcohol intake on blood pressure are unclear, the hypertensive effect of alcohol has been shown in observational studies (Fuchs et al. 2001; Marmot et al. 1994) as well as in randomized clinical trials of reduction (Xin et al. 2001) and increase

(McFadden et al. 2005) in alcohol intake. In the INTERSALT study, men who drank three to five drinks per day had a 2.7 mm Hg higher systolic blood pressure and 1.6 mm Hg higher diastolic blood pressure than nondrinkers, independently of other factors (Marmot et al. 1994). In the ARIC study, participants who drank three or more drinks per day were 1.2 to 2.3 times more likely to develop high blood pressure after six years of follow-up (Fuchs et al. 2001). Also, a low to moderate alcohol intake (up to three drinks per day) was associated with higher incidence of high blood pressure or increased blood pressure in African Americans, but not in whites, suggesting higher alcohol sensitivity among African Americans.

Interestingly, in two large cohort studies, Sesso et al. (2008) found that women who consumed from one drink per month to one drink per day were about 10% less likely, those who drank two to three drinks per day were as likely, and those who drank four or more drinks per day were 53% more likely to develop high blood pressure than never drinkers. In contrast, light-to-moderate alcohol intake did not change the risk of high blood pressure in men, but consumption of one or more drinks per day increased the risk by at least 20%. These levels of alcohol intake correspond to a population-attributable risk of 5.0% in women and 15.5% in men. A lower blood pressure following a reduction in alcohol intake has been demonstrated in randomized clinical trials (Xin et al. 2001).

Physical Activity

An inverse relationship has been observed between leisure time physical activity and blood pressure. Reduced stroke volume, systemic arterial resistance, sympathetic activity, urinary sodium retention, and insulin resistance may explain how long-term physical activity lowers blood pressure. In a cohort study of more than 8,000 men, Hu et al. (2004) found that those who reported a moderate or high level of physical activity were on average about 40% less likely to develop high blood pressure after 11 years of follow-up.

Some (Hu et al. 2004; Katzmarzyk et al. 2000; Levenstein et al. 2001) but not all (Folsom et al. 1990; Haapanen et al. 1997; Pereira et al. 1999) cohort studies have shown a lower risk of high blood pressure among physically active women. In addition, no beneficial effects of physical activity on blood pressure were observed in African Americans from the ARIC and the Coronary Artery Risk Development in (Young) Adults (CARDIA) cohorts (Dyer et al. 1999; Pereira et al. 1999). These inconsistencies may be attributable to lack of accuracy in the measurement of physical activity in women and African Americans. Although two meta-analyses of randomized clinical trials have shown that aerobic physical training was associated with reductions in systolic and diastolic blood pressure (Fagard 2001; Whelton et al. 2002b), the evidence from randomized clinical trials in women and African Americans is inconclusive. If the effect of physical activity observed in white men also applies to women and individuals of other races, low physical activity carries a population-attributable risk for high blood pressure of about 17% (Table 13-4).

Evidence-Based Interventions

Prevention of high blood pressure can and should be implemented at the individual and population levels. At the individual level, primary prevention is aimed at persons at high risk, with the goal of limiting the risk of becoming hypertensive, and secondary prevention is aimed at hypertensive and prehypertensive subjects, with the goal of avoiding the cardiovascular, neurological, renal, and ocular complications of high blood pressure. The strategy of population prevention is aimed at a collection of individuals, with the goal of shifting the whole blood pressure distribution to lower values (Whelton et al. 2002a). A change in the average blood pressure in the population would likely be small, but should result in a large reduction in the incidence of hypertension-related complications and mortality (Stamler 1991).

Prevention

Primary prevention at the population level complements the detection and treatment of high blood pressure at the individual level. The aim of public health interventions is to lower the average blood pressure in the whole population. Even modest decreases in the average blood pressure can delay the onset of high blood pressure and substantially reduce hypertension-related morbidity and mortality. Using data from observational studies and clinical trials, Cook et al. (1995) have shown that a reduction of 2 mm Hg in the average diastolic blood pressure in the U.S. population would result in a 17% decrease in the prevalence of high blood pressure, a 6% lower risk of coronary heart disease, and a 15% lower risk of stroke. Because the number of persons with normal blood pressure is considerably larger than the number of those with hypertension, more cases could be prevented in the first group. Therefore, from a public health perspective, it is useful to focus efforts toward the lowering of blood pressure not only in individuals with hypertension and prehypertension, but also in individuals with blood pressure within the "normal range" (MacMahon 2000; van den Hoogen et al. 2000).

Lifestyle modifications recommended for primary prevention in individuals are also recommended as interventions to reduce blood pressure in the general population (Eckel et al. 2014; Go et al. 2014; Brook et al. 2013). During the past few decades, community-based programs have been an effective means to raise awareness, increase knowledge, and promote lifestyle changes to improve blood pressure control (Kotchen 2007). Community-based demonstration projects funded by the National Heart, Lung, and Blood Institute (NHLBI) in the 1970s and early 1980s tested different educational strategies and showed significant but inconsistent reductions in average blood pressure (Welch and Hill 2002). In 1972, the NHLBI established the National High Blood Pressure Education Program as a cooperative effort to translate research into practice. This program has developed and promulgated several guidelines for the evaluation and management of high blood pressure. Although there has been no empiric evaluation of the program, since its inception, there has been a large increase in public and professional knowledge on high blood pressure.

A framework for prevention of high blood pressure was set by the Department of Health and Human Services as part of Healthy People 2010 (USDHHS 2008). Two main blood pressure–related goals were to reduce the prevalence of high blood pressure to 16% and to increase the proportion of adults with controlled hypertension to 50% by 2010. In recent years, the prevalence of hypertension has remained stable at around 32%. However, the overall proportion of adults with controlled blood pressure is now more than 50% in all patients with hypertension and more than 65% in those receiving drug treatment, although important age, gender, and racial disparities still remain. More prevention efforts are clearly needed. Improved access to care, additional education of health care professionals and the general public, promoting adherence to drug treatment, providing support for those attempting to change their lifestyle, reducing the burden and obstacles associated with those changes, and implementing goal-oriented treatment initiatives with feedback of target achievement are essential for making progress in the prevention of high blood pressure (Whelton 2015).

Lifestyle Modifications (Non-pharmacological Interventions)

Primary prevention of high blood pressure resides in the detection and management of modifiable risk factors through lifestyle changes. The efficacy of lifestyle changes in decreasing blood pressure and reducing the incidence of high blood pressure has been shown in randomized clinical trials. The JNC 7 guidelines recommended the use of lifestyle modifications in prehypertensive and hypertensive subjects and also encouraged their use in persons with normal blood pressure (Chobanian et al. 2003). Lifestyle modifications known to effectively reduce blood pressure—weight reduction, salt-intake reduction, dietary potassium increase, moderation of alcohol intake, physical activity, and change in dietary pattern—are discussed in the next paragraphs.

In a meta-analysis of 25 randomized clinical trials of weight control through increased physical activity or decreased energy intake, bodyweight reduction of 1 kilogram was associated with a decrease of approximately 1 mm Hg in both systolic and diastolic blood pressure (Table 13-5; Neter et al. 2003). Similar to other interventions, the beneficial effect of weight loss tended to be larger in hypertensive patients. In the Trials of Hypertension Prevention, 181 men and women with high–normal blood pressure were randomly assigned to an 18-month lifestyle modification intervention aimed at either weight loss or dietary sodium reduction or to a usual-care control group (He et al. 2000). By the end of the intervention, there was a net intervention-to-control difference of −3.5 kg in body weight, −5.8 mm Hg in systolic blood pressure, and −3.2 mm Hg in diastolic blood pressure. After seven years of follow-up, body weight was similar in both treatment groups, but the incidence of high blood pressure was still 77% lower in the weight loss intervention group. Randomized clinical trials also suggest that patients require less intensive antihypertensive drug therapy if they follow a weight-reducing diet (Whelton et al. 1998; Mulrow et al. 2000). The American Heart Association recommends maintaining a body mass index of less than 25 kg/m^2 in adults aged older than 20 years (Lloyd-Jones et al. 2010).

Large cohort studies (Mente et al. 2014; Ascherio et al. 1992; Ascherio et al. 1996) and numerous randomized clinical trials support a blood pressure–lowering effect of reduced salt intake. In a meta-analysis of 40 trials, an average urinary sodium decrease of 77 mmol per day (about 4.5 grams of salt per day) resulted in a reduction of 2.5 and 2.0 mm Hg in diastolic and systolic blood pressure, respectively (Table 13-5; Geleijnse et al. 2003).

Table 13-5. Effects of Lifestyle Interventions to Reduce Blood Pressure, Quantified in Randomized Controlled Trials

Intervention	Change	Reduction in Blood Pressure (mm Hg)		Recommended Level
		Systolic	Diastolic	
Weight loss[a]	−1 kg	1.0	1.0	BMI 18.5–24.9 kg/m²
Reduce sodium intake[b]	−77 mmol/day urinary sodium	2.0	2.5	100 mmol/day (5.7 g salt/day)
Increase potassium Intake[c]	75 mmol/day (supplement)	3.1	2.0	120 mmol/day (4.7 g/day, diet)
Moderation in alcohol intake[d]	−25%	3.3	2.0	≤2 drinks/day in men ≤1 drink/day in women
Aerobic physical activity[e]	≥3 sessions/week 30–60 minutes	3.5	2.5	30 minutes/day, most days of the week
DASH diet[f]	Diet rich in fruits, vegetables, and low-fat dairy products and low in saturated and total fat	5.5	3.0	Regularly

Source: [a]Neter et al. (2003); [b]Geleijnse et al. (2003); [c]Geleijnse et al. (2003) and Whelton et al. (1997); [d]Xin et al. (2001); [e]Fagard (2001) and Whelton et al. (2002b); [f]Appel et al. (1997) and Svetkey et al. (1999).

Note: BMI=body mass index; DASH=Dietary Approach to Stop Hypertension

Blood pressure reduction was at least two times larger in hypertensive than in normotensive subjects (systolic blood pressure: −5.24 vs. −1.26 mm Hg; diastolic blood pressure: −3.69 vs. −1.14 mm Hg). In the Trials of Hypertension Prevention, a difference of 33.3 mmol per day in urinary sodium excretion between intervention and control groups by the end of the intervention resulted in significant reductions of 3.3 mm Hg in systolic blood pressure and 1.7 mm Hg in diastolic blood pressure (He et al. 2000). After seven years of follow-up, urinary sodium excretion was similar but incidence of high blood pressure was still 35% lower in the sodium reduction arm. A lower need of antihypertensive medication in patients following a low-salt diet has also been demonstrated in randomized trials (Whelton et al. 1998). The American Heart Association currently recommends a maximum sodium intake of 1.5 grams per day (3.8 grams per day of salt) in all persons with hypertension, all middle-aged and older adults, and all African Americans, and a maximum of 2.3 grams per day (5.8 grams per day of salt) in the rest of the population (Lloyd-Jones et al. 2010; Whelton et al. 2012).

A consistently inverse relationship between increased potassium intake and blood pressure has been demonstrated in meta-analyses of randomized trials (Table 13-5; Geleijnse et al. 2003; Whelton et al. 1997) and more recently in a very large international cohort study (Mente et al. 2014). In one of these meta-analyses, potassium supplementation (median: 75 mmol/d) reduced systolic and diastolic blood pressure by 3.1 and 2.0 mm Hg, respectively (Whelton et al. 1997). The average effect size was larger in hypertensive subjects, and in African Americans. Similar results were obtained in a meta-analysis of trials in normotensive persons (Geleijnse et al. 2003). Moreover, the effect of potassium supplementation on blood pressure is larger in the context of a concurrent high intake of sodium, and vice versa (Morris et al. 1999). Based on findings from randomized clinical trials, the American Heart Association sets the recommended potassium intake level at about 4.7 grams per day in healthy individuals (Appel et al. 2006). Importantly, this level of potassium intake can and should be achieved through consumption of fruits, vegetables, and nuts in the diet, instead of diet pill supplements.

A dose-dependent association between high alcohol intake (≥1 drink/day) and risk of high blood pressure has been documented in observational and experimental studies. Light-to-moderate alcohol consumption seems to decrease hypertension risk in women and increase it in men, with cutpoint for harmful effects of four or more drinks per day in women and only one or more drinks per day in men (Sesso et al. 2008). Also, results from a meta-analysis of randomized trials suggest that an average reduction of about 25% in alcohol intake lowers systolic and diastolic blood pressure by 3.3 mm Hg and 2.0 mm Hg, respectively (Table 13-5; Xin et al. 2001). Although the effect was similar in normotensive and hypertensive subjects, the effect of the intervention was larger in those with higher baseline blood pressure. Alcohol intake should be limited to no more than two drinks per day in most men and no more than one drink per day in women and lighter-weight persons (one drink equals 12 ounces of regular beer, 5 ounces of wine, or 1.5 ounce of 80-proof distilled spirits; Appel et al. 2006).

Regular physical activity lowers blood pressure and prevents the development of high blood pressure. Two meta-analyses of randomized clinical trials have shown that aerobic physical training is associated with reductions in systolic and diastolic blood pressure of about 3.5 mm Hg and 2.5 mm Hg, respectively (Table 13-5; Fagard 2001; Whelton et al. 2002b). The effect of physical activity on blood pressure seems to be slightly greater in hypertensive subjects, independent of baseline body weight and weight loss. Unfortunately, there is currently inconclusive evidence on the effect of physical activity among women and African Americans. The influence of resistance training, such as weight lifting, on blood pressure is currently uncertain. The American Heart Association recommends 150 or more minutes per week of moderate-intensity, 75 minutes per week of vigorous-intensity, or 150 minutes or more per week of moderate- plus vigorous-intensity physical activity (Staessen et al. 1999). The JNC 7 guidelines recommend at least 30 minutes per day of aerobic physical activity of moderate intensity, such as quick walking, most days of the week (Chobanian et al. 2003).

A considerable proportion of the between-population variability in blood pressure could be explained not by differences in single nutrients but by large variations in dietary patterns. The effect of three dietary patterns on blood pressure was evaluated in the Dietary Approach to Stop Hypertension (DASH) Trial, a controlled dietary intervention study (Appel et al. 1997; Sacks et al. 2001). The DASH Trial included 133 hypertensive and 326 normotensive adults who received carefully controlled diets for 11 weeks. One group received a control diet low in fruits, vegetables, and dairy products, with a fat content typical of the average diet in the United States; the second group received a diet rich in fruits and vegetables; and the third group received the DASH diet (i.e., a combination diet rich in fruits, vegetables, and low-fat dairy products and with reduced saturated and total fat). The DASH diet significantly reduced systolic and diastolic blood pressure by 5.5 and 3.0 mm Hg more, respectively, than the control diet (Table 13-5). The effect of the DASH diet was significantly larger among participants with high blood pressure (reductions of 11.4 and 5.5 mm Hg in systolic and diastolic blood pressure, respectively) and among African Americans compared to whites (6.9 vs. 3.3 mm Hg in systolic blood pressure and 3.7 vs. 2.4 mm Hg in diastolic blood pressure, respectively; Appel et al. 1997; Svetkey et al. 1999). Importantly, the effect of the DASH diet was evident within the first two weeks of the trial. The DASH diet is currently recommended by the American Heart Association and by JNC 7 as a way to prevent and treat high blood pressure (Staessen et al. 1999; Chobanian et al. 2003; Appel et al. 2006).

Prevention at the Population Level

Screening

Screening for high blood pressure has a substantial net benefit, because blood pressure can be reliably and safely measured, and treating hypertensive patients significantly reduces their risk of cardiovascular morbidity and mortality. In adults, blood pressure should be measured at every routine clinic visit, then re-measured in two years in those with normal blood pressure and in one year in those with prehypertension (USPSTF 2007; Chobanian et al. 2003). In addition to blood pressure measurement, screening for high blood pressure should identify high-risk patients—those with a family history of hypertension, African American ancestry, overweight or obesity, a sedentary lifestyle, and a high alcohol intake (Whelton et al. 2002a). High salt and low potassium intake are also risk factors for high blood pressure, but they are difficult to identify in the context of a regular clinic visit. As a consequence of regular screening, hypertension awareness has improved progressively in the United States (Whelton 2015), from 68% in 1990–2000 to 76% in 2003–2004 (Ong et al. 2007) to 83% in 2011–2012 (Nwankwo et al. 2013).

Treatment

Secondary prevention interventions are aimed at prehypertensive and hypertensive individuals with the goal of avoiding the development and complications of high blood pressure. Blood pressure–lowering lifestyle modifications are now recommended for all prehypertensive persons (Table 13-6) and were justified for a number of reasons (Chobanian et al. 2003). First, prehypertensive individuals are several times more likely than normotensive individuals to become hypertensive within a few years (Vasan et al. 2001b; Winegarden 2005) and about 1.5 to 2.5 times more likely to develop cardiovascular disease (Vasan et al. 2001b; Hsia et al. 2007). Second, prehypertension is highly prevalent. About a quarter of the U.S. population were prehypertensive, 20% of women and 31% of men (NHANES, 1999–2004). Third, randomized clinical trials had documented that changes in lifestyle significantly reduce blood pressure in normotensive persons. In fact, the DASH study gave support to the JNC 7 recommendation for proactive management of prehypertension. There are at present no intervention studies with cardiovascular endpoints to support antihypertensive drug therapy in prehypertensive individuals. However, there is now evidence that the risk of stroke is significantly reduced with antihypertensive therapy in cohorts with prehypertensive blood pressure levels and a history of cardiovascular events (Sipahi et al. 2012). This has led to the recommendation for comparative effectiveness research as a necessary next step in building evidence for or against pharmacologic treatment of prehypertension (Selassie et al. 2011; Green et al. 2008). In contrast to the JNC 7 guidelines, the guidelines from the European Society of

Table 13-6. Management of High Blood Pressure According to JNC 7

BP Stage	Systolic BP (mm Hg)		Diastolic BP (mm Hg)	Starting Treatment
Normal	<120	and	<80	Encourage lifestyle modifications
Prehypertension	120–139	or	80–89	Lifestyle modifications
Stage 1 hypertension	140–159	or	90–99	Lifestyle modifications + 1 drug
Stage 2 hypertension	≥160	or	≥100	Lifestyle modifications + 2 drugs

Note: BP=blood pressure; JNC 7=Seventh report of the Joint National Committee on Prevention, Detection, Evaluation, and Treatment of High Blood Pressure. All patients with BP≥120/80 mm Hg and a compelling indication (heart failure, post–myocardial infarction, high risk of coronary heart disease, diabetes, chronic kidney disease, or recurrent stroke) should receive drugs for the compelling indication independently of their BP level. In these cases, the antihypertensive drug selected will depend on the compelling indication (Chobanian et al. 2003).

Cardiology and the European Society of Hypertension call for initiation of lifestyle modification in prehypertensive persons only if they have one or two additional cardiovascular risk factors (Mancia et al. 2007).

Although antihypertensive drugs reduce cardiovascular risk in almost all patients, the level of blood pressure at which drug treatment should be initiated and the target blood pressure levels that should be achieved through treatment are still controversial (Touyz and Dominiczak 2016). Though a discussion of the merits of different blood pressure management guidelines is beyond the scope of this chapter, it is worth noting some major differences in management guidelines. These differences pertain to patients without target organ damage and at low risk of cardiovascular events. The JNC 7 guidelines, the most widely used in the United States, and the Japanese Society of Hypertension Guidelines (Shimamoto et al. 2014) call for pharmacologic treatment of all patients with high blood pressure (≥ 140/90 mm Hg) without consideration of other risk factors (Table 13-6; Chobanian et al. 2003). In contrast, the Canadian Hypertension Education Program recommends drug treatment if blood pressure is greater than or equal to 160/100 mm Hg. The European Societies of Hypertension and Cardiology (Task Force for the Management of Arterial Hypertension of the ESH and ESC 2013) recommend starting drug treatment in patients with blood pressure greater than or equal to 140/90 mm Hg only if blood pressure remains elevated after several months of lifestyle modification, in patients with blood pressure 160 to 179/100 to 109 mm Hg after several weeks of lifestyle modification, and immediately in patients with blood pressure greater than or equal to 180/110 mm Hg. In this group of patients, the treatment goal is to reduce systolic and diastolic blood pressures to less than 140/90 mm Hg, but systolic blood pressure should be the primary focus (Chobanian et al. 2003; Task Force for the Management of Arterial Hypertension of the ESH and ESC 2013; Daskalopoulou et al. 2015; Krause et al. 2011). Also, all guidelines, except JNC 7, recommend a target of 150/90 mm Hg in patients aged 80 years and older.

Recent data from the Systolic Blood Pressure Intervention Trial (The SPRINT Research Group 2015) showed that patients treated to a target systolic blood pressure of less than 120 mm Hg compared to less than 140 mm Hg had a 25% reduction in the risk of cardiovascular diseases and a 27% reduction in all-cause mortality. Only 61 patients would need to be treated to a lower blood pressure target to prevent one cardiovascular event and only 90 patients to prevent one death from any cause. These findings are supported by three meta-analyses of trials showing that relative and absolute reductions in the risk of cardiovascular events were proportional to the magnitude of systolic blood pressure reductions achieved (Thomopoulos et al. 2016; Ettehad et al. 2016; Xie et al. 2016). These findings suggest that, at least in hypertensive patients at high risk of cardiovascular events, a therapeutic target of systolic blood pressure less than 120 mm Hg could be appropriate (Perkovic and Rodgers 2015). Also, they will likely lead to important changes in clinical practice, particularly in regard to blood pressure thresholds for defining hypertension and starting treatment and therapeutic targets in low- and high-risk patients (Perkovic and Rodgers 2015; Touyz and Dominiczak 2016; Jones et al. 2016).

There is irrefutable evidence that treatment of hypertensive patients with commonly used drugs (thiazide diuretics, long-acting calcium channel blockers, angiotensin-converting enzyme inhibitors, angiotensin type I receptor blockers, and ß-blockers) greatly reduces the risk of cardiovascular events, and that the reduction in risk is proportional to the reduction in blood pressure (Psaty et al. 2003; Turnbull 2003; Thomopoulos et al. 2015a; Thomopoulos et al. 2015b; Casas et al. 2010). The cardiovascular benefits of antihypertensive drugs have been documented in a recent meta-analysis of placebo-controlled randomized clinical trials in patients with hypertension and without renal or cardiovascular complications (Thomopoulos et al. 2015a). Treatment effects varied significantly with type of antihypertensive drugs and cardiovascular outcome (Table 13-7). Overall, the risk of stroke was reduced from 9% to 37% and 39 to 136 patients had to be treated for five years to prevent one stroke event, depending on the type of antihypertensive drug used. Corresponding figures were 6% to 26% and 111 to 455 for coronary heart disease; 10% to 49% and 35 to 194 for congestive heart failure; 9% to 29% and 34 to 64 for all major cardiovascular events; and 11% to 29% and 79 to 182 for cardiovascular deaths.

A weaker effect of calcium-channel blockers, angiotensin-converting enzyme inhibitors, and angiotensin receptor blockers could be partly explained by the concomitant use of other antihypertensive drugs in most of the trials for these drugs (Thomopoulos et al. 2015a). In fact, a meta-analysis of active controlled randomized trials showed that there were no significant differences between antihypertensive drug classes for most outcomes (Thomopoulos et al. 2015b). A particular drug could be preferred in patients with specific conditions or when prevention of a specific cardiovascular event is a therapeutic goal, though in most cases the type of outcome cannot be predicted (Mancia and Zanchetti 2008).

Even though the recommended drug of choice to start treatment in hypertensive patients without compelling indications for a particular drug vary significantly across management guidelines (Chobanian et al. 2003; Ernst and Bergus 2003; James et al. 2014; Weber et al. 2014; Krause et al. 2011; Shimamoto et al. 2014; Task Force for the Management of Arterial

Table 13-7. Effects of Pharmacologic Interventions to Reduce Blood Pressure, Ascertained in Randomized Placebo-Controlled Trials for Primary Prevention of Cardiovascular Outcomes

| Intervention | % Reduction in Risk of Outcome / No. Needed to Treat to Prevent One Event | | | | | |
	Stroke	CHD	CHF	CV Events	CV Deaths	Total Mortality
Diuretics	37/67	16/148	49/60	29/41	18/129	11/118
β-blockers	23/136	12[a]/194	43/35	21/64	15[a]/79	6[a]/273
Calcium antagonists	37/39	26/143	32/194	26/34	29/84	23/61
Angiotensin-converting enzyme inhibitors	20/116	13/111	21/84	17/35	11[a]/182	8[a]/135
Angiotensin II type I receptor blockers	9/114	6[a]/455	10/144	9/50		

Source: Data from Thomopoulos et al. (2015a).

Note: CHD=coronary heart disease; CHF=congestive heart failure; CV events=cardiovascular events (stroke+CHD+CHF); CV deaths=cardiovascular deaths. The number needed to treat refers to five years of treatment.

[a]Not statistically significant.

Hypertension of the ESH and ESC 2013), target therapeutic blood pressure may be more important for reducing cardiovascular risk than type of anti-hypertensive drug (Thomopoulos et al. 2015b; The SPRINT Research Group 2015; Thomopoulos et al. 2016; Ettehad et al. 2016; Xie et al. 2016). In fact, reducing systolic blood pressure by 12 mm Hg over 10 years results in pre-venting one death for every 25, 20, and 10 treated patients with stage 1, stage 2, and stage 3 hypertension (JNC 6 1997) and without additional risk factors, respectively. The number of patients needed to treat decreases to 10, 9, and 8, respectively, in patients with similar blood pressure and target organ damage, cardiovascular disease, or diabetes (Ogden et al. 2000).

In spite of the proven benefit of blood pressure lowering, current rates of high blood pressure treatment and control in the United States are still unsatisfactory, particularly in young people, men, minority groups, and those with low socio-economic status (Whelton 2015). During 2011 to 2014, 83.8% of all hypertensive adults in the United States were aware of their condition, 75.2% were receiving pharmacologic treatment, and 51.8% of all people with hypertension and 67.8% of all treated people with hypertension had their blood pressure controlled.

These results are very similar to those from 2011 to 2012 (Nwankwo et al. 2013). In a multivariate analysis, the probability of being aware was 40% higher in individuals aged 50 years and older ($p < .001$) and 21% lower in men than in women, but was not independently associated with race. Among those with hypertension, the probability of being treated was 45% lower in men than in women in those aged younger than 50 years ($p < .001$) and 18% lower in those aged 50 years and older ($p < .001$). Correspondingly, older age (≥ 50 years) increased the probability of being treated by 46% in women ($p < .001$) and by 116% in men ($p < .001$). Moreover, the probability of being treated was signifi-cantly lower (26%) only among Asians, compared to whites ($p < .001$). Blood pressure control was 45% lower ($p < .001$) in men than in women among young individuals (aged < 50 years) and similar among those who were older ($p = .55$). Correspondingly, older age had no effect among women, but increased blood pressure control by 54% ($p < .001$) among men. Compared to whites, blood pressure control was 20% to 26% lower in Mexicans ($p = .049$), African Ameri-cans ($p = .013$), and Asians ($p = .004$), and 15% lower in Hispanics ($p = .091$). Among treated individuals, blood pressure control was significantly lower in older compared to younger individuals (33%; $p < .001$) and in African Amer-icans compared to Whites (24%; $p < .001$). These results are consistent with those from previous studies (Ong et al. 2007).

Failure by patients to use medications as prescribed is a major contributor to poor blood pressure control. Studies based on pharmacy claims databases and cohort studies have shown that 32% to 53% of newly treated people with hypertension stop using their medication by the end of the first year of treatment (Bourgault et al. 2005; Perreault et al. 2005; Bautista et al. 2012). In a study based on NHANES data, stopping treatment (non-persistence) was 12 times higher in patients aged younger than 30 years than in those aged 50 years and older ($p < .001$), 31% higher in men than in women ($p = .01$), and 43% higher in Hispanics compared to other racial groups ($p = .03$; Bautista 2008). Moreover, non-persistence rates were almost twice as high in patients with low income ($p < .001$) and those without insurance ($p < .001$), and 10 times as high in patients who did not visit their doctor during the past year ($p < .001$). Also, patients with symptoms of anxiety and depression are at increased risk of becoming non-adherent to antihypertensive medication (Bautista et al. 2012).

Areas of Future Research

In spite of significant progress in the diagnosis and management of high blood pressure in the past few decades, hypertension prevalence remains high in middle- and high-income countries and it is increasing in low-income countries (Danaei et al. 2012; Anand and Yusuf 2011). Knowledge of factors driving the increase and persistence of high blood pressure in most world populations is needed to develop and implement ethnic/racial and culturally appropriate interventions. Little is known about heterogeneity on the prevalence and effect of established risk factors, such as obesity and increased salt intake across diverse populations (Bernabé-Ortiz et al. 2016; Ebrahim et al. 2013). Research efforts should also be focused on the identification of genetic, environmental, and behavioral factors that lead to a persistent impaired pressure natriuresis early in life, even before the diagnosis of high blood pressure. Promising avenues include the role of vascular oxidative stress, adhesion molecules, and inflammatory cytokines on blood pressure regulation (DeSouza et al. 1997; Dinh et al. 2014).

Poor medication adherence, which occurs in about 50% of newly treated hypertensive patients within the first year of treatment (Bautista et al. 2012), is a main cause of uncontrolled hypertension, which in turn increases overall mortality, hospitalization, and cost of care (Mazzaglia et al. 2009). Although some risk factors for poor adherence have been identified in prospective studies (Bautista et al. 2012; Tedla and Bautista 2016; Dezii 2000), further research on factors useful to predict short- and long-term adherence could have a significant impact on designing adherence-enhancing interventions, targeting patients who may benefit from those interventions, and blood pressure control.

Further knowledge on issues related to the diagnosis and treatment of hypertension is also needed. It is now well established that prehypertension is highly prevalent and has a large impact on cardiovascular health (Vasan et al. 2001b; Winegarden 2005; Hsia et al. 2007). Also, there is clear evidence that treating hypertensive patients to lower blood pressure targets results in a large (about 25%) reduction in the risk of cardiovascular and all-cause mortality (The SPRINT Research Group 2015; Thomopoulos et al. 2016; Ettehad et al. 2016; Xie et al. 2016). This begs the question of whether current cutpoints to define hypertension and blood pressure therapeutic targets should be lowered as a way to improve cardiovascular prevention. On a related issue, further research is also needed on the population-specific incremental cost-effectiveness ratio of treatment to target overall cardiovascular risk (benefit-based tailored treatment) as compared to treatment to target blood pressure in the management of hypertension (Sussman et al. 2013). Finally, more data are needed on the population-specific cost-effectiveness of the use of ambulatory blood pressure monitoring and home blood pressure monitoring for both diagnosis and management of high blood pressure (Goldberg and Levy 2016).

Resources

American Heart Association, http://www.heart.org/HEARTORG

American Society of Hypertension, http://www.ash-us.org

Centers for Disease Control and Prevention, High blood pressure program, http://www.cdc.gov/bloodpressure/index.htm

National Heart, Lung, and Blood Institute, http://www.nhlbi.nih.gov

Suggested Reading

Anand SS, Yusuf S. Stemming the global tsunami of cardiovascular disease. *Lancet.* 2011;377(9765):529–532.

Chobanian AV, Bakris GL, Black HR, et al. The Seventh Report of the Joint National Committee on Prevention, Detection, Evaluation, and Treatment of High Blood Pressure: The JNC 7 Report. *JAMA.* 2003;289(19):2560–2572.

Chow CK, Teo KK, Rangarajan S. Prevalence, awareness, treatment, and control of hypertension in rural and urban communities in high-, middle-, and low-income countries. *JAMA*. 2013;310(9):959–968.

Cloutier L, Schiffrin EL. Hypertension prevalence and control: impact of method of blood pressure measurement. *Curr Cardiovasc Risk Reports*. 2012;6(4):2 67–273.

Danaei G, Finucane MM, Lin JK, et al. National, regional, and global trends in systolic blood pressure since 1980: systematic analysis of health examination surveys and epidemiological studies with 786 country-years and 5.4 million participants. *Lancet*. 2012;377 (9765):568–577.

Daskalopoulou SS, Rabi DM, Zarnke KB, et al. The 2015 Canadian Hypertension Education Program recommendations for blood pressure measurement, diagnosis, assessment of risk, prevention, and treatment of hypertension. *Can J Cardiol*. 2015;31(5):549–568.

James PA, Oparil S, Carter BL. 2014 evidence-based guideline for the management of high blood pressure in adults: report from the panel members appointed to the Eighth Joint National Committee (JNC 8). *JAMA*. 2014;311(5):507–520.

Krause T, Lovibond K, Caulfield M, McCormack T, Williams B. Management of hypertension: summary of NICE guidance. *BMJ*. 2011;343:d4891.

Lim SS, Vos T, Flaxman AD, et al. A comparative risk assessment of burden of disease and injury attributable to 67 risk factors and risk factor clusters in 21 regions, 1990–2010: a systematic analysis for the Global Burden of Disease Study 2010. *Lancet*. 2010; 380(9859):2224–2260.

Mancia G. New threshold and target blood pressures in the hypertension guidelines. Which implications for the hypertensive population? *J Hypertens*. 2015;33(4):702–703.

The SPRINT Research Group. A randomized trial of intensive versus standard blood-pressure control. *N Eng J Med*. 2015;373:2103–2116.

Task Force for the Management of Arterial Hypertension of the European Society of Hypertension, Task Force for the Management of Arterial Hypertension of the European Society of Cardiology. 2013 ESH/ESC Guidelines for the Management of Arterial Hypertension. *Blood Press*. 2013;22(4):193–278.

Whelton PK. The elusiveness of population-wide high blood pressure control. *Annu Rev Public Health*. 2015;36:109–130.

World Health Organization. *Global Status Report on Noncommunicable Diseases 2010*. Geneva, Switzerland: World Health Organization; 2011.

References

Anand SS, Yusuf S. Stemming the global tsunami of cardiovascular disease. *Lancet.* 2011;377(9765):529–532.

Appel LJ, Brands MW, Daniels SR, Karanja N, Elmer PJ, Sacks FM. Dietary approaches to prevent and treat hypertension: a scientific statement from the American Heart Association. *Hypertension.* 2006;47(2):296–308.

Appel LJ, Moore TJ, Obarzanek E, et al. A clinical trial of the effects of dietary patterns on blood pressure. DASH Collaborative Research Group. *N Engl J Med.* 1997;336(16): 1117–1124.

Asayama K, Ohkubo T, Hoshide S, et al. From mercury sphygmomanometer to electric device on blood pressure measurement: correspondence of Minamata Convention on Mercury. *Hypertens Res.* 2016;39(4):179–182.

Ascherio A, Hennekens C, Willett WC, et al. Prospective study of nutritional factors, blood pressure, and hypertension among US women. *Hypertension.* 1996;27(5):1065–1072.

Ascherio A, Rimm EB, Giovannucci EL, et al. A prospective study of nutritional factors and hypertension among US men. *Circulation.* 1992;86(5):1475–1484.

Bautista LE. High blood pressure. In: Remington PL, Brownson RC, Wegner MV, ed. *Chronic Disease Epidemiology and Control.* 3rd ed. Washington, DC: American Public Health Association; 2010:336.

Bautista LE. Predictors of persistence with antihypertensive therapy: results from the NHANES. *Am J Hypertens.* 2008;21(2):183–188.

Bautista LE, Vera-Cala LM, Colombo C, Smith P. Symptoms of depression and anxiety and adherence to antihypertensive medication. *Am J Hypertens.* 2012;25(4):505–511.

Bazzano LA, He J, Whelton P. Blood pressure in westernized and isolated populations. In: Lip GYH, Hall JE, eds. *Comprehensive Hypertension.* 1st ed. Philadelphia, PA: Mosby Elsevier; 2007:20–30.

Bernabé-Ortiz A, Carrillo-Larco RM, Gilman RH, et al. Contribution of modifiable risk factors for hypertension and type-2 diabetes in Peruvian resource-limited settings. *J Epidemiol Community Health.* 2016;70(1):49–55.

Bourgault C, Senecal M, Brisson M, Marentette MA, Gregoire JP. Persistence and discontinuation patterns of antihypertensive therapy among newly treated patients: a population-based study. *J Hum Hypertens.* 2005;19(8):607–613.

Bowman TS, Gaziano JM, Kase CS, Sesso HD, Kurth T. Blood pressure measures and risk of total, ischemic, and hemorrhagic stroke in men. *Neurology.* 2006;67(5):820–823.

Brook RD, Appel LJ, Rubenfire M, et al. Beyond medications and diet: alternative approaches to lowering blood pressure: a scientific statement from the American Heart Association. *Hypertension.* 2013;61(6):1360–1383.

Burgess SE, MacLaughlin EJ, Smith PA, Salcido A, Benton TJ. Blood pressure rising: differences between current clinical and recommended measurement techniques. *J Am Soc Hypertens.* 2011;5(6):484–488.

Burt VL, Cutler JA, Higgins M, et al. Trends in the prevalence, awareness, treatment, and control of hypertension in the adult US population. Data from the Health Examination Surveys, 1960 to 1991. *Hypertension.* 1995;26(1):60–69.

Campbell NR, Berbari AE, Cloutier L, et al. Policy statement of the World Hypertension League on noninvasive blood pressure measurement devices and blood pressure measurement in the clinical or community setting. *J Clin Hypertens (Greenwich).* 2014; 16(5):320–322.

Casas JP, Chua W, Loukogeorgakis S, et al. Effect of inhibitors of the renin–angiotensin system and other antihypertensive drugs on renal outcomes: systematic review and meta-analysis. *Lancet.* 2010;366(9502):2026–2033.

Centers for Disease Control and Prevention (CDC), National Center for Health Statistics. National Health and Nutrition Examination Survey Data 1999–2000. US Department of Health and Human Services, CDC. Available at: https://wwwn.cdc.gov/Nchs/Nhanes/Search/Nhanes99_00.aspx. Accessed August 31, 2016.

Centers for Disease Control and Prevention (CDC), National Center for Health Statistics. National Health and Nutrition Examination Survey Data 2001–2002. US Department of Health and Human Services, CDC. Available at: https://wwwn.cdc.gov/Nchs/Nhanes/Search/Nhanes01_02.aspx. Accessed August 31, 2016.

Centers for Disease Control and Prevention (CDC), National Center for Health Statistics. National Health and Nutrition Examination Survey Data 2003–2004. US Department of Health and Human Services, CDC. Available at: https://wwwn.cdc.gov/Nchs/Nhanes/Search/Nhanes03_04.aspx. Accessed August 31, 2016.

Centers for Disease Control and Prevention (CDC), National Center for Health Statistics. National Health and Nutrition Examination Survey Data 2011–2012. US Department of Health and Human Services, CDC. Available at: https://wwwn.cdc.gov/nchs/nhanes/search/nhanes11_12.aspx. Accessed August 31, 2016.

Centers for Disease Control and Prevention (CDC), National Center for Health Statistics. National Health and Nutrition Examination Survey Data 2013–2014. US Department of Health and Human Services, CDC. Available at: https://wwwn.cdc.gov/Nchs/Nhanes/Search/Nhanes13_14.aspx. Accessed August 31, 2016.

Chae CU, Pfeffer MA, Glynn RJ, Mitchell GF, Taylor JO, Hennekens CH. Increased pulse pressure and risk of heart failure in the elderly. *JAMA*. 1999;281(7):634–639.

Chobanian AV, Bakris GL, Black HR, et al. Seventh report of the Joint National Committee on Prevention, Detection, Evaluation, and Treatment of High Blood Pressure. *Hypertension*. 2003;42(6):1206–1252.

Chow CK, Teo KK, Rangarajan S, et al. Prevalence, awareness, treatment, and control of hypertension in rural and urban communities in high-, middle-, and low-income countries. *JAMA*. 2013;310(9):959–968.

Cook NR, Cohen J, Hebert PR, Taylor JO, Hennekens CH. Implications of small reductions in diastolic blood pressure for primary prevention. *Arch Intern Med*. 1995; 155(7):701–709.

Cutler JA, Follmann D, Allender PS. Randomized trials of sodium reduction: an overview. *Am J Clin Nutr*. 1997;65(2 suppl):643S–651S.

Danaei G, Finucane MM, Lin JK, et al. National, regional, and global trends in systolic blood pressure since 1980: systematic analysis of health examination surveys and epidemiological studies with 786 country-years and 5.4 million participants. *Lancet*. 2012;377(9765):568–577.

Daskalopoulou SS, Rabi DM, Zarnke KB, et al. The 2015 Canadian Hypertension Education Program recommendations for blood pressure measurement, diagnosis, assessment of risk, prevention, and treatment of hypertension. *Can J Cardiol*. 2015; 31(5):549–568.

de la Sierra A. Definition of white coat hypertension: ambulatory blood pressure, self-measured blood pressure, or both? *Hypertension*. 2013;62(1):16–17.

DeSouza CA, Dengel DR, Macko RF, Cox K, Seals DR. Elevated levels of circulating cell adhesion molecules in uncomplicated essential hypertension. *Am J Hypertens*. 1997;10(12 pt 1):1335–1341.

Dezii CM. A retrospective study of persistence with single-pill combination therapy vs. concurrent two-pill therapy in patients with hypertension. *Manag Care*. 2000; 9(suppl 9):2–6.

Dinh QN, Drummond GR, Sobey CG, Chrissobolis S. Roles of inflammation, oxidative stress, and vascular dysfunction in hypertension. *Biomed Res Int*. 2014;2014:406960.

D'Agostino RB, Grundy S, Sullivan LM, Wilson, P. Validation of the Framingham coronary heart disease prediction scores: results of a multiple ethnic groups investigation. *JAMA*. 2001;286(2):180–187.

Dyer AR, Elliott P, Shipley M, Stamler R, Stamler J. Body mass index and associations of sodium and potassium with blood pressure in INTERSALT. *Hypertension*. 1994; 23(6 pt 1):729–736.

Dyer AR, Liu K, Walsh M, Kiefe C, Jacobs DR II, Bild DE. Ten-year incidence of elevated blood pressure and its predictors: the CARDIA study. Coronary Artery Risk Development in (Young) Adults. *J Hum Hypertens*. 1999;13(1):13–21.

Ebrahim S, Pearce N, Smeeth L, Casas JP, Jaffar S, Piot P. Tackling non-communicable diseases in low- and middle-income countries: is the evidence from high-income countries all we need? *PLoS Med*. 2013;10(1):e1001377.

Eckel RH, Jakicic JM, Ard JD, et al. 2013 AHA/ACC guideline on lifestyle management to reduce cardiovascular risk: a report of the American College of Cardiology/American Heart Association Task Force on Practice Guidelines. *JACC*. 2014;63(25 pt B):2960–2984.

Environmental Working Group. Protecting by degrees—what hospitals can do to reduce mercury pollution. Washington, DC: Environmental Working Group; 2000.

Ernst ME, Bergus GR. Ambulatory blood pressure monitoring. *South Med J*. 2003; 96(6):563–568.

Ettehad D, Emdin CA, Kiran A, et al. Blood pressure lowering for prevention of cardio-vascular disease and death: a systematic review and meta-analysis. *Lancet*. 2016;387(10022):957–967.

Evans JG, Rose G. Hypertension. *Br Med Bull*. 1971;27(1):37–42.

Fagard RH. Exercise characteristics and the blood pressure response to dynamic physical training. *Med Sci Sports Exerc*. 2001;33(6 suppl):S484–S492.

Field AE, Coakley EH, Must A, et al. Impact of overweight on the risk of developing common chronic diseases during a 10-year period. *Arch Intern Med*. 2001;161(13):1581–1586.

Fogari R, Corradi L, Zoppi A, Lusardi P, Poletti L. Repeated office blood pressure controls reduce the prevalence of white-coat hypertension and detect a group of white-coat normotensive patients. *Blood Press Monit*. 1996;1(1):51–54.

Folsom AR, Prineas RJ, Kaye SA, Munger RG. Incidence of hypertension and stroke in relation to body fat distribution and other risk factors in older women. *Stroke*. 1990;21(5):701–706.

Fox CS, Larson MG, Leip EP, Culleton B, Wilson PW, Levy D. Predictors of new-onset kidney disease in a community-based population. *JAMA*. 2004;291(7):844–850.

Franklin SS, Larson MG, Khan SA, et al. Does the relation of blood pressure to coronary heart disease risk change with aging? The Framingham Heart Study. *Circulation*. 2001; 103(9):1245–1249.

Fuchs FD, Chambless LE, Whelton PK, Nieto FJ, Heiss G. Alcohol consumption and the incidence of hypertension: the Atherosclerosis Risk in Communities study. *Hypertension*. 2001;37(5):1242–1250.

Ga VM. Oscillometric blood pressure measurement: progress and problems. *Blood Press Monit*. 2001;6(6):287–290.

Gallen IW, Rosa RM, Esparaz DY, et al. On the mechanism of the effects of potassium restriction on blood pressure and renal sodium retention. *Am J Kidney Dis*. 1998;31(1):19–27.

Geleijnse JM, Kok FJ, Grobbee DE. Blood pressure response to changes in sodium and potassium intake: a metaregression analysis of randomised trials. *J Hum Hypertens*. 2003;17(7):471–480.

Go AS, Bauman MA, Coleman King SM, et al. An effective approach to high blood pressure control: a science advisory from the American Heart Association, the American College of Cardiology, and the Centers for Disease Control and Prevention. *Hypertension*. 2014; 63(4):878–885.

Goff DC, Howard G, Russell GB, Labarthe DR. Birth cohort evidence of population influences on blood pressure in the United States, 1887–1994. *Ann Epidemiol*. 2001;11(4):271–279.

Goldberg EM, Levy PD. New approaches to evaluating and monitoring blood pressure. *Curr Hypertens Rep*. 2016;18(6):1–7.

Gorostidi M, Vinyoles E, Banegas JR, de la Sierra A. Prevalence of white-coat and masked hypertension in national and international registries. *Hypertens Res*. 2015; 38(1):1–7.

Green BB, Cook AJ, Ralston JD, et al. Effectiveness of home blood pressure monitoring, web communication, and pharmacist care on hypertension control: a randomized controlled trial. *JAMA*. 2008;299(24):2857–2867.

Grim CE, Grim CM. Auscultatory BP: still the gold standard. *J Am Soc Hypertens*. 2016;10(3):191–193.

Haapanen N, Miilunpalo S, Vuori I, Oja P, Pasanen M. Association of leisure time physical activity with the risk of coronary heart disease, hypertension and diabetes in middle-aged men and women. *Int J Epidemiol*. 1997;26(4):739–747.

Haider AW, Larson MG, Franklin SS, Levy D. Systolic blood pressure, diastolic blood pressure, and pulse pressure as predictors of risk for congestive heart failure in the Framingham Heart Study. *Ann Intern Med*. 2003:138(1):10–16.

Hajjar I, Kotchen TA. Trends in prevalence, awareness, treatment, and control of hypertension in the United States, 1988–2000. *JAMA*. 2003a;290(2):199–206.

Hajjar I, Kotchen TA. Regional variations of blood pressure in the United States are associated with regional variations in dietary intakes: The NHANES-III data. *J Nutr.* 2003b;133(1):211–214.

Haroun MK, Jaar BG, Hoffman SC, Comstock GW, Klag MJ, Coresh J. Risk factors for chronic kidney disease: a prospective study of 23,534 men and women in Washington County, Maryland. *J Am Soc Nephrol.* 2003;14(11):2934–2941.

Harrap SB, Stebbing M, Hopper JL, Hoang HN, Giles GG. Familial patterns of covariation for cardiovascular risk factors in adults: The Victorian Family Heart Study. *Am J Epidemiol.* 2000;152(8):704–715.

He FJ, MacGregor GA. Effect of longer-term modest salt reduction on blood pressure. *Cochrane Database Syst Rev.* 2004;(3):CD004937.

He J, Whelton PK, Appel LJ, Charleston J, Klag MJ. Long-term effects of weight loss and dietary sodium reduction on incidence of hypertension. *Hypertension.* 2000;35(2):544–549.

Hopkins PN, Hunt SC. Genetics of hypertension. *Genet Med.* 2003;5(6):413–429.

Hsia J, Margolis KL, Eaton CB, et al. Prehypertension and cardiovascular disease risk in the Women's Health Initiative. *Circulation.* 2007;115(7):855–860.

Hu G, Barengo NC, Tuomilehto J, Lakka TA, Nissinen A, Jousilahti P. Relationship of physical activity and body mass index to the risk of hypertension: a prospective study in Finland. *Hypertension.* 2004;43(1):25–30.

Inoue R, Ohkubo T, Kikuya M, et al. Predicting stroke using 4 ambulatory blood pressure monitoring-derived blood pressure indices: the Ohasama Study. *Hypertension.* 2006: 48(5):877–882.

James PA, Oparil S, Carter BL. 2014 evidence-based guideline for the management of high blood pressure in adults: report from the panel members appointed to the eighth Joint National Committee (JNC 8). *JAMA.* 2014;311(5):507–520.

[No authors listed.] Report of the Joint National Committee (JNC) on detection, evaluation, and treatment of high blood pressure. A cooperative study. *JAMA.* 1977;237(3):255–261.

[No authors listed.] The fifth report of the Joint National Committee (JNC 5) on Detection, Evaluation, and Treatment of High Blood Pressure. *Arch Intern Med.* 1993;153(2):154–183.

[No authors listed.] The sixth report of the Joint National Committee (JNC 6) on Prevention, Detection, Evaluation, and Treatment of High Blood Pressure. 1997;157(21): 2413–2446.

Jones DW, Appel LJ, Sheps SG, Roccella EJ, Lenfant C. Measuring blood pressure accurately: new and persistent challenges. *JAMA*. 2003;289(8):1027–1030.

Jones DW, Chambless LE, Folsom AR, et al. Risk factors for coronary heart disease in African Americans: the Atherosclerosis Risk in Communities study, 1987–1997. *Arch Intern Med*. 2002;162(22):2565–2571.

Jones DW, Weatherly L, Hall JE. SPRINT: what remains unanswered and where do we go from here? *Hypertension*. 2016;67(2):261–262.

Kannel WB. Blood pressure as a cardiovascular risk factor: prevention and treatment. *JAMA*. 1996;275(20):1571–1576.

Kannel WB, Gordon T, Schwartz MJ. Systolic versus diastolic blood pressure and risk of coronary heart disease. The Framingham Study. *Am J Cardiol*. 1971;27(4):335–346.

Kannel WB, Ho K, Thom T. Changing epidemiological features of cardiac failure. *Br Heart J*. 1994;72(suppl 2):S3–S9.

Kannel WB, Wolf PA, McGee DL, Dawber TR, McNamara P, Castelli WP. Systolic blood pressure, arterial rigidity, and risk of stroke. The Framingham study. *JAMA*. 1981;245(12):1225–1229.

Katzmarzyk PT, Rankinen T, Perusse L, Malina RM, Bouchard C. 7-year stability of blood pressure in the Canadian population. *Prev Med*. 2000;31(4):403–409.

Kearney PM, Whelton M, Reynolds K, Muntner P, Whelton PK, He J. Global burden of hypertension: analysis of worldwide data. *Lancet*. 2005;365(9455):217–223.

Keren S, Leibowitz A, Grossman E, Sharabi Y. Limited reproducibility of 24-h ambulatory blood pressure monitoring. *Clin Exp Hypertens*. 2015;37(7):599–603.

Kershaw KN, Diez Roux AV, Carnethon M, et al. Geographic variation in hypertension prevalence among blacks and whites: the Multi-Ethnic Study of Atherosclerosis. *Am J Hypertens*. 2010;23(1):46–53.

Khaw KT, Bingham S, Welch A, et al. Blood pressure and urinary sodium in men and women: the Norfolk Cohort of the European prospective investigation into cancer (EPIC-Norfolk). *Am J Clin Nutr*. 2004;80(5):1397–1403.

Kiefe CI, Williams OD, Bild DE, Lewis CE, Hilner JE, Oberman A. Regional disparities in the incidence of elevated blood pressure among young adults: the CARDIA study. *Circulation*. 1997;96(4):1082–1088.

Kikuya M, Hansen TW, Thijs L, et al. Diagnostic thresholds for ambulatory blood pressure monitoring based on 10-year cardiovascular risk. *Circulation*. 2007;115(16): 2145–2152.

Kittner SJ, White LR, Losonczy KG, Wolf PA, Hebel JR. Black–white differences in stroke incidence in a national sample. The contribution of hypertension and diabetes mellitus. *JAMA*. 1990; 264:1267–1270.

Klag MJ, Whelton PK, Randall BL, et al. Blood pressure and end-stage renal disease in men. *N Engl J Med*. 1996;334(1):13–18.

Klag MJ, Whelton PK, Randall BL, Neaton JD, Brancati FL, Stamler J. End-stage renal disease in African-American and white men. 16-year MRFIT findings. *JAMA*. 1997;277(16):1293–1298.

Kotchen TA. Hypertension control: trends, approaches, and goals. *Hypertension*. 2007; 49(1):19–20.

Krakoff LR. Blood pressure out of the office: its time has finally come. *Am J Hypertens*. 2015;29(3):289–295.

Krause T, Lovibond K, Caulfield M, McCormack T, Williams B. Management of hypertension: summary of NICE guidance. *BMJ*. 2011;343:d4891.

Kurella M, Lo JC, Chertow GM. Metabolic syndrome and the risk for chronic kidney disease among nondiabetic adults. *J Am Soc Nephrol*. 2005;16(7):2134–2140.

Landgraf J, Wishner SH, Kloner RA. Comparison of automated oscillometric versus auscultatory blood pressure measurement. *Am J Cardiol*. 2010;106(3): 386–388.

Lawes CM, Bennett DA, Feigin VL, Rodgers A. Blood pressure and stroke: an overview of published reviews. *Stroke*. 2004; 35(4):1024.

Leitschuh M, Cupples LA, Kannel W, Gagnon D, Chobanian A. High-normal blood pressure progression to hypertension in the Framingham Heart Study. *Hypertension*. 1991;17(1):22–27.

Levenstein S, Smith MW, Kaplan GA. Psychosocial predictors of hypertension in men and women. *Arch Intern Med*. 2001;161(10):1341–1346.

Levey AS, Coresh J, Balk E, et al. National Kidney Foundation practice guidelines for chronic kidney disease: evaluation, classification, and stratification. *Ann Intern Med*. 2003;139(2):137–147.

Levy D, Larson MG, Vasan RS, Kannel WB, Ho KK. The progression from hypertension to congestive heart failure. *JAMA*. 1996;275(20):1557–1562.

Lewington S, Clarke R, Qizilbash N, Peto R, Collins R. Age-specific relevance of usual blood pressure to vascular mortality: a meta-analysis of individual data for one million adults in 61 prospective studies. *Lancet*. 2002;360(9349):1903–1913.

Li C, Engstrom G, Hedblad B, Berglund G, Janzon L. Blood pressure control and risk of stroke: a population-based prospective cohort study. *Stroke*. 2005;36(4):725–730.

Lim SS, Vos T, Flaxman AD, et al. A comparative risk assessment of burden of disease and injury attributable to 67 risk factors and risk factor clusters in 21 regions, 1990–2010: a systematic analysis for the Global Burden of Disease study 2010. *Lancet*. 2010; 380(9849):2224–2260.

Lloyd-Jones DM, Hong Y, Labarthe D, et al. Defining and setting national goals for cardiovascular health promotion and disease reduction: the American Heart Association's strategic impact goal through 2020 and beyond. *Circulation*. 2010;121(4):586–613.

MacMahon S. Blood pressure and the risk of cardiovascular disease. *N Engl J Med*. 2000;342(1):50–52.

MacMahon S, Peto R, Cutler J, et al. Blood pressure, stroke, and coronary heart disease. Part 1, Prolonged differences in blood pressure: prospective observational studies corrected for the regression dilution bias. *Lancet*. 1990:335(8692):765–774.

Mancia G, De Backer G, Dominiczak A, et al. 2007 Guidelines for the Management of Arterial Hypertension: The Task Force for the Management of Arterial Hypertension of the European Society of Hypertension (ESH) and of the European Society of Cardiology (ESC). *J Hypertens*. 2007;25(6):1105–1187.

Mancia G, Facchetti R, Bombelli M, Grassi G, Sega R. Long-term risk of mortality associated with selective and combined elevation in office, home, and ambulatory blood pressure. *Hypertension*. 2006;47(5):846–853.

Mancia G, Verdecchia P. Clinical value of ambulatory blood pressure: evidence and limits. *Circ Res*. 2015;116(6):1034–1045.

Mancia G, Zanchetti A. Choice of antihypertensive drugs in the European Society of Hypertension–European Society of Cardiology guidelines: specific indications rather than ranking for general usage. *J Hypertens*. 2008;26(2):164–168.

Marmot MG, Elliott P, Shipley MJ, et al. Alcohol and blood pressure: the INTERSALT study. *BMJ*. 1994;308(6939):1263–1267.

Mazzaglia G, Ambrosioni E, Alacqua M, et al. Adherence to antihypertensive medications and cardiovascular morbidity among newly diagnosed hypertensive patients. *Circulation*. 2009;120(16):1598–1605.

McFadden CB, Brensinger CM, Berlin JA, Townsend RR. Systematic review of the effect of daily alcohol intake on blood pressure. *Am J Hypertens*. 2005;18(2 pt 1):276–286.

McNeill AM, Katz R, Girman CJ, et al. Metabolic syndrome and cardiovascular disease in older people: The Cardiovascular Health Study. *J Am Geriatr Soc*. 2006;54:1317–1324.

Mentari E, Rahman M. Blood pressure and progression of chronic kidney disease: importance of systolic, diastolic, or diurnal variation. *Curr Hypertens Rep*. 2004;6(5): 400–404.

Mente A, O'Donnell MJ, Rangarajan S, et al. Association of urinary sodium and potassium excretion with blood pressure. *N Engl J Med*. 2014;371(7):601–611.

Morris RC Jr, Sebastian A, Forman A, Tanaka M, Schmidlin O. Normotensive salt sensitivity: effects of race and dietary potassium. *Hypertension*. 1999;33(1):18–23.

Mozaffarian, Benjamin EJ, Go AS, et al. Executive Summary: Heart disease and stroke statistics—2016 update: a report from the American Heart Association. *Circulation* 2016;133(4):447–454.

Mulrow CD, Chiquette E, Angel L, et al. Dieting to reduce body weight for controlling hypertension in adults. *Cochrane Database Syst Rev*. 2000;(2):CD000484.

Myers MG, Valdivieso M, Kiss A. Use of automated office blood pressure measurement to reduce the white coat response. *J Hypertens*. 2009;27(2):280–286.

National Center for Health Statistics (NCHS). Analytic and reporting guidelines: The Third National Health and Nutrition Examination Survey, NHANES III (1988–94). Atlanta, GA: NCHS, Centers for Disease Control and Prevention; 1996.

National Center for Health Statistics (NCHS). Analytic and reporting guidelines. The National Health and Nutrition Examination Survey (NHANES). Atlanta, GA: NCHS, Centers for Disease Control and Prevention; 2006.

National Center for Health Statistics (NCHS), Centers for Disease Control and Prevention. *Health, United States, 2013, With Special Feature on Prescription Drugs*. Washington, DC: US Government Printing Office; 2015.

National Clinical Guideline Centre (UK). *Hypertension: The Clinical Management of Primary Hypertension in Adults: Update of Clinical Guidelines 18 and 34*. London, England: Royal College of Physicians; 2011. NICE Clinical Guidelines, no. 127. Available at: http://www.ncbi.nlm.nih.gov/books/NBK83274. Accessed August 31, 2016.

Neter JE, Stam BE, Kok FJ, Grobbee DE, Geleijnse JM. Influence of weight reduction on blood pressure: a meta-analysis of randomized controlled trials. *Hypertension*. 2003;42(5):878–884.

Nielsen WB, Lindenstrom E, Vestbo J, Jensen GB. Is diastolic hypertension an independent risk factor for stroke in the presence of normal systolic blood pressure in the middle-aged and elderly? *Am J Hypertens*. 1997:10(6):634–639.

Nwankwo T, Yoon SS, Burt V, Gu Q. Hypertension among adults in the United States: National Health and Nutrition Examination Survey, 2011–2012. *NCHS Data Brief*. 2013;(133):1–8.

O'Brien O. European Society of Hypertension recommendations for conventional, ambulatory and home blood pressure measurement. *J Hypertens.* 2003;21(5):821.

O'Brien E, Parati G, Stergiou G. Ambulatory blood pressure measurement: what is the international consensus? *Hypertension.* 2013;62(6):988–994.

Ogden LG, He J, Lydick E, Whelton PK. Long-term absolute benefit of lowering blood pressure in hypertensive patients according to the JNC VI risk stratification. *Hypertension.* 2000;35(2):539–543.

Ogedegbe G, Pickering TG, Clemow L, et al. The misdiagnosis of hypertension: the role of patient anxiety. *Arch Intern Med.* 2008;168(22):2459–2465.

Ohira T, Shahar E, Chambless LE, Rosamond WD, Mosley TH Jr, Folsom AR. Risk factors for ischemic stroke subtypes: the Atherosclerosis Risk in Communities study. *Stroke.* 2006:37:2493–2498.

Ohkubo T, Imai Y, Tsuji I, et al. Reference values for 24-hour ambulatory blood pressure monitoring based on a prognostic criterion: the Ohasama Study. *Hypertension.* 1998;32(2):255–259.

Olives C, Myerson R, Mokdad AH, Murray CJ, Lim SS. Prevalence, awareness, treatment, and control of hypertension in United States counties, 2001–2009. *PLoS One.* 2013;8(4):e60308.

Ong KL, Cheung BM, Man YB, Lau CP, Lam KS. Prevalence, awareness, treatment, and control of hypertension among United States adults 1999–2004. *Hypertension.* 2007;49(1):69–75.

Otiniano ME, Du XL, Maldonado MR, Ray L, Markides K. Effect of metabolic syndrome on heart attack and mortality in Mexican-American elderly persons: findings of 7-year follow-up from the Hispanic established population for the epidemiological study of the elderly. *J Gerontol A Biol Sci Med Sci.* 2005;60(4):466–470.

Palatini P, Mormino P, Canali C, et al. Factors affecting ambulatory blood pressure reproducibility. Results of the HARVEST Trial. Hypertension and Ambulatory Recording Venetia Study. *Hypertension.* 1994;23(2):211–216.

Parati G, Stergiou G, O'Brien E, et al. European Society of Hypertension practice guidelines for ambulatory blood pressure monitoring. *J Hypertens.* 2014;32(7): 1359–1366.

Parati G, Stergiou GS, Asmar R, et al. European Society of Hypertension guidelines for blood pressure monitoring at home: a summary report of the Second International Consensus Conference on Home Blood Pressure Monitoring. *J Hypertens.* 2008; 26(8): 1505–1526.

Pereira MA, Folsom AR, McGovern PG, et al. Physical activity and incident hypertension in black and white adults: the Atherosclerosis Risk in Communities study. *Prev Med.* 1999;28(3):304–312.

Perkovic V, Rodgers A. Redefining blood-pressure targets—SPRINT starts the marathon. *N Engl J Med.* 2015;373(22):2175–2178.

Perreault S, Lamarre D, Blais L, et al. Persistence with treatment in newly treated middle-aged patients with essential hypertension. *Ann Pharmacother.* 2005;39(9): 1401–1408.

Pickering T. Recommendations for the use of home (self) and ambulatory blood pressure monitoring. American Society of Hypertension Ad Hoc Panel. *Am J Hypertens.* 1996;9(1):1–11.

Pickering TG, Hall JE, Appel LJ, et al. Recommendations for blood pressure measurement in humans and experimental animals: part 1: blood pressure measurement in humans: a statement for professionals from the Subcommittee of Professional and Public Education of the American Heart Association Council on High Blood Pressure Research. *Circulation.* 2005;111(5):697–716.

Pickering TG, James GD, Boddie C, Harshfield GA, Blank S, Laragh JH. How common is white coat hypertension? *JAMA.* 1988;259(2):225–228.

Pickering TG, White WB, on behalf of the American Society of Hypertension Writing Group. ASH position paper: home and ambulatory blood pressure monitoring when and how to use self (home) and ambulatory blood pressure monitoring. *J Clin Hypertens (Greenwich).* 2008;10(11):850–855.

Piper MA, Evans CV, Burda BU, Margolis KL, O'Connor E, Whitlock EP. Diagnostic and predictive accuracy of blood pressure screening methods with consideration of rescreening intervals: a systematic review for the U.S. Preventive Services Task Force blood pressure screening methods and consideration of rescreening intervals. *Ann Intern Med.* 2015;162(3):192–204.

Psaty BM, Furberg CD, Kuller LH, et al. Association between blood pressure level and the risk of myocardial infarction, stroke, and total mortality: The Cardiovascular Health Study. *Arch Intern Med.* 2001;161(9):1183–1192.

Psaty BM, Lumley T, Furberg CD, et al. Health outcomes associated with various antihypertensive therapies used as first-line agents: a network meta-analysis. *JAMA.* 2003;289(19):2534–2544.

Qureshi AI, Suri MF, Mohammad Y, Guterman LR, Hopkins LN. Isolated and borderline isolated systolic hypertension relative to long-term risk and type of stroke: a 20-year follow-up of the National Health and Nutrition Survey. *Stroke.* 2002:33(12):2781–2788.

Redon J, Lurbe E. Ambulatory blood pressure monitoring is ready to replace clinic blood pressure in the diagnosis of hypertension: con side of the argument. *Hypertension.* 2014;64(6):1169–1174.

Reid CM, Ryan P, Miles H, et al. Who's really hypertensive? Quality control issues in the assessment of blood pressure for randomized trials. *Blood Press.* 2005;14(3):133–138.

Ritchie LD, Campbell NC, Murchie P. New NICE guidelines for hypertension. *BMJ.* 2011;343:d5644.

Rosamond W, Flegal K, Friday G, et al. Heart disease and stroke statistics—2007 update: a report from the American Heart Association Statistics Committee and Stroke Statistics Subcommittee. *Circulation.* 2007;115 (5):e69–171.

Sacks FM, Svetkey LP, Vollmer WM, et al. Effects on blood pressure of reduced dietary sodium and the dietary approaches to stop hypertension (DASH) diet. DASH-Sodium Collaborative Research Group. *N Engl J Med.* 2001;344(1):3–10.

Sega R, Facchetti R, Bombelli M, et al. Prognostic value of ambulatory and home blood pressures compared with office blood pressure in the general population: follow-up results from the Pressioni Arteriose Monitorate e Loro Associazioni (PAMELA) Study. *Circulation.* 2005;111(14):1777–1783.

Selassie A, Wagner CS, Laken ML, Ferguson ML, Ferdinand KC, Egan BM. Progression is accelerated from prehypertension to hypertension in blacks. *Hypertension.* 2011; 58(4):579–587.

Sesso HD, Cook NR, Buring JE, Manson JE, Gaziano JM. Alcohol consumption and the risk of hypertension in women and men. *Hypertension.* 2008;51(4):1080–1087.

Shimamoto K, Ando K, Fujita T, et al. The Japanese Society of Hypertension guidelines for the management of hypertension (JSH 2014). *Hypertens Res.* 2014;37(4):253–387.

Shimbo D, Kuruvilla S, Haas D, Pickering TG, Schwartz JE, Gerin W. Preventing misdiagnosis of ambulatory hypertension: algorithm using office and home blood pressures. *J Hypertens.* 2009;27(9):1775–1783.

Sipahi I, Swaminathan A, Natesan V, Debanne SM, Simon DI, Fang JC. Effect of antihypertensive therapy on incident stroke in cohorts with prehypertensive blood pressure levels: a meta-analysis of randomized controlled trials. *Stroke.* 2012;43(2):432–440.

Siu AL; US Preventive Services Task Force. Screening for high blood pressure in adults: U.S. Preventive Services Task Force recommendation statement. *Ann Intern Med.* 2015;163(10):778–786.

The SPRINT Research Group. A randomized trial of intensive versus standard blood-pressure control. *N Engl J Med.* 2015;373(22):2103–2116.

Staessen JA, Thijs L, Fagard R. Predicting cardiovascular risk using conventional vs ambulatory blood pressure in older patients with systolic hypertension. *JAMA.* 1999; 282(6):539–546.

Staessen JA, Wang J, Bianchi G, Birkenhager WH. Essential hypertension. *Lancet.* 2003;361(9369):1629–1641.

Stamler J. The INTERSALT study: background, methods, findings, and implications. *Am J Clin Nutr.* 1997;65(2 suppl):626S–642S.

Stamler R. Implications of the INTERSALT study. *Hypertension.* 1991;17(suppl 1): I16–I20.

Stergiou GS, Lourida P, Tzamouranis D, Baibas NM. Unreliable oscillometric blood pressure measurement: prevalence, repeatability and characteristics of the phenomenon. *J Hum Hypertens.* 2009a;23(12):794–800.

Stergiou GS, Nasothimiou EG, Giovas PP, Rarra VC. Long-term reproducibility of home vs. office blood pressure in children and adolescents: the Arsakeion school study. *Hypertens Res.* 2009b;32(4):311–315.

Stergiou GS, Parati G, Asmar R, O'Brien E. Requirements for professional office blood pressure monitors. *J Hypertens.* 2012;30(3):537–542.

Stergiou GS, Salgami EV, Tzamouranis DG, Roussias LG. Masked hypertension assessed by ambulatory blood pressure versus home blood pressure monitoring: is it the same phenomenon? *Am J Hypertens.* 2005;18(6):772–778.

Stergiou GS, Skeva II, Baibas NM, Kalkana CB, Roussias LG, Mountokalakis TD. Diagnosis of hypertension using home or ambulatory blood pressure monitoring: comparison with the conventional strategy based on repeated clinic blood pressure measurements. *J Hypertens.* 2000;18(12):1745.

Stranges S, Donahue RP. Health-related quality of life and risk of hypertension in the community. *J Hypertens.* 2015;33(4):720–726.

Sussman J, Vijan S, Hayward R. Using benefit-based tailored treatment to improve the use of antihypertensive medications. *Circulation.* 2013;128(21):2309–2317.

Svetkey LP, Simons-Morton D, Vollmer WM, et al. Effects of dietary patterns on blood pressure: subgroup analysis of the dietary approaches to stop hypertension (DASH) randomized clinical trial. *Arch Intern Med.* 1999;159(3):285–293.

Szklo M, Nieto FJ. *Epidemiology. Beyond the Basics.* 3rd ed. Burlington, MA: Jones and Barlett Learning; 2007.

Task Force for the Management of Arterial Hypertension of the European Society of Hypertension, Task Force for the Management of Arterial Hypertension of the European Society of Cardiology (Task Force for the Management of Arterial Hypertension of the ESH and ESC). 2013 ESH/ESC Guidelines for the Management of Arterial Hypertension. *Blood Press.* 2013;22(4):193–278.

Tedla YG, Bautista LE. Drug side effect symptoms and adherence to antihypertensive medication. *Am J Hypertens.* 2016;29(6):772–779.

Thomas O, Shipman KE, Day K, Thomas M, Martin U, Dasgupta I. Prevalence and determinants of white coat effect in a large UK hypertension clinic population. *J Hum Hypertens.* 2016;30(6):386–391.

Thomopoulos C, Parati G, Zanchetti A. Effects of blood pressure lowering on outcome incidence in hypertension: 4. Effects of various classes of antihypertensive drugs—overview and meta-analyses. *J Hypertens.* 2015a;33(2):195–211.

Thomopoulos C, Parati G, Zanchetti A. Effects of blood pressure-lowering on outcome incidence in hypertension: 5. Head-to-head comparisons of various classes of antihypertensive drugs—overview and meta-analyses. *J Hypertens.* 2015b;33(7): 1321–1341.

Thomopoulos C, Parati G, Zanchetti A. Effects of blood pressure lowering on outcome incidence in hypertension: 7. Effects of more vs. less intensive blood pressure lowering and different achieved blood pressure levels—updated overview and meta-analyses of randomized trials. *J Hypertens.* 2016;34(4):613–622.

Tobe SW, Izzo J. How should BP be measured in the office? *J Am Soc Hypertens.* 2016;10(3):189–190.

Touyz RM, Dominiczak AF. Hypertension guidelines: is it time to reappraise blood pressure thresholds and targets? *Hypertension.* 2016;67(4):688–689.

Turnbull F. Effects of different blood-pressure-lowering regimens on major cardiovascular events: results of prospectively-designed overviews of randomised trials. *Lancet.* 2003;362(9395):1527–1535.

US Department of Health and Human Services (USDHHS), Indian Health Service. *Regional Differences in Indian Health, 2000–2001 Edition.* Washington, DC: Indian Health Service; Rockville, MD: Division of Community and Environmental Health; 2001.

US Preventive Services Task Force (USPSTF). Screening for high blood pressure: U.S. Preventive Services Task Force reaffirmation recommendation statement. *Ann Intern Med.* 2007;147(11):783–786.

Vaccarino V, Holford TR, Krumholz HM. Pulse pressure and risk for myocardial infarction and heart failure in the elderly. *J Am Coll Cardiol.* 2000;36(1):130–138.

van den Hoogen PC, Feskens EJ, Nagelkerke NJ, Menotti A, Nissinen A, Kromhout D. The relation between blood pressure and mortality due to coronary heart disease among men in different parts of the world. Seven Countries Study Research Group. *N Engl J Med.* 2000;342(1):1–8.

van der Steen MS, Lenders JW, Graafsma SJ, den Arend J, Thien T. Reproducibility of ambulatory blood pressure monitoring in daily practice. *J Hum Hypertens.* 1999; 13(5):303.

Vasan RS, Beiser A, Seshadri S, et al. Residual lifetime risk for developing hypertension in middle-aged women and men: The Framingham Heart Study. *JAMA.* 2002;287(8): 1003–1010.

Vasan RS, Larson MG, Leip EP, et al. Impact of high-normal blood pressure on the risk of cardiovascular disease. *N Engl J Med.* 2001a;345(18):1291–1297.

Vasan RS, Larson MG, Leip EP, Kannel WB, Levy D. Assessment of frequency of progression to hypertension in non-hypertensive participants in the Framingham Heart Study: a cohort study. *Lancet.* 2001b;358(9294):1682–1686.

Villegas I, Arias IC, Botero A, Escobar A. Evaluation of the technique used by health-care workers for taking blood pressure. *Hypertension.* 1995;26(6 pt 2):1204–1206.

Wan Y, Heneghan C, Stevens R, et al. Determining which automatic digital blood pressure device performs adequately: a systematic review. *J Hum Hypertens.* 2010;24(7): 431–438.

Weber MA, Schiffrin EL, White WB, et al. Clinical practice guidelines for the management of hypertension in the community: a statement by the American Society of Hypertension and the International Society of Hypertension. *J Hypertens.* 2014; 32(1):3–15.

Wei M, Mitchell BD, Haffner SM, Stern MP. Effects of cigarette smoking, diabetes, high cholesterol, and hypertension on all-cause mortality and cardiovascular disease mortality in Mexican Americans. The San Antonio Heart Study. *Am J Epidemiol.* 1996;144(11):1058–1065.

Welch VL, Hill MN. Effective strategies for blood pressure control. *Cardiol Clin.* 2002;20(2):321–33,vii.

Whelton PK. Epidemiology of hypertension. *Lancet.* 1994;344(8915):101–106.

Whelton PK. The elusiveness of population-wide high blood pressure control. *Annu Rev Public Health.* 2015;36:109–130.

Whelton PK, Appel LJ, Espeland MA, et al. Sodium reduction and weight loss in the treatment of hypertension in older persons: a randomized controlled trial of nonpharmacologic interventions in the elderly (TONE). TONE Collaborative Research Group. *JAMA*. 1998;279(11):839–846.

Whelton PK, Appel LJ, Sacco RL, et al. Sodium, blood pressure, and cardiovascular disease: further evidence supporting the American Heart Association sodium reduction recommendations. *Circulation*. 2012;126(24):2880–2889.

Whelton SP, Chin A, Xin X, He J. Effect of aerobic exercise on blood pressure: a meta-analysis of randomized, controlled trials. *Ann Intern Med*. 2002b;136(7): 493–503.

Whelton PK, He J, Appel LJ, et al. Primary prevention of hypertension: clinical and public health advisory from the National High Blood Pressure Education Program. *JAMA*. 2002a;288(15):1882–1888.

Whelton PK, He J, Cutler JA, et al. Effects of oral potassium on blood pressure. Meta-analysis of randomized controlled clinical trials. *JAMA*. 1997;277(20):1624–1632.

Williams SA, Kasl SV, Heiat A, Abramson JL, Krumholz HM, Vaccarino V. Depression and risk of heart failure among the elderly: a prospective community-based study. *Psychosom Med*. 2002;64(1):6–12.

Winegarden CR. From "prehypertension" to hypertension? Additional evidence. *Ann Epidemiol*. 2005;15(9):720–725.

Wolf-Maier K, Cooper RS, Banegas JR, et al. Hypertension prevalence and blood pressure levels in 6 European countries, Canada, and the United States. *JAMA*. 2003;289(18):2363–2369.

Woodiwiss AJ, Molebatsi N, Maseko MJ, et al. Nurse-recorded auscultatory blood pressure at a single visit predicts target organ changes as well as ambulatory blood pressure. *J Hypertens*. 2009;27(2):287–297.

World Health Organization (WHO). *Global Health Risks: Mortality and Burden of Disease Attributable to Selected Major Risks*. Geneva, Switzerland: WHO; 2009.

World Health Organization (WHO). *Global Status Report on Noncommunicable Diseases 2010*. Geneva, Switzerland: WHO; 2011.

World Health Organization (WHO). A global brief on hypertension: silent killer, global public health crisis: World Health Day 2013. Geneva, Switzerland: WHO; 2013.

Xie X, Atkins E, Lv J, et al. Effects of intensive blood pressure lowering on cardiovascular and renal outcomes: updated systematic review and meta-analysis. *Lancet*. 2016; 3 87(10017):435–443.

Xin X, He J, Frontini MG, Ogden LG, Motsamai OI, Whelton PK. Effects of alcohol reduction on blood pressure: a meta-analysis of randomized controlled trials. *Hypertension*. 2001;38(5):1112–1117.

Yamagata K, Ishida K, Sairenchi T, et al. Risk factors for chronic kidney disease in a community-based population: a 10-year follow-up study. *Kidney Int*. 2007;71(2):159–166.

Yarows SA, Staessen JA. How to use home blood pressure monitors in clinical practice. *Am J Hypertens*. 2002;15(1 pt 1):93–96.

Yoon SS, Gu Q, Nwankwo T, Wright JD, Hong Y, Burt V. Trends in blood pressure among adults with hypertension: United States, 2003 to 2012. *Hypertension*. 2015;65(1):54–61.

Zanchetti A, Mancia G. Longing for clinical excellence: a critical outlook into the NICE recommendations on hypertension management—is nice always good? *J Hypertens*. 2012;30(4):660–668.

14

DYSLIPIDEMIA

Carla I. Mercado, PhD, MS, and Fleetwood Loustalot, PhD, FNP

Introduction

For almost 100 years, cardiovascular disease (CVD) has been the leading cause of death in the United States, responsible for 30.8% of all deaths in 2013 (Mozaffarian et al. 2016). One of the major risk factors for CVD is dyslipidemia (Stone et al. 2014), a condition in which one or more lipid profile measures are in the abnormal range. Primary lipid profile measures consist of total cholesterol (TC) and its major individual parts: low-density lipoprotein cholesterol (LDL-C), high-density lipoprotein cholesterol (HDL-C), and triglycerides (TGs), a measure of fat. Risk of CVD increases with increasing levels of TC, LDL-C, or TGs, or with decreasing levels of HDL-C. Mixed dyslipidemia, when HDL-C is low and TGs are high, despite the level of LDL-C, has also been associated with increased CVD risk (Cziraky and Thomas 2010). Abnormal lipid profile measures can result from an unhealthy lifestyle, other metabolic factors, certain medications, or heredity (Figure 14-1); however, lipid management can be achieved through lifestyle modifications and, if required, an appropriate medication regimen.

Significance

Dyslipidemia has been associated with an increased risk of coronary heart disease (CHD) and myocardial infarction (Isomaa et al. 2001). In addition to lower TC being associated with lower ischemic heart disease mortality, adults with the highest measures had the highest ischemic heart disease mortality (Lewington et al. 2007). From 2005 to 2012, 36.7% or 78.1 million U.S. adults aged 21 years and older were considered eligible for cholesterol-lowering management (currently on treatment or newly eligible based on condition

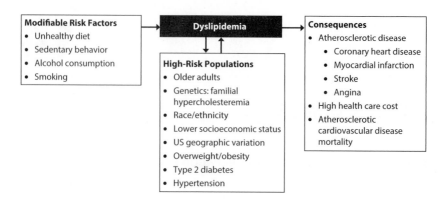

Figure 14-1. Dyslipidemia: Causes, Consequences, and High-Risk Groups

or risk), yet only 46.6% of those reported making lifestyle modifications and 55.5% were taking cholesterol-lowering medication (Mercado et al. 2015). Almost 68% of U.S. adults eligible for cholesterol-lowering management but not taking any medication were not aware of their condition. Dyslipidemia prevention and management deserves increased attention from the clinical and public health communities with dyslipidemia's high burden, significant association with CVD, underutilized treatment, and high cost ($34.5 billion in 2013; USDHHS 2013).

Pathophysiology

Cholesterol is a waxy, fat-like substance present in every cell membrane. It is also carried through the blood, used to make some hormones, and used to help digest fatty foods. If there is too much cholesterol in the blood, it can begin to build up on the walls of the blood vessels and produce deposits called plaque that can lead to atherosclerosis (Nakashima et al. 2007; Otsuka et al. 2015), a condition in which the plaque build-up can produce inflammation and scar tissue limiting or blocking the flow of blood.

The amount of cholesterol in the blood comes from two sources: made by the body and consumed through diet. The body's production of cholesterol is sufficient to sustain the functions for which cholesterol is needed. Dietary cholesterol can be found in foods from animal sources and these foods contain higher amounts of cholesterol as the fat content increases (Martin et al. 2014).

Cholesterol travels in the blood on proteins called lipoproteins, mainly LDL-C and HDL-C. Because LDL-C is responsible for the plaque buildup in the blood vessels that develops into atherosclerosis and HDL-C helps to manage LDL-C storage and clear the cholesterol out of the bloodstream, they have been labeled as "bad" and "good" cholesterol, respectively. Another type of fat found in the blood and part of the lipid profile measures are TGs. Based on the Friedewald equation, TC is equal to the sum of LDL-C, HDL-C, and 20% of TGs (Friedewald et al. 1972; Fukuyama et al. 2008).

Total cholesterol associated with CVD had been the main focus of lipid research in the past. However, TC assumes an additive effect of LDL-C, HDL-C, and TGs and cannot distinguish the protective effect of HDL-C or the inverse association of TGs with HDL-C (Kolovou et al. 2009). As the effects of HDL-C and non–HDL-C on ischemic heart disease mortality are independent of each other, the ratio of HDL-C to non–HDL-C tends to be more informative than either one alone (Lewington et al. 2007), with an ideal ratio of greater than 0.29 for men and greater than 0.35 for women (Kim et al. 2013). The TC-to-HDL-C ratio (ideal ratio of < 3.89 for women and < 4.39 for men [Kim et al. 2013]) has also been found to be highly correlated with severity of coronary artery calcification (CAC), a proxy measure for the amount of atherosclerosis in the arteries of the heart, and associated with increasing CVD event rates (Martin et al. 2014). Although HDL-C continues to show benefit to CHD risk at increasing levels with a potential threshold of benefit at very high levels (Wilkins et al. 2014), the HDL-C-to-non–HDL-C ratio shows no evidence of a threshold effect where higher levels are no longer associated with lower CHD risk (Eliasson et al. 2014). Therefore, each lipid profile measure and their individual and combined role in contributing to CVD has become the focus in treatment, research, and public health efforts.

With atherosclerosis responsible for the majority of atherosclerotic CVD (ASCVD; Arguelles et al. 2014; Martin et al. 2014; Mozaffarian et al. 2016), CAC has been positively associated with cardiovascular events (Greenland et al. 2004; Budoff et al. 2009; Polonsky et al. 2010; Criqui et al. 2014). Risk for ASCVD increases with multiple abnormal lipid profile measures because of their individual significant associations with incidence of CAC, a positive association with LDL-C and TGs, and a negative association with HDL-C (Kronmal et al. 2007). Although the risk of ASCVD may vary on the basis of which one or combination of abnormal lipid profile measures are present, having abnormal values for all measures tends to result in the highest risk for incident ASCVD (Table 14-1; Andersson et al. 2014).

Table 14-1. Combination of Abnormal Lipid Profile Measures and Risk of Cardiovascular Disease

Lipid Profile Measures			
HDL-C	LDL-C	Triglycerides	HR (95% CI)
Normal	Normal	Normal	Reference group
Normal	High	Normal	1.28 (1.03, 1.59)
Normal	Normal	High	1.35 (0.91, 1.98)
Normal	High	High	1.53 (1.13, 2.08)
Low	Normal	High	1.74 (1.28, 2.38)
Low	High	Normal	1.83 (1.35, 2.50)
Low	Normal	Normal	1.93 (1.38, 2.71)
Low	High	High	2.30 (1.75, 3.02)

Source: Data from Andersson et al. (2014).
Note: CI = confidence interval; HDL-C = high-density lipoprotein cholesterol; HR = hazard ratio; LDL-C = low-density lipoprotein cholesterol.

Familial Hypercholesterolemia

Familial hypercholesterolemia (FH) is a genetic disorder in which the capacity to clear LDL-C from the blood is decreased (Bouhairie and Goldberg 2016). Because FH is an autosomal-dominant condition with a dose effect, people who are homozygous have much higher LDL-C and earlier onset of CVD than those who are heterozygous (Hopkins et al. 2011; Robinson and Goldberg 2011; Nordestgaard et al. 2013). The LDL-C can range from 155 to 500 milligrams per deciliter (mg/dL) among untreated heterozygotes and can be greater than 500 mg/dL in untreated homozygotes (Hopkins et al. 2011; Raal and Santos 2012; Nordestgaard et al. 2013). People with heterozygous FH may or may not be asymptomatic during childhood and early adulthood; however, FH is responsible for 20% of heart attacks that occur in those aged younger than 45 years (Hopkins et al. 2011).

Descriptive Epidemiology

High-Risk Populations

Familial Hypercholesterolemia

Although the prevalence of FH varies in different populations (Benn et al. 2012; Raal and Santos 2012; Sjouke et al. 2015), the number of people with heterozygous FH in the United States has been projected to range from 620,000 to 1,500,000 people based on a prevalence of 1 in 250 to 500 (Goldberg et al. 2011). Among U.S. children and adolescents (aged 2 to 20 years) in a health care system from various regions of the United States, prevalence of diagnosed LDL-C greater than 190 mg/dL in 2012 was 0.08% and LDL-C from 130 to 190 mg/dL was 1.4% (Zachariah et al. 2015). In addition, incidence of diagnosed LDL-C greater than 190 mg/dL increased among children and adolescents from 0.03% to 0.06% during 2002 to 2012 ($p=.03$). However, these prevalence estimates are most likely an underestimation because not all children and adolescents had been tested for cholesterol. When only those who had a cholesterol test are considered, the prevalence of LDL-C greater than 190 mg/dL was 0.71% and LDL-C from 130 to 190 mg/dL was 12.58% in 2012.

Gender and Age Differences

Dyslipidemia presents differently in men and women and it changes during different life stages. During 2011 to 2014 in the United States, the prevalence of TC of 240 mg/dL or higher was greater for women (13%) than men (11%), but prevalence of low HDL-C (<40 mg/dL) was higher among men (28%) than women (10%; Carroll et al. 2015). The prevalence of LDL-C of 130 mg/dL or higher was similar between men (31%) and women (32%) in the United States during 2009 to 2012 (Mozaffarian et al. 2016). Although women also tend to have greater TC than men, on average women had lower TGs and TC-to-HDL-C ratio as well as greater HDL-C than men (Kolovou et al. 2009; Palacios et al. 2011; Bennasar-Veny et al. 2013; Melmer et al. 2013; Ali et al. 2014; Jenkins and Ofstedal 2014). Because of these differences, it is estimated that men are twice as likely to have both high TGs and low HDL-C compared with women (Kolovou et al. 2009).

Aside from gender differences, lipid levels change with age. Total cholesterol tends to increase with age with a potential threshold around age 50 to 59 years (Figure 14-2; Hatmi et al. 2011). Coinciding with TC, LDL-C also increases with age with greatest values anticipated among adults aged 60 years and older. Unlike TC and LDL-C, TGs tend to peak at about age 40 to 49 years and then start to decline. However, when comparisons were made between younger (aged 18–29 years) versus older (aged ≥ 70 years) adults, older age groups tended to have greater TGs and HDL-C than their younger counterparts (Sumner et al. 2012). Still, a decrease in TC lowers the risk of ischemic

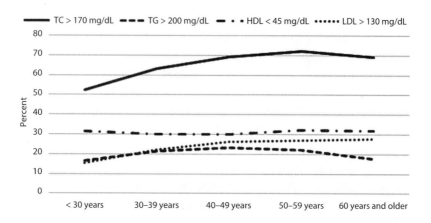

Source: Data from Hatmi et al. (2011).

Figure 14-2. Percentage of Adults with At-Risk Values for Lipid Profile Measures by Age Categories

heart disease mortality to a greater extent for younger adults than for older adults (Lewington et al. 2007). Although lipid profile measures change with age, there are greater changes (increases in TC, LDL-C, and TGs and decreases in HDL-C) in women during menopause independent of the aging effect (Stevenson et al. 1993; Anagnostis et al. 2015).

Gender difference in lipid measures among children and adolescents is more complex because of the expression of hormones during puberty resulting in multiple changes at different stages of childhood. In 2011 to 2014, among children and adolescents (aged 6–19 years) in the United States, the prevalence of TC of 200 mg/dL or higher was greater for girls (8.9%) than boys (5.9%; Nguyen et al. 2015). Similarly, girls had greater prevalence of non–HDL-C of 145 mg/dL or higher (9.4%) compared to boys (7.5%). However, the prevalence of HDL-C less than 40 mg/dL was higher among boys (14.8%) than girls (12%). For the most part, mean serum TC, TGs, and LDL-C were on average higher among girls than boys (Lambert et al. 2008; Vaisto et al. 2014). Nonetheless, the mean lipid levels may be greater in boys and girls (Lambert et al. 2008; Margolis et al. 2014; Vaisto et al. 2014; Nguyen et al. 2015) depending on the age distribution of study populations, which may reflect lipid levels at a different stage of childhood. Levels of HDL-C decrease with increasing age in boys and remained similar through ages 3 to 19 years in girls (Margolis et al. 2014). Levels of TGs tend to be higher among girls than boys before the age of 12 years, then decrease to similar levels from ages 12 to 19 years.

Race/Ethnicity

Disparities in dyslipidemia are seen among racial/ethnic groups. In 2011 to 2014, the prevalence of TC of 240 mg/dL or higher was lowest among non-Hispanic blacks (8.6%) compared to other race/ethnicities (non-Hispanic whites [12.5%], non-Hispanic Asians [11%], or Hispanics [13%]; Carroll et al. 2015). The prevalence of low HDL-C (< 40 mg/dL) was higher among Hispanics (21%) and non-Hispanic whites (19%) compared to non-Hispanic Asians (15%) and non-Hispanic blacks (14%). About 10% of non-Hispanic Asian adults in the United States during 2011 to 2012 had TC of 240 mg/dL or higher and 14% had low HDL-C (<40 mg/dL; Aoki et al. 2014). Although some studies show less desirable lipid profiles for Hispanics with higher LDL-C and TGs compared to other racial/ethnic groups (Bild et al. 2005), there is great variation within subtypes of Hispanics with the prevalence of LDL-C of 130 mg/dL or higher ranging from 32% to 45% and a TG level of 200 mg/dL or higher ranging from 8% to 70% (Rodriguez et al. 2014). Similarly, there are differences in mean lipid profile measures among Asian subtypes (Frank et al. 2014). This information needs to be considered when one is targeting interventions for specific populations.

On average, non-Hispanic blacks have lower TG levels than non-Hispanic whites, Hispanics, and Chinese (Bild et al. 2005). In a study comparing non-Hispanic whites, Hispanics, non-Hispanic blacks, and Chinese, LDL-C was lowest among Chinese and HDL-C was lowest among Hispanics (Bild et al. 2005). The TC-to-HDL-C ratio tends to be lower for non-Hispanic blacks compared to non-Hispanic whites (Jenkins and Ofstedal 2014). Although non-Hispanic blacks are more likely to have better lipid profiles than other racial/ethnic groups in the United States, both Hispanics and non-Hispanic blacks with abnormal LDL-C are less likely to have their condition under control compared to non-Hispanic whites (Upadhyay et al. 2010). Along with dyslipidemia presenting differently among racial/ethnic subgroups, the association between lipids and CVD risk differs by race/ethnicity. For example, previous research has shown a significant interaction between TC and race/ethnicity related to CVD events, with the risk of a CVD events increasing to a greater extent for every unit increase in TC among non-Hispanic blacks (140% higher) compared to non-Hispanic whites (Gijsberts et al. 2015).

Interestingly, the racial/ethnic differences in dyslipidemia seen in adults also occur among children and adolescents. Among U.S. children and adolescents (aged 6–19 years), non-Hispanic Asians (11%) and non-Hispanic blacks

(10%) had a greater prevalence of TC of greater than or equal to 200 mg/dL than Hispanics (6.3%) and non-Hispanic whites (7.3%) in 2011 to 2014 (Nguyen et al. 2015). However, non-Hispanic whites (14%) and Hispanics (16%) had greater prevalence of HDL-C less than 40 mg/dL compared to non-Hispanic blacks (7%) and non-Hispanic Asians (8%). Along with significantly higher HDL-C in non-Hispanic black children and adolescents, TGs were significantly lower compared to non-Hispanic whites and Mexican Americans (Kant and Graubard 2012). There was no significant difference in the prevalence of non–HDL-C greater than or equal to 145 mg/dL (Nguyen et al. 2015) or mean LDL-C (Kant and Graubard 2012) across racial/ethnic subgroups.

Socioeconomic Status

Socioeconomic status (SES) has been associated with health disparities, including dyslipidemia. Adults in professional occupations on average had higher HDL-C than those in manual labor occupations (Shohaimi et al. 2014). Similarly, HDL-C on average increased with greater educational attainment (Mosca et al. 2013; Everage et al. 2014; Shohaimi et al. 2014). Number of years in school was significantly negatively associated with TC-to-HDL-C ratio for women and positively associated with HDL-C for both men and women in a study that examined the association between SES and cardiovascular risk factors between men and women (Jenkins and Ofstedal 2014). Level of LDL-C was negatively associated with educational attainment (Upadhyay et al. 2010; Shohaimi et al. 2014). Income level was also negatively associated with TC-to-HDL-C ratio in men and positively associated with HDL-C in women (Jenkins and Ofstedal 2014).

Geographic Distribution

Although dyslipidemia is a more common condition in developed countries than in developing countries (Oya et al. 2015; Rankinen et al. 2015), the association between ischemic heart disease mortality and cholesterol do not differ between countries after differences in age distribution are taken into account (Lewington et al. 2007).

U.S. Prevalence and Distribution

The prevalence of TC of 240 mg/dL or higher among U.S. adults aged 20 years and older during 2011 to 2014 was approximately 12% (Carroll et al. 2015).

In 2009 to 2012, the prevalence of TC greater than or equal to 200 mg/dL, LDL-C greater than or equal to 130 mg/dL, HDL-C less than 40 mg/dL, and TGs greater 150 mg/dL in adults aged 20 years and older was 43%, 32%, 20%, and 25% respectively (Mozaffarian et al. 2016). Although the prevalence of having at least one abnormal lipid profile measure is close to 50% among adults (Ghandehari et al. 2008), there are variations among U.S. states in cholesterol screening, awareness, and in prescribing cholesterol medication (CDC 2012; Hsia et al. 2013). U.S. states that have older populations and populations with higher rates of Medicare-insured populations are more likely to perform cholesterol screenings and prescribe medication (Hsia et al. 2013). However, the geographic pattern of self-reported high cholesterol was not consistent with the geographic pattern of cholesterol screening (Figure 14-3; CDC 2012).

Time Trends

Population TC has declined in developing countries during the past 20 years with the distribution curve shifting toward the left while HDL-C has slightly increased (Hulman et al. 2014). The prevalence of TC of greater than or equal to 240 mg/dL has significantly decreased in the United States from 18% in 1999 to 11% in 2014, while the prevalence of HDL-C less than 40 mg/dL has decreased from 22% in 2007 to 20% in 2014 (Carroll et al. 2015). When one looks at trends in the mean serum lipid profile measures from 1976 to 2006 in the United States, TC declined (from 210 mg/dL to 200 mg/dL), LDL-C declined (from 134 mg/dL to 119 mg/dL), HDL-C increased (from 50 mg/dL to 53 mg/dL), and TGs increased (from 137 mg/dL to 146 mg/dL; Cohen et al. 2010). Triglycerides increased from 1976 to 2006, but declined to 110 mg/dL in 2007 to 2010 (Figure 14-4; Carroll et al. 2012). Not all racial/ethnic groups observed significant changes among cholesterol components. Mexican Americans and non-Hispanic blacks did not have significant changes in mean HDL-C or TGs. Although lipid profile measures have improved during the past few years, among those who had ever been screened for high blood cholesterol, the percentage of U.S. adults (aged ≥ 18 years) who have ever been told by a health care provider that they had high blood cholesterol has increased from 33% in 2005 to 35% in 2009 (CDC 2012).

Because the prevalence of TC less than 200 mg/dL without cholesterol medication use in U.S. adults aged 20 years and older (about 46%) has not changed from 1988 to 2010 (Yang et al. 2012), the decline in mean TC and

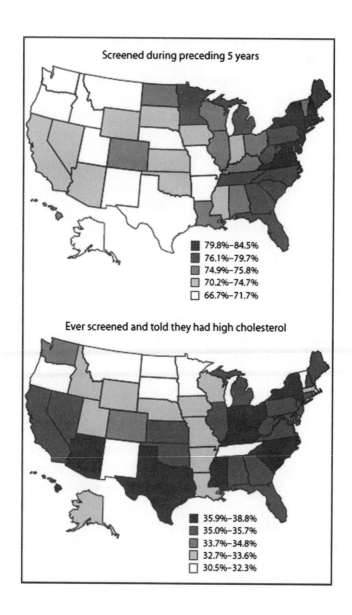

Source: Reprinted from CDC (2012).
*Age-adjusted to the 2000 U.S. standard population; weighted estimates.

Figure 14-3. Age-Adjusted* Percentage of Adults Aged 18 Years and Older Who Had Been Screened for High Blood Cholesterol During the Preceding Five Years and Percentage Who Had Ever Been Screened for Cholesterol and Were Told by a Health-Care Provider that They Had High Blood Cholesterol—Behavioral Risk Factor Surveillance System, United States, 2009

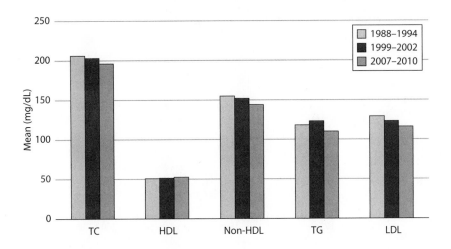

Source: Data from Carroll et al. (2012).

Figure 14-4. Age-Adjusted Mean Lipid Profile Measure among U.S. Adults Aged 20 Years and Older

LDL-C are likely attributable to decreases among those who had high levels because of the increase in medication use and population-level dietary changes (Ford and Capewell 2013). Although there has been a small decrease in the intake of saturated fat and cholesterol in the past three decades, the decline in TC and LDL-C levels during this time is more likely attributable to increased use of cholesterol-lowering medication than to individual dietary changes (Ford and Capewell 2013). From 1988 to 2010, cholesterol-lowering medication use in U.S. adults aged 20 years and older increased from 3.4% to 15.5% (Figure 14-5; Carroll et al. 2012). By 2012, cholesterol-lowering medication use increased to 28% among all U.S. adults aged 40 years and older (Gu et al. 2014). Nearly all of this increase was attributable to increased use of 3-hydroxy-3-methyl-glutaryl-coenzyme A (HMG-CoA) reductase inhibitors (statins; Gu et al. 2014).

Similar to adults, U.S. children and adolescents have also experienced improvements in their lipid profile measures during the past few decades. Among children and adolescents aged 6 to 19 years, there has been a significant decrease in TC (from 165 mg/dL to 160 mg/dL), non–HDL-C (from 115 mg/dL to 107 mg/dL), LDL-C (from 95 mg/dL to 90 mg/dL), and TGs (from 82 mg/dL to 73 mg/dL) from 1988 to 2010 (Kit et al. 2012). Levels of HDL-C significantly increased from 50.5 mg/dL in 1988 to 1994 to 52.2 mg/dL in 2007 to 2010.

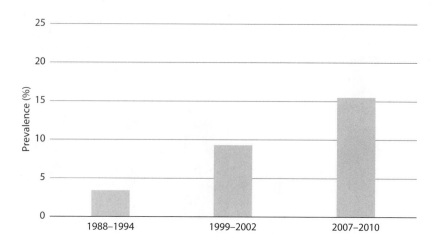

Source: Data from Carroll et al. (2012).

Figure 14-5. Age-Adjusted Prevalence of Lipid-Lowering Medication Use among U.S. Adults Aged 20 Years and Older

The prevalence of TC greater than or equal to 200 mg/dL decreased among children and adolescents (aged 8 to 17 years) from 11% to 8% and HDL-C less than 40 mg/dL decreased from 18% to 13% during 1999 to 2012 (Kit et al. 2015).

Causes

Risk Factors

Overweight or Obesity

Being overweight or obese is associated with increased risk of CVD as well as CVD risk factors such as hypertension, type 2 diabetes, and dyslipidemia (Mozaffarian et al. 2016). Categories of overweight or obesity have been associated with lower levels of HDL-C and higher levels of LDL-C and TGs in a dose–response relationship in which the various lipid levels worsen with higher levels of obesity (Upadhyay et al. 2010; Slagter et al. 2013; Slagter et al. 2014). Body mass index (BMI), which is a measure of weight status that takes height into account, is not always the measure best associated with lipid values, as lipid measures are affected by weight distribution in the body. Abdominal and visceral adiposity are positively associated with higher levels of LDL-C and TGs, whereas BMI was only associated with higher levels of TGs (Rosito et al. 2008;

Ali et al. 2014). When different weight distribution measures were compared, waist-to-hip ratio was the better estimator of HDL-C and LDL-C than was BMI, waist-to-height ratio, and body adiposity index (Melmer et al. 2013). Waist-to-hip ratio, waist-to-height ratio, and BMI were all significant estimators of TG levels. Although BMI is a commonly used measure of weight classification in epidemiologic and surveillance studies, the obesity measure that is a better predictor or more strongly associated with lipid measures may vary on the basis of the population because of different body compositions among various races/ ethnicities (Palacios et al. 2011; Bennasar-Veny et al. 2013).

Unlike adults, the better overweight or obesity predictor measure associated with dyslipidemia in children and adolescents is BMI. Body mass index percentiles are significantly associated with HDL-C and LDL-C, but visceral or subcutaneous adiposity are not associated with HDL-C or LDL-C among children and adolescents (Ali et al. 2014). Although BMI, obesity classes, or obese versus not obese are associated with greater levels of LDL-C, TGs, TG-to-HDL-C ratio, and lower HDL-C, subcutaneous adiposity was only associated with TG levels (Hamidi et al. 2006; Zhang et al. 2008; Pereira et al. 2009; Simsek et al. 2010; Di Bonito et al. 2014; Lima et al. 2015). The prevalence of HDL-C less than 40 mg/dL increases with the degree of overweight or obesity (6.8% for normal weight, 14.8% for overweight, and 33.2% for obese) among children, as does non–HDL-C greater than or equal to 145 mg/dL (5.7% for normal weight, 9.7% for overweight, and 16.7% for obese; Nguyen et al. 2015).

Dietary Intake

An unhealthy diet has been associated with a variety of chronic diseases and their risk factors including dyslipidemia (Table 14-2). Many studies investigating associations of diet with lipid profile measures have focused on dietary fat intake, and have found that, although the effect of a low-fat diet versus a high-fat diet is associated with a decline in serum TC and LDL-C, it has also been associated with a decrease in HDL-C and an increase in TGs (Schwingshackl and Hoffmann 2013). However, the type of fat consumed matters. When saturated fatty acid (SFA) intake was compared with that of polyunsaturated fatty acid (PUFA) on changes in cardiometabolic risk factors, there were significant declines in LDL-C-to-HDL-C and TC-to-HDL-C ratios with PUFA consumption versus an increase with SFA intake (Iggman et al. 2014). Although reducing SFA consumption results in decreases in TC and LDL-C, it is unclear if

Table 14-2. Lipid Changes Associated with Type of Dietary Changes

Type of Dietary Change	Lipid Profile Measures			
	Total Cholesterol	HDL-C	LDL-C	Triglycerides
Low-fat diet versus high-fat diet	↓	↓	↓	↑
Polyunsaturated fatty acid (PUFA) versus saturated fatty acid	↓	↑	↓	
Low-carbohydrate and increasing PUFA versus high-carbohydrate		↑	↓	↓
Mediterranean diet versus non-Mediterranean diet		↑		↓
Increasing fruit and vegetable consumption		↑		

Source: Compiled from Schwingshackl and Hoffmann (2013); Iggman et al. (2014); Blekkenhorst et al. (2015); Hooper et al. (2015); Larsson et al. (2012); Rajaie et al. (2014); Nordmann et al. (2006); Goff et al. (2013); USDA (2015); Estruch et al. (2013); Martinez-Gonzalez and Bes-Rastrollo (2014); Steffen et al. (2014).

Note: HDL-C = high-density lipoprotein cholesterol; LDL-C = low-density lipoprotein cholesterol.

reduction in SFA consumption alone is associated with any changes in HDL-C or TGs (Blekkenhorst et al. 2015; Hooper et al. 2015). Nonetheless, risk of stroke has been positively associated with dietary cholesterol and negatively associated with long-chain omega-3 fatty acids (one type of PUFA) in women (Larsson et al. 2012). In addition, monounsaturated fatty acid (MUFA) intake, another type of unsaturated fat, was associated with a decreased risk of ASCVD mortality, whereas SFA was associated with an increased risk (Hooper et al. 2015). When a diet with reduced SFA intake was compared with usual diet, a reduction of SFA consumption was associated with a 17% reduction in cardiovascular events.

Although a reduction in SFA intake can improve cardiovascular health, many times this dietary change results in an increase in carbohydrate consumption (Austin et al. 2011), which also has an effect on lipid profile measures. When a high-carbohydrate diet was compared with a moderately restricted–carbohydrate diet by increasing dietary fat (specifically MUFAs and PUFAs), a significant decline in the levels of TGs and TG-to-HDL-C ratio was observed after two weeks with the moderately restricted–carbohydrate diet and no change in the high-carbohydrate diet group (Rajaie et al. 2014). However, a low-carbohydrate diet is more effective in increasing HDL-C and decreasing

TGs compared to low-fat diets, and a low-fat diet is favorable in decreasing TC and LDL-C (Nordmann et al. 2006). Although a low-carbohydrate diet tends to lead to weight loss (Mansoor et al. 2016), which in itself can improve lipid profile measures, a low glycemic index diet (similar to a low-carbohydrate diet) has been shown to reduce TGs and LDL-C independent of weight loss (Goff et al. 2013).

While it is important to monitor the consumption of macronutrients including dietary fat and carbohydrates, focusing on the complete dietary pattern will reduce chronic disease risk and improve overall health. The 2015–2020 Dietary Guidelines for Americans recommend aiming to increase intake of nutrient-dense foods such as fruits and vegetables while limiting consumption of foods high in SFA, added sugar, and sodium (USDA 2015). Current Dietary Guidelines recommend that less than 10% of daily calories should come from SFA and that healthy oils such as MUFAs and PUFAs should be used instead. The Mediterranean diet, one commonly including plant-based foods, whole grains, nuts, legumes, fish and poultry, herbs and spices, and olive oil, has been identified as one type of heart-healthy dietary pattern that is low in SFA and red meat while focusing more on MUFA and PUFA intake along with fruits, vegetables, and whole grains (Estruch et al. 2013; Martinez-Gonzalez and Bes-Rastrollo 2014). Following a Mediterranean dietary pattern has been associated with lower risk of having TG levels greater than or equal to 150 mg/dL or HDL-C levels less than 50 mg/dL (Steffen et al. 2014). Also, meeting the guidelines for fruit and vegetable consumption was associated with higher levels of HDL-C compared to those who did not meet the guidelines (Everage et al. 2014).

Physical Activity

Physical activity has many health benefits, including a positive effect on lipid profile measures. Frequent moderate-intensity physical activity is inversely associated with TC-to-HDL-C ratio and positively associated with HDL-C (Jenkins and Ofstedal 2014). Aside from the frequency of being physical active, the intensity and the amount of time spent in physical activity has been associated with increases in HDL-C and decreases in TGs (Hu et al. 2015). Along with greater physical activity, fitness levels are also associated with higher levels of HDL-C and lower TGs (Camhi et al. 2013). Sedentary behavior (hours/day) has been associated with a decrease in HDL-C (Altenburg et al. 2014).

Although most of the physical activity evidence associated with dyslipidemia is related to HDL-C and TGs, the impact it has on LDL-C and TC remains unclear (Hu et al. 2015).

The Physical Activity Guidelines for Americans recommend that adults be active for at least 150 minutes a week of moderate-intensity or 75 minutes a week of vigorous-intensity aerobic physical activity or an equivalent combination to achieve or maintain good health (USDHHS 2008). For children and adolescents, physical activity should be done on a daily basis for 60 minutes or more (USDHHS 2008). People who do not meet the guidelines for physical activity tend to have lower HDL-C than those meeting the guidelines (Everage et al. 2014). Also, maintaining a physically active lifestyle from adolescence to young adulthood has a beneficial impact on HDL-C during adulthood (Rangul et al. 2012).

For children and adolescents, evidence exists of physical activity's impact on all lipid profile measures. Total physical activity (minutes/day) is significantly associated with lower TGs and LDL-C as well as greater HDL-C (Martinez-Vizcaino et al. 2014; Vaisto et al. 2014). In contrast, sedentary behavior (minutes/day) was associated with higher levels of TG and lower HDL-C in children and adolescents (Cliff et al. 2013; Vaisto et al. 2014). Even light physical activity is associated with higher HDL-C than no activity (Cliff et al. 2013).

Alcohol Consumption and Smoking

Alcohol consumption (drinks per day) has been positively associated with HDL-C and inversely associated with LDL-C and TC-to-HDL-C ratio (Shimomura and Wakabayashi 2013; Jenkins and Ofstedal 2014). The type of alcohol consumed (beer, wine, or spirits or mixed drinks) does not affect the positive association with HDL-C (Slagter et al. 2014). However, beer consumption has been associated with higher levels of TGs, most likely because of its carbohydrate content. The Dietary Guidelines for Americans recommend that, if drinking alcohol, adults should drink in moderation, up to one drink per day for women and up to two drinks per day for men (USDA 2015).

Along with being a risk factor for CVD and stroke, smoking is also associated with lipid profile levels. Smokers tend to have lower HDL-C and a higher TC-to-HDL-C ratio than nonsmokers (Everage et al. 2014; Jenkins and Ofstedal 2014; Slagter et al. 2014). There is a dose–response association with smoking and the decreasing of HDL-C and increasing of TGs (Slagter et al. 2013; Slagter et al. 2014). Although former smokers have similar HDL-C levels as nonsmokers, former smokers tend to have higher levels of LDL-C and TC compared to nonsmokers and even current smokers (Slagter et al. 2013). The higher LDL-C among former smokers compared to nonsmokers is irrespective of duration of cessation (Ogawa et al. 2015). The favorable association between alcohol consumption and HDL-C has been shown to be attenuated by active smoking in that a current smoker with moderate alcohol consumption has been shown to have similar HDL-C levels as someone who is a nonsmoker and nondrinker (Slagter et al. 2014).

Comorbidities

Other chronic conditions that tend to coexist with dyslipidemia because of similar upstream risk factors, such as type 2 diabetes and hypertension, further increase CVD risk. The prevalence of dyslipidemia among those with type 2 diabetes was twice that of adults with normal glucose tolerance (Isomaa et al. 2001). Although an increase of one standard deviation of LDL-C (26–29 mg/dL depending on hospitalization subgroup) was associated with a 50% increase risk of CVD hospitalization among adults with type 2 diabetes (Nichols et al. 2013), other lipid profile measures may be more of a problem in diabetic adults. Although LDL-C has been associated with CVD and tends not to be associated with CHD rates unless levels are greater than 3.0 millimoles per liter (mmol/L; >116.0 mg/dL) among adults with type 2 diabetes, non–HDL-C-to-HDL-C ratio had a consistent increasing linear association with CHD rate in this group (Eliasson et al. 2014). Non–HDL-C-to-HDL-C ratio was a better predictor of CHD than LDL-C alone among diabetic adults, potentially attributable to the fact that LDL-C alone does not include the role of other lipid types, such as TGs and HDL-C, in increasing or decreasing the risk of CHD (Eliasson et al. 2011).

Although among people with type 2 diabetes, non–HDL-C is a better measure in identifying those at greater risk for CHD, there are differences in the specific measure between men and women (Sone et al. 2012). For women with type 2 diabetes, TG level was the better measure of identifying those at greater risk for CHD (Sone et al. 2012) and the TC-to-HDL-C ratio was better for any CVD event (Tohidi et al. 2010). For diabetic men, LDL-C was a better measure in predicting any CVD events. Although adults with type 2 diabetes are at increased risk for dyslipidemia and ASCVD, diabetic adults with a history of CVD tend to have better lipid management, with 38% having LDL-C levels greater than or equal to 100 mg/dL versus 58% in diabetic adults with no history of CVD (Vazquez-Benitez et al. 2015).

Aside from type 2 diabetes, hypertension is independently associated with both increased ASCVD risk and lipid measures. Systolic blood pressure is about 2.4 millimeters of mercury (mm Hg) higher for every 1 mmol/L increase of TC after taking into account age, sex, and study population (Lewington et al. 2007). In children and adolescents, having blood pressure levels in the 95th percentile or higher was associated with an increased likelihood of having abnormal levels of TC and non–HDL-C compared to those with an average blood pressure reading, independent of BMI (Margolis et al. 2014). Furthermore, there is a significant effect modification between systolic blood pressure and TC in the association with ischemic heart disease mortality; at higher levels of systolic blood pressure, the association between increased TC and ischemic heart disease mortality is stronger than at lower systolic blood pressure readings, and having greater systolic blood pressure is more detrimental at greater levels of TC versus lower TC levels (Lewington et al. 2007).

Combined Risk and Risk Scores

Because dyslipidemia along with other ASCVD risk factors and comorbidities can occur together, efforts have been made to quantify the risk of an ASCVD event on the basis of a risk score that considers multiple risk factors. Risk equations have been designed to calculate the 10-year risk of an event for an individual to help inform and identify those at highest risk in the clinical setting. One of the first gender-specific 10-year CVD risk equations developed was based on the Framingham Heart Study and considered age, diabetes status, smoking status, blood pressure medication use, TC, and HDL-C (D'Agostino et al. 2008). However, this risk estimator did not take into account racial/ethnic differences when estimating 10-year CVD risk (Goff et al. 2014). The Pooled-Cohort ASCVD risk equation not only takes into account all the same predictors as the Framingham risk calculator, but also has a different predictive equation for each gender and race (white and African American) subgroup (Goff et al. 2014). The calculator is available at http://my.americanheart.org/cvriskcalculator.

Although the Pooled-Cohort equations incorporate additional important risk factors compared to the Framingham risk calculator, there are still limitations to these equations. For example, traditional risk equations may underestimate risk in certain populations (e.g., those with HIV/AIDS; Krikke et al. 2016), and may or may not be applicable to diverse subgroup populations across the United States, such as heterogeneous Hispanic and Asian groups. Studies have continued to investigate the validity of these equations among diverse populations. Validation of the Pooled-Cohort 10-year ASCVD risk equation performed with a diverse U.S. adult population found that at increasing percentage of ASCVD risk, LDL-C levels slightly increased from mean of 115.9 mg/dL for those with ASCVD risk less than 5% to 118.4 mg/dL for ASCVD risk greater than or equal to 10% whereas HDL-C (59.5 to 49.7 mg/dL) and TC (197.2 to 194.6 mg/dL) levels decreased (Muntner et al. 2014). However, the Pooled-Cohort equations tend to overestimate risk, specifically for those adults with a Pooled-Cohort calculated 10-year ASCVD risk greater than or equal to 10% and among subgroups of Asian populations (Chia et al. 2014).

Population-Attributable Risk

Elevated blood cholesterol levels are estimated to be responsible for 2.6 million deaths globally each year (Alwan 2011) and for 18% of global cerebrovascular disease and 56% of global ischemic heart disease (Guilbert 2003). Depending on which abnormal lipid profile measures are present, 3% to 7.5% of incidence of CVD events are attributed to dyslipidemia (Andersson et al. 2014). However, population-attributable risk of dyslipidemia varies on the basis of populations with comorbidities or history of CVD (Vazquez-Benitez et al. 2015). Among diabetic adults with no CVD history, 20% of myocardial infarction and acute coronary syndrome, 14% of ischemic stroke, 4% of heart failure, and 13% of all CVD events were attributable to LDL-C greater than or equal to 100 mg/dL. Among diabetic adults with a CVD history, only 5% of myocardial infarction and acute coronary syndrome, 6% of ischemic stroke, and 3% of all CVD events were attributable to LDL-C greater than or equal to 100 mg/dL.

Evidence-Based Interventions

Prevention

For the prevention and management of dyslipidemia and its downstream complications, following a lifestyle that promotes cardiovascular health is essential. Lifestyle modifications are critical for improving lipid profile measures and reducing ASCVD risk. Interventions focusing on lifestyle modification that include dietary changes, physical activity, and participation in a comprehensive cardiovascular risk factor reduction program have resulted in significant decreases in all lipid profile measures, with a range of -8% to -13% over a 30-day period (Rankin et al. 2012). Longer lifestyle modification interventions, from 12 to 24 weeks, among obese children and adolescents have resulted in significant decreases in LDL-C, TGs, and TC while increasing HDL-C (Kelishadi et al. 2012; Ryder et al. 2013). Aside from a healthy lifestyle being associated with lower LDL-C, lower CVD risk, and higher HDL-C, consistency in following a healthy lifestyle for approximately 20 years beginning in young adulthood was associated with low CVD risk (Liu et al. 2012) and changes in subclinical atherosclerotic measures of CAC and carotid intima- media thickness (CIMT; Spring et al. 2014). Specifically, greater positive change in healthy lifestyle was associated with a smaller percent change in CAC and CIMT compared to the greatest negative change in healthy lifestyle being associated with the largest percent change in CAC and CIMT.

Because fatty streaks in arteries can be found during childhood and the presence of abnormal lipid levels increases the risk of developing atherosclerosis in the presence of fatty streaks, dyslipidemia is of concern among children and adolescents in the United States. During 2011 to 2014, more than 7% of children and adolescents (aged 6 to 19 years) had TC greater than or equal to 200 mg/dL, 13% had HDL-C less than 40 mg/dL, and 8% had non–HDL-C greater than or equal to 145 mg/dL (Nguyen et al. 2015). As a result, 21% of U.S. children and adolescents have at least one abnormal cholesterol measure. Triglycerides, LDL-C, and TC are positively associated and HDL-C is negatively associated with CIMT and early development of atherosclerosis in children and adolescents (Simsek et al. 2010). Measures associated with CVD morbidity and mortality in adulthood (Velagaleti et al. 2014; Zile et al. 2014), including CIMT (Pacifico et al. 2014), concentric left ventricular remodeling and left ventricular hypertrophy (Di Bonito et al. 2014), and cardiometabolic risk factors (Di Bonito et al. 2015), are associated with increasing TG-to-HDL-C ratio in children and adolescents. Therefore, it is important to check lipid profile measures and provide lifestyle modification assistance when necessary during childhood and young adulthood to reduce the burden of ASCVD later in life.

Screening

In the United States, it is recommended that all adults aged 20 years and older have a fasting lipid profile tested once every five years and more frequently for people at increased CVD risk (NCEP Adult Treatment Panel III 2002). Among U.S. adults aged 18 years and older, 76% were screened for high blood cholesterol in 2009 (CDC 2012). Although more than half of the people who had their cholesterol tested were screened because of a health care provider recommendation, differences exist between those who have and have not had their cholesterol tested. People who do not have their cholesterol tested are more likely to smoke, have sedentary behavior, have high alcohol consumption, and have low fruit intake (Filippidis et al. 2014). In addition, men were less likely, and older adults were more likely, to have ever had a cholesterol screening than their counterparts (Kenik et al. 2014). In women, the prevalence of cholesterol screening was higher for nonsmokers, non-Hispanic blacks, those having health insurance, and those who have seen a health care provider within the recommended screening period of five years (Robbins et al. 2011). Non-Hispanic blacks were more likely and Hispanics less likely to report having their cholesterol checked in the past five years compared to Asian/Pacific Islanders and American Indians (Liao et al. 2011).

Almost all disparities related to cholesterol screening among minority populations can be explained by SES, access to care factors, and language barriers (Kenik et al. 2014). Lower income, fewer years of education, and not having health insurance or a personal doctor were significant factors associated with never having a cholesterol screening. Nonetheless, insurance coverage and cholesterol screening have increased after the Patient Protection and Affordable Care Act because of increased access, utilization of medical care, and preventive screening coverage (Lau et al. 2014).

There are also disparities in the awareness of having dyslipidemia. Adults without a routine place of care, with no health insurance, aged younger than 40 years, or with low income are less likely to be aware of having a TC greater than or equal to 240 mg/dL compared to their counterparts (Nguyen et al. 2011; Fisher-Hoch et al. 2012). Awareness of having elevated LDL-C levels that meet eligibility for cholesterol-lowering medication is less likely among younger adults than older ones (Upadhyay et al. 2010). Adults with some college or more education are more likely to be aware of their elevated LDL-C condition than adults with a high-school education or less. In the United States, foreign-born adults are more likely to have undiagnosed elevated LDL-C levels than adults born in the United States (Zallman et al. 2013). Once age, gender, income, and education are taken into account, the main reason for the difference between foreign- and U.S.-born adults was having health insurance (Zallman et al. 2013).

For children and adolescents, universal screening is recommended at ages 9 to 11 years and 17 to 21 years (Expert Panel on Integrated Guidelines for Cardiovascular Health and Risk Reduction in Children and Adolescents, NHLBI 2011). Of children and adolescents, those more likely to be screened for cholesterol were at increasing age, greater BMI and blood pressure percentiles, and girls (Margolis et al. 2014). However, the proportion of children and adolescents aged 2 to 20 years having lipid testing has declined from 2002 to 2012 (Zachariah et al. 2015). The U.S. Preventive Services Task Force periodically updates U.S. recommendations for lipid screening and treatment and should be reviewed for the most up-to-date information (see http://www.uspreventiveservicestaskforce.org). In addition, the American Academy of Pediatrics and Bright Futures provides regular updates on screening guidelines for cholesterol, among other screening and health assessments (Committee on Practice and Ambulatory Medicine and Bright Futures Periodicity Schedule Workgroup 2016).

Treatment

Along with lifestyle modification, cholesterol-lowering medication may be recommended for some people with dyslipidemia or who are at increased risk for ASCVD. There is a variety of types of cholesterol-lowering medications including statins, bile acid sequestrants, fibrates, niacin, cholesterol-absorption inhibitors, omega-3 fatty acids, and combination medicines. Because the majority of evidence from randomized clinical trials demonstrates that the most efficient way to reduce ASCVD risk is through lowering LDL-C, and the type of cholesterol-lowering medication most effective in lowering LDL-C is statins (Stone et al. 2014), the majority of people on cholesterol-lowering medications ($\geq$ 80%) are using statins. Current guidelines on medication recommendations for blood cholesterol also focus on maintaining a healthy lifestyle while considering ASCVD risk and LDL-C levels (Table 14-3 and Table 14-4).

Cholesterol-lowering medication use has greatly increased in the past 20 to 30 years and is predominantly responsible for decreasing population levels in TC and LDL-C (Hulman et al. 2014). Because statins have a dose–response relationship with the reduction of LDL-C (Law et al. 2003), adults at highest ASCVD risk are recommended to take high-intensity statins rather than moderate-intensity statins, resulting in greater declines of LDL-C levels. On average, an LDL-C reduction of 1.0 mmol/L (38.7 mg/dL) attributable to statins tends to be associated with a 1.2 mmol/L (46.4 mg/dL) reduction in TC. Depending on

Table 14-3. 2013 American College of Cardiology/American Heart Association Guideline on the Treatment of Blood Cholesterol

Statin medication recommended for the following four groups:
1. Clinical ASCVD[a] established.
2. LDL-C levels ≥190 mg/dL.
3. Adults aged 40–75 years with diabetes and LDL-C levels 70–189 mg/dL.
4. Adults aged 40–75 years without diabetes having a 10-year Pooled-Cohort ASCVD risk score ≥7.5% and LDL-C levels 70–189 mg/dL.

Source: Data from Stone et al. (2014).

Note: ASCVD = atherosclerotic cardiovascular disease; LDL-C = low-density lipoprotein cholesterol.

[a]Acute coronary syndrome, history of myocardial infarction, stable and unstable angina, coronary or other arterial revascularization, stroke, transient ischemic attack, or peripheral arterial disease.

statin type and dosage, statins can reduce LDL-C anywhere from 10% to 58%, and because high-intensity statins are recommended for high-risk adults who tend to be at the high end of the population LDL-C distribution, cholesterol-lowering medication has played a role in the population-level decrease in LDL-C and TC. Furthermore, the percentage reduction is independent of the pretreatment LDL-C concentration level. However, as with other chronic disease medications, adherence and persistence of cholesterol-lowering medication regimens can be a challenge given the side effects experienced by some individuals (Ho et al. 2009; Maningat et al. 2013).

Although statins on average increase HDL-C by about 0.07 mmol/L (2.7 mg/dL), the increase tends to be constant with no difference on the basis of dosage. Although adults on cholesterol-lowering medication tend to have lower TC-to-HDL-C ratios than those not on medication, HDL-C levels tend to be lower among those on cholesterol-lowering medication versus those not on medication even after accounting for the slight increase in HDL-C associated with statins (Jenkins and Ofstedal 2014).

Examples of Evidence-Based Interventions

With significant evidence existing for the benefits of lifestyle modifications and statin therapy on cholesterol management and control (Stone et al. 2014), and the steadily increasing use of cholesterol-lowering medication in the United States (Gu et al. 2014), the new eligibility determinations in the latest guidelines are likely going to continue to increase statin use. Adherence to chronic disease

Table 14-4. Recommended Treatment among Those with Diabetes

Additional Risk Factors	Lifestyle Modification[a]	Statin Recommended
None and aged < 40 years	Yes	No
TGs ≥ 150 mg/dL or HDL-C < 40 mg/dL (men) or HDL-C < 50 mg/dL (women)	Yes, intensify	No
None and aged ≥ 40 years	Yes	Yes
Acute coronary syndrome and LDL > 50 mg/dL and aged ≥ 40 years	Yes	Yes
Acute coronary syndrome and aged > 75 years	Yes	Yes
ASCVD risk factors[b]	Yes	Yes
History of ASCVD	Yes	Yes

Source: Data from ADA (2016).

Note: ASCVD = atherosclerotic cardiovascular disease; HDL-C = high-density lipoprotein cholesterol; LDL-C = low-density lipoprotein cholesterol; TGs = triglycerides.

[a]Lifestyle modification to manage or improve lipid profile includes maintaining a healthy weight; reducing saturated fat, trans fat, and cholesterol intake; increasing omega-3 fatty acids, fiber, and fruit and vegetable intake; and increasing physical activity.

[b]ASCVD risk factors: LDL ≥ 100 mg/dL, high blood pressure, smoking, overweight or obese, and family history of premature ASCVD.

medications is a challenge (Viswanathan et al. 2012). Efforts to promote adherence to cholesterol-lowering medications include interventions and supports for the patient, health professionals, and the health care system (Maningat et al. 2013).

Several historic intervention programs, such as the Minnesota Heart Health Program (Luepker et al. 1994), Stanford Five-City Project (Fortmann et al. 1995), Pawtucket Heart Health Program (Carleton et al. 1995), the North Karelia Project (Puska 2002), and the Franklin County, Maine, programs (Record et al. 2015) have provided considerable evidence for a wide range of interventions that promote cardiovascular health through diverse and persistent community programs and complementary clinical efforts. A guide for the promotion of cardiovascular health has been updated by the American Heart Association (Pearson et al. 2013) and is an excellent resource for audiences ranging from individuals to policymakers. The Centers for Disease Control and Prevention published a strategy and vision document that outlines the prevention and management of chronic disease through enhanced surveillance, environmental approaches, health system interventions, and community–clinical linkages (Bauer et al. 2014). Diverse use of evidence-based strategies are needed to have an impact on chronic disease, including dyslipidemia, ranging from individual-to population-level interventions (Frieden 2010), and selections of appropriate strategies are dependent upon access, reach, and resources.

Areas of Future Research

Dyslipidemia is a well-known risk factor for CVD, yet recent and impending changes in guidelines, screening, and treatment provide many opportunities for epidemiologic and implementation research. For example, recent updates to guidelines for the management of cholesterol have migrated away from target-based treatment (e.g., LDL-C < 100 mg/dL) while incorporating ASCVD risk scores, highlighting the need for health systems to be able to accurately and efficiently assess ASCVD risk during clinic visits, and focusing on the use of lifestyle modifications and statin therapy on those eligible for treatment (Stone et al. 2014). Recent research has found the gap between those eligible and those currently taking medications to be significant (Mercado et al. 2015), emphasizing the need to support and assess the uptake of guidelines in clinical practice. Although screening estimates for cholesterol are relatively high for the general population, disparities in screening are evident (CDC 2012). Efforts to promote improved screening and management through all available avenues (e.g., community health workers, team-based care, patient-centered care, and shared decision-making) should be explored. Primary prevention of ASCVD with statin therapy is also being considered by the U.S. Preventive Services Task Force, and the expanded use of cholesterol-lowering therapy among varied populations warrants additional research (USPSTF 2015).

The prevention, screening, and management of dyslipidemia are influenced by a multitude of factors, from individual-level dietary choices to national guidelines and systems of medical care. There are many intervention points for public health practitioners and selection of areas to target is dependent upon the setting, population, and program. The use of evidence-based recommendations to maximize impact is encouraged.

Acknowledgment

The findings and conclusions in this chapter are those of the authors and do not necessarily represent the official position of the Centers for Disease Control and Prevention.

Resources

2013 American College of Cardiology/American Heart Association Guideline on the Treatment of Blood Cholesterol, http://www.ncbi.nlm.nih.gov/pubmed/24222016

American Heart Association, Heart disease and stroke statistics—2016 update, http://www.ncbi.nlm.nih.gov/pubmed/26673558

Centers for Disease Control and Prevention, Cholesterol, http://www.cdc.gov/cholesterol

National Institutes of Health, National Heart, Lung, and Blood Institute, http://www.nhlbi.nih.gov/health/health-topics/topics/hbc

Guide to Community Preventive Services, Cardiovascular disease prevention and control: interventions engaging community health workers, http://www.thecommunityguide.org/cvd/CHW.html

US Department of Health and Human Services, Healthy People 2020, http://www.healthypeople.gov

US Department of Health and Human Services, Million Hearts Initiative, http://millionhearts.hhs.gov

US Department of Health and Human Services, US Department of Agriculture, *US Dietary Guidelines for Americans 2015–2020, 8th Edition,* http://health.gov/dietaryguidelines/2015/guidelines

US Preventive Services Task Force, Cholesterol screening and treatment recommendations, http://www.uspreventiveservicestaskforce.org

References

Ali O, Cerjak D, Kent JW Jr, James R, Blangero J, Zhang Y. Obesity, central adiposity and cardiometabolic risk factors in children and adolescents: a family-based study. *Pediatr Obes.* 2014;9(3):e58–e62.

Altenburg TM, Lakerveld J, Bot SD, Nijpels G, Chinapaw MJ. The prospective relationship between sedentary time and cardiometabolic health in adults at increased cardiometabolic risk—the Hoorn Prevention Study. *Int J Behav Nutr Phys Act.* 2014;11:90.

Alwan A. *Global Status Report on Noncommunicable Diseases 2010.* Geneva, Switzerland: World Health Organization; 2011.

American Diabetes Association (ADA). *Standards of Medical Care in Diabetes—2016.* 2016;39(suppl 1). Available at: http://care.diabetesjournals.org/content/suppl/2015/12/21/39.Supplement_1.DC2/2016-Standards-of-Care.pdf. Accessed August 25, 2016.

Anagnostis P, Stevenson JC, Crook D, Johnston DG, Godsland IF. Effects of menopause, gender and age on lipids and high-density lipoprotein cholesterol subfractions. *Maturitas.* 2015;81(1):62–68.

Andersson C, Lyass A, Vasan RS, Massaro JM, D'Agostino RB, Robins SJ. Long-term risk of cardiovascular events across a spectrum of adverse major plasma lipid combinations in the Framingham Heart Study. *Am Heart J.* 2014;168(6):878–883.e1.

Aoki Y, Yoon SS, Chong Y, Carroll MD. Hypertension, abnormal cholesterol, and high body mass index among non-Hispanic Asian adults: United States, 2011–2012. *NCHS Data Brief.* 2014;(140):1–8.

Arguelles W, Llabre MM, Penedo FJ, et al. Relationship of change in traditional cardiometabolic risk factors to change in coronary artery calcification among individuals with detectable subclinical atherosclerosis: the Multi-Ethnic Study of Atherosclerosis. *Int J Cardiol.* 2014;174(1):51–56.

Austin GL, Ogden LG, Hill JO. Trends in carbohydrate, fat, and protein intakes and association with energy intake in normal-weight, overweight, and obese individuals: 1971–2006. *Am J Clin Nutr.* 2011;93(4):836–843.

Bauer UE, Briss PA, Goodman RA, Bowman BA. Prevention of chronic disease in the 21st century: elimination of the leading preventable causes of premature death and disability in the USA. *Lancet.* 2014;384(9937):45–52.

Benn M, Watts GF, Tybjaerg-Hansen A, Nordestgaard BG. Familial hypercholesterolemia in the Danish general population: prevalence, coronary artery disease, and cholesterol-lowering medication. *J Clin Endocrinol Metab.* 2012;97(11):3956–3964.

Bennasar-Veny M, Lopez-Gonzalez AA, Tauler P, et al. Body adiposity index and cardiovascular health risk factors in Caucasians: a comparison with the body mass index and others. *PLoS One.* 2013;8(5):e63999.

Bild DE, Detrano R, Peterson D, et al. Ethnic differences in coronary calcification: the Multi-Ethnic Study of Atherosclerosis (MESA). *Circulation.* 2005;111(10):1313–1320.

Blekkenhorst LC, Prince RL, Hodgson JM, et al. Dietary saturated fat intake and atherosclerotic vascular disease mortality in elderly women: a prospective cohort study. *Am J Clin Nutr.* 2015;101(6):1263–1268.

Bouhairie VE, Goldberg AC. Familial hypercholesterolemia. *Endocrinol Metab Clin North Am.* 2016;45(1):1–16.

Budoff MJ, Nasir K, McClelland RL, et al. Coronary calcium predicts events better with absolute calcium scores than age-sex-race/ethnicity percentiles: MESA (Multi-Ethnic Study of Atherosclerosis). *J Am Coll Cardiol.* 2009;53(4):345–352.

Camhi SM, Katzmarzyk PT, Broyles S, et al. Association of metabolic risk with longitudinal physical activity and fitness: Coronary Artery Risk Development in Young Adults (CARDIA). *Metab Syndr Relat Disord.* 2013;11(3):195–204.

Carleton RA, Lasater TM, Assaf AR, Feldman HA, McKinlay S. The Pawtucket Heart Health Program: community changes in cardiovascular risk factors and projected disease risk. *Am J Public Health.* 1995;85(6):777–785.

Carroll MD, Fryar CD, Kit BK. Total and high-density lipoprotein cholesterol in adults: United States, 2011–2014. *NCHS Data Brief.* 2015;(226):1–8.

Carroll MD, Kit BK, Lacher DA, Shero ST, Mussolino ME. Trends in lipids and lipoproteins in US adults, 1988–2010. *JAMA.* 2012;308(15):1545–1554.

Centers for Disease Control and Prevention (CDC). Prevalence of cholesterol screening and high blood cholesterol among adults—United States, 2005, 2007, and 2009. *MMWR Morb Mortal Wkly Rep.* 2012;61(35):697–702.

Chia YC, Lim HM, Ching SM. Validation of the pooled cohort risk score in an Asian population—a retrospective cohort study. *BMC Cardiovasc Disord.* 2014;14:163.

Cliff DP, Okely AD, Burrows TL, et al. Objectively measured sedentary behavior, physical activity, and plasma lipids in overweight and obese children. *Obesity (Silver Spring).* 2013;21(2):382–385.

Cohen JD, Cziraky MJ, Cai Q, et al. 30-year trends in serum lipids among United States adults: results from the National Health and Nutrition Examination Surveys II, III, and 1999–2006. *Am J Cardiol.* 2010;106(7):969–975.

Committee on Practice and Ambulatory Medicine and Bright Futures Periodicity Schedule Workgroup. 2016 recommendations for preventive pediatric health care. *Pediatrics.* 2016;137(1):1–3.

Criqui MH, Denenberg JO, Ix JH, et al. Calcium density of coronary artery plaque and risk of incident cardiovascular events. *JAMA.* 2014;311(3):271–278.

Cziraky MJ, Thomas T. Attainment of combined optimal lipid values: a paradigm shift in the management of dyslipidemia. *Clin Lipidol.* 2010;5(4):527–541.

D'Agostino RB, Vasan RS, Pencina MJ, et al. General cardiovascular risk profile for use in primary care: the Framingham Heart Study. *Circulation.* 2008;117(6):743–753.

Di Bonito P, Moio N, Sibilio G, et al. Cardiometabolic phenotype in children with obesity. *J Pediatr.* 2014;165(6):1184–1189.

Di Bonito P, Valerio G, Grugni G, et al. Comparison of non-HDL-cholesterol versus triglycerides-to-HDL-cholesterol ratio in relation to cardiometabolic risk factors and preclinical organ damage in overweight/obese children: the CARITALY study. *Nutr Metab Cardiovasc Dis.* 2015;25(5):489–494.

Eliasson B, Cederholm J, Eeg-Olofsson K, et al. Clinical usefulness of different lipid measures for prediction of coronary heart disease in type 2 diabetes: a report from the Swedish National Diabetes Register. *Diabetes Care.* 2011;34(9):2095–2100.

Eliasson B, Gudbjornsdottir S, Zethelius B, Eeg-Olofsson K, Cederholm J; National Diabetes Register (NDR). LDL-cholesterol versus non-HDL-to-HDL-cholesterol ratio and risk for coronary heart disease in type 2 diabetes. *Eur J Prev Cardiol.* 2014;21(11): 1420–1428.

Estruch R, Ros E, Salas-Salvado J, et al. Primary prevention of cardiovascular disease with a Mediterranean diet. *N Engl J Med.* 2013;368(14):1279–1290.

Everage NJ, Linkletter CD, Gjelsvik A, McGarvey ST, Loucks EB. Social and behavioral risk marker clustering associated with biological risk factors for coronary heart disease: NHANES 2001–2004. *Biomed Res Int.* 2014;2014:389853.

Expert Panel on Integrated Guidelines for Cardiovascular Health and Risk Reduction in Children and Adolescents; National Heart, Lung, and Blood Institute (NHLBI). Expert Panel on Integrated Guidelines for Cardiovascular Health and Risk Reduction in Children and Adolescents: summary report. *Pediatrics.* 2011;128(suppl 5):S213–S256.

Filippidis FT, Gerovasili V, Majeed A. Association between cardiovascular risk factors and measurements of blood pressure and cholesterol in 27 European countries in 2009. *Prev Med.* 2014;67:71–74.

Fisher-Hoch SP, Vatcheva KP, Laing ST, et al. Missed opportunities for diagnosis and treatment of diabetes, hypertension, and hypercholesterolemia in a Mexican American population, Cameron County Hispanic Cohort, 2003–2008. *Prev Chronic Dis.* 2012;9: 110298.

Ford ES, Capewell S. Trends in total and low-density lipoprotein cholesterol among US adults: contributions of changes in dietary fat intake and use of cholesterol-lowering medications. *PLoS One.* 2013;8(5):e65228.

Fortmann SP, Flora JA, Winkleby MA, Schooler C, Taylor CB, Farquhar JW. Community intervention trials: reflections on the Stanford Five-City Project Experience. *Am J Epidemiol.* 1995;142(6):576–586.

Frank AT, Zhao B, Jose PO, Azar KM, Fortmann SP, Palaniappan LP. Racial/ethnic differences in dyslipidemia patterns. *Circulation.* 2014;129(5):570–579.

Frieden TR. A framework for public health action: the Health Impact Pyramid. *Am J Public Health.* 2010;100(4):590–595.

Friedewald WT, Levy RI, Fredrickson DS. Estimation of the concentration of low-density lipoprotein cholesterol in plasma, without use of the preparative ultracentrifuge. *Clin Chem.* 1972;18(6):499–502.

Fukuyama N, Homma K, Wakana N, et al. Validation of the Friedewald equation for evaluation of plasma LDL-cholesterol. *J Clin Biochem Nutr.* 2008;43(1):1–5.

Ghandehari H, Kamal-Bahl S, Wong ND. Prevalence and extent of dyslipidemia and recommended lipid levels in US adults with and without cardiovascular comorbidities: the National Health and Nutrition Examination Survey 2003–2004. *Am Heart J.* 2008; 156(1):112–119.

Gijsberts CM, Groenewegen KA, Hoefer IE, et al. Race/ethnic differences in the associations of the Framingham risk factors with carotid IMT and cardiovascular events. *PLoS One.* 2015;10(7):e0132321.

Goff LM, Cowland DE, Hooper L, Frost GS. Low glycaemic index diets and blood lipids: a systematic review and meta-analysis of randomised controlled trials. *Nutr Metab Cardiovasc Dis.* 2013;23(1):1–10.

Goff DC Jr, Lloyd-Jones DM, Bennett G, et al. 2013 ACC/AHA guideline on the assessment of cardiovascular risk: a report of the American College of Cardiology/American Heart Association Task Force on Practice Guidelines. *J Am Coll Cardiol.* 2014;63(25 pt B): 2935–2959.

Goldberg AC, Hopkins PN, Toth PP, et al. Familial hypercholesterolemia: screening, diagnosis and management of pediatric and adult patients: clinical guidance from the National Lipid Association Expert Panel on Familial Hypercholesterolemia. *J Clin Lipidol.* 2011;5(3 suppl):S1–S8.

Greenland P, LaBree L, Azen SP, Doherty TM, Detrano RC. Coronary artery calcium score combined with Framingham score for risk prediction in asymptomatic individuals. *JAMA.* 2004;291(2):210–215.

Gu Q, Paulose-Ram R, Burt VL, Kit BK. Prescription cholesterol-lowering medication use in adults aged 40 and over: United States, 2003–2012. *NCHS Data Brief.* 2014; (177):1–8.

Guilbert JJ. The World Health Report 2002—reducing risks, promoting healthy life. *Educ Health (Abingdon).* 2003;16(2):230.

Hamidi A, Fakhrzadeh H, Moayyeri A, et al. Obesity and associated cardiovascular risk factors in Iranian children: a cross-sectional study. *Pediatr Int.* 2006;48(6):566–571.

Hatmi ZN, Mahdavi-Mazdeh M, Hashemi-Nazari SS, Hajighasemi E, Nozari B, Mahdavi A. Trend of lipid ratios associated with well known risk factors of coronary artery disease in different age: a population based study of 31,999 healthy individuals. *Int J Cardiol.* 2011;151(3):328–332.

Ho PM, Bryson CL, Rumsfeld JS. Medication adherence: its importance in cardiovascular outcomes. *Circulation.* 2009;119(23):3028–3035.

Hooper L, Martin N, Abdelhamid A, Davey Smith G. Reduction in saturated fat intake for cardiovascular disease. *Cochrane Database Syst Rev.* 2015;(6):CD011737.

Hopkins PN, Toth PP, Ballantyne CM, Rader DJ. Familial hypercholesterolemias: prevalence, genetics, diagnosis and screening recommendations from the National Lipid Association Expert Panel on Familial Hypercholesterolemia. *J Clin Lipidol.* 2011;5(3 suppl):S9–S17.

Hsia SH, Desnoyers ML, Lee ML. Differences in cholesterol management among states in relation to health insurance and race/ethnicity across the United States. *J Clin Lipidol.* 2013;7(6):675–682.

Hu B, Liu XY, Zheng Y, et al. High physical activity is associated with an improved lipid profile and resting heart rate among healthy middle-aged Chinese people. *Biomed Environ Sci.* 2015;28(4):263–271.

Hulman A, Tabak AG, Nyari TA, et al. Effect of secular trends on age-related trajectories of cardiovascular risk factors: the Whitehall II longitudinal study 1985–2009. *Int J Epidemiol.* 2014;43(3):866–877.

Iggman D, Rosqvist F, Larsson A, et al. Role of dietary fats in modulating cardiometabolic risk during moderate weight gain: a randomized double-blind overfeeding trial (LIPOGAIN study). *J Am Heart Assoc.* 2014;3(5):e001095.

Isomaa B, Almgren P, Tuomi T, et al. Cardiovascular morbidity and mortality associated with the metabolic syndrome. *Diabetes Care.* 2001;24(4):683–689.

Jenkins KR, Ofstedal MB. The association between socioeconomic status and cardiovascular risk factors among middle-aged and older men and women. *Women Health.* 2014; 54(1):15–34.

Kant AK, Graubard BI. Race–ethnic, family income, and education differentials in nutritional and lipid biomarkers in US children and adolescents: NHANES 2003–2006. *Am J Clin Nutr.* 2012;96(3):601–612.

Kelishadi R, Malekahmadi M, Hashemipour M, et al. Can a trial of motivational lifestyle counseling be effective for controlling childhood obesity and the associated cardiometabolic risk factors? *Pediatr Neonatol.* 2012;53(2):90–97.

Kenik J, Jean-Jacques M, Feinglass J. Explaining racial and ethnic disparities in cholesterol screening. *Prev Med.* 2014;65:65–69.

Kim SW, Jee JH, Kim HJ, et al. Non-HDL-cholesterol/HDL-cholesterol is a better predictor of metabolic syndrome and insulin resistance than apolipoprotein B/apolipoprotein A1. *Int J Cardiol.* 2013;168(3):2678–2683.

Kit BK, Carroll MD, Lacher DA, Sorlie PD, DeJesus JM, Ogden C. Trends in serum lipids among US youths aged 6 to 19 years, 1988–2010. *JAMA*. 2012;308(6):591–600.

Kit BK, Kuklina E, Carroll MD, Ostchega Y, Freedman DS, Ogden CL. Prevalence of and trends in dyslipidemia and blood pressure among US children and adolescents, 1999–2012. *JAMA Pediatr*. 2015;169(3):272–279.

Kolovou GD, Anagnostopoulou KK, Damaskos DS, et al. Gender differences in the lipid profile of dyslipidemic subjects. *Eur J Intern Med*. 2009;20(2):145–151.

Krikke M, Hoogeveen RC, Hoepelman A, Visseren F, Arends JE. Cardiovascular risk prediction in HIV-infected patients: comparing the Framingham, atherosclerotic cardiovascular disease risk score (ASCVD), Systematic Coronary Risk Evaluation for the Netherlands (SCORE-NL) and Data Collection on Adverse Events of Anti-HIV Drugs (D:A:D) risk prediction models. *HIV Med*. 2016;17(4):289–297.

Kronmal RA, McClelland RL, Detrano R, et al. Risk factors for the progression of coronary artery calcification in asymptomatic subjects: results from the Multi-Ethnic Study of Atherosclerosis (MESA). *Circulation*. 2007;115(21):2722–2730.

Lambert M, Delvin EE, Levy E, et al. Prevalence of cardiometabolic risk factors by weight status in a population-based sample of Quebec children and adolescents. *Can J Cardiol*. 2008;24(7):575–583.

Larsson SC, Virtamo J, Wolk A. Dietary fats and dietary cholesterol and risk of stroke in women. *Atherosclerosis*. 2012;221(1):282–286.

Lau JS, Adams SH, Park MJ, Boscardin WJ, Irwin CE Jr. Improvement in preventive care of young adults after the affordable care act: the Affordable Care Act is helping. *JAMA Pediatr*. 2014;168(12):1101–1106.

Law MR, Wald NJ, Rudnicka AR. Quantifying effect of statins on low density lipoprotein cholesterol, ischaemic heart disease, and stroke: systematic review and meta-analysis. *BMJ*. 2003;326(7404):1423.

Lewington S, Whitlock G, Clarke R, et al. Blood cholesterol and vascular mortality by age, sex, and blood pressure: a meta-analysis of individual data from 61 prospective studies with 55,000 vascular deaths. *Lancet*. 2007;370(9602):1829–1839.

Liao Y, Bang D, Cosgrove S, et al. Surveillance of health status in minority communities—Racial and Ethnic Approaches to Community Health Across the US (REACH US) Risk Factor Survey, United States, 2009. *MMWR Surveill Summ*. 2011;60(6):1–44.

Lima MC, Romaldini CC, Romaldini JH. Frequency of obesity and related risk factors among school children and adolescents in a low-income community. A cross-sectional study. *Sao Paulo Med J*. 2015;133(2):125–130.

Liu K, Daviglus ML, Loria CM, et al. Healthy lifestyle through young adulthood and the presence of low cardiovascular disease risk profile in middle age: the Coronary Artery Risk Development in (Young) Adults (CARDIA) study. *Circulation*. 2012;125(8): 996–1004.

Luepker RV, Murray DM, Jacobs DR Jr, et al. Community education for cardiovascular disease prevention: risk factor changes in the Minnesota Heart Health Program. *Am J Public Health*. 1994;84(9):1383–1393.

Maningat P, Gordon BR, Breslow JL. How do we improve patient compliance and adherence to long-term statin therapy? *Curr Atheroscler Rep*. 2013;15(1):291.

Mansoor N, Vinknes KJ, Veierod MB, Retterstol K. Effects of low-carbohydrate diets v. low-fat diets on body weight and cardiovascular risk factors: a meta-analysis of randomised controlled trials. *Br J Nutr*. 2016;115(3):466–479.

Margolis KL, Greenspan LC, Trower NK, et al. Lipid screening in children and adolescents in community practice: 2007 to 2010. *Circ Cardiovasc Qual Outcomes*. 2014;7(5): 718–726.

Martin SS, Blaha MJ, Blankstein R, et al. Dyslipidemia, coronary artery calcium, and incident atherosclerotic cardiovascular disease: implications for statin therapy from the Multi-Ethnic Study of Atherosclerosis. *Circulation*. 2014;129(1):77–86.

Martinez-Gonzalez MA, Bes-Rastrollo M. Dietary patterns, Mediterranean diet, and cardiovascular disease. *Curr Opin Lipidol*. 2014;25(1):20–26.

Martinez-Vizcaino V, Sanchez-Lopez M, Notario-Pacheco B, et al. Gender differences on effectiveness of a school-based physical activity intervention for reducing cardiometabolic risk: a cluster randomized trial. *Int J Behav Nutr Phys Act*. 2014;11:154.

Melmer A, Lamina C, Tschoner A, et al. Body adiposity index and other indexes of body composition in the SAPHIR study: association with cardiovascular risk factors. *Obesity (Silver Spring)*. 2013;21(4):775–781.

Mercado C, DeSimone AK, Odom E, Gillespie C, Ayala C, Loustalot F. Prevalence of cholesterol treatment eligibility and medication use among adults—United States, 2005–2012. *MMWR Morb Mortal Wkly Rep*. 2015;64(47):1305–1311.

Mosca I, Bhuachalla BN, Kenny RA. Explaining significant differences in subjective and objective measures of cardiovascular health: evidence for the socioeconomic gradient in a population-based study. *BMC Cardiovasc Disord*. 2013;13:64.

Mozaffarian D, Benjamin EJ, Go AS, et al. Heart disease and stroke statistics—2016 update: a report from the American Heart Association. *Circulation*. 2016;133(4):e38–e60.

Muntner P, Colantonio LD, Cushman M, et al. Validation of the atherosclerotic cardiovascular disease Pooled Cohort risk equations. *JAMA*. 2014;311(14):1406–1415.

Nakashima Y, Fujii H, Sumiyoshi S, Wight TN, Sueishi K. Early human atherosclerosis: accumulation of lipid and proteoglycans in intimal thickenings followed by macrophage infiltration. *Arterioscler Thromb Vasc Biol.* 2007;27(5):1159–1165.

National Cholesterol Education Program (NCEP) Expert Panel on Detection, Evaluation, and Treatment of High Blood Cholesterol in Adults (Adult Treatment Panel III). Third Report of the National Cholesterol Education Program (NCEP) Expert Panel on Detection, Evaluation, and Treatment of High Blood Cholesterol in Adults (Adult Treatment Panel III) final report. *Circulation.* 2002;106(25):3143–3421.

Nguyen D, Kit B, Carroll M. Abnormal cholesterol among children and adolescents in the United States, 2011–2014. *NCHS Data Brief.* 2015;(228):1–8.

Nguyen QC, Waddell EN, Thomas JC, Huston SL, Kerker BD, Gwynn RC. Awareness, treatment, and control of hypertension and hypercholesterolemia among insured residents of New York City, 2004. *Prev Chronic Dis.* 2011;8(5):A109.

Nichols GA, Joshua-Gotlib S, Parasuraman S. Independent contribution of A1C, systolic blood pressure, and LDL cholesterol control to risk of cardiovascular disease hospitalizations in type 2 diabetes: an observational cohort study. *J Gen Intern Med.* 2013;28(5):691–697.

Nordestgaard BG, Chapman MJ, Humphries SE, et al. Familial hypercholesterolaemia is underdiagnosed and undertreated in the general population: guidance for clinicians to prevent coronary heart disease: consensus statement of the European Atherosclerosis Society. *Eur Heart J.* 2013;34(45):3478a–3490a.

Nordmann AJ, Nordmann A, Briel M, et al. Effects of low-carbohydrate vs low-fat diets on weight loss and cardiovascular risk factors: a meta-analysis of randomized controlled trials. *Arch Intern Med.* 2006;166(3):285–293.

Ogawa K, Tanaka T, Nagoshi T, et al. Increase in the oxidised low-density lipoprotein level by smoking and the possible inhibitory effect of statin therapy in patients with cardiovascular disease: a retrospective study. *BMJ Open.* 2015;5(1):e005455.

Otsuka F, Kramer MC, Woudstra P, et al. Natural progression of atherosclerosis from pathologic intimal thickening to late fibroatheroma in human coronary arteries: a pathology study. *Atherosclerosis.* 2015;241(2):772–782.

Oya J, Vistisen D, Christensen DL, et al. Geographic differences in the associations between impaired glucose regulation and cardiovascular risk factors among young adults. *Diabetic Med.* 2015;32(4):497–504.

Pacifico L, Bonci E, Andreoli G, et al. Association of serum triglyceride-to-HDL cholesterol ratio with carotid artery intima-media thickness, insulin resistance and nonalcoholic fatty liver disease in children and adolescents. *Nutr Metab Cardiovasc Dis.* 2014;24(7): 737–743.

Palacios C, Perez CM, Guzman M, Ortiz AP, Ayala A, Suarez E. Association between adiposity indices and cardiometabolic risk factors among adults living in Puerto Rico. *Public Health Nutr.* 2011;14(10):1714–1723.

Pearson TA, Palaniappan LP, Artinian NT, et al. American Heart Association Guide for Improving Cardiovascular Health at the Community Level, 2013 update: a scientific statement for public health practitioners, healthcare providers, and health policy makers. *Circulation.* 2013;127(16):1730–1753.

Pereira A, Guedes AD, Verreschi IT, Santos RD, Martinez TL. Obesity and its association with other cardiovascular risk factors in school children in Itapetininga, Brazil. *Arq Bras Cardiol.* 2009;93(3):253–260.

Polonsky TS, McClelland RL, Jorgensen NW, et al. Coronary artery calcium score and risk classification for coronary heart disease prediction. *JAMA.* 2010;303(16):1610–1616.

Puska P. Successful prevention of non-communicable diseases: 25 year experiences with North Karelia Project in Finland. *Public Health Med.* 2002;4(1):5–7.

Raal FJ, Santos RD. Homozygous familial hypercholesterolemia: current perspectives on diagnosis and treatment. *Atherosclerosis.* 2012;223(2):262–268.

Rajaie S, Azadbakht L, Khazaei M, Sherbafchi M, Esmaillzadeh A. Moderate replacement of carbohydrates by dietary fats affects features of metabolic syndrome: a randomized crossover clinical trial. *Nutrition.* 2014;30(1):61–68.

Rangul V, Bauman A, Holmen TL, Midthjell K. Is physical activity maintenance from adolescence to young adulthood associated with reduced CVD risk factors, improved mental health and satisfaction with life: the HUNT Study, Norway. *Int J Behav Nutr Phys Act.* 2012;9:144.

Rankin P, Morton DP, Diehl H, Gobble J, Morey P, Chang E. Effectiveness of a volunteer-delivered lifestyle modification program for reducing cardiovascular disease risk factors. *Am J Cardiol.* 2012;109(1):82–86.

Rankinen T, Sarzynski MA, Ghosh S, Bouchard C. Are there genetic paths common to obesity, cardiovascular disease outcomes, and cardiovascular risk factors? *Circ Res.* 2015;116(5):909–922.

Record NB, Onion DK, Prior RE, et al. Community-wide cardiovascular disease prevention programs and health outcomes in a rural county, 1970–2010. *JAMA.* 2015; 313(2):147–155.

Robbins CL, Dietz PM, Bombard JM, Gibbs F, Ko JY, Valderrama AL. Blood pressure and cholesterol screening prevalence among US women of reproductive age opportunities to improve screening. *Am J Prev Med.* 2011;41(6):588–595.

Robinson JG, Goldberg AC. Treatment of adults with familial hypercholesterolemia and evidence for treatment: recommendations from the National Lipid Association Expert Panel on Familial Hypercholesterolemia. *J Clin Lipidol.* 2011;5(3 suppl):S18–S29.

Rodriguez CJ, Daviglus ML, Swett K, et al. Dyslipidemia patterns among Hispanics/Latinos of diverse background in the United States. *Am J Med.* 2014;127(12):1186–1194.e1.

Rosito GA, Massaro JM, Hoffmann U, et al. Pericardial fat, visceral abdominal fat, cardiovascular disease risk factors, and vascular calcification in a community-based sample: the Framingham Heart Study. *Circulation.* 2008;117(5):605–613.

Ryder JR, Vega-Lopez S, Ortega R, Konopken Y, Shaibi GQ. Lifestyle intervention improves lipoprotein particle size and distribution without weight loss in obese Latino adolescents. *Pediatr Obes.* 2013;8(5):e59–e63.

Schwingshackl L, Hoffmann G. Comparison of effects of long-term low-fat vs high-fat diets on blood lipid levels in overweight or obese patients: a systematic review and meta-analysis. *J Acad Nutr Diet.* 2013;113(12):1640–1661.

Shimomura T, Wakabayashi I. Inverse associations between light-to-moderate alcohol intake and lipid-related indices in patients with diabetes. *Cardiovasc Diabetol.* 2013; 12:104.

Shohaimi S, Boekholdt MS, Luben R, Wareham NJ, Khaw KT. Distribution of lipid parameters according to different socio-economic indicators—the EPIC-Norfolk prospective population study. *BMC Public Health.* 2014;14:782.

Simsek E, Balta H, Balta Z, Dallar Y. Childhood obesity-related cardiovascular risk factors and carotid intima-media thickness. *Turk J Pediatr.* 2010;52(6):602–611.

Sjouke B, Kusters DM, Kindt I, et al. Homozygous autosomal dominant hypercholesterolaemia in the Netherlands: prevalence, genotype–phenotype relationship, and clinical outcome. *Eur Heart J.* 2015;36(9):560–565.

Slagter SN, van Vliet-Ostaptchouk JV, Vonk JM, et al. Associations between smoking, components of metabolic syndrome and lipoprotein particle size. *BMC Med.* 2013;11:195.

Slagter SN, van Vliet-Ostaptchouk JV, Vonk JM, et al. Combined effects of smoking and alcohol on metabolic syndrome: the LifeLines cohort study. *PLoS One.* 2014;9(4):e96406.

Sone H, Tanaka S, Tanaka S, et al. Comparison of various lipid variables as predictors of coronary heart disease in Japanese men and women with type 2 diabetes: subanalysis of the Japan Diabetes Complications Study. *Diabetes Care.* 2012;35(5):1150–1157.

Spring B, Moller AC, Colangelo LA, et al. Healthy lifestyle change and subclinical atherosclerosis in young adults: Coronary Artery Risk Development in Young Adults (CARDIA) study. *Circulation.* 2014;130(1):10–17.

Steffen LM, Van Horn L, Daviglus ML, et al. A modified Mediterranean diet score is associated with a lower risk of incident metabolic syndrome over 25 years among young adults: the CARDIA (Coronary Artery Risk Development in Young Adults) study. *Br J Nutr.* 2014;112(10):1654–1661.

Stevenson JC, Crook D, Godsland IF. Influence of age and menopause on serum lipids and lipoproteins in healthy women. *Atherosclerosis.* 1993;98(1):83–90.

Stone NJ, Robinson JG, Lichtenstein AH, et al. 2013 ACC/AHA guideline on the treatment of blood cholesterol to reduce atherosclerotic cardiovascular risk in adults: a report of the American College of Cardiology/American Heart Association Task Force on Practice Guidelines. *Circulation.* 2014;129(25 suppl 2):S1–S45.

Sumner AD, Sardi GL, Reed JF III. Components of the metabolic syndrome differ between young and old adults in the US population. *J Clin Hypertens (Greenwich).* 2012;14(8):502–506.

Tohidi M, Hatami M, Hadaegh F, Safarkhani M, Harati H, Azizi F. Lipid measures for prediction of incident cardiovascular disease in diabetic and non-diabetic adults: results of the 8.6 years follow-up of a population based cohort study. *Lipids Health Dis.* 2010;9:6.

Upadhyay UD, Waddell EN, Young S, et al. Prevalence, awareness, treatment, and control of high LDL cholesterol in New York City, 2004. *Prev Chronic Dis.* 2010;7(3):A61.

US Department of Agriculture (USDA), Agricultural Research Service. USDA Food and Nutrient Database for Dietary Studies 2011–2012. 2014. Available at: http://www.ars.usda.gov/ba/bhnrc/fsrg. Accessed August 25, 2016.

US Department of Agriculture (USDA). *2015–2020 Dietary Guidelines for Americans.* 8th ed. Washington, DC: USDA; 2015.

US Department of Health and Human Services (USDHHS). *2008 Physical Activity Guidelines for Americans.* Washington, DC: USDHHS; 2008.

US Department of Health and Human Services (USDHHS), Agency for Healthcare Research and Quality. Table 3: Total expenses and percent distribution for selected conditions by type of service: United States, 2013. Available at: https://meps.ahrq.gov/data_stats/tables_compendia_hh_interactive.jsp?_SERVICE=MEPSSocket0&_PROGRAM=MEPSPGM.TC.SAS&File=HCFY2013&Table=HCFY2013_CNDXP_C&_Debug=. Accessed August 25, 2016.

US Preventive Services Task Force (USPSTF). Draft recommendation statement. Statin use for the primary prevention of cardiovascular disease in adults: preventive medication. Rockville, MD: USPSTF; 2015.

Vaisto J, Eloranta AM, Viitasalo A, et al. Physical activity and sedentary behaviour in relation to cardiometabolic risk in children: cross-sectional findings from the Physical Activity and Nutrition in Children (PANIC) Study. *Int J Behav Nutr Phys Act.* 2014;11:55.

Vazquez-Benitez G, Desai JR, Xu S, et al. Preventable major cardiovascular events associated with uncontrolled glucose, blood pressure, and lipids and active smoking in adults with diabetes with and without cardiovascular disease: a contemporary analysis. *Diabetes Care.* 2015;38(5):905–912.

Velagaleti RS, Gona P, Pencina MJ, et al. Left ventricular hypertrophy patterns and incidence of heart failure with preserved versus reduced ejection fraction. *Am J Cardiol.* 2014;113(1):117–122.

Viswanathan M, Golin CE, Jones CD, et al. Closing the quality gap: revisiting the state of the science (vol. 4: medication adherence interventions: comparative effectiveness). *Evid Rep Technol Assess (Full Rep).* 2012;(208.4):1–685.

Wilkins JT, Ning H, Stone NJ, et al. Coronary heart disease risks associated with high levels of HDL cholesterol. *J Am Heart Assoc.* 2014;3(2):e000519.

Yang Q, Cogswell ME, Flanders WD, et al. Trends in cardiovascular health metrics and associations with all-cause and CVD mortality among US adults. *JAMA.* 2012;307(12):1273–1283.

Zachariah JP, McNeal CJ, Copeland LA, et al. Temporal trends in lipid screening and therapy among youth from 2002 to 2012. *J Clin Lipidol.* 2015;9(5 suppl):S77–S87.

Zallman L, Himmelstein DH, Woolhandler S, et al. Undiagnosed and uncontrolled hypertension and hyperlipidemia among immigrants in the US. *J Immigr Minor Health.* 2013;15(5):858–865.

Zhang CX, Tse LA, Deng XQ, Jiang ZQ. Cardiovascular risk factors in overweight and obese Chinese children: a comparison of weight-for-height index and BMI as the screening criterion. *Eur J Nutr.* 2008;47(5):244–250.

Zile MR, Gaasch WH, Patel K, Aban IB, Ahmed A. Adverse left ventricular remodeling in community-dwelling older adults predicts incident heart failure and mortality. *JACC Heart Fail.* 2014;2(5):512–522.

PART IV. DOWNSTREAM CHRONIC DISEASES

15

CARDIOVASCULAR DISEASE

Longjian Liu, MD, PhD, MSc, Craig J. Newschaffer, PhD, and Julianne Nelson, MPH

Introduction

Cardiovascular disease (CVD) refers to a wide variety of heart and blood vessel diseases, including coronary heart disease (CHD), cerebrovascular disease (also referred to as stroke), heart failure, and peripheral arterial disease (PAD; Figure 15-1). In the United States today, CVD is of paramount public health importance because of its widespread nature and the potential for intervention. Risk factors for each of these heart and blood vessel diseases overlap a great deal. Presence of risk factors such as obesity, hypertension, and diabetes can lead to a range of cardiovascular diseases. The prevalence and severity of CVDs also differ by age, sex, and race resulting in an increase in targeted prevention and treatment public health programs. The consequences of these diseases are beyond the physical (disability and death) and also include a significant economic burden (health care costs and loss of income).

Cardiovascular disease death rates have declined precipitously over the past 15 years; from 2000 to 2014, death rates attributable to CVD declined 35.64%. In the same 15-year period, the actual number of CVD deaths per year declined by 8.9%. Yet, in 2014, CVD still accounted for 30.6% (803,227) of all 2,626,418 deaths, or about one of every three deaths in the United States. This decline has been driven by continuing reductions in mortality from both CHD and stroke (Figure 15-2). Cardiovascular disease remains a major public health challenge with heart disease still the first, and cerebrovascular disease the fourth, leading overall causes of death in the United States (Mozaffarian et al. 2016).

Significance

Death rates for CVD vary markedly by age, race, and sex (Lloyd-Jones et al. 2009; Mozaffarian et al. 2016). In 2013, the death rates were 269.8 per

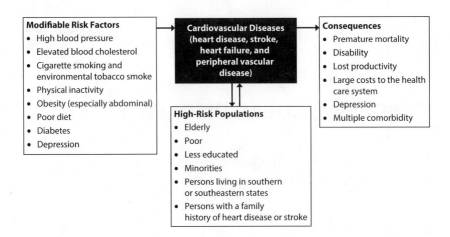

Source: Adapted from Newschaffer et al. (2010).

Figure 15-1. Cardiovascular Diseases: Causes, Consequences, and High-Risk Groups

100,000 for men and 184.8 for women. The rates were 270.6 for non-Hispanic white men, 356.7 for non-Hispanic black men, 197.4 for Hispanic men, 183.8 for non-Hispanic white women, 246.6 for non-Hispanic black women, and 136.4 for Hispanic women. The leading causes of death for both men and women aged 65 years or older were (1) diseases of the heart, (2) cancer, (3) chronic lower respiratory disease, and (4) stroke. Hispanics and Asian Americans appear to be at lower risk of heart disease and stroke mortality than whites. However, CVD-related diseases remain the leading contributors to mortality for these racial and ethnic groups (CDC NCHS 2013; Mozaffarian et al. 2016).

Yet mortality alone captures only a portion of the health burden imposed by CVD. Cardiovascular disease was a primary diagnosis for more than 7.8 million inpatient hospital discharges in 2010, and 4.6 million emergency department encounters. The total number of inpatient cardiovascular operations and procedures increased 28%, from 5.9 million in 2000 to 7.6 million in 2010. American adults self-reported heart trouble, stroke, or high blood pressure as the main reason for their disability in 2005 (CDC NCHS 2013). Cardiovascular disease accounted for 15% of total health expenditures in 2011 to 2012, more than any other major diagnostic group. The annual direct and indirect cost of CVD and stroke in the United States is an estimated

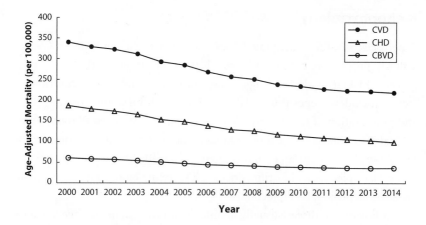

Source: Data from CDC NCHS (2015). Data are from the multiple cause of death files, 2000–2014, as compiled from data provided by the 57 vital statistics jurisdictions through the Vital Statistics Cooperative Program.

Note: CBVD = cerebrovascular disease; CHD = coronary heart disease; CVD = cardiovascular disease. Directly standardized to the age distribution of the 2000 U.S. standard population.

Figure 15-2. Age-Adjusted Cardiovascular Disease Mortality by Year, 2000–2014

$316.6 billion. This figure includes $193.1 billion in direct costs (which include the cost of physicians and other professionals, hospital services, prescribed medication, and home health care, but not the cost of nursing home care) and $123.5 billion in indirect costs (lost future productivity attributed to premature CVD and stroke mortality in 2011 to 2012; Mozaffarian et al. 2016). Mortality rates from CVD remain higher in the United States than in many other industrialized nations; however, reflective of the worldwide spread of CVD, the United States ranked 165th out of 192 nations in 2004 age-adjusted CVD mortality data in the World Health Organization Global Burden of Disease database (WHO 2008). The term "burden of disease" indicates the gap between actual and ideal health status. It is measured in disability-adjusted life years, a combination of years of life lost because of premature mortality and time lived in less than full health. Although CVD mortality is expected to continue to decline in the developed world, in the developing world, projections suggest that heart disease mortality will increase 120% for women and 137% for men from 1990 to 2020 with a tripling of both heart disease and stroke mortality expected in Latin America, the Middle East, and sub-Saharan Africa (Leeder et al. 2012).

Pathophysiology

Atherosclerosis, the underlying disease process of the major forms of CVD, is a slowly progressive condition in which the inner layers of the artery walls become thick, irregular, and rigid. The process is complex, with contributing factors including deposition of fat and cholesterol, inflammation, migration and proliferation of smooth muscle cells, formation of raised fibrous lesions, and calcification. With the progression of atherosclerosis, the arteries narrow, the blood flow is decreased, and there is greater likelihood that the built-up material, or plaque, will disrupt, creating a traveling blood clot (or embolism; see also Chapter 14, Dyslipidemia).

Cardiovascular disease usually manifests clinically in middle age or later—the lifetime risk for incident CVD for 40-year-old men is about 66% and just over 50% for like-aged women (Lloyd-Jones et al. 2009). However, atherosclerosis typically initiates in childhood and there is growing speculation that fetal factors may also be etiologically significant. Atherosclerosis is associated with several modifiable risk factors including those well known as risk factors for CVD: high blood cholesterol, high blood pressure, cigarette smoking, physical inactivity, diabetes, and obesity (Labarthe 2011; Liu et al. 2014; Liu and Nunez 2010). The advent of noninvasive means of evaluating atherosclerosis has fostered the epidemiologic study of asymptomatic CVD. Control of modifiable risk factors, at both the population and individual levels, remains the key to primary and secondary prevention of CVD.

Coronary heart disease, congestive heart failure, cerebrovascular disease (stroke), and PAD share, but are not influenced equally by, many of the same CVD risk factors. Coronary heart disease is rarely found in populations without elevated cholesterol and body mass index (BMI). In contrast, stroke is a disease most strongly associated with high blood pressure with less contribution coming from cholesterol and other risk factors. Diabetes and smoking are most strongly associated with PAD. This chapter provides a more detailed discussion of each of these four major types of CVD.

CORONARY HEART DISEASE

Significance

Coronary heart disease is the single largest killer of American men and women today, accounting for nearly 364,593 deaths in 2014. It represents almost half (more than 45%) of the CVD deaths and more than 13% of all-cause mortality (NCHS 2015). Each year there are more than 735,000 new or recurrent heart attacks and it is estimated that approximately 21% of these heart attacks are silent. The American Heart Association estimates that, among American adults aged 20 years and older, 12% have a family history of CHD. About 1.3 million hospital admissions each year involve diagnoses of CHD, and the costs associated with medical care, lost earnings, and lost productivity attributable to CHD were estimated at $204.4 billion for 2010 (Mozaffarian et al. 2016).

Pathophysiology

Coronary heart disease, also called ischemic heart disease or coronary artery disease, is a term used to identify several disorders that reduce the blood supply to the heart muscle. This impairment of circulation to the heart is most frequently the result of narrowing of the coronary arteries by atherosclerosis. The onset, and much of the progression, of atherosclerosis is subclinical (i.e., without symptoms), with the most common emergent clinical manifestations of coronary atherosclerosis being angina pectoris (chest pain), myocardial infarction (MI, heart attack), and sudden death.

Historically, CHD epidemiology has been dependent on studies of these clinical manifestations as endpoints. However, the incorporation of new technologies into epidemiologic investigations, such as the B-mode ultrasound of the carotid arteries used in the Atherosclerosis Risk in Communities (ARIC) studies, is allowing new insights about risk factors for early-stage CHD. Those implicated through these studies thus far include conventional CHD risk factors, genetic changes at the cellular level, circulating markers of inflammation, infectious agents, micronutrients, and hemostatic factors (de Andrade et al. 1995; Folsom et al. 1994; Folsom et al. 1993; Ma et al. 1995; Nieto et al. 1996).

Descriptive Epidemiology

High-Risk Populations

Throughout life, men have much higher CHD mortality rates than women. Overall, the age-adjusted death rate for CHD in the United States is almost twice as high for men as it is for women (NCHS 2015). The incidence of CHD in women lags behind men by 7 to 10 years for total CHD and by 20 years for more serious clinical events such as MI and sudden death

(Maas and Appelman 2010; Mozaffarian et al. 2016). However, in women, CHD is still the single greatest mortality risk, with the age-adjusted mortality rate more than three times greater than that for breast cancer (Anderson et al. 1997; NCHS 2015).

Coronary heart disease risk increases with age independent of known CHD risk factors. Almost 10 per 1,000 Americans aged 65 years or older will experience heart failure and 92% of the people who die of heart attacks are aged older than 65 years (Mozaffarian et al. 2016; NCHS 2015). Coronary heart disease is the leading cause of death for men and women aged older than 65 years and the third leading cause of disability in older men and women (CDC 2009a; NCHS 2015). For men, major increases in CHD risk begin around age 45 years, whereas for women, the marked increase is delayed until after menopause, around age 55 years (NHLBI 2016). Coronary heart disease incident rates in women after menopause are two to three times those of women the same age before menopause. Subclinical CHD is more prevalent in older than in younger individuals and has been shown to be associated with the same risk factors linked to clinical disease at younger ages, thereby suggesting that risk factor modification in older individuals may still be a very cost-effective public health strategy (Corti et al. 1996).

For men and women combined, CHD death rates are higher among African Americans than whites until age 85 years and older, at which point they are higher among whites. African-American men experience a slightly higher death rate from CHD than white men. In 2014, the overall age-adjusted CHD death rate was 133.5 per 100,000 population, with death rates of 134.6 for white men and 147.9 per 100,000 for African-American men. The racial gap in CHD mortality is closing, and in 2005 the rate for white women was 111.7 compared to 140.9 per 100,000 for African-American women. By 2014, both rates declined with the age-adjusted CHD mortality rate per 100,000 being 71.1 for white women and 87.8 for African-American women (NCHS 2015).

Although national data on CHD mortality among Americans of Hispanic origin are limited, existing data suggest that age-adjusted death rates in 2014 for CHD were 75.3 per 100,000 for Hispanics or Latinos, 76.4 per 100,000 for American Indians or Alaska Natives, and 55.1 for Asians or Pacific Islanders (NCHS 2015).

A family history of premature CHD increases the risk of CHD. The clustering of CHD in families is not fully understood but is believed to be a combination of genetics and higher levels of risk factors within these families (e.g., similar dietary patterns).

Coronary heart disease incidence and mortality rates are higher among people of lower socioeconomic status (SES) than among those in the middle or upper classes (Benderly et al. 2013). The greatest declines in CHD mortality over time among all races in the United States have been among those with the highest levels of income (NCHS 2015). Not surprisingly, the gradient of CHD mortality associated with SES is similar to the gradient of risk factors; for example, cigarette smoking, obesity, and high blood pressure are more common among people with lower income and education levels (Benderly et al. 2013).

In addition, neighborhood SES effects may persist above those related to differing distributions of individual-level risk factors. In general, living in a low-SES neighborhood is associated with increased risk of CHD and increased levels of risk factors. However, complex interactions between individual- and neighborhood-level SES on CHD risk factors in African-American men have been observed. For example, one analysis of African-American men living in Jackson, Mississippi, found that lower individual SES was associated with increased serum cholesterol in higher-SES neighborhoods and decreased serum cholesterol in lower-SES neighborhoods (Diez-Roux et al. 1997).

Geographic Distribution

In the United States, age-adjusted CHD death rates show striking variation by geographic region. In 2014, the age-adjusted death rates in the United States varied from a high of 144 per 100,000 in Oklahoma to a low of 60.8 per 100,000 in Minnesota (NCHS 2015). The CHD death rate for the United States is approximately midway between those of other industrialized countries. A World Health Organization study of CHD death rates from between 1995 and 2009 showed extremely high rates in Eastern Europe and Central Asia. Low rates were noted in certain Caribbean and South American countries as well as France, Portugal, and Japan. In the countries studied, the highest CHD death rate observed was as much as 20 times the lowest rate (Finegold et al. 2013).

Time Trends

Coronary heart disease has been the leading cause of death in the United States for most of this century, with death rates from CHD peaking in 1963. In recent years, the decline in CHD mortality has been accelerating with the largest rate of decline observed in older populations ($\geq$ 65 years) and in women

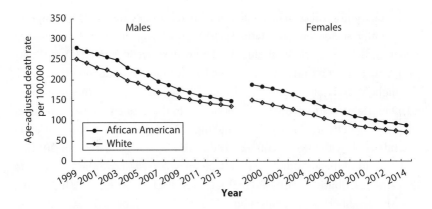

Source: Data from CDC NCHS (2015). Data are from the Multiple Cause of Death files, 1999–2014, as compiled from data provided by the 57 vital statistics jurisdictions through the Vital Statistics Cooperate Program.
Note: Rates are age-adjusted to 2000 standard.

Figure 15-3. Age-Adjusted Death Rates for Coronary Heart Disease by Sex and Race in the United States from 1999 to 2014

(Kulshreshtha et al. 2010). From 1980 to 2014, the age-adjusted death rate of CHD fell from 542.9 to 145.9 deaths per 100,000 population among men aged 25 to 84 years and from 263.3 to 66.5 deaths per 100,000 population among women aged 25 to 84 years. In 1980, a total of 462,984 deaths among people in this age group were recorded as attributable to CHD. By 2014, that had dropped to 230,781 recorded CHD deaths (NCHS 2015). Had the age-specific death rates from 1980 remained in 2000, an additional 598,680 deaths from CHD would have occurred (Ford et al. 2007; NCHS 2015). Declines in age-adjusted mortality since 1999 have been comparable across race/sex subgroups (CDC NCHS 2015; Figure 15-3).

Factors responsible for the decline in CHD mortality are not fully understood, but changes in lifestyle, reductions in risk factor prevalence, and improvements in medical care and treatment of CHD are thought to have contributed. However, not all groups have benefitted equally from these improvements (Gillespie et al. 2013; Goldman and Cook 1988). A study by Ford and colleagues indicates that approximately 47% of the decline in the CHD death rate from 1980 to 2000 was attributed to evidence-based medical treatments, including secondary preventive therapies after MI or revascularization (11%), initial treatment for acute MI or unstable angina (10%), treatments for heart failure (9%), revascularization for chronic angina (5%), and other therapies (12%). Approximately 44% was attributed to changes in major risk factors, including reductions in total cholesterol (24%), systolic blood pressure (20%), smoking prevalence (12%), and physical inactivity (5%). These reductions were partially offset by increases in the BMI and the prevalence of diabetes, which accounted for an increased number of CHD deaths (8% and 10%, respectively; Ford et al. 2007).

Causes

Coronary risk factors can be classified as either modifiable or nonmodifiable. Among modifiable risk factors, the major independent risk factors for CHD are high blood pressure, elevated blood cholesterol, cigarette smoking, physical inactivity, abdominal obesity, low daily fruit and vegetable consumption, and diabetes (Figure 15-1). Other modifiable risk factors include elevated blood C-reactive protein (CRP), fibrinogen, homocysteine, and secondhand smoke. Alcohol overconsumption and stress may also contribute to CHD risk. Nonmodifiable risk factors are discussed under the previous heading of "High-Risk Populations." Note, however, that not all high-risk groups are defined by nonmodifiable factors. Improved SES, for example, although it is not typically a direct goal of medical or public health intervention, certainly is a legitimate objective for social and economic policy.

Modifiable Risk Factors

High blood pressure, or hypertension (see Chapter 13), is a strong independent risk factor for morbidity and mortality from CHD (Hennekens et al. 1988). People with elevated blood pressure are two to four times as susceptible to CHD as are people with normal blood pressure (Table 15-1; Jenkins 1988). However, it is important to note that risk of CHD generally increases as levels of systolic or diastolic blood pressure rise whether or not one is looking at a population group above or below a particular hypertension cutpoint. Therefore, blood pressure reduction by individuals labeled "normotensive" by conventional definitions can also be beneficial. Studies suggest that a prolonged reduction of only 5 to 6 millimeters of mercury (mm Hg) in diastolic blood pressure results in a 20% to 25% reduction in CHD (MacMahon 1996).

Although drug therapy to reduce high blood pressure has resulted in lower overall rates of CVD deaths, major studies of drug treatment for high blood

Table 15-1. Modifiable Risk Factors for Coronary Heart Disease, United States

Magnitude	Risk Factor	Best Estimate (%) of PAR (Range)
Strong (relative risk > 4)	None	
Moderate (relative risk 2–4)	High blood pressure (≥ 140/90 mmHg)	25 (20–29)
	Cigarette smoking	22 (17–25)
	Elevated cholesterol (≥ 200 mg/dL)	43 (39–47)
	Diabetes (fasting glucose ≥ 140mg/dL)	8 (1–15)
Weak (relative risk < 2)	Obesity[a]	17 (7–32)
	Physical inactivity	35 (23–46)
	Secondhand smoke exposure	18 (8–23)
	Elevated C-reactive protein (> 3.0 mg/L)	19 (11–25)
	Elevated fibrinogen (> 3.74 g/L)	21 (17–25)
	Elevated homocysteine (> 15 μmol/L)	5 (2–9)
Possible	Psychological factors	
	Alcohol use[b]	
	Elevated plasma homocysteine	
	Infectious agents	
	Helicobacter pylori	
	Herpes simplex type 1	
	Chlamydia pneumoniae	
	Cytomegalovirus	
	Trimethylamine-N-oxide (TMAO)	
	Sleep disorders	

Source: Data from Abbott et al. (1987), CDC (1993), Cheng et al. (2014), Danesh et al. (2004), Ellis (1997), Fibrinogen Studies Collaboration et al. (2005), Fox (2010), He et al. (1996), Heidrich et al. (2007), Hennekens et al. (1988), Howard et al. (1998), Kawachi et al. (1997), Khalili et al. (2014), Kovar et al. (1987), Lam et al. (2000), Nilsson et al. (2006), Nygård et al. (1995), Powell and Blair (1994), Ridker (2006), Roivainen et al. (2000), Stamler et al. (1986), Stampfer et al. (1992), and Thom et al. (2006).
[a]Based on BMI > 27.8 kg/m^2 for men and > 27.3 kg/m^2 for women.
[b]Moderate to heavy alcohol use may increase risk, whereas light use may reduce risk.

pressure have failed to demonstrate a reduction in CHD deaths, possibly as a result of the untoward effects of antihypertensive therapy on other risk factors (Collins et al. 1990). Another possible explanation is that low diastolic blood pressure can increase the risk of coronary events such as MI among those with CHD (Franklin et al. 2015; Peralta et al. 2014).

Tobacco use (see Chapter 7) is a major cause of CHD among both men and women. Smokers have twice the risk of heart attack as nonsmokers. Smoking is also the major risk factor for sudden death from heart attack, with smokers having

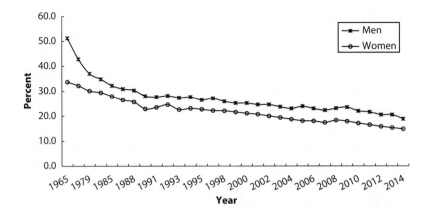

Source: Data from CDC NCHS (2013). Additional data are from 2004–2010, 2005–2012, 2006, 2007, 2008, 2009, 2011, and 2014.

Figure 15-4. Prevalence of Cigarette Smoking among Men and Women, United States, 1965–2014

two to four times the risk of nonsmokers. The risk increases with the number of cigarettes smoked (Caswell 2005; USDHHS 1983). Following the first Surgeon General's report on smoking in 1964, cigarette smoking declined sharply for men and at a slower pace for women (NCHS 2009; Figure 15-4). Overall, cigarette smokers are two to four times more likely to develop CHD compared to nonsmokers, and have CHD death rates 70% higher. Heavy smokers (i.e., those who smoke two or more packs per day) die from CHD at a rate two to three times that of nonsmokers. Studies have shown, however, that people who stop smoking experience a rapid and substantial reduction in CHD mortality. For people who have smoked a pack or less per day, within 10 years of quitting, death rates from CHD drop to the level of people who have never smoked (Caswell 2005; USDHHS 1983).

In addition, a number of studies suggest that exposure to environmental tobacco smoke (also called passive smoking or secondhand smoke) increases the risk of CHD (Caswell 2005; Glantz and Parmley 1991; Steenland 1992). For example, follow-up of a very large group of never-smoking U.S. women showed that those with regular exposure to secondhand smoke at home or at work had a 90% increased risk of developing CHD compared with those unexposed (Kawachi et al. 1997). An estimated 33,951 nonsmokers die from heart disease each year as a result of exposure to secondhand smoke (CDC 2016a). The association between secondhand smoke exposure and CHD mortality is elevating the importance of this critical public health issue to new heights.

Cholesterol (see Chapter 14) is the blood lipid most strongly associated with CHD. The risk of CHD increases steadily as blood cholesterol levels increase in a population. Studies have shown that a 10% decrease in total cholesterol levels may result in an estimated 30% reduction in incidence of CHD (CDC 2000). For people with cholesterol levels in the 250 to 300 milligrams per deciliter (mg/dL) range, each 1% reduction in cholesterol level results in about a 2% reduction in CHD morbidity and mortality (Sempos et al. 1989).

Cholesterol is transported in the blood by low-density lipoproteins (LDLs), very-low-density lipoproteins, and high-density lipoproteins (HDLs; NHLBI 2002). High levels of LDL are a leading factor in the progression of atherosclerosis and in the subsequent development of CHD (Blackburn 1992; NHLBI 2002). The very-low-density lipoproteins, which are composed primarily of triglyceride, comprise 10% to 15% of the total serum cholesterol. The role of triglycerides in development of CHD has been slower to be confirmed with recent studies finding a similar pattern of elevated triglycerides in patients with CHD as seen with elevated LDL. More recently, a causal link between high triglycerides and CHD has been reported (Do et al. 2013).

The level of HDL is inversely related to CHD; the lower the level of HDL, the higher the risk of CHD, particularly at levels below 35 mg/dL (NHLBI 2002; Rifkind 1990). The HDL level correlates inversely with LDL size and triglyceride level, and this, coupled with the complex metabolic interrelationships of these particles, makes it more difficult to separate the independent contributions of various lipids to CHD. It is quite possible that all play a role; one hypothesis is that LDL may be more important in early stage atherogenesis, whereas low HDL and triglyceride elevation develops closer to the clinical onset of CHD (Sharrett et al. 1994).

C-reactive protein is an inflammatory biomarker that is strongly associated with CHD, inflammation, and the metabolic syndrome. Although CRP, synthesized primarily in the liver, was discovered in 1930 (Ridker 2006), this protein has received substantial attention in recent years as a promising biological predictor of atherosclerotic disease (Pearson et al. 2003). An evolving body of work suggests that even small increases in CRP within the normal range are predictive of future vascular events in apparently healthy, asymptomatic individuals (Hackam and Anand 2003).

Danesh et al. (2004; 2000) reported a meta-analysis of 14 prospective long-term studies of CRP and the risk of nonfatal MI or death from CHD. The analysis comprised 2,557 cases with a mean age at entry of 58 years and a mean follow-up of eight years. The combined adjusted risk ratio was 1.9 (95% confidence interval [CI] = 1.5, 2.3) for the development of CHD among individuals in the top third of baseline CRP concentrations compared with those in the bottom third. A number of prospective studies have demonstrated that CRP also predicts recurrent events and increased mortality in patients with acute coronary syndromes, chronic stable angina, ischemic stroke, and peripheral vascular disease (Hackam and Anand 2003).

Fibrinogen is a circulating glycoprotein that acts at the final step in the coagulation response to vascular and tissue injury. Epidemiological data support an independent association between elevated levels of fibrinogen and CHD (Fibrinogen Studies Collaboration et al. 2005; Lam et al. 2000). Two meta-analyses involving 18 and 22 prospective, long-term studies demonstrated strong, statistically significant risk for individuals in the upper third of baseline fibrinogen concentration compared with those in the lower third (relative risk = 1.8; 95% CI = 1.6, 2.0; Danesh and Lewington 1998; Fibrinogen Studies Collaboration et al. 2005; Hackam and Anand 2003; Maresca et al. 1999).

Another plasma constituent, homocysteine, is receiving increased attention as a potentially modifiable risk factor for acute CHD events. Plasma homocysteine levels have been found to be positively associated with risk of CHD events (Nygård et al. 1997; Stampfer et al. 1992). A recent review conducted by Humphrey and colleagues (2008) searching MEDLINE (between 1966 and March 2006) identified 26 articles of good or fair quality. The results indicated that most studies found elevations of 20% to 50% in CHD risk for each increase of 5 micromoles per liter (μmol/L) in homocysteine level. A meta-analysis yielded a combined risk ratio for coronary events of 1.18 (95% CI = 1.10, 1.26) for each increase of 5 μmol/L in homocysteine level. The association between homocysteine and CHD was similar when analyzed by sex, length of follow-up, outcome, study quality, and study design (Humphrey et al. 2008).

Although the underlying mechanisms linking diabetes (see Chapter 12) and CHD are complex and still not fully understood, diabetes is generally considered a major CHD risk factor. Among people with diabetes, CHD is the most common cause of morbidity and mortality, and individuals with diabetes experience CHD at rates two to four times greater than those without the disease (National Research Council 1989). Data from national studies showed a disproportionately high prevalence of diabetes in African Americans (13.2%) compared with whites (7.6%; ADA 2014). The 2014 overall death rate per 100,000 population from diabetes was 20.9. Death rates were 24.1 for white men, 42.7 for African American men, 15.3 for white women, and 33.1 for African American women (NCHS 2015). At least 65% of people with diabetes die of some form of heart or blood vessel disease (Thom et al. 2006).

Obesity has widely been defined by using BMI (weight [kg]/height [m²]). A BMI of 25 and higher indicates overweight, and 30 or higher indicates obesity in adults (Thom et al. 2006). Obesity and overweight have significant associations with increases in blood pressure, serum total cholesterol, and glucose, and with decreases in serum HDL levels. In addition, obesity has been well documented as an independent risk factor for CVD and diabetes (see Chapter 12). Recent studies have observed a J-shaped relationship between BMI and CHD mortality and note that even small increases in BMI can result in increased risk of CHD (Canoy et al. 2013).

Recent studies suggest that the distribution of fat deposits on the body may also affect CHD risk. Upper body or abdominal fat ("central obesity" or "apple shape") appears to increase risk more than lower body fat (pear shape). Men and women in the upper quintile of subscapular skin fold as well as men with a waist-to-hip ratio greater than 1.0 and women with a ratio greater than 0.8 experience increased CHD risk (Barrett-Connor and Orchard 1985; USPSTF 1989; Freedman et al. 1995; Lawson 2013). The tendency toward abdominal disposition of body fat seems to increase CHD risk across all levels of BMI (Després 2012).

Physical inactivity (see Chapter 9) is increasingly recognized as a major risk factor for CHD. About 51% of U.S. adults do not engage in the recommended amount of regular leisure-time physical activity (defined as light to moderate activity for 30 minutes, five times per week or vigorous activity for 20 minutes, three times per week; CDC 2016b; Thom et al. 2006). Physical activity decreases body weight, decreases blood pressure, and improves insulin sensitivity (Balkau et al. 2008; USDHHS 1996). Mounting evidence suggests that small amounts of physical activity can also have a significant impact on heart disease mortality (Blair et al. 1989; Hakim et al. 1998). The greatest benefits appear to occur with the move from a completely sedentary lifestyle to very modest levels of activity.

Moderate to heavy alcohol consumption is known to raise blood pressure levels and to increase CHD mortality. However, in most studies, light regular drinking (two or fewer drinks per day) has been associated with modest reductions in CHD risk. The pathway for this protection appears to be through changes in HDL-cholesterol, fibrinogen, and hemoglobin A1C (Ruidavets et al. 2010). The relationship to other risk factors and the social consequences of alcohol use, however, preclude any public health recommendation for alcohol use (see Chapter 10).

Psychological factors and stress also have been studied in relation to the development of CHD. Perhaps the earliest studied is the Type A behavior pattern, characterized by excessive competitiveness, hostility, impatience, fast speech, and quick motor movements, although this is not as widely studied anymore (Ikeda et al. 2008). Considerable attention has been devoted to the exploration of specific psychological factors, including anger, job stress, anxiety, and social support (Richardson et al. 2012; Roest et al. 2010). Causal connections among these specific psychological risk factors and CHD have yet to be clearly established, but evidence supporting a causal role for anger, both as an event trigger and a long-term risk factor, and social support, particularly important in extending survival among those with disease, is mounting (Greenwood et al. 1996; Kawachi et al. 1996; Williams et al. 2000).

Lastly, risk factors for heart disease tend to cluster; that is, individuals with CHD are likely to have more than one risk factor. The greater the level of any single risk factor, the greater the chance of developing CHD. Moreover, the likelihood of developing CHD increases markedly when risk factors manifest simultaneously. There is at least an additive contribution to CHD risk for the major risk factors of high blood pressure, high LDL-cholesterol, and fibrinogen, as evident in the findings of the Prospective Cardiovascular Münster (PROCAM) study (Abbott et al. 1987; CDC 1989; Heinrich et al. 1994; Kovar et al. 1987; NHBPEP 1991; Powell and Blair 1994; Stamler et al. 1986).

Population-Attributable Risk

Coronary heart disease is a multifactorial disease, and precisely quantifying the contribution of each risk factor to overall heart disease is difficult. We can, however, roughly gauge the importance of risk factors by estimating population-attributable risk, which is the percentage of CHD that could be prevented by eliminating a particular risk factor in the population. There are several things that need to be remembered when one is considering population-attributable risks, with the two most important being (1) when there are many factors contributing to a disease, as is the case with CHD, these percentages will sum to more than 100%, and (2) when risk factors are continuous, like blood pressure or cholesterol level, the population-attributable risk estimated depends greatly on the cutpoint chosen to designate who is at high risk. Table 15-1 shows the proportion of CHD mortality that can be attributed to the risk factors discussed previously.

Evidence-Based Interventions

Prevention

Because of the multiple risk factors involved in CHD, modest changes in one or more risk factors can have a large public health impact. Primary prevention of CHD involves controlling the major preventable risk factors: hypertension, high blood cholesterol, tobacco use, diet, and physical inactivity (see Chapters 13, 14, 7, 8, and 9, respectively). Other effective methods of prevention include diabetes control, weight management, and limitations in alcohol consumption (see Chapters 12, 11, and 10, respectively).

The multifactorial nature of CHD etiology calls for multiple intervention strategies. In addition to the early detection and control of risk factors in adults, prevention approaches may include early and systematic health education regarding the importance of lifestyle behaviors in young people, such as avoiding tobacco, eating a healthy diet, and performing adequate physical activity. Other prevention interventions can include policy-related or environmental changes such as improved food choices in schools, improved food labeling in grocery stores, elimination of cigarette vending machines, and provision of smoke-free environments. (The multifaceted approach to risk reduction is discussed in Chapter 3 on intervention strategies.)

When one is considering prevention strategies, it is also important to recognize that CHD is affected by the social and economic characteristics of a community, including levels of income and education and occupations. Positive changes in public health are, therefore, often the result of general social and economic development policies, rather than public health policies per se. Research has even found that when risk factors are held constant, those with lower SES have a higher risk of heart disease (Franks et al. 2011; Wing et al. 1988).

Screening

The principal methods of early detection for CHD include screening for high blood pressure and elevated serum cholesterol, and assessing behavioral factors such as tobacco use, dietary fat intake, and physical activity level.

Screening electrocardiograms are not recommended for the general population but may be appropriate for individuals at increased risk of CHD. This group includes men aged older than 40 years with two or more CHD risk factors, high-risk sedentary men planning to begin an exercise program, and people who would endanger the safety of others if they were to experience sudden cardiac events (USPSTF 1989). Newer screening technologies include coronary artery calcium scoring and noninvasive angiography with computed tomography and may be useful tools for those who are at risk for CHD, specifically those with diabetes (Bax et al. 2007). However, many argue against such screening tools stating that there is insufficient evidence for their use on high-risk persons and it is expensive and potentially harmful in comparison to currently available alternatives (Ebell 2012).

Treatment

Advances in the treatment of CHD have contributed substantially to major reductions in mortality over the past four decades. Treatment for CHD is tailored to each patient, depending on the cause and severity of the coronary artery disease. Treatment options mainly include (1) healthy lifestyle programs, (2) medications, and (3) surgical and other invasive procedures. Of them, adopting a healthy lifestyle is one of the best treatments for CHD. Either by itself or in combination with medical treatment, a healthy lifestyle can prevent or attenuate disease progression.

When medications and lifestyle adjustments cannot relieve the chest pain symptomatic of CHD, surgery may be necessary to restore adequate function to the heart. Patients may benefit from one or more of these surgical treatment options:

1. Catheter-assisted procedures: A thin, flexible tube (catheter) is inserted into the patient's artery, usually in the leg, and then is threaded through the arteries to the heart.
2. Coronary angioplasty and stents: Angioplasty opens blocked coronary arteries to allow blood to flow more freely to the heart. When the catheter tip reaches a blocked artery, a small balloon expands in the artery to push open the blood vessel.
3. Radiation brachytherapy: In cases in which coronary artery blockage reoccurs, the patient may benefit from brachytherapy. In this procedure,

the coronary artery segment is reopened during angioplasty and exposed to radiation.

4. Atherectomy: A catheter is inserted into the blocked artery and one of several types of small devices removes plaque build-up.

5. Coronary artery bypass surgery: Bypass surgery, also called coronary artery bypass grafting, creates a detour around a blocked coronary artery with a new blood vessel, or graft.

Gene therapy is another one of the newest potential treatment modalities, but its effectiveness is still under investigation. Gene therapists are attempting to introduce into the heart a gene that codes for a blood vessel growth factor, to stimulate and repair adequate blood vessel growth (Goldstein et al. 2006; Mayo Foundation 2009). Finally, cardiac rehabilitation—prevention of CHD complications through diet, exercise, weight control, and smoking cessation—has reduced mortality and improved functional capacity and quality of life among patients with clinical CHD (Oldridge et al. 1988).

Examples of Evidence-Based Interventions

Two major primary prevention strategies have been used in attempts to reduce cardiovascular mortality rates: the high-risk and the community-based (or population-based) approaches. The high-risk approach aims to identify high-risk individuals through population screening and to refer them for treatment. The Healthy Hearts program (Richardson et al. 2008), Emerging Risk Factors Collaboration (Tikkanen et al. 2013), and the Multiple Risk Factor Intervention Trial (Stamler et al. 1993) are examples of this approach. Recently there has been a study of and interest in using genetic markers to create a CHD risk score and identify those in the population who should be directed toward additional screening and intervention programs (Tikkanen et al. 2013).

Community-based interventions are a cornerstone of the public health approach to CHD prevention. They are defined as programs that attempt to modify the prevalence of one or more CHD risk factors (i.e., hypertension, smoking, hyperlipidemia, physical inactivity, and unhealthy diet), CHD mortality, or both within a specifically identified, circumscribed community. Community-based interventions have typically used education or environmental change to promote and facilitate changes in the lifestyles and other behaviors of a population (Papadakis and Moroz 2008).

Largely because of a strong favorable but unanticipated secular trend in CHD risk factors in control communities, these interventions tended to have less power to demonstrate overall effectiveness at the community level than originally anticipated. However, within each intervention program, individual components frequently were shown to be successful in analyses of intermediate or process measures and in analyses of principal endpoints that were limited to subpopulations most likely to be exposed to the component (e.g., schoolchildren participating in school-based program with a home component; Simon et al. 2008). In addition, success has been found in intervention programs that are designed for the specific community. An example of this is the Partnership for an Active Community Environment committee, which, as a means to improve cardiovascular health in the area, installed a walking path and playground in a low-income neighborhood in New Orleans (Gustat et al. 2012). A recent review of 21 published major community-based CVD intervention programs worldwide showed positive impact on CHD risk factors within a distinct population (Papadakis and Moroz 2008).

More recent community-based CHD prevention programs have focused on discrete populations including the socioeconomically deprived, ethnic minorities, and rural communities (Papadakis and Moroz 2008). In 2012 the National Heart, Lung, and Blood Institute directed its efforts at reducing heart health disparities by funding nine strategic champions. This program is aimed at new community health worker projects in African American, American Indian, Filipino American, and Hispanic/Latin American communities. An example of this type of focused community-based program was recently conducted in California and directed toward Latina women. The pilot program for this intervention found that a targeted community-based prevention program was effective at improving cardiac health in the selected population (Altman et al. 2014).

In addition, existing community-based interventions may not have the same impact when applied to different at-risk populations. This has been observed with the Exercise and Nutrition Interventions for Cardiovascular Health (ENCORE) study. The ENCORE study was designed to test the effect of two different dietary patterns on risk factors for CHD: the Dietary Approaches to Stop Hypertension (DASH) diet alone and the DASH diet plus weight management (Hinderliter et al. 2014). Although the DASH diet has been found to be effective, adherence to the DASH diet is not the same across races, and thus this intervention has different results when applied to different racial at-risk groups (Epstein et al. 2012).

Community-based interventions have been evolving in recent years to be able to take advantage of the shifting use of technology in our lives and how this can be used in health interventions. An example of this is the mobile phone–based health (mHEALTH) intervention. Participants in the intervention received monthly motivational calls and weekly text messages that included diet and exercise information. Evaluations of the mHEALTH intervention found reductions in weight and improvement in healthy eating habits among those in the intervention group compared to standard care (Rubinstein et al. 2016). Programs such as these have an added benefit of being cost-effective and able to reach many more people than in-person community-based interventions.

Coronary heart disease and related mortality is not just an issue in the United States but is also on the rise in low- and middle-income countries. Recently there was an evaluation of the Secondary Prevention of Coronary Events After Discharge from Hospital (SPREAD) community health worker–based intervention that occurred in India, where rates of CHD-related mortality have been increasing. In this study, patients discharged from the hospital after a coronary event were placed in either a standard care group or the community health worker–based intervention group. The study found that those in the community health worker–based intervention had better medication adherence and lifestyle changes resulting in significant reductions in blood pressure, BMI, and tobacco use, and significant improvement in physical activity and diet compared to those in standard care (Xavier et al. 2016).

A report by Chen et al. (2008) described two successful community-based CVD intervention programs in China—the Capital Steel and Iron Company cardiovascular intervention program (CSICIP) and the Beijing Fangshan cardiovascular prevention program (BFCP). The two programs each included more than 110,000 participants. The CSICIP, a work site–based intervention, began with a cardiovascular health survey covering 60,000 employees in 1974, and grew to 110,000 persons by 1995. The program targeted altering diet (particularly reducing salt and fat intake), keeping alcohol consumption to modest levels, and quitting smoking, together with a strategy of controlling high risks such as hypertension. The BFCP was a comprehensive prevention trial in the Fangshan rural area during 1991 to 1999. It covered a total of 120,000 residents in five rural communities, including three serving as intervention communities with a total of 66,000 residents and two as control communities with a total of 54,000 residents.

In the CSICIP, significant reductions in blood pressure occurred in both intervention and control sites, with greater reductions at the intervention site.

In addition, intervention sites experienced a marked additional reduction in salt intake and better overall control of hypertension. In the BFCP, blood pressure fell in all communities to a more modest degree than that in the CSICIP. In the intervention communities of BFCP, participants had greater blood pressure declines and higher smoking cessation rates, and also kept alcohol consumption to more modest levels than those in the control communities (Chen et al. 2008).

In sum, there were numerous insights gained from these pioneering community CVD prevention interventions, relating to the following: effective use of mass media; building on existing settings or institutions; creating strategies for making a healthy heart lifestyle "doable"; developing approaches to support environmental, legislative, and policy changes; and establishing and maintaining community coalitions. One of the most important common threads in the truly exemplary prevention and control programs was their reliance on multiple channels and multiple levels. This strategy appears to be critical in effecting lasting change.

A model exemplifying this approach is the Multilevel Approach to Community Health (MATCH) model (CDC 1998). Under the model, the four specific channels suggested are work sites, schools, health care, and community sites. Interventions can be directed to the individual, organizational, or policy level in any of these sites. Simons-Morton and colleagues (1988) gave an example of an organizational-level MATCH intervention in the "school" channel. Other multilevel models that appear to be successful include the Spectrum of Prevention, used successfully in California for its tobacco control program, and the social ecology approach being used in other countries, such as Australia.

Public health leaders are now approaching consensus on high-yield strategies to help change social or community norms regarding other critical CHD risk factors, including physical activity and nutrition. As these strategies are tested and refined, various experts are recommending that they be implemented through the population-based approach like MATCH (CDC 1998; King et al. 1995; Sallis et al. 2002; Schmid et al. 1995; Simons-Morton et al. 1988). However, to date, large variability has also been noted in the success of population-level CHD prevention trials. Developing an in-depth understanding of best practice derived from experiences to date with community-based intervention trials is essential for the design of future population-level cardiovascular prevention interventions. The burgeoning epidemics of chronic disease will necessitate the application of population health interventions to effectively address a multiplicity of issues, disease states, and management challenges. It is also important that these interventions be delivered appropriately (Papadakis and Moroz 2008).

Areas of Future Research

Epidemiologic research on CHD will likely focus on emerging, yet not completely understood, modifiable factors, including plasma CRP, fibrinogen, homocysteine, and known, but complex, risk factors such as serum cholesterol. Studies focusing on subclinical endpoints will be important in revealing undiscovered risk factors potentially significant in primary prevention. For example, further exploration of the importance of infection and inflammation in increasing the risk of atherosclerosis may prove fruitful. Population-based studies devising novel means of using information on known risk factors may also be crucial to advancing secondary prevention strategies.

A new area of CHD research is exploring the genetic factors that can contribute to developing CHD. It is suspected that these unknown genetic risk factors account for 40% to 60% of CHD risk. It is still unclear what role genetics will serve in the future of CHD prevention, but it is already being studied for its potential as a screening tool (Roberts and Stewart 2012; Tikkanen et al. 2013).

There is also growing interest and recognition of the importance of conducting more research and demonstration efforts involving policy and environmental approaches to reduce CHD risk factors. Partnerships with nontraditional partners will be essential for success. Population-based prevention research should focus on CHD research in special populations such as women, children, older adults, and racial and ethnic minorities, addressing the applicability of current knowledge to these populations and designing population-specific interventions, like the Multi-Ethnic Study of Atherosclerosis (MESA; Bild et al. 2002) and The Hispanic Community Health Study/ Study of Latinos (HCHS/SOL; Hispanic Community Health Study 2007). The MESA is designed to study the prevalence, correlation, and progression of subclinical CVD in multiple ethnicities (white, African American, Hispanic, and Chinese; Bild et al. 2002). The HCHS/SOL is a multicenter epidemiologic study in Hispanic/Latino populations to determine the role of acculturation in the prevalence and development of disease and to identify risk factors playing a protective or harmful role in Hispanics/Latinos (Hispanic Community Health Study 2007). Finally, despite the huge potential for public health benefits, CHD control efforts have been modest at many state and local health department levels. Both levels would benefit from an infusion of resources and expertise to build capacity and expand activities in CHD control.

CEREBROVASCULAR DISEASE

Significance

Cerebrovascular disease (also referred to as stroke) is the fifth leading cause of death in the United States, behind heart disease, cancer, chronic lower respiratory diseases, and unintentional injury. In 2013, stroke led to the death of almost 130,000 of the 800,000 Americans who die of cardiovascular disease each year, which is one out of every 19 deaths from all causes. More than 795,000 people have a stroke each year in the United States. Of those, 610,000 are first or new strokes; 185,000 or nearly one in four are recurrent strokes; about 25% die at the time of the stroke event or soon after; 15% to 30% remain permanently disabled, and their families live with the disabling effects of stroke. Worldwide, the burden of stroke has also posed a serious public health problem. In 2010, there were an estimated 11.6 million events of incident ischemic stroke and 5.3 million events of incident hemorrhagic stroke, 63% and 80%, respectively, in low- and middle-income counties (Krishnamurthi et al. 2013; Mozaffarian et al. 2016).

Stroke-associated societal costs, including direct costs associated with medical care and indirect costs because of lost productivity, were estimated at $33 billion in 2012 (total direct costs of $17.2 billion and indirect costs of $15.8 billion). Transport of stroke patients to the hospital results in faster treatment. However, one third of stroke patients do not call 9-1-1 and use emergency medical services (EMS) to get to the hospital. Gaps remain in the quality of care provided to acute stroke patients (CDC Stroke Registry 2016; Mozaffarian et al. 2016).

Pathophysiology

Stroke occurs when an artery in the brain is either ruptured or clogged by a blood clot resulting in an interruption or a severe restriction of blood supply used to provide oxygen and nutrients to brain tissue. Two major types of stroke include ischemic and hemorrhagic. Ischemic strokes account for approximately 87% of all strokes and are caused by blockage attributable to a blood clot (thrombus), a wandering clot (embolus), or narrowing of the artery because of atherosclerotic plaque (Lloyd-Jones et al. 2009). The major form of ischemic stroke, cerebral thrombosis, is caused when a blood clot forms and blocks blood flow in the cerebral artery. This is generally the result of atherosclerosis in the cerebral vessels. Cerebral embolism occurs when a clot breaks loose from another part of the body, often the heart, and lodges in a cerebral artery.

Transient ischemic attacks (TIAs) or "ministrokes" exhibit symptoms similar to ischemic strokes but are "transient" in nature with a thrombus or embolus quickly dislodging, allowing restored blood flow. Typically, a TIA does not result in lasting neurological impairment or deficits. However, TIAs are important in predicting future strokes, as about 10% of ischemic strokes are preceded by a TIA and about 40% of TIAs lead to stroke (Furie et al. 2011; Mozaffarian et al. 2016; Sacco et al. 2006).

The other type of stroke, hemorrhagic, is caused by intracerebral or subarachnoid hemorrhaging. The rupturing of blood vessels because of head injury or a burst aneurysm can lead to bleeding into brain tissue (intracerebral hemorrhage) or into the space between the brain and the skull (subarachnoid hemorrhage). The severity of hemorrhagic stroke is dependent on the location and amount of bleeding. Although subarachnoid hemorrhaging is life-threatening with mortality averaging 40% within the first month of bleeding, those who survive the initial stroke and the following critical period often make remarkable recoveries. Hemorrhagic strokes account for 13% of all strokes (Lloyd-Jones et al. 2009).

Descriptive Epidemiology

High-Risk Populations

Age is a strong risk factor for stroke. After age 55 years, the rate of stroke incidence doubles in each successive decade. Stroke mortality also increases sharply with age. In 2005, the stroke death rate ranged from 33 per 100,000 in those aged 55 to 64 years to 1,142 per 100,000 in people aged 85 years and older (Lloyd-Jones et al. 2009). Data from the Brain Attack Surveillance in Corpus Christi (BASIC) Project for 2000 through 2010 demonstrated that ischemic stroke rates declined significantly in people aged 60 years or older but remained largely unchanged over time in those aged 45 to 59 years (Morgenstern et al. 2013; Mozaffarian et al. 2016).

Men generally have higher stroke mortality rates than women between the ages of 35 to 85 years. Women, however, represent approximately 60% of all strokes each year and generally surpass male incidence of stroke after age 85 years. The Framingham Heart Study examined sex differences in stroke incidence and estimated lifetime risk as one in five for women (20%–21%) and one in six for men (14%–17%; Petrea et al. 2009). The increased lifetime risk for women can be explained in large part by the longer life expectancy of women. Study researchers found women to be significantly older (75.1 years) than men (71.1 years) at first-ever stroke event (Petrea et al. 2009).

In the United States, distinct differences in stroke incidence, prevalence, and mortality rates exist among racial groups. In the Reasons for Geographic and Racial Differences in Stroke (REGARDS) cohort, in 27,744 participants followed up for 4.4 years (2003–2007), the overall age- and sex-adjusted black–white incidence rate ratio was 1.51, but for ages 45 to 54 years, it was 4.02 (Howard et al. 2011; Mozaffarian et al. 2016). Over 2006 to 2010, data from the Behavioral Risk Factor Surveillance System show that the overall self-reported stroke prevalence did not change. Older adults, blacks, people with lower levels of education, and people living in the southeastern United States had higher stroke prevalence (CDC 2012). In 2013, although age-adjusted stroke death rates for adults aged 18 years and older declined by about 50% or more among all racial groups, rates remained higher among blacks (65.7 per 100,000) than other races, including whites (46.9 per 100,000) and Asians (39.6 per 100,000; Mozaffarian et al. 2016).

Results from the BASIC study suggest that Mexican Americans have two-fold higher cumulative incidence for stroke (first-ever, recurrent, and TIA) compared with non-Hispanic whites in younger populations (aged 42–59 years; Morgenstern et al. 2004). The crude three-year cumulative incidence (2000–2002) was 16.8 per 1000 in Mexican Americans and 13.6 per 1000 in non-Hispanic whites. Specifically, Mexican Americans had a higher cumulative incidence of ischemic stroke at younger ages (45–59 years: rate ratio [RR] = 2.04 [95% CI = 1.55, 2.69]; 60–74 years: RR = 1.58 [95% CI = 1.31, 1.91]) but not at older ages (≥ 75 years: RR = 1.12 [95% CI = 0.94, 1.32]; Morgenstern et al. 2004). Despite the higher incidence rates of stroke for Hispanics compared with non-Hispanic whites in younger populations, Hispanic stroke survivors tend to live longer as evidenced by an approximately 15% to 20% decrease in mortality compared with non-Hispanic whites in 2005 (Kung et al. 2008; Lloyd-Jones et al. 2009). However, caution should be taken when one is interpreting Hispanic mortality rates because of potential reporting inconsistencies on death certificates and surveys.

Risk of stroke is greatly increased among people who have previously had a stroke or a TIA. Approximately one third to one half of people who have had one or more TIAs will later have a stroke (Kleindorfer et al. 2005; Lloyd-Jones et al. 2009). Risk of TIA increases with age and occurs more often in men. After TIA, the 90-day risk of stroke ranges from 9% to 17%. People who have had TIAs are nearly 10 times more likely to have a stroke than are people of the same age and sex who have not had a TIA. However, only about 15% of all strokes are preceded by TIAs (Lloyd-Jones et al. 2009).

The risk for stroke is higher for people with a family history of stroke. Positive paternal family history is associated with a doubling of stroke risk, whereas maternal family history increases stroke risk about 40%. The effect of family history appears to be about the same in African Americans and whites (Kim et al. 2004). In the Framingham Heart Study, a documented parental ischemic stroke by the age of 65 years was associated with a three-fold increase in ischemic stroke risk in offspring, even after adjustment for other known stroke risk factors. The absolute magnitude of the increased risk was greatest in those in the highest quintile of the Framingham Risk Score. By age 65 years, people in the highest quintile with an early parental ischemic stroke had a 25% risk of stroke compared with a 7.5% risk of ischemic stroke for those without such a history (Mozaffarian et al. 2016; Seshadri et al. 2010).

The "stroke belt" is represented by a group of states clustered in the Southeast with some of the highest stroke rates in the country: Alabama, Arkansas, Georgia, Louisiana, Mississippi, North Carolina, South Carolina, Oklahoma, Tennessee, and Virginia. In 2014, among 50 states plus the District of Columbia, Mississippi had the highest age-adjusted stroke mortality (48.8 per 100,000), followed by Alabama (48.34), Tennessee (45.77), Louisiana (45.56), Arkansas (45.45), South Carolina (44.18), North Carolina (43.02), Oklahoma (43.02), Georgia (42.63), and Virginia (37.03). The national average age-adjusted stroke mortality was 36.47 in 2014 (Figure 15-5).

Causes

The major modifiable risk factors for stroke include high blood pressure, atrial fibrillation (AF), PAD, cigarette smoking, diabetes, dyslipidemia, obesity, and physical inactivity (Table 15-2), with nutrition, high blood pressure, physical inactivity, diabetes, and AF contributing the highest population-attributable risk percentages in those aged 80 to 89 years (Table 15-2). As most of the risk factors are also associated with atherosclerotic cerebrovascular disease, treatment, management, and primary and secondary prevention of stroke remain targeted at reduction of these factors. Some studies suggest a possible increased risk associated with sleep-disordered breathing and comorbid chronic kidney disease (Broadley et al. 2007; Redline et al. 2010). Some studies also show possible increased risk associated with race and genetic factors including increased risk for stroke in identical twins when one has suffered a stroke.

Modifiable Risk Factors

High blood pressure remains the single most significant modifiable and treatable risk factor for stroke and has been shown to increase stroke risk for persons with blood pressures as low as 110/75 mm Hg, well within the normal range (Lewington et al. 2002). The risk increases with increasing blood pressure, both systolic and diastolic. In clinical trials, antihypertensive therapy has

Table 15-2. Modifiable Risk Factors for Stroke

Relative Magnitude Risk	Risk Factor	Estimated PAR, %
Strong		
4	Hypertension and diabetes	49.5
4	Hypertension (age 50 years)	40
4	Atrial fibrillation (age 50–59 years)	1.5
Moderate		
2.0	Peripheral arterial disease	3.0
1.8	Cigarette smoking	12–18
1.8–6	Diabetes	5–27
2.0	Dyslipidemia (high total cholesterol)	15
1.75–2.37	Obesity	12–20
Possible		
2.7	Physical inactivity	30
1.5–2.5	Dyslipidemia (low HDL-cholesterol)	10
1.4	Postmenopausal hormone therapy	7
1.5	Sodium intake > 2,300 mg	
1.4	Potassium < 4,700 mg	

Source: Data from Sacco et al. (2006) and Willey et al. (2014).
Note: PAR = population-attributable risk.

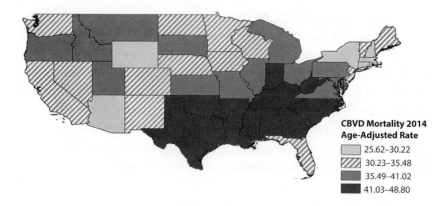

CBVD Mortality 2014
Age-Adjusted Rate

- 25.62–30.22
- 30.23–35.48
- 35.49–41.02
- 41.03–48.80

Source: Data from CDC NCHS (2015). Data are from the multiple cause of death files, 2000–2014, as compiled from data provided by the 57 vital statistics jurisdictions through the Vital Statistics Cooperative Program.

Figure 15-5. Age-Adjusted Cerebrovascular Disease (Stroke) Mortality (per 100,000 Population) by State, United States, 2014

been associated with reductions in stroke incidence, with an average 41% reduction in stroke risk with systolic blood pressure reductions of 10 mm Hg (Mozaffarian et al. 2016).

Several studies have shown significantly lower rates of recurrent stroke with lower blood pressure levels. Most recently, the blood pressure reduction component of the Secondary Prevention of Small Subcortical Strokes trial showed that targeting a systolic blood pressure less than 130 mm Hg was likely to reduce recurrent stroke by about 20% ($p = .08$) and significantly reduced intracerebral hemorrhagic stroke by two thirds (SPS3 Study Group 2013).

Because of the recognized significant role of high blood pressure in stroke, the American Heart Association and American Stroke Association (AHA/ASA) issued updated guidelines with recommendations for antihypertensive treatment for all patients with ischemic stroke, TIA, and acute ischemic stroke (Powers et al. 2015). Goals for target blood pressure level or reduction from pretreatment baseline are uncertain and should be individualized, but it is reasonable to achieve a systolic pressure less than 140 mm Hg and a diastolic pressure less than 90 mm Hg, and to have goals for people with diabetes of maintaining blood pressure less than 130/80 mm Hg, with caution in lowering the blood pressure in the elderly (Kernan et al. 2014).

Diabetes is also an independent risk factor for stroke (Liu et al. 2011; Liu et al. 2014; Mozaffarian et al. 2016; Yamori et al. 2006). Uncontrolled diabetes leads to arterial damage and increased risk for dyslipidemia, atherosclerosis, and hypertension—all of which confer high risk for stroke. The occurrence of stroke is two to five times higher among people with diabetes than among those without it.

Data from the U.S. Nationwide Inpatient Sample revealed that, from 1997 to 2006, the absolute number of acute ischemic stroke hospitalizations declined by 17% (from 489,766 in 1997 to 408,378 in 2006); however, the absolute number of acute ischemic stroke hospitalizations with comorbid diabetes rose by 27% (from 97,577 [20%] in 1997 to 124,244 [30%] in 2006). The rise in comorbid diabetes was more pronounced in individuals who were relatively younger, black or "other" race, on Medicaid, or admitted to hospitals located in the South. Factors independently associated with higher odds of diabetes in acute ischemic stroke patients were black or "other" (vs. white) race, congestive heart failure, peripheral vascular disease, and history of MI, renal disease, or hypertension (Mozaffarian et al. 2016; Towfighi et al. 2012). A few studies (and subsequently the AHA/ASA 2006 guidelines) have suggested intensive therapy and aggressive glycemic control to a hemoglobin A1c less than 7% are associated with a decrease in microvascular and cardiovascular complications; however, these studies are limited on macrovascular complications, and the risks of hypoglycemic complications in elderly patients seem to outweigh the benefits of tight control.

Atrial fibrillation is associated with worse outcomes such as mortality (two times more likely) or more severe disability (with 30-day mortality of 25% vs. 14% in AF vs. non-AF strokes, respectively), lower functional status, and greater rates of recurrences of stroke (Lin et al. 1996). In addition, the risk of stroke attributable to AF increases with age from 1.5% in those aged 50 to 59 years to 23.5% in those aged 80 to 89 years (Lloyd-Jones et al. 2009). Because AF is often asymptomatic and likely frequently undetected clinically, the stroke risk attributed to AF may be substantially underestimated.

Several studies have shown the association of cigarette smoking with an increased risk of stroke. The Framingham Heart Study in 1988 assessed cigarette smoking as a risk factor for stroke and found that the risk increase is dose-dependent. Cigarette smoking has also been shown to be strongly associated with carotid stenosis (Wilson et al. 1997). Current smokers have a two to four times increased risk of stroke compared with nonsmokers or those who have quit for greater than 10 years (Mozaffarian et al. 2016; Shah and Cole 2010). Smoking cessation, but not necessarily reduction, resulted in decreased risk and incidence of strokes and sustained ex-smokers' risk for stroke was not significantly different from never-smokers' risk (Bjartveit and Tverdal 2009). Several studies have shown that exposure to secondhand smoke is a risk factor for stroke (Liu et al. 2000; Mozaffarian et al. 2016). Smoking has also been identified as a risk factor for aneurysm formation, rupture of which results in hemorrhagic stroke.

Physical activity level is inversely proportional to stroke risk. Several studies including the Physicians' Health Study (Lee et al. 1999), the EPIC-Norfolk study (Myint et al. 2009), the Nurses' Health Study (Hu et al. 2000), the Northern Manhattan Stroke Study (Sacco et al. 2006), and the national REGARDS (McDonnell et al. 2013), support this relationship. For example, results from REGARDS found that participants reporting physical activity fewer than four times per week had a 20% increased risk of incident stroke over a mean of 5.7 years compared with those exercising four or more times per week. This relationship, which was more pronounced in men than in women, may be explained in large part by the effect of physical activity on reducing traditional risk factors, such as obesity and diabetes (McDonnell et al. 2013; Mozaffarian et al. 2016).

A number of studies have demonstrated that a certain diet pattern or nutrients are associated with risk reduction for stroke (Kernan et al. 2014; Mozaffarian et al. 2016; Yamori et al. 2006). Adherence to a Mediterranean-style diet that was higher in nuts and olive oil was associated with a reduced risk of stroke (hazard ratio = 0.54; 95% CI = 0.35, 0.84) in a randomized clinical trial conducted in Spain. The protective benefit of the Mediterranean diet observed was greater for strokes than for MI, but stroke subtype was not available (Estruch et al. 2013). In the Nurses Health and Health Professionals Follow-up Studies, each one-serving increase in sugar-sweetened soda was associated with a 13% increased risk of ischemic stroke, but not hemorrhagic stroke. Each one-serving increase in low-calorie or diet soda was associated with a 7% increased risk of ischemic stroke and 27% increased risk of hemorrhagic stroke (Bernstein et al. 2012).

A significant association between elevated serum cholesterol concentration and risk of ischemic stroke has been reported in several studies (ESCHD Collaborative Research Group 1998; Kurth et al. 2007), but not others (Prospective Studies Collaboration 1995). Elevated total cholesterol is inversely associated with stroke in the World Health Organization–Cardiovascular Comparison (CARDIAC) Study and several other studies (Yamori et al. 2006). In an analysis by the Emerging Risk Factors Collaboration of individual records on 302,430 people without initial vascular disease from 68 long-term prospective studies, hazard ratio (i.e., relative risk) for ischemic stroke was 1.12 (95% CI = 1.04, 1.20) with non-HDL cholesterol (ERF Collaboration et al. 2009).

Population-Attributable Risk

As shown in Table 15-3, an estimated 40% (varies by age group) of stroke deaths are attributed to elevated blood pressure and when comorbid with diabetes represents the greatest population-attributable risk percentage (49.5%). Smoking population-attributable risk varies from 12% to 18% with risk differences varied by age and sex (Goldstein et al. 2006). It is important to note that modifiable risk factors often interact or are accompanied by nonmodifiable risk factors (e.g., age, sex, and genetic factors). Such individuals are at greater risk and benefit from targeted prevention screenings and treatment of modifiable risk factors. Although the population-attributable risk for diabetes, ranging from 5% to 27%, is less than that observed for hypertension, the increasing prevalence and incidence of diabetes suggests the rise of future comorbid cases. Effective lifestyle modifications and interventions will be necessary to combat the growing obesity epidemic and the associated sedentary lifestyle (12%–20% and 30% population-attributable risk, respectively; Goldstein et al. 2006).

Evidence-Based Interventions

As described earlier, there is a number of primary risk factors associated with first and recurrent stroke. Risk assessment tools, such as the Framingham Stroke Profile, can be used to identify and classify individuals on the basis of risk score (Table 15-3; Goldstein et al. 2006). In 2011, the American Heart Association created a new set of central Strategic Impact Goals to drive organizational priorities for reaching Healthy People 2020 goals—to improve the cardiovascular health of all Americans by 20%, while reducing deaths from CVD and stroke by 20%. These goals introduce a new concept of cardiovascular health, characterized by seven metrics ("Life's Simple 7"), including health behaviors (diet quality, physical activity, smoking, BMI) and health factors (blood cholesterol, blood pressure, blood glucose). The "Life's Simple 7" is

Table 15-3. Modified Framingham Stroke Risk Profile

	Points										
	0	+1	+2	+3	+4	+5	+6	+7	+8	+9	+10
Men											
Age (years)	54-56	57-59	60-62	63-65	66-68	69-72	73-75	76-78	79-81	82-84	85
Untreated systolic blood pressure (mm Hg)	97-105	106-115	116-125	126-135	136-145	146-155	156-165	166-175	176-185	186-195	196-205
Treated systolic blood pressure (mm Hg)	97-105	106-112	113-117	118-123	124-129	130-135	136-142	143-150	151-161	162-176	177-205
History of diabetes	No		Yes								
Cigarette smoking	No			Yes							
Cardiovascular disease	No				Yes						
Atrial fibrillation	No				Yes						
Left ventricular hypertrophy on electrocardiogram	No					Yes					

(Continued)

Table 15-3. (Continued)

	Points										
	0	+1	+2	+3	+4	+5	+6	+7	+8	+9	+10
Women											
Age (years)	54-56	57-59	60-62	63-64	65-67	68-70	71-73	74-76	77-78	79-81	82-84
Untreated systolic blood (mm Hg)		95-106	107-118	119-130	131-143	144-155	156-167	168-180	181-192	193-204	205-216
Untreated systolic blood pressure (mm Hg)		95-106	107-118	119-130	131-143	144-155	156-167	168-180	181-192	193-204	205-216
Treated systolic blood pressure (mm Hg)		95-106	107-113	114-119	120-125	126-131	132-139	140-148	149-160	161-204	205-216
History of diabetes	No			Yes							
Cigarette smoking	No			Yes							
Cardiovascular disease	No		Yes								
Atrial fibrillation	No						Yes				
Left ventricular hypertrophy on electrocardiogram	No				Yes						

Source: Data from Sacco et al. (2006).

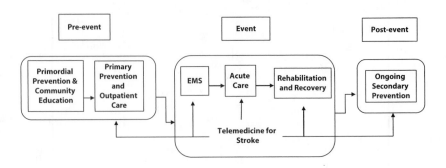

Source: Reprinted from CDC Stroke Registry (2016).

Figure 15-6. The Components of a Stroke System of Care

expected to play a pivotal role in stroke intervention at the population and community level (Mozaffarian et al. 2016; Willey et al. 2014). Meanwhile, three major components of a stroke system of care (pre-event, event, and post-event) have been addressed by the Centers for Disease Control and Prevention (CDC) State Heart Disease and Stroke Prevention Programs to highlight a comprehensive care of a stroke from primordial prevention to tertiary prevention (Figure 15-6; CDC Stroke Registry 2016; Schwamm et al. 2005).

Screening

Survivors of stroke or TIA are at increased risk for another stroke. All survivors should be monitored for hypertension on a routine basis. In addition to routine monitoring, antihypertensive treatment is recommended for prevention of recurrent stroke and other vascular events (Sacco et al. 2006). The National Institutes of Health (NIH) developed a scale known as the NIH Stroke Scale (NIHSS) to help diagnose stroke on the basis of the person's level of consciousness, eye muscle and visual impairments, facial muscle deficits, extremity muscle deficits, sensory deficits, and language and speech deficits. There are 11 criteria resulting in a total possible score ranging from 0 to 42. The NIHSS is one of the most widely used and validated scales. Adams et al. (1999) found that the baseline NIHSS score strongly predicted ischemic stroke outcome at seven days and three months. Previously, Goldstein et al. confirmed the reliability of the NIHSS score for both non-neurologists and neurologists (Goldstein et al. 2006; Goldstein and Samsa 1997).

Screening for AF (a powerful predictor for stroke) also plays a pivotal role in identifying patients at subclinical stages. Because it is often asymptomatic and likely frequently undetected clinically, studies have shown that screening for AF in patients with cryptogenic stroke or TIA by use of outpatient telemetry for 21 to 30 days has resulted in an AF detection rate of 12% to 23 (Durrant et al. 2013; Mozaffarian et al. 2016).

Treatment

Long-term effects of stroke can be devastating; therefore, initial assessment and proper management are crucial to minimizing complications and preventing recurrence. Some common medical complications of stroke include heart attack, heart failure, difficulty swallowing, aspiration pneumonia, deep vein thrombosis or pulmonary embolism, and residual paralysis. Regardless of whether an individual has a history of hypertension, it is important to acknowledge the severity of complications as approximately half of deaths after strokes are attributable to medical complications.

Treatment is also associated with a reduction of approximately 10 mm Hg systolic and 5 mm Hg diastolic blood pressure (Sacco et al. 2006). For survivors with diabetes, particular attention is placed in controlling blood pressure, lipids, glucose, and hemoglobin A1c (>7%). Stroke survivors with comorbid coronary artery disease or elevated cholesterol levels are similarly monitored to ensure proper lipid management following lifestyle modifications, dietary guidelines, and treatment recommendations (Sacco et al. 2006). Statin agents, in particular, are recommended in lowering cholesterol to reduce the risk of vascular events. Further research is needed to determine the efficacy of lipid management in preventing recurrent stroke or TIA events.

The landmark trial of thrombolytic therapy tissue plasminogen activator (t-PA) conducted by the National Institute of Neurological Disorders and Stroke Recombinant t-PA Stroke Study Group found that sufferers of ischemic stroke treated with t-PA within three hours after the onset of symptoms were at least 30% more likely than patients given placebo to have minimal or no disability at three months and one year. Current guidelines for the management of patients with acute ischemic stroke published by the American Heart Association Stroke Council include specific recommendations for the administration of intravenous recombinant tissue plasminogen activator (rtPA; Adams et al. 2007). Despite its effectiveness in improving neurological outcomes, the majority of patients with ischemic stroke are not treated with rtPA, largely because they arrive after the currently approved three-hour time limit for administration of the medication. One of the potential approaches for an increased treatment opportunity has been the designation of a longer time window for treatment. A recent prospective study, the European Cooperative Acute Stroke Study-3, has provided new data on rtPA treatment in the 3- to 4.5-hour window (Hacke et al. 2008).

Long-term goals include minimizing the physical manifestations of neurological deficits through physical therapy, speech and swallowing therapy, and occupational therapy, and minimizing the risk of recurrence of stroke, including antiplatelet or anticoagulation therapy as necessary, and strict control or modification of risk factors such as diabetes, dyslipidemia, hypertension, arrhythmias, and smoking cessation. As mentioned, equally important to the individual's recovery and long-term prognosis is addressing and preventing the common medical complications.

Examples of Evidence-Based Interventions

In 1998, Congress funded CDC to establish the National Heart Disease and Stroke Prevention Program, which helps build state- and local-level comprehensive heart disease and stroke programs. In 2001, following the death of Senator Paul Coverdell from a stroke, Congress funded CDC to establish the Paul Coverdell National Acute Stroke Registry (PCNASR). As of July 2015, CDC is funding nine states through the PCNASR program (California, Georgia, Massachusetts, Michigan, Minnesota, New York, Ohio, Washington, and Wisconsin). The goal of the PCNASR is to ensure that all stroke patients receive the highest quality acute stroke care available to reduce untimely deaths, prevent disability, and avoid recurrent strokes. The funded states are working on improving the care given to patients experiencing a stroke from the onset of stroke symptoms.

States will be working with EMS agencies to improve EMS care for suspected cases of stroke, the transition from EMS to hospital care, and the transition from the hospital to the next care setting. States are required to evaluate the effectiveness of implemented in-hospital and EMS quality improvement interventions and the transition from EMS to the hospital and transition-of-care protocols from hospital to transition-of-care systems (e.g., long-term care facility, rehabilitation center, primary care provider). Figure 15-6 depicts the components of a stroke system of care (CDC Stroke Registry 2016; Schwamm et al. 2005).

In 2007, CDC, The Joint Commission's Primary Stroke Center Certification program, and the AHA/ASA's Get With the Guidelines Stroke Program jointly released a set of standardized stroke performance measures to be used by all three programs. To enhance prevention efforts, several focused programs for heart and stroke risk reduction have been conducted. For example, the Mississippi Delta Health Collaborative (MDHC) is designed to prevent heart disease, stroke, and related chronic diseases. The MDHC targets the "ABCs" of heart and stroke prevention:

1. **A**spirin: Increase low-dose aspirin therapy according to recognized guidelines.
2. Hemoglobin **A**1c: Monitor and control blood glucose.
3. **B**lood pressure: Prevent and control high blood pressure.
4. **C**holesterol: Prevent and control high LDL-cholesterol.
5. **S**moking: Prevent initiation and increase cessation of smoking, and increase the percentage of the population protected by smoke-free air laws or regulations (CDC Coverdell 2011).

Areas of Future Research

Despite decreasing stroke incidence during the second half of the 20th century, stroke continues to be a major cause of death and disability worldwide. There has been increasing recognition that early risk factor detection and lifestyle modification can prevent or reduce stroke disease burden. Future research to detect surrogate and other potentially modifiable risk factors, including elevated cholesterol, BMI, and specific dietary patterns, is being defined. Further refinement is needed to promote specific interventions to high-risk populations (using risk assessment and other diagnostic tools). Guidelines are needed to tailor interventions to a variety of subpopulations. Creative methods to encourage lifestyle interventions such as diet and occupational and leisure physical activity along with appropriate treatment to reduce first or recurrent stroke and TIA is desired to combat the multifactoral nature of the disease. National initiatives partnered with community-based research will provide individual and population-level support to ensure that patients are properly screened, treated, and monitored for primary risk factors. As the world's population ages, development of effective methods of primary and secondary prevention of stroke will be crucial to reduce long-term disability and disease burden.

HEART FAILURE

Significance

Heart failure represents a new epidemic of CVD, affecting about 5.7 million Americans aged 20 years and older. It is estimated that about 915,000 new heart failure cases occur annually according to data from ARIC 2002–2012 (Mozaffarian et al. 2016). In 2013, heart failure any-mention mortality was 300,122 (140,126 men and 159,996 women) and heart failure was the underlying cause in 65,120 of those deaths (Mozaffarian et al. 2016). In contrast to other CVDs, the prevalence, incidence, and mortality from heart failure are increasing, and prognosis remains poor (Hunt et al. 2009; Liu 2011). Heart failure results in high hospitalization rates and mortality (up to 40% of patients die within one year of first hospitalization) making the survival rate bleaker than that for nearly all cancers.

In addition to the cost in human suffering, care for patients with heart failure places a large economic strain on the health care system, including the Medicare program. In 2012, total cost for heart failure was estimated to be $30.7 billion. Of this total, 68% was attributable to direct medical costs. Projections show that by 2030, the total cost of heart failure will increase almost 127% to $69.7 billion from 2012. This equals about $244 for every U.S. adult (Heidenreich et al. 2013; Mozaffarian et al. 2016).

Pathophysiology

Heart failure is a multisystem disorder characterized by abnormalities of cardiac function, skeletal muscle, renal function, stimulation of the sympathetic nervous system, and a complex pattern of neuro-hormonal changes that impairs the ability of either ventricle to fill with or eject blood (Jackson et al. 2000; Mann 1999). The cardinal manifestations of heart failure are dyspnea and fatigue, which may limit exercise tolerance, and fluid retention, which may lead to pulmonary and peripheral edema. Both abnormalities can impair the functional capacity and quality of life of affected individuals, but they may not necessarily dominate the clinical picture at the same time (Hunt et al. 2009).

Three clinical pathophysiological models (hypotheses) for heart failure have been suggested:

1. The cardio-renal model, in which heart failure is viewed as a problem of excessive salt and water retention that is caused by abnormalities of renal blood flow.
2. The cardio-circulatory, or hemodynamic, model, in which heart failure is thought to arise largely as a result of abnormalities in the pumping capacity of the heart and excessive peripheral vasoconstriction.
3. The neuro-hormonal model, in which heart failure progresses as a result of the overexpression of biologically active molecules that are capable of exerting toxic effects on the heart and circulation (Batlle et al. 2007; Mann and Bristow 2005).

In terms of left ventricular dysfunction, there are two mechanisms of reduced cardiac output: systolic dysfunction and diastolic dysfunction. Systolic dysfunction refers to impaired ventricular contraction. It is defined by a left-ventricular ejection fraction of less than 50%. The most common causes of systolic dysfunction are ischemic heart disease, idiopathic dilated cardiomyopathy, hypertension, and valvular heart disease. Diastolic dysfunction results from impaired myocardial relaxation, with increased stiffness in the ventricular wall and reduced left ventricular compliance, leading to impairment of diastolic ventricular filling. Diastolic dysfunction can occur in many of the same conditions that lead to systolic dysfunction. The most common causes of diastolic dysfunction are hypertension, ischemic heart disease, hypertrophic cardiomyopathy, and restrictive cardiomyopathy (Figueroa and Peters 2006; Liu 2011; Liu et al. 2009).

Descriptive Epidemiology

High-Risk Populations

Heart failure disproportionately affects the older population. The incidence of heart failure approaches 10 per 1,000 population after age 65 years, and approximately 80% of patients hospitalized with heart failure are aged older than 65 years (Hunt et al. 2009; Liu 2011; Liu et al. 2014; Liu et al. 2011). People with coronary artery disease, hypertension, and diabetes are at particular risk of developing heart failure. About 7 of 10 people with heart failure had high blood pressure before being diagnosed. About 22% of men and 46% of women will develop heart failure within six years of having a heart attack (Thom et al. 2006).

African Americans with heart failure are an average of 10 years younger than whites, have more hospital admissions and readmissions, and suffer a different spectrum of disease that predisposes them to heart failure. Specifically, African Americans have a higher incidence of hypertension, left ventricular hypertrophy, and diabetes (Liu et al. 2013; Yancy 2005; Yancy 2001). In MESA, African Americans had the highest risk of developing heart failure, followed by Hispanic, white, and Chinese Americans (4.6, 3.5, 2.4, and 1.0 per 1,000 person-years, respectively; Bahrami et al. 2008; Mozaffarian et al. 2016). Data from the ARIC study of the National Heart, Lung, and Blood Institute showed age-adjusted annual hospitalized heart failure incidence was highest for black men (15.7 per 1,000), followed by black women (13.3 per 1,000), white men (12.3 per 1000), and white women (9.9 per 1,000). This higher risk reflected differences in the prevalence of hypertension, diabetes, and low SES (Bahrami et al. 2008).

Geographic Distribution

Age-adjusted mortality rates for heart failure among all ages vary substantially across the United States. One study of fee-for-service Medicare beneficiaries aged 65 years and older who resided in the United States, Puerto Rico, or the U.S. Virgin Islands during the years 2000 to 2006 showed the average annual age-adjusted heart failure hospitalization rate per 1,000 Medicare beneficiaries was 21.5 per 1,000, and ranged from 7 to 61 per 1,000 among counties in the United States. For the total study population, a clear East–West gradient was evident, with the highest rates located primarily along the lower Mississippi River Valley and the Ohio River Valley, including the Appalachian region. Similar patterns were observed for blacks and whites, although the pattern for Hispanics differed (Casper et al. 2010).

Time Trends

Most current information on the epidemiology of heart failure is derived from several epidemiologic studies in the United States published since 1993 (Gillum 1993; Kannel 2000a; Liu et al. 2014). There have been several consistent findings, including a sharp increase in prevalence with age and strong male preponderance. The prevalence of heart failure has increased in the United States since 1980 in both sexes (Kannel 2000b; Kannel 2000a). From 1990 to 1999, the annual number of hospitalizations has increased from approximately 810,000 to more than one million for heart failure as a primary diagnosis and from 2.4 to 3.6 million for heart failure as a primary or secondary diagnosis (Haldeman et al. 1999; Hunt et al. 2009).

The aging of the post–World War II "baby boom" generation is likely to swell the number of patients with heart failure further (Young 2004). Data from the National Hospital Discharge Surveys between 1980 and 2006 suggested that of three major forms of cardiovascular disease, age-adjusted hospitalization rates in patients aged 65 years and older with primary diagnosis of CHD significantly decreased from early 1990s, and age-adjusted hospitalization rates in patients aged 65 years and older with a primary diagnosis of cerebrovascular disease significantly decreased from mid-1980s in both men and women. However, heart failure hospitalization rates have significantly increased, with an estimated annual rate increase of 1.20% in men and 1.55% in women (Liu et al. 2014).

Causes

Modifiable Risk Factors

The most common causes of heart failure are coronary artery disease, hypertension, diabetes, heart rhythm disorders (arrhythmias), congenital heart disease, and heart muscle disease (cardiomyopathy). Other risk factors associated with these diseases in general also contribute to heart failure by putting extra stress on the heart, including high cholesterol, cigarette smoking, alcohol abuse, and a family history of heart failure or other CVDs.

The odds of developing heart failure are especially high in people who have more than one of these risk factors. For example, a study of the predictors of heart failure among women with CHD found that those with diabetes had the highest risk of developing heart failure. Among diabetic participants with no additional risk factors, the annual incidence of heart failure was 3.0% compared with 8.2% among those with diabetes and at least three additional risk factors. Diabetic persons with fasting glucose greater than 300 mg/dL had a threefold adjusted risk of developing heart failure, compared with diabetic persons with controlled fasting blood sugar levels (Bibbins-Domingo et al. 2004; Liu et al. 2009; Thom et al. 2006). Multiple-comorbidity in patients with heart failure poses a serious clinical issue. In one study, of six selected comorbidities, about 50% of men and 40% of women with heart failure had coexisting CHD, the next common comorbidities being chronic obstructive pulmonary disease, diabetes, renal failure, and pneumonia (Liu 2011). Diet-related factors have been suggested as risk factors for heart failure, including vitamin D and leptin (Liu et al. 2010).

Population-Attributable Risk

Data from the Framingham Heart Study indicate that hypertension is one of the major predisposing risk factors for the development of heart failure in the general population. In terms of population-attributable risk, hypertension accounts for 39% of heart failure events in men and 59% in women. Myocardial infarction, despite only a 3% to 10% prevalence in the population, accounts for 34% of heart failure in men and 13% in women. Prevalence of diabetes in the Framingham cohort study was 8% in men and 5% in women. Diabetes accounted for 6% of heart failure in men and 12% in women (Kannel 2000b).

Evidence-Based Interventions

Early identification of heart failure risk factors and appropriate prevention and treatment will have the greatest impact in reducing progression of the disease.

Table 15-4. Heart Failure Classification

Level	Description	Simple Description
I	Cardiac disease without resulting limitations of physical activity.	Asymptomatic
II	Slight limitation of physical activity— comfortable at rest, but ordinary physical activity results in fatigue, dyspnea, or anginal pain.	Symptomatic with moderate exertion
III	Marked limitation in physical activity— comfortable at rest, but less than ordinary physical activity causes fatigue, dyspnea, or anginal pain.	Symptomatic with minimal exertion
IV	Inability to carry on any physical activity without discomfort of symptoms at rest.	Symptomatic at rest

Source: Compiled from Hunt et al. (2005) and Chavey et al. (2001).

Earlier guidelines for heart failure health care emphasized the functional status and appropriate treatment of patients with heart failure. According to the New York Heart Association Functional Classification, heart failure is classified into four classes that range from patients with asymptomatic left ventricular dysfunction (Class I) to those with severe symptoms at rest or with minimal exertion (Class IV; Table 15-4). This classification helps clinicians assess the severity of a patient's symptoms, guides the choice of therapy, and helps with subjective documentation of response or lack of response to therapy (Caboral and Mitchell 2003).

In 2001, to further emphasize prevention of heart failure, the American College of Cardiology (ACC) and the AHA created a new conceptual framework to help health professionals understand the continuum of disease progression in heart failure (Hunt et al. 2005). Rather than replacing the New York Heart Association classification, the framework defines disease progression in four stages—A, B, C, and D—beginning with patients who have risk factors for developing heart failure all the way to patients with end-stage disease (Hunt et al. 2009; Rasmusson et al. 2007). The ACC and AHA addressed these four stages in the development of heart failure and recommendations for preventing and treating heart failure by stages (Caboral and Mitchell 2003; Hunt et al. 2009; Rasmusson et al. 2007).

Patients in Stage A do not have any diagnosed structural heart disease but have risk factors that can lead to heart failure. At this stage, patient education is key, given that lifestyle modifications that reduce the risk of developing CVD include maintaining an appropriate diet, regular exercise, maintaining a normal BMI, smoking cessation, and limiting alcohol consumption.

Like patients in Stage A, those at Stage B are asymptomatic, but have either structural heart disease or evidence of left ventricular dysfunction. Treatments for Stage B are added to all those mentioned for Stage A, in an attempt to prevent the development of overt, symptomatic heart failure. Medications are requested for patients when appropriate.

Patients in Stage C have structural heart disease and current or previous symptoms of heart failure, such as reduced activity tolerance, dyspnea, and fluid retention. Recommended therapies for patients with Stage C are the same as those for patients with Stages A and B. But because these patients are symptomatic, most patients receive medications (such as a diuretic and digoxin along with angiotensin-converting enzyme inhibitors, angiotensin-receptor blockers, and ß blockers). Other important measures include sodium restriction, administration of the influenza and pneumococcal vaccine, and physical activity, except for patients in an acute decompensated state.

Stage D is reserved for patients with end-stage heart failure. These patients are markedly symptomatic, despite maximal tolerated therapy. In addition to the care outlined for patients in Stages A to C, these patients usually require specialized interventions to control and manage their heart failure such as mechanical assist devices (biventricular pacemaker or left ventricular assist device).

Because of the clear-cut relationship between preventable difficulties such as coronary heart disease and the tremendous burdens of heart failure medications, comorbidity, and mortality (Stages C and D), a great deal of attention should be focused on preventing the development of ventricular dysfunction in the first place. Clearly, early identification and prevention for patients at risk for heart failure (Stages A and B) are critical to control heart failure.

Examples of Evidence-Based Interventions

As the overwhelming majority of heart failure cases are traced to three preventable and treatable conditions (hypertension, coronary artery disease, and diabetes), prevention and treatment of these conditions and risk factors is the focus of efforts to reduce incidence of heart failure (Baker 2002). For example, several studies have shown that treating elevated blood pressure can dramatically decrease the risk of developing heart failure (Baker 2002; Dahlöf et al. 1991; Kostis et al. 1997). Results from the Swedish Trial in Old Patients with Hypertension indicated that treatment of hypertension reduced the risk of developing heart failure from 4.8% to 2.3%, a 52% relative reduction in those who received active treatment compared with the placebo (Dahlöf et al. 1991). Among patients with diabetes, controlling hypertension and hyperglycemia is also critical for preventing heart failure. In the U.K. Prospective Diabetes Study Group, for example, effective blood pressure control reduced the relative risk of developing heart failure by a dramatic 56%, compared with those who received less-effective blood pressure control (U.K. Prospective Diabetes Study Group 1998).

Areas of Future Research

Over the past decade, although there have been many studies on the etiology of heart failure and advances in the care of patients with heart failure, the causes remain poorly understood and the prognosis remains poor. Further research should include

1. Identifying heart failure risk factors to develop more effective methods of primary prevention, including studies of diet and particular nutrients.
2. Continued studies of secondary prevention of heart failure to reduce the mortality of heart failure and to improve quality of life for patients with heart failure.
3. Continued studies using multidisciplinary approaches, including pharmacoepidemiology, because patients with heart failure are typically older adults with complex drug regimens for heart failure, multiple concurrent diagnoses, and resulting polypharmacy.
4. Community-based studies, along with regional, national, and international cooperative studies, to identify specific prevention and treatment strategies for heart failure among different populations.

PERIPHERAL ARTERIAL DISEASE

Significance

Peripheral arterial disease causes functional morbidity and increases the risk for other CVD morbidity and mortality. It is associated with intermittent claudication, a classic presentation that involves calf pain and other symptoms (Herrington et al. 2016; Mozaffarian et al. 2016). However, intermittent claudication is now believed to be present in only approximately 10% of the estimated eight million U.S. adults with PAD (Mozaffarian et al. 2016; Roger et al. 2011). Large numbers of individuals with PAD report different constellations of leg symptoms and a substantial subgroup (estimated at 40%) presents without pain (Mozaffarian et al. 2016). However, when present, the pain of PAD is strongly associated with diminished functional status and quality of life.

Individuals with asymptomatic PAD have also been found to be at significant risk for decline in lower limb functioning (McDermott 2006). Peripheral arterial disease is a leading cause of lower limb amputation in the United States and accounted for $3.9 billion worth of health care expenses by the Medicare program in 2001, most of it going toward inpatient hospital stays (Hirsch et al. 2008). Annual Medicare spending for PAD is comparable with annual spending for congestive heart failure and cerebrovascular disease.

The major public health burden of PAD stems from its strong association with CVD mortality—individuals with PAD are more than three times more likely to experience CVD death than like-aged non-PAD patients (Heald et al. 2006). This excess risk of CVD mortality in PAD patients is independent of the effects of other CVD risk factors (McDermott 2006) and represents a very large attributable mortality risk because baseline CVD death rates are high in the older age groups most affected by PAD. The five-year all-cause mortality rate in PAD patients is higher than that among those with either breast cancer or Hodgkin's disease (Criqui 2001). Finally, in addition to the morbidity associated with lower limb function and the mortality burden, there is a growing body of evidence linking PAD with cognitive decline (Rafnsson et al. 2009).

Pathophysiology

Peripheral arterial disease is a condition involving atherosclerosis of the lower extremities, which is common in older populations. Peripheral arterial disease is caused by atherosclerosis of the arteries—consequently, its pathophysiology is not unique from that of other atherosclerosis-related CVDs. The presence of PAD is, therefore, a strong indication that there are also atherosclerotic manifestations in other vascular territories—particularly the heart or brain.

In epidemiologic studies, PAD is typically confirmed with the ankle–brachial index (ABI)—a ratio of Doppler-recorded systolic blood pressure in the upper compared with the lower extremities. An ABI below 0.90 is the conventional cutpoint for PAD case confirmation. Confirmed coronary atherosclerosis is found in very large proportions of patients diagnosed with PAD and also in patients with borderline ABI values (McDermott 2006). Peripheral arterial disease appears to be more frequently associated with disease at multiple vascular territories than either coronary artery disease or cerebrovascular disease (Steg et al. 2007) and, moreover, the coronary atherosclerosis present in patients with concomitant PAD tends to be more severe than that found in patients with coronary disease alone (Brevetti et al. 2009).

Descriptive Epidemiology

Prevalence of ABI-defined PAD in individuals aged 40 years or older was estimated at 4.3%, according to NHANES 2000 data (Selvin and Erlinger 2004).

Prevalence is strongly associated with age, even within older age groups (Ostchega et al. 2007) and approximately doubles with each successive decade after age 40 (Allison et al. 2007). The prevalence estimates for the U.S. population aged 65 years or older range from 12% to 20% (Lloyd-Jones et al. 2009). Strong sex differences in PAD prevalence have not been consistently documented. However, data from the Chronic Renal Insufficiency Cohort showed that female chronic kidney disease patients had a higher PAD risk compared with male chronic kidney disease patients at younger ages (Wang et al. 2016).

Peripheral arterial disease prevalence in African Americans aged 50 years or older is at least two-fold higher than in non-Hispanic whites (Allison et al. 2007). Prevalence in Hispanic Americans is similar to, or perhaps modestly higher, than that for non-Hispanic whites (Allison et al. 2007; Criqui et al. 2005). Globally, PAD disproportionately affects low- or middle-income counties (LMIC). It is estimated that 202 million people were living with PAD in 2010, 69.7% of them in low- or middle-income counties, including 54.8 million in Southeast Asia and 45.9 million in the Western Pacific Region. During the preceding decade, the number of individuals with PAD increased by 28.7% in low- or middle-income counties and 13.1% in high-income countries (Fowkes et al. 2013).

Prevalence of PAD may be underestimated because individuals with PAD who have undergone revascularization procedures may have normal ABIs and because up to 25% of individuals with ABIs in the 0.90 to 0.99 range, above the conventional cutpoint for defining PAD, may actually have disease (Allison et al. 2007).

Causes

Individuals with diabetes, hypertension, and renal disease have a higher prevalence of PAD. According to NHANES 2000 data for individuals aged older than 40 years, prevalence of PAD was more than 10% among those with diabetes and nearly 7% in those with hypertension (Selvin and Erlinger 2004). Patients with renal insufficiency also appear to have at least double the PAD prevalence of those with normal kidney function (Selvin and Erlinger 2004) and prospective data from the ARIC cohort suggest that individuals with chronic kidney disease had a 1.5-fold higher risk for developing incident PAD than do those with normal kidney function (Wattanakit et al. 2007).

In addition to age and the high-risk groups noted in the previous paragraphs, the constellation of risk factors for PAD is similar to those for other

CVDs. Smoking has a particularly strong effect. A cohort study of PAD inci-dence suggested a 2.55 increased PAD risk associated with current smoking (Newman et al. 1993), and case–control studies estimating current smoking relative risks yield even higher estimates (Cole et al. 1993). The prevalence ratio of PAD in current compared with never smokers is nearly seven (Selvin and Erlinger 2004). In a study of individuals with diabetes, and therefore already at high risk for PAD, active smoking was still associated with a doubling of PAD incidence (Wattanakit et al. 2007). Hypertension and dyslipidemia rel-ative risks are more modest than those for smoking or diabetes (Criqui 2001; Selvin and Erlinger 2004).

A recent, large, cross-sectional study of patients with PAD in France suggested that isolated systolic hypertension occurred more commonly among patients with PAD than coronary artery disease or CVD—a finding worthy of follow-up in epidemiologic studies (Safar et al. 2009). Findings from a recent meta-analysis of 22 studies from high-income countries and 12 from low- or middle-income countries suggest that smoking had the strongest effect on PAD, with meta-odds ratio for current smoking of 2.72 (95% CI = 2.39, 3.09) in high-income countries and 1.42 (95% CI = 1.25, 1.62) in low- or middle-income counties, followed by diabetes (1.88; 95% CI = 1.66, 2.14 vs. 1.47; 95% CI = 1.29, 1.68), hypertension (1.55; 95% CI = 1.42, 1.71 vs. 1.36; 95% CI = 1.24, 1.50), and hypercholesterol-emia (1.19; 95% CI = 1.07, 1.33 vs. 1.14; 95% CI = 1.03, 1.25; Fowkes et al. 2013).

Two less-traditional PAD risk factors worth considering as research moves forward are inflammatory biomarkers and genetics. Prospective studies of large cohorts have suggested that CRP, interleukin 6 (IL-6), tumor necrosis factor-alpha (TNF-α), and certain other circulating markers of inflamma-tion, are significant predictors of symptomatic PAD incidence (McDermott and Lloyd-Jones 2009; Pradhan et al. 2008; Ridker et al. 2001). In large cross-sectional studies, CRP levels were significantly different in those with and without prevalent PAD (Selvin and Erlinger 2004). Inflammatory bio-markers also have been significantly associated with all-cause mortality risk through two years of follow-up in a small cohort of PAD patients (Vidula et al. 2008). While not directly modifiable risk factors, CRP and other inflam-matory factors may ultimately prove useful as component biomarkers in the assessment of subclinical PAD, PAD severity, or treatment responsiveness.

As with other CVDs, genetic susceptibility likely plays a role in PAD eti-ology, but the mechanisms are complex, involving multiple genes and gene–environment interactions. The limited number of family studies of PAD completed to date do support a role for heritable genetics in PAD etiology—it is estimated that heritability of PAD ranges from 20% to 45%—but candidate gene studies have not yielded putative PAD risk genes (Knowles et al. 2007; McDermott and Lloyd-Jones 2009). Larger candidate gene studies are now underway with researchers also now contemplating the optimal strategies needed to mount large genome-wide association studies that could potentially reveal common genetic variants associated with PAD.

Evidence-Based Interventions

Strategies for primary prevention of PAD do not differ from those for any atherosclerotic chronic disease and will not be discussed here in detail. With respect to treatment, the foundational intervention for the management of symptomatic PAD is exercise. Exercise is hypothesized to improve PAD symptoms via adaptive responses of the muscle or increasing collateral blood flow in the affected limbs (Carman and Fernandez 2006). Higher levels of physical activity have been associated with increased survival among PAD patients (Garg et al. 2006). Smoking cessation is also advised for the improvement of leg pain symptoms of PAD (Hankey et al. 2006).

More recently, options for pharmacological therapy of symptomatic PAD have become available including statins, clopidogrel, and cilostazol (Camm et al. 2012; Garg et al. 2006; Hankey et al. 2006; Rooke et al. 2011).

By far, the single biggest issue related to PAD prevention and control, from a public health perspective, is secondary prevention. Given the high risk of mortality from CVD-related events among patients with PAD, individuals diagnosed with PAD are obvious candidates for interventions designed to reduce CHD and stroke risks. The pursuit of appropriate atherothrombotic risk factor reduction is a cornerstone of PAD treatment guidelines. Smoking cessation, blood pressure control, and cholesterol lowering have been linked with decreased CVD mortality, and blood glucose control and weight loss have been connected with other benefits. Antiplatelet therapy, including aspirin, has been demonstrated in multiple studies to prevent progression of atherosclerosis in patients with PAD, and in some studies to prevent CVD mortality.

Peripheral arterial disease researchers have advocated the use of more formal clinical staging approaches for PAD patients to guide intensity of intervention (Haugen et al. 2007). However, at the same time, studies have shown that physician awareness of the strong link between PAD and future cardiovascular events is low (Banerjee et al. 2010; Gornik and Creager 2006). Also well documented is the fact that PAD patients are less likely to receive CVD risk reduction pharmacotherapy than patients with atherosclerotic disease in other vascular beds (Bennett et al. 2009; Cacoub et al. 2009). This suggests that patients diagnosed with PAD are not receiving potentially effective interventions as often as indicated.

The REACH Registry, an international, prospective, observational registry of more than 68,000 patients with coronary artery disease, cerebrovascular disease, or PAD, recently reported that PAD patients had significantly fewer CVD risk factors under control than did the patients in either of the other two diagnostic groups (Cacoub et al. 2009). Moreover, as mentioned earlier, a large proportion of PAD is currently undiagnosed, implying a pressing need to improve disease detection. The ABI measure, though inexpensive and noninvasive, unfortunately has not been found sufficiently sensitive to be used as a population-based screening tool (Hankey et al. 2006) and secondary prevention in asymptomatic PAD patients is largely still a function of direct recognition of adverse CVD risk factor profiles. As a consequence, the vigilant monitoring of and intervention on classic CVD risk factors remains the most promising path for secondary prevention of PAD moving forward (Fowkes et al. 2013).

In instances in which limb pain is severely disabling or the limb is threatened because of ulceration or gangrene, endovascular surgical procedures, such as angioplasty with and without stents and arterial bypass surgery, are recommended; however, it has been argued that the evidence supporting efficacy of such procedures for PAD is much weaker than that for coronary artery disease (Cao and De Rango 2009). Despite this, endovascular procedures for PAD are one of the fastest growing surgical procedures in the United States (Almahameed and Bhatt 2006).

Resources

American College of Cardiology, http://www.acc.org

American Diabetes Association, http://www.diabetes.org

American Heart Association, http://www.heart.org/HEARTORG

American Stroke Association, http://www.strokeassociation.org/STROKEORG

American Society of Hypertension, http://www.ash-us.org

Centers for Disease Control and Prevention, Division for Heart Disease and Stroke Prevention, http://www.cdc.gov/DHDSP

Framingham Heart Study, http://www.framinghamheartstudy.org

Heart Failure Online, http://www.heartfailure.org

Heart Failure Society of America, http://www.hfsa.org

National Heart, Lung, and Blood Institute, http://www.nhlbi.nih.gov

National Institute of Neurological Disorders and Stroke, http://www.ninds.nih.gov

National Center for Health Statistics Fast Stats, http://www.cdc.gov/nchs/fastats/ heart-disease.htm and http://www.cdc.gov/nchs/fastats/stroke.htm

World Health Organization, cardiovascular diseases, http://www.who.int/topics/ cardiovascular_diseases/en

Suggested Reading

Heidenreich PA, Albert NM, Allen LA, et al. Forecasting the impact of heart failure in the United States: a policy statement from the American Heart Association. *Circ Heart Fail.* 2013,6(3):606–619.

Labarthe DR. *Epidemiology and Prevention of Cardiovascular Diseases—A Global Challenge.* 2nd ed. Burlington, MA: Jones and Bartlett Publishers; 2011.

Lloyd-Jones D, Adams R, Carnethon M, et al. Heart disease and stroke statistics—2009 update: a report from the American Heart Association Statistics Committee and Stroke Statistics Subcommittee. *Circulation.* 2009,119(3):480–486.

McMurray JJ, Stewart S. Epidemiology, aetiology, and prognosis of heart failure. *Heart.* 2000,83(5):596–602.

Mozaffarian D, Benjamin EJ, Go AS, et al. Executive summary: heart disease and stroke statistics—2016 update. A report from the American Heart Association. *Circulation.* 2016:133(4):447–454.

O'Donnell CJ, Elosua R. Cardiovascular risk factors. Insights from Framingham Heart Study [in Spanish]. *Rev Esp Cardiol.* 2008,61(3):299–310. Available in English at: http:// www.revespcardiol.org/en/factores-riesgo-cardiovascular-perspectivas-derivadas/ articulo/13117552.

Rooke TW, Hirsch AT, Misra S, et al. 2011 ACCF/AHA focused update of the guideline for the management of patients with peripheral artery disease (updating the 2005 guideline): a report of the American College of Cardiology Foundation/American Heart Association Task Force on Practice Guidelines. *J Am Coll Cardiol.* 2011,58(19): 2020–2045.

References

Abbott RD, Donahue RP, MacMahon SW, Reed DM, Yano K. Diabetes and the risk of stroke. The Honolulu Heart Program. *JAMA.* 1987;257(7):949–952.

Adams H, Davis P, Leira E, et al. Baseline NIH Stroke Scale score strongly predicts outcome after stroke: a report of the Trial of Org 10172 in Acute Stroke Treatment (TOAST). *Neurology.* 1999;53(1):126–126.

Adams HP, del Zoppo G, Alberts MJ, et al. Guidelines for the early management of adults with ischemic stroke: a guideline from the American Heart Association/American Stroke Association Stroke Council, Clinical Cardiology Council, Cardiovascular Radiology and Intervention Council, and the Atherosclerotic Peripheral Vascular Disease and Quality of Care Outcomes in Research Interdisciplinary Working Groups: the American Academy of Neurology affirms the value of this guideline as an educational tool for neurologists. *Circulation.* 2007;115(20):e478–e534.

Allison MA, Ho E, Denenberg JO, et al. Ethnic-specific prevalence of peripheral arterial disease in the United States. *Am J Prev Med.* 2007;32(4):328–333.

Almahameed A, Bhatt DL. Contemporary management of peripheral arterial disease: III. Endovascular and surgical management. *Cleve Clin J Med.* 2006;73(suppl 4):S45–S51.

Altman R, Nunez de Ybarra J, Villablanca AC. Community-based cardiovascular disease prevention to reduce cardiometabolic risk in Latina women: a pilot program. *J Womens Health.* 2014;23(4):350–357.

American Diabetes Association (ADA). Statistics about diabetes. 2014. Available at: http://www.diabetes.org/diabetes-basics/statistics. Accessed August 26, 2016.

Anderson RN, Kochanek KD, Murphy SL. Report of final mortality statistics, 1995. *Mon Vital Stat Rep.* 1997;45(11 suppl 2):1–40.

Bahrami H, Kronmal R, Bluemke DA, et al. Differences in the incidence of congestive heart failure by ethnicity: the Multi-Ethnic Study of Atherosclerosis. *Arch Intern Med.* 2008;168(19):2138–2145.

Baker DW. Prevention of heart failure. *J Card Fail.* 2002;8(5):333–346.

Balkau B, Mhamdi L, Oppert J-M, et al. Physical activity and insulin sensitivity. *Diabetes.* 2008;57(10):2613–2618.

Banerjee A, Fowkes FG, Rothwell PM. Associations between peripheral artery disease and ischemic stroke: implications for primary and secondary prevention. *Stroke.* 2010;41(9):2102–2107.

Barrett-Connor E, Orchard T. Diabetes and heart disease. In: National Diabetes Data Group, ed. *Diabetes in America: Diabetes Data Compiled 1984.* Bethesda, MD: National Institute of Arthritis, Diabetes, and Digestive and Kidney Diseases; 1985;16:1–41.

Batlle M, Perez-Villa F, Garcia-Pras E, et al. Down-regulation of matrix metalloproteinase-9 (MMP-9) expression in the myocardium of congestive heart failure patients. *Transplant Proc.* 2007;39(7):2344–2346.

Bax JJ, Young LW, Frye RL, et al. Screening for coronary artery disease in patients with diabetes. *Diabetes Care.* 2007;30(10):2729–2736.

Benderly M, Haim M, Boyko V, Goldbourt U. Socioeconomic status indicators and incidence of heart failure among men and women with coronary heart disease. *J Card Fail.* 2013;19(2):117–124.

Bennett PC, Silverman S, Gill P. Hypertension and peripheral arterial disease. *J Hum Hypertens.* 2009;23(3):213–215.

Bernstein AM, de Koning L, Flint AJ, Rexrode KM, Willett WC. Soda consumption and the risk of stroke in men and women. *Am J Clin Nutr.* 2012;95(5):1190–1199.

Bibbins-Domingo K, Lin F, Vittinghoff E, et al. Predictors of heart failure among women with coronary disease. *Circulation.* 2004;110(11):1424–1430.

Bild DE, Bluemke DA, Burke GL, et al. Multi-Ethnic Study of Atherosclerosis: objectives and design. *Am J Epidemiol.* 2002;156(9):871–881.

Bjartveit K, Tverdal A. Health consequences of sustained smoking cessation. *Tob Control.* 2009;18(3):197–205.

Blackburn H. Ancel Keys Lecture. The three beauties. Bench, clinical, and population research. *Circulation.* 1992;86(4):1323–1331.

Blair SN, Kohl HW III, Paffenbarger RS II, et al. Physical fitness and all-cause mortality. A prospective study of healthy men and women. *JAMA.* 1989;262(17):2395–2401.

Brevetti G, Sirico G, Giugliano G, et al. Prevalence of hypoechoic carotid plaques in coronary artery disease: relationship with coexistent peripheral arterial disease and leukocyte number. *Vasc Med.* 2009;14(1):13–19.

Broadley SA, Jørgensen L, Cheek A, et al. Early investigation and treatment of obstructive sleep apnoea after acute stroke. *J Clin Neurosci.* 2007;14(4):328–333.

Caboral M, Mitchell J. New guidelines for heart failure focus on prevention. *Nurse Pract.* 2003;28(1):13,16, 22–23; quiz 24–15.

Cacoub PP, Abola MTB, Baumgartner I, et al. Cardiovascular risk factor control and outcomes in peripheral artery disease patients in the Reduction of Atherothrombosis for Continued Health (REACH) Registry. *Atherosclerosis.* 2009;204(2):e86–e92.

Camm AJ, Lip GY, De Caterina R, et al. 2012 focused update of the ESC Guidelines for the management of atrial fibrillation. *Eur Heart J.* 2012;33(21):2719–2747.

Canoy D, Cairns BJ, Balkwill A, et al. Body mass index and incident coronary heart disease in women: a population-based prospective study. *BMC Med.* 2013;11:87.

Cao P, De Rango P. Endovascular treatment of peripheral artery disease (PAD): so old yet so far from evidence! *Eur J Vasc Endovasc Surg.* 2009;37(5):501–503.

Carman TL, Fernandez BB II. Contemporary management of peripheral arterial disease: II. Improving walking distance and quality of life. *Cleve Clin J Med.* 2006; 73(suppl 4):S38–S44.

Casper M, Nwaise I, Croft JB, et al. Geographic disparities in heart failure hospitalization rates among Medicare beneficiaries. *J Am Coll Cardiol.* 2010;55(4):294–299.

Caswell J. When risk factors unite. American Heart Association. *Stroke Connection Magazine.* January/February 2005:18–21.

Centers for Disease Control and Prevention (CDC). Chronic disease reports: coronary heart disease mortality—United States, 1986. *MMWR Morb Mortal Wkly Rep.* 1989;38(16):285–288.

Centers for Disease Control and Prevention (CDC). Public health focus: physical activity and the prevention of coronary heart disease. 1993. Available at: http://www.cdc.gov/mmwr/preview/mmwrhtml/00021477.htm. Accessed May 26, 2016.

Centers for Disease Control and Prevention (CDC). Changes in mortality from heart failure—United States, 1980–1995. *MMWR Morb Mortal Wkly Rep.* 1998;47(30):633–637.

Centers for Disease Control and Prevention (CDC). State-specific cholesterol screening trends—United States, 1991–1999. *MMWR Morb Mortal Wkly Rep.* 2000;49(33):750–755.

Centers for Disease Control and Prevention (CDC). Prevalence and most common causes of disability among adults—United States, 2005. *MMWR Morb Mortal Wkly Rep.* 2009a;58(16):421–426.

Centers for Disease Control and Prevention (CDC). Prevention: prevalence of stroke—United States, 2006–2010. *MMWR Morb Mortal Wkly Rep.* 2012;61(20):379–382.

Centers for Disease Control and Prevention (CDC). Tobacco-related mortality. 2016a. Available at: https://www.cdc.gov/tobacco/data_statistics/fact_sheets/health_effects/tobacco_related_mortality. Accessed August 26, 2016.

Centers for Disease Control and Prevention (CDC). Early release of selected estimates based on data from the National Health Interview Survey, 2014. 2016b. Available at: http://www.cdc.gov/nchs/data/nhis/earlyrelease/earlyrelease201506.pdf. Accessed August 26, 2016.

Centers for Disease Control and Prevention (CDC) Coverdell. National Heart Disease and Stroke Prevention Program. 2011. Available at: http://www.cdc.gov/dhdsp/programs/spha/docs/orientation_manual.pdf. Accessed August 26, 2016.

Centers for Disease Control and Prevention, National Center for Health Statistics (CDC NCHS). Mortality multiple cause micro-data files, 2013, public-use data file and documentation. NHLBI Tabulations. 2013. Available at: http://www.cdc.gov/nchs/data_access/Vitalstatsonline.htm#Mortality_. Accessed March, 15, 2016.

Centers for Disease Control and Prevention, National Center for Health Statistics (CDC NCHS). Underlying cause of death 1999–2014 on CDC WONDER online database. Multiple cause of death files. 2015. Available at: http://wonder.cdc.gov/ucd-icd10.html. Accessed August 16, 2016.

Centers for Disease Control and Prevention (CDC) Stroke Registry. CDC State Heart Disease and Stroke Prevention Programs. 2016. Available at: http://www.cdc.gov/dhdsp/programs/stroke_registry.htm. Accessed February 16, 2016.

Chavey WE II, Blaum CS, Bleske BE, Harrison RV, Kesterson S, Nicklas JM. Guideline for the management of heart failure caused by systolic dysfunction: part I. Guideline development, etiology, and diagnosis. *Am Fam Physician.* 2001:64(5):769–774.

Chen J, Wu X, Gu D. Hypertension and cardiovascular diseases intervention in the Capital Steel and Iron Company and Beijing Fangshan community. *Obes Rev.* 2008;9(suppl 1):142–145.

Cheng S, Claggett B, Correia A, et al. Temporal trends in the population attributable risk for coronary heart disease: Atherosclerosis Risk in Communities Study. *Circulation.* 2014;130(10):820–828.

Cole CW, Hill G, Farzad E, et al. Cigarette smoking and peripheral arterial occlusive disease. *Surgery.* 1993;114(4):753–753.

Collins R, Peto R, MacMahon S, et al. Blood pressure, stroke, and coronary heart disease. Part 2, Short-term reductions in blood pressure: overview of randomised drug trials in their epidemiological context. *Lancet.* 1990;335(8693):827–838.

Corti MC, Guralnik JM, Bilato C. Coronary heart disease risk factors in older persons. *Aging (Milan)*. 1996;8(2):75–89.

Criqui MH. Peripheral arterial disease—epidemiological aspects. *Vasc Med*. 2001; 6(1 suppl):3–7.

Criqui MH, Vargas V, Denenberg JO, et al. Ethnicity and peripheral arterial disease the San Diego Population Study. *Circulation*. 2005;112(17):2703–2707.

Dahlöf B, Lindholm LH, Hansson L, Scherstén B, Ekbom T, Wester PO. Morbidity and mortality in the Swedish Trial in Old Patients With Hypertension (STOP-Hypertension). *Lancet*. 1991;338(8778):1281–1285.

Danesh J, Lewington S. Plasma homocysteine and coronary heart disease: systematic review of published epidemiological studies. *J Cardiovasc Risk*. 1998;5(4):229–232.

Danesh J, Wheeler JG, Hirschfield GM, et al. C-reactive protein and other circulating markers of inflammation in the prediction of coronary heart disease. *N Engl J Med*. 2004;350(14):1387–1397.

Danesh J, Whincup P, Walker M, et al. Low grade inflammation and coronary heart disease: prospective study and updated meta-analyses. *BMJ*. 2000;321(7255):199–204.

de Andrade M, Thandi I, Brown S, Gotto A II, Patsch W, Boerwinkle E. Relationship of the apolipoprotein E polymorphism with carotid artery atherosclerosis. *Am J Hum Genet*. 1995;56(6):1379–1390.

Després J-P. Body fat distribution and risk of cardiovascular disease. *Circulation*. 2012;126(10):1301–1313.

Diez-Roux AV, Nieto FJ, Muntaner C, et al. Neighborhood environments and coronary heart disease: a multilevel analysis. *Am J Epidemiol*. 1997;146(1):48–63.

Do R, Willer CJ, Schmidt EM, et al. Common variants associated with plasma triglycerides and risk for coronary artery disease. *Nat Genet*. 2013;45(11):1345–1352.

Durrant J, Lip GY, Lane DA. Stroke risk stratification scores in atrial fibrillation: current recommendations for clinical practice and future perspectives. *Expert Rev Cardiovasc Ther*. 2013;11(1):77–90.

Eastern Stroke and Coronary Heart Disease (ESCHD) Collaborative Research Group. Blood pressure, cholesterol, and stroke in eastern Asia. *Lancet*. 1998;352(9143):1801–1807.

Ebell MH. Should family physicians use coronary artery calcium scores to screen for coronary artery disease? *Am Fam Physician*. 2012;86(5):405–406.

Ellis RW. Infection and coronary heart disease. *J Med Microbiol*. 1997;46(7):535–539.

Emerging Risk Factors (ERF) Collaboration, Di Angelantonio E, Sarwar N, et al. Major lipids, apolipoproteins, and risk of vascular disease. *JAMA*. 2009;302(18):1993–2000.

Epstein DE, Sherwood A, Smith PJ, et al. Determinants and consequences of adherence to the DASH diet in African American and white adults with high blood pressure: results from the ENCORE trial. *J Acad Nutr Diet*. 2012;112(11):1763–1773.

Estruch R, Ros E, Salas-Salvadó J, et al. Primary prevention of cardiovascular disease with a Mediterranean diet. *N Engl J Med*. 2013;368(14):1279–1290.

Fibrinogen Studies Collaboration, Danesh J, Lewington S, et al. Plasma fibrinogen level and the risk of major cardiovascular diseases and nonvascular mortality: an individual participant meta-analysis. *JAMA*. 2005;294(14):1799–1809.

Figueroa MS, Peters JI. Congestive heart failure: diagnosis, pathophysiology, therapy, and implications for respiratory care. *Respir Care*. 2006;51(4):403–412.

Finegold JA, Asaria P, Francis DP. Mortality from ischaemic heart disease by country, region, and age: statistics from World Health Organisation and United Nations. *Int J Cardiol*. 2013;168(2):934–945.

Folsom AR, Eckfeldt JH, Weitzman S, et al. Relation of carotid artery wall thickness to diabetes mellitus, fasting glucose and insulin, body size, and physical activity. Atherosclerosis Risk in Communities (ARIC) Study Investigators. *Stroke*. 1994;25(1):66–73.

Folsom AR, Wu KK, Shahar E, Davis CE. Association of hemostatic variables with prevalent cardiovascular disease and asymptomatic carotid artery atherosclerosis. The Atherosclerosis Risk in Communities (ARIC) Study Investigators. *Arterioscler Thromb*. 1993;13(12):1829–1836.

Ford ES, Ajani UA, Croft JB, et al. Explaining the decrease in US deaths from coronary disease, 1980–2000. *N Engl J Med*. 2007;356(23):2388–2398.

Fowkes FG, Rudan D, Rudan I, et al. Comparison of global estimates of prevalence and risk factors for peripheral artery disease in 2000 and 2010: a systematic review and analysis. *Lancet*. 2013;382(9901):1329–1340.

Fox CS. Cardiovascular disease risk factors, type 2 diabetes mellitus, and the Framingham Heart Study. *Trends Cardiovasc Med*. 2010;20(3):90–95.

Franklin SS, Gokhale SS, Chow VH, et al. Does low diastolic blood pressure contribute to the risk of recurrent hypertensive cardiovascular disease events? The Framingham Heart Study. *Hypertension*. 2015;65(2):299–305.

Franks P, Winters PC, Tancredi DJ, Friscella KA. Do changes in traditional coronary heart disease risk factors over time explain the association between socio-economic status and coronary heart disease? *BMC Cardiovasc Disord*. 2011;11:28.

Freedman DS, Williamson DF, Croft JB, Ballew C, Byers T. Relation of body fat distribution to ischemic heart disease. The National Health and Nutrition Examination Survey I (NHANES I) Epidemiologic Follow-up Study. *Am J Epidemiol.* 1995;142(1):53–63.

Furie KL, Kasner SE, Adams RJ, et al. Guidelines for the prevention of stroke in patients with stroke or transient ischemic attack: a guideline for healthcare professionals from the American Heart Association/American Stroke Association. *Stroke.* 2011;42(1): 227–276.

Garg PK, Tian L, Criqui MH, et al. Physical activity during daily life and mortality in patients with peripheral arterial disease. *Circulation.* 2006;114(3):242–248.

Gillespie CD, Wigington C, Hong Y. Coronary heart disease and stroke deaths— United States, 2009. *MMWR Suppl.* 2013;62(3):157–160.

Gillum RF. Epidemiology of heart failure in the United States. *Am Heart J.* 1993;126(4): 1042–1047.

Glantz SA, Parmley WW. Passive smoking and heart disease. Epidemiology, physiology, and biochemistry. *Circulation.* 1991;83(1):1–12.

Goldman LE, Cook F. Reasons for the decline in coronary heart disease mortality: medical interventions versus life-style changes. In: Higgins MW, Luepker RV, eds. *Trends in Coronary Heart Disease Mortality: The Influence of Medical Care.* New York, NY: Oxford University Press; 1988:67–75.

Goldstein LB, Adams R, Alberts MJ, et al. Primary prevention of ischemic stroke: a guideline from the American Heart Association/American Stroke Association Stroke Council: cosponsored by the Atherosclerotic Peripheral Vascular Disease Interdisciplinary Working Group; Cardiovascular Nursing Council; Clinical Cardiology Council; Nutrition, Physical Activity, and Metabolism Council; and the Quality of Care and Outcomes Research Interdisciplinary Working Group: the American Academy of Neurology affirms the value of this guideline. *Stroke.* 2006;37(6):1583–1633.

Goldstein LB, Samsa GP. Reliability of the National Institutes of Health Stroke Scale extension to non-neurologists in the context of a clinical trial. *Stroke.* 1997;28(2):307–310.

Gornik HL, Creager MA. Contemporary management of peripheral arterial disease: I. Cardiovascular risk-factor modification. *Cleve Clin J Med.* 2006;73(suppl 4):S30–S37.

Greenwood DC, Muir KR, Packham CJ, Madeley RJ. Coronary heart disease: a review of the role of psychosocial stress and social support. *J Public Health Med.* 1996;18(2):221–231.

Gustat J, Rice J, Parker KM, Becker AB, Farley TA. Effect of changes to the neighborhood built environment on physical activity in a low-income African American neighborhood. *Prev Chronic Dis.* 2012;9:110165.

Hackam DG, Anand SS. Emerging risk factors for atherosclerotic vascular disease: a critical review of the evidence. *JAMA*. 2003;290(7):932–940.

Hacke W, Kaste M, Bluhmki E, et al. Thrombolysis with alteplase 3 to 4.5 hours after acute ischemic stroke. *N Engl J Med*. 2008;359(13):1317–1329.

Hakim AA, Petrovitch H, Burchfiel CM, et al. Effects of walking on mortality among nonsmoking retired men. *N Engl J Med*. 1998;338(2):94–99.

Haldeman GA, Croft JB, Giles WH, Rashidee A. Hospitalization of patients with heart failure: national Hospital Discharge Survey, 1985 to 1995. *Am Heart J*. 1999;137(2):352–360.

Hankey GJ, Norman PE, Eikelboom JW. Medical treatment of peripheral arterial disease. *JAMA*. 2006;295(5):547–553.

Haugen S, Casserly IP, Regensteiner JG, Hiatt WR. Risk assessment in the patient with established peripheral arterial disease. *Vasc Med*. 2007;12(4):343–350.

He, Y, Lam TH, Li LS, et al. The number of stenotic coronary arteries and passive smoking exposure from husband in lifelong non-smoking women in Xi'an, China. *Atherosclerosis* 1996,127(2):229–238.

Heald C, Fowkes F, Murray G, Price J; Ankle–Brachial Index Collaboration. Risk of mortality and cardiovascular disease associated with the ankle–brachial index: systematic review. *Atherosclerosis*. 2006;189(1):61–69.

Heidenreich PA, Albert NM, Allen LA, et al. Forecasting the impact of heart failure in the United States: a policy statement from the American Heart Association. *Circ Heart Fail*. 2013;6(3):606–619.

Heidrich J, Wellmann J, Heuschmann PU, Kraywinkel K, Keil U. Mortality and morbidity from coronary heart disease attributable to passive smoking. *Eur Heart J*. 2007;28(20):2498–2502.

Heinrich J, Balleisen L, Schulte H, Assmann G, van de Loo J. Fibrinogen and factor VII in the prediction of coronary risk. Results from the PROCAM study in healthy men. *Arterioscler Thromb Vasc Biol*. 1994;14(1):54–59.

Hennekens CH, Satterfield S, Hebert PR. Treatment of elevated blood pressure to prevent coronary heart disease. In: Higgins MW, Luepker RV, eds. *Trends in Coronary Heart Disease Mortality: The Influence of Medical Care*. New York, NY: Oxford University Press; 1988:103–108.

Herrington W, Lacey B, Sherliker P, Armitage J, Lewington S. Epidemiology of atherosclerosis and the potential to reduce the global burden of atherothrombotic disease. *Circ Res*. 2016;118(4):535–546.

Hinderliter L, Andrew Sherwood A, Craighead LW, et al. The long-term effects of lifestyle change on blood pressure: one-year follow-up of the ENCORE Study. *Am J Hypertens.* 2014;27(5):734–741.

Hirsch AT, Hartman L, Town RJ, Virnig BA. National health care costs of peripheral arterial disease in the Medicare population. *Vasc Med.* 2008;13(3):209–215.

Hispanic Community Health Study. Hispanic Community Health Study/Study of Latinos. 2007. Available at: https://www2.cscc.unc.edu/hchs. Accessed September 1, 2016.

Howard G, Wagenknecht LE, Burke GL, et al. Cigarette smoking and progression of atherosclerosis: The Atherosclerosis Risk in Communities (ARIC) Study. *JAMA.* 1998,279(2):119–124.

Howard VJ, Kleindorfer DO, Judd SE, et al. Disparities in stroke incidence contributing to disparities in stroke mortality. *Ann Neurol.* 2011;69(4):619–627.

Hu FB, Stampfer MJ, Colditz GA, et al. Physical activity and risk of stroke in women. *JAMA.* 2000;283(22):2961–2967.

Humphrey LL, Fu R, Rogers K, Freeman M, Helfand M. Homocysteine level and coronary heart disease incidence: a systematic review and meta-analysis. *Mayo Clin Proc.* 2008;83(11):1203–1212.

Hunt SA, Abraham WT, Chin MH, et al. ACC/AHA 2005 Guideline Update for the Diagnosis and Management of Chronic Heart Failure in the Adult: a report of the American College of Cardiology/American Heart Association Task Force on Practice Guidelines (Writing Committee to Update the 2001 Guidelines for the Evaluation and Management of Heart Failure): developed in collaboration with the American College of Chest Physicians and the International Society for Heart and Lung Transplantation: endorsed by the Heart Rhythm Society. *Circulation.* 2005;112(12):e154–e235.

Hunt SA, Abraham WT, Chin MH, et al. 2009 focused update incorporated into the ACC/AHA 2005 Guidelines for the Diagnosis and Management of Heart Failure in Adults: a report of the American College of Cardiology Foundation/American Heart Association Task Force on Practice Guidelines: developed in collaboration with the International Society for Heart and Lung Transplantation. *Circulation.* 2009;119(14):e391–e479.

Ikeda, Iso H, Kawachi I, Inoue M, Tsugane S. Type A behaviour and risk of coronary heart disease: the JPHC Study. *Int J Epidemiol.* 2008;37(6):1395–1405.

Jackson G, Gibbs CR, Davies MK, Lip GY. ABC of heart failure. Pathophysiology. *BMJ.* 2000;320(7228):167–170.

Jenkins CD. Epidemiology of cardiovascular diseases. *J Consult Clin Psychol.* 1988; 56(3):324–332.

Kannel WB. Vital epidemiologic clues in heart failure. *J Clin Epidemiol*. 2000a;53(3): 229–235.

Kannel WB. Incidence and epidemiology of heart failure. *Heart Fail Rev*. 2000b;5(2): 167–173.

Kawachi I, Colditz GA, Speizer FE, et al. A prospective study of passive smoking and coronary heart disease. *Circulation*. 1997;95(10):2374–2379.

Kawachi I, Sparrow D, Spiro A III, Vokonas P, Weiss ST. A prospective study of anger and coronary heart disease. The Normative Aging Study. *Circulation*. 1996;94(9):2090–2095.

Kernan WN, Ovbiagele B, Black HR, et al. Guidelines for the prevention of stroke in patients with stroke and transient ischemic attack: a guideline for healthcare professionals from the American Heart Association/American Stroke Association. *Stroke*. 2014;45(7):2160–2236.

Khalili D, Sheikholeslami FH, Bakhtiyari M, Azizi F, Momenan AA, Hadaegh F. The incidence of coronary heart disease and the population attributable fraction of its risk factors in Tehran: a 10-year population-based cohort study. *PLoS One*. 2014;9(8):e105804.

Kim H, Friedlander Y, Longstreth WT Jr, Edwards KL, Schwartz SM, Siscovick DS. Family history as a risk factor for stroke in young women. *Am J Prev Med*. 2004;27(5): 391–396.

King AC, Jeffery RW, Fridinger F, et al. Environmental and policy approaches to cardiovascular disease prevention through physical activity: issues and opportunities. *Health Educ Q*. 1995;22(4):499–511.

Kleindorfer D, Panagos P, Pancioli A, et al. Incidence and short-term prognosis of transient ischemic attack in a population-based study. *Stroke*. 2005;36(4):720–723.

Knowles JW, Assimes TL, Li J, Quertermous T, Cooke JP. Genetic susceptibility to peripheral arterial disease: a dark corner in vascular biology. *Arterioscler Thromb Vasc Biol*. 2007;27(10):2068–2078.

Kostis JB, Davis BR, Cutler J, et al. Prevention of heart failure by antihypertensive drug treatment in older persons with isolated systolic hypertension. SHEP Cooperative Research Group. *JAMA*. 1997;278(3):212–216.

Kovar MG, Harris MI, Hadden WC. The scope of diabetes in the United States population. *Am J Public Health*. 1987;77(12):1549–1550.

Krishnamurthi RV, Feigin VL, Forouzanfar MH, et al. Global and regional burden of first-ever ischaemic and haemorrhagic stroke during 1990–2010: findings from the Global Burden of Disease Study 2010. *Lancet Glob Health*. 2013;1(5):e259–e281.

Kulshreshtha A, Veledar E, Goyal A, Vaccarino V. Recent trends in coronary heart disease (CHD) deaths among the elderly in the United States. 2010. Available at: http://professional.heart.org/idc/groups/ahaecc-internal/@wcm/@sop/documents/downloadable/ucm_323623.pdf. Accessed September 1, 2016.

Kung H-C, Hoyert DL, Xu J, Murphy SL. Deaths: final data for 2005. *Natl Vital Stat Rep.* 2008;56(10):1–120.

Kurth T, Everett BM, Buring JE, Kase CS, Ridker PM, Gaziano JM. Lipid levels and the risk of ischemic stroke in women. *Neurology.* 2007;68(8):556–562.

Labarthe DR. *Epidemiology and Prevention of Cardiovascular Diseases—A Global Challenge.* 2nd ed. Burlington, MA: Jones and Bartlett Publishers; 2011.

Lam TH, Liu LJ, Janus ED, Lau CP, Hedley AJ. Fibrinogen, angina and coronary heart disease in a Chinese population. *Atherosclerosis.* 2000;149(2):443–449.

Lawson H. *Food Oils and Fats: Technology, Utilization and Nutrition.* Berlin, Germany: Springer Science and Business Media; 2013.

Lee I-M, Hennekens CH, Berger K, Buring JE, Manson JE. Exercise and risk of stroke in male physicians. *Stroke.* 1999;30(1):1–6.

Leeder S, Raymond S, Greenberg H, Liu H, Esson K. *A Race Against Time: The Challenge of Cardiovascular Disease in Developing Economies 2004.* New York, NY: Trustees of Columbia University; 2012.

Lewington S, Clarke R, Qizilbash N, Peto R, Collins R. Prospective studies collaboration. Age-specific relevance of usual blood pressure to vascular mortality: a meta-analysis of individual data for one million adults in 61 prospective studies. *Lancet.* 2002;360(9349): 1903–1913.

Lin HJ, Wolf PA, Kelly-Hayes M, et al. Stroke severity in atrial fibrillation. The Framingham Study. *Stroke.* 1996;27(10):1760–1764.

Liu L. Changes in cardiovascular hospitalization and comorbidity of heart failure in the United States: findings from the National Hospital Discharge Surveys 1980–2006. *Int J Cardiol.* 2011;149(1):39–45.

Liu L, Eisen HJ. Epidemiology of heart failure and scope of the problem. *Cardiol Clin.* 2014;32(1):1–8.

Liu L, Hankins SR, Watson RA, Weinstock PJ, Eisen HJ. Serum 25-hydroxyvitamin D concentration, heart failure mortality, and premature death from all-cause in US adults: an eight-year follow-up study. *J Card Fail.* 2010;16(8):S7.

Liu L, Ma J, Yin X, Kelepouris E, Eisen HJ. Global variability in angina pectoris and its association with body mass index and poverty. *Am J Cardiol.* 2011;107(5):655–661.

Liu L, Miura K, Fujiyoshi A, et al. Impact of metabolic syndrome on the risk of cardio-vascular disease mortality in the United States and in Japan. *Am J Cardiol.* 2014;113(1): 84–89.

Liu L, Nettleton JA, Bertoni AG, Bluemke DA, Lima JA, Szklo M. Dietary pattern, the metabolic syndrome, and left ventricular mass and systolic function: the Multi-Ethnic Study of Atherosclerosis. *Am J Clin Nutr.* 2009;90(2):362–368.

Liu L, Nguyen C, Ariola K, et al. Action-oriented participatory intervention and out-comes in patients with heart failure: findings from the African American Heart Fail-ure (Pilot) Study. *Circ Cardiovasc Qual Outcomes.* 2013;6(suppl 1):A310–A310.

Liu L, Nunez AE. Cardiometabolic syndrome and its association with education, smoking, diet, physical activity, and social support: findings from the Pennsylvania 2007 BRFSS Survey. *J Clin Hypertens (Greenwich).* 2010;12(7):556–564.

Liu L, Wu K, Lin X, et al. Passive smoking and other factors at different periods of life and breast cancer risk in Chinese women who have never smoked—a case–control study in Chongqing, People's Republic of China. *Asian Pac J CancerPrev.* 2000;1(2):131–137.

Lloyd-Jones D, Adams R, Carnethon M, et al. Heart disease and stroke statistics—2009 update: a report from the American Heart Association Statistics Committee and Stroke Statistics Subcommittee. *Circulation.* 2009;119(3):480–486.

Ma A, Folsom R, Melnick SL, et al. Associations of serum and dietary magnesium with cardiovascular disease, hypertension, diabetes, insulin, and carotid arterial wall thick-ness: the ARIC study. Atherosclerosis Risk in Communities Study. *J Clin Epidemiol.* 1995;48(7):927–940.

Maas AH, Appelman YE, gender differences in coronary heart disease. *Neth Heart J.* 2010;18(12):598–602.

MacMahon S. Blood pressure and the prevention of stroke. *J Hypertens.* 1996;14(12): S39–S46.

Mann DL. Mechanisms and models in heart failure: a combinatorial approach. *Circu-lation.* 1999;100(9):999–1008.

Mann DL, Bristow MR. Mechanisms and models in heart failure: the biomechanical model and beyond. *Circulation.* 2005;111(21):2837–2849.

Maresca G, Di Blasio A, Marchioli R, Di Minno G. Measuring plasma fibrinogen to predict stroke and myocardial infarction: an update. *Arterioscler Thromb Vasc Biol.* 1999;19(6):1368–1377.

Mayo Foundation for Medical Education and Research. Coronary artery disease treatment. 2009. Available at: http://www.mayoclinic.org/diseases-conditions/coronary-artery-disease/diagnosis-treatment/treatment/txc-20165340. Accessed August 26, 2016.

McDermott M. The magnitude of the problem of peripheral arterial disease: epidemiology and clinical significance. *Cleve Clin J Med*. 2006;73(suppl 4):S2–S7.

McDermott M, Lloyd-Jones D. The role of biomarkers and genetics in peripheral arterial disease. *J Am Coll Cardiol*. 2009;54(14):1228–1237.

McDonnell MN, Hillier SL, Hooker SP, Le A, Judd SE, Howard VJ. Physical activity frequency and risk of incident stroke in a national US study of blacks and whites. *Stroke*. 2013;44(9):2519–2524.

Morgenstern LB, Smith MA, Lisabeth LD, et al. Excess stroke in Mexican Americans compared with non-Hispanic whites: the Brain Attack Surveillance in Corpus Christi Project. *Am J Epidemiol*. 2004;160(4):376–383.

Morgenstern LB, Smith MA, Sánchez BN, et al. Persistent ischemic stroke disparities despite declining incidence in Mexican Americans. *Ann Neurol*. 2013;74(6):778–785.

Mozaffarian D, Benjamin EJ, Go AS, et al. Heart disease and stroke statistics—2016 update: a report from the American Heart Association. *Circulation*. 2016;133(4): 447–454.

Myint PK, Luben RN, Wareham NJ, Bingham SA, Khaw K-T. Combined effect of health behaviours and risk of first ever stroke in 20 040 men and women over 11 years' follow-up in Norfolk cohort of European Prospective Investigation of Cancer (EPIC Norfolk): prospective population study. *BMJ*. 2009;338:b349.

National Center for Health Statistics (NCHS). *Health, United States, 2008*. Atlanta, GA: National Center for Health Statistics; 2009.

National Center for Health Statistics (NCHS). *Health, United States, 2014: With Special Feature on Adults Aged 55–64*. Atlanta, GA: National Center for Health Statistics; 2015.

National Heart, Lung and Blood Institute (NHLBI). *Third Report of the Expert Panel on Detection, Evaluation, and Treatment of High Blood Cholesterol in Adults (ATP III Final Report)*. 2002. Available at: https://www.nhlbi.nih.gov/files/docs/resources/heart/atp-3-cholesterol-full-report.pdf. Accessed September 1, 2016.

National Heart, Lung, and Blood Institute (NHLBI). Coronary heart disease risk factors. 2016. Available at: https://www.nhlbi.nih.gov/health/health-topics/topics/hd. Accessed September 1, 2016.

National Research Council. *Diet and Health: Implications for Reducing Chronic Disease Risk*. Washington, DC: National Academy Press; 1989.

Newman AB, Siscovick DS, Manolio TA, et al. Ankle–arm index as a marker of atherosclerosis in the Cardiovascular Health Study. Cardiovascular Heart Study (CHS) Collaborative Research Group. *Circulation*. 1993;88(3):837–845.

National High Blood Pressure Education Program (NHBPEP). National Education Programs Working Group report on the management of patients with hypertension and high blood cholesterol. *Ann Intern Med.* 1991;114(3):224–237.

Newschaffer CJ, Liu L, Sim A. Cardiovascular disease. In: Remington PL, Brownson RC, Wegner MV, ed. *Chronic Disease Epidemiology and Control.* 3rd ed. Washington, DC: American Public Health Association; 2010:383.

Nieto FJ, Adam E, Sorlie P, et al. Cohort study of cytomegalovirus infection as a risk factor for carotid intimal-medial thickening, a measure of subclinical atherosclerosis. *Circulation.* 1996;94(5):922–927.

Nilsson P, Nilsson JA, Berglund G. Population-attributable risk of coronary heart disease risk factors during long-term follow-up: the Malmö Preventive Project. *J Intern Med.* 2006;260(2):134–141.

Nygård O, Nordrehaug JE, Refsum H, Ueland PM, Farstad M, Vollset SE. Plasma homocysteine levels and mortality in patients with coronary artery disease. *N Engl J Med.* 1997;337(4):230–236.

Nygård O, Vollset SE, Refsum H, et al. Total plasma homocysteine and cardiovascular risk profile: the Hordaland Homocysteine Study. *JAMA.* 1995;274(19):1526–1533.

Oldridge NB, Guyatt GH, Fischer ME, Rimm AA. Cardiac rehabilitation after myocardial infarction. Combined experience of randomized clinical trials. *JAMA.* 1988;260(7):945–950.

Ostchega Y, Paulose-Ram R, Dillon CF, Gu Q, Hughes JP. Prevalence of peripheral arterial disease and risk factors in persons aged 60 and older: data from the National Health and Nutrition Examination Survey 1999–2004. *J Am Geriatr Soc.* 2007;55(4):583–589.

Papadakis S, Moroz I. Population-level interventions for coronary heart disease prevention: what have we learned since the North Karelia project? *Curr Opin Cardiol.* 2008;23(5):452–461.

Pearson TA, Mensah GA, Alexander RW, et al. Markers of inflammation and cardiovascular disease: application to clinical and public health practice. A statement for healthcare professionals from the Centers for Disease Control and Prevention and the American Heart Association. *Circulation.* 2003;107(3):499–511.

Peralta CA, Katz R, Newman AB, Psaty BM, Odden MC. Systolic and diastolic blood pressure, incident cardiovascular events, and death in elderly persons the role of functional limitation in the cardiovascular health study. *Hypertension.* 2014;64(3):472–480.

Petrea RE, Beiser AS, Seshadri S, Kelly-Hayes M, Kase CS, Wolf PA. Gender differences in stroke incidence and poststroke disability in the Framingham Heart Study. *Stroke.* 2009;40(4):1032–1037.

Powell KE, Blair SN. The public health burdens of sedentary living habits: theoretical but realistic estimates. *Med Sci Sports Exerc.* 1994;26(7):851–856.

Powers WJ, Derdeyn CP, Biller J, et al. 2015 American Heart Association/American Stroke Association focused update of the 2013 Guidelines for the Early Management of Patients With Acute Ischemic Stroke Regarding Endovascular Treatment: A Guideline for Healthcare Professionals from the American Heart Association/American Stroke Association. *Stroke.* 2015;46(10):3020–3035.

Pradhan AD, Shrivastava S, Cook NR, Rifai N, Creager MA, Ridker PM. Symptomatic peripheral arterial disease in women nontraditional biomarkers of elevated risk. *Circulation.* 2008;117(6):823–831.

Prospective Studies Collaboration. Cholesterol, diastolic blood pressure, and stroke: 13000 strokes in 450000 people in 45 prospective cohorts. *Lancet.* 1995;346(8991):1647–1653.

Rafnsson SB, Deary IJ, Fowkes F. Peripheral arterial disease and cognitive function. *Vasc Med.* 2009;14(1):51–61.

Rasmusson KD, Hall JA, Renlund DG. The intricacies of heart failure. *Nurs Manage.* 2007;38(5):33–40; quiz 40–41.

Redline S, Yenokyan G, Gottlieb DJ, et al. Obstructive sleep apnea—hypopnea and incident stroke: the Sleep Heart Health Study. *Am J Respir Crit Care Med.* 2010;182(2): 269–277.

Richardson G, van Woerden HC, Morgan L, et al. Healthy Hearts—a community-based primary prevention programme to reduce coronary heart disease. *BMC Cardiovasc Disord.* 2008;8:18.

Richardson S, Shaffer JA, Falzon L, Krupka D, Davidson KW, Edmondson D. Meta-analysis of perceived stress and its association with incident coronary heart disease. *Am J Cardiol.* 2012;110(12):1711–1716.

Ridker PM, Rifai N. *C-Reactive Protein and Cardiovascular Disease.* St Laurent, QC: MediEdition; 2006.

Ridker PM, Stampfer MJ, Rifai N. Novel risk factors for systemic atherosclerosis: a comparison of C-reactive protein, fibrinogen, homocysteine, lipoprotein (a), and standard cholesterol screening as predictors of peripheral arterial disease. *JAMA.* 2001;285(19):2481–2485.

Rifkind BM. High-density lipoprotein cholesterol and coronary artery disease: survey of the evidence. *Am J Cardiol.* 1990;66(6):3A–6A.

Roberts R, Stewart A. The genetics of coronary artery disease. *Curr Opin Cardiol.* 2012;27(3):221–227.

Roest AM, Martens EJ, Jonge PD, Denollet J. Anxiety and risk of incident coronary heart disease. *J Am Coll Cardiol.* 2010;56(1):38–46.

Roger VL, Go AS, Lloyd-Jones DM, et al. Heart disease and stroke statistics—2011 update: a report from the American Heart Association. *Circulation.* 2011;123(4):e18–e209.

Roivainen M, Viik-Kajander M, Palosuo T, et al. Infections, inflammation, and the risk of coronary heart disease. *Circulation.* 2000;101(3):252–257.

Rooke TW, Hirsch AT, Misra S, et al. 2011 ACCF/AHA focused update of the guideline for the management of patients with peripheral artery disease (updating the 2005 guideline): a report of the American College of Cardiology Foundation/American Heart Association Task Force on Practice Guidelines. *J Am Coll Cardiol.* 2011;58(19):2020–2045.

Rubinstein J, Miranda J, Beratarrechea A, et al. Effectiveness of an mHealth intervention to improve the cardiometabolic profile of people with prehypertension in low-resource urban settings in Latin America: a randomised controlled trial. *Lancet Diabetes Endocrinol.* 2016;4(1):52–63.

Ruidavets J-B, Ducimetiere P, Evans A, et al. Patterns of alcohol consumption and ischaemic heart disease in culturally divergent countries: the Prospective Epidemiological Study of Myocardial Infarction (PRIME). *BMJ.* 2010;341:c6077.

Sacco RL, Adams R, Albers G, et al. Guidelines for prevention of stroke in patients with ischemic stroke or transient ischemic attack: a statement for healthcare professionals from the American Heart Association/American Stroke Association Council on Stroke: co-sponsored by the council on cardiovascular radiology and intervention: the American Academy of Neurology affirms the value of this guideline. *Circulation.* 2006;113(10):e409–e449.

Safar M, Priollet P, Luizy F, et al. Peripheral arterial disease and isolated systolic hypertension: the ATTEST study. *J Hum Hypertens.* 2009;23(3):182–187.

Sallis JF, Owen N, Rimer BK. Ecological models of health behavior. In: Glanz K, Lewis FM, eds. *Health Behavior and Health Education: Theory, Research, and Practice.* Vol. 3. San Francisco, CA: Jossey-Bass Publishers; 2002:462–484.

Schmid TL, Pratt M, Howze E. Policy as intervention: environmental and policy approaches to the prevention of cardiovascular disease. *Am J Public Health.* 1995;85(9):1207–1211.

Schwamm LH, Pancioli A, Acker JE, et al. Recommendations for the establishment of stroke systems of care recommendations from the American Stroke Association's Task Force on the Development of Stroke Systems. *Stroke.* 2005;36(3):690–703.

Selvin ET, Erlinger P. Prevalence of and risk factors for peripheral arterial disease in the United States results from the National Health and Nutrition Examination Survey, 1999–2000. *Circulation.* 2004;110(6):738–743.

Sempos C, Fulwood R, Haines C, et al. The prevalence of high blood cholesterol levels among adults in the United States. *JAMA*. 1989;262(1):45–52.

Seshadri S, Beiser A, Pikula A, et al. Parental occurrence of stroke and risk of stroke in their children the Framingham study. *Circulation*. 2010;121(11):1304–1312.

Shah RS, Cole JW. Smoking and stroke: the more you smoke the more you stroke. *Expert Rev Cardiovasc Ther*. 2010;8(7):917–932.

Sharrett AR, Patsch W, Sorlie PD, Heiss G, Bond MG, Davis CE. Associations of lipoprotein cholesterols, apolipoproteins A-I and B, and triglycerides with carotid atherosclerosis and coronary heart disease. The Atherosclerosis Risk in Communities (ARIC) Study. *Arterioscler Thromb*. 1994;14(7):1098–1104.

Simon C, Schweitzer B, Oujaa M, et al. Successful overweight prevention in adolescents by increasing physical activity: a 4-year randomized controlled intervention. *Int J Obes*. 2008;32(10):1489–1498.

Simons-Morton DG, Simons-Morton BG, Parcel GS, Bunker JF. Influencing personal and environmental conditions for community health: a multilevel intervention model. *Fam Community Health*. 1988;11(2):25–35.

SPS 3 Study Group. Blood-pressure targets in patients with recent lacunar stroke: the SPS3 randomised trial. *Lancet*. 2013;382(9891):507–515.

Stamler J, Wentworth D, Neaton JD. Is relationship between serum cholesterol and risk of premature death from coronary heart disease continuous and graded? Findings in 356,222 primary screenees of the Multiple Risk Factor Intervention Trial (MRFIT). *JAMA*. 1986;256(20):2823–2828.

Stamler O, Vaccaro J, Neaton D, Wentworth D. Diabetes, other risk factors, and 12-yr cardiovascular mortality for men screened in the multiple risk factor intervention trial. *Diabetes Care*. 1993;16(2):434–444.

Stampfer MJ, Malinow MR, Willett WC, et al. A prospective study of plasma homocyst(e)ine and risk of myocardial infarction in US physicians. *JAMA*. 1992;268(7):877–881.

Steenland K. Passive smoking and the risk of heart disease. *JAMA*. 1992;267(1):94–99.

Steg PG, Bhatt DL, Wilson PW, et al. One-year cardiovascular event rates in outpatients with atherothrombosis. *JAMA*. 2007;297(11):1197–1206.

Thom T, Haase N, Rosamond W, et al. Heart disease and stroke statistics—2006 update: a report from the American Heart Association Statistics Committee and Stroke Statistics Subcommittee. *Circulation*. 2006;113(6):e85–e151.

Tikkanen E, Havulinna AS, Palotie A, Salomaa V, Ripatti S. Genetic risk prediction and a 2-stage risk screening strategy for coronary heart disease. *Arterioscler Thromb Vasc Biol.* 2013;33(9):2261–2266.

Towfighi A, Markovic D, Ovbiagele B. Current national patterns of comorbid diabetes among acute ischemic stroke patients. *Cerebrovasc Dis.* 2012;33(5):411–418.

UK Prospective Diabetes Study Group. Intensive blood-glucose control with sulphonylureas or insulin compared with conventional treatment and risk of complications in patients with type 2 diabetes (UKPDS 33). *Lancet.* 1998;352(9131):837–853.

US Department of Health and Human Services (USDHHS). *The Health Consequences of Smoking: Cardiovascular Disease. A Report of the Surgeon General.* Rockville, MD: USDHHS, Public Health Service; 1983. DHHS Publication no. (PHS) 84-50204;

US Department of Health and Human Services (USDHHS). *Physical Activity and Health: A Report of the Surgeon General.* Atlanta, GA: Centers for Disease Control and Prevention; 1996.

US Preventive Services Task Force (USPSTF). *Guide to Clinical Preventive Services: An Assessment of the Effectiveness of 169 Interventions. Report of the US Preventive Services Task Force.* Baltimore, MD: Williams and Wilkins; 1989.

Vidula H, Tian L, Liu K, et al. Biomarkers of inflammation and thrombosis as predictors of near-term mortality in patients with peripheral arterial disease: a cohort study. *Ann Intern Med.* 2008;148(2):85–93.

Wang GJ, Shaw PA, Townsend RR, et al. Sex differences in the incidence of peripheral artery disease in the chronic renal insufficiency cohort. *Circ Cardiovasc Qual Outcomes.* 2016;9(2 suppl 1):S86–S93.

Wattanakit K, Folsom AR, Selvin E, Coresh J, Hirsch AT, Weatherley BD. Kidney function and risk of peripheral arterial disease: results from the Atherosclerosis Risk in Communities (ARIC) Study. *J Am Soc Nephrol.* 2007;18(2):629–636.

Willey JZ, Moon YP, Kahn E, et al. Population attributable risks of hypertension and diabetes for cardiovascular disease and stroke in the northern Manhattan study. *J Am Heart Assoc.* 2014;3(5):e001106.

Williams JE, Paton CC, Siegler IC, Eigenbrodt ML, Nieto FJ, Tyroler HA. Anger proneness predicts coronary heart disease risk prospective analysis from the Atherosclerosis Risk in Communities (ARIC) study. *Circulation.* 2000;101(17):2034–2039.

Wilson PW, Hoeg JM, D'Agostino RB, et al. Cumulative effects of high cholesterol levels, high blood pressure, and cigarette smoking on carotid stenosis. *N Engl J Med.* 1997;337(8):516–522.

Wing S, Casper M, Riggan W, Hayes C, Tyroler HA. Socioenvironmental characteristics associated with the onset of decline of ischemic heart disease mortality in the United States. *Am J Public Health*. 1988;78(8):923–926.

World Health Organization (WHO). The Global Burden of Disease: 2004 update. Geneva, Switzerland: WHO; 2008.

Xavier D, Gupta R, Kamath D, et al. Community health worker–based intervention for adherence to drugs and lifestyle change after acute coronary syndrome: a multicentre, open, randomised controlled trial. *Lancet Diabetes Endocrinol*. 2016;4(3):244–253.

Yamori Y, Liu L, Mizushima S, Ikeda K, Nara Y; CARDIAC Study Group. Male cardiovascular mortality and dietary markers in 25 population samples of 16 countries. *J Hypertens*. 2006;24(8):1499–1505.

Yancy CW. Heart failure in blacks: etiologic and epidemiologic differences. *Curr Cardiol Rep*. 2001;3(3):191–197.

Yancy CW. Heart failure in African Americans. *Am J Cardiol*. 2005;96(7B):3i–12i.

Young JB. The global epidemiology of heart failure. *Med Clin North Am*. 2004;88(5): 1135–1143, ix.

16

CANCER

Maria Mora Pinzon, MD, MS, Corinne Joshu, PhD, MPH, MA, and Ross C. Brownson, PhD

Introduction

Cancer is now the leading cause of death among adults aged 40 to 79 years (Siegel et al. 2016) and the second-leading cause of death overall in the United States, accounting for 1.5 million new cases and 582,600 deaths in 2012 (Table 16-1; Murphy et al. 2015; Howlader et al. 2015; US Cancer Statistics Working Group 2015). It is estimated that in 2016, 1.6 million people will develop cancer and 595,700 people will die from the disease (ACS 2016a).

The most recent U.S. data show declines in overall incidence and mortality, yet with some variations by sex and type of cancer: among men, overall cancer incidence decreased by 1.4% per year, and among women, overall rates were stable (Ryerson et al. 2016). Men have a 42% lifetime probability of developing cancer and women have a 38% lifetime probability (Siegel et al. 2016). The five-year relative survival has also increased, from 49% for those diagnosed between 1975 and 1977 to 69% for those diagnosed between 2005 and 2011 (ACS 2016a).

Regarding cancer death rates, these increased steadily from 1930 (when nationwide mortality was first compiled) to 1990, mainly because of a sharp rise in lung cancer rates. However, cancer death rates began to decline in the early 1990s, and between 2003 and 2012 they decreased 1.5% per year. Among men, the rates declined 1.8% per year, and among women 1.4% per year (Ryerson et al. 2016). If these trends continue, cancer will overtake heart disease as the leading cause of death among men and women (Figure 16-1; CDC 2014a).

Significance

Although cancer occurs more frequently with advancing age, it is also the second leading cause of death attributable to disease among U.S. children aged

Table 16-1. Public Health Impact of Major Cancers, United States, 2012

Cancer Type (*ICD-10* Code)	Number of New Cases[a]	Number of Deaths[b]	Five-Year Survival[c]	Number of Hospital Days[d]
All sites (C00–C97)	1,529,078	582,607	68.7	8,965
Lung (C34)	210,828	157,423	18.4	957
Colon and rectum (C18–C20)	134,784	51,516	66.1	1,027
Breast (C50)	226,272	41,555	90.7	177
Pancreas (C25)	43,213	38,797	7.8	315
Prostate (C61)	177,489	27,244	99.4	221
Leukemia (C91–C95)	44,396	23,309	61.7	618
Non-Hodgkin's lymphoma (C82–C85, C96)	63,419	20,388	71.9	109
Bladder (C67)	69,974	15,245	79.0	212
Stomach (C16)	22,623	11,191	29.9	266
Skin—melanoma (C43)	67,753	9,251	93.1	
Oral cavity (C00–C14)	39,879	8,924	66.3	83
Uterine corpus (C54)	49,154	5,099	83.3	151
Uterine cervix (C53)	12,042	4,074	69.3	76
Hodgkin's lymphoma (C81)	8,273	1,130	88.3	73

Source: Data from US Cancer Statistics Working Group (2015), Howlader et al. (2015), and CDC (2010).

Note: ICD-10=International Statistical Classification of Diseases and Related Health Problems, Tenth Revision (WHO 2005).

[a]Data are from selected statewide and metropolitan area cancer registries that meet the data quality criteria for all invasive cancer sites combined (US Cancer Statistics Working Group 2015).

[b]Data are from the National Vital Statistics System (US Cancer Statistics Working Group 2015).

[c]Five-year relative survival rate (%) for 2005–2011, based on follow-up of patients into 2012 (Howlader et al. 2015).

[d]Days of care for discharges by first-listed diagnostic category, number in thousands, based on the 2010 National Hospital Discharge Survey (CDC 2010).

1 to 14 years (ACS 2016a). Similarly, racial and ethnic groups are not affected equally by cancer (Figure 16-2). African-American men have the highest overall cancer incidence and mortality rate for most cancers, followed by non-Hispanic white men (Howlader et al. 2015). The higher overall cancer death rate in blacks is attributable to breast and colorectal cancer in women, and prostate, lung, and colorectal cancer in men (ACS 2016b).

The causes of these inequalities are not related to race per se, but rather are a reflection of socioeconomic disparities in income, housing, education, cigarette smoking, poor nutrition, and inadequate access to health care, which

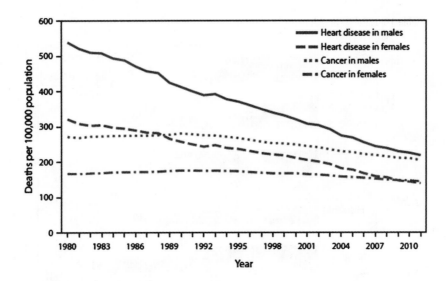

Source: Reprinted from CDC (2014b).

Figure 16-1. Age-Adjusted Death Rates for Heart Disease and Cancer by Sex, United States, 1980–2011

can delay cancer diagnosis and treatment (Ghafoor et al. 2002), resulting in more advanced stages at diagnosis. For example, in 2014, African Americans had an uninsured rate of 11.8% (Smith and Medalia 2015), accounted for 26.2% of those living in poverty (DeNavas-Walt and Proctor 2015), but only 13.2% of the total U.S. population (US Census Bureau 2010).

People of Hispanic origin represent 16% of the total U.S. population, and have overall lower incidence of cancer than non-Hispanic whites (ACS 2015a). Those cancers that are higher among the Hispanic population tend to be associated with infectious etiologies, such as cancers of the cervix (i.e., human papillomavirus [HPV]), stomach (i.e., *Helicobacter pylori*), and liver (i.e., hepatitis B and C viruses), which may be the consequence of poor sanitary conditions and lack of preventive services (Howe et al. 2006).

As with African Americans, Hispanics are more likely to be poor in the United States, having an uninsured rate of 19.9% (Smith and Medalia 2015), and accounting for 23.6% of those living in poverty (DeNavas-Walt and Proctor 2015). Hispanics are less likely to be screened, and more likely to be diagnosed at later stages. Cancer risk among Hispanics also varies by country origin (Howe et al. 2006) and acculturation, which refers to the process of

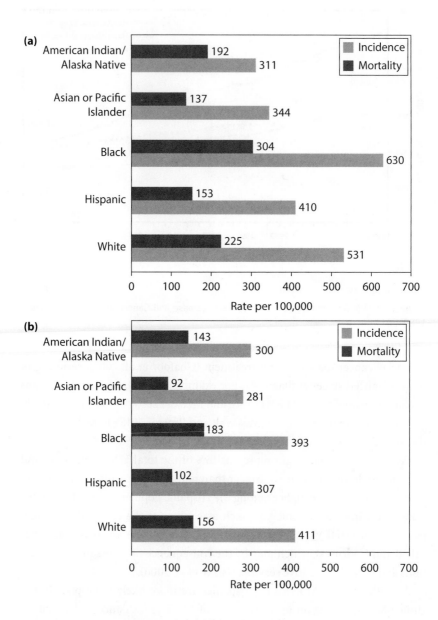

Source: Adapted from SEER (2015).

Figure 16-2. Cancer Incidence and Mortality Rates (a) per 100,000 Men and (b) per 100,000 Women, by Race and Ethnic Group, United States, 2009–2013

assimilating the behaviors of their new culture: U.S.-born Hispanic men have cancer death rates 22% higher than foreign-born Hispanic men (ACS 2015a). Thus, future prevention efforts may need to target country of origin rather than generalizing to the entire Hispanic population.

The estimated direct medical costs of cancer in 2013 were $74.8 billion (ACS 2016a). Indirect costs such as lost work productivity were estimated at $115.8 billion in 2000, and may increase to $147.6 billion by 2020 because of population growth and aging (Yabroff et al. 2011). In contrast to the huge cost of cancer treatment, the total national resources dedicated to early detection activities, such as screening for breast, cervical, and colorectal cancer, are considerably smaller. The allocation of national resources to the primary prevention of cancer (e.g., tobacco control, dietary intervention) is even smaller.

Pathophysiology

Cancer has a complex set of "upstream" causes and "downstream" consequences (Figure 16-3), Cancer occurs as a result of alterations in the mechanisms that control normal cell behavior. Cancer cells are different than normal cells as they (1) acquire inappropriate growth properties and (2) generally lose their ability to serve the functions they normally have in a given tissue. Cancer is a diverse group of diseases characterized by uncontrolled growth and spread of these abnormal cells. Tumors, or abnormal enlargements of tissue, may be either benign or malignant. Benign tumors are generally innocuous and

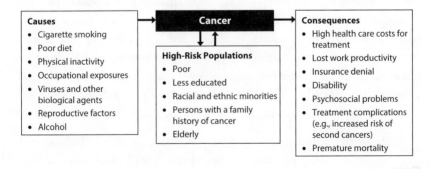

Source: Compiled from Colditz et al. (2000); EPA (1992); Miller (1992); and Rothenberg et al. (1987).

Figure 16-3. Cancer: Causes, Consequences, and High-Risk Groups

slow-growing, whereas malignant tumors (commonly called cancers) contain abnormal genetic material and grow more rapidly. The principal danger of a cancer is its tendency to invade neighboring tissues or organs, or to metastasize and to grow in other areas of the body. If this spread remains untreated, cancer cells invade vital organs or cause dysfunction by displacing normal tissue.

Different cancer types have widely varying induction periods—that is, the time between exposure to cancer-causing agents and cancer occurrence. For example, the induction period for some types of leukemia may be as short as a few years, compared with induction periods as long as four or five decades for some types of bladder cancer.

Cancers are classified according to their organ or tissue of origin (site code) and according to their histologic features (morphology code). The most widely used classification schemes are the *International Statistical Classification of Disease and Related Health Problems, Tenth Revision* (*ICD-10*; WHO 2005) and the *International Classification of Diseases for Oncology* (*ICD-O-3*; WHO 2000). The existence of hundreds of cancer varieties is readily apparent with 43 organs of origin and multiple histologic types for each organ (Giordano 2006).

In addition to being grouped by site and histologic features, cancers are classified according to their stage at diagnosis, or the extent to which the cancer has grown locally or invaded other tissues or organs. Cancer cells may remain at their original site (local stage), spread to an adjacent area of the body (regional stage), or spread (metastasize) throughout the body (distant stage).

Cancer registries collect detailed information on patients with cancer through hospitals and medical clinics (see also Chapter 3). Cancer registry data have many valuable uses, such as evaluation of cancer incidence patterns, cancer risk factors, effects of prevention and early detection efforts, survival patterns, and treatment effects. In the United States, the National Cancer Institute's Surveillance, Epidemiology, and End Results (SEER) Program has collected population-based data on newly diagnosed cancers since 1973, covering approximately 30% of the U.S. population (NCI 2016a). The SEER Program is designed to accomplish the following goals:

1. To assemble and report, on a periodic basis, estimates of cancer incidence, mortality, survival, and prevalence in the United States.
2. To monitor annual cancer incidence trends to identify unusual changes in specific forms of cancer occurring in population subgroups defined by geographic and demographic characteristics.

3. To provide continuing information on trends over time in the extent of disease at diagnosis, trends in therapy, and associated changes in patient survival.

4. To promote studies designed to identify factors amenable to cancer control interventions.

5. To provide research resources and training materials for the research community.

6. To conduct quality control and improvement of the collection of data (NCI 2016b).

The Centers for Disease Control and Prevention (CDC) has established the National Program of Cancer Registries (NPCR; Public Law 102-515) and has funded 45 states, the District of Columbia, and three U.S. territories to develop registries or to enhance current registries. The NPCR provides cancer incidence information on 96% of the U.S. population, and the data are designed to (CDC 2015):

1. Monitor cancer trends over time.
2. Determine cancer patterns in various populations.
3. Guide planning and evaluation of cancer control programs (e.g., determine whether prevention, screening, and treatment efforts are making a difference).
4. Help set priorities for allocating health resources.
5. Advance clinical, epidemiologic, and health services research.

Causes

Several studies have been conducted to estimate the proportion of overall cancer deaths attributable to various modifiable causes (Doll and Peto 1981; Miller 1992; Harvard Report on Cancer Prevention 1996; Danaei et al. 2005). The Harvard Center for Cancer Prevention (Harvard Report on Cancer Prevention 1996) and Danaei et al. (2009) provide a useful benchmark on which to base preventive efforts (Table 16-2). These findings suggest the following priorities for cancer prevention and control:

1. Eliminating use of tobacco.
2. Consuming a prudent diet that includes an abundant distribution of fruits and vegetables and achieves a balance between energy intake and regular physical activity.

3. Reducing exposures to occupational carcinogens.
4. Controlling exposures to microbial agents that may be sexually transmitted or transmitted by sharing contaminated needles or personal articles, or prevented by immunization.
5. Limiting consumption of alcohol.
6. Avoiding overexposure to sunlight (Greenwald and Sondik 1986; Colditz et al. 2002).

In 1985, the National Cancer Institute set a goal of reducing cancer mortality by 50% by the year 2000 through the systematic application of existing cancer control technologies (Greenwald and Sondik 1986). Although this 50% goal was overly ambitious and was not achieved, it was extremely beneficial in focusing cancer control efforts at all levels of public health practice. A recent initiative, named National Cancer Moonshot Initiative, was launched in January 2016 to accelerate cancer research. It aims to make more therapies available to more patients, while also improving our ability to prevent cancer and detect it at an early stage (NCI 2016c).

In addition to these goals by the National Cancer Institute, the U.S. Public Health Service has established a variety of objectives related to cancer prevention and control through the use of evidence-based measures in Healthy People 2020 (USDHHS 2016). It has been noted that, without a stronger U.S. commitment to cancer prevention, public health goals for cancer prevention are unlikely to be achieved (Bailar and Gornik 1997; Byers et al. 1999).

Table 16-2. Distribution of Cause-Specific Death Attributable to Risk Factors by Age Group and Sex

Risk Factor	30–45 y, % (95% CI)	45–69 y, % (95% CI)	≥70 y, % (95% CI)	Males, % (95% CI)	Females, % (95% CI)
Overweight-obesity (high BMI)	2 (2, 3)	42 (38, 47)	55 (51, 60)	40 (36, 46)	60 (54, 64)
High dietary salt	5 (1, 8)	36 (21, 52)	59 (43, 74)	58 (40, 73)	42 (27, 60)
Low intake of fruits and vegetables	3 (2, 5)	56 (39, 71)	41 (25, 58)	62 (47, 76)	38 (24, 53)
Alcohol use	5 (4, 6)	55 (49, 61)	40 (34, 46)	64 (58, 69)	36 (31, 42)
Physical inactivity	5 (3, 7)	42 (35, 50)	53 (45, 60)	24 (18, 29)	76 (71, 82)
Tobacco smoking	1 (0, 2)	43 (42, 44)	56 (55, 57)	61 (60, 62)	39 (38, 40)

Source: Data from Danaei (2009).

Note: BMI = body mass index; CI = confidence interval.

Evidence-Based Interventions

As noted by Alciati et al. (1995), public health agencies at the federal, state, and local levels are vital entities in translating cancer control technologies into practice. The federal support for cancer control activities in state health agencies only began in 1986 when the National Cancer Institute initiated its Technical Development in Health Agencies Program. Cancer Control P.L.A.N.E.T. (AHRQ et al. 2016) is an initiative that provides data and resources to program staff, public health officials, and researchers to design, implement, and evaluate evidence-based programs. Similarly, *The Guide to Community Preventive Services: What Works to Promote Health?* (CPSTF 2016), provides systematic reviews of selected population-based interventions.

Meissner et al. (1992) summarized internal and external factors contributing to success in controlling cancer in public health settings. Internal factors include (1) commitment of the organization's leadership to cancer control, (2) existence of appropriate data to monitor and evaluate programs, (3) appropriately trained staff, and (4) the ability to obtain funds for future activities. External factors include (1) successful linkages and coalitions, (2) an established cancer control plan, (3) access to outside health experts, (4) an informed state legislature, and (5) diffusion of initially successful programs to other sites. The basic steps linking cancer surveillance and research on the etiology of cancer with cancer prevention and control interventions requires ethics, accountability, empowerment, and efficiency, to determine what information is available, what is useful, and how interventions can be implemented (Hiatt and Rimer 2006). Public health agencies that take all of the issues mentioned are more likely to be successful in controlling cancer through evidence-based interventions.

Describing each cancer site in detail in this chapter would be impractical. Therefore, we have limited this discussion to cancers that have one or more of the following characteristics: (1) they account for a major proportion of all cancer cases, (2) they can be reduced through scientifically proven prevention and control measures, or (3) they are frequently encountered in public health practice. Because of their importance, cancers of the lung, colon and rectum, breast, and cervix are discussed in detail. Shorter descriptions are provided for prostate cancer, lymphoma, leukemia, bladder cancer, cancer of the oral cavity, and skin melanoma.

LUNG CANCER

Significance

Lung cancer is the leading cause of cancer deaths in the United States, which will account for an estimated 26% of all cancer mortality in 2016, or a total of 158,080 deaths (Siegel et al. 2016). Lung cancer is also the most common cause of cancer death worldwide. This high mortality rate results from both a high incidence rate and a low survival rate: only 17.8% (ALA 2014a) of U.S. lung cancer patients survive five years after diagnosis. There has been some improvement in lung cancer survival over the past half century, as the survival rate for lung cancer was only 6% in the early 1950s (Spitz et al. 2006).

Pathophysiology

More than 90% of lung cancers are believed to originate in the basal cells of the lung epithelium, or the lining surfaces of the lung. A series of changes, over a period of years, occurs as lung cancer develops. These involve an increase in the number of cells, structural changes in certain epithelial cells that lead to abnormal function, appearance of patient signs and symptoms, and cancer spread. The major cell types of lung cancer are adenocarcinoma (approximately 43% of cases), squamous cell cancer (approximately 22% of cases), small-cell cancer (approximately 13% of cases), and large-cell cancer (approximately 2% of cases; Howlader et al. 2015). Lung cancer growth rates vary on the basis of the cell type involved. Of the major cell types, small-cell cancer appears to grow and spread the most rapidly.

Numerous genetic factors affect susceptibility to lung cancer. These are likely to involve a variety of cellular pathways including DNA repair, cell cycle, metabolism, and inflammation. Among the most studied genetic factors are the cytochrome P-450 enzymes (e.g., CYP1A1), which are known to metabolize many carcinogenic compounds (e.g., polycyclic aromatic hydrocarbons). The internal dose of tobacco smoke and other carcinogens to which the lung tissue is exposed are modulated by gene polymorphisms encoding for enzymes that affect activation and detoxification of cancer-causing chemicals (Spitz et al. 2006).

Descriptive Epidemiology

Because lung cancer is so strongly associated with cigarette smoking, its descriptive epidemiology is largely explained by smoking patterns and trends (see Chapter 7).

High-Risk Populations

Although lung cancer mortality rates remain 1.8 times higher among men than among women, lung cancer surpassed breast cancer as the leading cause of cancer deaths in women in 1987. Mortality rates are 1.1 times higher among African Americans than among whites (Howlader et al. 2015). This racial difference is attributable to large differences in mortality between African American and white men, as rates are nearly identical in African American and white women. Lung cancer mortality rates are approximately 60% lower among people of Hispanic origin than among non-Hispanics. Lung cancer rates increase with age, with 60 years being the average age of diagnosis. People of lower socioeconomic status are at higher risk for lung cancer, reflecting the higher prevalence of smoking among these populations.

Geographic Distribution

Lung cancer tends to cluster in areas with high smoking rates. In the United States, lung cancer rates are generally highest in the Southern and Lower-Midwestern states. Kentucky has the highest lung cancer death rate followed by West Virginia and Arkansas. Utah has by far the lowest mortality rate, followed by Hawaii and New Mexico (Howlader et al. 2015). Worldwide, lung cancer is most common in developed countries in North America and Europe (especially Central and Eastern Europe). Eastern Asia also demonstrates higher incidence rates compared to other world areas (Torre et al. 2015).

Time Trends

The lung cancer mortality rate in the United States increased dramatically over the past 60 years, from 7 per 100,000 in 1940 to 45 per 100,000 in 2004 (Howlader et al. 2015). The major increase in lung cancer mortality rates in men occurred from 1940 to 1979. In the 1980s, the rate of increase slowed, and from 1991 to 2003, the male lung cancer mortality rate declined 1.9% per year (ACS 2014b). In contrast, a sharp increase in lung cancer mortality rates was observed among women in the 1960s, although female lung cancer mortality rates are now approaching a plateau.

Causes

Modifiable Risk Factors

The strongest risk factor for lung cancer is cigarette smoking (Table 16-3). The association between smoking and lung cancer is one of the most widely studied and clearly defined relationships in chronic disease epidemiology. The relative risk of lung cancer attributable to current smoking is approximately 23 for men and 7 for women (Pesch et al. 2012), although the relative risk for women has been increasing over time as women have begun smoking more cigarettes per day and have started smoking at increasingly younger ages.

Exposure to lung carcinogens in the workplace increases lung cancer risk. Asbestos exposure among nonsmokers accounts for a relative risk of about five (Saracci 1987). When asbestos exposure is combined with cigarette smoking, the risk increases markedly to approximately 50-fold. Occupational exposure to radon accounts for a 20-fold increase in lung cancer risk (Lubin et al. 1994). Radon also interacts with smoking to greatly increase the risk. Increases in lung cancer risk have also been documented for exposure to inorganic arsenic, polycyclic hydrocarbons, chloromethyl ethers, chromium, and nickel (Spitz et al. 2006).

Table 16-3. Modifiable Risk Factors for Lung Cancer, United States

Magnitude	Risk Factor	Best Estimate (%) of Population-Attributable Risk (Range)
Strong (relative risk > 4)	Cigarette smoking	82
	Occupation[a]	13 (10–20)
Moderate (relative risk 2–4)	None	
Weak (relative risk < 2)	Residential radon exposure	1.4 (-2.0–4.8)
	Secondhand smoke exposure	9.9 (1.3–18.5)
	Five or more servings of fruits and vegetables per day[b]	
	Residence near large city for 10+ years	

Source: Data from Miller (1992); USEPA (1992); Colditz et al. (2000); Alavanja et al. (1995); and Rothenberg et al. (1987).
[a]Includes occupational exposures to asbestos, aluminum, beryllium, bis(chloromethyl) ether and chloromethyl ether, cadmium, chromium, coke, mustard gas, radon, silica, or sulfuric acid mist.
[b]Eating five or more servings of fruits and vegetables per day reduces risk.

Exposure to radon gas in the home, especially in combination with cigarette smoking, increases the risk of lung cancer. In addition, exposure to secondhand tobacco smoke (also called environmental tobacco smoke) elevates lung cancer risk slightly in nonsmokers (i.e., a 20% to 30% excess risk among nonsmokers associated with secondhand smoke exposure; USDHHS 2006). Among dietary factors, the most consistent association is that between a low intake of fresh fruits and vegetables and higher risk of lung cancer (Spitz et al. 2006). Intake of high-dose supplements of beta-carotene—normally considered to be a cancer-reducing vitamin—actually increases lung cancer risk in smokers (WCRF/AICR 2007).

Population-Attributable Risk

An estimated 90% of lung cancer deaths are attributable to cigarette smoking (Table 16-3). The smoking-associated attributable risk is 90% among men and 80% among women (ALA 2014a). Occupational exposures are estimated to contribute to an additional 13% of lung cancers. Extrapolations from risks among underground miners indicate that exposure to indoor radon may account for up to 10% of lung cancer deaths (ALA 2014a), although quantifying this risk factor accurately is extremely difficult. Exposure to secondhand smoke accounts for approximately 2% of U.S. lung cancer cases (about 3,000 deaths per year; NCI 2004).

Evidence-Based Interventions

Prevention

Numerous interventions address primary prevention of lung cancer by reducing smoking rates. Smoking cessation drastically reduces the risk of lung cancer, although a former smoker's risk does not drop back to that of a lifetime nonsmoker (USDHHS 2004). Smoking is usually adopted early in life; therefore, prevention of tobacco use among youths is critical to the overall goal of reducing smoking prevalence (see Chapter 7). Workers exposed to lung carcinogens (e.g., asbestos workers, uranium miners) should also be targeted for intervention, as many of their exposures interact with smoking to increase dramatically the risk of lung cancer. Dietary changes to increase consumption of fresh fruits and vegetables may decrease lung cancer risk. These changes are consistent with dietary guidelines discussed in other sections and chapters.

Evidence-based interventions can be found in numerous sources. Among these, *The Guide to Community Preventive Services: What Works to Promote Health* uses a systematic review process to highlight effective approaches (CPSTF 2016). Numerous effective interventions exist for tobacco control. These are also embodied in CDC's *Best Practices for Comprehensive Tobacco Control* (CDC 2014b).

Screening

Several randomized trials have assessed the role of chest x-rays and examination of cells in the sputum (sputum cytology) in detecting lung cancer in the early stages. Although these tests are able to detect early lesions, trials have not demonstrated a reduction in lung cancer mortality. Low-dose spiral computed tomography (CT) scanning has shown that improved detection by CT will result in 20% reduction in lung cancer mortality (NLSTRT et al. 2011). The U.S. Preventive Services Task Force recommends annual screening for lung cancer with low-dose CT in adults aged 55 to 80 years who have a 30 pack-year smoking history and currently smoke or have quit within the past 15 years. Screening should be discontinued once a person has not smoked for 15 years or develops a health problem that substantially limits life expectancy or the ability or willingness to have curative lung surgery (Moyer 2014).

Treatment

Lung cancer treatment is largely determined by the cell type and stage at diagnosis. Treatment options include surgery, radiation therapy, and chemotherapy. Lung cancer mortality could be reduced by an estimated 20% through early application of existing state-of-the-art treatments (NLSTRT 2011).

Examples of Evidence-Based Interventions

Public health interventions that are likely to affect lung cancer rates include the National Cancer Institute's American Stop Smoking Intervention Study (ASSIST) for Cancer Prevention (NCI 2005), the CDC's National Tobacco Control Program (CDC 2014b), and dedicated state tobacco taxes, such as those in California and Massachusetts (see Chapter 7; Chaloupka et al. 2012). A common element to all these programs involves a comprehensive approach, using price increases (e.g., through excise taxes), clean indoor air laws, mass media campaigns, restricting youth access, and providing low- or no-cost smoking cessation services.

Areas of Future Research

First, effective smoking prevention and cessation techniques must be targeted to high-risk and difficult-to-reach populations such as youths, minorities, the economically disadvantaged, and heavy smokers. Second, the roles of risk factors such as occupational exposures and residential radon exposure and their interactions with cigarette smoking must be further examined. Third, the role of dietary factors in the prevention of lung cancer needs to be further evaluated. Finally, experiences with lung cancer screening need to be evaluated and improved over time.

COLORECTAL CANCER

Significance

Cancer of the colon and rectum, also known as colorectal cancer, is the third most commonly diagnosed cancer and the third leading cause of cancer death in men and women in the United States (ACS 2016a). In 2016, it is estimated that approximately 70,820 new cases of colon and rectum cancer will be diagnosed in men and 63,670 new cases will be diagnosed in women. The overall five-year survival rate for colorectal cancer is 65%, with a rate of 90% for cancers identified in the local stage (Siegel et al. 2016). However, only 39% of cases are diagnosed at local stage (Siegel et al. 2016).

Pathophysiology

Colorectal cancer develops from conventional adenomas and sessile serrated polyps or adenomas (Strum 2016). The predominant cell type seen in colorectal cancer is adenocarcinoma. The prevalence of adenomas has been reported to be as high as 50% in asymptomatic persons who undergo screening, and an estimated 3% to 7% of detected adenomas are advanced (Strum 2016). Although only around 10% of adenomas progress into cancer, several factors increase the likelihood including larger size (greater than or equal to 1 centimeter in surface diameter), multiplicity, degree of dysplasia, and villous histology (Giovannucci and Kana 2006).

A family history of colorectal cancer or adenomas and inherited genetic conditions (familial adenomatous polyposis and hereditary nonpolyposis colorectal cancer) increase risk of colorectal cancer (ACS 2016a). Familial adenomatous polyposis is very rare and characterized by multiple adenomas, usually 100 at the minimum, that turn cancerous if left untreated. Hereditary nonpolyposis colorectal cancer is also rare, and is characterized by adenomas more likely to have characteristics associated with progression to cancer. A personal history of chronic inflammatory bowel disease, ulcerative colitis, Crohn's disease, and diabetes also elevates risk (ACS 2016a).

Descriptive Epidemiology

High-Risk Populations

More than one third all colorectal cancer deaths occur in adults aged 80 years or older (Siegel et al. 2014). Incidence and death rates are higher in men than women, and highest in blacks and lowest in Asians/Pacific Islanders (Siegel et al. 2014). Colorectal mortality in black male patients was 50% higher than in non-Hispanic white male patients between 2006 and 2010 (Siegel et al. 2014).

Time Trends

Since the mid-1980s, colorectal cancer incidence has declined overall, with steeper declines between 2008 and 2012, which has been attributed to changes in risk factors, such as the decrease in smoking, and increases in colorectal cancer screening. However, among those aged younger than 50 years, incidence rates have been increasing by 1.8% per year, and the reasons for this increase are unknown. Like incidence rates overall, colorectal cancer mortality rates have also been decreasing over time, 2.8% per year between 2003 and 2012 (Howlader et al. 2015).

Causes

Modifiable Risk Factors

There is now considerable evidence that several lifestyle factors influence colorectal cancer risk (Table 16-4). Body and abdominal fatness increase risk,

Table 16-4. Modifiable Risk Factors for Colorectal Cancer, United States

Magnitude	Risk Factor	Best Estimate (%) of Population-Attributable Risk (Range)
Strong (relative risk > 4)	None	
Moderate (relative risk 2–4)	None	
Weak (relative risk < 2)	Physical inactivity[a]	26 (17–35)
	Age > 50 years not screened with appropriate method	17
	Obesity[b]	27 (0–43)
	No dietary milk or calcium supplement on most days	13
	Three or more red meat servings per week	9
	Alcohol consumption[c]	< 1
	Multivitamin use[d]	
	Aspirin use[d]	35 (-3–64.0)

Source: Data from Ballard-Barbash et al. (2006) and Lee and Oguma (2006).
[a]Includes occupational and recreational physical activities, population activity prevalence estimated for adults aged 45 to 64 years.
[b]Body mass index greater than 30.
[c]Two or more drinks per day.
[d]Use of multivitamin or aspirin may decrease risk (Giovannucci and Kana 2006).

whereas physical activity decreases risk (WCRF/AICR 2011). Up to half of colorectal cancer cases may be related to obesity and physical inactivity (see Chapters 9 and 11). With regard to diet, consuming foods high in dietary fiber decreases risk, whereas consuming alcohol, red meat, and processed meat increases risk (WCRF/AICR 2011). The International Agency for Research on Cancer classified red meat as a probable carcinogen to humans and processed meat as a carcinogen to humans largely on the basis of the associations with colorectal cancer (IARC 2015). Use of aspirin can also reduce the risk of colorectal cancer (Chan and Giovannucci 2010). Recently, the U.S. Preventive Services Task force released a draft recommendation for low-dose aspirin use for the primary prevention of cardiovascular disease and colorectal cancer in adults aged 50 to 59 years who have a 10% or greater 10-year cardiovascular disease risk, are not at increased risk for bleeding, have a life expectancy of at least 10 years, and are willing to take low-dose aspirin daily for at least 10 years (Dehmer et al. 2015; USPSTF 2015a).

Evidence-Based Interventions

Prevention

Current evidence suggests that primary prevention strategies that improve diet and reduce sedentary behavior could reduce colorectal cancer incidence. Although the relationship of diet to colorectal cancer is not completely understood, some dietary recommendations can be made, such as limiting intake of red meat, processed meat, and alcohol. Aspirin use may also provide a benefit for those not at increased risk for bleeding and with a greater than 10-year life expectancy. Furthermore, increasing physical activity and maintenance of a healthy weight can also reduce risk (see Chapters 8, 9, and 11).

Screening

The principal screening tests for early detection of colorectal cancer are colonoscopy, sigmoidoscopy, stool tests for occult blood, CT colonography, and multi-targeted stool DNA tests. The U.S. Preventive Services Task Force recommends colorectal screening for average-risk adults aged 50 to 75 years (USPSTF 2015b). Follow-up screens are determined on the basis of screening results and methodology. Adults aged 76 to 85 years should consult with a health professional to determine whether or not to be screened; those who have never been screened, and those who are healthy enough to undergo treatment if cancer is found and do not have comorbid conditions that significantly limit life expectancy, are most likely to benefit (USPSTF 2015b). Despite the benefit of screening, just under 60% of those aged between 50 and 75 years in the United States report having had a recent colorectal cancer screening test; rates are particularly low for those without insurance (Sabatino et al. 2015). Improving access to colorectal cancer screening across all populations could have an important impact on colorectal cancer incidence and mortality in the United States (Siegel et al. 2014).

Treatment

Surgery is the most common method of treating colorectal cancer. After treatment, colorectal cancer patients need to be followed closely, because they are at a high risk of having recurrent or new cancers in the colon and rectum.

BREAST CANCER

Significance

Breast cancer is the most common cancer type among women in the United States and the second leading cause of cancer death (ACS 2016a). It is estimated that in 2016 there will be 249,260 new cases of invasive cancer and 40,890 deaths. Breast cancer rarely occurs in men, accounting for 1% of breast cancer cases in the United States (ACS 2015b). Approximately one of every eight women will develop breast cancer at some time during her lifetime, with an overall five-year survival rate of 89%. However, survival can range from 26% for distant-stage cancer to 99% for local-stage cancer (NCI 2015).

Pathophysiology

Breast cancer develops as cells lose their normal regulatory control, and transition from noninvasive cancer, to invasive cancer, and finally metastatic disease. Noninvasive lesions can be confined to the duct (ductal carcinoma in situ) or to the lobule (lobular carcinoma in situ), and some of their forms can be considered precursor lesions of invasive carcinoma (Houghton et al. 2003).

The predominant cell type of breast cancer is adenocarcinoma (approximately 95% of cases). Among invasive tumors, the number of lymph nodes involved is the best prognostic indicator of survival. Hormones, both endogenous and exogenous, play a role in breast cancer pathogenesis as they increase cell proliferation in the breast and the opportunity for random genetic errors during cell division deaths (Colditz et al. 2006). Proliferation is mediated by hormone receptors. Estrogen and progesterone receptors are often present in breast cancer tumors. When receptors are present above a certain threshold value, the tumor is considered receptor-positive. Receptor-positive women respond better to hormonal therapy and show increased survival rates.

Women with a first-degree relative with breast cancer have a 1.5- to 3-times increased risk of developing the disease (Yang et al. 1998). Mutations in *BRCA1* (breast cancer 1) or *BRCA2* (breast cancer 2) may correspond with up to an 80% lifetime risk of developing breast cancer (Easton et al. 1993). These germ line mutations likely account for 2% to 5% of all breast cancers. Previous diagnosis of high-risk breast lesions is associated with significant 10-year risks: Lobular carcinoma in situ is associated with 23.7% risk, atypical ductal hyperplasia with 17.3% risk, atypical lobular hyperplasia with 20.7% risk, and 26.0% risk with severe atypical ductal hyperplasia (Coopey et al. 2012).

Descriptive Epidemiology

High-Risk Populations

Incidence and mortality increase with age, with the risk of being diagnosed going from 1 in 227 (0.44%) at age 30 to 1 in 26 (3.89%) at age 70 (Howlader et al. 2015). Other non-modifiable factors are family history of breast cancer, genetic predispositions (*BRCA1* and *BRCA2*), history of radiation exposure, early menarche, late menopause, null parity, and race (Hunt et al. 2012).

Although the incidence of breast cancer is higher in whites, mortality rates are 35% higher among African-American women than among white women (ACS 2014a). Disparities in health outcomes are attributed to tumor behavior, psychosocial or behavioral factors, socioeconomic status, variation in access to care, and screening and treatment differences (Wheeler et al. 2013).

Geographic Distribution

Breast cancer mortality rates in the United States are generally higher in Eastern states and lower in Western states. These variations vary according to race and ethnicity—among white women, mortality rate is highest in Nevada (24.5) and lowest in Vermont (18.7), whereas for black women, the highest death rate is seen in Oklahoma (35.4), and the lowest in Minnesota (21.7) (ACS 2015b).

Breast cancer rates show wide international variations—the highest incidence rates are seen in North America and Europe and the lowest are seen in Middle Africa and Eastern Asia (Ferlay et al. 2013). However, when one considers the mortality rate, the lowest rate is seen in Eastern Asia, and the highest is seen in Western Africa.

Time Trends

Breast cancer incidence rates in the United States rose sharply throughout the 1980s, in part because of the increase in use of mammography screening.

Later, this trend reversed as incidence rates decreased from 132 per 100,000 in 1990 to 124 per 100,000 in 2004, remaining stable since 2004 for white women, and slightly increased for black women (119 per 100,000 in 1990 to 118 per 100,000 in 2004; ACS 2015b).

Mortality attributable to breast cancer remained relatively stable in the first half of the 1900s. Between 1973 and 1990, breast cancer mortality rates increased 2% among U.S. women overall and 21% among African-American women (USDHHS 1995). Since 1990, the overall mortality rate has decreased by 36%, with data from 2003 to 2010 establishing the decrease at a rate of 1.9% per year among white women, and 1.4% among African Americans (ACS 2016b).

Causes

Modifiable Risk Factors

Through numerous epidemiologic studies, an array of modifiable breast cancer risk factors has been established (Table 16-5). Despite the large number of risk factors, few are strongly associated with the development of breast cancer,

Table 16-5. Modifiable Risk Factors for Breast Cancer, United States

Magnitude	Risk Factor	Best Estimate (%) of Population-Attributable Risk (Range)
Strong (relative risk > 4)	None	
Moderate (relative risk 2–4)	Ionizing radiation	
Weak (relative risk < 2)	Never having children	5 (1–9)
	Physical Activity	15.7 (-6.5–33.7)
	Weight gain since age 18[a]	21.3 (13.1–29.3)
	First full-term pregnancy after age 30	7 (1–13)
	Obesity after menopause	11 (4–37)
	Alcohol consumption	6.1 (2.1–10.3)
	High-caloric or high-fat diet	16–24
	Lack of breast-feeding	4 (2–11)
	Postmenopausal hormone use	4.6 (-3.5–11.9)

Source: Data from Ballard-Barbash et al. (2006); Lee and Oguma (2006); Sprague et al. (2008).
[a]Among postmenopausal women.
[b]Prevalence estimate for women aged 40 to 44 years.

and no single factor or combination of factors can predict the occurrence of breast cancer in any one individual.

The risk associated with reproductive variables—never having children, being of a late age at first birth, having an early menarche, having a late menopause—is related to the hormonal environment to which the breast is exposed (e.g., during pregnancy or during a long menstrual history; USDHHS 1996; Colditz et al. 2006). Conversely, lactation is associated with a 4.3% decrease in risk for every 12 months of breast-feeding (Collaborative Group on Hormonal Factors in Breast Cancer 2002).

In Western populations, body fat is associated with an increased risk among postmenopausal women and decreased risk among premenopausal women (Colditz et al. 2006). Physical activity has an inverse, dose–response effect on breast cancer risk.

Investigation of endogenous hormones has shown an increased risk of breast cancer among premenopausal women with high blood levels of insulin-like growth factor I and among postmenopausal women with high blood estrogens. Exogenous hormones, such as oral contraceptive and postmenopausal hormones have been associated with an increased risk of breast cancer (Beral et al. 2003, Chen et al. 2002). Although current and recent users of oral contraceptives may have a slight elevation in risk, these women tend to be younger with a low absolute risk. Likewise, current users of postmenopausal hormones and those with the longest duration of use are also at an increased risk of breast cancer, though this risk is mitigated if hormone use has stopped for five or more years, regardless of previous duration.

Several dietary factors have also been examined in relation to breast cancer risk. Current evidence regarding fat and fruit and vegetable intake has been inconclusive or unsupportive of a relationship to breast cancer risk (Colditz et al. 2006). However, beta-carotene and folate intake do appear to be protective against breast cancer. Moderate-to-heavy alcohol consumption is associated with an increased risk of breast cancer (Longnecker 1994). High intake of folic acid may protect against the risk associated with alcohol intake (Zhang et al. 2003).

Population-Attributable Risk

Several established risk factors each account for relatively small proportions of overall breast cancer incidence (Table 16-5).

Evidence-Based Interventions

Prevention

Although challenging, there is sufficient evidence that the risk of breast cancer could be reduced by maintaining healthy weight (especially after menopause), being physically active, breast-feeding, and perhaps avoiding alcohol use. However, given the small attributable risk for these factors, and challenges in making changes, public health practitioners should also focus attention on secondary prevention—that is, early detection.

Screening

Recommendations for screening vary according to the age group and organization that created the guidelines (Table 16-6): American Cancer Society (Oeffinger et al. 2015), USPSTF (Nelson et al. 2016), the American Academy of Family Physicians (AAFP 2013), American Congress of Obstetricians and Gynecologists (ACOG 2011), and National Comprehensive Cancer Network (NCCN 2014).

Differences in screening recommendations are based on the evidence and a process used to compare and contrast the harms and benefits of screening. However, according to recent research, 69% of recommendation statements either did not quantify harms or presented them in an asymmetric manner, which limits the ability to compare the trade-offs of the interventions (Caverly et al. 2016).

Breast self-examination and clinical breast examination are no longer recommended by the American Cancer Society, because of the lack of evidence that their use is associated with improved outcomes (Kösters and Gøtzsche 2003), and moderate quality evidence that adding clinical breast examination to mammography screening increased the false-positive rate (Oeffinger et al. 2015).

Breast cancer mortality is reduced with mammography screening, with which the magnitudes of effect are small for younger ages, and with a 25% to 31% risk reduction for women aged 50 to 69 years. Higher stage tumors are also reduced with screening for women aged 50 years and older. False-positive results are common in all age groups, and are higher for younger women and those with risk factors (Nelson et al. 2016). Approximately 10% to 30% of cases may be overdiagnosed and overtreated, which means that for every 2,000 women

Table 16-6. Screening Recommendations for Breast Cancer among Women with Average Risk

Source	<40 Years	40–44 Years	45–54 Years	≥55 Years	Age of Discontinuance
U.S. Preventive Services Task Force[a]		Individual decision based on the potential benefit and harms among women aged 40 to 49 years—Evidence C		Biennial mammography starting at age 50 years—Evidence B	Insufficient evidence to assess the benefits of screening on women aged 75 years or older
American Cancer Society[b]		Women should have the choice to start mammography	Yearly mammography	Biennial mammography	For as long as the woman is in good health, and expected to live 10 more years
American Academy of Family Physicians[c]		Individualized decision, considering risk factors		Biennial mammography starting at age 50 years	No screening after age 75 years
American Congress of Obstetricians and Gynecologists[d]	Clinical Breast examination every year for women aged 19 years or older	Yearly mammography and clinical breast examination			
American College of Radiology[e]		Yearly mammography			Individual basis
National Comprehensive Cancer Network[f]		Yearly mammography, clinical breast examination, and breast awareness			

Source: Compiled from Nelson (2016)[a]; Oeffinger (2015)[b]; AAFP (2013)[c]; ACOG (2011)[d]; ACR (2013)[e]; and NCCN (2014).[f]

invited for screening throughout 10 years, 10 will be treated unnecessarily, and more than 200 will experience important psychological distress because of false-positive findings (Gøtzsche and Jørgensen 2013).

There is no evidence that the use of ultrasonography as an adjunct for mammography for breast cancer screening provides additional benefit (Gartlehner et al. 2013).

For women who are at increased risk for breast cancer and at low risk for adverse medication effects, clinicians should offer to prescribe risk-reducing medications, such as tamoxifen or raloxifene (Nelson et al. 2009). In addition, those women with family history of breast cancer should receive genetic counseling and, if indicated, *BRCA* testing (Nelson et al. 2013).

Treatment

Depending on the stage of cancer and the patient's medical history, breast cancer treatment may require lumpectomy (local removal of the cancer), mastectomy (surgical removal of the breast), radiation therapy, chemotherapy, or hormone therapy. Two or more treatment methods are often used in combination. Cancer support groups such as the American Cancer Society's Reach to Recovery Program can provide valuable information and emotional support to breast cancer patients.

Examples of Evidence-Based Interventions

At the population level, there are strategies that can be used to increase screening (Guide to Community Preventive Services 2015):

1. Client reminders: Written or telephone messages advising people that they are due for skin cancer screening provided a median increase of 14 percentage points compared with baseline appointments. When added to other types of interventions, the median incremental effect for client reminders was an increase of 5.0 percentage points (Sabatino et al. 2012).
2. Use of videos and printed materials such as letters, brochures, and newsletters to inform and motivate people to be screened.
3. Group education by a health professional or trained laypeople who use presentations or teaching aids, with information on indications, benefits, and ways to overcome barriers to screening.

4. One-on-one education by a health care worker or other professional in person or over the phone, often accompanied by supporting materials via printed or audio media.

5. Reducing structural barriers to access screening, such as reducing time or distance between service delivery, modifying hours of service to meet client needs, using alternative or non-clinical settings, and eliminating or simplifying administrative procedures and other obstacles.

6. Reducing client out-of-pocket costs to minimize economic barriers that make it difficult for clients to access cancer screening services.

Areas of Future Research

In light of the differences of guidelines for screening and the controversy associated with them, more research is required to determine the ideal interval for mammography screening and follow-up after treatment and to characterize the benefits and harms that should be accounted in the decision-making process. This will facilitate an individualized experience that considers quality of life and increases patient satisfaction. In addition, the use of new technologies such as tomosynthesis and magnetic resonance imaging should be further explored.

Although several possible risk factors for breast cancer—diet, alcohol use, physical inactivity—are amenable to primary prevention, more research is required to identify the best policies or interventions at a population level (Ferrini et al. 2015). Other modifiable risk factors, such as reproductive timing and breast-feeding duration, are influenced by social norms and may be affected by policy interventions such as support for childcare, breast-feeding in the workplace, or longer maternity leaves (Colditz et al. 2006).

CERVICAL CANCER

Significance

Invasive cancer of the uterine cervix, commonly known as cervical cancer, will have an estimated 12,990 new cases and 4,120 deaths among women in the United States in 2016 (Siegel et al. 2016). In situ cervical cancer—that is, detected in the earliest, premalignant stage—is much more common, accounting for about 60,000 U.S. cases per year. Cervical cancer is the 21st most common cancer in the United States, yet it is the fourth most common cancer among women worldwide, with an estimated 527,600 incident cases in 2012 (Torre et al. 2015). The overall five-year survival rate for cervical cancer is 68%; however, survival approaches 92% for cervical cancers detected in situ (Siegel et al. 2016).

Pathophysiology

Because of advances in molecular biology, researchers now identify cervical cancer as a multi-step process. As described later in this chapter, nearly all cases of cervical cancer are believed to result from persistent infection with one of about 15 genotypes of carcinogenic HPV (Schiffman et al. 2007). There are four major steps in cervical cancer development: (1) infection of metaplastic epithelium at the cervical transformation zone, (2) viral persistence, (3) progression of persistently infected epithelium to cervical precancer, and (4) invasion through the basement membrane of the epithelium.

It is believed that early stages of cervical cancer are characterized by dysplasia, or the presence of cells that are altered in size, shape, and organization. Pre-clinical, pre-invasive changes in the cervix are called cervical intraepithelial neoplasia. These early cervical cancer changes can easily be detected through the Papanicolaou (Pap) test. The Pap test involves collecting and analyzing a small sample of cells from the cervix. Clinical manifestations of cervical cancer may involve bleeding or other vaginal discharges. The major cell types observed for invasive cervical cancer are squamous cell cancer (approximately 65% of cases) and adenocarcinoma (approximately 28% of cases; Howlader et al. 2015).

Descriptive Epidemiology

High-Risk Populations

Cervical cancer incidence increases sharply until age 45 and peaks around that age. The incidence of cervical cancer is 54% higher among African Americans as it is among whites, and mortality rates are approximately two times higher among African Americans (Howlader et al. 2015). Elevated cervical cancer rates are also observed for Hispanics, American Indians, and Hawaiian natives. Women of lower socioeconomic status are at higher risk of cervical cancer. Several religious groups—Catholic nuns, Amish, Mormons, and Jews—have very low rates of cervical cancer, probably because of marital and sexual risk factors.

Geographic Distribution

Cervical cancer mortality rates in the United States are generally higher in Southeastern states and lower in Western (Rocky Mountain) and Upper-Midwestern states. Arkansas has the highest cervical cancer mortality rate, and North Dakota and Vermont have the lowest (Howlader et al. 2015). Internationally, cervical cancer incidence rates are highest in Africa, Melanesia, and parts of Central and South America (Torre et al. 2015).

Time Trends

Incidence and mortality rates of invasive cervical cancer have been decreasing steadily over the past 50 years. Between 1975 and 2012, invasive cervical cancer incidence has decreased in half (14.8 per 100,000 to 6.7 per 100,000; ACS 2016a). In women aged younger than 50 years, however, these rates have remained steady from 2008 to 2012. From 1950 to 2004, cervical cancer incidence and mortality in the United States have shown a larger annual percentage decrease than have any other major cancer among women (Ries et al. 2007). However, this decline has been due to squamous cell carcinoma, and there is concern that cervical adenocarcinoma rates have risen in the past few decades in several countries, including the United States (Schiffman and Hildesheim 2006).

Causes

Modifiable Risk Factors

The primary risk factor for cervical cancer is infection with HPV—it is now accepted to be the central, necessary cause of virtually all cases of cervical cancer (Schiffman and Hildesheim 2006). There are likely more than 100 types of HPV. About 30 of these are transmitted by sexual contact, and approximately 20 of these are causally related to cervical cancer. The relative risk estimate for HPV-DNA and cervical cancer was estimated at 158 (95% confidence interval = 113,221) in the IARC multicenter study (Munoz et al. 2003), among the highest effect sizes observed for any human cancer (Bosch and de Sanjose 2003).

There are other established risk factors for cervical cancer including long-term use of hormonal contraceptives, cigarette smoking, five or more pregnancies, and several sexual risk factors: partners with greater than six other sexual partners and HPV infection in a male partner (Bosch and de Sanjose 2003).

Population-Attributable Risk

Estimates of attributable risk for HPV infection and cervical cancer range from 90% to 98%, suggesting that nearly all cases of cervical cancer are attributable to HPV infection.

Evidence-Based Interventions

Prevention

Several behavioral changes will reduce the risk of cervical cancer. These include limiting the number of sexual partners, delaying intercourse until a later age, avoiding sexually transmitted diseases, and eliminating cigarette smoking.

Three vaccines have been approved by the U.S. Food and Drug Administration for the prevention of the HPV infection (NCI 2016d). If given before individuals begin to engage in sexual activity, they are considered highly effective in preventing the HPV infection. It is recommended that female individuals receive the vaccine between ages 13 and 26 years and male individuals between ages 13 and 21 years. The vaccine must be given in a series of three shots. These vaccines prevent infection with the two types of HPV that cause approximately 70% of cervical cancers, and the two types of HPV that cause 90% of genital warts (NCI 2007). The approved vaccine provides protection against infection with these HPV types for at least eight years.

Screening

The principal screening test for cervical cancer over the past six decades has been the Pap test—it is the oldest and most established early detection test (Hiatt et al. 2002). Decreases in cervical cancer incidence and mortality over the past 60 years are mainly the result of early detection through widespread use of the Pap test. Despite the availability and frequent use of the Pap test, subgroups of high-risk women—for example, those of lower education and income—either have never been screened or are screened infrequently. Pap testing is especially important in these high-risk groups and in women who no longer see a physician for obstetric needs. Both the U.S. Preventive Services Task Force and the American Cancer Society agree on their recommendations for screening guidelines. Women should have their first Pap test by the age of 21 years. These should occur every three years until the age of 30 years, when women should have both a Pap test and HPV test every five years until the age of 65 years. This interval is less often than the annual screening recommendation that was the standard for many decades. Women aged older than 65 years do not need regular screenings if they have a history of normal results from previous screenings (Vesco et al. 2011; Saslow et al. 2012).

Treatment

Depending on the stage at diagnosis, cervical cancer is usually treated by surgery or radiation or both. In situ cancers can be treated by cryotherapy (cell destruction by extreme cold), electrocoagulation (cell destruction by intense heat), or local surgery.

Examples of Evidence-Based Interventions

The National Cancer Institute and the CDC began funding a series of cervical cancer research and application projects in 1985 (NIH 1991). Most of these projects sought to increase the use of the Pap test in high-risk populations through "in-reach," or increasing use in women who attend clinics, and "outreach," or offering community-wide screening programs. In 2005, the Gynecologic Cancer Education and Awareness Act was passed to target women and health professionals through media campaigns, research, and outreach organizations. These efforts are headed up by the CDC's Inside Knowledge: Get the Facts about Gynecologic Cancer Campaign (CDC 2016).

In addition, the CDC is sponsoring large-scale cervical cancer screening projects as part of the Breast and Cervical Cancer Mortality Prevention Act of 1990 (Henson et al. 1996). This law has become an effective screening program across the United States serving a large number of low-income women in the 25 years of its existence (Lee et al. 2014).

Areas of Future Research

Further research into the causes of cervical cancer will lead to increased opportunities for primary prevention. A better understanding of the interaction among multiple risk factors is also needed. Given the high rates of cervical cancer mortality among minority and economically disadvantaged women, better targeting of proven cervical cancer control technologies is clearly needed.

PROSTATE CANCER

Significance

Prostate cancer is the most common cancer diagnosed among men in the United States and the second-most-common cause of cancer death among men. In 2016, it is estimated that approximately 180,890 new prostate cancer cases will be diagnosed, and 26,120 prostate cancer deaths will occur (Siegel et al. 2016).

Descriptive Epidemiology

The risk of prostate cancer is 70% higher in black men than in non-Hispanic white men (ACS 2016a). Furthermore, black men are more than two times more likely to die of prostate cancer than any other group (ACS 2016a). The reasons underlying these differences are not well understood. Prostate cancer incidence rates increased dramatically in the early 1990s with the detection of asymptomatic prostate cancer via the widespread use of prostate-specific antigen (PSA) screening (Siegel et al. 2016). Routine PSA screening is no longer recommended because of concerns about high rates of overdiagnosis (Hayes and Barry 2014; Lin et al. 2011). Recently, incidence rates have declined 4.0% per year (ACS 2016a). Mortality rates have also been decreasing, 3.5% between 2003 and 2012 (ACS 2016a). Over the past two decades, the five-year survival rate has increased to 99% (ACS 2016a), primarily because of a combination of better treatments, early detection, and overdiagnosis of PSA-detected indolent cancers.

Causes

The causes of prostate cancer are largely unknown. The only conclusive risk factors are not modifiable, and include older age, being African American, and family history of prostate cancer (Platz and Giovannucci 2006). Although obesity and smoking do not appear to increase risk overall, both increase the risk of aggressive or fatal disease (Cao and Ma 2011; USDHHS 2014).

Evidence-Based Interventions

Because its causes are not clearly understood, prostate cancer is not currently amenable to primary prevention, although men may benefit from smoking cessation and maintaining a healthy weight with respect to the development of aggressive or fatal disease. The U.S. Preventive Services Task Force recommended against routine screening with PSA testing (Moyer 2012), although this recommendation is currently undergoing an update. The American Cancer Society recommends that men discuss the potential benefits and harms of prostate cancer screening with a health care provider to make an informed decision about whether to be tested for prostate cancer (ACS 2016d). Research continues intensively on ways to improve the use of PSA as a screening test and to identify other biomarkers that may be a better screening test for early prostate cancer.

LYMPHOMA

Significance

Lymphomas are cancers that affect lymphocytes, primarily in the lymph nodes, spleen, and thymus. Lymphomas are generally classified as either Hodgkin's lymphoma or non-Hodgkin's lymphoma.

Hodgkin's Lymphoma

In 2015, an estimated 9,050 cases of Hodgkin's lymphoma were reported, and 1,150 deaths. The overall risk of being diagnosed with Hodgkin's lymphoma over a lifetime is 0.2% (Howlader et al. 2015).

Non-Hodgkin's Lymphoma

In 2015, an estimated 71,850 persons were diagnosed with non-Hodgkin's lymphoma and 19,790 deaths (Howlader et al. 2015). Approximately 2.1% of men and women will be diagnosed with non-Hodgkin's lymphoma at some point during their lifetime, based on 2010–2012 data (Howlader et al. 2015).

Descriptive Epidemiology

Hodgkin's Lymphoma

The incidence has been higher among whites than African Americans, and among male than female individuals (Mueller et al. 2006). The age distribution of Hodgkin's lymphoma is bimodal; one peak in early adulthood, and a second after age 60. The leading cause of death among long-term Hodgkin's lymphoma survivors is second malignancies. It is associated with AIDS.

Non-Hodgkin's Lymphoma

The incidence of non-Hodgkin's lymphoma is higher among men compared with women and is higher among whites compared with African Americans. Age-specific incidence and mortality rates increase with age. The U.S. incidence rate has remained stable over 2003 to 2012, and death rates have been falling on average 2.5% each year (Howlader et al. 2015).

The five-year survival rates for non-Hodgkin's lymphoma (70%) and Hodgkin's lymphoma (86%) are also markedly different.

Causes

The causes of the lymphomas are not well understood, in part because of the diversity of histologic forms of cancer in these diagnoses. Immune system disorders, infection with HIV or Epstein-Barr virus, and treatment with immunosuppressive drugs (e.g., in transplant patients) increase risk of non-Hodgkin's lymphoma (Hartge et al. 2006). There is also some evidence that exposure to certain herbicides and pesticides elevates non-Hodgkin's lymphoma risk, including phenoxy acid–based herbicides (such as 2,4-dichloro-phenoxyacetic acid) and chlorophenols.

An infectious origin has been suggested for Hodgkin's lymphoma on the basis of its epidemiologic features, age at onset, and spatial clustering. Current evidence indicates the Epstein-Barr virus is a causal factor in a considerable proportion of Hodgkin's lymphoma cases (Mueller et al. 2006).

Evidence-Based Interventions

Because the causes of lymphoma are not fully understood, clear prevention strategies are unavailable. Given the growing evidence of an association between pesticide use and non-Hodgkin's lymphoma, however, prudent use of these chemicals is warranted. No screening tests are yet available for the early detection of lymphoma. Although the five-year survival for Hodgkin's lymphoma is high, treatment for Hodgkin's lymphoma appears to result in a high rate of fatal secondary malignancies (Mueller et al. 2006). The development of effective treatments that do not lead to secondary cancers is an important area for future research.

LEUKEMIA

Significance

Leukemia comprises a variety of cancers that arise in the bone marrow, lymph nodes, or other lymphoid tissue with immune function. Leukemia affects both children and adults and accounts for about 27% of cancers among children (4,884 new cases per year; Leukemia and Lymphoma Society 2016) and 2% of adult cancer cases (new cases per year). There are four main types of leukemia: acute myeloid (including acute monocytic) leukemia, acute lymphocytic leukemia, chronic lymphocytic leukemia, and chronic myeloid leukemia. In the United States, acute lymphocytic leukemia accounts for 75% of leukemia cases among children (ACS 2016a). The most common leukemia types among adults are acute myeloid leukemia and chronic lymphocytic leukemia.

From a public health standpoint, leukemia is important not only for its health impact on the population but also because of the frequency of public inquiries regarding leukemia, the emotional nature of these inquiries, and the media impact. State and local health departments respond to more than 1,000 inquiries per year about suspected cancer clusters (Thun and Sinks 2004). These inquiries frequently concern apparent spatial clustering of childhood leukemia cases. Use of an established protocol aids in response to these concerns about cancer clusters (Goodman et al. 2014).

Descriptive Epidemiology

Leukemia is 76% more common among men in the United States than among women and is slightly more common in whites than in African Americans (Siegel et al. 2016; Howlader et al. 2015). Among adults, leukemia mortality has declined over the past 30 years. In the mid-1970s, the five-year survival rate for leukemia was around 41%. That rate has increased to 70% from 2005 to 2011 (Siegel et al. 2016). In contrast, survival among children with acute lymphocytic leukemia has increased dramatically (58%–87%) over the past few decades as the result of improvements in therapy (ACS 2016a).

Causes

The major causes of leukemia are unknown; however, several risk factors have been identified, including genetic abnormalities such as Down syndrome, exposure to ionizing radiation, and workplace exposure to benzene and other related solvents (Linet et al. 2006). Adult T-cell leukemia is strongly associated with infection by human T-lymphotrophic virus, type I, in endemic areas (Blattner 1993). Increasing evidence suggests that cigarette smoking is a causative risk factor for some forms of leukemia (USDHHS 2014). Some studies have suggested that residential exposure to magnetic fields among children and occupational exposure among adults may increase risk, but more recent literature suggests that the evidence for magnetic fields as a risk factor is weak (Linet et al. 2006).

Evidence-Based Interventions

Because the causes of leukemia are largely undetermined, primary prevention is difficult. Reducing occupational and environmental exposures to radiation and leukemogenic chemicals and eliminating cigarette smoking may reduce leukemia incidence. Because symptoms often appear late, diagnosing leukemia early is difficult and no routine screening test exists.

BLADDER CANCER

Significance

Bladder cancer is the most common cancer of the urinary tract, estimated to account for 76,960 new cases and 16,390 deaths in the United States in 2016 (ACS 2016a).

Descriptive Epidemiology

The incidence rate of bladder cancer is almost four times higher among men than women, and two times higher among whites than blacks (ACS 2016a). However, five-year survival is higher among whites (80%), than blacks (64%; ACS 2015c). The reasons for the striking differences in incidence and survival by sex and race are not well established. After decades of slight increases, incidence rates of bladder cancer declined by 0.5% between 2003 and 2012 (ACS 2016a). Since the late 1980s, mortality rates have been stable among men, and decreasing 0.4% annually among women (ACS 2016c).

Causes

Cigarette smoking is the best-established cause of bladder cancer. Bladder cancer risk for a current smoker is approximately three times that of a nonsmoker (Al-Zalabani et al. 2016), and smoking is estimated to account for 50% to 65% of cases in men and 20% to 30% of cases in women (Silverman et al. 2006). More than 40 occupational groups and exposures have been associated with bladder cancer, yet only a few of these are well established (Al-Zalabani et al. 2016). Among these, bladder cancer incidence was highest for workers exposed to aromatic amines and polycyclic aromatic hydrocarbons, including tobacco and dye workers, and chimney sweeps (Cumberbatch et al. 2015). Bladder cancer mortality was highest for workers exposed to heavy metals and polycyclic aromatic hydrocarbons, including chemical and metal workers (Cumberbatch et al. 2015).

Evidence-Based Interventions

Primary prevention of bladder cancer should focus on eliminating cigarette smoking and minimizing exposure to hazardous chemicals in the workplace. Currently, no routine screening test is available for early detection of bladder cancer.

ORAL AND PHARYNGEAL CANCER

Significance

Cancer of the oral cavity—that is, lip, salivary gland, mouth, and pharynx—accounted for an estimated 45,780 new cases and 8,650 U.S. deaths in 2015 (Howlader et al. 2015).

Descriptive Epidemiology

Oral cancer age-adjusted mortality rates are 2.6 times higher among men in the United States than among women, and 1.5 times higher among African Americans than among whites. These rates have remained stable over 2003 to 2012. The overall five-year survival rate for oral cancer in the United States is 63%, although survival for cancer diagnosed in the local stage is 83% (Howlader et al. 2015).

Causes

The use of tobacco in any form—cigarettes, cigars, and pipes, as well as the use of chewing tobacco and snuff—substantially elevates the risk of cancer of the tongue, mouth, and pharynx (Mayne et al. 2006), being responsible for up to 30% of oral cancer cases (Petti 2009). Cigarette smokers have a three-times-greater risk of oral cancer than do nonsmokers (Olson et al. 2013). Excessive alcohol consumption is also associated with cancer of the oral cavity. Smoking and drinking are independent risk factors for oral cancer and also interact synergistically to multiply risk (Blot et al. 1988). Fruit and vegetable intake, as well as certain nutrients including vitamin C and carotene and other carotenoids have been shown to have an inverse relationship with oral cancer risk (Leoncini et al. 2015).

Infection with HPV has been associated with oropharyngeal cancer among younger patients, and white race, in the absence of other risk factors such as heavy tobacco and alcohol use, where the age difference is likely related to higher prevalence of oral sex among younger populations (Moore and Mehta 2015).

Evidence-Based Interventions

Oral and pharyngeal cancers are largely preventable. Oral cancer death rates could be reduced significantly through primary prevention and early detection. Eliminating smoking and smokeless tobacco use and reducing heavy alcohol consumption would substantially reduce oral cancer incidence.

The U.S. Preventive Services Task Force concluded there is insufficient evidence to recommend screening of the general or high-risk population for oral cancer in the United States (Olson et al. 2013), and acknowledges that more research is required to establish a definition of a high-risk patient, on whom screening by dental hygienist, dentists, or other trained experts in U.S. settings might have a role. Similarly, a Cochrane Review that further randomized clinical trials is recommended to assess the efficacy and cost-effectiveness of a visual examination (Brocklehurst et al. 2013).

In contrast, the American Cancer Society recommends self-examination of the oral cavity for abnormal lesions on a monthly basis, and by a health care professional as part of periodic health examinations (ACS 2014a; ACS 2014b).

MELANOMA OF THE SKIN

Significance

Melanoma is a common diagnosis, expected to be the sixth-most-common cancer in 2016, with an estimate of 76,380 new cases and 10,130 deaths (Howlader et al. 2015). Regarding prevalence, in 2013, there were an estimated 1,034,460 people living with melanoma of the skin in the United States.

Descriptive Epidemiology

Between 2003 and 2012, there was an increased incidence for both sexes, and the increase in mortality affected mostly among men (Siegel et al. 2016). The overall probability of developing melanoma over the lifetime is 3.0% for men and 1.9% for women (Siegel et al. 2016). The overall five-year survival for melanoma is 91% (Howlader et al. 2015), and melanoma incidence increases with age, male sex, and white races (Siegel et al. 2016). Other risk factors for melanoma include childhood cancer history, immunosuppression, Parkinson's disease, and use of indoor tanning (Mayer et al. 2014).

Mortality rates also increase with age, and men have a higher risk than women. African Americans are more likely to die from the disease, with a five-year survival rate of 74% compared with 93% for whites (Siegel et al. 2016).

Causes

Sun exposure accounts for an estimated 90% of melanoma cases (Gruber et al. 2006). Recreational sun exposure, especially intense, repeated, blistering overdoses during childhood, increase risk for melanoma. Risk is highest among fair-skinned people who sunburn easily. A family history of melanoma increases the risk by two to eight times. Both benign acquired nevi (e.g., moles) and atypical nevi (e.g., moles with irregular pigmentation and borders) are markers of increased melanoma risk and precursors of melanoma in some cases.

More recently, indoor tanning and artificial sunlamps have been associated with an increased melanoma risk, which is higher if the first use of sunbeds occurred before age 35 years (Boniol et al. 2012).

Evidence-Based Interventions

Prevention of melanoma should include avoiding all forms of ultraviolet radiation exposure, including the sun during peak exposure periods (10:00 A.M.–4:00 P.M.), wearing protective clothing, and wearing sunscreen (AHRQ 2006). However, wearing sunscreen alone could increase risk of melanoma if it also increases the amount of time spent in the sun. Recent research suggesting benefits from moderate sun exposure may lead to confusing messages for the public.

The U.S. Preventive Task Services Force concluded that there is insufficient evidence to recommend routine screening with whole body examination (Wolff et al. 2009), but they recommended counseling of children, adolescents, and young adults aged 10 to 24 years who have fair skin about minimizing their exposure to ultraviolet radiation to reduce risk for skin cancer (Lin et al. 2011).

Some organizations, such as the American Cancer Society, recommend that adults should perform monthly skin self-examinations, especially those people with heavy occupational or recreational sun exposure or with other significant risk factors (Gruber et al. 2006).

Regarding population-level measures to decrease skin cancer overall, the Guide to Community Preventive Services recommends

1. The use of multicomponent community-wide interventions combining individual-directed strategies, mass media campaigns, and environmental and policy changes across multiple settings within a defined geographic area (Guide to Community Preventive Services 2012a).

2. Use of child care center, primary school–, and middle school–based interventions that include sun protection policies, education of staff and parents, and environmental changes such as clothing guidelines and restrictions of outdoor activities during peak hours (Guide to Community Preventive Services 2013a; Guide to Community Preventive Services 2012b).

3. Interventions in outdoor occupational settings to promote sun protective behaviors (Guide to Community Preventive Services 2013b).

4. Interventions in outdoor recreational settings among visitors to promote education about skin cancer prevention or providing free sunscreen (Guide to Community Preventive Services 2014).

Resources

American Cancer Society, http://www.cancer.org

Division of Cancer Prevention and Control, Centers for Disease Control and Prevention, http://www.cdc.gov/cancer

Guide to Community Preventive Services, Community Guide Branch, National Center for Health Marketing, Centers for Disease Control and Prevention, http://www.thecommunityguide.org/index.html

National Cancer Institute, Cancer Information Service, http://www.cancer.gov

World Health Organization, Cancer, http://www.who.int/cancer/en

References

Agency for Healthcare Research and Quality (AHRQ). *The Guide to Clinical Preventive Services 2006: Recommendations of the US Preventative Services Task Force.* Rockville, MD: AHRQ; 2006. AHRQ Publication 06-0588.

Agency for Healthcare Research and Quality (AHRQ), American Cancer Society, Centers for Disease Control and Prevention, The Commission on Cancer, National Cancer Institute, Substance Abuse and Mental Health Services Administration. Cancer Control P.L.A.N.E.T. 2016. Available at: http://cancercontrolplanet.cancer.gov. Accessed April 16, 2016.

Alavanja MC, Brownson RC, Benichou J, Swanson C, Boice JD Jr. Attributable risk of lung cancer in lifetime nonsmokers and long-term ex-smokers (Missouri, United States). *Cancer Causes Control.* 1995;6(3):209–216.

Alciati M, Marconi J, Greenwalk P, Kramer B, Weed D. The public health potential for cancer prevention and control. In: Greenwald P, Kramer B, Weed D, eds. *Cancer Prevention and Control.* New York, NY: Marcel Dekker; 1995:435–449.

Al-Zalabani AH, Stewart KF, Wesselius A, Schols AM, Zeegers MP. Modifiable risk factors for the prevention of bladder cancer: a systematic review of meta-analyses. *Eur J Epidemiol.* 2016; Epub ahead of print March 21, 2016.

American Academy of Family Physicians (AAFP). Updated AAFP breast cancer screening recommendations stress communication. 2013. Available at: http://www.aafp.org/online/en/home/publications/news/news-now/clinical-care-research/20100115aafp-brca-recs.html. Accessed April 12, 2016.

American Cancer Society (ACS). Cancer facts & figures 2014. Atlanta, GA: American Cancer Society; 2014a. Available at: http://www.cancer.org/research/cancerfactsstatistics/cancerfactsfigures2014. Accessed August 30, 2016.

American Cancer Society (ACS). Can oral cavity and oropharyngeal cancers be found early? 2014b. Available at: http://www.cancer.org/cancer/oralcavityandoropharyngeal cancer/detailedguide/oral-cavity-and-oropharyngeal-cancer-detection. Accessed April 25, 2016.

American Cancer Society (ACS). Cancer facts & figures for Hispanics/Latinos 2015–2017. Atlanta, GA: ACS; 2015a.

American Cancer Society (ACS). Breast cancer facts & figures 2015–2016. Atlanta, GA: ACS; 2015b.

American Cancer Society (ACS). Cancer facts and figures 2015. Special section: breast carcinoma in situ. Atlanta, GA: ACS; 2015c.

American Cancer Society (ACS). Cancer facts & figures 2016. Atlanta, GA: ACS; 2016a.

American Cancer Society (ACS). Cancer facts & figures for African Americans 2016–2018. Atlanta, GA: ACS; 2016b.

American Cancer Society (ACS). Cancer facts and figures 2016. Special section: cancer in Asian Americans, Native Hawaiians, and Pacific Islanders. Atlanta, GA: ACS; 2016c.

American Cancer Society (ACS). American Cancer Society recommendations for prostate cancer early detection. Atlanta, GA: ACS; 2016d. Available at: http://www. cancer.org/cancer/prostatecancer/moreinformation/prostatecancerearlydetection/ prostate-cancer-early-detection-acs-recommendations. Accessed August 30, 2016.

American College of Radiology (ACR). *ACR Practice Guideline for the Performance of Screening and Diagnostic Mammography.* 2013. Available at: http://www.acr.org/ quality-safety/standards-guidelines/practice-guidelines-by-modality/breast-imaging. Accessed August 30, 2016.

American Congress of Obstetricians and Gynecologists (ACOG). Breast cancer screening. *Obstet Gynecol.* 2011;118(2 pt 1):372–382.

American Lung Association (ALA). Trends in lung cancer morbidity and mortality. 2014a. Available at: http://www.lung.org/assets/documents/research/lc-trend-report. pdf. Accessed April 10, 2016.Bailar JC III, Gornik HL. Cancer undefeated. *N Engl J Med.* 1997;336(22):1569–1574.

Ballard-Barbash R, Friedehreich C, Slattery M, Thune I. Obesity and body composition. In: Schottenfeld M, Fraumeni JF Jr, eds. *Cancer Epidemiology and Prevention.* 3rd ed. New York, NY: Oxford University Press; 2006:422–448.

Beral V; Million Women Study Collaborators. Breast cancer and hormone-replacement therapy in the Million Women Study [erratum in: *Lancet.* 2003;362(9390):1160]. *Lancet.* 2003;362(9382):419–427.

Blattner W. T-cell lymphotrophic viruses and cancer causation. In: deVita VT, Hellman S, Rosenberg SA, eds. *Cancer: Principles and Practice of Oncology.* Philadelphia, PA: Lippincott; 1993.

Blot WJ, McLaughlin JK, Winn DM, et al. Smoking and drinking in relation to oral and pharyngeal cancer. *Cancer Res.* 1988;48(11):3282–3287.

Boniol M, Autier P, Boyle P, Gandini S. Cutaneous melanoma attributable to sunbed use: systematic review and meta-analysis. *BMJ.* 2012;345:e4757.

Bosch FX, de Sanjose S. Chapter 1: human papillomavirus and cervical cancer—burden and assessment of causality. *J Natl Cancer Inst Monogr.* 2003;(31):3–13.

Brocklehurst P, Kujan O, O'Malley LA, Ogden G, Shepherd S, Glenny AM. Screening programmes for the early detection and prevention of oral cancer. *Cochrane Database Syst Rev.* 2013;(11):CD004150.

Byers T, Mouchawar J, Marks J, et al. The American Cancer Society challenge goals. How far can cancer rates decline in the US by the year 2015? *Cancer.* 1999;86(4):715–727.

Cao Y, Ma J. Body mass index, prostate cancer-specific mortality, and biochemical recurrence: a systematic review and meta-analysis. *Cancer Prev Res (Phila).* 2011;4(4):486–501.

Caverly TJ, Hayward RA, Reamer E, Zikmund-Fisher BJ, Connochie D, Heisler M, Fagerlin A. presentation of benefits and harms in US cancer screening and prevention guidelines: systematic review. *J Natl Cancer Inst.* 2016;108(6):djv436.

Centers for Disease Control and Prevention (CDC). National Hospital Discharge Survey. 2010. Data highlights—selected tables. Average length of stay and days of care. 2010. Available at: http://www.cdc.gov/nchs/nhds/nhds_tables.htm#average. Accessed March 21, 2016.

Centers for Disease Control and Prevention (CDC). QuickStats: age-adjusted death rates for heart disease and cancer, by sex—United States, 1980–2011. *MMWR Morbid Mortal Wkly Rep.* 2014a;63(37):827.

Centers for Disease Control and Prevention (CDC). *Best Practices for Comprehensive Tobacco Control Programs—2014.* Atlanta, GA: National Center for Chronic Disease Prevention and Health Promotion, Office on Smoking and Health; 2014b.

Centers for Disease Control and Prevention (CDC). National Program of Cancer Registries. National Center for Chronic Disease Prevention and Health Promotion, Division of Cancer Prevention and Control. 2015. Available at: http://www.cdc.gov/cancer/npcr/about.htm. Accessed March 23, 2016.

Centers for Disease Control and Prevention (CDC). About the Inside Knowledge Campaign. 2016. Available at: http://www.cdc.gov/cancer/knowledge/about.htm. Accessed April 10, 2016.

Chaloupka F, Yurekli A, Fong G. Tobacco taxes as a tobacco control strategy. *Tob Control.* 2012;21(2):172–180.

Chan AT, Giovannucci EL. Primary prevention of colorectal cancer. *Gastroenterology.* 2010;138(6):2029–2043.e10.

Chen C, Weiss NS, Newcomb P, Barlow W, White E. Hormone replacement therapy in relation to breast cancer. *JAMA.* 2002;287(6):734–741.

Collaborative Group on Hormonal Factors in Breast Cancer. Breast cancer and breast-feeding: collaborative reanalysis of individual data from 47 epidemiological studies in 30 countries, including 50,302 women with breast cancer and 96,973 women without the disease. *Lancet.* 2002:360(9328):187–195.

Colditz GA, Atwood KA, Emmons K, et al. Harvard Report on Cancer Prevention. Vol. 4: Harvard Cancer Risk Index. Risk Index Working Group, Harvard Center for Cancer Prevention. *Cancer Causes Control.* 2000:11(6):477–488.

Colditz GA, Baer HJ, Tamimi RM. Breast cancer. In: Schottenfeld D, Fraumeni JF Jr, eds. *Cancer Epidemiology and Prevention.* 3rd ed. New York, NY: Oxford University Press; 2006:995–1012.

Colditz GA, Samplin-Salgado M, Ryan CT, et al. Harvard report on cancer prevention. Vol. 5: fulfilling the potential for cancer prevention: policy approaches. *Cancer Causes Control.* 2002;13(3):199–212.

Community Preventive Services Task Force (CPSTF). *The Guide to Community Preventive Services: What Works to Promote Health?* 2016. Available at: http://www.thecommunityguide.org/index.html. Accessed April 10, 2016.

Coopey SB, Mazzola E, Buckley JM, et al. The role of chemoprevention in modifying the risk of breast cancer in women with atypical breast lesions. *Breast Cancer Res Treat.* 2012;136(3):627–633.

Cumberbatch MG, Cox A, Teare D, Catto JW. Contemporary occupational carcinogen exposure and bladder cancer: a systematic review and meta-analysis. *JAMA Oncol.* 2015;1(9):1282–1290.

Danaei G, Ding EL, Mozaffarian D, et al. The preventable causes of death in the United States: comparative risk assessment of dietary, lifestyle, and metabolic risk factors. *PLoS Med.* 2009;6(4):e1000058.

Danaei G, Vander Hoorn S, Lopez AD, et al. Causes of cancer in the world: comparative risk assessment of nine behavioural and environmental risk factors. *Lancet.* 2005;366(9499):1784–1793.

Dehmer SP, Maciosek MV, Flottemesch TJ. *Aspirin Use to Prevent Cardiovascular Disease and Colorectal Cancer: A Decision Analysis: Technical Report.* Rockville, MD: Agency for Healthcare Research and Quality; 2015.

DeNavas-Walt C, Proctor BD. US Census Bureau. Current Population Reports, P60-252, Income and poverty in the United States: 2014. Washington, DC: US Government Printing Office; 2015.

Doll R, Peto R. *The Causes of Cancer. Quantitative Estimates of Avoidable Risks of Cancer in the United States Today.* New York, NY: Oxford University Press; 1981.

Easton DF, Bishop DT, Ford D, Crockford GP. Genetic linkage analysis in familial breast and ovarian cancer: results from 214 families. The Breast Cancer Linkage Consortium. *Am J Hum Genet.* 1993:52(4):678–701.

Ferlay J, Soerjomataram I, Ervik M, et al. GLOBOCAN 2012 v1.0, Cancer Incidence and Mortality Worldwide: IARC CancerBase No. 11. Lyon, France: International Agency for Research on Cancer; 2013. Available at: http://globocan.iarc.fr. Accessed April 6, 2016.

Ferrini K, Ghelfi F, Mannucci R, Titta L. Lifestyle, nutrition and breast cancer: facts and presumptions for consideration. *Ecancermedicalscience.* 2015;23(9):557.

Gartlehner G, Thaler K, Chapman A, et al. Mammography in combination with breast ultrasonography versus mammography for breast cancer screening in women at average risk. *Cochrane Database Syst Rev.* 2013;(4):CD009632.

Ghafoor A, Jemal A, Cokkinides V, et al. Cancer statistics for African Americans. *CA Cancer J Clin.* 2002;52(6):326–341.

Giordano TJ. Morphologic and molecular classification of human cancer. In: Schottenfeld D, Fraumeni JF Jr, eds. *Cancer Epidemiology and Prevention.* 3rd ed. New York, NY: Oxford University Press; 2006:10–20.

Giovannucci E, Kana W. Cancers of the colon and rectum. In: Schottenfeld D, Fraumeni JF Jr, eds. *Cancer Epidemiology and Prevention.* 3rd ed. New York, NY: Oxford University Press; 2006:809–829.

Goodman M, LaKind JS, Fagliano JA, et al. Cancer cluster investigations: review of the past and proposals for the future. *Int J Environ Res Public Health.* 2014;11(2):1479–1499.

Gøtzsche PC, Jørgensen KJ. Screening for breast cancer with mammography. *Cochrane Database Syst Rev.* 2013;(6):CD001877.

Greenwald P, Sondik E. *Cancer Control Objectives for the Nation: 1985–2000.* Bethesda, MD: US Department of Health and Human Services, National Institutes of Health; 1986. NIH Publication 86-2880.

Gruber SB, Armstrong BK. Cutaneous ocular melanoma. In: Schottenfeld D, Fraumeni JF Jr, eds. *Cancer Epidemiology and Prevention.* 3rd ed. New York, NY: Oxford University Press; 2006:1196–1229.

Guide to Community Preventive Services. Preventing skin cancer: multicomponent community-wide interventions. 2012a. Available at: http://www.thecommunityguide.org/cancer/skin/community-wide/multicomponent.html. Accessed April 10, 2016.

Guide to Community Preventive Services. Preventing skin cancer: primary and middle school interventions. 2012b. Available at: http://www.thecommunityguide.org/cancer/skin/education-policy/primaryandmiddleschools.html. Accessed April 10, 2016.

Guide to Community Preventive Services. Preventing skin cancer: child care center-based interventions. 2013a. Available at: http://www.thecommunityguide.org/cancer/skin/education-policy/childcarecenters.html. Accessed April 10, 2016.

Guide to Community Preventive Services. Preventing skin cancer: interventions in outdoor occupational settings. 2013b. Available at: http://www.thecommunityguide.org/cancer/skin/education-policy/outdooroccupations.html. Accessed April 10, 2016.

Guide to Community Preventive Services. Preventing skin cancer: interventions in outdoor recreational and tourism settings. 2014. Available at: http://www.thecommunityguide.org/cancer/skin/education-policy/outdoorrecreation.html. Accessed April 10, 2016.

Guide to Community Preventive Services. Cancer prevention and control: client-oriented interventions to increase breast, cervical, and colorectal cancer screening. 2015. Available at: http://www.thecommunityguide.org/cancer/screening/client-oriented/index.html. Accessed April 10, 2016.

Hartge P, Bracci PM, Wang SS, et al. Non-Hodgkin's lymphoma. In: Schottenfeld D, Fraumeni JF Jr, eds. *Cancer Epidemiology and Prevention.* 3rd ed. New York, NY: Oxford University Press; 2006:898–918.

Harvard Report on Cancer Prevention. Vol. 1: causes of human cancer. *Cancer Causes Control.* 1996;7(suppl 1):S3–S59.

Hayes JH, Barry MJ. Screening for prostate cancer with the prostate-specific antigen test: a review of current evidence. *JAMA.* 2014;311(11):1143–1149.

Henson RM, Wyatt SW, Lee NC. The National Breast and Cervical Cancer Early Detection Program: a comprehensive public health response to two major health issues for women. *J Public Health Manag Pract.* 1996;2(2):36–47.

Hiatt RA, Klabunde C, Breen N, Swan J, Ballard-Barbash R. Cancer practices from National Health Interview Surveys: past, present, and future. *J Natl Cancer Inst.* 2002;94(24):1837–1846.

Hiatt R, Rimer B. Principles and applications of cancer prevention and control interventions. In: Schottenfeld D, Fraumeni JF Jr, eds. *Cancer Epidemiology and Prevention.* 3rd ed. New York, NY: Oxford University Press; 2006:1283–1291.

Houghton J, George WD, Cuzick J, et al. Radiotherapy and tamoxifen in women with completely excised ductal carcinoma in situ of the breast in the UK, Australia, and New Zealand: randomised controlled trial. *Lancet.* 2003;362(9378):95–102.

Howe HL, Wu X, Ries LA, et al. Annual report to the nation on the status of cancer, 1975–2003, featuring cancer among US Hispanic/Latino populations. *Cancer.* 2006;107(8):1711–1742.

Howlader N, Noone AM, Krapcho M, et al., eds. *SEER Cancer Statistics Review, 1975–2012.* National Cancer Institute. 2015. Available at: http://seer.cancer.gov/csr/1975_2012. Accessed March 15, 2016.

Hunt K, Green M, Buchholz T. Diseases of the breast. In: Townsend C, Beauchamp R, Evers B, Mattox K, eds. *Sabiston Textbook of Surgery.* 19th ed. Philadelphia, PA: Saunders; 2012:824–869.

International Agency for Research on Cancer (IARC). IARC Monographs evaluate consumption of red meat and processed meat. WHO. Lyon, France: IARC; 2015.

Kösters JP, Gøtzsche PC. Regular self-examination or clinical examination for early detection of breast cancer. *Cochrane Database Syst Rev.* 2003;(2):CD003373.

Lee IM, Oguma Y. Physical activity. In: Schottenfeld D, Fraumeni JF Jr, eds. *Cancer Epidemiology and Prevention.* 3rd ed. New York, NY: Oxford University Press; 2006:449–467.

Lee NC, Wong FL, Jamison PM, et al. Implementation of the National Breast and Cervical Cancer Early Detection Program: the beginning. *Cancer.* 2014;120(suppl 16):2540–2548.

Leoncini E, Nedovic D, Panic N, Pastorino R, Edefonti V, Boccia S. Carotenoid intake from natural sources and head and neck cancer: a systematic review and meta-analysis of epidemiological studies. *Cancer Epidemiol Biomarkers Prev.* 2015;24(7):1003–1011.

Leukemia and Lymphoma Society. Childhood blood cancer facts and statistics. 2016. Available at: https://www.lls.org/http%3A/llsorg.prod.acquia-sites.com/facts-and-statistics/facts-and-statistics-overview/facts-and-statistics/childhood-blood-cancer-facts-and-statistics. Accessed April 8, 2016.

Lin K, Croswell JM, Koenig H, Lam C, Maltz A. *Prostate-Specific Antigen-Based Screening for Prostate Cancer: An Evidence Update for the US Preventive Services Task Force.* Rockville, MD: US Preventive Services Task Force; 2011.

Linet MS, Devesa SS, Morgan GJ. The leukemias. In: Schottenfeld D, Fraumeni JF Jr, eds. *Cancer Epidemiology and Prevention.* 3rd ed. New York, NY: Oxford University Press; 2006:841–871.

Longnecker MP. Alcoholic beverage consumption in relation to risk of breast cancer: meta-analysis and review. *Cancer Causes Control.* 1994;5(1):73–82.

Lubin JH, Boice JD II. Estimating Rn-induced lung cancer in the United States. *Health Phys.* 1989;57(3):417–427.

Lubin JH, Boice JD Jr, Edling C, et al. Radon and lung cancer risk: a joint analysis of 11 underground miners studies. Bethesda, MD: US Department of Health and Human Services, National Institutes of Health; 1994. NIH Publication 94-3644.

Mayer JE, Swetter SM, Fu T, Geller AC. Screening, early detection, education, and trends for melanoma: current status (2007–2013) and future directions: part I. Epidemiology, high-risk groups, clinical strategies, and diagnostic technology. *J Am Acad Dermatol.* 2014;71(4):599.e1–599.e12; quiz 610, 599.e512.

Mayne ST, Morse DE, Winn DM. Cancers of the oral cavity and pharynx. In: Schottenfeld D, Fraumeni JF Jr, eds. *Cancer Epidemiology and Prevention.* 3rd ed. New York, NY: Oxford University Press; 2006:674–696.

Meissner HI, Bergner L, Marconi KM. Developing cancer control capacity in state and local public health agencies. *Public Health Rep.* 1992;107(1):15–23.

Miller A. Planning cancer control strategies. *Chronic Dis Can.* 1992;13(1):S1–S40.

Moore KA, Mehta V. The growing epidemic of HPV-positive oropharyngeal carcinoma: a clinical review for primary care providers. *J Am Board Fam Med.* 2015; 28(4):498–503.

Moyer VA. Screening for prostate cancer: US Preventive Services Task Force recommendation statement. *Ann Intern Med.* 2012;157(2):120–134.

Moyer VA, US Preventive Services Task Force. Screening for lung cancer: US Preventive Services Task Force recommendation statement. *Ann Intern Med.* 2014;160(5):330–338.

Mueller NE, Grufferman S. Hodgkin's lymphoma. In: Schottenfeld D, Fraumeni JF Jr, eds. *Cancer Epidemiology and Prevention*. 3rd ed. New York, NY: Oxford University Press; 2006:872–897.

Munoz N, Bosch FX, de Sanjose S, et al. Epidemiologic classification of human papillomavirus types associated with cervical cancer. *N Engl J Med*. 2003;348(6):518–527.

Murphy SL, Kochanek KD, Xu JQ, Arias E. Mortality in the United States, 2014. Hyattsville, MD: National Center for Health Statistics; 2015. NCHS Data Brief, no 229.

National Cancer Institute (NCI). *Cancer Progress Report 2003*. Rockville, MD: US Department of Health and Human Services, Public Health Service, National Institutes of Health; 2004.

National Cancer Institute (NCI). ASSIST: shaping the future of tobacco prevention and control. Tobacco Control Monograph No. 16. Bethesda, MD: US Department of Health and Human Services, National Institutes of Health, NCI; 2005. NIH Publication 05-5645.

National Cancer Institute (NCI). Cervical cancer prevention (PDQ). National Cancer Institute. 2007. Available at: http://www.cancer.gov/cancertopics/pdq/prevention/cervical/Patient/page2#Section_14. Accessed April 2, 2016.

National Cancer Institute (NCI). SEER cancer statistics factsheets: female breast cancer. 2015. Available at: http://seer.cancer.gov/statfacts/html/breast.html. Accessed March 20, 2016.

National Cancer Institute (NCI). About the SEER Program—SEER. 2016a. Available at: http://seer.cancer.gov/about/overview.html. Accessed April 10, 2016.

National Cancer Institute (NCI). Goals of the SEER Program—about SEER. 2016b. Available at: http://seer.cancer.gov/about/goals.html. Accessed April 10, 2016.

National Cancer Institute (NCI). Vice President Biden's cancer initiative. 2016c. Available at: http://www.cancer.gov/research/key-initiatives/moonshot-cancer-initiative. Accessed April 10, 2016.

National Cancer Institute (NCI). Human papillomavirus (HPV) vaccines. 2016d. Available at: http://www.cancer.gov/about-cancer/causes-prevention/risk/infectious-agents/hpv-vaccine-fact-sheet. Accessed April 10, 2016.

National Comprehensive Cancer Network (NCCN). *NCCN Clinical Practice Guidelines in Oncology: Breast Cancer Screening and Diagnosis*. 2014. Available at: http://www.nccn.org/professionals/physician_gls/f_guidelines.asp. Accessed March 30, 2016.

National Institutes of Health (NIH). *Cervical Cancer Control: Status and Directions*. Bethesda, MD: National Institutes of Health; 1991. NIH Publication 91-3223.

National Lung Screening Trial Research Team (NLSTRT), Aberle DR, Adams AM, et al. Reduced lung-cancer mortality with low-dose computed tomographic screening. *N Engl J Med*. 2011;365(5):395–409.

Nelson HD, Cantor A, Humphrey L, et al. Screening for breast cancer: a systematic review to update the 2009 US Preventive Services Task Force Recommendation. Evidence Synthesis no. 124. Rockville, MD: Agency for Healthcare Research and Quality; 2016. AHRQ Publication no. 14-05201-EF-1.

Nelson HD, Fu R, Goddard K, et al. Risk assessment, genetic counseling, and genetic testing for BRCA-related cancer: systematic review to update the US Preventive Services Task Force Recommendation. Evidence Synthesis no. 101. Rockville, MD: Agency for Healthcare Research and Quality; 2013. AHRQ Publication no. 12-05164-EF-1.

Nelson HD, Fu R, Humphrey L, Smith ME, Griffin JC, Nygren P. Comparative effectiveness of medications to reduce risk of primary breast cancer in women. Comparative Effectiveness Review no. 17. (Prepared by Oregon Evidence-Based Practice Center under Contract no. 290-2007-10057-1.) Agency for Healthcare Research and Quality. 2009. Available at: http://www.effectivehealthcare.ahrq.gov/reports/final.cfm. Accessed April 1, 2016.

Oeffinger KC, Fontham EH, Etzioni R, et al. Breast cancer screening for women at average risk: 2015 guideline update from the American Cancer Society. *JAMA*. 2015;314(15):1599–1614.

Olson CM, Burda BU, Beil T, Whitlock EP. Screening for oral cancer: a targeted evidence update for the US Preventive Services Task Force. Evidence Synthesis no. 102. Rockville, MD: Agency for Healthcare Research and Quality; 2013. AHRQ Publication no. 13-05186-EF-1.

Pesch B, Kendzia B, Gustavsson P, et al. Cigarette smoking and lung cancer—relative risk estimates for the major histological types from a pooled analysis of case–control studies. *Int J Cancer*. 2012;131(5):1210–1219.

Petti S. Lifestyle risk factors for oral cancer. *Oral Oncol*. 2009;45(4–5):340–350.

Platz EA, Giovannucci E. Prostate cancer. In: Schottenfeld D, Fraumeni JF Jr, eds. *Cancer Epidemiology and Prevention*. 3rd ed. New York, NY: Oxford University Press; 2006:1128–1150.

Ries L, Melbert D, Krapcho M, et al., eds. *SEER Cancer Statistics Review, 1975–2004*. Bethesda, MD: National Cancer Institute; 2007.

Rothenberg R, Nasca P, Mikl J, et al. Cancer. In: Amler R, Dull H, eds. *Closing the Gap: The Burden of Unnecessary Illness*. New York, NY: Oxford University Press; 1987:30–42.

Ryerson AB, Eheman CR, Altekruse SF, et al. Annual Report to the Nation on the Status of Cancer, 1975–2012, featuring the increasing incidence of liver cancer. *Cancer.* 2016;122(9):1312–1337.

Sabatino SA, Lawrence B, Elder R, et al. Effectiveness of interventions to increase screening for breast, cervical, and colorectal cancers: nine updated systematic reviews for the guide to community preventive services. *Am J Prev Med.* 2012;43(1):765–786.

Sabatino SA, White MC, Thompson TD, Klabunde CN. Cancer screening test use—United States, 2013. *MMWR Morb Mortal Wkly Rep.* 2015;64(17):464–468.

Saracci R. The interactions of tobacco smoking and other agents in cancer etiology. *Epidemiol Rev.* 1987;9:175–193.

Saslow D, Solomon D, Lawson HW, et al. American Cancer Society, American Society for Colposcopy and Cervical Pathology, and American Society for Clinical Pathology screening guidelines for the prevention and early detection of cervical cancer. *Am J Clin Pathol.* 2012;137(4):516–542.

Schiffman M, Hildesheim A. Cervical cancer. In: Schottenfeld D, Fraumeni JF Jr, eds. *Cancer Epidemiology and Prevention.* 3rd ed. New York, NY: Oxford University Press; 2006:1044–1067.

Schiffman M, Castle PE, Jeronimo J, Rodriguez AC, Wacholder S. Human papillomavirus and cervical cancer. *Lancet.* (2007):370(9590):890–907.

Surveillance, Epidemiology, and End Results Program (SEER). SEER Cancer Statistics Factsheets: Cancer of any site. National Cancer Institute. 2015. Available at: http://seer.cancer.gov/statfacts/html/all.html. Accessed August 30, 2016.Siegel R, Desantis C, Jemal A. Colorectal cancer statistics, 2014. *CA Cancer J Clin.* 2014;64(2):104–117.

Siegel RL, Miller KD, Jemal A. Cancer statistics, 2016. *CA Cancer J Clin.* 2016;66(1):7–30.

Silverman D, Devesa S, Moore L, Rothman N. Bladder cancer. In: Schottenfeld D, Fraumeni JF Jr, eds. *Cancer Epidemiology and Prevention.* 3rd ed. New York, NY: Oxford University Press; 2006:1101–1127.

Smith JC, Medalia C. US Census Bureau, Current Population Reports, P60-253, Health insurance coverage in the United States: 2014. Washington, DC: US Government Printing Office; 2015.

Spitz MR, Wu X, Wilkinson A, Wei Q. Cancer of the lung. In: Schottenfeld D, Fraumeni JF Jr, eds. *Cancer Epidemiology and Prevention.* 3rd ed. New York, NY: Oxford University Press; 2006:638–658.

Sprague BL, Trentham-Dietz A, Egan KM, Titus-Ernstoff L, Hampton JM, Newcomb PA. Proportion of invasive breast cancer attributable to risk factors modifiable after menopause. *Am J Epidemiol.* 2008;168(4):404–411.

Strum WB. Colorectal adenomas. *N Engl J Med*. 2016;374(11):1065–1075.

Thun MJ, Sinks T. Understanding cancer clusters. *CA Cancer J Clin*. 2004;54(5):273–280.

Torre L, Bray F, Siegel R, Ferlay J, Lortet-Tieulent J, Jemal A. Global cancer statistics, 2012. *CA Cancer J Clin*. 2015;65(2):87–108.

US Cancer Statistics Working Group. United States cancer statistics: 1999–2012 incidence and mortality Web-based report. Atlanta, GA: US Department of Health and Human Services, Centers for Disease Control and Prevention and National Cancer Institute; 2015. Available at: http://www.cdc.gov/uscs. Accessed April 10, 2016.

US Census Bureau. Population Estimates Program (PEP). 2010. Available at: http://www.census.gov/popest. Accessed March 21, 2016.

US Department of Health and Human Services (USDHHS). *Cancer Rates and Risks*. 4th ed. Washington, DC: USDHHS; 1996. Publication 96–691.

US Department of Health and Human Services (USDHHS). *The Health Consequences of Smoking: A Report of the Surgeon General*. Washington, DC: USDHHS, Centers for Disease Control and Prevention; 2004.

US Department of Health and Human Services (USDHHS). *The Health Consequences of Involuntary Exposure to Tobacco Smoke: A Report of the Surgeon General*. Rockville, MD: USDHHS, Centers for Disease Control and Prevention, Coordinating Center for Health Promotion, National Center for Chronic Disease Prevention and Health Promotion, Office on Smoking and Health; 2006.

US Department of Health and Human Services (USDHHS). *The Health Consequences of Smoking—50 Years of Progress: A Report of the Surgeon General, 2014*. Atlanta, GA: USDHHS, Centers for Disease Control and Prevention, National Center for Chronic Disease Prevention and Health Promotion, Office on Smoking and Health; 2014.

US Department of Health and Human Services (USDHHS). Cancer, Healthy People 2020. 2016. Available at: https://www.healthypeople.gov/2020/topics-objectives/topic/cancer. Accessed March 15, 2016.

US Environmental Protection Agency (USEPA). *Respiratory Health Effects of Passive Smoking: Lung Cancer and Other Disorders*. Washington, DC: USEPA; 1992.

US Preventive Services Task Force (USPTF). Aspirin use to prevent cardiovascular disease and colorectal cancer: preventive medication. 2015a. Available at: http://www.uspreventiveservicestaskforce.org/Page/Document/UpdateSummaryDraft/aspirin-to-prevent-cardiovascular-disease-and-cancer?ds=1&s=aspirin. Accessed April 5, 2016.

US Preventive Services Task Force (USPTF). *Draft Recommendation Statement on Colorectal Cancer Screening*. 2015b. Available at: http://www.uspreventiveservicestaskforce.

org/Page/Document/draft-recommendation-statement38/colorectal-cancer-screening2. Accessed April 5, 2016.

Vesco KK, Whitlock EP, Eder M, et al. *Screening for Cervical Cancer: A Systematic Evidence Review for the US Preventive Services Task Force. Evidence Syntheses, No. 86.* Agency for Healthcare Research and Quality. 2011. Available at: http://www.ncbi.nlm. nih.gov/books/NBK66099. Accessed April 10, 2016.

Wheeler SB, Reeder-Hayes KE, Carey LA. Disparities in breast cancer treatment and outcomes: biological, social, and health system determinants and opportunities for research. *Oncologist*. 2013;18(9):986–993.

Wolff T, Tai E, Miller T. Screening for skin cancer: an update of the evidence for the U.S. Preventive Services Task Force. Agency for Healthcare Research and Quality. 2009. Available at: http://www.ncbi.nlm.nih.gov/books/NBK34051. Accessed August 30, 2016.

World Cancer Research Fund/American Institute for Cancer Research (WCRF/AICR). *Food, Nutrition, Physical Activity, and the Prevention of Cancer: A Global Perspective.* Washington, DC: AICR; 2007.

World Cancer Research Fund/American Institute for Cancer Research (WCRF/AICR). *Continuous Update Project. Food, Nutrition, Physical Activity, and the Prevention of Colorectal Cancer.* Washington, DC: AICR; 2011.

World Health Organization (WHO). *International Classification of Diseases for Oncology.* 3rd ed. Geneva, Switzerland: WHO; 2000.

World Health Organization (WHO). *WHO's International Statistical Classification of Diseases and Related Health Problems.* 2nd ed., 10th rev. Geneva, Switzerland: WHO; 2005.

Yabroff KR, Lund J, Kepka D, Mariotto A. Economic burden of cancer in the US: estimates, projections, and future research. *Cancer Epidemiol Biomarkers Prev.* 2011; 20(10):2006–2014.

Yang Q, Khoury MJ, Rodriguez C, Calle EE, Tatham LM, Flanders WD. Family history score as a predictor of breast cancer mortality: prospective data from the Cancer Prevention Study II, United States, 1982–1991. *Am J Epidemiol.* 1998;147(7): 652–659.

Zhang SM, Willett WC, Selhub J, et al. Plasma folate, vitamin B6, vitamin B12, homocysteine, and risk of breast cancer. *J Natl Cancer Inst.* 2003;95(5):373–380.

17

CHRONIC RESPIRATORY DISEASES

Henry A. Anderson, MD, Carrie Tomasallo, PhD, MPH,
and Mark A. Werner, PhD

Introduction

Chronic respiratory diseases include a broad range of conditions marked by variability in the range of symptoms, causative and exacerbating factors, and diagnostic criteria. The "upstream" causes and "downstream" consequences of chronic respiratory diseases are complex, and related to the specific type of disease (Figure 17-1). According to the Centers for Disease Control and Prevention's (CDC's) National Center for Health Statistics, chronic lower respiratory diseases were the third leading cause of death in the United States in 2013, responsible for 5.7% of U.S. deaths (Xu et al. 2016). Hospitalization is a frequent adverse outcome of a chronic respiratory disease diagnosis, with the average duration of a hospitalization of 4.5 days for chronic bronchitis and 3.6 days for asthma in 2010 (CDC 2012a). Population-based national health surveys have found that approximately 12% of adults reported obstructive lung disease, including chronic bronchitis, emphysema, and asthma in 2014 (Blackwell and Lucas 2015).

Significance

The primary consequence of chronic respiratory diseases that contributes to morbidity is dyspnea, or pathologic breathlessness (Stulberg and Adams 2000). Depending on the severity, dyspnea may result in restrictions ranging from inability to climb stairs to constant breathlessness and difficulty in sleeping. Effects of dyspnea include impaired respiratory tract clearance mechanisms, excessive mucus production, and reduced lung capacity, which likely contribute to more frequent, severe, and prolonged acute viral and bacterial respiratory

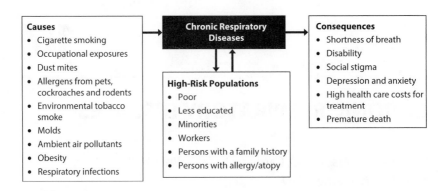

Source: Adapted from Anderson and Werner (2010).

Figure 17-1. Chronic Respiratory Diseases: Causes, Consequences, and High-Risk Groups

infections (Mahler and Meija 1999). Dyspnea is also a common clinical feature in chronic nonpulmonary conditions such as heart disease, obesity, and muscular diseases. Cough, chest pain, excessive phlegm or sputum production, wheezing, and coughing of blood (or hemoptysis) are other commonly observed symptoms of respiratory disease (Mason et al. 2000). As is the case for dyspnea, these symptoms can manifest variously in different respiratory and nonrespiratory disorders.

Among the challenges of describing symptoms commonly observed in respiratory disease is that terminology can differ greatly among clinicians describing similar patterns of respiratory impairment. The use of the term chronic obstructive pulmonary disease (COPD) can describe sets of symptoms that are alternately described as chronic bronchitis, emphysema, or asthma; as such, assigning a definition based on clinical, physiologic, or pathologic criteria may be problematic (Figure 17-2). Clinicians may also use the term COPD to describe nonspecific respiratory symptoms in cases in which airflow impairment may be either absent or present. The *International Classification of Diseases (ICD)*-9 and -10 codes and the definitions used in this chapter are presented in Table 17-1.

Both cystic fibrosis (CF) and sleep apnea are chronic diseases affecting multiple systems with principal effects on the respiratory system. Cystic fibrosis is an inherited disease characterized by the production of abnormally thick and sticky mucus, resulting in respiratory infections and pancreatic obstruction, and is a major source of severe chronic lung disease in children and an increasingly important cause of morbidity and mortality from chronic lung disease in young adults (Boucher et al. 2000). Obstructive sleep apnea is characterized by

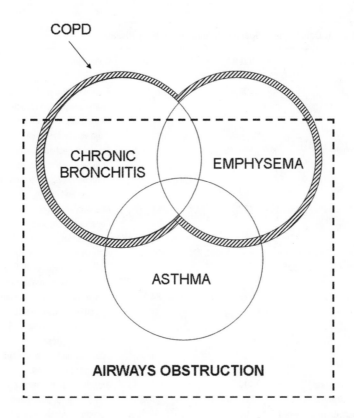

Source: Based on Snider (1988).
Note: Chronic obstructive pulmonary disease (COPD) includes patients with chronic bronchitis and emphysema, and a subset of patients with asthma. Patients with COPD found outside the box for airways obstruction would have clinical or radiographic features of chronic bronchitis or emphysema.

Figure 17-2. Schema of Chronic Obstructive Pulmonary Disease (COPD)

sleep-disordered breathing associated with daytime symptoms, such as excessive sleepiness, and intermittent upper respiratory tract obstruction (Caples et al. 2005). The condition has been estimated to be present in 3% to 7% of men and 2% to 5% of women (Punjabi 2008).

Pathophysiology

The diagnostic tests and associated criteria for definition differ among various chronic respiratory diseases. Chronic bronchitis is diagnosed by clinical signs and reported symptom history, whereas asthma and other forms of COPD are

Table 17-1. Definitions of Specific Chronic Respiratory Diseases

Disease	ICD-9	ICD-10	Definition
Asthma	493	J45–J46	Reversible airway obstruction with airway inflammation and increased airways responsiveness to a variety of stimuli.
Bronchitis[a]	490–491	J40–J42	Excessive tracheobronchial mucus production associated with narrowing of the bronchial airways and cough.
Emphysema[a]	492	J43	Alveolar destruction and associated airspace enlargement.
Other chronic obstructive pulmonary diseases	491.21–491.22, 493.2, 496	J44	Asthma with chronic obstructive pulmonary disease and other chronic airway obstruction.
Cystic fibrosis	277.00, 277.01	E84	Genetic disease with exocrine gland dysfunction resulting in pancreatic insufficiency, chronic progressive lung disease, and elevated sweat chloride production.
Bronchiectasis	494	J47	Bronchial wall destruction.
Pneumoconioses (and other externally induced alveolar diseases)	500–504, 506.4, 507.1, 507.8, 515, 516.3	J60–J67	Dust-, fume- or mist-induced pneumoconiosis or lung injury (not immunologically mediated).
Sleep apnea	780.51, 780.53, 780.57	G47.3	Repetitive cessation of breathing during sleep.

Note: ICD-9 = International Classification of Diseases, Ninth Revision; ICD-10 = International Classification of Diseases, Tenth Revision.
[a]Bronchitis and emphysema are the major conditions falling under the classification of chronic obstructive pulmonary disease.

diagnosed by clinical evaluation and spirometric tests of lung function (GINA 2015; GOLD 2016). Emphysema is defined in histopathologic terms (i.e., study of lung tissue) and is diagnosed with certainty only with lung biopsy or autopsy, although computerized axial tomography (CT) scanning of the chest can be informative. A further complication is that the symptoms of gastroesophageal reflux, a digestive condition, can occasionally be similar to those of various airways diseases, and the two conditions are often confused (Guill 1995).

One manifestation of the occupation-related pneumoconioses, or dust-induced lung conditions, is a fibrotic response to deposition of inorganic material. Diagnosis requires an exposure history and x-ray assessment (ILO 2002). In a heterogeneous group of lung disorders, interstitial lung diseases, the chest x-ray, and occasionally CT of the chest can assist in the evaluation and monitoring of disease status and are used in conjunction with other methods of assessing respiratory function, such as spirometry.

Spirometric testing is simple and inexpensive and is a sensitive and noninvasive method of assessing obstructive lung diseases as well as different fibrotic or restrictive lung diseases. Spirometry measures the expired volume as a function of time. Forced vital capacity (FVC) and forced expiratory volume in the first one second (FEV1) are less variable than many other tests of lung function (Gold 2000a). Using the FVC or FEV1, or the ratio of FEV1 to FVC, lung disorders can be categorized into those with airflow obstruction (ratio of FEV1 to FVC less than 0.75) or restriction (FVC less than 80% of predicted) or into mixed disorders (decreases in both FEV1 to FVC ratio and FVC).

In addition to spirometry, other lung function tests can include measurement of total lung capacity, functional residual capacity, carbon monoxide diffusing capacity, and cardiopulmonary exercise testing. Assessment of lung function following bronchoprovocation with methacholine or histamine may indicate airway hyperreactivity and is sometimes performed if asthma is suspected but spirometry is inconclusive.

The chest radiograph is of most help in the clinical evaluation of chronic lung diseases. However, its role in the screening or epidemiologic study of lung diseases is limited by expense, feasibility, and technical considerations. A uniform method of chest radiograph interpretation has been developed by the International Labour Office (ILO) for use in selected clinical settings (e.g., disability assessment for occupational lung disease) and for research purposes (ILO 2002; ILO 2011). The system categorizes opacities and pleural changes on the chest radiograph by their shape, size, location, and density (ILO 2002; ILO 2011). Physicians who obtain additional training in ILO interpretation of the chest x-ray and pass an examination are called B readers. Methods similar to the ILO scheme for the chest x-ray have been developed for standardized interpretation of CT images of the chest (Tamura et al. 2015).

This chapter not only discusses the two major chronic lung diseases, asthma and COPD, but also includes shorter descriptions of a variety of occupationally induced chronic lung diseases, including coal workers' pneumoconiosis, silicosis, asbestosis, byssinosis, and occupational asthma; lung diseases associated with exposure to organic dusts; a diverse group of diseases resulting in fibrosis of the lung (i.e., interstitial lung disease); CF; and obstructive sleep apnea.

ASTHMA

According to results of the 2014 National Health Interview Survey, approximately 7.7% of the general population currently has asthma (current prevalence), and 12.9% have received a diagnosis of asthma during their lifetime (lifetime prevalence; CDC 2016a). Although much effort has been made in recent years to develop standardized diagnostic criteria for asthma, estimates of asthma prevalence continue to vary with different data collection approaches, such as self-reported and physician-reported data. International asthma prevalence estimates vary widely, ranging from less than 2% in Nepal to 16% in Isle of Man (GINA 2015). In 2013, 3,630 people in the United States died from asthma (Xu et al. 2016).

Significance

Asthma was responsible for an estimated 17.3 million ambulatory care visits in 2010, including visits to physician offices, emergency departments, and hospital outpatient departments (CDC 2012b). Appropriate medical management may limit the degree to which asthma affects productivity of children and adults; however, asthma remains a significant cause of missed days of work or school. In 2013, U.S. children missed an estimated 13.8 million days of school because of asthma (CDC 2013).

Pathophysiology

Historically, asthma has been classified into two categories: allergic or atopic (extrinsic) and nonallergic or nonatopic (intrinsic) asthma. Atopy is defined as the capacity to produce abnormal amounts of immunoglobulin E (IgE) in response to environmental allergen exposure. Between the two categories, asthma appears to be more commonly classified as allergic in children than in adults (Pearce et al. 1999; Knudsen et al. 2009). However, many individuals have asthmatic responses that are characteristic of both categories and the basis for this classification has been under question. The introduction of newer information about the role of genetics in asthma and observations of higher IgE levels in patients of all age groups has added weight to the proposal of a unifying hypothesis for both types of asthma (White and Kaliner 1991; Meyers et al. 2004).

Asthma primarily manifests itself in the airways, and patients with asthma show evidence of mucosal edema, epithelial disruption, infiltration with inflammatory cells, and excessive amounts of mucus in airways (Boushey et al. 2000). The development of the changes responsible for airway obstruction and hyperresponsiveness is primarily attributable to inflammatory responses in the airways of patients. In allergic asthma, IgE–antigen complexes bind to the membranes of various connective tissue cells, causing the release of signaling chemical agents responsible for an asthmatic response. Positive response to skin test batteries for common allergens is more prevalent among those with extrinsic asthma than those with intrinsic asthma, and more common among people with asthma as a category than among people without asthma (Pearce et al. 1999).

Symptoms of asthma, such as intermittent wheezing or shortness of breath triggered by specific environmental exposures or exercise, frequently appear in children before the age of five years. About 50% of adults who were diagnosed with asthma as children no longer have the condition, with about half of these becoming totally symptom-free (Barbee and Murphy 1998). Conversely, about one fourth of childhood asthma cases persist with a similar degree of severity into adulthood, and the remaining one fourth may experience a temporary cessation in symptoms, with symptoms returning in adulthood (Sears 1991).

Descriptive Epidemiology

High-Risk Populations

Although there is a range of factors that are useful for describing the distribution of asthma and asthma-related adverse health outcomes among populations, the most important determinants of asthma and related morbidity and mortality are race/ethnicity, age, and sex. Racial disparities for asthma are found for a range of endpoints, most notably prevalence, mortality, and hospitalizations (Figure 17-3). Data from the 2014 National Health Interview Survey found significantly higher values of current asthma prevalence for non-Hispanic African Americans than for non-Hispanic whites (9.9% vs. 7.6%;

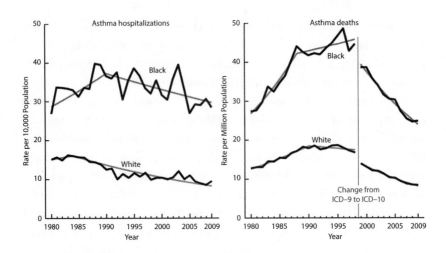

Source: Reprinted from Moorman et al. (2012).
Note: Population-based rates age-adjusted to the 2000 standard population. Rates based on asthma as the first-listed diagnosis or as the underlying cause of death. Straight lines show the modeled trend estimated by Joinpoint. Inflection points represent a change in the annual percent change.
Figure 17-3. Asthma Hospitalization Rates and Asthma Death Rates (Population-Based), by Race, United States, 1980–2009

CDC 2016a). When the data were limited to children, the disparity was even more striking (13.4% vs. 7.6%; CDC 2016a). Across all race groups, Hispanic ethnicity is not associated with higher asthma prevalence. As a subset of the Hispanic population, however, those of Puerto Rican descent have an asthma prevalence rate of 16.5% for all age groups and 23.5% among children. Asthma prevalence tends to be higher in children than adults. Data from the 2014 National Health Interview Survey show similar prevalence among white children and adults (7.6%) but higher prevalence among children versus adults for African Americans (13.4% vs. 9.9%), and among Hispanics (8.5% vs. 6.7%; CDC 2016a).

For health care utilization, rates of inpatient hospitalization and emergency department use related to asthma are significantly higher for African Americans than for whites. In 2010, the inpatient hospitalization rate for asthma among African Americans was 29.9 per 10,000 population compared to 8.7 per 10,000 for whites (CDC 2016b). The emergency department visit rate for asthma among African Americans and whites per 10,000 population was 182.1 and 51.0, respectively, in 2009 (Moorman et al. 2012). Differences in asthma health care utilization for persons with current asthma by age, sex, and race are depicted in Figure 17-4 (Moorman et al. 2012). Rates for the population with asthma take into account differences in asthma prevalence among demographic groups. In 2014, the asthma mortality rate for non-Hispanic African Americans was three times higher compared to that for non-Hispanic whites (2.5 vs. 0.9 per 1,000,000 population, respectively; CDC 2015).

Among the striking features of the epidemiology of asthma is the observed trend by which prevalence shifts according to sex among age groups. By sex, asthma prevalence is higher in boys than in girls (Moorman et al. 2012). In 2014, asthma prevalence among boys and girls was 10.1% and 7.0%, respectively (CDC 2016a). Among adults, however, this trend is reversed, with 2014 asthma prevalence rates for men and women of 5.1% and 9.6%, respectively

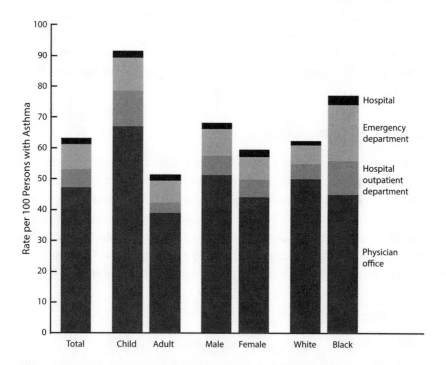

Source: Reprinted from Moorman et al. (2012).

Note: Crude risk-based rates (per 100 persons with current asthma) are presented.

Figure 17-4. Asthma Physician Office Visit, Hospital Outpatient Department, Emergency Department and Hospitalization Rates by Age, Sex, and Race: United States, Average Annual 2007–2009

(CDC 2016a). This trend is borne out in health care utilization rates (inpatient admissions, emergency department visits, and ambulatory care visits) and for mortality rates. No clear explanation for this observation has emerged.

The degree to which the racial disparity in asthma prevalence and adverse health outcomes can be explained by socioeconomic differences is a subject of some controversy. Factors such as access to high-quality health care and housing conditions are likely to account for some of the racial disparities seen with asthma. Some ecologic studies of national databases indicate that controlling for family income can diminish or decrease the racial difference in asthma prevalence (Weitzman et al. 1992; Smith et al. 2005), whereas others have found that racial and ethnic disparities in asthma prevalence and health care utilization persist after accounting for income and other socioeconomic factors (Bhan et al. 2015; Law et al. 2011).

As described earlier, approximately 30% to 50% of the general population can be classified as atopic, and most asthmatics fall into this category (Pearce et al. 1999). Because of growing knowledge that atopy is strongly influenced by genetics, it follows that some aspects of asthma development may be under genetic control. Indeed, those with a family history of asthma have long been known to be at increased risk for developing the disease (Burke et al. 2003).

Geographic Distribution

Data from the National Health Interview Survey from 2008 to 2010 suggest that regional differences exist in the United States for asthma prevalence. Based on standard U.S. census regions, asthma prevalence is highest in the Northeast (8.8%), followed by the Midwest (8.7%), West (8.0%), and South (7.6%; Moorman et al. 2012). Average annual emergency department visit rate estimates for the period 2007 to 2009 are highest in the Northeast (10.2 per 100 persons with current asthma), followed by the South (8.7), Midwest (8.0), and West (5.5; Moorman et al. 2012).

Time Trends

Although the range of data sources available for asthma surveillance has changed over time, observed increases in patient encounter measures for asthma have been predicated by increased asthma prevalence in recent decades (Moorman et al. 2012). Based on survey responses regarding whether a family member had asthma in the past 12 months, asthma prevalence increased from 3.1% in 1980 to 5.5% in 1996, an increase of 3.8% per year. This increase occurred among all age, sex, and race subgroups. Although changes in survey questions make comparisons from 1997 to 2000 with newer national prevalence data problematic, current asthma prevalence rates increased from 7.3% in 2001 to 8.4% in 2010, an increase of 1.5% per year. Data on asthma mortality suggest that death rates increased from 1980 through 1989, remained stable from 1989 to 1998, and have declined by 4.9% per year from 1999 to 2009 (Moorman et al. 2012).

Seasonal trends have been consistently exhibited for both asthma morbidity and mortality. Asthma hospitalization rates reflect a seasonal variation whereby the highest rates occur in early spring and early fall, and rates are lowest in the summer (Weiss 1990). Studies on asthma mortality have suggested that asthma mortality in children and young adults may peak in summer, whereas mortality among older adults peaks in winter. Potential explanations for this observed seasonality include plant allergens, acute respiratory infections, cold weather, and air pollution. For school-age children, the onset of school in September has been found to contribute to increased emergency department visits for asthma (Silverman et al. 2005).

Causes

Modifiable Risk Factors

The bulk of the published literature on asthma epidemiology and risk factors has focused on the identification of asthma triggers—specific exposures that often precipitate symptoms in individuals with asthma. Common asthma triggers include dust mites, allergens from pets, cockroaches and rodents, secondhand smoke, molds, ambient air pollutants, cold conditions, and exercise (GINA 2015). There are, by contrast, relatively few conclusive findings about what risk factors contribute to the development of the condition itself, and the factors that cause asthma remain largely unidentified (Taussig et al. 2003).

As discussed in the previous section, atopic individuals are more likely to be diagnosed with asthma than others, and atopy is a significant risk factor for developing asthma. One study found that most people with asthma are atopic (Arbes et al. 2007). Although the relationship to atopy suggests that there is a strong genetic component among the factors related to the etiology of asthma, environmental factors appear to play a role as well. One longitudinal study in children found that although IgE levels in umbilical cord blood were not predictive of subsequent development of asthma, IgE blood levels in blood samples taken at age one year were predictive (Martinez et al. 1995). This finding suggests that exposures within the first year of life may be substantial contributors to the risk of developing asthma in childhood.

Although exposures to dogs and cats in the home can be an asthma trigger for some people with asthma, results from studies on the effect of the presence of dogs and cats in the home environment on the development of asthma have been mixed. One longitudinal study found a decreased likelihood for developing wheezing among children without maternal asthma in homes with one or more indoor dogs, but no effect related to cats in the home (Remes et al. 2001). Another study found increased likelihood of cat sensitization and development of severe asthma among children reporting the presence of cats in the home before the age of two years (Melen et al. 2001).

Although breast-feeding practices in childhood may also affect the risk of developing asthma in children, the results of studies on this question have also been mixed. In one longitudinal study, atopic children with asthmatic mothers were more likely to have asthma if they were exclusively breast-fed as infants (Wright et al. 2001). In the same study, however, exclusive breast-feeding was associated with reduced likelihood of recurrent wheeze in the first two years of life regardless of atopy status or whether the child's mother had asthma.

Secondhand smoke has clearly been established as a risk factor for asthma exacerbations (Chilmonczyk et al. 1993; Witorsch and Witorsch 2000). There is also increasing evidence that exposure to secondhand smoke may contribute to the development of asthma, both in adults and children (Gold 2000b; Jaakkola et al. 2003). For children, the risk associated with secondhand smoke may be confounded by effects of maternal smoking that may have been incurred during pregnancy.

The relationship between asthma and obesity has received increased attention in recent years. Because obesity is associated with a generalized increase in inflammatory response, a causal role in asthma has been postulated (Beuther et al. 2006). Increased incidence of asthma and poorer asthma control have been observed at higher rates among people with elevated body mass index (BMI) values (Akinbami and Fryar 2016). In children, the impact of obesity on incident asthma was shown to be more pronounced among girls than boys (Gold et al. 2003). Because of the possibility that reduced physical activity among people with asthma could contribute to the likelihood of obesity, the relationship between asthma and obesity is likely to be complex in nature.

Ambient air pollutants have been shown to be important asthma triggers (GINA 2015). Associations between asthma and exposure to ozone and particulate matter have been commonly observed, but other pollutants such as nitrogen dioxide and volatile organic compounds, and community traffic density and proximity to heavily traveled roads have also been found to be associated with adverse asthma-related health outcomes (Sarnat and Holguin 2007). The role of air pollution in the development of asthma is less certain. In a study of southern California schoolchildren, residence within 75 meters of a major road was found to be associated with increased risk of lifetime asthma, with effects more pronounced in girls than in boys (McConnell et al. 2006). Incidence of asthma was also associated with traffic-related air pollution exposure from roadways near homes and schools (McConnell et al. 2010). Among school-age children active in sports, incidence of asthma was found to be higher in children living in communities with high ozone concentrations than among other children (McConnell et al. 2002).

Population-Attributable Risk

The development of asthma clearly appears to be related to both genetic and environmental factors. As such, quantifying the relative contribution of genetics and environment is a difficult proposition. Specific genes related to atopy and asthma development have begun to be identified (Ober and Yao 2011). Although it appears increasingly apparent that some specific environmental factors play a role in asthma development, there is a substantial amount of variability among individuals with asthma as to the triggers causing exacerbations. It is likely that the list of environmental and occupational exposures that may contribute to the development will be highly individual-specific as well.

Evidence-Based Interventions

Prevention

Because of the considerable uncertainty about how specific genetic and environmental factors contribute to the development of asthma at both the individual and population levels, there are few clear recommendations to offer by way of preventing the development of asthma. For potentially susceptible populations, such as siblings and children of people with asthma, there may be benefit in extending environmental control measures applied to the individual with asthma (such as limiting exposure to pests and mold) to other members of the household. For example, dust mites can be effectively controlled by encasing mattresses and pillows in airtight covers, washing bedding every week, and removing wall-to-wall carpeting, especially in bedrooms. Given the increased evidence regarding secondhand smoke and air pollutants as contributors to developing asthma, public policy efforts to ban smoking in public places and establish appropriate air pollutant restrictions for ozone and particulate matter may have benefit in reducing future asthma incidence and prevalence.

Rather than focus on poorly informed efforts on asthma prevention, public health activity on asthma has focused primarily on means by which individuals with asthma can reduce or eliminate exacerbations that may pose a threat to a patient's health or limit his or her quality of life. This has been done by promoting regular interaction with appropriate health care providers, providing and disseminating guidance about appropriate use of controller medications to patients and health care providers, and by educating patients about the nature of asthma as a chronic disease and how to identify and avoid asthma triggers that may cause exacerbations. Because secondhand smoke is a known asthma trigger, efforts to discourage tobacco use in homes and other indoor environments or focusing smoking cessation efforts on people with asthma and their families may be worthwhile approaches to consider. Because influenza may have a considerable impact on asthma-related morbidity, it is recommended that people with asthma obtain a yearly flu shot. Whether people with asthma constitute a risk category on par with the elderly or other groups for targeting flu shots when resources are scarce remains an open question (Bueving et al. 2005). Exposure to ambient airborne particulates and irritants has been associated with asthma exacerbations and increased inpatient hospitalization and emergency department visit rates for asthma. In addition to efforts to decrease ambient concentrations of these pollutants, state and national public health alerts are issued when pollution concentrations exceed standards and could pose a threat to sensitive populations, including people with asthma.

Screening

Because effective management can minimize the frequency and severity of asthma exacerbations, applying a proper diagnosis to individuals who have asthma is an important step in controlling the disease and reducing asthma-related adverse health outcomes. However, mild to moderate cases of asthma may be difficult to diagnose, especially among young children. In such cases, symptoms can often be confused with recurrent respiratory infections or bronchitis, and, as such, may not be recognized as a chronic condition.

Because of its impact on school attendance, as a major cause of hospitalization in children, and the preventable nature of asthma-related morbidity, the notion of population-based screening for asthma has received much attention as a potential intervention. Many organizations, including the American Thoracic Society, have refrained from endorsing such screening efforts because of the lack of evidence that such approaches result in measurable improvements in health outcomes (Gerald et al. 2007). Population-based screening may be most effective in areas where there is likely to be a high prevalence of undiagnosed asthma and where access to high-quality care is likely to be available for newly diagnosed patients.

Treatment

The primary goal of asthma treatment is to control the condition and minimize exacerbations to avoid adverse asthma-related health outcomes. Most asthma medications can be described as controller medications or reliever (rescue) medications (GINA 2015). Controller medications are generally taken daily on a long-term basis to achieve control of inflammation. Common types of controller medications include inhaled corticosteroids such as fluticasone, leukotriene modifiers such as montelukast, and long-acting $\beta2$-agonists such as salmeterol. Reliever medications act quickly to address bronchoconstriction. These include rapid-acting $\beta2$-agonists and systemic glutocorticosteroids. Frequent use of reliever medications (e.g., on a daily basis) may signify that a patient's asthma is not being well controlled and his or her treatment plan should be re-evaluated. Some medications in both classes are not recommended as stand-alone therapies, but are generally prescribed only when other controller medications are included in the patient's therapy plan.

Examples of Evidence-Based Interventions

Over the past decade, substantial effort has been made in designing, implementing, and evaluating public health interventions to address asthma. Common objectives for intervention efforts include educating patients about asthma, controlling exposure to triggers in the home and work environments, and enhancing communication across different parts of the health care system about patients with asthma. Sites where interventions have been implemented to address asthma include health care facilities (clinics, hospitals, and emergency departments), pharmacies, homes, schools, and workplaces. The focus of such interventions has ranged from patients and parents to teachers and health care providers, and effective programs have taken approaches such as modifying the home environment during pregnancy to reduce the likelihood of developing asthma in childhood (Custovic et al. 2001), assessing the quality of patients' interaction with pharmacists (Barbanel et al. 2003), and ensuring that health education messages are culturally appropriate for patients (Brotanek et al. 2007).

Reducing exposure to secondhand smoke through state smoke-free policies has been associated with a lower risk of asthma health care utilization (Mackay et al. 2010; Millett et al. 2013). A systematic review of public health interventions for asthma found that skills-based asthma self-management education is effective for both children and adults (Labre et al. 2012). Furthermore, a Guide to Community Preventive Services review indicated that home-based, multi-trigger, multi-component environmental interventions are effective in children and demonstrate a modest return on investment (Guide to Community Preventive Services 2012). Guidelines have been established for asthma management and prevention at both the national and international levels, setting the stage for more uniform practices for the evaluation, dissemination, and adaptation of effective public health interventions for asthma (GINA 2015; NHLBI 2007).

Areas of Future Research

Risk factors for the development of childhood asthma have not been fully assessed, and further work to develop appropriate animal models for asthma research is needed (Coleman 1999). Longitudinal cohorts of asthma patients are recommended to further understand the origins of asthma and the relationships between exposures and developmental changes over the lifespan (Levy et al. 2015). A broader description of the genetic determinants of asthma will help enable the identification of high-risk individuals for whom particular interventions to prevent asthma might be recommended. Although effective medications for asthma control exist, there remain concerns about long-term side effects, such as growth restrictions in children, for which more data are required. Although home-based multicomponent interventions to reduce exposure to asthma triggers in the home have been shown to be effective in children with asthma, the evidence demonstrating effectiveness for adults with asthma remains tenuous (Guide to Community Preventive Services 2012). Further data on the effectiveness of such interventions for adults with asthma would be of great benefit.

CHRONIC OBSTRUCTIVE PULMONARY DISEASE

Chronic obstructive pulmonary disease (COPD) has been defined as a disease chiefly marked by airway obstruction that is not fully reversible (Rabe et al. 2007). The condition is usually progressive in nature and is associated with an abnormal inflammatory response of the lungs to noxious particles and gases (Shapiro et al. 2000). Conditions such as chronic bronchitis and emphysema that are obstructive in nature are frequently grouped together under the broader heading of COPD. Because there can be a significant overlap of symptoms and manifestations of different forms of COPD, distinctions among the various diagnoses within the broader COPD category can be difficult to make successfully.

Significance

In National Health Interview Survey findings from 2007 to 2009, self-reported prevalence for chronic bronchitis (in the past 12 months) or emphysema (lifetime) was estimated at 5.1% (Akinbami and Liu 2011). Findings from the Behavioral Risk Factor Surveillance System indicate that 6.3% of adults in the United States reported having been given a diagnosis of COPD by a physician or other health professional (CDC 2012c). For adults aged 40 to 79 years, population projections based on spirometry data from physical examinations from the National Health and Nutrition Examination Survey (NHANES) from 2007 to 2010 place the prevalence of mild and moderate obstructive pulmonary disease between 10.2% and 20.9% (Tilert et al. 2013). These findings suggest that prevalence estimates based on self-reported data may significantly underestimate actual COPD prevalence. Inpatient hospitalization rates in the United States for COPD of 33.4 (women) and 31.6 (men) per 10,000 population were observed in 2010 (Ford et al. 2013), with a national mortality rate for that year of 63.1 per 100,000 population. For all health endpoints related to COPD, however, imprecise and variable definitions make the quantification of prevalence, morbidity, and mortality difficult.

An estimate of the economic costs of COPD in the United States was placed at $36 billion—including $32.1 billion for direct medical costs and $3.9 billion for absenteeism (Ford et al. 2015). Primary payers of direct costs included Medicare (51%), Medicaid (25%), and private insurance (18%).

In addition to being a common primary diagnosis for hospitalization, COPD is a common comorbidity for inpatient hospitalizations. It was found to be present as a comorbid condition in 12% of hospital discharge records (Merrill and Elixhauser 2005).

Pathophysiology

Initial pathologic changes of COPD occur in the proximal and peripheral airways, lung parenchyma, and pulmonary vasculature (Hogg 2004). These pathologic changes consist of inflammatory responses and associated increases in goblet cell number and mucous gland size. This inflammation appears to be an amplification of normal inflammatory responses to toxic gases and particulates. This response is most commonly observed as ongoing exposure to tobacco smoke (Rabe et al. 2007).

Emphysema is best characterized by the destruction of the bronchioles, alveolar ducts, and alveoli that constitute gas exchange air spaces. The mechanism for this destruction is inflammatory in nature, most commonly resulting from ongoing exposure to tobacco smoke (Shapiro et al. 2000). The chief physiological result in emphysema is the obstruction of expiratory airflow and reduced gas transfer capacity. It is increasingly recognized that elastases play an important role in the pathophysiology of emphysema. Elastases are enzymes that digest and degrade elastin, an elastic substance that supports the structure of the lungs. It is theorized that exposure to toxic gases and particulates alters the balance between proteinase and antiproteinase activity in the lungs, resulting in the degradation of lung tissue that leads to the symptoms of emphysema (Shapiro et al. 2000).

In adults, the onset of COPD often begins with a moderate decline in lung function capacity before age 50 years. In many cases, COPD would be observable by spirometry, but medical attention may not be sought until symptoms such as dyspnea are observed. Among smokers, a characteristic cough may provide early evidence of the onset of COPD. In the typical case, the decline in lung function accelerates after the age of 50 years (Shapiro et al. 2000; GOLD 2016). As the disease progresses, the damage to the lung ultimately results in inadequate oxygen delivery. Chronic obstructive pulmonary disease is a common comorbid condition among patients presenting with cardiovascular disease and a range of other systemic conditions.

Descriptive Epidemiology

High-Risk Populations

Although describing the epidemiological burden of COPD is complicated by variable diagnostic criteria and differences between self-reported data and results from physical examinations, certain groups are at greater risk for COPD than others. Smokers and ex-smokers constitute the most distinct high-risk group for COPD, and the prevalence of tobacco smoking is the best predictor of COPD prevalence across the globe (GOLD 2016). The prevalence of COPD also increases with age, especially after the age of 40 years (Halbert et al. 2006). This increase in risk with age is attributable to both increased cumulative tobacco smoke exposure among smokers and a generally observed decline in lung function with age across populations. While the U.S. death rate from COPD remained steady among women from 1999 to 2010, it decreased moderately for men over the same period (from 88 per 100,000 to 74 per 100,000; Ford et al. 2013). Although observed COPD prevalence by sex closely follows expectations based on patterns of tobacco smoking, decline in lung function consistent with COPD appears to be more strongly affected by smoking in women than in men (Connett et al. 2003). Improvements in lung function upon tobacco cessation also appear to be greater among women than among men.

A small number of patients with COPD have a deficiency of the protein alpha-1 antitrypsin. The genetic variation leading to this deficiency is seen most commonly in whites of Scandinavian descent, and is estimated to be present in some degree in roughly one of every 2,500 to 5,000 newborns in Western Europe (Fregonese and Stolk 2008). This protein acts to inhibit the destructive capabilities of the white blood cell elastase responsible for degradation of lung tissue, and deficiencies of alpha-1 antitrypsin have been associated with emphysema. Other high-risk groups may be defined based on low birthweight, respiratory infections in childhood, and occupational exposure to dusts (described later in this chapter). In addition, there is some evidence that physician-diagnosed asthma increases one's risk of developing the irreversible airway obstruction seen in COPD (Silva et al. 2004).

Geographic Distribution

By state, COPD mortality rates tend to be higher in some parts of the West and South, including Appalachia. Mortality data from 2010 showed the highest age-adjusted COPD mortality rates among adults aged 25 years and older in Oklahoma (102.6 per 100,000 population), West Virginia (95.1), Kentucky (90.7) and Wyoming (89.6), whereas the lowest rates were found in Hawaii (24.8 per 100,000), the District of Columbia (37.7), and Connecticut (43.6; Ford et al. 2013). Although comparison with state-specific smoking-attributable mortality rates explains COPD mortality rates for Appalachian states, it does not explain elevated rates in Western states (Weinhold 2000). Although theories regarding population migration, ambient air pollutants, and diagnostic differences have been postulated, this discrepancy has yet to be fully explained.

Time Trends

Unlike the period of 1990 to 1998, when COPD prevalence increased among women in the United States (Mannino et al. 2002), COPD prevalence was largely stable over the period 1999 to 2010 (Ford et al. 2013). Declines were seen over this period for COPD inpatient hospitalizations and Medicare hospital discharge claims overall, among men, and among enrollees aged 65 to 74 years (Ford et al. 2013).

Causes

Modifiable Risk Factors

The most commonly encountered risk factor for the development of COPD is cigarette smoking. This risk is dose-related, and factors such as age of starting to smoke, total pack-years smoked, and current smoking status are all predictive of COPD mortality (GOLD 2016). As has been increasingly found for other smoking-related health outcomes, exposure to secondhand smoke may also contribute to the risk of developing COPD (Eisner et al. 2005). Further study has indicated that exposure to secondhand smoke in childhood is associated with COPD and related respiratory symptoms in adulthood (Johannessen et al. 2012).

Occupational exposure to organic and inorganic dusts and fumes may contribute to the development of COPD (Trupin et al. 2003; Blanc et al. 2009).

In an analysis of data from the NHANES, occupations found to be associated with an increased risk of developing COPD included records processing and construction trades workers (Hnizdo et al. 2002). There is growing literature that indoor pollution from the burning of biomass in poorly ventilated dwellings can contribute to the development of COPD, especially in developing countries (Ezzati 2005; Orozco-Levi et al. 2006; Hu et al. 2010). Although outdoor air pollution can contribute to COPD exacerbations, its role in the development of COPD remains unclear.

Population-Attributable Risk

Cigarette smoking is by far the most commonly encountered risk factor for COPD, and estimates of the fraction of cases attributable to smoking range from 45% to 90% (Marsh et al. 2006). The American Thoracic Society concluded that the population-attributable fraction of COPD attributable to cigarette smoking is no more than 80% (Eisner et al. 2010). Estimates for the population-attributable fraction for secondhand smoke in the home and work environments have been derived to account for 9% and 7% of COPD cases, respectively (Eisner et al. 2005). Other factors for which quantifiable fractions of COPD may be derived include occupational exposures, exposure to biomass smoke, and exposure to traffic and outdoor air pollutants (Eisner et al. 2010).

Evidence-Based Interventions

Prevention

Because of the primacy of tobacco smoking as a risk factor for COPD, prevention of tobacco smoking is the single most important preventive activity to reduce the burden of COPD. Because the effect of tobacco smoking on COPD is dose-related, any reduction in smoking may bring about a reduction in related COPD morbidity. When a smoker quits, the age-related rate of decline in FEV1 can approach the rate of lung function decline in never smokers, but it does not return to the level of lung function seen in never smokers.

For individuals exposed to multiple risk factors, the effect of the collective set of risk factors appears to be additive. As such, identifying individuals with multiple risk factors, such as smoking and occupational exposures, may provide an important avenue for COPD prevention.

Screening

Because interventions aimed at reducing harmful exposures can be effective in slowing the progression of COPD, early detection of disease is beneficial for patients. The primary mode of screening for COPD is to measure airflow obstruction with spirometry or peak airflow measurement. Because there is a large population that may be in the early stages of COPD without being aware of it, increasing awareness of the relationship between symptoms such as chronic cough and excessive sputum production and COPD may increase the fraction of patients who are appropriately diagnosed with COPD. Broad population-based screening should be limited to individuals at high risk for developing COPD, such as cigarette smokers. Screening for genetic markers for alpha-1 antitrypsin deficiency is available and is recommended for individuals for whom a genetic predisposition to the deficiency is suspected as well as infants displaying unusual hepatic symptoms (de Serres and Blanco 2006; Fregonese and Stolk 2008).

Treatment

The most effective treatment for COPD is to avoid exposure to causative and exacerbatory agents, such as cigarette smoke, workplace dusts, and ambient air pollutants. Once COPD has been diagnosed, the objectives of disease management are to relieve symptoms, improve exercise tolerance and health status, and prevent and treat complications and exacerbations (GOLD 2016). A range of medications, such as inhaled bronchodilators and glucocorticosteroids, can help alleviate some of the symptoms of COPD. When the progression of disease results in decreased blood oxygen, supplemental oxygen therapy has been shown to increase survival (Shapiro et al. 2000). Pulmonary rehabilitation efforts such as exercise training and breathing retraining have been shown to decrease dyspnea, increase exercise tolerance, and improve patients' quality of life (GOLD 2016). Surgical approaches, such removal of emphysematous lung or lung transplantation, can be effective in increasing survival in selected circumstances. Pneumococcal and influenza vaccination are recommended for people diagnosed with COPD (GOLD 2016).

Examples of Evidence-Based Interventions

Effective tobacco prevention and control efforts (as discussed in Chapter 7) represent the most important avenue for interventions achieving a reduction in the burden of COPD. Policies prohibiting tobacco smoking in workplaces such as taverns and restaurants are now commonplace in the United States and may decrease exposures that can precipitate COPD exacerbations.

Governmental agencies such as the Occupational Safety and Health Administration (OSHA) and the Mine Safety and Health Administration (MSHA) have established enforceable occupational exposure limits to reduce harmful workplace exposures that may contribute to COPD development. The Environmental Protection Agency (EPA) and various state and local agencies have adopted emissions limits for ambient air pollutants. Public health and environmental agencies routinely issue alerts when air pollutant levels exceed guidelines to advise individuals with COPD and other high-risk groups to avoid activities that may increase the risk of an exacerbation.

Areas of Future Research

Although the primary risk factors for COPD are well established, differences in regional COPD mortality rates that remain unexplained by tobacco smoking patterns may offer an opportunity to better understand the epidemiology of COPD. Additional studies of the cellular basis of COPD and identification of more sensitive and specific biochemical, genetic, and molecular markers of COPD may lead to better approaches for the diagnosis and control of COPD (Petty and Weinmann 1997; Thomashow et al. 2014). Additional epidemiologic studies assessing the interaction between cigarette smoking and exposures from environmental and occupational sources may aid in assessing the relative efficacy of various avenues for intervention. Longitudinal epidemiology studies may help identify and quantify risk factors that contribute to the development of COPD, either independently or in tandem with established COPD risk factors.

CYSTIC FIBROSIS

Significance

Cystic fibrosis is an inherited disease characterized by the production of abnormally thick and sticky mucus resulting in respiratory infections and pancreatic obstruction, and is a major source of severe chronic lung disease in children and an increasingly important cause of morbidity and mortality from chronic lung disease in young adults (Boucher et al. 2000). Although CF continues to result

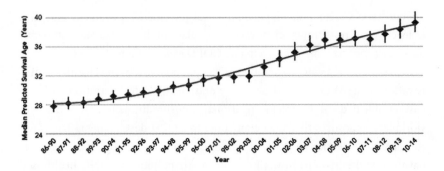

Source: Reprinted with permission from CFF (2015).
Note: Cystic fibrosis patients under care at CF Foundation–accredited care centers in the United States, who consented to have their data entered.

Figure 17-5. Median Predicted Survival Age for Individuals with Cystic Fibrosis, 1986–2014 (Five-Year Intervals)

in premature death from its effects on the respiratory, gastrointestinal, and endocrine systems, major strides in screening and treatment in recent decades have improved patient outcomes and survival for patients with CF (Figure 17-5; Strausbaugh and Davis 2007; MacKenzie et al. 2014). There are an estimated 30,000 patients in the United States with CF, and the current median projected survival for patients born and diagnosed with CF in 2010 is estimated at 37 years for female and 40 years for male patients (MacKenzie et al. 2014).

Pathophysiology

The primary genetic defect associated with CF affects a transmembrane conductance regulator protein that acts as a chloride channel. This genetic defect has been localized to chromosome seven, and more than 1,500 specific mutations have been identified and recorded. Levels of the functional regulator protein are substantially reduced in patients with CF, affecting ion transport in sweat ducts, airways, pancreatic ducts, and elsewhere. The severity and level of organ involvement in CF is directly related to tissue levels of the protein. The primary manifestation of CF in the respiratory tract is abnormally thick and copious mucus in the airways that impairs microbial and mucociliary clearance. This often contributes to progressive cycles of respiratory infection and inflammation (Strausbaugh and Davis 2007; Flume and Van Devanter 2012). Impaired ion transport may result in depletion of periciliary liquid on airway surfaces, resulting in impaired clearance by both cough and ciliary mechanisms (Boucher 2004). As more patients survive into adulthood, extrarespiratory effects such as CF-induced diabetes and fibrotic and cirrhotic liver disease are increasingly observed. Lung disease, however, remains the primary cause of morbidity and mortality from CF.

Descriptive Epidemiology

High-Risk Populations

Cystic fibrosis is among the most common lethal genetic defects affecting whites in the United States. Incidence varies greatly in the United States on the basis of ethnicity, with incidence at 1 in 3,200 births for whites, 1 in 15,000 births for African Americans, and 1 in 31,000 births for Asian Americans (Orenstein et al. 2000). It is inherited in an autosomal recessive fashion, and the estimates of the prevalence of the heterozygous form in individuals of Northern European descent ranges from 2% to 4% (Tsui and Buchwald 1991; Schulz et al. 2006). Individuals with the heterozygous form are not affected with CF.

A review of CF mortality records from 10 countries found that the median age of death was consistently highest in the United States. Although increases in life span were observed in all 10 countries over time, all 10 showed a shorter life span for women with CF than for men with CF (Fogarty et al. 2000).

Causes

Risk for developing CF is based on genetics. However, there are several classes of specific mutations within the target gene that can lead to the condition, and there are observed differences in disease severity associated with the different classes (Strausbaugh and Davis 2007). Among patients with CF, decrease in FEV1 and use of nutritional intervention have been established as markers for mortality risk (Kerem et al. 1992; Belkin et al. 2004).

Evidence-Based Interventions

Prevention

Aside from genetic counseling and education for prospective parents, the prevention of CF is a difficult proposition. Gene therapy approaches, whereby copies of the normal *CFTR* gene could be incorporated and expressed in affected cells, remain a promising line of inquiry. The approach in this regard would be to place a copy of the gene for normal transmembrane conductance regulator protein in affected cells, resulting in production of the normal protein. Although clinical trials have shown some early success, many hurdles remain to the use of gene therapy approaches in routine treatment of CF (Griesenbach and Alton 2012).

Screening

Newborn screening for CF is now undertaken in all 50 states. The most common method used for screening is measurement of immunoreactive trypsinogen on dried blood spots, followed by direct gene analysis approach for confirmation. Among the reported benefits of early screening is the ability to begin nutritional interventions that may reduce the risk of growth failure and prolonged vitamin deficiency that can be associated with CF (Castellani 2003; Dunn et al. 2011).

SLEEP APNEA

Significance

Sleep apnea is a chronic condition characterized by recurrent episodes of partial or complete collapse of the upper airway during sleep (Punjabi 2008). It is one of the leading causes of excessive daytime sleepiness in adults, and contributes to the development of conditions such as hypertension and cardiovascular disease. Obstructive sleep apnea is the most common form of the condition. In obstructive sleep apnea, airflow is restricted because of occlusion at the oropharyngeal level, which leads to arousal and obstruction relief. The observed arousal does not always lead to complete awakening, but may interfere with sleep efficiency and contribute to daytime sleepiness.

Pathophysiology

Apnea is defined as a total cessation of airflow; hypopnea occurs when there is a decrease in airflow at the nose and mouth (Caples et al. 2005). A small number of apnea and hypopnea events occur in all people during sleep; the number of apneas and hypopneas considered abnormal depends on the population being tested and indications for testing. The frequency with which airflow reductions occur is termed the apnea–hypopnea index. The index is used as a quantitative characterization of the severity of sleep apnea (Caples et al. 2005). An apnea–hypopnea index of five or more is indicative of mild sleep apnea, whereas an index value of 15 or more indicates sleep apnea of moderate severity.

Depending on the severity of the condition, sleepiness may be observed during passive activities such as reading or, in more severe cases, activities such as operating motor vehicles. Aside from daytime sleepiness, commonly observed symptoms of sleep apnea include snoring, poor memory, and impaired psychomotor function (Young et al. 2002).

Descriptive Epidemiology

High-Risk Populations

Estimates of the prevalence of obstructive sleep apnea can vary greatly depending on the methodology used. Because obtaining an assessment of an individual's apnea–hypopnea index requires an overnight visit to an appropriate sleep laboratory, data to support measurements of the prevalence of obstructive sleep apnea can be scarce. Available data from population-based studies place the prevalence of sleep apnea in the range of 5% to 7% for men and 2% to 5% for women (Punjabi 2008). However, because of the intensive nature of the assessment needed to diagnose sleep apnea, it is thought that the majority of cases of sleep apnea go undiagnosed (Young et al. 1997).

Obstructive sleep apnea has been implicated as a contributor to the development of a range of conditions, including hypertension, and cardiovascular and cerebrovascular diseases (Young et al. 2002). Specific outcomes such as acute myocardial infarction incidence and mortality (He et al. 1988; Hung et al. 1990) and stroke (Mooe et al. 2001) have been observed at increased levels among people with sleep apnea. Injury-related outcomes observed with increased frequency in people with sleep apnea include motor vehicle crashes and occupational injuries (Young et al. 2002). In one study, individuals with sleep apnea were found to be about 2.5 times more likely to have had an automobile accident than individuals without the syndrome (Karimi et al. 2015).

Causes

Factors contributing to the development of obstructive sleep apnea include age, excess body weight, smoking, alcohol consumption, nasal congestion, and habitual snoring (Wetter et al. 1994; Young et al. 2002; Punjabi 2008). Other factors for which a causative role is suspected include certain craniofacial features and hypothyroidism.

Evidence-Based Interventions

Screening

Certain features of obstructive sleep apnea, such as its high prevalence and its low recognition as a public health problem, have generated interest in using screening approaches to address the condition. Applying screening approaches to certain occupational populations such as long-distance truck drivers and hazardous duty personnel may be warranted (Baumel et al. 1997). Concern about public safety led to the issuance of specific screening recommendations for sleep apnea in commercial motor vehicle operators (Hartenbaum et al. 2006). Validated screening tools such as the STOP-Bang questionnaire (Chung et al. 2008; Chung et al. 2013) have been developed for application in identifying surgical patients at risk for postoperative complications as a result of undiagnosed sleep apnea.

Examples of Evidence-Based Interventions

The use of continuous positive airway pressure (CPAP) via a nasal mask is a well established and effective means of therapy for obstructive sleep apnea (Caples et al. 2005). Certain oral appliances worn overnight may be useful in some cases. In some cases where the habitual use of CPAP does not improve the condition, surgical options to remove soft palate tissue may be considered.

Addressing known risk factors such as body weight has been shown to reduce apnea–hypopnea index in affected patients, and population-based weight reduction interventions may address diagnosed and undiagnosed cases of obstructive sleep apnea. Increased awareness of sleep apnea as a focus for attention in primary care settings and referral of individuals with suspected cases of sleep apnea to sleep specialists may help reduce the burden of this condition.

INTERSTITIAL LUNG DISEASE

Interstitial lung disease refers to diseases that manifest in the interstitium, which includes the spaces between the pulmonary capillary cells and the pulmonary alveoli, the connective tissue surrounding blood vessels and bronchi, and the connective tissue of the pleura. Specific descriptors of this category of disease include pulmonary fibrosis, alveolitis, and pneumonitis. Although exposure to occupational dusts and fumes can be associated with this form of disease, most cases of interstitial lung disease cannot be attributed to occupational exposures (Coultas et al. 1994). Non-occupational contributors to this class of disease include medications, therapeutic radiation exposure, infections, and toxic gas inhalations (Raghu et al. 2004).

During the initial assessment of individuals with interstitial lung disease, it is important to look for connective tissue disease or malignancy, and to consider medication use, symptom duration, and the history of exposure to different organic and inorganic dusts. Progressive dyspnea is the most common presenting complaint. Pulmonary function testing, although it may show abnormalities with a restrictive defect with decreased FVC, is more helpful in following the course of the disease than in the initial diagnostic evaluation. The location and type of opacities on the chest radiograph can be helpful in diagnosing interstitial lung diseases (Coultas et al. 1994). A lung biopsy is sometimes required if the diagnosis remains in doubt or if the disease process is severe or rapidly progressive.

Descriptive Epidemiology

Aside from specific agents and processes described elsewhere in this chapter, literature on the epidemiology of interstitial lung diseases is scarce. Diagnosis of interstitial lung disease can often be a diagnosis of exclusion. In many cases, a diagnosis of idiopathic interstitial fibrosis may be applied in the absence of a thorough investigation of occult occupational exposures. In a population-based registry in an urban county, the prevalence of interstitial lung disease in adults aged older than 18 years was 80.9 per 100,000 population in men, and 67.2 per 100,000 population in women (Mannino et al. 1996). Occupational and environmental causes were the most frequent in men (20.8 per 100,000) with idiopathic pulmonary fibrosis as the second-most-likely diagnosis (20.2 per 100,000). In women, pulmonary fibrosis was the most common diagnosis (14.3 per 100,000 individuals) with idiopathic pulmonary fibrosis second (13.2 per 100,000 individuals; Mannino et al. 1996). In a retrospective cohort study of idiopathic pulmonary fibrosis using health plan records from 1996 to 2000, national U.S. prevalence and incidence rates were estimated at 14.0 and 6.8 per 100,000, respectively (Raghu et al. 2006).

Causes

Risk factors for developing many of the interstitial lung diseases remain poorly understood. An autopsy study on the risk factors for idiopathic pulmonary fibrosis found that laundry workers, barbers, beauticians, painters, production metalworkers, and production woodworkers were at greater risk for developing the disease (Scott et al. 1990). Other studies on environmental factors and idiopathic pulmonary fibrosis have found increased odds ratios for exposure to wood dust, textile dust, metal dust, agricultural dust, and damp, moldy environments (Hubbard et al. 1996; Mapel et al. 1996; Baumgartner et al. 1997; Taskar and Coultas 2008). Smoking has been found to be a risk factor for idiopathic pulmonary fibrosis in several studies (Scott et al. 1990; Hubbard et al. 1996; Baumgartner et al. 1997). In a case–control study, a history of having ever smoked increased the risk for idiopathic pulmonary fibrosis by 60% (Hubbard et al. 1996).

Occupational exposure to artificial food flavorings such as butter flavoring (diacetyl) applied to many different food products such as microwave popcorn has been associated with bronchiolitis obliterans (CDC 2007). Exposure to diacetyl and other diketones has been observed from the commercial grinding and roasting of unflavored coffee beans (Gaffney et al. 2015). These findings highlight the need for vigilance as the use of synthetic chemicals use evolves to new settings and the need to establish and maintain surveillance for illness associated with emerging industries and product use.

Evidence-Based Interventions

For interstitial lung diseases that develop from inhaling organic or inorganic dusts or fumes, limiting or avoiding the exposure will minimize or prevent the disease. Because of the important therapeutic benefits of medications and radiation therapy, addressing these exposures as risk factors for interstitial lung disease is difficult. For many of the interstitial diseases, treatment is primarily supportive, treating the complications of respiratory and right heart failure. Preventive care should include influenza and pneumococcal vaccines. Public health surveillance and clinician reporting of unusual diseases associated with occupational exposures is critical to early identification of emerging problems when intervention has the greatest potential for interrupting the emergence of disease.

OCCUPATIONAL LUNG DISEASES

This section covers coal workers' pneumoconiosis, silicosis, asbestosis, byssinosis, occupational asthma, and organic dust–related lung disease.

Significance

It is estimated that, in 1999, 14 occupational illnesses generated $14.5 billion of health expenditures, including $2.2 billion attributed to COPD and $1.5 billion to asthma (Leigh et al. 2003). One of the most common occupational lung diseases, occupational chronic bronchitis (see COPD earlier in the chapter), along with the symptom of cough, is the least specific response to occupational exposures and is often the first indication of work-related pulmonary pathology. Given a sufficient dose and duration of exposure, nearly all respirable agents can contribute to the development or aggravation of chronic lung diseases. It is not uncommon to have multiple occupational lung diseases present in the same workforce or even the same person. This is especially true for occupational bronchitis and occupational asthma.

Many chronic occupational lung diseases are defined by the agent associated with the specific disease and often named after the agent (i.e., silica inhalation causes silicosis, asbestos fiber inhalation causes asbestosis). Several distinct pathological processes have been associated with exposure to specific respirable dusts present in the occupational environment. Only a few of these diseases result from acute exposures. Most, especially pneumoconiosis, result from multiple years of exposure and are associated with an important hallmark of the disease process known as the "disease latency period." This means that disease does not appear immediately, and typically at least 10, and commonly 20 or more, years pass between first exposure and the recognition of clinical disease. Some of these diseases may first appear and even progress many years after exposure has ended.

Occupational dusts are classified as either inorganic (e.g., coal dust, silica, asbestos) or organic (e.g., cotton dust, grain dust, mold spores). The respiratory conditions associated with most inorganic dusts are called pneumoconioses and result from the direct effect of the dust on lung tissue. Chest x-ray is the primary diagnostic tool used to identify these diseases. Guidelines on how to classify chest radiographs for persons with pneumoconioses have been published by the World Health Organization ILO since 1950. These guidelines describe and codify the radiographic abnormalities of the pneumoconioses in a simple, reproducible manner by using two sets of standard comparison films. The guidelines were issued in 1971 and 1980, revised in 2000, and published in 2002 (ILO 2002). In 2011, the ILO revised the guidelines to extend the classification to use with digital radiographic images (ILO 2011).

From 1968 to 2010, a total of 145,750 deaths from pneumoconiosis were recorded among U.S. residents (NIOSH 2016a). The U.S. OSHA has established national permissible exposure limits for all inorganic dusts associated with disease. Diseases resulting from exposure to most organic dusts are immunologically mediated. One exception to this latter classification is the condition related to cotton dust exposure; cotton dust is organic, but the condition is probably not immunologically mediated and is related to endotoxins present in the cotton dust.

Cigarette smoking increases the risk of lung disease in occupationally exposed workers. In most cases, the disease risks are additive—that is, the total disease risk is the sum of the risk from cigarette smoking and the risk from the occupational exposure. An exception to this is the multiplicative risk between asbestos exposure and cigarette smoking in the occurrence of lung cancer (discussed in Chapter 2).

The following sections briefly describe some important occupation-related chronic lung diseases.

COAL WORKERS' PNEUMOCONIOSIS

Coal workers' pneumoconiosis (CWP), first described in 1831 in a British coal miner, is known as black lung disease and is identified by a pattern of x-ray abnormalities and an exposure history. Through greater mechanization, coal production has increased while the workforce has declined. However, greater mechanization has led to dustier conditions. In 2013, there were approximately 123,000 coal mining sector employees in the United States.

Between 1968 and 2010, 73,849 U.S. deaths occurred with coal workers' pneumoconiosis noted on the death certificates. Deaths have significantly declined from a high of 2,870 in 1972 to 486 in 2010. For the decade from 1990 to 1999, more than three fourths of all CWP decedents were residents of Pennsylvania, West Virginia, Virginia, and Kentucky. Pennsylvania alone accounted for about half of all CWP deaths in this period (NIOSH 2016a). Mining machine operators had the highest proportionate mortality ratio among occupations (NIOSH 2016a). Although CWP has declined in the United States, the threat of CWP has significantly increased in developing countries seeking inexpensive sources of energy and where dust control measures are often rudimentary and regulatory frameworks ineffective. Since the enactment of the U.S. Black Lung Compensation Program in 1969, through 2004, approximately $41 billion has been paid for CWP benefits. In 2012, 52,296 beneficiaries received $376,497,000 in benefits (NIOSH 2016b).

Descriptive Epidemiology

The prevalence of CWP increases with increasing exposure to coal dust. In studies of CWP, years of mining are often used as a surrogate for dust exposure because information on dust exposure for individual miners is rarely complete.

Coal workers' pneumoconiosis is classified as simple CWP if rounded opacities less than one centimeter are seen on the chest radiograph (ILO opacities "p," "q," or "r"; ILO 2002). It is typical for the opacities to first appear in the upper lung fields of the chest x-ray and then to progress to involve all lung fields. The National Study of Coal Workers' Pneumoconiosis is maintained by NIOSH. Data from that ongoing surveillance program shows that, among U.S. underground coal miners with 25 or more years of mining surveyed between 1973 and 1978, 34% had simple CWP. The prevalence of simple CWP declined to 4% during survey years 1996 to 1999 (NIOSH 2004). It is uncommon in simple CWP for the radiographic abnormalities to progress after the individual has left the dusty environment.

Complicated CWP, often described as massive progressive fibrosis, is often preceded by recurrent infection, especially tuberculosis. Radiographically, it is defined as small opacities and the presence of large opacities (greater than one centimeter) on the chest x-ray. Data from the national study suggest that the incidence of both simple and complicated CWP is declining, largely attributed to dust standards in mines being enforced, but may be increasing among younger individuals. In addition, although CWP prevalence in working coal miners declined substantially from 1970 to 1994, it increased from 1995 to 2006 (Figure 17-6; Attfield et al. 2009; NIOSH 2016b).

Chronic exposure to coal dust can lead to the development of COPD, even in the absence of radiographic changes (Oxman et al. 1993). Coal miners with COPD have increased rates of dyspnea, cough, and phlegm production. The magnitude of the deficit in lung function attributable to chronic coal dust exposure is between 150 and 450 milliliters over an average lifetime of work in a coal mine, with a smaller percentage of individuals having deficits of greater than one liter (Lewis et al. 1996).

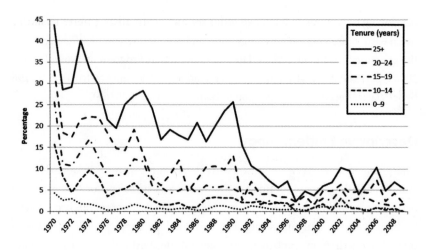

Source: Reprinted from NIOSH (2016b).

Figure 17-6. Percentage of Examined Underground Miners with Coal Workers' Pneumoconiosis (International Labour Office [ILO] Category 1/0+) by Tenure in Mining, 1970–2009

Causes

Coal workers' pneumoconiosis is related to the total dust burden in the lungs. The type of coal (known as coal rank, which is determined by the carbon content of the coal) is also important; the higher the rank, the greater the disease risk and dust biologic activity. Anthracite coal has the highest rank, followed by bituminous, subbituminous, and lignite. Coal workers' pneumoconiosis is caused by respirable coal mine dust (generally defined as dust particles less than five microns in aerodynamic diameter). Usually, 10 or more years of exposure to coal dust must have elapsed before CWP can be diagnosed by a chest x-ray. Coal dust also may contain other harmful mineral dusts, such as silica dust, which increase the risk of other chronic lung diseases such as silicosis. The radiographic appearance of silicosis can be indistinguishable from CWP. The risk of CWP diagnosed by x-ray increases with the higher rank of coal, in part explaining the higher occurrence in miners from the eastern coal-producing regions of the United States compared to western areas. Miners who work underground, where dust control is problematic, are at higher risk than aboveground or surface miners.

Risk factors for the development of COPD in coal miners are the duration and extent of dust exposure, previous dust exposure, and the presence of other risk factors for obstructive lung disease, especially cigarette smoking. The average lifetime coal dust exposure among coal miners with symptoms of chronic lung disease was found to result in a loss in lung function equivalent to that associated with smoking 20 cigarettes per day over a lifetime (Lewis et al. 1996). Coal miners working in jobs with higher silica exposure, such as surface coal mine drillers, are at higher risk for the development of COPD.

Evidence-Based Interventions

Coal workers' pneumoconiosis can best be prevented by reducing coal dust exposure in mines and the workplace, comprehensive industrial hygiene monitoring to measure dust suppression, educating workers about disease risk and safe work practices, and, when excessive exposure circumstances are unavoidable, providing respiratory protection. Medical monitoring of coal miners is required, and periodic chest radiographs are intended to identify individuals who have CWP in its preliminary phases, thus enabling them to avoid further exposure and possibly preventing the disease's progression to more advanced stages. The use of the ILO pneumoconiosis grading system is critically important to allow quantification of changes over time and assessment of progression.

The Federal Coal Mine Health and Safety Act passed in 1969 and its amendments set limits on the amount of worksite respirable coal dust in the United States. For coal dust with less than 5% silica, the standard is 2 milligrams per cubic meter of air (mg/m^3). Although there is evidence that the current dust standards have contributed to the decrease in the occurrence of CWP, the MSHA monitoring data from the 1980s through 1999 show little change in the level of coal dust exposure exceedances. More than 8% of the 794,000 samples exceeded the permissible exposure limit. In 1995, NIOSH adopted a recommended exposure level of 1 mg/m^3, which was adopted because of concerns that the current standard did not protect against other lung conditions. Between 1995 and 2003, one fourth of coal mine dust exposures recorded by MSHA exceeded the recommended exposure level (NIOSH 2016b).

SILICOSIS

Silicons comprise almost 28% of the earth's crust. It is the crystalline forms that are most toxic. It exists as five polymorphs, the most common being quartz. Silica has many industrial applications. Occupational exposures occur worldwide, and although the disease is decreasing in the developed countries, it is increasing in developing countries. In the United States, excessive exposures continue and are most frequently found in small operations that are seldom visited by regulatory agencies. Chronic inhalation of respirable particles of crystalline silica is the cause of silicosis. Like CWP, silicosis is characterized by a predominance of small, rounded x-ray abnormalities predominantly in the upper lung fields indicative of fibrosis. The histopathologic hallmark is the formation of silicotic nodules containing birefringent particles. Also like CWP, silicosis can be divided into simple silicosis and complicated silicosis, or progressive massive fibrosis, based on the size of the opacities on the chest x-ray.

Unlike CWP, silicosis is also characterized as acute, accelerated, or chronic. Fortunately, acute silicosis is uncommon today and occurs after high levels of exposure as can occur in silica flour mills or in the now-outlawed use of silica for sandblasting. It is defined as silicosis that appears in less than five years from first exposure. The acute form is often life-threatening and characterized by pulmonary edema, accumulation of proteinaceous fluid within alveoli, and interstitial inflammation. The most common form of the disease is chronic silicosis, which is defined as silicosis that appears 10 or more years after first exposure.

In its initial phases, the disease is not associated with declines in lung function, although cough and phlegm production are common. Chronic exposure to silica dust can also result in COPD, even without the x-ray manifestations of silicosis (Hnizdo and Vallyathan 2003). The disease may slowly progress over 20 to 40 years to the point of respiratory failure. Individuals with silicosis are at increased risk of developing tuberculosis (Snider 1978). On the basis of analyses of nine studies showing increased rates of lung cancer, silica is now categorized as a probable human carcinogen by the International Agency for Cancer Research (Smith et al. 1995; IARC 1997; IARC 19972012). Although deaths in the United States attributed to silicosis have decreased from more than 1,000 per year before 1971 to less than 200 in the late 1990s (NIOSH 2016a), an estimated 2,000 cases of silicosis are diagnosed each year in the United States (Weeks et al. 1991).

Descriptive Epidemiology

Hazardous exposure to respirable silica occurs in many different occupational settings including surface and underground mining of ores containing silica, surface drilling, ceramics manufacturing, stone cutting, construction, silica flour mills, foundries, cement production, abrasive manufacturing and use, and sandblasting. In 2013, when OSHA proposed a revised silica standard, they estimated that approximately 2.2 million workers were currently exposed to respirable crystalline silica including 1.85 million workers in the construction industry and 320,000 workers in general industry and maritime workplaces (OSHA 2016), As with CWP deaths, silicosis listed as a cause of death on a death certificate has declined from more than 1,000 annual deaths in the 1960s to less than 200 per year in the 1990s and to 101 in 2010 (NIOSH 2016a). Pennsylvania alone accounted for nearly 18% of all reported silicosis deaths from 1990 to 1999. Construction and mining industries accounted for more than one third of deaths from silicosis during that same period. Short-stay, nonfederal hospital-reported discharges listing silicosis decreased from approximately 6,000 per year in 1970 to 1,000 in 2000 (NIOSH 2016b).

The prevalence of nonfatal silicosis in the United States is unknown. There are no national registries for the disease, and only a few states have surveillance requirements. By extrapolating from national mortality data, the Michigan state-based surveillance system and capture–recapture methodology estimated that from 1987 through 1996, 3,600 to 7,300 cases of silicosis occurred annually (Rosenman et al. 2003). The U.S. Department of Labor estimated in 1980 that 59,000 of the workers who were then exposed to silica would eventually develop silicosis (Bates et al. 1992).

Silicosis is most prevalent among workers involved in the dry drilling or grinding of rock with high silica content and other activities that generate large quantities of respirable particles. Largely reflecting the exposed workforce, silicosis is nine times more common in men than in women and more common among African American than white males. The most common industrial environments where silicosis occurs among men are mines, foundries, quarries, and silica flour mills (NIOSH 2016b). Among women, silicosis occurs most commonly in the ceramics industry.

Causes

Silicosis is caused by acute or chronic inhalation of crystalline silica, which is present in quartz. A more toxic form of silica may be produced when quartz is heated or with freshly fractured quartz particles (Vallyathan et al. 1995). Foundry workers who are in occupations involving both heating and grinding quartz may be at greater risk of silicosis. A disturbing trend has been the continuing occurrence of silicosis deaths in young adults (aged 15–44 years) and reports of new occupations and tasks that place workers at risk for silicosis, such as fabricators and installers of quartz-containing engineered stone products and most recently workers employed to extract natural gas by hydraulic fracturing exposed to the silica used in that process (Mazurek et al. 2015).

Evidence-Based Interventions

The most effective method for preventing silicosis is primary prevention—eliminating exposure to respirable silica—and, in settings where silica dust occurs, verifying exposure reduction and maintenance through an industrial hygiene monitoring program. A secondary line of defense is worker education and training, use of protective equipment, and regulatory inspections and enforcement of existing work site standards. The OSHA regulatory exposure limits for silica concentrations in the work environment were 0.1 mg/m^3 from 1989 to 1993. In 1993, this limit was modified (and effectively raised) based on a formula with a default limit of 5 mg/m^3 that is reduced as the silica content in a dust sample increases. NIOSH and American Conference of Governmental Industrial Hygienists (ACGIH) recommended an exposure limit of 0.05 mg/m^3. Under development by OSHA since 2013, a revised silica standard became effective on June 23, 2016, reduces the permissible exposure limit for respirable crystalline silica to 50 micrograms per cubic meter of air, averaged over an eight-hour shift. It is estimated to prevent nearly 900 cases of silicosis each year and 600 deaths per year (OSHA 2016). As with medical screening for conditions associated with other inorganic dusts, x-ray screening may identify individuals who have minimal disease, enabling these people to avoid additional exposure and possibly preventing progression to more advanced phases.

ASBESTOSIS

There are four main types of commercially used asbestos fiber—chrysotile (serpentine mineral), and the amphibole minerals amosite, crocidolite, and anthophyllite. Another fibrous amphibole, tremolite, is a frequent contaminant of chrysotile ores as well as vermiculite. An estimated 27,500,000 workers were exposed to asbestos between 1940 and 1979 (American Thoracic Society 2004a). Asbestos was widely used in construction materials, especially those used for insulation and acoustical products in many public, residential, and commercial buildings.

Most uses of asbestos have been eliminated and many countries, but not the United States, have banned all use of asbestos (Collegium Ramazzini 2011). Although its use in Europe, United States, and many other countries has significantly decreased, the mining production of asbestos has been growing. Raw fiber continues to be used in less-developed countries (LaDou 2004). Current concerns in the United States focus on the potential for exposure to widely distributed, in-place asbestos-containing materials. The risk of adverse health effects from these sources of asbestos to workers or to building occupants depends on many factors, most specifically the status of the material—whether it is releasing asbestos fibers into the indoor environment, whether it is frequently disturbed, and how well contained fiber releases are from maintenance activities.

Adverse health effects from exposure to asbestos include pleural effusions, pleural thickening, and plaques with and without calcification, malignant mesothelioma, lung cancer, and asbestosis. Of these, asbestosis is the most prevalent chronic lung condition. Approximately 107,000 asbestos-related deaths (from cancer or other diseases) occur worldwide each year (Collegium Ramazzini 2016). For each year since 1998, asbestosis deaths outnumbered CWP deaths, displacing CWP as the most frequent type of pneumoconiosis death.

In its early stages, asbestosis is often clinically characterized by dry rales, or whistling or crackling noises, at the end of each inspiration. Often, clinical signs and pulmonary function abnormalities appear before chest x-ray abnormalities become apparent. Eventually, diffuse fibrosis can result in decreased lung capacity, decreased gas exchange, and severe shortness of breath. The x-ray abnormalities evident in people with asbestosis are predominantly small, irregular opacities in the lower lung fields (ILO "s," "t," and "u"). In addition, pleural thickening or pleural plaques, often with calcification, can occur alone or in combination with asbestosis. Unlike CWP or silicosis, asbestosis deaths were increasing, from fewer than 100 in 1968 to more than 1,250 in 1999, but between 2000 and 2010, U.S. death numbers leveled out at around 1,400 deaths per year (NIOSH 2016a).

Descriptive Epidemiology

In various surveys, between 6% and 40% of asbestos textile or insulation workers have detectable x-ray lung abnormalities. Results from the NHANES indicate that 2.3% of U.S. men and 0.2% of U.S. women have pleural thickening upon chest x-ray (Rogan et al. 1987). In a study of 17,800 insulation workers in the United States, asbestosis was identified as the cause of death in 7% of the workers who died (Selikoff et al. 1979; Markowitz et al. 2013).

Asbestos had thousands of uses, each of which presented the possibility of exposure. Occupations and workers at risk span the life cycle of asbestos from removal from the ground to product manufacturing to installation of products to maintenance and removal, and finally disposal. Although most uses of asbestos in newly manufactured products in the United States have been eliminated, today's exposure threats come from the long life of asbestos-containing products still present in building materials, which may pose a risk to workers during maintenance, repair, renovation, and demolition. A long latency period usually exists between exposure and the development of asbestosis resulting in current cases seen today being a result of the legacy of exposures in the 1940s to 1970s (Selikoff and Lee 1978).

Causes

Asbestosis is caused by exposure to airborne asbestos fibers. The magnitude of the risk of asbestosis depends on both the duration and the intensity of the exposure to asbestos dust. The more intense and prolonged the exposure, the greater the risk of developing the disease. Brief, but very heavy exposure can also cause the disease.

Asbestos is unique among the pneumoconiosis-causing agents. Non-occupational exposure to family members of workers bringing dust home on their clothes and those living in residences near mines and manufacturing facilities using asbestos have been associated with the occurrence of asbestos-associated disease (Anderson et al. 1976; NIOSH 1995). Most recently, an environmental disaster was identified in Libby, Montana, where a large vermiculite mine and processing facility had been operating since the mid-1920s. The facility closed in 1990 and the community health impacts of the vermiculite asbestiform amphibole present in concentrations as high as 26% have been investigated. Six hundred and ninety-four decedents were identified as having at least one asbestos-related cause of death and residing within the study area boundary. Workers, family members of workers, and community residents had significant excesses of asbestos-associated disease (Naik et al. 2016).

Evidence-Based Interventions

Asbestosis can be prevented by eliminating exposure to asbestos. New asbestos-containing product manufacturing has been largely eliminated from the work environment in the United States and the European Union countries, but its release from existing materials must be controlled. Containment of asbestos in buildings may be initially less expensive than removal; however, containment is only a temporary solution, because product aging and deterioration will continue and ongoing maintenance and repair can result in a further release of asbestos and eventual enforced removal under U.S. EPA regulations. National legislation requires accreditation of contractors who work with asbestos and training for asbestos abatement workers to ensure safety as well as to prevent "bystander" exposure. Safe work practices include identifying materials that contain asbestos; implementing rigorous operating procedures, such as wetting asbestos-containing materials; and wearing a self-contained breathing apparatus.

X-ray and pulmonary function screening may also help in protecting workers. Results from these examinations can encourage the workers to avoid additional exposure, make them more aware of the need for strict work practices, and encourage them to participate in special health surveillance programs.

BYSSINOSIS

Byssinosis is both an acute and chronic airways disease caused by exposure to cotton dust. The acute phase of byssinosis is sometimes called "Monday morning syndrome," in which chest tightness or shortness of breath occurs when workers return to cotton dust exposure following a weekend or days off. Symptoms usually resolve the second day. Progression of the disease is characterized by chronic cough and a decline in lung function. After more than 10 years of exposure, overall pulmonary function is often seen to decline. Byssinosis is similar in pathology to chronic bronchitis. A grading system has been developed for byssinosis (Bouhuys et al. 1977). In the United States, approximately 500,000 workers are potentially at risk for byssinosis (Glindmeyer et al. 1991; Lai and Christiani 2013), although the disease is rarely fatal, claiming fewer than 10 lives per year between 1995 and 2005 (NIOSH 2016a).

Descriptive Epidemiology

It is estimated that more than 60 million people worldwide work in the textile or clothing industry and are at risk for developing byssinosis. The prevalence of byssinosis varies from a few percent to as high as 47% in some surveys (Zuskin et al. 1991). In 1970, it was estimated that approximately 35,000 workers in the cotton textile mills had byssinosis (Glindmeyer et al. 1991). Since regulation of cotton dust began in 1978, the degree of lung function impairment in cotton textile workers may have decreased (Glindmeyer et al. 1991). There is no evidence of sex or race differences in risk of developing byssinosis.

Causes

Byssinosis results from exposure to the dust of cotton, flax, or hemp. Much has been learned about the causal agent of byssinosis, but the precise etiology is still being investigated. Evidence supports that it is not the cotton itself that is the causal agent but a bacterial endotoxin present in cotton dust (Rylander 2002; Shi et al. 2010). Among cotton workers, the risk is highest among workers involved in the initial stages of processing: opening, picking, carding, stripping, and grinding raw cotton.

Evidence-Based Interventions

The best way to prevent byssinosis is to avoid exposure to cotton dust. Cotton dust concentrations in the workplace must be kept below OSHA's permissible exposure level. A technique known as "cotton washing" is effective but may not be feasible on a large scale. Employers must treat the acute phase of byssinosis as a sentinel health event, using it as an opportunity to reduce exposure among other workers with early symptoms.

OCCUPATIONAL ASTHMA

Although the incidence of occupational respiratory diseases already discussed in this chapter is decreasing, occupational asthma is increasing and is rapidly becoming the most common occupational lung disorder in the developed countries (ATS 2004b). Work-related asthma includes occupational asthma and asthma aggravated by work or the work environment, and is characterized by episodes of bronchoconstriction, airway inflammation, and airway hyperresponsiveness to agents or conditions present in the work environment (Tarlo 2016). Primary occupational asthma is distinguished from exacerbations of existing asthma by the presence of a workplace sensitizing agent or acute exposure event and diagnosis by a specific case definition (Beach et al. 2007). The overall prevalence of occupational asthma varies from region to region with estimates for the United States ranging between 10% and 23% of all adults with asthma (ATS 2004b). In the United States, it was estimated that 15% of all asthma cases in the 1978 Social Security Disability Survey were occupationally related (Smith et al. 1989). Between 50% and 90% of individuals with occupational asthma will continue to have symptoms even after being removed from the source of the exposure (Blanc 1987).

In diagnosing occupational asthma, it is important to establish the presence of airflow obstruction (Tarlo et al. 2008). If the preliminary spirometry is normal, a repeat test, following inhalation challenge with methacholine or histamine, may be indicated. It may be difficult to establish that asthma is caused by an occupational exposure. The fact that initial symptoms may occur only at home or after work can be misleading (Blanc 1987). To document a change in airflow obstruction related to work, it may be helpful to measure the peak expiratory flow rate several times a day for two to three weeks. Skin testing with the suspected compound may also be of diagnostic value in selected cases. Specific inhalation challenge with the suspected compound is not routinely performed because it is expensive, time-consuming, not widely available, and carries the risk of a potentially serious reaction (Alberts and Brooks 1992; Tarlo et al. 2008).

Reactive airways dysfunction syndrome occurs hours after a single exposure to high levels of irritant gases and results in cough, wheezing, and shortness of breath (Tarlo et al. 2008). Reactive airways dysfunction syndrome is not usually considered a form of occupational asthma because there is no latency period between the exposure and the development of symptoms. In occupational asthma, symptoms usually do not appear until a few weeks to as long as several years after the first exposure (Alberts and Brooks 1992). Byssinosis is another condition that may be confused with occupational asthma.

Descriptive Epidemiology

Several mechanisms have been identified that are associated with the development of work-related asthma; they include the following: sensitization; reactive airways dysfunction syndrome (associated with a single, high exposure to irritant agents with onset of symptoms within hours); nonimmunologic airway irritation of preexisting asthma; and poor indoor environments with biologic contaminants (ATS 2004b; Tarlo et al. 2008). Agents are classified as high-molecular-weight compounds or low-molecular-weight compounds (Chan-Yeung and Malo 1999).

The high-molecular-weight compounds are proteins, polysaccharides, and peptides, which induce an allergic response by stimulating the production of specific IgE and sometimes IgG antibodies. Depending on the level of exposure, the prevalence of asthma from these compounds can be high. Asthma has been reported in 3% to 30% of animal handlers; 10% to 45% of workers exposed to biologic enzymes that are used, for example, in laundry detergents and other cleaning agents; 20% of bakers; and in 70% of flight crews dispersing sterile irradiated screwworm flies (Blanc 1987).

Examples of the low-molecular-weight compounds are isocyanates, wood dusts, metals, and drugs (Chan-Yeung 1990). An allergic response involving IgE occurs less frequently in the development of asthma from the low-molecular-weight compounds than from the high-molecular-weight compounds. Work-related asthma has been reported in 4% of workers exposed to the dust of western red cedar (Chan-Yeung et al. 1982), in 5% to 10% of workers exposed to toluene diisocyanate, in 29% to 40% of workers using epoxy resins, and in 70% of workers exposed to platinum salts in such processes as metallurgy and photography (Mapp et al. 2005).

Causes

Several groups have developed and applied criteria to characterize chemicals as asthmagens (AOEC 2008; Crewe et al. 2016). The AOEC list was updated in 2015 and designated 327 substances as asthma agents. Among these 173 (52.9%) were coded as sensitizers, and 113 (34.6%) proposed as sensitizers but not yet reviewed (Rosenman and Beckett 2015).

Materials having known or suspected allergic properties account for the majority of cases of occupational asthma. The risk of developing occupational asthma is usually related to the magnitude of exposure for many agents including western red cedar, toluene diisocyanate, baking products, and colophony fumes from soldering (Blanc 1987). Atopy, or allergy, is an important risk factor for developing asthma from the high-molecular-weight compounds but not for the low-molecular-weight compounds (Beach et al. 2007).

The risk for persistent symptoms in workers diagnosed with occupational asthma was examined in 125 western red cedar workers (Chan-Yeung et al. 1982). All workers who remained at work continued to have symptoms. Among workers who left the work, those who were older, had a longer duration of exposure, and had a longer duration of symptoms were at higher risk for having persistent symptoms. Workers who develop toluene diisocyanate–related asthma and continue to be exposed to the compound have been found to have continued deterioration in pulmonary function.

Evidence-Based Interventions

The only way to prevent occupational asthma is to avoid work and work sites where exposure to certain levels of agents occurs. Thus, it is important for facility managers to know what agents in their plant have been associated with asthma and to inform their workers and establish work practices that maintain exposures below known sensitization levels (Spagnolo et al. 2015). Material safety data sheets need to include information on components that may cause or exacerbate asthma. Workers need to be educated and trained on proper handling of materials and avoiding spills. Improved ventilation and the use of respirators when exposures are likely can decrease the risk of disease.

When sensitization occurs, often the only remedy for the affected worker is a transfer from the area of exposure. In cases where transfer is not possible, it is debatable whether the worker should be allowed to continue working with the suspected compound, even when protective measures are instituted (ATS 2004b; Tarlo et al. 2008). Deaths have been recorded when sensitized individuals have been re-exposed at the workplace. Desensitization before exposure has not been shown to be effective (Weeks et al. 1991).

ORGANIC DUST–RELATED LUNG DISEASE

A variety of chronic lung conditions can develop following short-term or long-term exposure to organic dusts (hypersensitivity pneumonitis) or toxic gases such as nitrogen oxides produced from the storage or decay of organic material (silo fillers disease). Although agricultural workers are most frequently impacted (Bang et al. 2006), as with occupational asthma, there are more than 200 agents known to cause hypersensitivity pneumonitis and among them industrial chemicals such as metal-working fluids (Kreiss and Cox-Ganser 1997).

In 2003, OSHA estimated that, in 1996, 92,000 grain elevator and 68,000 grain mill employees working in approximately 5,200 grain elevator firms and 1,500 grain mill firms were impacted by the OSHA (2003) grain dust standard. Grain dust is a mixture of different grains, bacteria and fungus, mites, inorganic material, and herbicides and pesticides. Grain-handlers' disease, caused by inhaling grain dust, is characterized by a drop in lung function over a work shift and by changes that persist over a harvest season (James et al. 1986). Chronic grain dust exposure can result in chronic cough, phlegm, wheezing, and dyspnea, and a permanent decline in lung function. Pulmonary fibrosis may occur but is uncommon in workers with chronic grain dust exposure (James et al. 1986).

Farmer's lung is caused by inhaling spores from moldy hay and is characterized by repeated attacks of fever, chills, malaise, coughing, and breathlessness (do Pico 1992). The condition is a type of hypersensitivity pneumonitis or extrinsic allergic alveolitis that results from inhaling many different organic dusts. Most commonly, thermophilic *Actinomyces* or other fungi are present. Testing patient serum for specific precipitating antibodies can help identify which organisms or agents may be contributing to the disease. In a well-controlled research setting, inhalation chamber challenges have been used to identify offending agents. Such testing is not a routine practice. The chronic form occurs in fewer than 5% of patients who develop the acute form of the disease (Speizer 1981). Lung function is abnormal in patients with the chronic form of the disease, with a decline in the FVC and a diffuse fibrosis on the chest x-ray.

Descriptive Epidemiology

Hypersensitivity pneumonitis is a rare disease with an increasing incidence and little is known about the distribution of the disease outside the agricultural sector (Bang et al. 2006; Spagnolo et al. 2015). Some of the increase may be attributable to changes in agricultural practices and the movement to large-scale production of livestock in confined feeding operations (Van Essen and Auvermann 2005). Symptoms are often similar to asthma, COPD, and bronchitis, and initial acute attacks are often mistaken for pneumonia. No single clinical or laboratory test exists to establish the diagnosis. Chronic lung disease from inhaling of grain dust is probably more common, but relatively little is known about its epidemiologic patterns.

Causes

Those at risk for the disease from inhaling biologically active organic dusts include farmers, grain handlers, wood workers, bird breeders, mushroom workers, and animal handlers, including workers who clean pens and handle laboratory animals (Bang et al. 2006). Environments where water-based machining fluids are used have also been associated with hypersensitivity pneumonitis, probably because of aerosolization of bacteria or fungi growing in the fluids (Kreiss and Cox-Ganser 1997).

Evidence-Based Interventions

Agricultural dusts are regulated in the United States; the NIOSH has proposed a limit of 4 mg/m^3 for grain dust. The concern over dust levels in grain handling facilities has, in part, been because of the risk of explosions (OSHA 2003). Improved design of grain elevators and livestock confinement spaces, proper ventilation, and education of farmworkers and rescue services can reduce the risk from dust and toxic gases (Speizer 1981). Self-contained breathing devices should be worn by workers entering closed or poorly ventilated spaces or tanks containing liquid manure. Diseases caused by molds can be minimized by proper grain storage techniques. A critical factor in control of disease is worker knowledge of the circumstances in which exposures are likely to occur so that preventive precautions can be taken.

Resources

American Lung Association, http://www.lungusa.org

Centers for Disease Control and Prevention, http://www.cdc.gov

- Agency for Toxic Substances and Disease Registry, http://www.atsdr.cdc.gov
- Case Studies in Environmental Medicine, http://www.atsdr.cdc.gov/csem/csem.html
- National Asthma Control Program, http://www.cdc.gov/asthma
- National Institute for Occupational Safety and Health, http://www.cdc.gov/niosh
- Toxicological Profiles, http://www.atsdr.cdc.gov/substances/index.asp
- Work-Related Lung Disease Surveillance System, http://wwwn.cdc.gov/eworld/Set/Work-Related_Respiratory_Diseases/88

Cystic Fibrosis Foundation, http://www.cff.org

Environmental Protection Agency (asthma and indoor environments), http://www.epa.gov/asthma

Global Initiative for Chronic Obstructive Lung Disease, http://www.goldcopd.com

National Heart, Lung, and Blood Institute, http://www.nhlbi.nih.gov

- Guidelines for the Diagnosis and Management of Asthma (EPR-3), http://www.nhlbi.nih.gov/health-pro/guidelines/current/asthma-guidelines
- Lung disease information for patients and the general public, http://www.nhlbi.nih.gov/health/public/lung/index.htm

National Sleep Foundation (obstructive sleep apnea), http://www.sleepfoundation.org

Suggested Reading

Chen JC, Mannino DM. Obstructive, occupational, and environmental diseases. Worldwide epidemiology of chronic obstructive pulmonary disease. *Curr Opin Pulm Med.* 1999;5(2):93–99.

Levy BS, Wagner GR, Rest KM, Weeks JL, eds. *Preventing Occupational Disease and Injury.* 2nd ed. Washington, DC: American Public Health Association; 2005.

Moorman JE, Akinbami LJ, Bailey CM, et al. National surveillance of asthma: United States, 2001–2010. National Center for Health Statistics. *Vital Health Stat.* 2012;3(35):1–58.

Morgan MT. *Environmental Health.* 3rd ed. Florence, KY: Brooks Cole; 2003.

Office of Disease Prevention and Health Promotion, Department of Health and Human Services. Healthy People 2020: respiratory diseases. Available at: https://www.healthypeople.gov/2020/topics-objectives/topic/respiratory-diseases. Accessed April 15, 2016.

Speizer FE, Horton S, Batt J, Slutsky AS. Respiratory diseases of adults. In: Jamison DT, Breman JG, Measham AR, et al., eds, *Disease Control Priorities in Developing Countries.* 2nd ed. New York, NY: Oxford University Press; 2006:681–694.

References

Akinbami LJ, Fryar CD. Asthma prevalence by weight status among adults: United States, 2001–2014. *NCHS Data Brief.* 2016;(239):1–8.

Akinbami LJ, Liu X. Chronic obstructive pulmonary disease among adults aged 18 and over in the United States, 1998–2009. *NCHS Data Brief.* 2011;(63):1–8.

Alberts W, Brooks S. Advances in occupational asthma. *Clin Chest Med*. 1992;13(2): 281–302.

American Thoracic Society. Diagnosis and initial management of nonmalignant disease related to asbestos. *Am J Respir Crit Care Med*. 2004a;170(6):691–715.

American Thoracic Society. Guidelines for assessing and managing asthma risk at work, school, and recreation. *Am J Respir Crit Care Med*. 2004b;169(7):873–881.

Anderson HA, Daum SM, Lilis R, Fischbein AS, Selikoff IJ. Household-contact asbestos neoplastic risk. *Ann N Y Acad Sci*. 1976;271:311–323.

Anderson HA, Werner M. Chronic respiratory diseases. In: Remington PL, Brownson RC, Wegner MV, ed. *Chronic Disease Epidemiology and Control*. 3rd ed. Washington, DC: American Public Health Association; 2010:470.

Arbes SJ, Gergen PJ, Vaughn B, Zeldin DC. Asthma cases attributable to atopy: results from the Third National Health and Nutrition Examination Survey. *J Allergy Clin Immunol*. 2007;120(5):1139–1145.

Association of Occupational and Environmental Clinics (AOEC). Revised protocol: Criteria for designating substances as occupational asthmagens on the AOEC list of exposure codes. Washington, DC: AOEC; 2008.

Attfield MD, Bang KM, Petsonk EL, Schleiff PL, Mazurek JM. Trends in pneumoconiosis mortality and morbidity for the United States, 1968–2005, and relationship with indicators of extent of exposure. *J Phys Conf Ser*. 2009;151:012051.

Bang K, Weissman D, Pinheiro G, Antao V, Wood J, Syamlal G. Twenty-three years of hypersensitivity pneumonitis mortality surveillance in the United States. *Am J Ind Med*. 2006;49(12):997–1004.

Barbanel D, Eldridge S, Griffiths C. Can a self-management programme delivered by a community pharmacist improve asthma control? A randomized trial. *Thorax*. 2003; 58(10):851–854.

Barbee R, Murphy S. Natural history of asthma. *J Allergy Clin Immunol*. 1998;102(4 pt 2): S65–S72.

Bates D, Gotsch A, Brooks S, Landrigan P, Hankinson J, Merchant J. Prevention of occupational lung disease. *Chest*. 1992;102(3 suppl):257S–276S.

Baumel M, Maislin G, Pack A. Population and occupational screening for obstructive sleep apnea: are we there yet? *Am J Respir Crit Care Med*. 1997;155(1):9–14.

Baumgartner K, Samet J, Stidley C, Colby T, Waldron J. Cigarette smoking: a risk factor for idiopathic pulmonary fibrosis. *Am J Respir Crit Care Med*. 1997;155(1):242–248.

Beach J, Russell K, Blitz S, et al. Systematic review of the diagnosis of occupational asthma. *Chest.* 2007;131(2):569–578.

Belkin NA, Henig NR, Singer LG, et al. Risk factors for death of patients with cystic fibrosis awaiting lung transplantation. *Am J Respir Crit Care Med.* 2004;173(6):659–666.

Beuther D, Weiss S, Sutherland E. Obesity and asthma. *Am J Respir Crit Care Med.* 2006;174(2):112–119.

Bhan N, Kawachi I, Glymour MM, Subramanian SV. Time trends in racial and ethnic disparities in asthma prevalence in the United States from the Behavioral Risk Factor Surveillance System (BRFSS) study (1999–2011). *Am J Public Health.* 2015;105(6):1269–1275.

Blackwell DL, Lucas JW. Tables of summary health statistics for US adults: 2014. National Health Interview Survey. 2015. Available at: http://www.cdc.gov/nchs/nhis/SHS/tables.htm. Accessed August 30, 2016.

Blanc P. Occupational asthma in a national disability survey. *Chest.* 1987;92(4):613–617.

Blanc PD, Iribarren C, Trupin L, et al. Occupational exposures and the risk of COPD: dusty trades revisited. *Thorax.* 2009;64(1):6–12.

Boucher R. New concepts of the pathogenesis of cystic fibrosis lung disease. *Eur Respir J.* 2004;23(1):146–158.

Boucher R, Knowles M, Yankaskas J. Cystic fibrosis. In: Mason R, Murray J, Broaddus V, Nadel J, eds. *Murray and Nadel's Textbook of Respiratory Medicine.* Philadelphia, PA: WB Saunders Co; 2000.

Bouhuys A, Schoenberg J, Beck G, Schilling R. Epidemiology of chronic lung disease in a cotton mill community. *Lung.* 1977;154(3):167–186.

Boushey H, Corry D, Fahy J, Burchard E, Woodruff P. Asthma. In: Mason R, Murray J, Broaddus V, Nadel J, eds. *Murray and Nadel's Textbook of Respiratory Medicine.* Philadelphia, PA: WB Saunders Co; 2000.

Brotanek J, Grimes K, Flores G. Leave no asthmatic child behind: the cultural competency of asthma education. *Ethn Dis.* 2007;17(4):742–748.

Bueving H, Thomas S, Wouden J. Is influenza vaccination in asthma helpful? *Curr Opin Allergy Clin Immunol.* 2005;5(4):65–70.

Burke W, Fesinmeyer M, Reed K, Hampson L, Carlsten C. Family history as a predictor of asthma risk. *Am J Prev Med.* 2003;24(2):160–169.

Caples S, Gami A, Somers V. Obstructive sleep apnea. *Ann Intern Med.* 2005;142(3):187–197.

Castellani C. Evidence for newborn screening for cystic fibrosis. *Paediatr Respir Rev.* 2003;4(4):278–284.

Centers for Disease Control and Prevention (CDC). Fixed obstructive lung disease among workers in the flavor-manufacturing industry—California 2004–2007. *MMWR Morb Mortal Wkly Rep.* 2007;56(16):389–393.

Centers for Disease Control and Prevention (CDC), National Center for Health Statistics. National Hospital Discharge Survey, 2010. 2012a. Available at: http://www.cdc.gov/nchs/data/nhds/2average/2010ave2_firstlist.pdf. Accessed April 10, 2016.

Centers for Disease Control and Prevention (CDC), National Center for Health Statistics. National Ambulatory Medical Care Survey, 2010 and National Hospital Ambulatory Medical Care Survey, 2010. 2012b. Available at: http://www.cdc.gov/nchs/ahcd/ahcd_products.htm. Accessed August 30, 2016.

Centers for Disease Control and Prevention (CDC). Chronic obstructive pulmonary disease among adults—United States, 2011. *MMWR Morb Mortal Wkly Rep.* 2012c;61(46): 938–943.

Centers for Disease Control and Prevention (CDC), National Center for Health Statistics. National Health Interview Survey. Asthma stats: asthma-related missed school days among children aged 5–17 years. 2013. Available at: http://www.cdc.gov/asthma/asthma_stats/aststatchild_missed_school_days.pdf. Accessed August 30, 2016.

Centers for Disease Control and Prevention (CDC), National Center for Health Statistics. Compressed Mortality File 1999–2014 on CDC WONDER online database. 2015. Available at: http://wonder.cdc.gov/cmf-icd10.html. Accessed April 16, 2016.

Centers for Disease Control and Prevention (CDC), National Center for Health Statistics (NCHS). National Health Interview Survey, 2014. 2016a. Available at: http://www.cdc.gov/asthma/nhis/2014/data.htm. Accessed August 30, 2016.

Centers for Disease Control and Prevention (CDC), National Center for Health Statistics. National Hospital Discharge Survey, 2010. 2016b. Available at: http://www.cdc.gov/asthma/most_recent_data.htm. Accessed April 16, 2016.

Chan-Yeung M. Clinician's approach to determine the diagnosis, prognosis, and therapy of occupational asthma. *Med Clin North Am.* 1990;74(3):811–822.

Chan-Yeung M, Lam S, Koener S. Clinical features and natural history of occupational asthma due to western red cedar (*Thuja plicata*). *Am J Med.* 1982;72(3):411–415.

Chan-Yeung M, Malo J. Natural history of occupational asthma. In: Bernstein I, Chan-Yeung M, Malo J, Bernstein D, eds. *Asthma in the Workplace.* 2nd ed. New York, NY: Marcel Dekker; 1999.

Chilmonczyk B, Salmun L, Megathlin K, et al. Association between exposure to environmental tobacco smoke and exacerbations of asthma in children. *N Engl J Med.* 1993;328(23):1665–1669.

Chung F, Yang X, Liao P. Predictive performance of the STOP-Bang score for identifying obstructive sleep apnea in obese patients. *Obes Surg.* 2013;23(12):2050–2057.

Chung F, Yegneswaran B, Liao P, et al. STOP questionnaire: a tool to screen patients for obstructive sleep apnea. *Clin Sci.* 2008;12:87–89.

Coleman R. Current animal models are not predictive for clinical asthma. *Pulm Pharmacol Ther.* 1999;12(2):87–89.

Collegium Ramazzini. Asbestos is still with us: repeat call for a universal ban. *Am J Ind Med.* 2011;54(2):168–173.

Collegium Ramazzini. The 18th Collegium Ramazzini statement: the global health dimensions of asbestos and asbestos-related diseases. *Scand J Work Environ Health.* 2016;42(1):86–90.

Connett J, Murray R, Buist S, et al. Changes in smoking status affect women more than men: results of the Lung Health Study. *Am J Epidemiol.* 2003;157(11):973–979.

Coultas D, Zumwalt R, Black W, Sobonya R. Epidemiology of interstitial lung diseases. *Am J Respir Crit Care Med.* 1994;150(4):967–972.

Crewe J, Carey R, Glass D, et al. A comprehensive list of asthmagens to inform health interventions in the Australian workplace. *Aust N Z J Public Health.* 2016;40(2):170–173.

Custovic A, Simpson B, Simpson A, Kissen P, Woodcock A. Effect of environmental manipulation in pregnancy and early life on respiratory symptoms and atopy during the first year of life: a randomized trial. *Lancet.* 2001;358(9277):188–193.

Cystic Fibrosis Foundation (CFF). Cystic Fibrosis Foundation patient registry 2014 annual data report. Bethesda, MD: CFF; 2015.

de Serres F, Blanco I. Estimating the risk for alpha 1-antitrypsin deficiency among COPD patients: evidence supporting targeted screening. *COPD.* 2006;3(3):133–139.

do Pico G. Hazardous exposure and lung disease among farm workers. *Clin Chest Med.* 1992;13(2):311–328.

Dunn CT, Skrypek MM, Powers ALR, Laguna TA. The need for vigilance: the case of a false-negative newborn screen for cystic fibrosis. *Pediatrics.* 2011;128(2):e446.

Eisner MJ, Anthonisen N, Coultas N, et al. An official American Thoracic Society public policy statement: novel risk factors and the global burden of chronic obstructive pulmonary disease. *Am J Respir Crit Care Med.* 2010;182(5):693–718.

Eisner M, Balmes J, Katz P, Trupin L, Yelin E, Blanc P. Lifetime environmental tobacco smoke exposure and the risk of chronic obstructive pulmonary disease. *Environ Health.* 2005;4(1):7–11.

Ezzati M. Indoor air pollution and health in developing countries. *Lancet.* 2005; 366(9480):104–106.

Flume PA, Van Devanter DR. State of progress in treating cystic fibrosis respiratory disease. *BMC Med.* 2012;10:88.

Fogarty A, Hubbard R, Britton J. International comparison of median age at death from cystic fibrosis. *Chest.* 2000;117(6):1656–1660.

Ford ES, Croft JB, Mannino DM, Wheaton AG, Zhang X, Giles WH. COPD surveillance—United States, 1999–2011. *Chest.* 2013;144(1):284–305.

Ford ES, Murphy LB, Khavjou O, Giles WH, Holt JB, Croft JB. Total and state-specific costs of CPOD among adults aged ≥18 years in the United States for 2010 and projections through 2020. *Chest.* 2015;147(1):31–45.

Fregonese L, Stolk J. Hereditary alpha-1-antitrypsin deficiency and its clinical consequences. *Orphanet J Rare Dis.* 2008;3:16.

Gaffney SH, Abelman A, Pierce JS, et al. Naturally occurring diacetyl and 2,3-pentanedione concentrations associated with roasting and grinding unflavored coffee beans in a commercial setting. *Toxicol Rep.* 2015;2:1171–1181.

Gerald L, Sockrider M, Grad R, et al. An official ATS workshop report: issues in screening for asthma in children. *Proc Am Thorac Soc.* 2007;4(2):133–141.

Glindmeyer H, Lefante J, Jones R, Rando R, Abdel Kader H, Weill H. Exposure-related declines in the lung function of cotton textile workers. *Am Rev Respir Dis.* 1991; 144(3 pt 1):675–683.

Global Initiative for Asthma (GINA). Global Strategy for Asthma Management and Prevention. 2015. Available at: http://ginasthma.org. Accessed August 30, 2016.

Global Initiative for Chronic Obstructive Lung Disease (GOLD). Global Strategy for the Diagnosis, Management and Prevention of COPD. 2016. Available at: http://goldcopd. org. Accessed August 30, 2016.

Gold W. Pulmonary function testing. In: Mason R, Murray J, Broaddus V, Nadel J, eds. *Murray and Nadel's Textbook of Respiratory Medicine.* Philadelphia, PA: WB Saunders Co; 2000a.

Gold D. Environmental tobacco smoke, indoor allergens, and childhood asthma. *Environ Health Perspect.* 2000b;108(suppl 4):643–651.

Gold D, Damokosh A, Dockery D, Berkey C. Body-mass index as a predictor of incident asthma in a prospective cohort of children. *Pediatr Pulmonol*. 2003;36(6): 514–521.

Griesenbach U, Alton EW. Progress in gene and cell therapy for cystic fibrosis lung disease. *Curr Pharm Des*. 2012;18(5):642–662.

Guide to Community Preventive Services. Asthma control: home-based multi-trigger, multicomponent interventions. 2012. Available at: http://www.thecommunityguide.org/asthma/multicomponent.html. Accessed February 2, 2016.

Guill M. Respiratory manifestations of gastroesophageal reflux in children. *J Asthma*. 1995;32(3):173–179.

Halbert R, Natoli J, Gano A, Badamgarav E, Buist A, Mannino D. Global burden of COPD: systemic review and meta-analysis. *Eur Respir J*. 2006;28(3):523–532.

Hartenbaum N, Collop N, Rosen I, et al. Sleep apnea and commercial motor vehicle operators: statement from the joint task force of the American College of Chest Physicians, American College of Occupational and Environmental Medicine, and the National Sleep Foundation: executive summary. *J Occup Environ Med*. 2006;48(suppl):1–3.

He J, Kryger M, Zorick F, Conway W, Roth T. Mortality and apnea index in obstructive sleep apnea: experience in 385 male patients. *Chest*. 1988;94(1):9–14.

Hnizdo E, Sullivan P, Bang KM, Wagner G. Association between chronic obstructive pulmonary disease and employment by industry and occupation in the US population: a study of data from the Third National Health and Nutrition Examination Survey. *Am J Epidemiol*. 2002;156(8):738–746.

Hnizdo E, Vallyathan V. Chronic obstructive pulmonary disease due to occupational exposure to silica dust: a review of epidemiological and pathological evidence. *Occup Environ Med*. 2003;60(4):237–243.

Hogg J. Pathophysiology of airflow limitation in chronic obstructive respiratory disease. *Lancet*. 2004;364(9435):709–721.

Hu G, Zhou Y, Tian J, et al. Risk of COPD from exposure to biomass smoke: a meta-analysis. *Chest*. 2010;138(1):20–31.

Hubbard R, Lewis S, Richards K, Britton J, Johnston I. Occupational exposure to metal or wood dust and aetiology of cryptogenic alveolitis. *Lancet*. 1996;347(8997): 284–289.

Hung J, Whitford E, Parsons R, Hillman D. Association of sleep apnoea with myocardial infarction in men. *Lancet*. 1990;336(8710):261–264.

International Agency for Research on Cancer (IARC). Monograph on the Evaluation of the Carcinogenic Risk of Chemicals to Humans: Silica, some silicates, coal dust, and para-aramid fibres. Lyon, France: IARC; 1997.

International Agency for Research on Cancer (IARC). IARC Monographs on the Evaluation of Carcinogenic Risks to Humans. Volume 100C: A review of human carcinogens: arsenic, metals, fibres, and dusts. IARC, World Health Organization. 2012. Available at: http://monographs.iarc.fr/ENG/Monographs/vol100C/index.php. Accessed August 30, 2016.

International Labour Office (ILO). Guidelines for the use of ILO International Classification of Radiographs of Pneumoconioses. Occupational safety and health series (no. 22). Geneva, Switzerland: ILO; 2002.

International Labour Office (ILO). Guidelines for the use of ILO International Classification of Radiographs of Pneumoconioses. Occupational safety and health series (no. 22). Geneva, Switzerland: ILO; 2011.

Jaakkola M, Piipari R, Jaakkola N, Jaakkola J. Environmental tobacco smoke and adult-onset asthma: a population-based incident case–control study. *Am J Public Health*. 2003;93(12):2055–2060.

James A, Cookson W, Buters G, et al. Symptoms and longitudinal changes in lung function in young seasonal grain handlers. *Br J Ind Med*. 1986;43(9):587–591.

Johannessen A, Bakke PS, Hardie JA, Eagan TM. Association of exposure to environmental tobacco smoke in childhood with chronic obstructive pulmonary disease and respiratory symptoms in adults. *Respirology*. 2012;17(3):499–505.

Karimi M, Hedner J, Häbel H, Nerman O, Grote L. Sleep apnea related risk of motor vehicle accidents is reduced by continuous positive airway pressure: Swedish Traffic Accident Registry data. *Sleep*. 2015;38(3):341–349.

Kerem E, Reisman J, Corey M, Canny G, Levison H. Prediction of mortality in patients with cystic fibrosis. *N Engl J Med*. 1992;326(18):1187–1191.

Knudsen TB, Thomsen SF, Nolte H, Backer V. A population-based clinical study of allergic and non-allergic asthma. *J Asthma*. 2009;46(1):91–94.

Kreiss K, Cox-Ganser J. Metalworking fluid-associated hypersensitivity pneumonitis: a workshop summary. *Am J Ind Med*. 1997;32(4):423–432.

Labre MP, Herman EJ, Dumitru GG, Valenzuela KA, Cechman CL. Public health interventions for asthma: an umbrella review, 1990–2010. *Am J Prev Med*. 2012;42(4):403–410.

LaDou J. The asbestos cancer epidemic. *Environ Health Perspect*. 2004;112(3):285–290.

Lai PS, Christiani DC. Long-term respiratory health effects in textile workers. *Curr Opin Pulm Med*. 2013;19(2):152–157.

Law HZ, Oraka E, Mannino DM. The role of income in reducing racial and ethnic disparities in emergency room and urgent care center visits for asthma—United States, 2001–2009. *J Asthma*. 2011;48(4):405–413.

Leigh J, Yasmeen S, Miller T. Medical costs of fourteen occupational illnesses in the United States in 1999. *Scand J Work Environ Health*. 2003;29(4):304–313.

Levy BD, Noel PJ, Freemer MM, et al. Future research directions in asthma: an NHLBI working group report. *Am J Respir Crit Care Med*. 2015;192(11):1366–1372.

Lewis S, Bennett J, Richards K, Britton J. A cross-sectional study of the independent effect of occupation on lung function in British coal miners. *Occup Environ Med*. 1996;53(2):125–128.

Mackay D, Haw S, Ayres JG, Fischbacher C, Pell JP. Smoke-free legislation and hospitalizations for childhood asthma. *N Engl J Med*. 2010;363(12):1139–1145.

MacKenzie T, Gifford AH, Sabadosa KA, et al. Longevity of patients with cystic fibrosis in 2000 and 2010 and beyond: survival analysis of the Cystic Fibrosis Foundation patient registry. *Ann Intern Med*. 2014;161(12):233–241.

Mahler D, Meija R. Dyspnea. In: Mason R, Murray J, Broaddus V, Nadel J, eds. *Murray and Nadel's Textbook of Respiratory Medicine*. Philadelphia, PA: WB Saunders Co; 1999.

Mannino D, Etzel R, Parrish R. Pulmonary fibrosis deaths in the United States, 1979–1991. An analysis of multiple-cause mortality data. *Am J Respir Crit Care Med*. 1996;153(5):1548–1552.

Mannino D, Homa D, Akinbami L, Ford E, Redd S. Chronic obstructive pulmonary disease surveillance—United States, 1971–2000. *MMWR Surveill Summ*. 2002;51(6):1–16.

Mapel D, Samet J, Coultas D. Corticosteroids and the treatment of idiopathic pulmonary fibrosis. *Chest*. 1996;110(4):1058–1067.

Mapp C, Boschetto P, Maestrelli P, Fabbri L. Occupational asthma. *Am J Respir Crit Care Med*. 2005;172(3):280–305.

Markowitz SB, Stephen M, Levin SM, Miller A, Morabia A. Asbestos, asbestosis, smoking, and lung cancer: new findings from the North American insulator cohort. *Am J Respir Crit Care Med*. 2013;188(1):90–96.

Marsh S, Aldington S, Shirtcliffe P, Weatherall M, Beasley R. Smoking and COPD: what really are the risks? *Eur Respir J*. 2006;28(4):883–884.

Martinez F, Wright A, Taussig L, Holberg C, Halonen M, Morgan W. Asthma and wheezing in the first six years of life. *N Engl J Med.* 1995;332(3):133–138.

Mason R, Murray J, Broaddus V, Nadel J, eds. *Murray and Nadel's Textbook of Respiratory Medicine.* Philadelphia, PA: WB Saunders Co; 2000.

Mazurek JM, Patricia L, Schleiff PL, Wood JM, Hendricks SA, Weston A. Update: silicosis mortality—United States, 1999–2013. *MMWR Morb Mortal Wkly Rep.* 2015;64(23):653–654.

McConnell R, Berhane K, Gilliland F, et al. Asthma in exercising children exposed to ozone: a cohort study. *Lancet.* 2002;359(9304):386–391.

McConnell R, Berhane K, Yao L, et al. Traffic, susceptibility and childhood asthma. *Environ Health Perspect.* 2006;114(5):766–772.

McConnell R, Islam T, Shankardass K, et al. Childhood incident asthma and traffic-related air pollution at home and school. *Environ Health Perspect.* 2010;118(7):1021–1026.

Melen E, Wickman M, Nordvall S, van Hage-Hamsten M, Lindfors A. Influence of early and current environmental exposure factors on sensitization and outcome of asthma in pre-school children. *Allergy.* 2001;56(7):646–652.

Merrill C, Elixhauser A. *Hospitalization in the United States, 2002: HCUP Fact Book No. 6.* Rockville, MD: Agency for Healthcare Research and Quality; 2005.

Meyers D, Larj M, Lange L. Genetics of asthma and COPD: similar results for different phenotypes. *Chest.* 2004;126(2 suppl):105–110.

Millett C, Lee JT, Laverty AA, Glantz SA, Majeed A. Hospital admissions for childhood asthma after smoke-free legislation in England. *Pediatrics.* 2013;131(2):e485–e501.

Mooe T, Franklin K, Holmström K, Rabben T, Wiklund U. Sleep-disordered breathing and coronary artery disease: long-term prognosis. *Am J Respir Crit Care Med.* 2001;164(10):1910–1913.

Moorman JE, Akinbami LJ, Bailey CM, et al. National surveillance of asthma: United States, 2001–2010. National Center for Health Statistics. *Vital Health Stat.* 2012;3(35):1–58.

Naik SL, Lewin M, Young R, Dearwent SM, Lee R. Mortality from asbestos-associated disease in Libby, Montana 1979–2011. *J Expo Sci Environ Epidemiol.* 2016; Epub ahead of print March 30, 2016.

National Heart, Lung, and Blood Institute (NHLBI). Guidelines for the diagnosis and management of asthma: National Asthma Education and Prevention Program Expert Panel Report 3. Bethesda, MD: NHLBI, National Institutes of Health; 2007.

National Institute for Occupational Safety and Health (NIOSH). Report to Congress: Workers' Home Contamination Study conducted under the Workers' Family Protection Act. Cincinnati, OH: NIOSH; 1995.

National Institute for Occupational Safety and Health (NIOSH). *Worker Health Chartbook—2004*. Cincinnati, OH: NIOSH; 2004.

National Institute for Occupational Safety and Health (NIOSH). National Occupational Respiratory Mortality System (NORMS). 2016a. Available at: http://webappa.cdc.gov/ords/norms.html. Accessed April 11, 2016.

National Institute for Occupational Safety and Health (NIOSH). Work-Related Lung Disease Surveillance System (eWoRLD). 2016b. Available at: http://wwwn.cdc.gov/eworld/Set/Work-Related_Respiratory_Diseases/88. Accessed April 11, 2016.

Ober C, Yao T-C. The genetics of asthma and allergic disease: a 21st century perspective. *Immunol Rev*. 2011;242(1):10–30.

Occupational Safety and Health Administration (OSHA). Grain handling facilities standard. *Fed Regist*. 2003;68:12301–12303.

Occupational Safety and Health Administration (OSHA). Occupational exposure to respirable crystalline silica. 2016. Available at: https://www.federalregister.gov/articles/2016/03/25/2016-04800/occupational-exposure-to-respirable-crystalline-silica. Accessed August 30, 2016.

Orenstein D, Rosenstein B, Stern R. Diagnosis of cystic fibrosis. In: Orenstein D, Rosenstein B, Stern R, eds. *Cystic Fibrosis Medical Care*. Philadelphia, PA: Lippincott, Williams and Wilkins; 2000:21–54.

Orozco-Levi M, Garcia-Aymerich J, Villar J, Ramirez-Sarmiento A, Anto J, Gea J. Wood smoke exposure and risk of chronic obstructive pulmonary disease. *Eur Respir J*. 2006;27(3):542–546.

Oxman A, Muir D, Shannon H, Stock S, Hnizdo E, Lange H. Occupational dust exposure and chronic obstructive pulmonary disease. *Am Rev Respir Dis*. 1993;148(1):38–48.

Pearce N, Pekkanen J, Beasley R. How much asthma is really attributable to atopy? *Thorax*. 1999;54(3):268–272.

Petty T, Weinmann G. Building a national strategy for the prevention and management of and research in chronic obstructive pulmonary disease. *JAMA*. 1997;277(3):246–253.

Punjabi NM. Epidemiology of adult obstructive sleep apnea. *Proc Am Thorac Soc*. 2008;5(2):136–143.

Rabe K, Hurd S, Anzueto A, et al. Global strategy for the diagnosis, management and prevention of chronic obstructive pulmonary disease: gold executive summary. *Am J Respir Crit Care Med.* 2007;176(6):532–555.

Raghu G, Nyberg F, Morgan G. The epidemiology of interstitial lung disease and its association with lung cancer. *Br J Cancer.* 2004;91(suppl 2):S3–S10.

Raghu G, Weycker D, Edelsberg J, Bradford WZ, Oster G. Incidence and prevalence of idiopathic pulmonary fibrosis. *Am J Respir Crit Care Med.* 2006;174(7):810–816.

Remes S, Castro-Rodriguez J, Holberg C, Martinez F, Wright A. Dog exposure in infancy decreases the subsequent risk of frequent wheeze but not of atopy. *J Allergy Clin Immunol.* 2001;108(4):509–515.

Rogan W, Gladen B, Ragan N, Anderson H. US prevalence of occupational pleural thickening: a look at chest x-rays from the First National Health and Nutrition Examination Survey. *Am J Epidemiol.* 1987;126(5):893–900.

Rosenman K, Reilly M, Henneberger P. Estimating the total number of newly-recognized silicosis cases in the United States. *Am J Ind Med.* 2003;44(2):141–147.

Rosenman KD, Beckett WS. Web based listing of agents associated with new onset work-related asthma. *Respir Med.* 2015;109(5):625–631.

Rylander R. Endotoxin in the environment: exposure and effects. *J Endotoxin Res.* 2002;8(4):241–252.

Sarnat J, Holguin F. Asthma and air quality. *Curr Opin Pulm Med.* 2007;13(1):63–66.

Schulz S, Jakubiczka S, Kropf S, Nickel I, Muschke P, Kleinstein J. Increased frequency of cystic fibrosis transmembrane conductance regulator gene mutations in infertile males. *Fertil Steril.* 2006;85(1):135–138.

Scott J, Johnston I, Britton J. What causes cryptogenic fibrosing alveolitis? A case-control study of environmental exposure to dust. *BMJ.* 1990;301(6759):1015–1017.

Sears M. Epidemiological trends in bronchial asthma. In: Kaliner M, Barnes P, Persson C, eds. *Asthma: Its Pathology and Treatment.* New York, NY: Marcel Dekker; 1991:1–49.

Selikoff I, Hammond E, Seidman H. Mortality experience of insulation workers in the United States and Canada, 1943–1976. *Ann N Y Acad Sci.* 1979;330:91–116.

Selikoff I, Lee D, eds. *Asbestos and Disease.* New York, NY: Academic Press; 1978.

Shapiro S, Snider G, Rennard SI. Chronic bronchitis and emphysema. In: Mason R, Murray J, Broaddus V, Nadel J, eds. *Murray and Nadel's Textbook of Respiratory Medicine.* Philadelphia, PA: WB Saunders Co; 2000.

Shi J, Mehta AJ, Hang J, et al. Chronic lung function decline in cotton textile workers: roles of historical and recent exposures to endotoxin. *Environ Health Perspect.* 2010;118(11):1620–1624.

Silva G, Sherrill D, Guerra S, Barbee R. Asthma as a risk factor for COPD in a longitudinal study. *Chest.* 2004;126(1):59–65.

Silverman R, Ito K, Stevenson L, Hastings H. Relationship of fall school opening and emergency department asthma visits in a large metropolitan area. *Arch Pediatr Adolesc Med.* 2005;159(9):818–823.

Smith A, Castellan R, Lewis D, Matte T. Guidelines for the epidemiologic assessment of occupational asthma. *J Allergy Clin Immunol.* 1989;84(5 pt 2):794–805.

Smith A, Lopipero P, Barroga V. Meta-analysis of studies of lung cancer among silicotics. *Epidemiology.* 1995;6(6):17–24.

Smith LA, Hatcher-Ross JL, Wertheimer R, Kahn RS. Rethinking race/ethnicity, income, and childhood asthma: racial/ethnic disparities concentrated among the very poor. *Public Health Rep.* 2005;120(2):109–116.

Snider D. Relationship between tuberculosis and silicosis. *Am Rev Respir Dis.* 1978;118(3):455–460.

Snider GL. Chronic bronchitis and emphysema. In: Murrary JF, Nadel JA, eds. *Textbook of Respiratory Medicine.* Philadelphia, PA: WB Saunders Company; 1988:1069–1106.

Spagnolo P, Rossi G, Cavazza A, et al. Hypersensitivity pneumonitis: a comprehensive review. *J Investig Allergol Clin Immunol.* 2015;25(4):237–250.

Speizer F. Epidemiology of environmentally-induced chronic respiratory disease. *Chest.* 1981;80(1 suppl):21S–23S.

Strausbaugh S, Davis P. Cystic fibrosis: a review of epidemiology and pathobiology. *Clin Chest Med.* 2007;28(2):279–288.

Stulberg M, Adams L. Symptoms of respiratory disease and their management. In: Mason R, Murray J, Broaddus V, Nadel J, eds. *Murray and Nadel's Textbook of Respiratory Medicine.* Philadelphia, PA: WB Saunders Co; 2000.

Tamura T, Suganuma N, Hering KG, et al. Relationships (I) of international classification of high-resolution computed tomography for occupational and environmental respiratory diseases with the ILO international classification of radiographs of pneumoconioses for parenchymal abnormalities. *Ind Health.* 2015;53(3):260–270.

Tarlo SM. Update on work-exacerbated asthma. *Int J Occup Med Environ Health.* 2016;29(3):369–374.

Tarlo SM, Balmes J, Balkissoon R, et al. American College of Chest Physicians. Diagnosis and management of work-related asthma: American College of Chest Physicians Consensus Statement. *Chest*. 2008;134(3 suppl):1S–41S.

Taskar V, Coultas D. Exposures and idiopathic lung disease. *Semin Respir Crit Care Med*. 2008;29(6):670–679.

Taussig L, Wright A, Holberg C, Halonen M, Morgan W, Martinez F. Tucson Children's Respiratory Study: 1980 to present. *J Allergy Clin Immunol*. 2003;111(4):661–675.

Thomashow BM, Walsh JW, Malanga EDF. The COPD Foundation: celebrating a decade of progress and looking ahead to a cure. *J COPD F*. 2014;1(1):4–16.

Tilert T, Dillon C, Paulose-Ram R, Hnizdo E, Doney B. Estimating the US prevalence of chronic obstructive pulmonary disease using pre- and post-bronchodilator spirometry: the National Health and Nutrition Examination Survey (NHANES) 2007–2010. *Respir Res*. 2013;14:103.

Trupin L, Earnest G, San Pedro M, et al. Occupational burden of chronic obstructive respiratory disease. *Eur Respir J*. 2003;22(3):462–469.

Tsui LC, Buchwald M. Biochemical and molecular genetics of cystic fibrosis. *Adv Hum Genet*. 1991;20(153–266):311–312.

Vallyathan V, Castronova V, Pack D, et al. Freshly fractured quartz inhalation leads to enhanced lung injury and inflammation. *Am J Respir Crit Care Med*. 1995;152(3):1003–1009.

Van Essen S, Auvermann B. Health effects from breathing air near CAFOs for feeder cattle or hogs. *J Agromedicine*. 2005;10(4):55–64.

Weeks J, Levy B, Wagner G, eds. *Preventing Occupational Disease and Injury*. Washington, DC: American Public Health Association; 1991.

Weinhold B. Death out West: the link to COPD. *Environ Health Perspect*. 2000;108(8):A350.

Weiss K. Seasonal trends in US asthma hospitalizations and mortality. *JAMA*. 1990;263(17):2323–2328.

Weitzman M, Gortmaker S, Sobol A, Perrin J. Recent trends in the prevalence and severity of childhood asthma. *JAMA*. 1992;268(19):2673–2677.

Wetter D, Young T, Bidwell T, Safwan Badr M, Palta M. Smoking as a risk factor for sleep-disordered breathing. *Arch Intern Med*. 1994;154(19):2219–2224.

White M, Kaliner M. Mast cells and asthma. In: Kaliner M, Barnes P, Persson C, eds. *Asthma: Its Pathology and Treatment*. New York, NY: Marcel Dekker; 1991:409–440.

Witorsch R, Witorsch P. Review: environmental tobacco smoke and respiratory health in children: a critical review and analysis of the literature from 1969 to 1998. *Indoor Built Environ.* 2000;9(5):246–264.

Wright A, Holberg C, Taussig L, Martinez F. Factors influencing the relation of infant feeding to asthma and recurrent wheeze in childhood. *Thorax.* 2001;56(3):192–197.

Xu JQ, Murphy SL, Kochanek KD, Bastian BA. Deaths: final data for 2013. *Natl Vital Stat Rep.* 2016;64(2):1–119.

Young T, Blustein J, Finn L, Palta M. Sleep-disordered breathing and motor vehicle accidents in a population-based sample of employed adults. *Sleep.* 1997;20(8):608–613.

Young T, Peppard P, Gottlieb D. Epidemiology of obstructive sleep apnea: a population health perspective. *Am J Respir Crit Care Med.* 2002;165(9):1217–1239.

Zuskin E, Ivankovic D, Schachter E, Witek T II. Ten-year follow-up study of cotton textile workers. *Am Rev Respir Dis.* 1991;143(2):301–305.

18

MENTAL DISORDERS

Elizabeth Stein, MD, MS, and Ron Manderscheid, PhD

Introduction

Traditionally, mental health care has been isolated from the rest of medicine. However, the public health community increasingly recognizes mental disorders as some of the most serious chronic diseases, rivaling heart disease and cancer in years and quality of life lost and having linkages with most other chronic diseases. In 2012, 18.6% of adults in the United States suffered from a mental illness in the past year (excluding substance use), and for 22% of these adults, the mental illness qualified as a serious mental illness resulting in severe functional impairment that significantly interfered with major life activities (SAMHSA 2013).

Despite research showing that treatment for such disorders can mitigate these life-shortening effects, people with mental illness, relative to other chronic disease, are more likely to go without treatment. For instance, studies show that, in the United States, 30% to 60% of people diagnosed with current mental illness received no treatment (SAMHSA 2013; Wang et al. 2007). In contrast, only about 3% of people diagnosed with diabetes went without care (Hill et al. 2011). Accompanying these issues of unmet need, a drastic change occurred in the mid-20th century in the way we care for people with serious mental illness as we transitioned from public state mental institutions to a model of community treatment. However, lack of purposeful and well-funded planning for this transition has resulted in a large population of people with severe mental illness who are homeless or incarcerated (Bassuk and Gerson 1978).

A growing body of research showing significant morbidity and mortality associated with poor mental health is generating momentum in the public health community to seek ways to help prevent mental disorders and connect persons with these disorders to treatment. Yet several barriers pose challenges to this endeavor. Improving the population's relatively low mental health

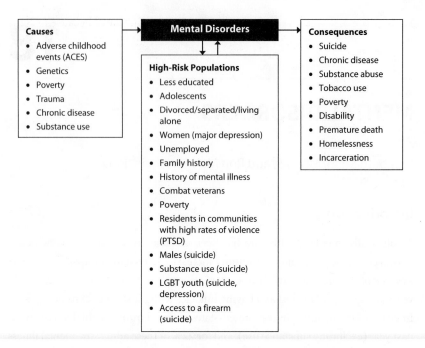

Figure 18-1. Mental Disorders: Causes, Consequences, and High-Risk Groups

treatment access—a problem that stems from stigma, underrecognition by medical providers, and inadequate community mental health resources—requires a multisector approach by the government, health care system, criminal justice system, and community leaders (SAMHSA 2009).

Recent efforts to increase access to treatment for mental disorders include federal legislation introduced by the Mental Health Parity and Addiction Equity Act of 2008 and the Patient Protection and Affordable Care Act of 2010 (ACA), which are leading to better access to health insurance and better integration of mental health treatment and primary care (Beronio et al. 2013). Despite these advances, much work remains to prevent, treat, and reduce the social burden of these debilitating chronic diseases.

Significance

Mental disorders, including substance abuse, are leading causes of death, disability, and human suffering in the United States and throughout the world (Mokdad et al. 2004; Ustun 1999). The false dichotomy between physical and mental illness (sometimes called the "Cartesian dichotomy" because of René Descartes' philosophy of mind–body dualism) continues to bedevil both medicine and public health, and it is clear that the burden of mental disorders will continue to be underestimated unless there is some appreciation for the contribution that mental illness makes to the burden of illness in the United States and in the world (Prince et al. 2007). Figure 18-1 summarizes the burden of mental illness to individuals and to society.

Morbidity and Mortality

Mental illness results in lost years of life because of its association with suicide and comorbid chronic or infectious diseases and in lost years of quality of life because of symptom burden. In the 2010 Global Burden of Disease study, mental illness ranked second in years lost because of morbidity and premature mortality. However, the authors go on to note that mental illness is inextricably linked to other chronic diseases, so that when someone with depression dies of heart disease, the heart disease will be documented as the cause of death. Thus, this method of calculating mortality associated with mental illness likely underestimates its true impact. In addition, data from this study and the World Health Organization show that mental illness is the leading cause of global disability, accounting for 23% to 31% of the years of life with a disability worldwide (Kessler et al. 2009; Vigo et al. 2016; Whiteford et al. 2015).

Although suicide among people with mental illness garners the most public attention, in reality, comorbid chronic diseases associated with mental illness account for more person-years of life lost than suicide. The cause of these comorbid diseases is multifactorial, stemming from the effect of psychiatric illness itself on physiology and human behavior and the effect of some psychiatric medications on human metabolism (Vigo et al. 2016).

In a growing body of literature, researchers point to an association between psychiatric conditions and alterations in immunity and metabolism as a cause of other chronic diseases. For instance, both stress and depression impair immune function, which could increase risk for both cancer and infectious diseases. States of stress and depression have been implicated in causing an inflammatory response; furthermore, inflammation itself may in turn induce the pathology of depression, initiating a feedback cycle that is hard to break (Leonard 2000).

In addition to altering immunity, mental disorders are sometimes associated with behavior that increases risk for infectious diseases. For instance,

Sartorius (2007) has noted that people with schizophrenia are more likely to die from infectious diseases such as tuberculosis and HIV, in addition to chronic diseases such as heart disease and diabetes. Impaired judgment and decision-making, characteristic of psychosis found in schizophrenia and bipolar disorder, may result in risky behaviors such as unsafe sexual practices and injection drug use, putting these patients at greater risk for communicable diseases such as HIV and hepatitis C (Beyer et al. 2007; Swartz et al. 2003). Depression and post-traumatic stress disorder (PTSD) also have associations with behaviors that increase comorbid disease risk and mortality, such as alcohol, tobacco, and substance use. In the 40-year Sterling County Study, participants who became depressed were more likely to start and less likely to quit smoking than those who had never been depressed. As noted by Murphy et al. (2003) "when depression and smoking coexist, the quality and quantity of life are doubly assaulted."

In other cases, psychiatric medications increase the risk of developing chronic diseases. For instance, atypical antipsychotics significantly enhance the risk of diabetes and dyslipidemia through mechanisms causing weight gain and metabolic alterations (Newcomer and Haupt 2006). Despite the negative impact of these side effects, it is important to consider evidence showing that, relative to treated mental illness, untreated mental illness has significantly greater mortality and morbidity (Baxter et al. 2016).

Just as often as mental illness increases risk for comorbid diseases, many chronic diseases perceived as physical affect mental physiology and increase the risk for mental disorders. Thus, the relationship between mental illness and other chronic diseases can be bidirectional (Snoek et al. 2015). For example, depression occurs in 40% to 60% of patients who have experienced a heart attack, and one in four people with cancer suffers from depression (APA 2003). These associations are particularly concerning, with emerging research showing that in patients with cancer, cardiovascular disease, or diabetes, comorbid psychiatric illness leads to increased morbidity and mortality.

The disabling effects of mental illness are particularly striking in the large National Health Interview Survey of 2007. The researchers found that, among people who reported having serious mental illness in the general community-dwelling population, 35% had a history of homelessness or incarceration. Another disheartening finding of this study related to their treatment history, with fewer than two thirds of these adults with serious mental illness reporting that they had seen a mental health professional in the past year (Pratt 2012).

New research showing that treated mental illness can reduce or even eliminate the impact of these diseases on mortality and morbidity emphasizes the importance of connecting sufferers to treatment (Pratt et al. 2016). First, this study found that community-dwelling people with depression or anxiety died eight years earlier on average relative to people without these disorders. However, receipt of mental health services eliminated this disparity in age of death. Second, the study found that mediators between mental illness and early death, such as education, income, smoking, exercise, body mass, and comorbid chronic disease, explained the increased mortality risk. Of these factors, comorbid diseases and behaviors such as smoking, exercise, and body mass were the strongest mediators of earlier death, and socioeconomic factors contributed more modestly. Lastly, by the authors' calculations, 3.5% of all mortality in the United States can be attributed to untreated depression and anxiety. Later in this chapter, we will further discuss the role of the Recovery Movement and the National Association of Mental Illness in bringing hope to people with mental illness and helping them access effective treatment and support.

Finally, media attention has focused on the contribution of mental illness to violence, such as mass shootings, with many pointing to untreated mental illness as one of the drivers for these acts of violence (Metzl and MacLeish 2015). These assertions further stigmatize people with mental illness by fueling the public's pervasive belief that people with serious mental illnesses are far more dangerous than the general population, an idea that was debunked as early as the 1990s (Swanson et al. 2015). For instance, a seminal study using data from the National Institute of Mental Health Epidemiologic Catchment Area Study of 1990 found that only a small fraction of violent crime (4%) is attributable to serious mental illnesses such as schizophrenia and bipolar disorder (Swanson 1994). The other 96% of violent acts stem from other causes such as substance use and antisocial personality disorder.

More recent research using data from the National Epidemiologic Survey on Alcohol and Related Conditions found a similar pattern, estimating that people with serious mental illness and no comorbid substance use have a 12-month prevalence for violence of 2.9%, compared with 0.08% among people with no history of mental disorder or substance use (Van Dorn et al. 2012). Although the risk for violence is higher among people with serious mental illness, the absolute risk of violence in this population is very low relative to the public perception that serious mental illness accounts for a significant portion of our national violence problem.

Social Burden

Mental illness has tremendous economic costs to individuals and to society as a whole. Some of these increased costs are easier to measure—such as health care and social service costs. Other costs are less direct, stemming from the effect of mental illness on families and caregivers, reduced productivity or employment, and morbidity and mortality described previously (Sayers 2001). For the individuals with mental illness, longitudinal follow-up of the National Comorbidity Study showed that participants with mental illness at baseline had lower odds of gainful employment and academic achievement 10 years later (Mojtabai et al. 2015a; Mojtabai et al. 2015b). Another recent study of mental health and marital status found that people with mental disorders were less likely to get married. Among participants with mental illness that did marry, researchers found a positive association between divorce and all of the 18 mental disorders (Breslau et al. 2011).

Untreated mental illness, in particular, results in enormous social burden because of high volumes of people with mental illness who are homeless or incarcerated. Before the closing of public psychiatric hospitals in the second half of the 20th century, people with serious mental illness were institutionalized. The closing of these institutions shifted the burden to the community to care for people with serious mental disorders, but most communities lacked funding and resources to adequately meet their needs. Since this transition, the rate of people with mental illness in prisons and jails has tripled in most estimates—with 20% of people in state prisons having a serious mental illness, up from 5% to 10% in the 1980s (Slate et al. 2013). The prevalence of mental disorders is also high among people with unstable housing. For instance, in a study of Medicaid enrollees in Minnesota with unstable housing, half had a mental disorder (Diaz Vickery et al. 2016). Similarly, a 2012 survey by the National Alliance to End Homelessness described characteristics of people who are chronically homeless and estimated that 30% to 50% have a serious mental illness, most commonly schizophrenia or bipolar disorder (National Alliance to End Homelessness 2016) .

Pathophysiology

Mental disorders are commonplace, and more than 10 million adults in the United States have a serious mental disorder at any one time (Watanabe-Galloway and Zhang 2007). In the United States, mental disorders are defined by criteria outlined in the *Diagnostic and Statistical Manual of Mental Disorders* (*Fifth ed.*; *DSM-5*; APA 2013), published by the American Psychiatric Association (APA). The APA first released the *DSM* in 1952 and has published multiple updates since, most recently in 2013 with the release of the *DSM-5*. The goal of the *DSM* is to provide standard criteria for the classification of mental disorders for use by clinicians and researchers. In addition to the *DSM-5*, behavioral health providers refer to the World Health Organization's *International Statistical Classification of Diseases and Related Health Problems, Tenth Revision,* to obtain codes for billing purposes (*ICD-10*; WHO 1992). The *ICD-10*, a manual that describes mental disorders in addition to other diseases, is used by clinicians in most non-U.S. countries for both diagnostic and billing purposes. To assist U.S. behavioral health providers, who rely on two different manuals for diagnosis and billing, the *DSM-5* lists corresponding *ICD-10* codes for each disorder. The categories for each manual are presented in Table 18-1.

The biopsychosocial model, first described by George Engel in 1977, has helped shape our understanding of both the cause and the treatment of mental disorders. The model posits that mental illness has biological (e.g., genetics), psychological (e.g., learned behavior and conditioning), and social components (e.g., life stress, traumatic experiences, family and social support) that contribute to the development of the illness, all of which need to be addressed during treatment (Engel 1977). For instance, research shows that genetics accounts for about 30% to 40% of the variance in major depressive disorder, with environmental factors causing the remaining 60% to 70%. These individual-specific environmental factors include more remote adverse events in childhood and recent stressors such as divorce and unemployment (Hasler 2010). With the advent of the Human Genome Project, we have a greater appreciation for the biological and genetic underpinnings for most mental disorders. However, to truly prevent mental illness, we must continue to recognize the role of environment and life experiences in the pathophysiology of these diseases.

Common serious mental illnesses associated with high mortality, morbidity, and social burden include schizophrenia, mood disorders such as bipolar disorder and major depression, and anxiety or trauma-related disorders such as generalized anxiety disorder and PTSD. Thus, in this chapter, we will describe pathophysiology, epidemiology, prevention, and treatment in the context of each of these very different disorders along with suicide, one of the gravest potential consequences of these disorders. Substance use disorders are often included as mental health conditions; however, the magnitude of alcohol abuse

Table 18-1. Comparison of *ICD-10* and *DSM-5* Categories

ICD-10 Mental and Behavioral Disorders (F00–F99)[a]

- F00–F09 Organic, including symptomatic, mental disorders
- F10–F19 Mental and behavioral disorders due to psychoactive substance use
- F20–F29 Schizophrenia, schizotypal, and delusional disorders
- F30–F39 Mood [affective] disorders
- F40–F49 Neurotic, stress-related, and somatoform disorders
- F50–F59 Behavioral syndromes associated with physiological disturbances and physical factors
- F60–F69 Disorders of adult personality and behavior
- F70–F79 Mental retardation
- F80–F89 Disorders of psychological development
- F90–F98 Behavioral and emotional disorders with onset usually occurring in childhood and adolescence
- F99 Unspecified mental disorder

DSM-5 Categories

- **Neurodevelopmental Disorders**
  - Intellectual disabilities
  - Communication disorders
  - Autism spectrum disorder
  - Attention-deficit/hyperactivity disorder
  - Specific learning disorders
  - Motor disorders
  - Tic disorders
  - Other neurodevelopmental disorders
- **Schizophrenia Spectrum and Other Psychotic Disorders**
  - Bipolar and related disorders
  - Depressive disorders
  - Anxiety disorders
  - Obsessive–compulsive and related disorders
  - Trauma- and stressor-related disorders
  - Dissociative disorders
  - Somatic symptom and related disorders
  - Feeding and eating disorders
  - Elimination disorders
  - Sleep–wake disorders
    - Insomnia disorder
    - Hypersomnolence disorder
    - Narcolepsy
    - Breathing-related sleep disorders
    - Parasomnias
  - Sexual dysfunctions
  - Gender dysphoria
  - Disruptive, impulse-control, and conduct disorders

(Continued)

Table 18-1. (Continued)

- ○ Substance-related and addictive disorders (includes alcohol, covered in Chapter 10)
- ○ Neurocognitive disorders (categories covered in Chapter 19)
- ○ Personality disorders
- ○ Paraphilic disorders
- ○ Other mental disorders
- ○ Medication-induced movement disorders and other adverse effects of medications
- ○ Other conditions that may be a focus of clinical attention
  - ▪ Relational problems
  - ▪ Abuse and neglect
  - ▪ Educational and occupational problems
  - ▪ Housing and economic problems
  - ▪ Other problems related to the social environment
  - ▪ Problems related to crime or interaction with the legal system
  - ▪ Other health service encounters for counseling and medical advice
  - ▪ Problems related to other psychosocial, personal, and environmental circumstances
  - ▪ Other circumstances of personal history
  - ▪ Problems related to access to medical and other health care
  - ▪ Nonadherance to medical treatment

Note: DSM-5 = Diagnostic and Statistical Manual of Mental Disorders, Fifth Edition (APA 2013); ICD-10 = International Statistical Classification of Diseases and Related Health Problems, Tenth Revision (WHO 1992).
[a]*ICD-10 codes corresponding to DSM-5 disorders are specified in the original DSM-5.*

as a public health problem is significant enough that this problem is discussed in Chapter 10 and will not be included in this chapter. Likewise, although Alzheimer's disease and other dementias are included as mental disorders in the *ICD-10* and *DSM-5*, they are discussed in Chapter 19. Figure 18-1 summarizes populations at high risk for mental illness.

Schizophrenia

Schizophrenia is a chronic and complex neuropsychiatric disorder that, when untreated, causes social and occupational dysfunction attributable to psychotic symptoms (e.g., auditory hallucinations, delusions, and paranoia), disorganized speech and behavior, and negative symptoms (e.g., apathy, lack of motivation, and social withdrawal). To meet *DSM-5* criteria for schizophrenia, symptoms must be present for at least six months (APA 2013). The disorder most commonly develops in adolescence and young adulthood, usually developing in men between ages 18 and 24 years and in women between ages 25 and 35 years (Castle et al. 1993).

The symptoms of schizophrenia likely stem from interrupted brain development in adolescence and early adulthood, which results in dysfunction in the transmission of several neurotransmitters, especially dopamine. This neural disturbance has both a genetic and environmental cause, as evidenced by studies showing 40% to 60% concordance among monozygotic twins (Cardno and Gottesman 2000).

Because schizophrenia is a heterogeneous syndrome with many types, people with schizophrenia suffer diverse symptoms with varying degrees of severity. Although many people with schizophrenia struggle with disability, unemployment, or homelessness, many are able to treat their symptoms and go on to lead productive and full lives. For example, the late mathematician John Nash Jr., a Princeton professor memorialized in the movie *A Beautiful Mind*, spent several years in and out of psychiatric hospitals but was then able to manage his symptoms and make seminal contributions to the field of economics, artificial intelligence, and political science (Funaki 2009).

Mood Disorders

Within the category of mood disorders, major depressive disorder and bipolar disorder have the highest global burden in disability-adjusted life years (Whiteford et al. 2015). For a diagnosis of major depressive disorder, people have a loss of interest in activities and depressed mood on most days for at least two weeks. Accompanying loss of interest and low mood are at least four other depressive symptoms, such as fatigue, poor concentration, hopelessness, guilt, irritability, restlessness, sluggishness, appetite change, worthlessness, insomnia, and suicidal thoughts. Likewise, in bipolar disorder, people suffer from episodes of major depression, but unlike major depressive disorder, people with bipolar disorder must have experienced an episode of mania or hypomania as well. Manic episodes may include symptoms of reduced need for sleep, elevated or irritable mood, rapid speech, delusions of grandeur, and even psychotic symptoms such as auditory hallucinations. A hypomanic episode is similar but with less severe symptoms and never includes symptoms of psychosis (APA 2013).

Anxiety Disorders

Common anxiety disorders include generalized anxiety disorder, social anxiety disorder, and panic disorder. In generalized anxiety disorder, people suffer excess, exaggerated worry over everyday events to the extent that it affects their daily functioning. Social anxiety disorder is also marked by excess worry, but the worries are stimulated by fear of social interactions such as public speaking, meeting new people, or eating in front of people. In panic disorder, sufferers have panic attacks characterized by feelings of doom, racing heart, nausea, and shortness of breath, and they fear having future attacks to the degree that it affects their daily functioning (APA 2013).

Like most mental disorders, people with anxiety disorders have a genetic tendency to develop the disorder, but environment contributes as well, with stress and learned behavior playing a role. Anxiety disorders can develop at any point in the lifespan, but have different causes depending on the development stage. For children, school and social dynamics may be a source of anxiety, whereas older adults may develop anxiety in the context of dementia and stress from activities of daily living (Lenze and Wetherell 2011). The disorder is characterized by disturbances in neurotransmitters and overactivation of stress responses by the sympathetic nervous system. People with anxiety disorders often suffer from comorbid depression (APA 2013).

Post-traumatic Stress Disorder

The most serious of the trauma-related disorders is PTSD, an illness that occurs in people with symptoms of flashbacks of re-experiencing of the event, hypervigilance, avoidance, insomnia, panic, and numbing after directly experiencing trauma in which they felt as if their life or the life of a loved one was in danger. The symptoms continue for longer than a month (APA 2013).

In people who develop PTSD, traumatic exposures condition parts of the limbic system, including the amygdala, to activate even in the absence of threatening stimuli. The amygdala is a center for memory consolidation and feelings of fear and aggression, among other functions. When activated, the amygdala and its associated structures signal the activation of a neuroendocrine state that is characteristic of a flight-or-flight response. This includes an increase of adrenaline and the stress hormone cortisol—neurotransmitters and hormones that cause symptoms of PTSD. Chronic overactivation of these structures and the associated neuroendocrine response may lead to some of the negative health outcomes of PTSD such as increased risk for cognitive decline, diabetes, and heart disease. Like anxiety, comorbid depression commonly afflicts people with PTSD (Kessler et al. 1995; Stein et al. 2002).

Suicide

In the United States, firearms and intentional poisonings are the most commonly used methods for suicide in men and women, respectively, followed by hanging for both sexes (CDC 2013). Although suicide overtly results from the behavior and environmental condition of the victim, many studies have elucidated underlying unique physiology in patients after they attempt or complete suicide. These studies find that patients who attempted suicide have decreased levels of the neurotransmitter serotonin in their cerebrospinal fluid and that these reductions correlated with degree of lethality, planning, and damage of the suicide attempt (Bach and Arango 2012).

Descriptive Epidemiology

Three major psychiatric epidemiological surveys have been conducted in the United States: the Epidemiologic Catchment Area study (Robins and Regier 2001), the National Comorbidity Survey (Kessler et al. 1994), and the National Comorbidity Survey Replication (Kessler et al. 2005). These surveys were generally consistent in finding that 12-month mental disorders are highly prevalent, with 26% to 30% of the population meeting criteria for at least one *DSM-IV* disorder. The more recent National Comorbidity Survey Replication found that non-Hispanic blacks and Hispanics had a lower risk for mood and anxiety disorders relative to whites; however, when these disorders were present, these populations tended to have more persistent symptoms (Breslau et al. 2005).

Schizophrenia

According to meta-analyses of international epidemiological surveys, the median lifetime prevalence of schizophrenia is about 4 in 1,000, with an incidence of about 1.5 per 1,000 (McGrath et al. 2004; Saha et al. 2005). Although some studies have measured higher incidence rates among men, who were 1.4 times more likely to be diagnosed, recent prevalence estimates by Saha et al. (2005) found no gender differences in lifetime prevalence of the disorder (Aleman et al. 2003). The authors of one review proposed that higher suicide rates in men relative to women could explain the disparate findings in incidence and prevalence. The fact that the incidence data is based on clinical encounters rather than the epidemiological survey-based prevalence data may also explain this difference (Ochoa et al. 2012).

The onset of schizophrenia typically occurs in the teen or early adult years, but onset before adolescence is rare. Women tend to have later onset, more prominent mood symptoms, and a better prognosis (APA 2013). High-risk populations include people who are homeless and people in jails or prison. Other high-risk populations include migrants. According to a meta-analysis by Saha et al. (2005), migrant populations have a schizophrenia prevalence ratio of 1.8, relative to native-born populations. Other high-risk populations include the children of people with schizophrenia, who carry a six-fold higher risk of developing the disorder (Owen et al. 2016).

Mood Disorders

Depression is sometimes referred to as the "common cold of mental illness," a phrase that highlights the prevalence of this disorder. In 2012, about 6.9% of the community-dwelling, noninstitutionalized adults and 9.1% of youths aged 12 to 17 years had a major depressive episode in the past year. Recent estimates show that the lifetime prevalence for any *DSM-IV* mood disorder is 17.5% for people aged older than 13 years—14.4% for major depressive disorder and 2.5% for bipolar disorder (Kessler et al. 2012).

Depression risk differs between groups: women have higher risk than men (2.7:1 in the Epidemiologic Catchment Area study), adolescents have higher risk than adults and the elderly; people with less education have higher risk than people with more years of education; unemployed people have higher risk than employed; and separated or divorced people have nearly a three-fold higher risk for depression relative to single or married persons (Horwath et al. 2002). In addition, poverty is known to be a risk factor for major depressive disorder, with higher rates of depression found in current and recent welfare recipients (Siefert et al. 2000). People with a parent with major depression have three times the risk of developing it themselves, with both genetics and learned behavior likely having a causative role.

Like schizophrenia and major depressive disorder, genetic studies demonstrate that bipolar disorder is highly heritable. Bipolar disorder tends develop during young adulthood, is more prevalent in urban populations, and—unlike major depressive disorder—occurs about equally in men and women. Social class and ethnicity are not significant predictors of bipolar disorder. Individuals who cohabit, divorce, or never marry are more likely to have bipolar disorder than married individuals, and there is a dramatically higher prevalence rate for homeless people (Tohen and Angst 2002).

Anxiety

According to data from the 2005 National Comorbidity Study, Kessler et al. (2012) estimate that the lifetime prevalence for any anxiety disorder is 23.6%, excluding PTSD and obsessive–compulsive disorder (which are no longer categorized as anxiety disorders by the *DSM-5*). This lifetime prevalence of any anxiety disorder is accounted for by specific phobia (15.6%), social anxiety (10.7%), separation anxiety disorder (6.7%), generalized anxiety disorder (4.3%), panic disorder (3.8%), and agoraphobia (2.5%).

Anxiety is a common disorder affecting people across all phases of the lifespan, but there are certain groups at higher risk for developing an anxiety disorder. One group with higher rates of anxiety, especially generalized anxiety disorder, are older adults with functional disabilities, cognitive impairment, or caregiver burden. Other high-risk populations include people who are childless, people with trauma exposure, and low-income groups (Lenze and Wetherell 2011).

Post-traumatic Stress Disorder

Rates of PTSD differ depending on population studied, but the estimate for national lifetime prevalence among the U.S. community-dwelling population is 5.7 (Kessler et al. 2012). Although between 50% and 60% of people report having experienced a traumatic event in their lifetime, only about 7% go on develop PTSD (Kessler et al. 2005). Studies find that people who experience an early life trauma, such as combat exposure or child abuse, are more like to have subsequent traumatic exposures, and that genetics may confer traits of either resilience or risk (Jang et al. 2007; Stein et al. 2002). In addition to people with inherited risk, studies have identified several populations at high risk for PTSD because of environmental factors, including people in urban communities with high rates of violence, combat veterans, and first-responders.

In studies of combat veterans, about 15% develop PTSD, and risk factors include being from disadvantaged backgrounds, having traumatic brain injury, and repeated exposure to trauma (Dannefer 2003; Howlett and Stein 2016; Sachs-Ericsson et al. 2016). Other high-risk populations include people living in urban communities with high rates of violence. Studies of community-dwelling residents in Detroit find that blacks are two times more likely to develop PTSD relative to whites, a difference that was not significant after controlling for trauma exposure and central-city location. Most studies examining the apparent disparity of PTSD prevalence among whites and blacks attribute these differences to income, as evidenced by high rates of PTSD among white adults in low-income groups (Breslau et al. 2004; Parto et al. 2011).

Suicide

Suicide is the 10th leading cause of death in the United States, more common than homicide. Among people aged 15 to 24 years, it is the second leading cause of death, preceded by motor vehicle accidents. The mortality rate for suicide is 13.4 per 100,000 for all U.S. adults (Drapeau and McIntosh 2015). The risk for suicide is higher for male relative to female individuals, people with access to a firearm relative to people without firearm access, and people of white race relative to people of other races (Miller et al. 2012). Lesbian, gay, bisexual, and transgender youths also have higher risk of suicide, self-harm, and suicidal thoughts; however, protective factors such as social support from family and friends and school safety have been found to largely mediate this increased risk (Eisenberg and Resnick 2006; Russell and Joyner 2001). Other risk factors for suicide include being divorced or separated, having a history of previous suicide attempts, having a family history of suicide, experiencing a recent stressful life event, and substance use (Mościcki 1995; Vijayakumar et al. 2011).

Geographic Distribution

Considerable geographic variability exists in the degree of support people with mental illness receive. Psychiatric hospitalization in New York City, for example, has been shown to vary according to socioeconomic status and proximity to general hospitals with psychiatric beds. Other predictors of psychiatric hospitalization included living in a high-poverty area, being African American, and living alone. One study found that the highest hospital admission rates were concentrated in those areas of the city in which social and economic disadvantages were greatest (Almog et al. 2004). Another well-studied factor affecting the geographic distribution of mental illness is poverty, with one study finding that the odds for depression were more than twice as high for people living in low-income neighborhoods relative to high-income neighborhoods (Galea et al. 2007).

Time Trends

The 19th century witnessed dramatic growth in asylums in both Europe and the United States, and many psychiatrists argued forcefully at the time that serious mental illness was increasing. However, the extant data are for prevalence rather than incidence, and the dramatic changes that occurred during the century can be attributed just as easily to the confluence of a number of social, political, and economic forces. Most authorities (Bresnahan et al. 2003; Warner 1995) believe that the incidence of serious mental illness remained stable or declined slightly during the 20th century. In contrast, trends in the treatment of mental illness in United States show marked change over the past century, as the treatment of serious mental illness shifted from a model of public institutionalization to our current community health treatment model.

With the advent of antipsychotic medications that proved effective in treating many of the psychotic symptoms of serious mental illness, social and political forces favored treating people with mental illness in the community rather than housing them in public psychiatric institutions, a practice that was increasingly viewed as ostracizing and inhumane. This environment led to the Community Mental Health Centers and Mental Retardation Act of 1963, a pivotal event in mental health care in the United States. This piece of legislation called for the closure of most public psychiatric institutions in favor of a community treatment model, allocating funding to states to open centers to treat community-dwelling residents with serious mental illness. However, half of these centers never opened, and state mental health departments rarely receive adequate funding to care for these individuals. Experts in the field attribute this system overhaul to the increasing prevalence of people with serious mental illness among incarcerated populations and the increasing population of homeless individuals (Durham 1989; Pow et al. 2015; Slate et al. 2013).

More recently, The Mental Health Parity and Addiction Equity Act of 2008 and the ACA of 2010 have had an impact on the treatment of mental illness in the United States. The Mental Health Parity Act was intended to level the field between mental health and substance use insurance benefits and those of medical care. Specifically, this legislation was designed originally for private insurance plans of 50 or more enrollees that offered behavioral health insurance benefits. The concept of parity applied both to the actual insurance benefits and to how the benefits were managed. Two years later, the ACA extended parity to all insurance offered through the state health insurance marketplaces and to insurance offered through the state Medicaid expansions. The U.S. Department of Health and Human Services has estimated that the ACA extended parity to the health insurance of more than 62 million more Americans (Beronio et al. 2013).

Since the passage of the Mental Health Parity Act, advocates for mental health and policy experts have raised concerns that insurance companies are not being fully transparent about behavioral health and medical benefits, thus making it difficult for consumers to understand whether parity requirements actually are being followed. This concern has reached Congress, which has proposed draft legislation to enforce and monitor insurance parity.

Without any question, the ACA represented the most significant change to behavioral health care in the half century since the passage of the Community Mental Health Centers and Mental Retardation Act of 1963. The ACA sought to extend health insurance coverage to an additional 40 million Americans, while standardizing the categories of insurance benefits, including disease prevention and health promotion. It also eliminated all pre-existing condition exclusion clauses in health insurance, and permitted all young adults to remain on family policies until age 26.

To implement the new insurance coverage, state health insurance marketplaces were developed for all states. Because of federal–state controversy, about two thirds of these marketplaces are operated by the U.S. Department of Health and Human Services. In addition, the ACA provided for Medicaid expansions in all states to cover all persons up to 138% of the federal poverty level. To date, 31 states have undertaken a state Medicaid expansion (Han et al. 2015).

Other provisions of the ACA promoted the development of integrated behavioral health and primary care through medical and health homes, reform of financing systems away from encounter-based payments and toward case and capitation rates, and the implementation of consistent national performance measures. Many of the latter provisions of the ACA have not yet been fully realized (Caffrey 2014).

Causes

Modifiable Risk Factors

In the World Health Organization Summary Report (2004) entitled "Prevention of Mental Disorders," authors describe social, economic, and environmental factors that either increase risk for mental disorders or serve as protective factors. Although genetic inheritance explains much of the variance in the development of mental disorders, external factors account for at least half. Unlike genetic factors, social contributors to mental illness are modifiable and are therefore opportune targets for prevention. Figure 18-1 provides an outline of modifiable risk factors.

Some of these modifiable risk factors involve macro-level issues such as war, violence, poverty, and inequality—all of which increase the risk for mental disorders such as PTSD, alcohol use disorder, anxiety, and depression (Hosman et al. 2005; Yoshikawa et al. 2012). For example, one recent study found that U.S. women living in states with higher income inequality had an increased risk for developing depression (Pabayo et al. 2014). Urban violence is associated with the development of PTSD symptoms, with a recent study finding that 70% of black males in Baltimore suffered two or more symptoms of post-traumatic stress (Smith and Patton 2016).

Other modifiable risk factors stemming from the family and community context contribute to the development of mental illness. Studies show that adverse childhood experiences—such as lack of secure attachment and family support, child abuse, parental mental illness, or abuse by peer group—can increase the risk for depression and anxiety later in life (Beardslee et al. 2013; Khan et al. 2015; Solantaus and Salo 2005; Weersing et al. 2016). In addition, early maternal factors such as postpartum depression and low birthweight have long been identified as a risk factor for the later development of psychiatric disorder and behavioral problems (Botellero et al. 2016; Kersten-Alvarez et al. 2012).

Individual factors that are associated with mental illness are substance use and comorbid chronic diseases such as diabetes, heart disease, and cancer, and personal traits such as reduced resilience. A review studying the temporal associations between alcohol use disorder and mental illness concluded that alcohol use disorders frequently precede major depression and anxiety disorders (Falk et al. 2008). In patients who suffered a heart attack, one in five develop depression within three months of the event (Larsen 2013). Lastly, studies of people commonly exposed to trauma (e.g., soldiers, people living in Israel, paramedics) find that people with stronger resilience traits are less likely to develop PTSD (Shoshani and Slone 2015; Streb et al. 2014; Szivak and Kraemer 2015).

Population-Attributable Risk

Few studies have been conducted to understand the modifiable risk factors for mental disorders, thus making estimates of population-attributable risk difficult. One area in which such research has been done involves risk factors for suicide. These studies estimate that, for suicide, mental illness has a population-attributable fraction of 47% to 74% (Cavanagh et al. 2003; Li et al. 2011). Other studies counter that environmental factors such as firearm access and low socioeconomic status contribute equally or more to the population-attributable fraction for suicide deaths. For example, Australia and Switzerland had dramatic decreases in private firearm ownership in response to government policy changes, setting the stage for natural experiments on the population-attributable risk for suicide attributable to firearm ownership. Researchers found striking reductions in the suicide rate coinciding with the decrease in firearm ownership. In Switzerland, researchers estimated that only 22% of the prevented firearm suicides resulted in people committing suicide by another method, and in Australia, there was no evidence that people substituted other suicide methods (Chapman et al. 2006; Reisch et al. 2013). In another recent Australian study, Page et al. (2014) emphasized that poverty has an attributable risk fraction to suicide in young adults of 46% (males) and 58% (females), similar to the mental health population-attributable risk fraction of 48% (males) and 52% (females).

Evidence-Based Interventions

Two approaches to eliminating the morbidity and mortality of mental illness include (1) interventions to prevent the development of mental illness and (2) interventions to treat existing mental illness and promote recovery.

Prevention

Preventing the Development of Mental Illness

Interventions to prevent mental illness focus on decreasing or mitigating the effects of adverse childhood experiences, events shown to be associated with the later development of mental disorders. These early life interventions include enhancing social support, teaching parenting skills, improving early childhood education, and reducing—if not eliminating—school bullying. Poor social support, lack of good parenting, lack of quality early education, and child abuse all constitute risk factors for mental disorders. It is possible to enhance protective factors for children by promoting resilience, teaching social skills, and expanding a child's social network. The most successful primary prevention programs in mental health have a double focus—they work to reduce existing stressors and enhance the problem-solving competency of the children involved. As these children become more competent, they are better able to withstand or deal with those forces that would be likely to lead to deviancy, delinquency, or mental illness.

A meta-analysis of 177 primary prevention mental health programs for children and adolescents supported the general efficacy of these programs, demonstrating that they reduced problems, enhanced academic performance, increased general levels of competencies, and had a positive influence across multiple measures of functioning (Durlak and Wells 1998).

Interventions to Promote Recovery

In the 1990s, advocacy organizations such as National Alliance for Mental Illness began spearheading a recovery-oriented model to treatment of mental illness to promote the idea that people with mental illness can live full lives with meaning and purpose. This concept emerged much earlier in the treatment of people with physical disability, likely because people with mental illness face complex hurdles such as overcoming stigma and social problems associated with their disease such as unemployment (SAMHSA 2009).

For a mental health system to be recovery-oriented, many criteria must be met beyond providing good clinical care. The recovery-oriented model acknowledges the complex psychosocial determinants of mental health, recognizing that people with persistent psychiatric symptoms can still recover but have nonclinical needs that must be met. These needs may include peer support from others with a mental illness, social support through hobbies and activities, person-centered community supports such as childcare and transportation, and employment and educational opportunities. Moreover, recovery from mental illness requires a community with an integrated, multisector approach to mental health, where re-emergence of symptoms does not result in arrest, loss of employment, or housing instability (SAMHSA 2009).

Screening

In a summary report, the Center for Mental Health Services of the Substance Abuse and Mental Health Services Administration identified those programs in mental health and substance abuse prevention that hold the greatest promise in diminishing or preventing the development of a mental illness or a substance use disorder (Nitzkin and Smith 2004). The following programs are included:

- Universal screening of pregnant women for use of tobacco, alcohol, and illicit drugs.
- Home visitation for selected pregnant women, and some children up to age 5 years.
- Supplemental educational services for vulnerable infants from disadvantaged families.
- Screening children and adolescents for behavioral disorders.
- Screening adolescents for tobacco or alcohol use, depression, and anxiety.
- Screening adults for depression, anxiety, and use of tobacco or alcohol.
- Psychoeducation to increase early ambulation of surgical patients and enhance adherence to prescribed regimens of care for patients with chronic diseases.

The report then identifies the following three practices with the most potential for reducing overall health care costs:

- Screening pregnant women for use of tobacco, alcohol, and illicit drugs.
- Screening for depression in persons with major chronic medical disease.
- Psycho-education for persons scheduled for major surgical procedures, persons with major chronic diseases, and selected other heavy users of health care services.

The effect sizes for these preventive services in randomized controlled trials ranged from 5% to 30%. Nitzken and Smith (2004) explain that the identified interventions often reduce mental illness burden rather than completely prevent them and go on to assert, "The adverse consequences of the underlying disorders are such that the preventive services can be expected to pay for themselves in reduced health care costs and improved clinical and/or social outcomes."

More recently, the U.S. Preventive Services Task Force recommended depression screening for all adults by primary care providers with the resources to treat or refer these patients, citing sufficient evidence that this practice results in moderate benefits. Studies find improved outcomes in clinical morbidity for patients that screened positive for depression and were subsequently treated with psychotherapy or antidepressant therapy (Siu et al. 2016).

Treatment

As discussed, a major change that has occurred since the 1990s is an enhanced appreciation for the fact that many people with mental illness do recover and go on to function effectively in society. Moreover, recent studies show that mortality caused by mental illness can be reduced by mental health treatment. Harrison et al. (2001) analyzed projects by 69 investigators studying more than 1,000 individuals with schizophrenia from 14 countries around the world, with follow-up periods up to 25 years. The most important finding from this rigorous and well-designed investigation was that more than half of the participants were rated as recovered at the end of the 15- to 25-year follow-up period.

Despite the high likelihood of recovery with appropriate treatment, many people with mental illness do not get care relative to people with other chronic diseases. The President's New Freedom Commission (Mental Health Commission 2001) identified three obstacles that prevent Americans from getting good mental health care: stigma, unfair treatment limitations imposed by private health insurance companies, and a fragmented mental health service delivery system. In addition to calling for major reform of the U.S. health care system, this group underscored the importance of recovery and resilience, and the fact that recovery is possible.

The treatments that have been shown in controlled studies to be effective for mental illness and addictions vary across illness categories, and it is not possible to survey all treatments for all conditions within the confines of a chapter. However, the following general principles apply (Lehman et al. 2004):

- Medications effectively treat most mental illnesses. For severe mental illnesses, they are superior to psychosocial treatments alone.
- Combined treatments (medication plus psychosocial interventions) often produce the best results.

- Many psychotherapies are empirically supported, particularly cognitive–behavioral and interpersonal psychotherapies, and have equal efficacy vis-à-vis medication in mild-to-moderate cases of many conditions such as depression, anxiety, and PTSD.
- Other psychosocial treatments (e.g., family education, psychoeducation) and services (e.g., assertive community treatment [ACT] and supported employment for adults; multimodal treatment for children with conduct disorder) provide advantages for many conditions—particularly to promote rehabilitation and recovery in the most impaired individuals.

Examples of Evidence-Based Interventions

There are numerous examples of evidence-based interventions for both the prevention and treatment of mental illness, varying according to type of mental disorder and target population. We will focus on two areas—interventions for the prevention of depression and community psychiatry interventions for the treatment of serious mental illnesses. For more examples of evidence-based interventions, refer to SAMHSA's National Registry of Evidence Based Practices and Programs (http://nrepp.samhsa.gov) and the WHO summary report entitled "Prevention of Mental Disorders" (2004).

Interventions for Preventing Depression

Interventions for mental disorders, including depression, have three major approaches depending on the target population—universal, selective, and indicated interventions. In universal interventions, the program applies to an entire population, such as incorporating social–emotional skills training into an elementary school curriculum. Selective interventions, in contrast, target individuals at high risk, such as prenatal health and parenting education programs for low-income parents. Lastly, indicated interventions aim to reduce problem behavior and symptoms in children that are already displaying problems.

In a 2005 WHO summary report, the authors argue for community interventions that incorporate components of universal, selective, and indicated approaches to reduce the incidence of depression, citing literature reviews that find an overall 11% reduction in depressive symptoms post-intervention (Hosman et al. 2005). One promising approach is to improve parents' well-being and efficacy through therapy and education to improve the health of parents and transfer positive outcomes to the children of these individuals. A Cochrane review of indicated interventions for parents of young children with behavioral problems reported that behavioral and cognitive–behavioral group-based parenting interventions resulted in reduced child conduct problems and improved parental mental health and parenting skills. These interventions aim to help parents learn coping skills and cognitive reframing techniques that they can pass on to their children, as well parenting skills such as to use positive reinforcement to increase desired behavior in their children. The reviewers of these intervention studies concluded that the modest costs of such programs are worth the potential benefits in long-term health, social change, and academic outcomes (Furlong et al. 2013).

Intervention for Serious Mental Illness

The most powerful interventions for people living with serious mental illnesses such as schizophrenia and bipolar disorder succeed by taking a biopsychosocial approach with multidisciplinary teams, aiming to improve the lives of individuals beyond their psychiatric symptoms. Two widely used models with a true biopsychosocial approach are the Clubhouse Model and Assertive Community Treatment Model (Brown 2011).

The Clubhouse Model of Psychosocial Rehabilitation, forwarded by the International Center for Clubhouse Development in the 1970s, optimizes recovery in adults with mental disorders by engaging individuals as members of the Clubhouse. The Clubhouse includes day treatment facilities with access to education, psychiatric and general health care treatment, employment opportunities, social relationships, and housing. The members of the Clubhouse increase quality of life and gain a sense of purpose by participating in Clubhouse responsibilities such as clerical duties, reception, food service, and financial services. In this way, members become a critical part of the community and are granted access to outside jobs that often become permanent employment. The Clubhouse is staffed by multidisciplinary professionals with backgrounds in psychology, psychiatry, counseling, social work, and education. Membership is voluntary and the amount that members contribute varies depending on member choice; moreover, members that choose to end participation are granted the lifetime right of reentry. Studies of the Clubhouse model find that members have improved outcomes in the areas of employment, quality of life, and perceived recovery from a mental health problem

(Macias et al. 2006; Mowbray et al. 2009). For more information, visit the website of the world's first clubhouse, Fountain House of New York City (http://www.fountainhouse.org).

Assertive Community Treatment

Assertive Community Treatment (ACT) is another stellar example of a cost-effective treatment for persons with severe mental illness. Developed as a way to respond to the needs of the large numbers of mentally ill people released from state psychiatric hospitals in the 1970s as a result of deinstitutionalization, ACT is a team-based approach aimed at keeping clients connected with providers, reducing hospital admissions, and improving everyday functioning and quality of life. Assertive outreach, mobile treatment teams, and continuous treatment are essential components of ACT. Other important features include multidisciplinary staffing, integration of services, low client-to-staff ratios, home visits, a focus on ordinary problems in living, rapid access to needed services, and individualized treatment plans. This approach has been shown to be more effective than standard community care, hospital-based rehabilitation services, and typical case management. Multiple randomized clinical trials have documented that ACT, which targets the patients with the highest consumption of mental health services, reduces the costs associated with hospital care at the same time that it produces high levels of patient satisfaction (Burns et al. 2007).

Areas of Future Research

The needs of people with severe mental illness clearly exceed the capacity of the current mental health community to treat these needs. The Annapolis Coalition on the Behavioral Health Workforce has noted:

> Across the nation there is a high degree of concern about the state of the behavioral health workforce and pessimism about its future.... Most critically, there are significant concerns about the capability of the workforce to provide quality care. The majority of the workforce is uninformed about and unengaged in health promotion and prevention activities.... There is overwhelming evidence that the behavioral health workforce is not equipped in skills or in numbers to respond adequately to the changing needs of the American population (Annapolis Coalition 2007).

As discussed, behavioral health integration within primary care is gaining recognition as an approach to this workforce dilemma. This collaborative care approach has been shown to be cost-effective in the treatment of depression, and it results in greater adherence to treatment goals and patient satisfaction (Hunkeler et al. 2000; Katon et al. 1995; Katon et al. 1996). Moreover, this approach to chronic disease management has been shown to be both efficient and effective, holding great promise in addressing the mental health needs of the nation (Manderscheid and Kathol 2014).

Other future areas of research include public health approaches to caring for people with serious mental illness at risk for incarceration or housing instability and interventions to optimize reentry and recovery for persons with mental illness leaving prison (Slate et al. 2013). These developing areas of research include mental health courts and court-ordered outpatient treatment.

The National Institute for Mental Health released a strategic plan, outlined in Table 18-2, for future research that recognizes the importance of addressing

Table 18-2. National Institute of Mental Health (NIMH) Strategic Plan 2015

Strategic Objective 1: Define the mechanisms of complex behaviors.

1.1 Describe the molecules, cells, and neural circuits associated with complex behaviors.
1.2 Identify the genomic and non-genomic factors associated with mental illnesses.
1.3 Map the connectomes for mental illnesses.

Strategic Objective 2: Chart mental illness trajectories to determine when, where, and how to intervene.

2.1 Characterize the developmental trajectories of brain maturation and dimensions of behavior to understand the roots of mental illnesses across diverse populations.
2.2 Identify clinically useful biomarkers and behavioral indicators that predict change across the trajectory of illness.

Strategic Objective 3: Strive for prevention and cures.

3.1 Develop new treatments based on discoveries in genomics, neuroscience, and behavioral science.
3.2 Develop ways to tailor existing and new interventions to optimize outcomes.
3.3 Test interventions for effectiveness in community practice settings.

Strategic Objective 4: Strengthen the public health impact of NIMH-supported research.

4.1 Improve the efficiency and effectiveness of existing mental health services through research.
4.2 Establish research–practice partnerships to improve dissemination, implementation, and continuous improvement of evidence-based mental health service.
4.3 Develop innovative service delivery models to improve dramatically the outcomes of mental health services received in diverse communities and populations.
4.4 Develop new capacity for research that evaluates the public health impact of mental health services innovations.

Source: Adapted from NIMH (2015).

urgent mental health care needs at the same time as pursuing long-term basic science objectives. The National Institute for Mental Health also recognizes that advances in neuroscience and genomics should be considered within the context of environmental exposures and social factors known to influence mental health (USDHHS 2015).

Our understanding of mental disorders and their associations with increased morbidity and mortality has definitely advanced in recent years. Future research must focus on reducing the risk of early death for those with mental disorders by altering the mediators between mental illness and death, as well as through the provision of mental health services. Just as we have a national monitoring system for cancer, there is a need for a parallel system tracking early death relating to mental illness or substance use conditions. Specific mental disorders and the contributing factors to early death from these disorders must be assessed so we can track year-to-year progress in reducing the disparity in length of life.

Resources

National Alliance on Mental Illness, http://www.nami.org

National Institute of Mental Health: psychiatric epidemiology, http://www.nimh.nih.gov/about/director/bio/publications/psychiatric-epidemiology.shtml

Substance Abuse and Mental Health Services Administration, http://www.samhsa.gov

Substance Abuse and Mental Health Services Administration's National Registry of Evidence-Based Practices and Programs, http://nrepp.samhsa.gov

Surgeon General's Report on Mental Health (1999), http://www.surgeongeneral.gov/library/mentalhealth/home.html

Surgeon General's Report on Suicide Prevention (2012), http://www.surgeongeneral.gov/library/reports/national-strategy-suicide-prevention/index.html

Suggested Reading

Slate RN, Buffington-Vollum JK, Johnson WW. *The Criminalization of Mental Illness: Crisis and Opportunity for the Justice System: Second Edition*. Durham, NC: Carolina Academic Press; 2013.

Susser E, Schwartz S, Morabia A, Bromet EJ. *Psychiatric Epidemiology: Searching for the Causes of Mental Disorders*. New York, NY: Oxford University Press; 2006.

Vigo D, Thornicroft G, Atun R. Estimating the true global burden of mental illness. *Lancet Psychiatry.* 2016;3(2):171–178.

Wedding D, DeLeon PH, Olson P. Mental health care in the United States. In: Olson P, ed. *Mental Health Systems Compared.* Springfield, IL: Charles C. Thomas; 2006.

References

Aleman A, Kahn RS, Selten J-P. Sex differences in the risk of schizophrenia: evidence from meta-analysis. *Arch Gen Psychiatry.* 2003;60(6):565–571.

Almog M, Curtis S, Copeland A, Congdon P. Geographical variation in acute psychiatric admissions within New York City 1990–2000: growing inequalities in service use? *Soc Sci Med.* 2004:59(2):361–376.

American Psychiatric Association (APA). *Coexisting Severe Mental Disorders and Physical Illness.* Washington, DC: APA; 2003.

American Psychiatric Association (APA). *Diagnostic and Statistical Manual of Mental Disorders.* 5th ed. Washington, DC: APA; 2013.

Annapolis Coalition. *An Action Plan for Behavioral Health Workforce Development: A Framework for Discussion.* Rockville, MD: US Department of Health and Human Services: 2007. SAMHSA/DHHS Publication 280-02-0302.

Bach H, Arango V. Neuroanatomy of serotonergic abnormalities in suicide. In: Dwivedi Y, ed. *The Neurobiological Basis of Suicide.* Boca Raton, FL: CRC Press/Taylor and Francis; 2012.

Bassuk EL, Gerson S. Deinstitutionalization and mental health services. *Sci Am.* 1978;238(2):46–53.

Baxter AJ, Harris MG, Khatib Y, Brugha TS, Bien H, Bhui K. Reducing excess mortality due to chronic disease in people with severe mental illness: meta-review of health interventions. *Br J Psychiatry.* 2016;208(4):322–329.

Beardslee WR, Brent DA, Weersing VR, et al. Prevention of depression in at-risk adolescents: longer-term effects. *JAMA Psychiatry.* 2013;70(11):1161–1170.

Beronio K, Po R, Skopec L, Glied S. Affordable Care Act expands mental health and substance use disorder benefits and federal parity protections for 62 million Americans. 2013. Available at: https://aspe.hhs.gov/report/affordable-care-act-expands-mental-health-and-substance-use-disorder-benefits-and-federal-parity-protections-62-million-americans. Accessed August 29, 2016.

Beyer JL, Taylor L, Gersing KR, Ranga K, Krishnan R. Prevalence of HIV infection in a general psychiatric outpatient population. *Psychosomatics.* 2007:48(1):31–37.

Botellero VL, Skranes J, Bjuland KJ, et al. Mental health and cerebellar volume during adolescence in very-low-birth-weight infants: a longitudinal study. *Child Adolesc Psychiatry Mental Health.* 2016;10:6.

Breslau J, Kendler KS, Su M, Gaxiola-Aguilar S, Kessler RC. Lifetime risk and persistence of psychiatric disorders across ethnic groups in the United States. *Psychol Med.* 2005;35(3):317–327.

Breslau J, Miller E, Jin R, et al. A multinational study of mental disorders, marriage, and divorce. *Acta Psychiatr Scand.* 2011;124(6):474–486.

Breslau N, Wilcox HC, Storr CL, Lucia VC, Anthony JC. Trauma exposure and post-traumatic stress disorder: a study of youths in urban America. *J Urban Health.* 2004;81(4):530–544.

Bresnahan M, Boydell J, Murray R, Susser E. Temporal variation in the oncidence, course and outcome of schizophrenia. In: Murray RM, Jones PB, Susser E, van Os J, Cannon M, eds. *The Epidemiology of Schizophrenia.* Cambridge, UK: Cambridge University Press; 2003.

Brown LD. *Consumer-Run Mental Health: Framework for Recovery.* New York, NY: Springer Science & Business Media; 2011.

Burns T, Catty J, Dash M, Roberts C, Lockwood A, Marshall M. Use of intensive case management to reduce time in hospital in people with severe mental illness: systematic review and meta-regression. *BMJ.* 2007;335(7615):336.

Caffrey MK. Integrated treatment for diabetes, depression gains notice, with help from ACA. *Am J Manag Care.* 2014;20(10 spec no):E1.

Cardno AG, Gottesman II. Twin studies of schizophrenia: from bow-and-arrow concordances to Star Wars Mx and functional genomics. *Am J Med Genet.* 2000;97(1):12–17.

Castle DJ, Wessely S, Murray RM. Sex and schizophrenia: effects of diagnostic stringency, and associations with and premorbid variables. *Br J Psychiatry.* 1993;162:658–664.

Cavanagh JT, Carson AJ, Sharpe M, Lawrie SM. Psychological autopsy studies of suicide: a systematic review. *Psychol Med.* 2003;33(3):395–405.

Centers for Disease Control and Prevention (CDC). Web-based Injury Statistics Query and Reporting System (WISQARS). 2013. Available at: https://www.cdc.gov/injury/wisqars. Accessed August 29, 2016.

Chapman S, Alpers P, Agho K, Jones M. Australia's 1996 gun law reforms: faster falls in firearm deaths, firearm suicides, and a decade without mass shootings. *Inj Prev.* 2006;12(6):365–372.

Dannefer D. Cumulative advantage/disadvantage and the life course: cross-fertilizing age and social science theory. *J Gerontol B Psychol Sci Soc Sci.* 2003;58(6):S327–S337.

Diaz Vickery K, Guzman-Corrales L, Owen R, et al. Medicaid expansion and mental health: a Minnesota case study. *Fam Syst Health.* 2016;34(1):58–63.

Drapeau CW, McIntosh JL. USA suicide 2013: official final data. Washington, DC: American Association of Suicidology; 2015.

Durham ML. The impact of deinstitutionalization on the current treatment of the mentally ill. *Int J Law Psychiatry.* 1989;12(2):117–131.

Durlak J, Wells A. Evaluation of indicated preventive interventions (secondary prevention) mental health programs for children and adolescents. *Am J Community Psychol.* 1998;26(5):775–802.

Eisenberg ME, Resnick MD. Suicidality among gay, lesbian and bisexual youth: the role of protective factors. *J Adolesc Health.* 2006;39(5):662–668.

Engel GL. The need for a new medical model: a challenge for biomedicine. *Science.* 1977;196(4286):129–136.

Falk DE, Yi H-Y, Hilton ME. Age of onset and temporal sequencing of lifetime DSM-IV alcohol use disorders relative to comorbid mood and anxiety disorders. *Drug Alcohol Depend.* 2008;94(1–3):234–245.

Funaki T. Nash: genius with schizophrenia or vice versa? *Pac Health Dialog.* 2009;15(2): 129–137.

Furlong M, McGilloway S, Bywater T, Hutchings J, Smith SM, Donnelly M. Cochrane review: Behavioural and cognitive–behavioural group-based parenting programmes for early-onset conduct problems in children aged 3 to 12 years (Review). *Evid Based Child Health.* 2013;8(2):318–692.

Galea S, Ahern J, Nandi A, Tracy M, Beard J, Vlahov D. Urban neighborhood poverty and the incidence of depression in a population-based cohort study. *Ann Epidemiol.* 2007;17(3):171–179.

Han B, Gfroerer J, Kuramoto SJ, Ali M, Woodward AM, Teich J. Medicaid expansion under the Affordable Care Act: potential changes in receipt of mental health treatment among low-income nonelderly adults with serious mental illness. *Am J Public Health.* 2015;105(10):1982–1989.

Harrison G, Hopper K, Craig T, et al. Recovery from psychotic illness: a 15- and 25-year international follow-up study. *Br J Psychiatry.* 2001;178:506–517.

Hasler G. Pathophysiology of depression: do we have any solid evidence of interest to clinicians? *World Psychiatry.* 2010;9(3):155–161.

Hill SC, Miller GE, Sing M. Adults with diagnosed and untreated diabetes: who are they? How can we reach them? *J Health Care Poor Underserved.* 2011;22(4):1221–1238.

Horwath E, Cohen RS, Weissman MM. Epidemiology of depressive and anxiety disorders. In: Tsuang MT, Tohen M, eds. *Textbook in Psychiatric Epidemiology.* 2nd ed. Hoboken, NJ: John Wiley and Sons Inc; 2002.

Hosman C, Jane-Llopis E, Saxena S, eds. *Prevention of Mental Disorders: Effective Interventions and Policy Options.* Oxford, UK: Oxford University Press; 2005.

Howlett JR, Stein MB. Post-traumatic stress disorder: relationship to traumatic brain injury and approach to treatment. In: Laskowitz D, Grant G, eds. *Translational Research in Traumatic Brain Injury.* Boca Raton, FL: CRC Press/Taylor and Francis Group; 2016.

Hunkeler EM, Meresman JF, Hargreaves WA, et al. Efficacy of nurse telehealth care and peer support in augmenting treatment of depression in primary care. *Arch Fam Med.* 2000:9(8):700–708.

Jané-Llopis E, Barry M, Hosman C, Patel V. Mental health promotion works: a review. *Promot Educ.* 2005;12(suppl 2):9–25,61,67.

Jang KL, Taylor S, Stein MB, Yamagata S. Trauma exposure and stress response: exploration of mechanisms of cause and effect. *Twin Res Hum Genet.* 2007;10(4):564–572.

Katon W, Robinson P, Von Korff M, et al. A multifaceted intervention to improve treatment of depression in primary care. *Arch Gen Psychiatry.* 1996:53(10):924–932.

Katon W, Von Korff M, Lin E, et al. Collaborative management to achieve treatment guidelines: impact on depression in primary care. *JAMA.* 1995:273(13):1026–1031.

Kersten-Alvarez LE, Hosman CMH, Riksen-Walraven JM, van Doesum KTM, Smeekens S, Hoefnagels C. Early school outcomes for children of postpartum depressed mothers: comparison with a community sample. *Child Psychiatry Hum Dev.* 2012;43(2): 201–218.

Kessler RC, Aguilar-Gaxiola S, Alonso J, et al. The global burden of mental disorders: an update from the WHO World Mental Health (WMH) surveys. *Epidemiol Psichiatr Soc.* 2009;18(1):23–33.

Kessler RC, Berglund P, Demler O, Jin R, Merikangas KR, Walters EE. Lifetime prevalence and age-of-onset distributions of DSM-IV disorders in the national comorbidity survey replication. *Arch Gen Psychiatry.* 2005;62(6):593–602.

Kessler RC, McGonagle KA, Zhao S, et al. Lifetime and 12-month prevalence of DSM-III-R psychiatric disorders in the United States. Results from the National Comorbidity Survey. *Arch Gen Psychiatry.* 1994;51(1):8–19.

Kessler RC, Petukhova M, Sampson NA, Zaslavsky AM, Wittchen H-U. Twelve-month and lifetime prevalence and lifetime morbid risk of anxiety and mood disorders in the United States. *Int J Methods Psychiatr Res.* 2012;21(3):169–184.

Kessler RC, Sonnega A, Bromet E, Hughes M, Nelson CB. Posttraumatic stress disorder in the National Comorbidity Survey. *Arch Gen Psychiatry.* 1995;52(12):1048–1060.

Khan A, McCormack HC, Bolger EA, et al. Childhood maltreatment, depression, and suicidal ideation: critical importance of parental and peer emotional abuse during developmental sensitive periods in males and females. *Front Psychiatry.* 2015; 6:42.

Larsen KK. Depression following myocardial infarction—an overseen complication with prognostic importance. *Dan Med J.* 2013;60(8):B4689.

Lehman AF, Goldman HH, Dixon LB, Print RC. *Evidence-Based Mental Health Treatments and Services: Examples to Inform Public Policy.* New York, NY: Milbank Memorial Fund; 2004.

Lenze EJ, Wetherell JL. A lifespan view of anxiety disorders. *Dialogues Clin Neurosci.* 2011;13(4):381–399.

Leonard B. Stress, depression and the activation of the immune system. *World J Biol Psychiatry.* 2000;1(1):17–25.

Li Z, Page A, Martin G, Taylor R. Attributable risk of psychiatric and socio-economic factors for suicide from individual-level, population-based studies: a systematic review. *Soc Sci Med.* 2011;72(4):608–616.

Macias C, Rodican CF, Hargreaves WA, Jones DR, Barreira PJ, Wang Q. Supported employment outcomes of a randomized controlled trial of ACT and Clubhouse models. *Psychiatr Serv.* 2006;57(10):1406–1415.

Manderscheid R, Kathol R. Fostering sustainable, integrated medical and behavioral health services in medical settings. *Ann Intern Med.* 2014;160(1):61–65.

McGrath J, Saha S, Welham J, El Saadi O, MacCauley C, Chant D. A systematic review of the incidence of schizophrenia: the distribution of rates and the influence of sex, urbanicity, migrant status and methodology. *BMC Medicine.* 2004;2:13.

Mental Health Commission. *President's New Freedom Commission on Mental Health* (2001). Available at: http://govinfo.library.unt.edu/mentalhealthcommission/reports/FinalReport/toc.html. Accessed September 1, 2016.

Metzl JM, MacLeish KT. Mental illness, mass shootings, and the politics of American firearms. *Am J Public Health*. 2015;105(2):240–249.

Miller M, Azrael D, Barber C. Suicide mortality in the United States: the importance of attending to method in understanding population-level disparities in the burden of suicide. *Annu Rev Public Health*. 2012;33(1):393–408.

Mojtabai R, Stuart EA, Hwang I, Eaton WW, Sampson N, Kessler RC. Long-term effects of mental disorders on educational attainment in the National Comorbidity Survey ten-year follow-up. *Soc Psychiatry Psychiatr Epidemiol*. 2015a;50(10): 1577–1591.

Mojtabai R, Stuart EA, Hwang I, et al. Long-term effects of mental disorders on employment in the National Comorbidity Survey ten-year follow-up. *Soc Psychiatry Psychiatr Epidemiol*. 2015b;50(11):1657–1668.

Mokdad AH, Marks JS, Stroup DF, Gerberding JL. Actual causes of death in the United States, 2000. *JAMA*. 2004;291(10):1238–1245.

Mościcki EK. Epidemiology of suicide. *Int Psychogeriatr*. 1995;7(2):137–148.

Mowbray CT, Woodward AT, Holter MC, MacFarlane P, Bybee D. Characteristics of users of consumer-run drop-in centers versus clubhouses. *J Behav Health Serv Res*. 2009;36(3):361–371.

Murphy JM, Horton NJ, Monson RR, Laird NM, Sobol AM, Leighton AH. Cigarette smoking in relation to depression: historical trends from the Stirling County study. *Am J Psychiatry*. 2003;160(9):1663–1669.

National Alliance to End Homelessness. About homelessness: cost of homelessness. 2016. Available at: http://www.endhomelessness.org/pages/cost_of_homelessness. Accessed May 19, 2016.

National Institute of Mental Health (NIMH). The National Institute of Mental Health Strategic Plan. 2015. Available at: http://www.nimh.nih.gov/about/strategic-planning-reports/index.shtml. Accessed September 12, 2016.

Newcomer JW, Haupt DW. *Schizophrenia, Metabolic Disturbance, and Cardiovascular Risk. Medical and Psychiatric Comorbidity Over the Course of Life*. Arlington, VA: American Psychiatric Publishing; 2006:331–349.

Nitzkin J, Smith SA. *Clinical Preventive Services in Substance Abuse and Mental Health Update: From Science to Services*. Rockville, MD: Center for Mental Health Services, Substance Abuse and Mental Health Services Administration; 2004.

Ochoa S, Usall J, Cobo J, Labad X, Kulkarni J. Gender differences in schizophrenia and first-episode psychosis: a comprehensive literature review, gender differences in schizophrenia and first-episode psychosis: a comprehensive literature review. *Schizophr Res Treatment*. 2012;2012:e916198.

Owen MJ, Sawa A, Mortensen PB. Schizophrenia. *Lancet*. 2016;388(10039):86–97.

Pabayo R, Kawachi I, Gilman SE. Income inequality among American states and the incidence of major depression. *J Epidemiol Community Health*. 2014;68(2):110–115.

Page A, Morrell S, Hobbs C, et al. Suicide in young adults: psychiatric and socioeconomic factors from a case–control study. *BMC Psychiatry*. 2014;14:68.

Parto JA, Evans MK, Zonderman AB. Symptoms of posttraumatic stress disorder among urban residents. *J Nerv Ment Dis*. 2011;199(7):436–439.

Pow JL, Baumeister AA, Hawkins MF, Cohen AS, Garand JC. Deinstitutionalization of American public hospitals for the mentally ill before and after the introduction of antipsychotic medications. *Harv Rev Psychiatry*. 2015;23(3):176–187.

Pratt LA. Characteristics of adults with serious mental illness in the United States household population in 2007. *Psychiatr Serv*. 2012;63(10):1042–1046.

Pratt LA, Druss BG, Manderscheid RW, Walker ER. Excess mortality due to depression and anxiety in the United States: results from a nationally representative survey. *Gen Hosp Psychiatry*. 2016;39:39–45.

Prince M, Patel V, Saxena S, et al. No health without mental health. *Lancet*. 2007; 370(9590):859–877.

Reisch T, Steffen T, Habenstein A, Tschacher W. Change in suicide rates in Switzerland before and after firearm restriction resulting from the 2003 "Army XXI" reform. *Am J Psychiatry*. 2013;170(9):977–984.

Robins LN, Regier DA, eds. *Psychiatric Disorders in America: The Epidemiologic Catchment Area Study*. New York, NY: The Free Press; 2001.

Russell ST, Joyner K. Adolescent sexual orientation and suicide risk: evidence from a national study. *Am J Public Health*. 2001;91(8):1276–1281.

Sachs-Ericsson N, Joiner TE, Cougle JR, Stanley IH, Sheffler JL. Combat exposure in early adulthood interacts with recent stressors to predict PTSD in aging male veterans. *Gerontologist*. 2016;56(1):82–91.

Saha S, Chant D, Welham J, McGrath J. A systematic review of the prevalence of schizophrenia. *PLoS Med*. 2005;2(5):e141.

Sartorius N. Physical illness in people with mental disorders. *World Psychiatry*. 2007:6(1):3–4.

Sayers J. The world health report 2001 — Mental health: new understanding, new hope. *Bulletin of the World Health Organization.* 2001;79(11):1085.

Shoshani A, Slone M. The resilience function of character strengths in the face of war and protracted conflict. *Front Psychol.* 2015;6:2006.

Siefert K, Bowman PJ, Heflin CM, Danziger S, Williams DR. Social and environmental predictors of maternal depression in current and recent welfare recipients. *Am J Orthopsychiatry.* 2000;70(4):510–522.

Siu AL, US Preventive Services Task Force, Bibbins-Domingo K, et al. Screening for depression in adults: US Preventive Services Task Force recommendation statement. *JAMA.* 2016;315(4):380–387.

Slate RN, Buffington-Vollum JK, Johnson WW. *The Criminalization of Mental Illness: Crisis and Opportunity for the Justice System.* 2nd ed. Durham, NC: Carolina Academic Press; 2013.

Smith JR, Patton DU. Posttraumatic stress symptoms in context: examining trauma responses to violent exposures and homicide death among Black males in urban neighborhoods. *Am J Orthopsychiatry.* 2016;86(2):212–223.

Snoek FJ, Bremmer MA, Hermanns N. Constructs of depression and distress in diabetes: time for an appraisal. *Lancet Diabetes Endocrinol.* 2015;3(6):450–460.

Solantaus T, Salo S. Paternal postnatal depression: fathers emerge from the wings. *Lancet.* 2005;365(9478):2158–2159.

Stein MB, Jang KL, Taylor S, Vernon PA, Livesley WJ. Genetic and environmental influences on trauma exposure and posttraumatic stress disorder symptoms: a twin study. *Am J Psychiatry.* 2002;159(10):1675–1681.

Streb M, Häller P, Michael T. PTSD in paramedics: resilience and sense of coherence. *Behav Cogn Psychother.* 2014;42(4):452–463.

Substance Abuse and Mental Health Services Administration (SAMHSA). Guiding principles and elements of recovery-oriented systems of care. 2009. Available at: http://store.samhsa.gov/product/Guiding-Principles-and-Elements-of-Recovery-Oriented-Systems-of-Care/SMA09-4439. Accessed April 6, 2016.

Substance Abuse and Mental Health Services Administration (SAMHSA). Results from the 2012 National Survey on Drug Use and Health: mental health findings. Rockville, MD: SAMHSA; 2013. NSDUH Series H-47, HHS Publication no. (SMA) 13-4805.

Swanson JW. Mental disorder, substance abuse, and community violence: an epidemiological approach. In: Monahan J, Steadman H, eds. *Violence and Mental Disorder.* Chicago, IL: University of Chicago Press; 1994:101–136.

Swanson JW, McGinty EE, Fazel S, Mays VM. Mental illness and reduction of gun violence and suicide: bringing epidemiologic research to policy. *Ann Epidemiol.* 2015; 25(5):366–376.

Swartz MS, Swanson JW, Hannon MJ, et al. Five-Site Health and Risk Study Research Committee. Regular sources of medical care among persons with severe mental illness at risk of hepatitis C infection. *Psychiatr Serv.* 2003:54(6):854–859.

Szivak TK, Kraemer WJ. Physiological readiness and resilience: pillars of military preparedness. *J Strength Cond Res.* 2015;29(suppl 11):S34–S39.

Tohen M, Angst J. Epidemiology of bipolar disorder. In: Tsuang M, Tohen M, eds. *Textbook in Psychiatric Epidemiology.* 2nd ed. New York, NY: John Wiley and Sons; 2002.

US Department of Health and Human Services (USDHHS), National Institutes of Health, National Institute of Mental Health. NIMH Strategic Plan for Research. 2015. NIH Publication no. 02 2650. Available at: http://www.nimh.nih.gov/about/strategic-planning-reports/index.shtml. AccessedAugust 29, 2016.

Ustun TB. The global burden of mental disorders. *Am J Public Health.* 1999;89(9):1315–1318.

Van Dorn R, Volavka J, Johnson N. Mental disorder and violence: is there a relationship beyond substance use? *Soc Psychiatry Psychiatr Epidemiol.* 2012;47(3):487–503.

Vigo D, Thornicroft G, Atun R. Estimating the true global burden of mental illness. *Lancet Psychiatry.* 2016;3(2):171–178.

Vijayakumar L, Kumar MS, Vijayakumar V. Substance use and suicide. *Curr Opin Psychiatry.* 2011;24(3):197–202.

Wang PS, Aguilar-Gaxiola S, Alonso J, et al. Use of mental health services for anxiety, mood, and substance disorders in 17 countries in the WHO World Mental Health surveys. *Lancet.* 2007;370(9590):841–850.

Warner R. Time trends in schizophrenia: changes in obstetric risk factors with industrialization. *Schizophr Bull.* 1995;21(3):483–500.

Watanabe-Galloway S, Zhang W. Analysis of U.S. trends in discharges from general hospitals for episodes of serious mental illness, 1995–2002. *Psychiatr Serv.* 2007:58(4):496–502.

Weersing VR, Shamseddeen W, Garber J, et al. Prevention of depression in at-risk adolescents: predictors and moderators of acute effects. *J Am Acad Child Adolesc Psychiatry.* 2016;55(3):219–226.

Whiteford HA, Ferrari AJ, Degenhardt L, Feigin V, Vos T. The global burden of mental, neurological and substance use disorders: an analysis from the Global Burden of Disease study 2010. *PLoS One.* 2015;10(2):e0116820.

World Health Organization (WHO). *International Statistical Classification of Diseases and Related Health Problems, 10th Revision (ICD-10).* Geneva, Switzerland: WHO; 1992.

World Health Organization (WHO). *Prevention of Mental Disorders.* Geneva, Switzerland: WHO; 2004.

Yoshikawa H, Aber JL, Beardslee WR. The effects of poverty on the mental, emotional, and behavioral health of children and youth: implications for prevention. *Am Psychol.* 2012;67(4):272–284.

19

NEUROLOGICAL DISORDERS

Edwin Trevathan, MD, MPH

Introduction

Both high-income countries and low- and medium-income countries experience a major health burden from chronic neurological conditions, which are a leading cause of lost productivity, disability, and premature death (Whiteford et al. 2015). Complex neurological conditions are better understood than ever before, and classifications of neurological diseases are being changed—great news, but offering both opportunities and challenges for public health professionals.

Societies of high-income countries in the 21st century generally understand the brain as the organ that determines the manifestations of communication, cognition, behavior, socialization, intelligence, and even personality, while in many low-income countries the general population is just beginning to recognize neurological disease as distinct from spiritual matters. As a result, public health officials have growing demands to address neurological disorders in the growing elderly population and neurodevelopmental disorders among children. This chapter examines some of the more common neurological disorders from a public health perspective.

Unfortunately, among the most common neurological disorders, such as Alzheimer's disease, Parkinson's disease, multiple sclerosis (MS), and the epilepsies, primary prevention efforts are either not possible or very limited because we have not identified sufficient modifiable risk factors. Unintentional injuries resulting in traumatic brain injury (TBI) and spinal cord injury (SCI) offer significant opportunities for prevention. Likewise, the morbidity and loss of productivity caused by low back pain and carpal tunnel syndrome (CTS) offer prevention opportunities yet to be fulfilled. Thus, the need for public health–focused, genetic epidemiological research to identify modifiable risk factors for Alzheimer's disease, Parkinson's disease, MS, and epilepsy should be emphasized, while opportunities for prevention of injuries and health promotion among people with disabilities should be a public health priority (see Table 19-1).

Table 19-1. Neurological Diseases: Causes, Consequences, and High-Risk Groups

Disease	Causes	Consequences	High-Risk Groups
Epilepsy	Genetic factors	Increased risk of premature death	Family history
	Environmental exposures (often undefined)	Increased risk of falls, burns, or drowning	Central nervous system infections
	Cerebral malformations		Cerebral malaria survivors
	Trauma		Head injury
	Encephalitis or meningitis		Children with developmental delay
	Brain tumors or metastatic disease		Elderly with stroke
	Hypoxic injury		
	Strokes, vascular disease		
Parkinson's disease	Genetic factors	Motor impairment	Family history
	Environmental triggers	Cognitive decline	Men
	Viral infection	Depression	Whites
	Exposure to neurotoxins in the environment	Increased long-term care needs	Certain occupations (e.g., teachers, health care workers, firefighters, farmers, welders)
	Occupational exposures to heavy metals	Premature death	
Alzheimer's disease and other dementias	Genetic factors	Premature death	Family history
	Long-term survival of chronic disease	Cognitive decline	Elderly
	Traumatic brain injury	Increased long-term care needs	
	Multi-infarct strokes	Depression	
	Diabetes, hypertension		
Cerebral palsy	Prematurity	Feeding difficulties	Premature births
	Very low birthweight	Motor disability	Twins and multiple births
	High birthweight	Social isolation	Family history

(Continued)

Table 19-1. (Continued)

Disease	Causes	Consequences	High-Risk Groups
	Hypoxic–ischemic encephalopathy		Neonatal hyperbilirubinemia
	Multiple births		
Autism spectrum disorders	Genetic factors	Social isolation	Family history
	Potential environmental exposures	Anxiety	Males
		Impaired communication	Premature births
			Advanced parental age
ALS	Genetic factors	Progressive weakness	Family history
	Exposures to lead, mercury, and other heavy metals	Paralysis	Men
		Respiratory impairment	Older adults
		Premature death	
MS	Genetic factors	Intermittent motor, language, and/or cognitive impairment	Family history
	Viral or other infectious diseases	Long-term care needs	Females
		Depression	Young adults
		Premature death	
Guillain-Barré syndrome	Genetic factors	Temporary weakness and paralysis	Family history
	Autoimmune response triggered by a recent viral or bacterial infection	Respiratory failure	Whites
		Pneumonia	Living in northern latitudes
		Deep vein thrombosis	
Tic disorders and Tourette syndrome	Genetic factors	School failure—increased risk	Family history

(Continued)

Table 19-1. (Continued)

Disease	Causes	Consequences	High-Risk Groups
	Potential environmental exposures	Social isolation	Males
		Behavior problems	
Traumatic brain injury and spinal cord injury	Falls	Paralysis and death	Alcohol and drug abusers
	Transportation-related injuries and automobile crashes	Cognitive deficits[a]	Elderly
	Sports or recreation injuries	Epilepsy[a]	Children and adolescents
	Assaults	Dementia[a]	Men
	Alcohol and drug use	Depression	Lower social/economic persons
		Complications of immobility	Construction, farming, roofing, and logging occupations
		Deep vein thrombosis	Motorcyclists
			Those who fail to wear seat belts
ADHD	Genetic factors	Poor self-esteem	Males
	Potential environmental exposures, injuries	Anxiety	
		Conduct disorder	
		Depression	
		Sleep problems	
		Substance abuse	
Carpal tunnel syndrome	Repetitive hand or wrist movements	Impaired hand use	Workers who engage in repetitive fine-motor movements (e.g., typists)
		Lost income and job loss	Food-processing workers, roofers, carpenters, and mill workers
	Wrist trauma		Pregnant women
	Diabetes, hypothyroidism		

(Continued)

Table 19-1. (Continued)

Disease	Causes	Consequences	High-Risk Groups
	Pregnancy		
Low back pain	Heavy lifting	Disability	Occupations with heavy lifting (e.g., nursing, truck driving, warehouse, farming, lumber, construction work, mining)
	Abdominal obesity	Lost income	Caregivers of disabled
	Cigarette smoking	Time away from work	
	Premature menopause		
	Genetic factors		
Migraine and tension headaches	Genetic factors	School absence	Family history of headache
	Depression	Lost income	Women
	Stress	Time away from work	Low social and economic class
	Environmental triggers (e.g., food)	Depression	

Source: Adapted from Trevathan (2010).

Note: ADHD=attention-deficit/hyperactivity disorder; ALS=amyotrophic lateral sclerosis; MS=multiple sclerosis.

ªComplications of brain injury only.

EPILEPSY

Epilepsy is a category of diseases of the brain defined by any of the following three conditions: (1) at least two unprovoked (or reflex) seizures occurring more than 24 hours apart, (2) one unprovoked (or reflex) seizure and a high probability ($\geq 60\%$) of recurrent seizures, or (3) diagnosis of an epilepsy syndrome (Fisher et al. 2014). Epilepsy is the underlying condition that predisposes the individual to having repeated seizures, and is the most common serious neurological disorder among children worldwide (Kale 1997; WHO 2003). There are many people in low-income countries and poor neighborhoods of developed countries with epilepsy without adequate access to care (Meyer et al. 2010).

Significance

There are many types of epilepsy, each with different clinical manifestations, causes, possible outcomes, and comorbid conditions, and so the term "the epilepsies" is now being used to describe this heterogeneous group of brain disorders (England et al. 2012). For example, benign rolandic epilepsy tends to undergo spontaneous remission in almost all children who have this disorder, but it may also be associated with specific learning disorders (Panayiotopoulos et al. 2008). On the other end of the severity spectrum, Lennox-Gastaut syndrome is a profoundly severe epilepsy syndrome with affected children typically suffering multiple daily seizures that do not respond to treatment, and with almost universal intellectual disability and an increased risk of premature death (Shields 2004; Autry et al. 2010). The needs of people with severe epilepsy syndromes who have high risk of severe disability and premature death are great (Figure 19-1).

People with epilepsy frequently have comorbid conditions that interact with their epilepsy and make treatment of their epilepsy more complex, and

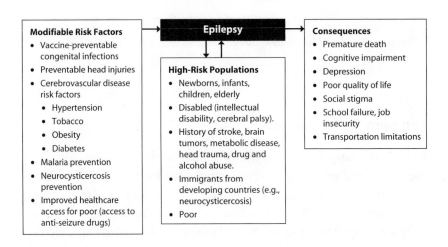

Note: For further information about high-risk populations for epilepsy, see England et al. (2012).

Figure 19-1. Epilepsy: Causes, Consequences, and High-Risk Groups

increase their risk of early disability and death. Although the mechanisms of the association between epilepsy and comorbid conditions is often unclear, studies have consistently demonstrated that people with epilepsy are up to eight times more likely to have comorbid conditions such as depression, anxiety, dementia, migraine, heart disease, arthritis, and obesity than the general population (Keezer et al. 2016).

Epilepsy with continued seizures in spite of treatment with antiseizure medication is associated with significant reductions in quality of life, associated with inability to drive an automobile, limitations at school and in the workplace, and stigma or discrimination in society. Improved quality of life among people with epilepsy is associated with cessation of seizures (Birbeck et al. 2002). Among people with seizures that cannot be stopped with medication or surgery, reducing the adverse effects of antiseizure medication and treating comorbid depression increases quality of life (Luoni et al. 2011).

That people with epilepsy have an increased risk of death, with elevated overall standardized mortality ratios on the order of 2.5, has been known for many decades. These mortality ratios are highest for childhood-onset symptomatic epilepsy syndromes including Lennox-Gastaut syndrome and other severe epilepsy syndromes associated with other neurological conditions such as cerebral palsy or intellectual disability (Autry et al. 2010). The reasons for excessive mortality among people with epilepsy are only partially understood. Seizures causing falls, burns, or drowning are not rare, especially in developing countries where adequate seizure control is hampered by limited access to basic antiseizure drugs (Tomson et al. 2008; Hughes 2009; Surges and Sander 2012).

Sudden unexpected death in epilepsy is second only to stroke among neurological disorders as the most common cause of the number of adult life years lost, with 1.16 deaths per 1,000 people with epilepsy (Nevalainen et al. 2015). In the United States and Europe alone, sudden death among those with epilepsy accounts for approximately 7,000 deaths per year (Thurman et al. 2014). Sudden death is most common among young adults with intractable epilepsy (ongoing seizures despite optimal antiseizure medication), and has an incidence of about 2 to 10 per 1,000 person-years—many times higher than the risk of sudden death among age-matched people in the general population without epilepsy (Thurman et al. 2014; Lhatoo et al. 2015). Maintaining seizure control, often with appropriate levels of antiseizure drugs, reduces the risk of sudden death (Hughes 2009; Surges and Sander 2012).

Pathophysiology

Excessive abnormal electrical discharges from cortical neurons and from specific structures adjacent to the cortex (e.g., the hippocampus) form the biological basis of seizures. Indeed, the manifestations of seizures are as varied as the functions of the cortex, defying simple rules for diagnosis, and often resulting in a delay in diagnosis of potentially serious epilepsy in some people, and among others the erroneous diagnosis of epilepsy (Jette and Wiebe 2016).

Seizures that begin in a single region of the brain are classified as *focal seizures* and seizures that start all over both hemispheres at the beginning of the seizure are classified as *generalized seizures*. People with generalized seizures tend to have altered consciousness at the onset of their seizures, whereas people with focal seizures often do not have altered consciousness until the electrical seizure has spread over the cortex (Duncan et al. 2006; Guerrini 2006; Berg et al. 2010).

Given the difficulties with accurate diagnosis of epilepsy noted among communities in both the United Kingdom (Chadwick and Smith 2002) and the United States, a few general observations regarding the diagnosis of epilepsy are important to note. First, the degree of alteration of conscious (or altered awareness) caused by a seizure is usually a function of the size of the cortical surface involved in the seizure; the larger the amount of cortex involved with the seizure, the greater the degree of altered awareness. If a large portion of the cortex is involved with the seizure, especially if both hemispheres are actively seizing, then consciousness is almost always impaired.

Second, if the seizure starts in a single region of the brain, the manifestation of the seizure is a direct result of the disordered function of that brain region. For example, if the seizure starts in a region of the brain that normally moves the left thumb and fingers, then the seizure onset is manifested by twitching of the thumb and fingers on the left hand. Then, as the seizure spreads along the cortical surface, the seizure manifests those other cortical functions. If the seizure starts in the area of brain that stores memories (e.g., the hippocampus within the temporal lobe), then the seizure onset is manifested by a sudden memory that emerges out of context—typically referred to as an *aura*. Seizures that begin in a specific region of the brain tend to be *stereotypic*, as that region of the brain when seizing has identical characteristics at the beginning of each seizure, helping experienced clinicians make a diagnosis (Duncan et al. 2006; Guerrini 2006; Berg et al. 2010).

The history, taken by an experienced clinician who hypothesizes the location of the seizure onset from listening to the patient and the observers, can then, in combination with an electroencephalogram (EEG), make a diagnosis and minimize delays in proper treatment. The EEG is often normal between seizures—especially among people with focal epilepsy whose seizures start in areas of cortex folded far from the scalp (Trevathan 2003; Duncan et al. 2006; Guerrini 2006).

Sudden deaths associated with epilepsy typically occur during sleep at night after an apparent seizure, in the prone position, and are unwitnessed, and yet the mechanism of death is unclear. Dysfunction of the brain's control of respirations related to seizures (or delayed recovery of respirations following a seizure), and genes that predispose to cardiac arrthymias during or after seizures are two potential mechanisms that contribute to sudden death (Lhatoo et al. 2015). Regardless, experts agree that having no seizures on antiseizure medication significantly reduces the risk of sudden death (Hughes 2009; Tomson et al. 2008).

Descriptive Epidemiology

The prevalence of epilepsy, with use of a variety of methods, has been estimated at about six to nine per 1,000 in developed countries of Europe, Asia, and in the United States. With use of different methods, the prevalence of epilepsy in both Rochester, Minnesota, and in Atlanta, Georgia, has been estimated at approximately seven per 1,000; extrapolated to the total U.S. population, an estimated two million Americans have active epilepsy (Yeargin-Allsopp et al. 2008). The prevalence of epilepsy in developing low-income countries has consistently been reported to be higher than in developed countries, with reported prevalence rates of 15 per 1,000 or even as high as 105 per 1,000 (Birbeck and Kalichi 2004; Prischich et al. 2008).

The highest incidence of new-onset epilepsy is among the very young and the elderly—important clues as to the two broad categories of etiologic factors. Between birth and age 65 years, the highest incidence occurs during the first year of life, with fairly high incidence during the first few years of life. Despite the fairly constant incidence of new-onset epilepsy between school age and age 65 years, the prevalence remains fairly constant, as the new cases tend to equal those in the general population who experience spontaneous remission, as well as an increased mortality rate experienced by people with severe epilepsy. Beginning at age 65 years, the incidence of new-onset epilepsy rises sharply, as the aging population develops epilepsy as a secondary condition—associated largely with strokes and vascular disease, dementias, and cancer (Hauser et al. 1996).

Epilepsy disproportionately affects the poor. In the United States, about half of adults with active epilepsy live in poverty (CDC 2016a). Adults living in the United States between 2010 and 2013 with active epilepsy were more likely to be uninsured or insured by Medicaid, less likely to have private health insurance, less likely to be employed, more likely to be disabled, and more likely to report barriers to health care access and medication access than the general population (Thurman et al. 2016).

Causes

Among infants and children who have onset of epilepsy, genetic risk factors are the most important class of risk factors. Some forms of epilepsy, such as childhood absence epilepsy, benign rolandic epilepsy, and juvenile myoclonic epilepsy are clearly genetic disorders, with probably a minimal role for environmental triggers (Lagae 2008). Still, other forms of epilepsy, such as partial epilepsy of mesial temporal lobe origin, are likely attributable to the combination of environmental triggers (mostly yet to be discovered) in genetically predisposed individuals (Aronica and Gorter 2007), or environmental–epigenetic interactions (Kobow and Blumcke 2014). Much has been learned about susceptibility genes over the past few years, and gene–environmental interactions among genetically susceptible people will require much more study over the next several decades (Petrovski and Kwan 2013).

In general, anything that damages, alters the structure, or inflames the cerebral cortex can cause epilepsy. Therefore, stroke, cerebral malformations, trauma, encephalitis, brain tumors or metastatic disease in the brain, and hypoxic injury to the cortex can all cause seizures and epilepsy. However, not all people who experience the same insult from a stroke or other injury to the cortex, or encephalitis, or tumor have seizures, and susceptibility genes appear to play a role in these situations as well (Yang et al. 2014; Diamond et al. 2015).

Epilepsy associated with developmental regression during the first 18 months of life is a devastating feature of many different neurodevelopmental disorders (Trevathan 2004), and the combination of developmental regression associated with new-onset epilepsy is often associated with a genetic susceptibility (McTague et al. 2016). For those disorders that are well known, a pattern of normal-appearing development preceding the regression typically occurs even when an obvious preexisting genetic or even cortical structural abnormality occurs, as in the case of Rett's syndrome (Nissenkorn et al. 2015). Over the past several years, vaccines occurring at or around the time of regression at 4 to 18 months have been blamed by some. However, the biologic plausibility of a vaccine-induced etiology is weak to nonexistent for almost all of these cases. For example, the myoclonic epilepsy and developmental regression (with encephalopathy) attributed by some in the 1980s to the pertussis vaccine is caused by the *SCN1A* gene mutation that causes severe myoclonic epilepsy of infancy (Dravet syndrome)—regardless of vaccine history (Berkovic et al. 2006; Verbeek et al. 2015).

Febrile seizures, especially febrile status epilepticus, are known to be associated with development of epilepsy—especially partial epilepsy of temporal lobe origin. However, most children with febrile seizures and febrile status epilepticus do not develop later epilepsy, and the relationship is apparently attributable to the underlying genes (or infections) causing the febrile seizures rather than the actual seizures themselves (Scheffer et al. 2007; Camfield and Camfield 2015).

Evidence-Based Interventions

Several vaccines are likely effective in preventing epilepsy such as those that prevent *Haemophilus influenzae* meningitis, meningococcal meningitis, pertussis, and rubella, with their associated cortical inflammation and injury or cortical malformations (e.g., rubella; Vezzani et al. 2016). Prevention of malaria in areas with endemic spread of *Plasmodium falciparum* may also prevent seizures and epilepsy (Boivin et al. 2015; Kariuki et al. 2015). Folic acid fortification of the grain supply and preconception supplementation has significantly reduced the incidence of neural tube defects and associated hydrocephalus (from Chiari II malformations) and is most effective where fortification is mandatory (Atta et al. 2016), but we still do not know if other brain malformations that increase the risk of seizures have been reduced by folic acid fortification and supplementation. Prevention of congenital infections such as cytomegalovirus, herpes, and toxoplasmosis also prevents serious brain damage with associated intellectual disabilities and epilepsy. Prevention of head injuries likely could, and perhaps already does, have an impact upon the onset of epilepsy and associated neurological comorbidities—especially among adolescents. Among older adults, preventing cerebrovascular disease could have major impact on the prevention of associated epilepsy.

Areas of Future Research

- Perhaps the greatest untapped opportunity for prevention of the consequences of serious epilepsy is improved rapid diagnosis and appropriate early treatment for epilepsy—especially among children (England et al. 2012).
- Identifying genetically susceptible individuals, and intervening early to prevent epilepsy is now a realistic possibility. Intervening early among those with tuberous sclerosis complex, for which there is an animal model, could be an important first step (Jeong and Wong 2016).
- Prevention of the excessive morbidity and mortality associated with status epilepticus by prompt treatment of prolonged seizures in emergency departments and in communities should be a priority, and following newly published guidelines may prevent status epilepticus–associated morbidity and mortality (Glauser et al. 2016).
- Epidemiological studies should emphasize the role of gene–environmental interactions and the identification of potentially modifiable risk factors for specific epilepsy syndromes (Larsen et al. 2015; Lal et al. 2016).

PARKINSON'S DISEASE

Parkinson's disease is a common age-related neurodegenerative disorder manifested by a resting tremor, slowness initiating movements, rigidity, postural instability, dystonia, and occasionally by other movement abnormalities such as chorea, tics, and myoclonus. Depression is a common comorbidity, and people with Parkinson's disease have an increased risk of psychosis. Dementia occurs in up to 80% of people with advanced Parkinson's disease, and most people with Parkinson's disease experience cognitive decline associated with dysfunction of prefrontal cortical regions (Gelb et al. 1999).

Significance

The prevalence of age-related neurodegenerative diseases, including Parkinson's disease, will continue to increase as populations age in high-income countries, and as mortality from other causes is reduced in low- and middle-income countries. Among neurological disorders, Parkinson's disease lags behind only epilepsy, migraine, and Alzheimer's disease in terms of age-standardized disability-adjusted life years (Whiteford et al. 2015).

Pathophysiology

The neuropathological basis of the classical motor features of Parkinson's disease is the unique neuronal loss within the *substantia nigra* and the targeted disruption of dopamine within the brain. The non-motor manifestations of Parkinson's disease, which include hyposmia, constipation, rapid eye movement sleep behavior disorder, orthostatic hypotension, dysphagia, cognitive impairment, and urinary urgency, may be manifest months to years before the development of the classic motor signs and symptoms. The pathognomonic α-synucleinopathy with Lewy bodies is often present outside of the nigrostriatal (motor) pathways, and appear to be markers of these non-motor manifestations of the disease (Adler and Beach 2016).

Descriptive Epidemiology

Worldwide, more than five million people suffer from Parkinson's disease, and the prevalence is expected to triple over the next half-century as the population ages (Whiteford et al. 2015). The average age-adjusted incidence rate in the United States is approximately 20 per 100,000 per year. Among those aged 65 to 84 years, the incidence is more than 500 per 100,000 per year and is very low before the age of 50 years. Rarely, Parkinson's disease occurs among people in their third decade. Several studies have reported that age-adjusted incidence and prevalence are higher among men than among women, and higher among whites than among African Americans (Elbaz et al. 2016). People with Parkinson's disease are at much higher risk of serious injury, and even death, associated with falls (Almeida et al. 2014).

Causes

A viral encephalitis epidemic in 1919, and a subsequent sequelae of parkinsonism provided the first demonstrated cause of selective damage to the *substantia nigra*, although other viral etiologies in Parkinson's disease have not been demonstrated (Tanner and Goldman 1996). A very rapidly developing cluster of Parkinson's disease among a few injection drug users who injected MPTP (1-methyl-4-phenyl-1,2,3,6 tetrahydropyridine), a synthetic compound with heroin-like clinical effects, demonstrated that environmental toxins could produce Parkinson's disease (Langston 1996). The search for pesticide exposures similar to MPTP that cause Parkinson's disease has yielded hypotheses, but has not identified modifiable risk factors. Paraquat exposure in Taiwan and increased brain levels of dieldrin, as well as exposure to other herbicides, insecticides, alkylated phosphates, wood preservatives, and organochlorines, have all been reported to be associated with a higher risk of Parkinson's disease (Hatcher et al. 2008). A recent meta-analysis has reported that there is some inconsistent evidence that rural living, drinking well water, and exposures to pesticides, herbicides, insecticides, fungicides, and paraquat are associated with an increased risk for Parkinson's disease (Breckenridge et al. 2016).

The prevalence of Parkinson's disease among male welders has been reported to be significantly higher than in controls from the general population. The clinical features of Parkinson's disease among welders has been found to be indistinguishable from idiopathic Parkinson's disease, other than age of onset, suggesting that an exposure experienced by welders might be a risk factor for Parkinson's disease (Racette et al. 2001). The reason for higher risk among welders is unclear, but some authors have hypothesized that excessive exposure to solvents, pesticides, iron, copper, or manganese may play a role, and that modifications in welding processes may lower risk (Sriram et al. 2015).

Genetic and hereditary susceptibility factors for Parkinson's disease have been important areas of research for several years. Twin studies have shown no difference in concordance between monozygotic and dizygotic twins. Some authors have suggested that the approximately 10% of people with Parkinson's disease who have one or more affected relatives may represent shared environmental influences rather than classic heritable disease. Yet genetic susceptibility to environmental neurotoxins could play an important etiologic role (Mullin and Schapira 2015). The genetic susceptibility of cognitive decline in Parkinson's disease is now known to have considerable overlap with cognitive decline genetic risks in Alzheimer's disease (Mata et al. 2014). Rare autosomal dominant forms have been found with linkage studies among large kindred with Parkinson's disease, and how these autosomal-dominant or autosomal-recessive genes contribute to the burden of disease in the general population is inadequately understood (Yang et al. 2009; Mullin and Schapira 2015).

Evidence-Based Interventions

There remains no primary treatment to reverse the degeneration of the *substantia nigra* neurons, although some experts have hypothesized that stem cell transplants may be effective (Barker et al. 2016). Replacing lost dopamine through administration of levodopa, or treatment with dopamine agonists (e.g., bromocriptine) can offer significant symptomatic relief. Unfortunately, over time, the dopamine agonists become less effective, and among some people with Parkinson's disease, long-term therapy with dopamine agonists can be associated with emergence of dyskinesias or psychiatric adverse effects (LeWitt and Fahn 2016).

Areas of Future Research

To prevent Parkinson's disease, interventions at least five to six years, or perhaps even 20 years, before the onset of motor symptoms occur, is required—probably before or during the early presentation of non-motor symptoms such as hyposmia, constipation, depression, and rapid eye movement sleep behavior disorder (Savica et al. 2010). The more than 11 Parkinson's disease susceptibility genes that have been discovered within the past 20 years (Corti et al. 2011), the recognition that mitochondrial dysfunction plays a key role in the disease process (Gautier et al. 2014), and efforts to better categorize the non-motor manifestations and early course of Parkinson's disease (Martino et al. 2016) should help better define high-risk individuals for preventive interventions. Among susceptible individuals, reducing risk through physical exercise (Paillard et al. 2015), aggressive treatment of early onset hypertension and prevention of obesity and diabetes (Kotagal et al. 2014), and treatment with antioxidants (Angeles et al. 2016) may modify the disease course or even prevent many of the disabling manifestations of Parkinson's disease.

A significant reduction in morbidity and premature mortality may be possible with appropriate accommodations in the built environment of people with Parkinson's disease and following recently published guidelines for reducing falls, especially among those without dementia (Almeida et al. 2014).

ALZHEIMER'S DISEASE AND DEMENTING DISORDERS

Alzheimer's disease is an age-related irreversible degenerative brain disease manifested by insidious onset of progressive memory loss, followed by loss of cognitive abilities, confusion, problems understanding visual images, behavioral abnormalities, and an inability to perform the simplest tasks of daily living. Alzheimer's disease is responsible for 60% to 80% of dementia in adults, and shares some etiologic factors and clinical manifestations with other forms of dementia such as frontotemporal dementia (Pick's disease), Lewy body dementia, and vascular dementia (Wilson et al. 2012). Individuals with Alzheimer's disease tend to first present with mild cognitive impairment, a condition manifested by measurable changes in thinking abilities, noticeable to the family and sometimes the individual, but which does not negatively affect the individual's ability to carry out everyday activities (Maioli et al. 2007).

Significance

The burden of dementing disorders upon society is enormous. Up to one in nine people aged 65 years and older and about one third of people aged 85 years and older in high-income countries have Alzheimer's disease. An estimated 5.3 million American suffer from the disease (Alzheimer's Association 2015). About half of people with Alzheimer's disease in high-income countries are probably undiagnosed, and even more people with Alzheimer's disease in middle- and low-income countries with Alzheimer's disease lack a diagnosis and access to appropriate services (Bradford et al. 2009). More than 15 million Americans alone provide unpaid care for people with Alzheimer's disease and related dementias, estimated in 2013 to be valued at $217.7 billion, approximately equal to the cost of all Alzheimer's disease medical care (Hurd et al. 2013). Figure 19-2 lists the major Alzheimer's disease causes, consequences, and high-risk groups.

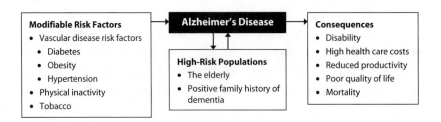

Note: For further information about high-risk populations for Alzheimer's disease, visit: http://www.alz.org.
Figure 19-2. Alzheimer's Disease: Causes, Consequences, and High-Risk Groups

Pathophysiology

Alzheimer's disease is associated with the accumulation of beta-amyloid plaques outside cortical neurons, as well as the accumulation of an abnormal form of the protein tau (or tau tangles) inside neurons. Early in the course of the disease, synaptic transmission in the hippocampus begins to fail, the number of synapses declines, and neurons eventually die, with associated atrophy of the affected cortical areas (Selkoe 2002). As with Parkinson's disease, the brain changes associated with Alzheimer's disease have their onset 20 or more years before clinical manifestations (Goudsmit 2016).

Descriptive Epidemiology

Assuming current trends continue, the prevalence will almost triple by 2050, with approximately 13.2 million having Alzheimer's disease in the United States by then (with estimates ranging from 11.3 million to 16 million; Ziegler-Graham et al. 2008). There is a slightly higher prevalence of Alzheimer's disease among women than among men (1.6:1) in several studies, and African Americans in the United States may have slightly higher prevalence rates of Alzheimer's disease than whites. The prevalence of Alzheimer's disease is high, but it reflects only about half of the overall burden of dementia from all causes upon society (Szekely et al. 2008).

Causes

Although the genetic risk factors for Alzheimer's disease have received considerable attention, probably less than 5% of Alzheimer's disease is associated with classic autosomal-dominant inheritance, and there is considerable complexity in the genetic susceptibility for Alzheimer's disease. There is a strong association between the presence of the epsilon 4 (E4) allele of the apolipoprotein E (*APOE*) gene and late-onset Alzheimer's disease. The E4 allele has been associated with increased beta-amyloid deposition in susceptible brain regions associated with Alzheimer's disease (Raber et al. 2004; Bertram and Tanzi 2008).

Vascular disease appears to be a risk factor for Alzheimer's disease, but the relationship is complex as there is often coexistence of neuropathological findings of multi-infarct dementia and Alzheimer's disease in the same patients (Knopman 2007; Norton et al. 2014). Insulin resistance syndrome and associated conditions (e.g., hypertension, type 2 diabetes mellitus) are associated with age-related memory impairment and Alzheimer's disease. Raising plasma insulin to levels associated with insulin resistance causes increased levels of beta-amyloid and inflammatory agents—the very pathological findings known to impair memory associated with Alzheimer's disease. Therefore, the potential causal relationship between insulin resistance and Alzheimer's disease seems biologically plausible (Craft et al. 2013).

Low to moderate amounts of alcohol likely reduce the accumulation of cardiovascular pathology, as well as potentially exert a protective effect on cognitive function and reduce risk for dementia (Neafsey and Collins 2011). Studies of cigarette smoking have not provided consistent results, with some studies showing no relationship, some studies showing a modest increase in risk, and still others suggesting a differential survival effect with smokers dying earlier and, therefore, having less time exposure to the risk of Alzheimer's disease with advanced age (Anstey et al. 2007). The issue of whether ingested aluminum might play a causal role in Alzheimer's disease is not yet settled, as some authors continue to argue that aluminum seems to play a role in amyloid aggregation and the potential pathogenic mechanisms of Alzheimer's disease (Drago et al. 2008; Pogue and Lukiw 2016).

Evidence-Based Interventions

Among those with the *APOE* E4 allele, non-steroidal anti-inflammatory drugs may be associated with reduced risk of Alzheimer's disease, and may deserve additional study (Sano et al. 2008), but no protective effect has been consistently documented in the general population. Studies of hormone replacement therapy in women have not demonstrated a consistent impact on the risk of developing Alzheimer's disease (Sano et al. 2008; Hu et al. 2016).

Some people with Alzheimer's disease pathology do not have a clinical diagnosis of dementia; the reasons why are not clear, but these protected individuals seem to have more cognitive reserve, and larger brain size. Studies to determine whether individuals with relative protection from clinical dementia who have Alzheimer's disease pathology have common potentially protective characteristics may be helpful (Whitwell 2010; Guo et al. 2013).

A robust literature has now developed regarding the potential protective effects of exercise in the prevention of Alzheimer's disease, potentially among those at higher risk for the disease (Beydoun et al. 2014; Norton et al. 2014; Paillard et al. 2015; Huang et al. 2016). When combined with interventions to reduce smoking and obesity, and to treat midlife hypertension, programs to increase physical activity have considerable potential to prevent Alzheimer's disease.

Areas of Future Research

Studies of interventions among those with mild cognitive impairment or with genetic susceptibility to Alzheimer's disease that consist of increased physical activity, smoking cessation, and modifying other risk factors for cerebrovascular disease are needed.

CEREBRAL PALSY

Cerebral palsy describes a broad category of nonprogressive, but often changing with developmental stage, motor impairment syndromes attributable to abnormalities of brain structure or function with onset during early stages of brain development (Yeargin-Allsopp et al. 2008; van Lieshout et al. 2016). The cerebral palsy syndromes each have different underlying neuropathology (Folkerth 2007). Most people with cerebral palsy have *spasticity*, or significant resistance to passive movement that becomes functionally worse as the velocity of movement increases. The spasticity alone can be limiting or disabling regardless of weakness, but typically the spasticity and weakness go hand in hand.

Between 18% and 45% of children with cerebral palsy have spastic diplegia, with *diplegia* referring to weakness of all four limbs, with the legs more severely affected than the arms. People with spastic diplegia typically have some trunk weakness and problems with balance, which, when combined with spasticity, place them at increased risk of falls and injuries. Infants with spastic diplegia often have normal or reduced muscle tone (resistance to passive movement) for the first few weeks or months of life and then develop obvious spasticity by the end of the first year (Stanley et al. 2000). Spastic diplegia is a clinical diagnosis, but often is associated with brain magnetic resonance imaging (MRI) abnormalities in the "watershed" region between the distribution of the anterior cerebral artery and the middle cerebral artery, or periventricular leukomalacia (Robinson et al. 2009).

Spastic hemiplegic cerebral palsy occurs in about a third of children with cerebral palsy and is characterized by hand and arm greater than leg weakness contralateral to the side of the brain lesion. Spastic hemiplegic cerebral palsy is often the result of an underlying intraventricular hemorrhage, or a stroke that occurred during intrauterine life, or very early in the neonatal period (Yeargin-Allsopp et al. 2008).

Spastic quadriplegic cerebral palsy accounts for about 10% to 30% of cases of cerebral palsy and is associated with severe impairment of both arms and legs—legs typically more severely affected. *Double hemiplegia* has been a term used to describe some people with quadriplegia whose arms bilaterally are more severely affected than their legs. Brain malformations are common causes of quadriplegia. Hypoxic–ischemic encephalopathy is a cause of a minority of cases of spastic quadriplegia cerebral palsy (Pakula et al. 2009).

Cerebral palsy is often associated with intellectual disability. The frequency of associated intellectual disability and the severity of the intellectual disability is typically less with the types of cerebral palsy that involve smaller areas of cortical abnormality (e.g., spastic diplegia) and almost uniformly present and severe among those whose cerebral palsy is a reflection of widespread cortical dysfunction or damage (e.g., spastic quadriplegia). Coexisting morbidities, including feeding problems, visual impairment, and epilepsy, often exacerbate the level of disability, complicate the medical management, and impair the community participation of people with cerebral palsy (Pakula et al. 2009; van Lieshout et al. 2016).

Significance

Cerebral palsy is associated with significant morbidity, including epilepsy and status epilepticus, feeding and swallowing difficulty with associated aspiration pneumonias, and severe orthopedic problems often requiring multiple surgeries (Yeargin-Allsopp et al. 2008). In many countries, having a child with cerebral palsy has a negative impact upon the entire family's economic well-being because of the increased care needs, and is associated with high rates of divorce and other family stresses. The Danish system for family support seems to have been successful in keeping parents working and living together with their affected child (Michelsen et al. 2015).

Descriptive Epidemiology

The prevalence of cerebral palsy among school-age children in recent reports has ranged from about two to four per 1,000, with the majority of studies reporting a prevalence of about two to three per 1,000. Boys are more likely to have cerebral palsy than are girls, with a sex ratio of 1.1:1 to 1.5:1. The relationship between race and the risk of cerebral palsy is complex. Studies in metropolitan Atlanta have demonstrated that African American children had lower prevalence rates of cerebral palsy than did white children if their birthweight was less than 2,500 grams, but higher rates if their birthweight was 2,500 grams or more. Cerebral palsy prevalence rates from three different states using a common methodology have recently been reported, with similar rates in Georgia, Wisconsin, and Alabama and an overall prevalence rate of 3.3 per 1,000. The prevalence rate of cerebral palsy among eight-year-old children in 2002 in Georgia was 3.8 per 1000, higher than the rates reported from Georgia in the 1990s. Ongoing surveillance to determine if the increase is a trend is essential (Yeargin-Allsopp et al. 2008).

Causes

Prematurity is the most common risk factor for cerebral palsy. A bimodal distribution of birthweight among children with cerebral palsy has been reported— one peak at about 1,000 grams, and a second peak at about 3,000 grams. About one fourth of children with cerebral palsy were born weighing less than 1,500 grams, compared with about 1% of the general population. About half of children with cerebral palsy were born weighing less than 2,500 grams, compared with about 5% of the general population. Children from multiple births have a high risk of cerebral palsy, primarily associated with their increased risk of prematurity. Death of a co-twin in utero is a significant risk factor for cerebral palsy. Children with cerebral palsy have higher rates of birth defects than do children in the general population (Yeargin-Allsopp et al. 2008; Allen 2008).

Acute chorioamnionitis and funisitis are significant risk factors for cerebral palsy, best documented among premature infants, but also among full-term infants (Shalak et al. 2002; Kim et al. 2015; Park et al. 2015).

Zika virus infection during pregnancy, and the resulting brain damage associated with microcephaly, cerebral palsy, and intellectual disability, has become a global public health emergency. Methods of prevention of Zika virus transmission, with an emphasis on the prevention of maternal infection, are a priority (Rasmussen et al. 2016).

Evidence-Based Interventions

Cerebral palsy primary prevention largely depends upon efforts to prevent prematurity (Pakula et al. 2009), but a few other opportunities for prevention exist. Magnesium sulfate given before preterm birth has been shown to offer neuroprotection to the fetus and seems to be a factor in reducing the rates of prematurity-associated cerebral palsy (Hirtz et al. 2015; Teela et al. 2015). A Cochrane Collaboration analysis suggested that the number of at-risk women needed to treat to prevent one baby from having cerebral palsy is 63 (95% confidence interval [CI] = 43, 87; Doyle et al. 2009). A preliminary report has suggested that, among infants less than 26 weeks gestational age, antenatal administration of magnesium sulfate may increase the risk of necrotizing enterocolitis and death; additional studies of the risks and benefits of magnesium sulfate administered antenatally is needed among very premature infants (Kamyar et al. 2016).

About 5% of cerebral palsy is preventable after neonatal encephalopathy with neonatal hypothermia treatment (Garfinkle et al. 2015). Placental inflammatory villitis is associated with poor neurological outcomes among infants who had hypoxic–ischemic encephalopathy and who underwent hypothermia therapy (Mir et al. 2015).

Children with cerebral palsy may benefit from physical therapy and from improved nutrition that considers their higher caloric requirements. For some children, the treatment of epilepsy and the management of speech and language impairment can significantly improve quality of life and enhance community participation.

Areas of Future Research

The risks and benefits of antenatal magnesium sulfate is an important ongoing area of research, as well as the prevention and treatment of chorioamnionitis and funisitis. The development of a Zika virus vaccine is a global health priority, as are other methods of maternal Zika virus infection prevention.

AUTISM SPECTRUM DISORDERS

Autism spectrum disorders are a group of disorders of the developing brain that tend to have the following characteristics: social problems that include difficulty interacting and communicating, repetitive and stereotypic behaviors with a limited range of interests or activities, and symptoms recognized during the first two years of life. Autism spectrum disorders, including autistic disorder, Asperger's syndrome, and pervasive developmental disorder–not otherwise specified, are a heterogeneous group of developing brain disorders, or neurodevelopmental disorders. People with autistic disorder have classic abnormalities of language, severe impairment of reciprocal social behavior, and severely restricted behaviors and interests. People with Asperger's syndrome have relative preservation of cognitive, language, and communication skills (Yeargin-Allsopp et al. 2008).

Significance

The burden of autism spectrum disorders on society is significant, and with the growing recognition of autism among adults, the cost of autism is not limited to schools, caregiver, and health care facilities, but also extends into the workforce and has significant impact on the economy of high-income countries (Leigh et al. 2016). The mortality risk among people with autism spectrum disorders is two-fold higher than that of the general population throughout young adulthood, with the highest increase in risk among those with epilepsy or intellectual disability comorbidities (Schendel et al. 2016).

Pathophysiology

Over the past two decades, neuroscience research has clearly demonstrated that autism is not primarily caused by mechanisms that cause brain damage, but rather by intricate genetic influences that may interact with environmental events, with resulting dysfunction of the widespread neural networks that interconnect language, social, emotional, and other regions of the cerebral cortex (Trevathan and Shinnar 2006; Yeargin-Allsopp et al. 2008).

Descriptive Epidemiology

The prevalence of autism spectrum disorders over the past few years has been reported at approximately 14 per 1,000 school-aged children, or about 1 in 68 eight-year-old children (Christensen et al. 2016a), and about 13 per 1,000 four-year-old children (Christensen et al. 2016b). All population-based studies have documented a significantly higher prevalence among boys than among girls. Debate exists regarding whether the prevalence of autism spectrum disorders now is higher than 20 years ago when the case definitions were different, when societal beliefs regarding the origins of behavioral abnormalities were different, and when special education programs for children with autism spectrum disorders were more limited, or simply nonexistent (Trevathan and Shinnar 2006; Yeargin-Allsopp et al. 2008). It will be very difficult, if not impossible, to determine whether the high prevalence rates of autism now are attributable only to increased recognition.

In the most comprehensive autism spectrum disorder prevalence studies, investigators have searched both health and educational records, with the highest reported prevalence rates occurring in studies in which educational records were abstracted (Christensen et al. 2016b), and some authors have suggested that some of the increased prevalence is attributed to diagnostic substitution related to educational services (Shattuck 2006). Regardless, it is now clear that the autism spectrum disorder prevalence among adults, at least in the United Kingdom, is similar to the prevalence among children (Brugha et al. 2011). Autism spectrum disorders represent a common group of neurodevelopmental disorders that constitute a significant public health and educational concern in the United States and throughout the world.

Causes

Children with autism may appear normal for the first few months of life, but almost all children with autism are predestined to have autism from before birth, as determined by their genetic predisposition to autism, and with the emergence of autism signs and symptoms when their abnormalities of brain development become manifest (Trevathan and Shinnar 2006; Yeargin-Allsopp et al. 2008). The four-to-one male-to-female ratio and twin studies have demonstrated evidence of the strong genetic component for autism. Likewise, known genetic disorders such as fragile X syndrome, tuberous sclerosis, untreated phenylketonuria, Down syndrome, and neurofibromatosis all have high rates of co-existing autism (Miles 2011).

Some parents who witness their normal-appearing children developmentally regress during the first two years of life, when vaccines are frequently administered, have blamed vaccines for their child's autism. Multiple studies have now been completed that have not demonstrated any causal relationship between autism and vaccines, and yet the concerns remain for some parents who find it difficult to believe that they witnessed a temporal relationship that was genetically driven and not caused by exposure to vaccines (Gerber and Offit 2009; Gadad et al. 2015; Jain et al. 2015). Andrew Wakefield's now discredited 1998 study that hypothesized a relationship between the measles, mumps, and rubella

(MMR) vaccine and autism was not replicated and was retracted by *The Lancet* (Editors 2010). Wakefield was sanctioned for "dishonestly and irresponsibly" conducting his research, in which study participants were referred to Wakefield by plaintiffs' lawyers, the published data were falsified, and Wakefield falsely claimed that the studies were approved by a university ethics committee (Offit 2008; GMC 2009; Godlee et al. 2011). Meanwhile, the number of studies documenting the genetic basis for autism has grown, so that several new susceptibility genes have been determined over the past few years—susceptibility genes that will need to be studied further to investigate other possible gene–environmental interactions (Miles 2011; de la Torre-Ubieta et al. 2016).

Parental age has recently received considerable attention as a risk factor for autism spectrum disorders (Durkin et al. 2008). Maternal diabetes may be associated with an increased risk of autism (Xiang et al. 2015). A variety of risk factors currently being investigated include various hormonal factors, immune mechanisms, and potential environmental toxins (Yeargin-Allsopp et al. 2008; Sandin et al. 2016).

Evidence-Based Interventions

At present, there are no proven ways to prevent or cure autism spectrum disorders. However, early identification of children with signs and symptoms of language delays or regression and social impairment, and enrollment in early intervention programs before the age of three years seems to offer improved developmental outcomes in some children. Therefore, community programs aimed at early diagnosis and intervention are currently a focus of public health, educational, and pediatric interventions (Estes et al. 2015; CDC 2016b). There is now evidence that parent-mediated interventions among high-risk infants could reduce the risk of autism (Green et al. 2015); more research is needed to reproduce and further define these potentially effective parenting interventions.

Areas of Future Research

Although additional genetic research will be helpful, and certainly will be done, further research on the implementation of potential interventions such as parent-mediated interventions of high-risk infants is especially important. In addition, further research to clarify the role of potentially modifiable risk factors such as maternal diabetes and parental age are important.

AMYOTROPHIC LATERAL SCLEROSIS AND MOTOR NEURON DISEASE

Amyotrophic lateral sclerosis (ALS), also known as Lou Gehrig's disease, is the most common motor neuron disease worldwide, with onset in adulthood of relentlessly progressive weakness leading to death from respiratory failure and related complications, typically within months to three years (Riva et al. 2016), although occasional patients survive for up to 20 years or longer with either pure upper-motor (termed primary lateral sclerosis) or pure lower-motor (termed progressive muscular atrophy) neuron involvement (Turner et al. 2013).

Significance

Amyotrophic lateral sclerosis is rare, with an incidence of about 2.8 per 100,000 person-years. However, because ALS often attacks adults during the peak of their working lives, the burden for affected families and local communities is significant (Bozzoni et al. 2016; Riva et al. 2016).

Pathophysiology

Amyotrophic lateral sclerosis is characterized by slow, steadily progressive, and selective cell death of motor neurons in the spinal cord and the lower brain stem, whose axons innervate skeletal muscles of the body and the face and oral pharynx. In addition, ALS is also associated with some motor neuron loss in the primary motor area of the cerebral cortex—the precentral gyrus, whose neurons project to the spinal cord motor neurons. The devastating clinical manifestations of the progressive cell death of spinal cord and precentral gyrus motor neurons are muscle wasting and weakness with fasciculations noted on electromyography that typically starts in one location and then spreads throughout the affected limb, then typically crosses over to affect the contralateral limb, and then spreads throughout the body. Non-motor signs, including impaired executive function and behavioral abnormalities are often present, and frontotemporal dementia may occur in up to 15% of people with ALS (Chio et al. 2013).

Descriptive Epidemiology

With the exception of the pockets of excessive rates of the Western Pacific variant of ALS, the incidence rates of ALS have been fairly constant throughout the world. An incidence rate of about 2.2 per 100,000 per year has been reported in several different studies in the United States and in Europe. The incidence of sporadic ALS in men is slightly higher than the incidence in women (about 1.2:1). The average age at diagnosis is 65 years. Population-based studies have demonstrated that the age-specific incidence rates increase with age (Chio et al. 2013). There are very few studies that have examined the racial and ethnic group–specific incidence rates.

Over the past few years, slightly higher rates of ALS have been reported than several decades ago. Several factors may together account for these recent slightly higher rates in the United Kingdom—the aging population, the improved diagnosis and case ascertainment in more recent studies (as neurological diagnostic expertise has become more uniformly available), a possible loss of competing causes of death in susceptible cohorts, and possibly increased reporting of ALS on death certificates (Kiernan et al. 2011; Chio et al. 2013).

Several authors classify ALS into three separate forms—a variant of ALS primarily occurring in the Western Pacific islands, a classic familial form of ALS, and a sporadic form of ALS. In the mid–20th century, epidemics of ALS were reported in Guam, New Guinea, and in the Kii Peninsula in the Western Pacific. Further epidemics of ALS in the Western Pacific have not been described. The Western Pacific variant of ALS has reported to have distinct pathological characteristics, and often co-occurs with a separate Parkinsonism–dementia complex, suggesting that the Pacific variant of ALS may have separate etiologic risk factors. Some authors have suggested that a nut from a cycad tree in the Western Pacific may serve as a toxin in susceptible individuals and be a risk factor for the Western Pacific variant of ALS (Chio et al. 2013; Turner et al. 2013).

Other forms of motor neuron disease occur less frequently among infants as well as older children and adolescents. Spinal muscular atrophy is an autosomal-recessive motor neuron disease, with a birth prevalence of approximately eight cases per 100,000 live births, and a high mortality during infancy with no known treatment. Death is caused by restrictive lung disease and respiratory failure (Lunn and Wang 2008).

Causes

Several genes have been identified for the familial forms of ALS, prompting many experts to hypothesize the presence of susceptibility genes for the sporadic forms of ALS. A gene for the familial form of ALS has been discovered on the X chromosome. Up to 20% of familial cases of ALS are attributed to mutations at the *SOD1* gene on chromosome 21. More than nine genes have now been discovered that are associated with dominant mutations linked to ALS, and there is evidence to suggest interplay among multiple genes (Turner et al. 2013). Susceptibility genes for adult sporadic forms of ALS have been hypothesized as being those involved in the development of infantile spinal muscular atrophy, such as the *SMN* gene and the neuronal apoptosis inhibitory protein (*NAIP*) gene. Infantile spinal muscular atrophy is generally recognized as a genetic disorder caused by homozygous disruption of the survival motor neuron 1 (*SMN1*) gene (Lunn and Wang 2008; Siddique and Siddique 2008; Rothstein 2009; Turner et al. 2013).

Several studies have investigated the potential relationships between environmental exposures and development of sporadic ALS, and overall there are inconclusive results. Some studies have reported an increased risk of ALS with high-level exposures to lead, mercury, and other heavy metals, with odds ratios as high as 1.5 to 6.0, but negative reports have also been published. Occupations that are involved with heavy metal exposure, such as welding, have been reported to have an increased risk of ALS, but the data at present are inconclusive (Bozzoni et al. 2016). In addition, the exposure to agricultural chemicals has also been reported to have an increased association with ALS. Some studies have investigated the relationship between electrical shock and exposures to electromagnetic fields. Many of these studies have some methodological limitations, including small sample size, selective reporting, recall bias, and inconsistent measurement of levels of exposures (Sumner 2007; Shaw and Höglinger 2008). Authors of a detailed systematic review recently concluded that only exposure to pesticides has been a consistent potentially modifiable environmental risk factor for ALS (Bozzoni et al. 2016).

Low dietary intake of exogenous antioxidants has been hypothesized to increase the risk of ALS. A diet high in fruits and vegetables might offer some reduction in the risk of ALS (Okamoto et al. 2009).

Evidence-Based Interventions and Areas of Future Research

Good pulmonary care and advances in mechanical ventilation have prolonged survival and improved the quality of life among people with motor neuron diseases, but unfortunately there is no effective treatment for the underlying disease process. Future epidemiological studies will need to examine the gene–environmental interactions among susceptible populations, especially with regard to pesticide exposures. The role of diet in ALS deserves additional study.

MULTIPLE SCLEROSIS

Multiple sclerosis is a demyelinating disease of the central nervous system characterized by abnormalities of the myelin sheath of axons, resulting in impaired transmission of electrical signals through axons; clinical symptoms are a reflection of the location of the damaged myelin within the brain and spinal cord. Typical symptoms at onset of the disease are highly variable but often include double vision, tremor, weakness, sensory disturbances, bladder or bowel dysfunction, impaired balance and coordination, and problems with speech, language, and cognitive processing. Typically, MS has a stuttering course with overall reduced neurological functioning over time, but with short-term remissions and exacerbations. Although the severity of the disease and the rate of progression vary considerably, the median survival following disease onset is approximately 30 years (Noseworthy et al. 2000).

Significance

Although MS is less common than Alzheimer's disease, epilepsy, Parkinson's disease, and migraine, MS contributes significantly to the global burden of neurological disorders (Whiteford et al. 2015). New medical therapies that allow more people with MS to achieve longer remissions are expensive, but because of the significant reduction in level of disability and the increased productivity demonstrated by people with MS who are treated with these drugs, new treatments for relapsing remitting MS tend to be cost-effective (Chevalier et al. 2016).

Pathophysiology

The pathological features of MS are white-matter plaques that vary in age and in distribution in the brain and spinal cord. This scattering of MS lesions in time and place was noted by Charcot in the mid-1800s and led to the basic neurological principle that the clinical symptoms needed to involve different areas of the central nervous system and have onset in different time periods to make the clinical diagnosis. We now know that the demyelinating lesions in MS also involve the cortical regions (Mahad et al. 2015). More recently, standardized diagnostic criteria and the use of brain MRI imaging, and spinal cord imaging, have greatly assisted diagnosis of MS (Gass et al. 2015; Matthews et al. 2016).

Descriptive Epidemiology

More than 400,000 people are estimated to live in the United States with MS, and probably more than 2.5 million people have MS worldwide. Incidence rates of MS have consistently been reported to be higher in colder climates (Kingwell et al. 2013). With onset typically in the early 30s, MS is the most common chronic progressive neurological disorder among adults between the ages of 20 and 50 years. Despite the prolonged survival compared with some other progressive neurological disorders, the contribution of MS to long-term disability and excessive morbidity is considerable. About half of people with MS will need assistance with walking within 15 years of diagnosis (Debouverie et al. 2008a; Debouverie et al. 2008b). Multiple sclerosis is significantly more common among women than men, and more common among whites than among African Americans within the United Kingdom. It has been reported to be more common among those of upper socioeconomic groups, but whether reduced access to specialty care and early diagnosis of MS among lower socioeconomic groups underestimate the rates of MS is unknown (Noseworthy et al. 2000).

The prevalence of MS in the United States and in other developed countries seems to be increasing, associated with longer survival rates (Gracia et al. 2009). There is some evidence that the incidence of MS is increasing as well in some studies—an increase that cannot be totally accounted for on the basis of improved diagnostic techniques, such as brain imaging with MRI (Alonso and Hernán 2008; Kingwell et al. 2013).

Causes

Classically, the MS prevalence and risk of death have increased with distance from the equator. The highest prevalence rates have been reported from the northern and north-midwestern regions of the United States, Northern Europe, and Canada, as well as Australia and New Zealand. Whites also have higher rates of MS than Africans, African Americans, and Asians. Incidence rates of MS have been reported to be lower in Africa and in Asia. Migration studies have repeatedly shown that people migrating from a high-risk to a low-risk area before age 15 years seem to adopt the lower risk of their new regional home, while those people who migrate to lower risk areas as adults retain a higher risk of MS. It seems unlikely that these results of migration studies are attributable totally to enhanced access to diagnostic services and technology in the more affluent and technologically advanced developed countries of the north compared with the developing countries near the equator. Growing evidence supports the impact of both susceptibility genes and migration effects to cooler climates as risk factors for MS (Smestad et al. 2008).

Aggregation of MS cases within families and higher rates of MS among whites have long suggested a genetic susceptibility to MS. Population-based twin studies of MS have reported much higher concordance rates among monozygotic than among dizygotic twin pairs. The risk of non-twin siblings of MS cases has been found to be similar to the risk of MS among dizygotic twins (Fagnani et al. 2015). Overall, the familial studies of MS have pointed to likely shared genes among affected family members rather than environmental factors, and that several genes likely contribute to MS susceptibility (Ramagopalan et al. 2008).

Whereas the pace of discovery of susceptibility genes for many chronic diseases has been extremely rapid over the last decade, the identification of MS susceptibility genes has been relatively limited. Recent studies have suggested that epigenetic modifications of germline susceptibility might play an important role (Ramagopalan et al. 2008). Epigenetic interactions with major histocompatibility complex may play important roles in MS (Küçükali et al. 2015). Whether genome-wide association studies will lead to other clues regarding the role of genetics in MS should be determined in the near future.

Because MS cases have tended to cluster in time and have varied with latitude, many investigators have focused on the roles of infectious diseases as risk factors for MS. Latent viral infections from childhood and early adolescence in genetically susceptible individuals that via unknown immunologic mechanisms initiate the disease process in early adulthood may be important in the pathogenesis of MS (McKay et al. 2015; McKay et al. 2016). For example, some authors have reported that rubella antibody titers are higher among patients with MS than among controls from the general population. The risk of MS seems to increase among people whose rubella infection occurred in later childhood or early adolescence. An oft-cited study is that of an epidemic of MS in the Faroe Islands a few years after World War II, following the arrival of British troops, consistent with the introduction of a new (but yet undetermined) infectious agent into the island population. Hypothesized, but not proven, associations between Epstein-Barr virus (Jilek et al. 2008) and other viruses such as herpes simplex virus I and II (Alvarez-Lafuente et al. 2008), varicella zoster (Sotelo et al. 2008), mumps, and cytomegalovirus have been reported (Hernán et al. 2001; Winkelmann et al. 2016). A possible association between *Chlamydia* infection and the risk of MS has received some recent attention in the literature (Parratt et al. 2008). Many of these studies of associations with infectious diseases are complicated by both potential recall bias and by inconsistent laboratory procedures for measurement of the infectious exposures.

The well-established modulation of the immune system by sex hormones, along with the variation in MS incidence by sex, has prompted the investigation of sex hormones as potential modulating factors in MS. Relapses of MS have long been recognized as being rare during pregnancy. Exacerbations of MS are often seen among women with MS weeks after delivery (Lee and O'Brien 2008). A recent possible association has been reported between oral contraceptives and MS, although the authors noted that an unmeasured confounder might explain the weak association (Hellwig et al. 2016).

Exacerbation of MS symptoms has been reported after cigarette smoking, and early cigarette smoking has been reported as a possible risk factor in case–control studies from Canada and the United Kingdom. It is also appears that cigarette smoking worsens the long-term prognosis among people with MS (Sundstrom et al. 2008; Fragoso 2014).

Evidence-Based Interventions

Although the clinical management of MS has improved with more people with MS experiencing remission of their symptoms, a cure for MS does not exist. However, the clinical management of MS has improved considerably (Winkelmann et al. 2016). As the treatment regimens for MS have become more complex, treatment guidelines that can be uniformly and consistently followed by patients who maintain long-term compliance have become a challenge. Strategies for effective long-term treatment require coordination between the primary care medical home and neurologists, with effective utilization of nursing and health education. The guidelines updated on a regular basis by the American Academy of Neurology are an important resource for clinicians (https://www.aan.com). The built environment and accessibility for people with motor disabilities is especially important for people who are disabled as a result of MS.

As with some other progressive neurological disorders, low concentrations of dietary antioxidants have been thought to be a potential risk factor by some authors. Although a protective role for vitamin D has been discussed in the literature (Sundström and Salzer 2015), the known variations in MS incidence by latitude could be an important confounding variable. Recent publications have highlighted the high rate of adverse health behaviors (e.g., smoking, lack of exercise) as well as obesity among people with MS, suggesting the need for targeted health promotion and chronic disease prevention activities (Hedström et al. 2015a; Hedström et al. 2015b).

Areas of Future Research

Better population-based surveillance data and epidemiological research of potential risk factors, including gene–environmental interaction studies, are needed to mount a public health response to MS in developing countries. The role of diet, hormonal factors, and latent viral infections with long-term immunologic responses continue to be important areas of investigation.

GUILLAIN-BARRÉ SYNDROME

Guillain-Barré syndrome is an acute post-infectious demyelinating disease of the peripheral nervous system affecting motor and sensory motor neurons throughout the body. The onset is characterized by progressive weakness over many hours to many days. Typically, the onset of weakness is accompanied by vague uncomfortable sensory complaints, with progression from the legs and arms to the trunk and chest muscles, then leading to requirements for mechanical ventilation. The rate of demyelination and associated clinical deterioration is often faster in children than among adults, with children recovering faster as well. Most people with Guillain-Barré syndrome have complete or near-complete recovery of their weakness. However, short-term mortality and morbidity remain significant. Standard case definitions for Guillain-Barré syndrome have improved both clinical research efforts and epidemic investigations (Willison et al. 2016).

Significance

Guillain-Barré syndrome has a highly variable course, with some patients requiring only short hospital stays, whereas others have prolonged periods of hospitalization followed by lengthy periods of rehabilitation. Although most people with Guillain-Barré syndrome eventually fully recover neurological function, mortality rates of more than 5% have been reported, often from complications of respiratory failure or autonomic dysfunction with associated cardiac arrthymias (Kalita et al. 2016).

Pathophysiology

Guillain-Barré syndrome results from an autoimmune response directed against the myelin sheath of peripheral nerves, typically triggered by a recent viral or bacterial infection, or less commonly a noninfectious agent (Willison et al 2016; Burns 2008; Pritchard 2008). Motor and sensory nerve function can be impacted by the demyelination, and some patients have bulbar involvement as well as autonomic dysfunction, which is associated with high rates of cardiac arrhythmias (Dimario and Edwards 2012; van den Berg et al. 2014).

Descriptive Epidemiology

The reported incidence of Guillain-Barré syndrome has varied considerably, with annual incidence rates in the United States ranging from less than 0.5 to more than 2 per 100,000 (Sejvar et al. 2011; Webb et al. 2015). Some studies have reported higher incidence rates for men than for women and higher rates for whites than for African Americans (Willison et al. 2016).

Causes

Infections that trigger peripheral nerve myelin-directed autoimmune responses have long been the focus of research and are thought to be the primary risk factors for Guillain-Barré syndrome. Gastrointestinal and upper respiratory infections a few weeks before onset of weakness are typical and are more common among Guillain-Barré syndrome cases than among controls. *Campylobacter* (Parker et al. 2015), Epstein-Barr virus, and cytomegalovirus have received the most attention from investigators (Taheraghdam et al. 2014) in the past, and more recently, 42 cases of Guillain-Barré syndrome occurred during a Zika virus outbreak (Watrin et al. 2016).

Concern regarding the increased risk of Guillain-Barré syndrome following the swine flu vaccine in 1976 and 1977 received considerable attention. Of interest is that the studies of swine flu vaccine administered after 1977 and Guillain-Barré syndrome have not shown any association, suggesting that there was a unique immunologic reaction from the vaccine used in 1976 and 1977 that has not occurred since that time (Kuwabara 2004; McGrogan et al. 2009).

Evidence-Based Interventions

Prevention of infectious triggers of Guillain-Barré syndrome and control of epidemics of *Campylobacter* are currently the best opportunities for primary prevention. Rapid diagnosis and supportive care, including respiratory care and mechanical ventilation if needed, remain the mainstay of treatment. If treated early in the course of the disease process, plasmapheresis or intravenous gamma globulin can shorten the course of the demyelinating disorder and may reduce the odds of requiring mechanical ventilation (Willison et al. 2016). Vigilance on the part of public health officials and rapid response to potential epidemics of Guillain-Barré syndrome remains important (Sejvar et al. 2011).

Areas of Future Research

Ongoing surveillance to detect outbreaks in order to mount a rapid public health response, as well as educational programs for primary health care providers that facilitates rapid diagnosis, may reduce the respiratory failure and mortality associated with Guillain-Barré syndrome.

TIC DISORDERS AND TOURETTE SYNDROME

Tics are stereotypic, purposeless, and sudden movements that, although they may be transiently suppressed and resemble purposeful movement, are involuntary. Tics have been generally classified as simple and chronic. Simple tic disorders are those in which a single motor tic manifestation occurs in an individual, such as eye blinks, jaw-jutting movements, or throat clearing, without evolution of multiple different motor tic manifestations and without vocal tics. Chronic multifocal tic disorders manifest multiple different simple and complex motor tics, often accompanied by vocal tics that are most commonly noises such as snorts or consonant sounds, but may also be involuntary expletive speech (coprolalia). Simple tics often undergo spontaneous remission, especially among children, within a year of onset. Chronic multifocal tics, when in association with vocal tics, that last for greater than a year are typically lifelong in duration and are classified as Tourette syndrome (Gunduz and Okun 2016).

Significance

Although most people with tics are not disabled, and often are not aware that their movements are abnormal, some people with Tourette syndrome are significantly impaired. Tourette syndrome is commonly associated with attention-deficit disorder or obsessive–compulsive disorder, as well as anxiety mood disorders and attention-deficit/hyperactivity disorder (ADHD; Kossoff and Singer 2001; Faridi and Suchowersky 2003; Lombroso and Scahill 2008; Hirschtritt et al. 2015; Gunduz and Okun 2016).

A major challenge for both clinical and epidemiological investigations is the lack of laboratory or radiographic diagnostic tests for tic disorders or Tourette syndrome. Furthermore, distinguishing Tourette syndrome from simple tic disorders by using medical record review and self-reported data is difficult at best.

Pathophysiology

The tics and other movement abnormalities in Tourette syndrome are considered to be a manifestation of disinhibition within the cortico-striato-thalamo circuits of the brain. The exact cause of the abnormality manifested by tics is not known, but is hypothesized to be an abnormality of the gamma-aminobutyric acid (GABA) system (Thenganatt and Jankovic 2016).

Descriptive Epidemiology

Tic disorders are very common among children, but the published estimates range considerably with the methods used. The prevalence of Tourette syndrome has been reported to be as low as five per 10,000 and as high as 3.8%. Overall, the best estimates for the prevalence of Tourette syndrome, including relatively mild cases, are approximately 1% of the childhood population between the ages of 5 and 18 years. Boys have a higher prevalence of Tourette syndrome than girls, with male-to-female ratios reported to be as high as 4.7 to 1. Tourette syndrome seems to occur worldwide (Hirschtritt et al. 2015).

Causes

Tourette syndrome has a strong familial predisposition, although parents are often diagnosed as a result of manifestations in their children, underscoring the likely underascertainment from medical record reviews (Faridi and Suchowersky 2003). Evidence of linkage to the centromeric region of chromosome five in a single large family with Tourette syndrome has been reported (Laurin et al. 2009). Recently a few candidate susceptibility genes have been reported (Bertelsen et al. 2016).

The association of simple tics with Group A beta-hemolytic streptococci has been reported, but this association has been questioned as a causal factor for chronic tic disorders (Harris and Singer 2006), and has also not been found to be a causal factor in exacerbations of tic and obsessive–compulsive symptoms (Leckman et al. 2011).

Evidence-Based Interventions

There are no proven methods for preventing tic disorders or Tourette syndrome. Management of the behavioral and learning (attention-deficit) comorbid conditions is important, and public health professionals should be aware of the mental health needs of people with Tourette syndrome (Gunduz and Okun 2016).

Areas of Future Research

Future epidemiological studies of Tourette syndrome will need to address the potential factors (genetic and environmental) that might have an impact on the severity of these tic disorders, with an emphasis on factors that may exacerbate tics in susceptible individuals.

TRAUMATIC BRAIN INJURY

Significance

Traumatic brain injury is a leading cause of long-term disability and death in the United States and worldwide. In the United States alone, more than 1.4 million people experience TBI, and more than 53,000 people die each year from TBI. Traumatic brain injury contributes to about 30% of all injury-related

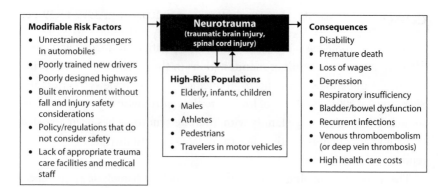

Figure 19-3. Neurotrauma: Causes, Consequences, and High-Risk Groups

deaths in the United States (Coronado et al. 2011). An estimated 7.7 million people in Europe and 5.3 million people in the United States are living with TBI-related disability (Horton 2012; Peeters et al. 2015). The disability-adjusted life year burden of abusive head trauma among children aged 0 to 4 years in the United States far exceeds the disability-adjusted life years burden for all severe burns in the United States (Miller et al. 2014).

The high estimates of disability after TBI are probably underestimates. For example, as we have learned from chronic traumatic encephalopathy in athletes, the clinical manifestations of cognitive decline, depression, and emotional disturbances may occur years to decades after the repeated traumatic insults occur (Pan et al. 2016). Because chronic traumatic encephalopathy is currently only diagnosed reliably at autopsy, it is certainly underdiagnosed. Figure 19-3 lists the major neurotroma causes, consequences, and high-risk groups.

Descriptive Epidemiology

Differences in TBI study methods make comparisons between studies difficult without careful consideration of inclusion and exclusion criteria for each study. The annual incidence of TBI in the United States is approximately 180 to 250 per 100,000. Male persons and people living in lower socioeconomic regions tend to have higher rates. The very young, adolescents, young adults, and the elderly are also at higher risk for TBI. The associated annual mortality rate in the United States decreased from 25 per 100,000 in 1979 to 19 per 100,000 in 1992 (Thurman et al. 1999; Bruns and Hauser 2003; Langlois et al. 2006; Coronado et al. 2011).

Causes

In the United States, firearms (34.8%), motor vehicle crashes (31.4%), and falls (16.7%) are the leading causes of TBI-related deaths (Coronado et al. 2011). Alcohol and drug use are interactive risk factors for motor vehicle crashes, falls, transportation-related injuries and automobile crashes, sports or recreation injuries, and assaults. Workers in specific occupations such as construction, farming, roofing, and logging are at especially high risk of TBI (Thurman et al. 1999; Bruns and Hauser 2003; Rutland-Brown et al. 2006).

Evidence-Based Interventions

Policies that promote evidence-based prevention have been the most helpful interventions for preventing TBI. Since 1980, overall there has been a decrease in TBI-related death in the United States. The largest decrease has been in motor vehicle crash–related deaths, primarily because of increased use of seat belts, airbags, child safety seats, and motorcycle helmets. Graduated licensing of young drivers, driver's education courses, and gradual improvements in public policy and safety laws have also contributed to declines in motor vehicle crash–related deaths (Liu et al. 2008; Coronado et al. 2011; Olsen et al. 2016). Primary prevention efforts for preventing TBI include both modifications of the built environment and policy changes (Olsen et al. 2016). Brain injury prevention through improved vehicle and road design, better separation between pedestrian walkways and major highways, prevention of falls (especially in the elderly), and prevention of work-related injuries are all important areas of intervention (Langlois et al. 2006; GBD Pediatrics Collaboration et al. 2016).

Preventing falls and reducing brain injuries among the elderly begins with making living areas safer by (1) removing tripping hazards (e.g., throw rugs), (2) using nonslip mats in bathtubs and showers, (3) installing handrails on both sides of stairways, (4) installing grab bars next to toilets and in showers and tubs, (5) enhancing the lighting throughout homes, and (6) providing opportunities for regular physical activity. Preventing falls among children also requires making living areas safer by (1) installing window guards to keep young children from falling out of open windows, (2) using safety gates at the top and the bottom of stairs when young children are present, and (3) building surfaces on playgrounds made of shock-absorbing material such as hardwood mulch or sand (Qin and Baccaglini 2016; Verma et al. 2016). Building codes and policies that require and enforce these prevention measures offer opportunities for brain injury prevention (Mack et al. 2015).

Policies that require and enforce the use of bicycle and motorcycle helmets, seatbelts, and speed limits have been proven to reduce serious head injuries. Children and parents should know that helmets should also be worn when playing contact sports (e.g., football, hockey, boxing, wrestling), using in-line skates or riding skateboards, batting or running bases in baseball or softball, riding a horse, or skiing and snowboarding (Liu et al. 2008; Benson et al. 2009; Mack et al. 2015).

Further reductions in brain injuries among young children can be achieved by following the evidence-based guidelines for preventing motor vehicle crash-related injuries (CIVPP and Durbin 2011). Likewise, public education efforts combined with policies that reduce alcohol- and drug-related crashes and injuries have been helpful, but can be improved.

SPINAL CORD INJURY

Significance

According to the Spinal Cord Injury Information Network at the University of Alabama, Birmingham, about 12,500 Americans sustain an SCI each year. Estimates from several years ago suggested that in the United States there were about 276,000 people with some form of disability attributable to previous SCI. Male patients account for about 80% of new SCI cases. The most common causes of SCI vary by age. Among people aged 65 years and older, most injury is caused by falls—many of which are preventable. Overall, the leading cause of SCI among people aged younger than 65 years is motor vehicle crashes. Sports and other recreational activities are responsible for about 20% of all SCI and are more common among adolescents and young adults (NSCISC 2015).

Secondary medical conditions and comorbidities are a major health issue for the developed world, where more people survive SCIs than in years past. Airway management problems, secondary pulmonary conditions and pneumonia, urinary tract infections, pressure sores, spasticity, deep vein thrombosis, osteoporosis, and scoliosis are all major secondary conditions that have their own opportunities for secondary prevention efforts (Meyers et al. 2000). The annual cost to the United States for SCIs is estimated at more than $10 billion. The average lifetime cost for a typical 25-year-old person with SCI varies by the severity (or spinal cord level) of the injury and has recently been estimated to be between $682,000 for an incomplete motor impairment and more than $3 million for a complete high-cervical (C1–C4) injury (NSCISC 2015).

Descriptive Epidemiology

The estimated incidence of SCI in the United States every year is about 40 per million. Worldwide, the incidence of SCI varies from 12 per million to about 60 per million. Throughout the world, the incidence of SCI shows a bimodal age distribution, with the first peak at ages 15 to 29 years, and a second peak among adults aged 65 years and older (van den Berg et al. 2010). The prevalence is estimated at 11 to 112 per 100,000, but recently emerging estimates suggest that these may be significant underestimates. Overall mortality from SCI is very high but has declined considerably over the past several decades. The reduction in SCI-associated mortality rates, as well as the rising prevalence estimates of people living with disability, is attributable in part to improvements in emergency medical services (especially emergency neurosurgical care), development of specialty centers for care, improved professional training, and reduction in the death rates from infections and other secondary conditions (van den Berg et al. 2010; Furlan et al. 2013; NSCISC 2015).

Causes

Spinal cord injury primarily occurs among adolescents and young adults. Over the past decade, approximately 75% of SCIs have occurred among male individuals. Since 2005, about 42% have been the result of motor vehicle crashes, with falls (27%), violence (15%), and sports and recreational injuries (7.4%) also significantly contributing to the total burden. As with TBI, alcohol and drug use significantly contribute to the risk of SCI (van den Berg et al. 2010). The three most common causes of SCI throughout the world are motor vehicle crashes, falls, and violence (Furlan 2013).

Evidence-Based Interventions

As noted in the prevention of TBI, improving the built environment, promoting policies that improve safety, and prevention education for the community can all lead to improved primary prevention of SCI.

For those with SCI, outcomes are better with skilled trauma care and with a well-coordinated emergency medical system—including emergency trauma center systems that cross state lines and national borders when saving time saves lives and improves outcomes (Rubiano et al. 2015). Emphasizing the coordination among public health surveillance, primary prevention programs, and emergency medical systems in any health care reform measures will enhance prevention efforts.

ATTENTION-DEFICIT/HYPERACTIVITY DISORDER

Attention-deficit/hyperactivity disorder is a syndrome defined by diagnostic criteria detailed in the 5th edition of *Diagnostic and Statistical Manual of Mental Disorders* (*DSM-5*), with onset during preschool years and characterized by problems with attention, impulsivity, and overactivity (APA 2013). Anxiety, conduct disorder, learning disorders, obsessive–compulsive disorder, epilepsy, tic disorders, depression, bipolar disorder, and sleep disorders all occur more commonly among children and adults with ADHD than in the general population. People with ADHD are more likely than their peers in the general population to have problems with substance abuse and to smoke cigarettes (McClernon and Kollins 2008; Thapar and Cooper 2016).

Significance

Attention-deficit/hyperactivity disorder is strongly associated with various behavior problems, including oppositional defiant behavior disorder and conduct disorders. The subgroup of children with ADHD and conduct disorder has higher risk for neurocognitive impairment (Jensen and Steinhausen 2015). Attention-deficit/hyperactivity disorder tends to persist into adulthood, and may predict serious antisocial behavior, involvement with police, and substance misuse in adolescence (Langley et al. 2010; Thapar and Cooper 2016).

The occurrence of comorbid conditions among adults with ADHD is beginning to receive attention by investigators. Adolescents and young adults with ADHD have high rates of suicidal ideations and suicide attempts compared to the general population (Chou et al. 2016). Treatment of ADHD with medication seems to reduce the risk of concurrent and subsequent depression (Chang et al. 2016).

Pathophysiology

Neural connections between the prefrontal cortex and the striatum of the brain (the caudate nuclei and the putamen) have been identified as areas of dysfunction among people with ADHD. Other studies have suggested that, although the frontal and prefrontal areas of the brain are clearly implicated in the pathophysiology of ADHD, more posterior regions of the brain are involved as well. Systems involving visual attention and orientation seem to be especially important (Amso and Scerif 2015; Thapar and Cooper 2016). When performing cognitive tasks, people with ADHD tend to activate broader regions of the cortex than do people who have less difficulty focusing—probably explaining the tendency of people with ADHD to have problems with distraction (Brennan and Arnsten 2008).

Descriptive Epidemiology

Attention-deficit/hyperactivity disorder occurs in about 3% to 4% of all school-age children (95% CI=2.6, 4.5) according to a recent meta-analysis, and is estimated to affect about 2% to 4% of adults in the United States. School-age boys are almost three times more likely to be diagnosed with ADHD as are girls. Trends in the true frequency of ADHD in the general population are difficult to determine, as the prevalence rates increase as community awareness is enhanced and as treatments for ADHD are made available and promoted. Although reported prevalence rates of ADHD among school-age children in the United States are higher than 30 years ago, it is clear that children with signs and symptoms were reported early in the 20th century (Still 1902), and prevalence rates now are not substantially different from those rates reported in the late 20th century (Thapar and Cooper 2016). Prevalence rates for ADHD vary by use of diagnostic criteria in different areas of the United States, with significant differences in treatment patterns from one part of the United States to the other. Once considered to be a disorder of childhood, ADHD is now known to occur commonly among adults—perhaps in as many as 4% of all adults (Stein and Shin 2008; Thapar and Cooper 2016).

Causes

Attention-deficit/hyperactivity disorder is a familial disorder, and the genetics of ADHD have been explored with both twin studies and traditional family genetic studies. About 76% of ADHD is said to be attributable to inherited genetic susceptibility, similar to what has been reported in autism and in schizophrenia (Thapar et al. 2013). Most cases of ADHD are multifactorial and involve the interaction of many different genes, or single nucleotide polymorphisms. However, there are genetic syndromes (e.g., fragile X syndrome, tuberous sclerosis complex, 22q11 microdeletion, and Williams syndrome) with very high rates of ADHD (Bastain et al. 2002). Recently a synaptosomal-associated protein (SNAP-25), a presynaptic plasma membrane protein expressed specifically in neuronal cells, has been found to have several polymorphisms associated with ADHD in both family studies and in case–control studies (Liu et al. 2016).

Evidence-Based Interventions

Primary prevention opportunities for ADHD are limited. However, given the high frequency of comorbid conditions among adolescents and adults who were diagnosed with ADHD as children, identification of children with ADHD identifies those who are at higher risk of cigarette smoking, substance abuse, depression, and other mental illnesses; therefore, opportunities for focused health promotion efforts should become an emphasis among public health professionals. The diagnosis and management of the child with ADHD has benefited in recent years by the development of consensus guidelines for diagnosis, evaluation, and treatment. Early diagnosis and treatment can prevent school failure and improve long-term academic and social outcomes (Thapar and Cooper 2016).

CARPAL TUNNEL SYNDROME

Carpal tunnel syndrome, the most common entrapment neuropathy, is caused by entrapment of the median nerve at the wrist as it passes under the transverse carpal ligament, and results in sensory changes (numb tingling, pain) and weakness of the muscles of the hand. Symptoms of CTS are exacerbated at night during sleep, and occur frequently among pregnant women and among workers who engage in repetitive fine motor movements of the fingers and wrists (e.g., typists). The diagnosis is made on the basis of typical history and examination findings consistent with an inflamed and dysfunctional median nerve distal to the wrist. Diagnosis of CTS is aided by abnormal median nerve conduction studies (LeBlanc and Cestia 2011; Osterman et al. 2012).

Significance

If untreated, CTS may result in hand numbness and weakness with lost productivity.

Descriptive Epidemiology

There appears to be increased reporting and diagnosis of CTS over the past few decades, possibly with the introduction of improved diagnostic techniques. In Rochester, Minnesota, the adjusted annual rates increased from 258 per 100,000 in 1981 through 1985 to 424 in 2000 through 2005. One study from Sweden reported a prevalence of about 3.8% in the general population of adults, and, across multiple studies, CTS prevalence is about 3% to 6% of adults (Atroshi et al. 1999; Gelfman et al. 2009; LeBlanc and Cestia 2011).

Causes

Wrist trauma is strongly associated with development of CTS. However, other risk factors, such as diabetes, hypothyroidism, pregnancy, and repetitive hand or wrist movements, probably account for a higher proportion of cases. Food-processing workers, roofers, carpenters, and mill workers seem to have especially high rates of CTS. Office workers who spend long hours typing are likewise at high risk for CTS, although recently published cohort studies do not show a relationship between computer work and new cases of CTS among workers in diverse jobs with varying job exposures. The increasing rates of obesity may contribute to the increasing rates of CTS (Farmer and Davis 2008; LeBlanc and Cestia 2011).

Evidence-Based Interventions

Enhancing worker safety programs and training in ergonomics hazard prevention in the workplace can prevent CTS. Screening tools to identify workers at risk have been used by many industries, and enhance targeted ergonomic interventions that can prevent CTS. Prevention of obesity and early diagnosis and nonsurgical management of CTS can reduce morbidity and time lost from work (LeBlanc and Cestia 2011).

LOW BACK PAIN

About two thirds of adults in the United States experience low back pain at some point in their lives, and it is one of the most common reasons adults consult a physician. Concern has been raised by many investigators about overtreatment of low back pain by physicians, with excessive use of expensive imaging studies that do not alter management, and perhaps excessive numbers of low back surgeries (Balagué et al. 2012).

Significance and Descriptive Epidemiology

Approximately 2% of all workers in the United States report disabling back pain each year. Reported rates of low back pain are higher in lower socioeconomic classes (Karahan et al. 2009; Balagué et al. 2012). Among people with acute low back pain, recovery usually occurs within a few weeks regardless of treatment. Low levels of pain and occasional disability persist from 3 to at least 12 months after onset of pain for some people with low back pain. Most people return to work one month after onset of low back pain, and about 90% of people return to work by three months after onset of low back pain. A majority of people with new-onset low back pain will have at least one recurrence within a year. Because low back pain is so common, a small percentage of people who have longer-term pain or significant disability account for a significant burden of disability, morbidity, and lost productivity (Balagué et al. 2012).

Causes

High-risk occupations include hospital nursing, prolonged truck driving, dock work, warehouse work, farm work, lumber work, mining, construction work, and other occupations that involve frequent heavy lifting. Cigarette smoking, premature menopause, and abdominal obesity all increase the risk of low back pain (Adera et al. 1994; Shiri et al. 2010a; Shiri et al.2010b). A genetic susceptibility, especially with a genetic interaction with obesity, is associated with low back pain and lumbar disc degeneration (Battie et al. 2007; Dario et al. 2015).

Evidence-Based Interventions

Generalized prevention efforts have not been proven effective in the general population. However, among those who have had an episode of low back pain, a combination of exercises that strengthen the paraspinous and abdominal muscles, maintaining correct posture, and lifting objects properly can help prevent injuries and recurrences of low back pain. Improvements in the built environment can reduce the risk of low back pain among workers in high-risk populations. Improved ergonomic design in vehicles and high-risk workplaces, as well as education on lifting techniques and strength conditioning may further reduce risk of back injuries (Balagué et al. 2012).

MIGRAINE AND TENSION-TYPE HEADACHE

Almost everyone experiences headache at some time. Headaches are a very common reason for adolescents and adults to visit a physician. About one third of men and approximately one half of women experience episodic tension-type headache. For most of these people, their headaches have minimal impact on their lives, but for the small percentage of people who have evolution of chronic daily headache, the degree of impairment and even disability can be significant. An estimated 20% of women and about 5% to 10% of men experience migraine (Schwedt 2014; Barnes 2015).

Significance

Migraine is among the more prevalent disabling neurological disorders. Children with migraine average twice as many days absent from school as children without migraine headaches (Mack 2009). Throughout the world, migraine is one of the leading causes of disability, especially among children and young adults (GBD Pediatrics Collaboration et al. 2016), and yet migraine is generally considered a low health care priority in most countries (WHO 2011).

Descriptive Epidemiology

The International Headache Society diagnostic criteria for migraine have become the gold standard used by clinicians (HCSIHS 2004). Yet the practical application of headache classification schemes in the general population is difficult, as the distinction between migraine and other types of headache is often blurred. Given these methodological issues, the average annual incidence of severe headache has been estimated at 0.5%. Migraine typically presents in childhood or adolescence, with new onset of migraine after age 40 years being very rare. Migraine prevalence is two to four times higher among women than men and is twice as high among low-income populations. Exacerbation of migraine headaches during or after menopause is common among women (Merikangas 2013).

Causes

A positive family history, depression, epilepsy, female sex, and low socioeconomic status are all risk factors for migraine headaches (Haan et al. 2008; Martin and Lipton 2008; Bigal et al. 2007). Given the high frequency of maternal migraine history among people with migraine, a mitochondrial DNA pattern of inheritance has long been hypothesized. Recent reports have verified that two common mitochondrial DNA polymorphisms are highly associated with migraine headache, and likely account for a very high proportion of familial cases of migraine (Zaki et al. 2009). Depression and stress have long been known to be important risk factors for other types of headaches (Jensen and Stovner 2008).

Among people with headaches, especially migraine, specific triggers that precipitate headaches are well defined and require that clinicians and patients become familiar with the triggers unique to each person affected. The most common triggers include onset of menses, dietary changes or specific foods (cheeses, chocolate, nuts), extreme fatigue, or variation in sleep patterns. Patient surveys have been developed to identify potential triggers in order to develop prevention strategies (Kelman 2007). Excessive use of painkillers, including narcotics for headache, can cause rather than cure or prevent headaches (Hawkes 2012).

Evidence-Based Interventions

Among people with migraine headaches, a medical home, sustained care, and education that allows them to learn their own triggers with the help of their physician offer the best opportunity for improving quality of life and preventing headaches. Although chronic stress is a major contributor to episodic tension-type headache, prevention of chronic stress involves major upstream interventions to address the social determinants of health. Proper diet and regular adequate sleep are important for minimizing headaches among most people with migraine.

People with frequent migraine headaches often benefit from daily prophylactic treatment; medications such as propranolol, tricyclic drugs, and cyproheptadine have all been helpful. Drugs that can abort migraine attacks if given early in the course of a headache, such as ergotamine tartrate and sumatriptan, can be helpful but require careful expert medical management to minimize adverse events (Diener et al. 2015; Richer et al. 2016). People with disabling episodic tension-type headache, especially those with chronic daily headache, benefit from stress management and psychophysiological techniques such as biofeedback (Smitherman et al. 2015); treatment for coexisting depression is sometimes important for people with chronic daily headaches (Zebenholzer et al. 2016).

Resources
Alzheimer's Disease

Alzheimer's Association, http://www.alz.org

Alzheimer's Foundation of America, http://www.alzfdn.org

Autism Spectrum Disorder

Autism Science Foundation, http://autismsciencefoundation.org

Autism Society of America, http://www.autism-society.org

The Interactive Autism Network Project, http://www.ianresearch.org

Simons Foundation Autism Research Initiative, http://sfari.org

Parkinson's Disease

American Parkinson Disease Association, http://www.apdaparkinson.org

Michael J. Fox Foundation for Parkinson's Research, https://www.michaeljfox.org

National Parkinson Foundation Inc., http://www.parkinson.org

Parkinson's Disease Foundation, http://www.pdf.org

Epilepsy

Citizens United for Research in Epilepsy, http://www.cureepilepsy.org

Epilepsy Foundation of America, http://www.epilepsyfoundation.org

Other Neurological Disorders

Brain Injury Association of America, http://www.biausa.org

Muscular Dystrophy Association, http://www.mda.org

National Headache Foundation, http://www.headaches.org

National Multiple Sclerosis Society, http://www.nationalmssociety.org

Paralyzed Veterans of America, Spinal Cord Research Foundation, http://www.pva.org

Tourette Syndrome Association of America, http://www.tourette.org

Suggested Readings

Alzheimer's Association. 2015 Alzheimer's disease facts and figures. *Alzheimers Dement.* 2015;11(3):332–384.

Boivin MJ, Kakooza AM, Warf BC, Davidson LL, Grigorenko EL. Reducing neurodevelopmental disorders and disability through research and interventions. *Nature.* 2015;527(7578):S155–S160.

England MJ, Liverman CT, Schultz AM, Strawbridge LM, eds. *Epilepsy Across the Spectrum: Promoting Health and Understanding.* Washington, DC: National Academies Press; 2012.

Estes A, Munson J, Rogers SJ, Greenson J, Winter J, Dawson G. Long-term outcomes of early intervention in 6-year-old children with autism spectrum disorder. *J Am Acad Child Adolesc Psychiatry.* 2015;54(7):580–587.

Garfinkle J, Wintermark P, Shevell MI, Platt RW, Oskoui M, Canadian Cerebral Palsy Registry. Cerebral palsy after neonatal encephalopathy: how much is preventable? *J Pediatr.* 2015;167(1):58–63.e51.

Global Burden of Disease Pediatrics Collaboration, Kyu HH, Pinho C, et al. Global and national burden of diseases and injuries among children and adolescents between 1990 and 2013: findings from the Global Burden of Disease 2013 study. *JAMA Pediatr.* 2016;170(3):267–287.

Hemphill D, Centers for Disease Control and Prevention. Surveillance for traumatic brain injury–related deaths—United States, 1997–2007. *MMWR Surveill Summ.* 2011; 60(5):1–32.

Kiernan MC, Vucic S, Cheah BC, Turner MR, Eisen A, Hardiman O, Burrell JR, Zoing MC. Amyotrophic lateral sclerosis. *Lancet.* 2011;377(9769):942–955.

Kim CJ, Romero R, Chaemsaithong P, Chaiyasit N, Yoon BH, Kim YM. Acute chorio-amnionitis and funisitis: definition, pathologic features, and clinical significance. *Am J Obstet Gynecol.* 2015; 213(4 suppl):S29–S52.

LeBlanc KE, Cestia W. Carpal tunnel syndrome. *Am Fam Physician.* 2011;83(8):952–958.

Mack KA, Liller KD, Baldwin G, Sleet D. Preventing unintentional injuries in the home using the Health Impact Pyramid. *Health Educ Behav.* 2015;42(1 suppl):115S–122S.

Olsen CS, Thomas AM, Singleton M, et al. Motorcycle helmet effectiveness in reducing head, face and brain injuries by state and helmet law. *Inj Epidemiol.* 2016;3:8.

Qin Z, Baccaglini L. Distribution, determinants, and prevention of falls among the elderly in the 2011–2012 California Health Interview Survey. *Public Health Rep.* 2016;131(2):331–339.

Thapar A, Cooper M. Attention deficit hyperactivity disorder. *Lancet.* 2016;387(10024): 1240–1250.

Thurman DJ, Hesdorffer DC, French JA. Sudden unexpected death in epilepsy: assessing the public health burden. *Epilepsia.* 2014;55(10):1479–1485.

World Health Organization. *Atlas of Headache Disorders and Resources in the World 2011.* Geneva, Switzerland: World Health Organization; 2011.

References

Adera T, Deyo RA, Donatelle RJ. Premature menopause and low back pain. A population-based study. *Ann Epidemiol.* 1994;4(5):416–422.

Adler CH, Beach TG. Neuropathological basis of nonmotor manifestations of Parkinson's disease. *Mov Disord.* 2016;31(8):1114–1119.

Allen MC. Neurodevelopmental outcomes of preterm infants. *Curr Opin Neurol* 2008;21(2):123–128.

Almeida LR, Valenca GT, Negreiros NN, Pinto EB, Oliveira-Filho J. Recurrent falls in people with Parkinson's disease without cognitive impairment: focusing on modifiable risk factors. *Parkinsons Dis.* 2014;2014:432924.

Alonso A, Hernán MA. Temporal trends in the incidence of multiple sclerosis: a systematic review. *Neurology.* 2008;71(2):129–135.

Alvarez-Lafuente R, Garcia-Montojo M, De Las Heras V, et al. Herpesviruses and human endogenous retroviral sequences in the cerebrospinal fluid of multiple sclerosis patients. *Mult Scler.* 2008;14(5):595–601.

Alzheimer's Association. 2015 Alzheimer's disease facts and figures. *Alzheimers Dement.* 2015;11(3):332–384.

American Psychiatric Association (APA). *Diagnostic and Statistical Manual of Mental Disorders.* 5th ed. Washington, DC: APA; 2013.

Amso D, Scerif G. The attentive brain: insights from developmental cognitive neuroscience. *Nat Rev Neurosci.* 2015;16(10):606–619.

Angeles DC, Ho P, Dymock BW, Lim KL, Zhou ZD, Tan EK. Antioxidants inhibit neuronal toxicity in Parkinson's disease-linked LRRK2. *Ann Clin Transl Neurol.* 2016;3(4):288–294.

Anstey KJ, von Sanden C, Salim A, O'Kearney R. Smoking as a risk factor for dementia and cognitive decline: a meta-analysis of prospective studies. *Am J Epidemiol.* 2007;166(4):367–378.

Aronica E, Gorter JA. Gene expression profile in temporal lobe epilepsy. *Neuroscientist.* 2007;13(2):100–108.Atroshi I, Gummesson C, Johnsson R, Ornstein E, Ranstam J, Rosen I. Prevalence of carpal tunnel syndrome in a general population. *JAMA.* 1999;282(2):153–158.

Atta CA, Fiest KM, Frolkis AD, et al. Global birth prevalence of spina bifida by folic acid fortification status: a systematic review and meta-analysis. *Am J Public Health.* 2016;106(1):e24–e34.

Autry AR, Trevathan E, Van Naarden Braun K, Yeargin-Allsopp M. Increased risk of death among children with Lennox-Gastaut syndrome and infantile spasms. *J Child Neurol.* 2010;25(4):441–447.

Balagué F, Mannion AF, Pellise F, Cedraschi C. Non-specific low back pain. *Lancet.* 2012;379(9814):482–491.

Barker RA, Parmar M, Kirkeby A, Bjorklund A, Thompson L, Brundin P. Are stem cell-based therapies for Parkinson's disease ready for the clinic in 2016? *J Parkinsons Dis.* 2016;6(1):57–63.

Barnes NP. Migraine headache in children. *BMJ Clin Evid.* 2015;2015:pii:0318.

Bastain TM, Lewczyk CM, Sharp WS, et al. Cytogenetic abnormalities in attention-deficit/hyperactivity disorder. *J Am Acad Child Adolesc Psychiatry.* 2002;41(7):806–810.

Battie MC, Videman T, Levalahti E, Gill K, Kaprio J. Heritability of low back pain and the role of disc degeneration. *Pain.* 2007;131(3):272–280.

Benson BW, Hamilton GM, Meeuwisse WH, McCrory P, Dvorak J. Is protective equipment useful in preventing concussion? A systematic review of the literature. *Br J Sports Med.* 2009;43(suppl 1):i56–i67.

Berg AT, Berkovic SF, Brodie MJ, et al. Revised terminology and concepts for organization of seizures and epilepsies: report of the ILAE Commission on Classification and Terminology, 2005–2009. *Epilepsia*. 2010;51(4):676–685.

Berkovic SF, Harkin L, McMahon JM, et al. De-novo mutations of the sodium channel gene SCN1A in alleged vaccine encephalopathy: a retrospective study. *Lancet Neurol*. 2006;5(6):488–492.

Bertelsen B, Stefansson H, Riff Jensen L, et al. Association of AADAC deletion and Gilles de la Tourette syndrome in a large European cohort. *Biol Psychiatry*. 2016;79(5):383–391.

Bertram L, Tanzi RE. Thirty years of Alzheimer's disease genetics: the implications of systematic meta-analyses. *Nat Rev Neurosci*. 2008;9(10):768–778.

Beydoun MA, Beydoun HA, Gamaldo AA, Teel A, Zonderman AB, Wang Y. Epidemiologic studies of modifiable factors associated with cognition and dementia: systematic review and meta-analysis. *BMC Public Health*. 2014;14:643.

Bigal ME, Lipton RB, Winner P, et al. Migraine in adolescents: association with socioeconomic status and family history. *Neurology* 2007:69(1):16–25.

Birbeck GL, Hays RD, Cui X, Vickrey BG. Seizure reduction and quality of life improvements in people with epilepsy. *Epilepsia*. 2002;43(5):535–538.

Birbeck GL, Kalichi EM. Epilepsy prevalence in rural Zambia: a door-to-door survey. *Trop Med Int Health*. 2004;9(1):92–95.

Boivin MJ, Kakooza AM, Warf BC, Davidson LL, Grigorenko EL. Reducing neurodevelopmental disorders and disability through research and interventions. *Nature*. 2015;527(7578):S155–S160.

Bozzoni V, Pansarasa O, Diamanti L, Nosari G, Cereda C, Ceroni M. Amyotrophic lateral sclerosis and environmental factors. *Funct Neurol*. 2016;31(1):7–19.

Bradford A, Kunik ME, Schulz P, Williams SP, Singh H. Missed and delayed diagnosis of dementia in primary care: prevalence and contributing factors. *Alzheimer Dis Assoc Disord*. 2009;23(4):306–314.

Breckenridge CB, Berry C, Chang ET, Sielken RL Jr, Mandel JS. Association between Parkinson's disease and cigarette smoking, rural living, well-water consumption, farming and pesticide use: systematic review and meta-analysis. *PLoS One*. 2016;11(4): e0151841.

Brennan AR, Arnsten AF. Neuronal mechanisms underlying attention deficit hyperactivity disorder: the influence of arousal on prefrontal cortical function. *Ann N Y Acad Sci*. 2008;1129:236–245.

Brugha TS, McManus S, Bankart J, et al. Epidemiology of autism spectrum disorders in adults in the community in England. *Arch Gen Psychiatry.* 2011;68(5):459–465.

Bruns J Jr, Hauser WA. The epidemiology of traumatic brain injury: a review. *Epilepsia.* 2003;44(suppl 10):2–10.

Burns TN. Guillain-Barré syndrome. *Semin Neurol.* 2008;28(2):152–167.

Camfield P, Camfield C. Febrile seizures and genetic epilepsy with febrile seizures plus (GEFS+). *Epileptic Disord.* 2015;17(2):124–133.

Centers for Disease Control and Prevention (CDC). About one-half of adults with active epilepsy and seizures have annual family incomes under $25,000: the 2010 and 2013 US National Health Interview Surveys. *Epilepsy Behav.* 2016a;58:33–34.

Centers for Disease Control and Prevention (CDC). Learn the signs. Act early. 2016b. Available at: http://www.cdc.gov/ncbddd/actearly/index.html. Accessed August 29, 2016.

Chadwick D, Smith D. The misdiagnosis of epilepsy. *BMJ.* 2002;324(7336):495–496.

Chang Z, D'Onofrio BM, Quinn PD, Lichtenstein P, Larsson H. Medication for attention-deficit/hyperactivity disorder and risk for depression: a nationwide longitudinal cohort study. *Biol Psychiatry.* 2016 [Epub ahead of print February 23, 2016].

Chevalier J, Chamoux C, Hammes F, Chicoye A. Cost-effectiveness of treatments for relapsing remitting multiple sclerosis: a French societal perspective. *PLoS One.* 2016;11(3):e0150703.

Chio A, Logroscino G, Traynor BJ, et al. Global epidemiology of amyotrophic lateral sclerosis: a systematic review of the published literature. *Neuroepidemiology.* 2013;41(2): 118–130.

Chou WJ, Liu TL, Hu HF, Yen CF. Suicidality and its relationships with individual, family, peer, and psychopathology factors among adolescents with attention-deficit/ hyperactivity disorder. *Res Dev Disabil.* 2016;53–54:86–94.

Christensen DL, Baio J, Braun KV, et al. Prevalence and characteristics of autism spectrum disorder among children aged 8 years—autism and developmental disabilities monitoring network, 11 sites, United States, 2012. *MMWR Surveill Summ.* 2016a;65(3): 1–23.

Christensen DL, Bilder DA, Zahorodny W, et al. Prevalence and characteristics of autism spectrum disorder among 4-year-old children in the autism and developmental disabilities monitoring network. *J Dev Behav Pediatr.* 2016b;37(1):1–8.

Committee on Injury, Violence, and Poison Prevention (CIVPP), Durbin DR. Child passenger safety. *Pediatrics.* 2011;127(4):788–793.

Coronado VG, Xu L, Basavaraju SV, et al. Surveillance for traumatic brain injury–related deaths—United States, 1997–2007. *MMWR Surveill Summ.* 2011;60(5):1–32.

Corti O, Lesage S, Brice A. What genetics tells us about the causes and mechanisms of Parkinson's disease. *Physiol Rev.* 2011;91(4):1161–1218.

Craft S, Cholerton B, Baker LD. Insulin and Alzheimer's disease: untangling the web. *J Alzheimers Dis.* 2013;33(suppl 1):S263–S275.

Dario AB, Ferreira ML, Refshauge KM, Lima TS, Ordonana JR, Ferreira PH. The relationship between obesity, low back pain, and lumbar disc degeneration when genetics and the environment are considered: a systematic review of twin studies. *Spine J.* 2015;15(5):1106–1117.

de la Torre-Ubieta L, Won H, Stein JL, Geschwind DH. Advancing the understanding of autism disease mechanisms through genetics. *Nat Med.* 2016;22(4):345–361.

Debouverie M, Pittion-Vouyovitch S, Brissart H, Guillemin F. Physical dimension of fatigue correlated with disability change over time in patients with multiple sclerosis. *J Neurol.* 2008a;255(5):633–636.

Debouverie M, Pittion-Vouyovitch S, Louis S, Guillemin F, Group L. Natural history of multiple sclerosis in a population-based cohort. *Eur J Neurol.* 2008b;15(9):916–921.

Diamond ML, Ritter AC, Failla MD, et al. IL-1beta associations with posttraumatic epilepsy development: a genetics and biomarker cohort study. *Epilepsia.* 2015;56(7):991–1001.

Diener HC, Charles A, Goadsby PJ, Holle D. New therapeutic approaches for the prevention and treatment of migraine. *Lancet Neurol.* 2015;14(10):1010–1022.

Dimario FJ Jr, Edwards C. Autonomic dysfunction in childhood Guillain-Barré syndrome. *J Child Neurol.* 2012;27(5):581–586.

Doyle LW, Crowther CA, Middleton P, Marret S, Rouse D. Magnesium sulphate for women at risk of preterm birth for neuroprotection of the fetus. *Cochrane Database Syst Rev.* 2009;(1):CD004661.

Drago D, Bolognin S, Zatta P. Role of metal ions in the abeta oligomerization in Alzheimer's disease and in other neurological disorders. *Curr Alzheimer Res.* 2008;5(6):500–507.

Duncan JS, Sander JW, Sisodiya SM, Walker MC. Adult epilepsy. *Lancet.* 2006;367(9516):1087–1100.

Durkin MS, Maenner MJ, Newschaffer CJ, et al. Advanced parental age and the risk of autism spectrum disorder. *Am J Epidemiol.* 2008;168(11):1268–1276.

Editors. Retraction—Ileal-lymphoid-nodular hyperplasia, non-specific colitis, and pervasive developmental disorder in children. *Lancet.* 2010;375(9713):445.

Elbaz A, Carcaillon L, Kab S, Moisan F. Epidemiology of Parkinson's disease. *Rev Neurol (Paris).* 2016;172(1):14–26.

England MJ, Liverman CT, Schultz AM, Strawbridge LM, eds. *Epilepsy Across the Spectrum: Promoting Health and Understanding.* Washington, DC: National Academies Press; 2012.

Estes A, Munson J, Rogers SJ, Greenson J, Winter J, Dawson G. Long-term outcomes of early intervention in 6-year-old children with autism spectrum disorder. *J Am Acad Child Adolesc Psychiatry.* 2015;54(7):580–587.

Fagnani C, Neale MC, Nistico L, et al. Twin studies in multiple sclerosis: a meta-estimation of heritability and environmentality. *Mult Scler.* 2015;21(11):1404–1413.

Faridi K, Suchowersky O. Gilles de la Tourette's syndrome. *Can J Neurol Sci.* 2003;30(suppl 1):S64–S71.

Farmer JE, Davis TR. Carpal tunnel syndrome: a case–control study evaluating its relationship with body mass index and hand and wrist measurements. *J Hand Surg Eur.* 2008;33(4):445–448.

Fisher RS, Acevedo C, Arzimanoglou A, et al. A practical clinical definition of epilepsy. *Epilepsia.* 2014;55(4):475–482.

Folkerth RD. The neuropathology of acquired pre- and perinatal brain injuries. *Semin Diagn Pathol.* 2007;24(1):48–57.

Fragoso YD. Modifiable environmental factors in multiple sclerosis. *Arq Neuropsiquiatr.* 2014;72(11):889–894.

Furlan JC. Databases and registries on traumatic spinal cord injury in Canada. *Can J Neurol Sci.* 2013;40(4):454–455.

Furlan JC, Sakakibara BM, Miller WC, Krassioukov AV. Global incidence and prevalence of traumatic spinal cord injury. *Can J Neurol Sci.* 2013;40(4):456–464.

Gadad BS, Li W, Yazdani U, et al. Administration of thimerosal-containing vaccines to infant rhesus macaques does not result in autism-like behavior or neuropathology. *Proc Natl Acad Sci U S A.* 2015;112(40):12498–12503.

Garfinkle J, Wintermark P, Shevell MI, Platt RW, Oskoui M, Canadian Cerebral Palsy Registry. Cerebral palsy after neonatal encephalopathy: how much is preventable? *J Pediatr.* 2015;167(1):58–63.e51.

Gass A, Rocca MA, Agosta F, et al. MRI monitoring of pathological changes in the spinal cord in patients with multiple sclerosis. *Lancet Neurol.* 2015;14(4):443–454.

Gautier CA, Corti O, Brice A. Mitochondrial dysfunctions in Parkinson's disease. *Rev Neurol (Paris)*. 2014;170(5):339–343.

Gelb DJ, Oliver E, Gilman S. Diagnostic criteria for Parkinson's disease. *Arch Neurol*. 1999;56(1):33–39.

Gelfman R, Melton LJ III, Yawn BP, Wollan PC, Amadio PC, Stevens JC. Long-term trends in carpal tunnel syndrome. *Neurology*. 2009;72(1):33–41.

General Medical Council (GMC). Fitness to Practise Panel Hearing—Dr Andrew Jeremy Wakefield (GMC Reference no. 2733564). London, UK: General Medical Council; 2009:1–95.

Gerber JS, Offit PA. Vaccines and autism: a tale of shifting hypotheses. *Clin Infect Dis*. 2009;48(4):456–461.

Glauser T, Shinnar S, Gloss D, et al. Evidence-based guideline: treatment of convulsive status epilepticus in children and adults: report of the Guideline Committee of the American Epilepsy Society. *Epilepsy Curr*. 2016;16(1):48–61.

Global Burden of Disease (GBD) Pediatrics Collaboration, Kyu HH, Pinho C, et al. Global and national burden of diseases and injuries among children and adolescents between 1990 and 2013: findings from the Global Burden of Disease 2013 study. *JAMA Pediatr*. 2016;170(3):267–287.

Godlee F, Smith J, Marcovitch H. Wakefield's article linking MMR vaccine and autism was fraudulent. *BMJ*. 2011;342:c7452.

Goudsmit J. The incubation period of Alzheimer's disease and the timing of tau versus amyloid misfolding and spreading within the brain. *Eur J Epidemiol*. 2016;31(2):99–105.

Gracia F, Castillo LC, Benzadon A, et al. Prevalence and incidence of multiple sclerosis in Panama (2000–2005). *Neuroepidemiology*. 2009;32(4):287–293.

Green J, Charman T, Pickles A, et al. Parent-mediated intervention versus no intervention for infants at high risk of autism: a parallel, single-blind, randomised trial. *Lancet Psychiatry*. 2015;2(2):133–140.

Guerrini R. Epilepsy in children. *Lancet*. 2006;367(9509):499–524.

Gunduz A, Okun MS. A review and update on Tourette syndrome: where is the field headed? *Curr Neurol Neurosci Rep*. 2016;16(4):37.

Guo LH, Alexopoulos P, Wagenpfeil S, Kurz A, Perneczky R; Alzheimer's Disease Neuroimaging Initiative. Brain size and the compensation of Alzheimer's disease symptoms: a longitudinal cohort study. *Alzheimers Dement*. 2013;9(5):580–586.

Haan J, van den Maagdenberg AM, Brouwer OF, Ferrari MD. Migraine and epilepsy: genetically linked? *Expert Rev Neurother.* 2008;8(9):1307–1311.

Harris K, Singer HS. Tic disorders: neural circuits, neurochemistry, and neuroimmunology. *J Child Neurol.* 2006;21(8):678–689.

Hatcher JM, Pennell KD, Miller GW. Parkinson's disease and pesticides: a toxicological perspective. *Trends Pharmacol Sci.* 2008;29(6):322–329.

Hauser WA, Annegers JF, Rocca WA. Descriptive epidemiology of epilepsy: contributions of population-based studies from Rochester, Minnesota. *Mayo Clin Proc.* 1996;71(6):576–586.

Hawkes N. Too frequent use of painkillers can cause rather than cure headaches. *BMJ.* 2012;345:e6281.

Headache Classification Subcommittee of the International Headache Society (HCSIHS). The International Classification of Headache Disorders. *Cephalalgia.* 2004;24(suppl 1): 1–160.

Hedström AK, Lima Bomfim I, Hillert J, Olsson T, Alfredsson L. Obesity interacts with infectious mononucleosis in risk of multiple sclerosis. *Eur J Neurol.* 2015a;22(3): 578–e38.

Hedström AK, Olsson T, Alfredsson L. Smoking is a major preventable risk factor for multiple sclerosis. *Mult Scler.* 2015b;22(8):1021–1026.

Hellwig K, Chen LH, Stancyzk FZ, Langer-Gould AM. Oral contraceptives and multiple sclerosis/clinically isolated syndrome susceptibility. *PLoS One.* 2016;11(3):e0149094.

Hernán MA, Zhang SM, Lipworth L, Olek MJ, Ascherio A. Multiple sclerosis and age at infection with common viruses. *Epidemiology.* 2001;12(3):301–306.

Hirschtritt ME, Lee PC, Pauls DL, et al. Lifetime prevalence, age of risk, and genetic relationships of comorbid psychiatric disorders in Tourette syndrome. *JAMA Psychiatry.* 2015;72(4):325–333.

Hirtz DG, Weiner SJ, Bulas D, et al. Antenatal magnesium and cerebral palsy in preterm infants. *J Pediatr.* 2015;167(4):834–839.e3.

Horton R. GBD 2010: understanding disease, injury, and risk. *Lancet.* 2012;380(9859): 2053–2054.

Hu Z, Yang Y, Gao K, Rudd JA, Fang M. Ovarian hormones ameliorate memory impairment, cholinergic deficit, neuronal apoptosis and astrogliosis in a rat model of Alzheimer's disease. *Exp Ther Med.* 2016;11(1):89–97.

Huang P, Fang R, Li BY, Chen SD. Exercise-related changes of networks in aging and mild cognitive impairment brain. *Front Aging Neurosci.* 2016;8:47.

Hughes JR. A review of sudden unexpected death in epilepsy: prediction of patients at risk. *Epilepsy Behav.* 2009;14(2):280–287.

Hurd MD, Martorell P, Langa KM. Monetary costs of dementia in the United States. *N Engl J Med.* 2013;369(5):489–490.

Jain A, Marshall J, Buikema A, Bancroft T, Kelly JP, Newschaffer CJ. Autism occurrence by MMR vaccine status among US children with older siblings with and without autism. *JAMA.* 2015;313(15):1534–1540.

Jensen CM, Steinhausen HC. Comorbid mental disorders in children and adolescents with attention-deficit/hyperactivity disorder in a large nationwide study. *Atten Defic Hyperact Disord.* 2015;7(1):27–38.

Jensen R, Stovner LJ. Epidemiology and comorbidity of headache. *Lancet Neurol* 2008;7(4):354-361.

Jeong A, Wong M. Tuberous sclerosis complex as a model disease for developing new therapeutics for epilepsy. *Expert Rev Neurother.* 2016;16(4):437–447.

Jette N, Wiebe S. Initial evaluation of the patient with suspected epilepsy. *Neurol Clin.* 2016;34(2):339–350.

Jilek S, Schluep M, Meylan P, et al. Strong EBV-specific CD8+ T-cell response in patients with early multiple sclerosis. *Brain.* 2008;131(pt 7):1712–1721.

Kale R. Bringing epilepsy out of the shadows. *BMJ.* 1997;315(7099):2–3.

Kalita J, Ranjan A, Misra UK. Outcome of Guillain-Barre syndrome patients with respiratory paralysis. *QJM.* 2016;109(5):319–323.

Kamyar M, Clark EA, Yoder BA, Varner MW, Manuck TA. Antenatal magnesium sulfate, necrotizing enterocolitis, and death among neonates < 28 weeks gestation. *AJP Rep.* 2016;6(1):e148–e154.

Karahan A, Kav S, Abbasoglu A, Dogan N. Low back pain: prevalence and associated risk factors among hospital staff. *J Adv Nurs.* 2009;65(3):516–524.

Kariuki SM, Kakooza-Mwesige A, Wagner RG, et al. Prevalence and factors associated with convulsive status epilepticus in Africans with epilepsy. *Neurology.* 2015;84(18):1838–1845.

Keezer MR, Sisodiya SM, Sander JW. Comorbidities of epilepsy: current concepts and future perspectives. *Lancet Neurol.* 2016;15(1):106–115.

Kelman L. The triggers or precipitants of the acute migraine attack. *Cephalagia.* 2007;27(5):394–402.

Kiernan MC, Vucic S, Cheah BC, et al. Amyotrophic lateral sclerosis. *Lancet.* 2011; 377(9769):942–955.

Kim CJ, Romero R, Chaemsaithong P, Chaiyasit N, Yoon BH, Kim YM. Acute chorioamnionitis and funisitis: definition, pathologic features, and clinical significance. *Am J Obstet Gynecol.* 2015;213(4 suppl):S29–S52.

Kingwell E, Marriott JJ, Jette N, et al. Incidence and prevalence of multiple sclerosis in Europe: a systematic review. *BMC Neurol.* 2013;13:128.

Knopman DS. Cerebrovascular disease and dementia. *Br J Radiol.* 2007;80(spec no 2): S121–S127.

Kobow K, Blumcke I. Epigenetic mechanisms in epilepsy. *Prog Brain Res.* 2014;213: 279–316.

Kossoff EH, Singer HS. Tourette syndrome: clinical characteristics and current management strategies. *Paediatr Drugs.* 2001;3(5):355–363.

Kotagal V, Albin RL, Muller ML, Koeppe RA, Frey KA, Bohnen NI. Modifiable cardiovascular risk factors and axial motor impairments in Parkinson disease. *Neurology.* 2014;82(17):1514–1520.

Küçükali CI, Kürtüncü M, Çoban A, Çebi M, Tüzün E. Epigenetics of multiple sclerosis: an updated review. *Neuromol Med.* 2015;17(2):83–96.

Kuwabara S. Guillain-Barré syndrome: epidemiology, pathophysiology and management. *Drugs.* 2004;64(6):597–610.

Lagae L. What's new in: "genetics in childhood epilepsy." *Eur J Pediatr.* 2008;167(7): 715–722.

Lal D, Reinthaler EM, Dejanovic B, et al. Evaluation of presumably disease causing SCN1A variants in a cohort of common epilepsy syndromes. *PLoS One.* 2016;11(3):e0150426.

Langley K, Fowler T, Ford T, et al. Adolescent clinical outcomes for young people with attention-deficit hyperactivity disorder. *Br J Psychiatry.* 2010;196(3):235–240.

Langlois JA, Rutland-Brown W, Wald MM. The epidemiology and impact of traumatic brain injury: a brief overview. *J Head Trauma Rehabil.* 2006;21(5):375–378.

Langston JW. The etiology of Parkinson's disease with emphasis on the MPTP story. *Neurology.* 1996;47(6 suppl 3):S153–S160.

Larsen J, Johannesen KM, Ek J, et al. The role of SLC2A1 mutations in myoclonic astatic epilepsy and absence epilepsy, and the estimated frequency of GLUT1 deficiency syndrome. *Epilepsia.* 2015;56(12):e203–e208.

Laurin N, Wigg KG, Feng Y, Sandor P, Barr CL. Chromosome 5 and Gilles de la Tourette syndrome: linkage in a large pedigree and association study of six candidates in the region. *Am J Med Genet B Neuropsychiatr Genet.* 2009;150B(1):95–103.

LeBlanc KE, Cestia W. Carpal tunnel syndrome. *Am Fam Physician.* 2011;83(8):952–958.

Leckman JF, King RA, Gilbert DL, et al. Streptococcal upper respiratory tract infections and exacerbations of tic and obsessive–compulsive symptoms: a prospective longitudinal study. *J Am Acad Child Adolesc Psychiatry.* 2011;50(2):108–118.e103.

Lee M, O'Brien P. Pregnancy and multiple sclerosis. *J Neurol Neurosurg Psychiatry.* 2008;79(12):1308–1311.

Leigh JP, Grosse SD, Cassady D, Melnikow J, Hertz-Picciotto I. Spending by California's Department of Developmental Services for persons with autism across demographic and expenditure categories. *PLoS One.* 2016;11(3):e0151970.

LeWitt PA, Fahn S. Levodopa therapy for Parkinson disease: a look backward and forward. *Neurology.* 2016;86(14 suppl 1):S3–S12.

Lhatoo S, Noebels J, Whittemore V, NINDS Center for SUDEP Research. Sudden unexpected death in epilepsy: identifying risk and preventing mortality. *Epilepsia.* 2015;56(11):1700–1706.

Liu BC, Ivers R, Norton R, Boufous S, Blows S, Lo SK. Helmets for preventing injury in motorcycle riders. *Cochrane Database Syst Rev.* 2008;(1):CD004333.

Lombroso PJ, Scahill L. Tourette syndrome and obsessive–compulsive disorder. *Brain Dev.* 2008;30(4):231–237.

Liu YS, Dai X, Wu W, et al. The association of SNAP25 gene polymorphisms in attention deficit/hyperactivity disorder: a systematic review and meta-analysis. *Mol Neurobiol.* 2016 [Epub ahead of print March 3, 2016].

Lunn MR, Wang CH. Spinal muscular atrophy. *Lancet.* 2008;371(9630):2120–2133.

Luoni C, Bisulli F, Canevini MP, et al. Determinants of health-related quality of life in pharmacoresistant epilepsy: results from a large multicenter study of consecutively enrolled patients using validated quantitative assessments. *Epilepsia.* 2011;52(12):2181–2191.

Mack KA, Liller KD, Baldwin G, Sleet D. Preventing unintentional injuries in the home using the Health Impact Pyramid. *Health Educ Behav.* 2015;42(1 suppl):115S–122S.

Mack KJ. New daily persistent headache in children and adults. *Curr Pain Headache Rep.* 2009;13(1):47–51.

Mahad DH, Trapp BD, Lassmann H. Pathological mechanisms in progressive multiple sclerosis. *Lancet Neurol.* 2015;14(2):183–193.

Maioli F, Coveri M, Pagni P, et al. Conversion of mild cognitive impairment to dementia in elderly subjects: a preliminary study in a memory and cognitive disorder unit. *Arch Gerontol Geriatr.* 2007;44(suppl 1):233–241.

Martin VT, Lipton RB. Epidemiology and biology of menstrual migraine. *Headache.* 2008;48(suppl 3):S124–S130.

Martino R, Candundo H, Lieshout PV, Shin S, Crispo JA, Barakat-Haddad C. Onset and progression factors in Parkinson's disease: a systematic review. *Neurotoxicology.* 2016 [Epub ahead of print April 5, 2016].

Mata IF, Leverenz JB, Weintraub D, et al. APOE, MAPT, and SNCA genes and cognitive performance in Parkinson disease. *JAMA Neurol.* 2014;71(11):1405–1412.

Matthews PM, Roncaroli F, Waldman A, et al. A practical review of the neuropathology and neuroimaging of multiple sclerosis. *Pract Neurol.* 2016;16(4):279–287.

McClernon FJ, Kollins SH. ADHD and smoking: from genes to brain to behavior. *Ann N Y Acad Sci.* 2008;1141:131–147.

McGrogan A, Madle GC, Seaman HE, de Vries CS. The epidemiology of Guillain-Barré syndrome worldwide. A systematic literature review. *Neuroepidemiology.* 2009;32(2):150–163.

McKay KA, Jahanfar S, Duggan T, Tkachuk S, Tremlett H. Factors associated with onset, relapses or progression in multiple sclerosis: a systematic review. *Neurotoxicology.* 2016 [Epub ahead of print April 1, 2016].

McKay KA, Kwan V, Duggan T, Tremlett H. Risk factors associated with the onset of relapsing-remitting and primary progressive multiple sclerosis: a systematic review. *Biomed Res Int.* 2015;2015:817238.

McTague A, Howell KB, Cross JH, Kurian MA, Scheffer IE. The genetic landscape of the epileptic encephalopathies of infancy and childhood. *Lancet Neurol.* 2016;15(3):304–316.

Merikangas KR. Contributions of epidemiology to our understanding of migraine. *Headache.* 2013;53(2):230–246.

Meyer AC, Dua T, Ma J, Saxena S, Birbeck G. Global disparities in the epilepsy treatment gap: a systematic review. *Bull World Health Organ.* 2010;88(4):260–266.

Meyers AR, Andresen EM, Hagglund KJ. A model of outcomes research: spinal cord injury. *Arch Phys Med Rehabil.* 2000;81(12 suppl 2):S81–S90.

Michelsen SI, Flachs EM, Madsen M, Uldall P. Parental social consequences of having a child with cerebral palsy in Denmark. *Dev Med Child Neurol.* 2015;57(8):768–775.

Miles JH. Autism spectrum disorders—a genetics review. *Genet Med.* 2011;13(4):278–294.

Miller TR, Steinbeigle R, Wicks A, Lawrence BA, Barr M, Barr RG. Disability-adjusted life-year burden of abusive head trauma at ages 0–4. *Pediatrics.* 2014;134(6):e1545–e1550.

Mir IN, Johnson-Welch SF, Nelson DB, Brown LS, Rosenfeld CR, Chalak LF. Placental pathology is associated with severity of neonatal encephalopathy and adverse developmental outcomes following hypothermia. *Am J Obstet Gynecol.* 2015;213(6):e841–e847.

Mullin S, Schapira AH. Pathogenic mechanisms of neurodegeneration in Parkinson disease. *Neurol Clin.* 2015;33(1):1–17.

National Spinal Cord Injury Statistical Center (NSCISC). Spinal cord injury (SCI) facts and figures at a glance. Birmingham, AL: University of Alabama Birmingham; 2015.

Neafsey EJ, Collins MA. Moderate alcohol consumption and cognitive risk. *Neuropsychiatr Dis Treat.* 2011;7:465–484.

Nevalainen O, Simola M, Ansakorpi H, et al. Epilepsy, excess deaths and years of life lost from external causes. *Eur J Epidemiol.* 2015;31(5):445–453.

Nissenkorn A, Levy-Drummer RS, Bondi O, et al. Epilepsy in Rett syndrome—lessons from the Rett networked database. *Epilepsia.* 2015;56(4):569–576.

Norton S, Matthews FE, Barnes DE, Yaffe K, Brayne C. Potential for primary prevention of Alzheimer's disease: an analysis of population-based data. *Lancet Neurol.* 2014;13(8):788–794.

Noseworthy JH, Lucchinetti C, Rodriguez M, Weinshenker BG. Multiple sclerosis. *N Engl J Med.* 2000;343(13):938–952.

Offit PA. *Autism's False Prophets: Bad Science, Risky Medicine, and the Search for a Cure.* New York, NY: Columbia University Press; 2008.

Okamoto K, Kihira T, Kobashi G, et al. Fruit and vegetable intake and risk of amyotrophic lateral sclerosis in Japan. *Neuroepidemiology.* 2009;32(4):251–256.

Olsen CS, Thomas AM, Singleton M, et al. Motorcycle helmet effectiveness in reducing head, face and brain injuries by state and helmet law. *Inj Epidemiol.* 2016;3:8.

Osterman M, Ilyas AM, Matzon JL. Carpal tunnel syndrome in pregnancy. *Orthop Clin North Am.* 2012;43(4):515–520.

Paillard T, Rolland Y, de Souto Barreto P. Protective effects of physical exercise in Alzheimer's disease and Parkinson's disease: a narrative review. *J Clin Neurol.* 2015;11(3):212–219.

Pakula AT, Van Naarden Braun K, Yeargin-Allsopp M. Cerebral palsy: classification and epidemiology. *Phys Med Rehabil Clin N Am.* 2009;20(3):425–452.

Pan J, Connolly ID, Dangelmajer S, Kintzing J, Ho AL, Grant G. Sports-related brain injuries: connecting pathology to diagnosis. *Neurosurg Focus.* 2016;40(4):E14.

Panayiotopoulos CP, Michael M, Sanders S, Valeta T, Koutroumanidis M. Benign childhood focal epilepsies: assessment of established and newly recognized syndromes. *Brain*. 2008;131(pt 9):2264–2286.

Park HW, Choi YS, Kim KS, Kim SN. Chorioamnionitis and patent ductus arteriosus: a systematic review and meta-analysis. *PLoS One*. 2015;10(9):e0138114.

Parker CT, Huynh S, Heikema AP, Cooper KK, Miller WG. Complete genome sequences of *Campylobacter jejuni* strains RM3196 (233.94) and RM3197 (308.95) isolated from patients with Guillain-Barré syndrome. *Genome Announc*. 2015;3(6):e1312–e1315.

Parratt J, Tavendale R, O'Riordan J, Parratt D, Swingler R. *Chlamydia pneumoniae*–specific serum immune complexes in patients with multiple sclerosis. *Mult Scler*. 2008;14(3): 292–299.

Peeters W, van den Brande R, Polinder S, et al. Epidemiology of traumatic brain injury in Europe. *Acta Neurochir (Wien)*. 2015;157(10):1683–1696.

Petrovski S, Kwan P. Unraveling the genetics of common epilepsies: approaches, platforms, and caveats. *Epilepsy Behavior*. 2013;26:229–233.

Pogue AI, Lukiw WJ. Aluminum, the genetic apparatus of the human CNS and Alzheimer's disease (AD). *Morphologie*. 2016;100(329):56–64.

Prischich F, De Rinaldis M, Bruno F, et al. High prevalence of epilepsy in a village in the Littoral Province of Cameroon. *Epilepsy Res*. 2008;82(2–3):200–210.

Pritchard J. What's new in Guillain-Barré syndrome? *Postgrad Med J*. 2008;84(996):532–538.

Qin Z, Baccaglini L. Distribution, determinants, and prevention of falls among the elderly in the 2011–2012 California Health Interview Survey. *Public Health Rep*. 2016;131(2):331–339.

Raber J, Huang Y, Ashford JW. ApoE genotype accounts for the vast majority of AD risk and AD pathology. *Neurobiol Aging*. 2004;25(5):641–650.

Racette BA, McGee-Minnich L, Moerlein SM, Mink JW, Videen TO, Perlmutter JS. Welding-related parkinsonism: clinical features, treatment, and pathophysiology. *Neurology*. 2001;56(1):8–13.

Ramagopalan SV, Dyment DA, Ebers GC. Genetic epidemiology: the use of old and new tools for multiple sclerosis. *Trends Neurosci*. 2008;31(12):645–652.

Rasmussen SA, Jamieson DJ, Honein MA, Petersen LR. Zika virus and birth defects—reviewing the evidence for causality. *N Engl J Med*. 2016;374(20):1981–1987.

Richer L, Billinghurst L, Linsdell MA, et al. Drugs for the acute treatment of migraine in children and adolescents. *Cochrane Database Syst Rev*. 2016;(4):CD005220.

Riva N, Agosta F, Lunetta C, Filippi M, Quattrini A. Recent advances in amyotrophic lateral sclerosis. *J Neurol.* 2016;263(6):1241–1254.

Robinson MN, Peake LJ, Ditchfield MR, Reid SM, Lanigan A, Reddihough DS. Magnetic resonance imaging findings in a population-based cohort of children with cerebral palsy. *Dev Med Child Neurol.* 2009;51(1):39–45.

Rothstein JD. Current hypotheses for the underlying biology of amyotrophic lateral sclerosis. *Ann Neurol.* 2009;65(suppl 1):S3–S9.

Rubiano AM, Carney N, Chesnut R, Puyana JC. Global neurotrauma research challenges and opportunities. *Nature.* 2015;527(7578):S193–S197.

Rutland-Brown W, Langlois JA, Thomas KE, Xi YL. Incidence of traumatic brain injury in the United States, 2003. *J Head Trauma Rehabil.* 2006;21(6):544–548.

Sandin S, Schendel D, Magnusson P, et al. Autism risk associated with parental age and with increasing difference in age between the parents. *Mol Psychiatry.* 2016;21(5):693–700.

Sano M, Grossman H, Van Dyk K. Preventing Alzheimer's disease: separating fact from fiction. *CNS Drugs.* 2008;22(11):887–902.

Sano M, Jacobs D, Andrews H, et al. A multi-center, randomized, double blind placebo-controlled trial of estrogens to prevent Alzheimer's disease and loss of memory in women: design and baseline characteristics. *Clin Trials.* 2008;5(5):523–533.

Savica R, Rocca WA, Ahlskog JE. When does Parkinson disease start? *Arch Neurol.* 2010;67(7):798–801.

Scheffer IE, Harkin LA, Grinton BE, et al. Temporal lobe epilepsy and GEFS+ phenotypes associated with SCN1B mutations. *Brain.* 2007;130(pt 1):100–109.

Schendel DE, Overgaard M, Christensen J, et al. Association of psychiatric and neurologic comorbidity with mortality among persons with autism spectrum disorder in a Danish population. *JAMA Pediatr.* 2016;170(3):243–250.

Schwedt TJ. Chronic migraine. *BMJ.* 2014;348:g1416.

Sejvar JJ, Baughman AL, Wise M, Morgan OW. Population incidence of Guillain-Barre syndrome: a systematic review and meta-analysis. *Neuroepidemiology.* 2011;36(2):123–133.

Selkoe DJ. Alzheimer's disease is a synaptic failure. *Science.* 2002;298(5594):789–791.

Shalak LF, Laptook AR, Jafri HS, Ramilo O, Perlman JM. Clinical chorioamnionitis, elevated cytokines, and brain injury in term infants. *Pediatrics.* 2002;110(4):673–680.

Shattuck PT. The contribution of diagnostic substitution to the growing administrative prevalence of autism in US special education. *Pediatrics.* 2006;117(4):1028–1037.

Shaw CA, Höglinger GU. Neurodegenerative diseases: neurotoxins as sufficient etiologic agents? *Neuromolecular Med.* 2008;10(1):1–9.

Shields WD. Diagnosis of infantile spasms, Lennox-Gastaut syndrome, and progressive myoclonic epilepsy. *Epilepsia.* 2004;45(suppl 5):2–4.

Shiri R, Karppinen J, Leino-Arjas P, Solovieva S, Viikari-Juntura E. The association between obesity and low back pain: a meta-analysis. *Am J Epidemiol.* 2010a;171(2):135–154.

Shiri R, Karppinen J, Leino-Arjas P, Solovieva S, Viikari-Juntura E. The association between smoking and low back pain: a meta-analysis. *Am J Med.* 2010b;123(1):87.e7–35.

Siddique N, Siddique T. Genetics of amyotrophic lateral sclerosis. *Phy Med Rehabil Clin N Am.* 2008;19(3):429–439.

Smestad C, Sandvik L, Holmoy T, Harbo HF, Celius EG. Marked differences in prevalence of multiple sclerosis between ethnic groups in Oslo, Norway. *J Neurol.* 2008;255(1):49–55.

Smitherman TA, Wells RE, Ford SG. Emerging behavioral treatments for migraine. *Curr Pain Headache Rep.* 2015;19(4):13.

Sotelo J, Martinez-Palomo A, Ordonez G, Pineda B. Varicella-zoster virus in cerebrospinal fluid at relapses of multiple sclerosis. *Ann Neurol.* 2008;63(3):303–311.

Sriram K, Lin GX, Jefferson AM, et al. Modifying welding process parameters can reduce the neurotoxic potential of manganese-containing welding fumes. *Toxicology.* 2015;328:168–178.

Stanley F, Blair E, Alberman E. *Cerebral Palsies: Epidemiology and Causal Pathways.* London, UK: MacKeith Press; 2000.

Stein MA, Shin D. Disorders of attention: diagnosis. In: Accardo PJ, ed. *Capute & Accardo's Neurodevelopmental Disabilities in Infancy and Childhood.* Vol. II. Baltimore, MD: Paul H. Brookes Publishing Co; 2008:639.

Still GF. The Goulstonian lectures on some abnormal psychical conditions in children. *Lancet.* 1902;159:1008–1013.

Sumner CJ. Molecular mechanisms of spinal muscular atrophy. *J Child Neurol.* 2007;22(8):979–989.

Sundström P, Nystrom L, Hallmans G. Smoke exposure increases the risk for multiple sclerosis. *Eur J Neurol.* 2008;15(6):579–583.

Sundström P, Salzer J. Vitamin D and multiple sclerosis—from epidemiology to prevention. *Acta Neurol Scan.* 2015;132(199):56–91.

Surges R, Sander JW. Sudden unexpected death in epilepsy: mechanisms, prevalence, and prevention. *Curr Opin Neurol.* 2012;25(2):201–207.

Szekely CA, Breitner JC, Fitzpatrick AL, et al. NSAID use and dementia risk in the Cardiovascular Health Study: role of APOE and NSAID type. *Neurology.* 2008;70(1):17–24.

Taheraghdam A, Pourkhanjar P, Talebi M, et al. Correlations between cytomegalovirus, Epstein-Barr virus, anti-ganglioside antibodies, electrodiagnostic findings and functional status in Guillain-Barré syndrome. *Iran J Neurol.* 2014;13(1):7–12.

Tanner CM, Goldman SM. Epidemiology of Parkinson's disease. *Neurol Clin.* 1996;2: 317–335.

Teela KC, De Silva DA, Chapman K, et al. Magnesium sulphate for fetal neuroprotection: benefits and challenges of a systematic knowledge translation project in Canada. *BMC Pregnancy Childbirth.* 2015;15:347.

Thapar A, Cooper M. Attention deficit hyperactivity disorder. *Lancet.* 2016;387(10024): 1240–1250.

Thapar A, Cooper M, Eyre O, Langley K. What have we learnt about the causes of ADHD? *J Child Psychol Psychiatry.* 2013;54(1):3–16.

Thenganatt MA, Jankovic J. Recent advances in understanding and managing Tourette syndrome. *F1000Res.* 2016;5.

Thurman DJ, Alverson C, Dunn KA, Guerrero J, Sniezek JE. Traumatic brain injury in the United States: a public health perspective. *J Head Trauma Rehabil.* 1999;14(6):602–615.

Thurman DJ, Hesdorffer DC, French JA. Sudden unexpected death in epilepsy: assessing the public health burden. *Epilepsia.* 2014;55(10):1479–1485.

Thurman DJ, Kobau R, Luo YH, Helmers SL, Zack MM. Health-care access among adults with epilepsy: the US National Health Interview Survey, 2010 and 2013. *Epilepsy Behav.* 2016;55:184–188.

Tomson T, Nashef L, Ryvlin P. Sudden unexpected death in epilepsy: current knowledge and future directions. *Lancet Neurol.* 2008;7(11):1021–1031.

Trevathan E. The diagnosis of epilepsy and the art of listening. *Neurology.* 2003;61(12): E13–E14.

Trevathan E. Seizures and epilepsy among children with language regression and autistic spectrum disorders. *J Child Neurol.* 2004;19(suppl 1):S49–S57.

Trevathan E, Shinnar S. Epidemiology of autism spectrum disorders. In: Tuchman R, Rapin I, editors. *Autism: A Neurological Disorder of Early Brain Development.* London, UK: MacKeith Press; 2006:20–36.

Turner MR, Hardiman O, Benatar M, et al. Controversies and priorities in amyotrophic lateral sclerosis. *Lancet Neurol.* 2013;12(3):310–322.

van den Berg B, Walgaard C, Drenthen J, Fokke C, Jacobs BC, van Doorn PA. Guillain-Barré syndrome: pathogenesis, diagnosis, treatment and prognosis. *Nat Rev Neurol.* 2014;10(8):469–482.

van den Berg ME, Castellote JM, Mahillo-Fernandez I, de Pedro-Cuesta J. Incidence of spinal cord injury worldwide: a systematic review. *Neuroepidemiology.* 2010;34(3): 184–192; discussion 192.

van Lieshout P, Candundo H, Martino R, Shin S, Barakat-Haddad C. Onset factors in cerebral palsy: a systematic review. *Neurotoxicology.* 2016 [Epub ahead of print April 1, 2016].

Verbeek NE, van der Maas NA, Sonsma AC, et al. Effect of vaccinations on seizure risk and disease course in Dravet syndrome. *Neurology.* 2015;85(7):596–603.

Verma SK, Willetts JL, Corns HL, Marucci-Wellman HR, Lombardi DA, Courtney TK. Falls and fall-related injuries among community-dwelling adults in the United States. *PLoS One.* 2016;11(3):e0150939.

Vezzani A, Fujinami RS, White HS, et al. Infections, inflammation and epilepsy. *Acta Neuropathol.* 2016;131(2):211–234.

Watrin L, Ghawche F, Larre P, Neau JP, Mathis S, Fournier E. Guillain-Barré syndrome (42 cases) occurring during a Zika virus outbreak in French Polynesia. *Medicine (Baltimore).* 2016;95(14):e3257.

Webb AJ, Brain SA, Wood R, Rinaldi S, Turner MR. Seasonal variation in Guillain-Barré syndrome: a systematic review, meta-analysis and Oxfordshire cohort study. *J Neurol Neurosurg Psychiatry.* 2015;86(11):1196–1201.

Whiteford HA, Ferrari AJ, Degenhardt L, Feigin V, Vos T. The global burden of mental, neurological and substance use disorders: an analysis from the Global Burden of Disease study 2010. *PLoS One.* 2015;10(2):e0116820.

Whitwell JL. The protective role of brain size in Alzheimer's disease. *Expert Rev Neurother.* 2010;10(12):1799–1801.

Willison HJ, Jacobs BC, van Doorn PA. Guillain-Barre syndrome. *Lancet.* 2016; 388(10045):717–727.

Wilson RS, Segawa E, Boyle PA, Anagnos SE, Hizel LP, Bennett DA. The natural history of cognitive decline in Alzheimer's disease. *Psychol Aging.* 2012;27(4):1008–1017.

Winkelmann A, Loebermann M, Reisinger EC, Hartung H-P, Zettl UK. Disease-modifying therapies and infectious risks in multiple sclerosis. *Nat Rev Neurol.* 2016;12(4):217–233.

World Health Organization (WHO). *WHO Global Campaign Against Epilepsy.* Geneva, Switzerland: ILAE/IBE/WHO; 2003.

World Health Organization (WHO). *Atlas of Headache Disorders and Resources in the World 2011*. Geneva, Switzerland: WHO; 2011.

Xiang AH, Wang X, Martinez MP, et al. Association of maternal diabetes with autism in offspring. *JAMA*. 2015;313(14):1425–1434.

Yang H, Song Z, Yang GP, et al. The ALDH2 rs671 polymorphism affects post-stroke epilepsy susceptibility and plasma 4-HNE levels. *PLoS One*. 2014;9(10):e109634.

Yang YX, Wood NW, Latchman DS. Molecular basis of Parkinson's disease. *Neuroreport*. 2009;20(2):150–156.

Yeargin-Allsopp M, Boyle C, van Naarden Braun K, Trevathan E. The epidemiology of developmental disabilities. In: Accardo PJ, ed. *Capute and Accardo's Neurodevelopmental Disabilities in Infancy and Childhood*. Vol. 1. Baltimore, MD: Paul H. Brookes Publishing Co; 2008:61–104.

Yeargin-Allsopp M, Van Naarden Braun K, Doernberg NS, Benedict RE, Kirby RS, Durkin MS. Prevalence of cerebral palsy in 8-year-old children in three areas of the United States in 2002: a multisite collaboration. *Pediatrics*. 2008;121(3):547–554.

Zaki EA, Freilinger T, Klopstock T, et al. Two common mitochondrial DNA polymorphisms are highly associated with migraine headache and cyclic vomiting syndrome. *Cephalagia* 2009;29(7):719–728.

Zebenholzer K, Lechner A, Broessner G, et al. Impact of depression and anxiety on burden and management of episodic and chronic headaches—a cross-sectional multicentre study in eight Austrian headache centres. *J Headache Pain*. 2016;17(1):15.

Ziegler-Graham K, Brookmeyer R, Johnson E, Arrighi HM. Worldwide variation in the doubling time of Alzheimer's disease incidence rates. *Alzheimers Dement*. 2008;4(5):316–323.

20

ARTHRITIS AND OTHER MUSCULOSKELETAL DISEASES

Huan J. Chang, MD, MPH, Daniel J. Finn, MPH,
Dorothy D. Dunlop, PhD, Diego Tamez, MD,
and Rowland W. Chang, MD, MPH

Introduction

Arthritis and osteoporosis are the most frequent causes of disability among adults in the United States (CDC 2009; CDC 2013, USDHHS 2004). More than 100 diseases make up the spectrum of arthritis and musculoskeletal disorders, with a variety of "upstream" causes and "downstream" consequences (Figure 20-1). Most of these diseases are uncommon, are of unknown cause, and allow little opportunity for primary or secondary prevention in the general population (Hirsch and Hochberg 2010). However, osteoarthritis (OA) accounts for a significant portion of overall disability and economic cost and is subject to primary and secondary prevention initiatives.

About 50 million U.S. adults—one in five—reported doctor-diagnosed arthritis and an estimated 13 million adults aged 50 years and older have osteoporosis (USDHHS 2004). About 21 million adults have arthritis-attributable activity limitations (CDC 2010), and in 2003, the costs attributable to arthritis totaled nearly 1% of that year's gross domestic product (Yelin et al. 2007). It is estimated that, among U.S. adults, nearly 27 million people have clinical OA (up from an estimated 21 million in 1995), up to three million have self-reported gout (up from an estimated 2.1 million in 1995), and five million have fibromyalgia (Lawrence et al. 2008). The number of U.S. adults with arthritis is expected to rise to 67 million by 2030 (Hootman et al. 2016).

As of 2012, more than one in five (22.7%) adults in the United States reported that they had arthritis as diagnosed by their primary care provider (CDC 2013). That percentage represents 52.5 million adults. Of those 52.5 million individuals,

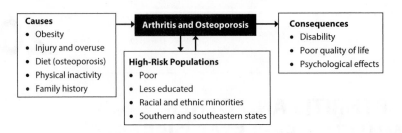

Source: Adapted from Hirsch and Hochberg (2010).
Note: For further information on obesity, see Chapter 11.

Figure 20-1. Arthritis: Causes, Consequences, and High-Risk Groups

22.7 million (9.8% of U.S. adults) have some activity limitation attributable to their arthritis (CDC 2013). Future projections predict that 78.4 million (25.9%) of U.S. adults aged older than 18 years will report doctor-diagnosed arthritis by 2040—a 49% increase. In addition, in the same timeframe, the number of individuals with activity limitations because of their arthritis will increase 52%, affecting 34.6 million (11.4%) of U.S. adults (Hootman et al. 2016).

The prevalence of arthritis was recently estimated by using data from the 2010–2012 National Health Interview Survey. Arthritis was defined as a "yes" response to "Have you ever been told by a doctor or other health professional that you have some form of arthritis, rheumatoid arthritis, gout, lupus, or fibromyalgia?" (Hootman et al. 2016). With this definition, the prevalence of arthritis is slightly higher in women than in men, and rises dramatically with increasing age. By age 65 years, more than 50% of adults have doctor-diagnosed arthritis (Figure 20-2).

Along with the increase in individuals reporting doctor-diagnosed arthritis are the increased costs associated with the rising prevalence and incidence. In fact, most states in the United States report that their annual costs related to arthritis and related conditions is greater than 1% of each state's gross domestic product (CDC 2009). Total arthritis-related costs varied greatly, ranging from $225 million in the District of Columbia to $12 billion in California (CDC 2009). Total costs attributed to arthritis and other rheumatic conditions in the United States reached approximately $128 billion in 2003, with $81 billion as direct costs and $47 billion as indirect costs (CDC 2009).

The Centers for Disease Control and Prevention (CDC) has taken steps to address the high total attributed costs related to the treatment and maintenance

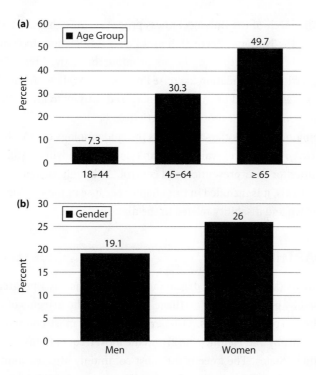

Source: Data are from National Health Interview Survey 2010-2012; CDC (2013).
*Answered yes to the question, "Have you ever been told by a doctor or other health professional that you have some form of arthritis, rheumatoid arthritis, gout, lupus, or fibromyalgia?"

Figure 20-2. Prevalence of Doctor-Diagnosed Arthritis* (a) by Age and (b) by Gender in the United States

of arthritic conditions through programs and support at both the state and national levels. At the state level, the CDC helps fund health departments to increase the scope of established physical activity programs through partnerships with community organizations. These partnerships enable local organizations to deliver physical activity and health education programming, in partnership with state arthritis programs, to all populations affected by arthritis (CDC 2016).

At the national level, the CDC partners with seven foundations (e.g., American Physical Therapy Foundation, Arthritis Foundation, National Association of Chronic Disease Directors) to increase access to physical activity programs, encourage the use of self-management materials, and to promote physical activity through walking (CDC 2016). Specific national organizations include The Y (http://www.ymca.net), which aims to support and broaden the reach of the EnhanceFitness program through local Y divisions. In addition, the National Recreation and Parks Association, in concert with the CDC and the Arthritis Foundation, promote the Active Living Every Day Program, Arthritis Foundation Exercise Program, or Walk with Ease Program across 32 states designed to encourage increased activity to lessen the burden of arthritis conditions for those who participate (CDC 2016).

The remainder of this chapter reviews the epidemiology of OA, rheumatoid arthritis (RA), gout, fibromyalgia, and ankylosing spondylitis (AS), as well as opportunities for their prevention and control. Although osteoporosis is not a form of arthritis, it is included in this chapter because of the significant public health burden and disability related to the disease.

OSTEOARTHRITIS

Osteoarthritis (known also as degenerative joint disease) is a progressive disease caused by gradual loss of cartilage. As a result, the margins of the joints develop bony spurs and cysts. Osteoarthritis is the most common type of arthritis (Murphy and Helmick 2012) and the most frequent cause of disability in the United States. The knee is the most commonly affected joint, specifically the medial compartment of the knee (Vincent et al. 2012a); however, OA can affect both weight-bearing and non–weight-bearing joints.

Osteoarthritis is characterized by pain in the involved joints, crepitus, stiffness after immobility, and limitation of movement (Bijlsma and Knahr 2007). It may develop in any joint, but mainly affects knees, hips, hands, feet, and spine. It is important to note that symptoms and radiographic changes are poorly correlated in OA (Litwic et al. 2013) and the prevalence of OA varies by the means used to define the disease (Felson and Zhang 1998), usually radiographic, symptomatic, or self-reported (Hannon et al. 1993).

Knee pain is an imprecise marker of radiographic knee OA, and vice versa. A systematic literature review found that the proportion of those with knee pain found to have radiographic OA ranged from 15% to 76%, and in those with radiographic knee OA the proportion with pain ranged from 15% to 81% (Bedson and Croft 2008). Figure 20-3 is a schematic that shows this discordance between self-reported arthritis, symptomatic knee pain, and radiographic knee OA. The American College of Rheumatology (ACR) also has established definitions for hand, hip, and knee OA (Altman et al. 1990; Arden and Nevitt 2006).

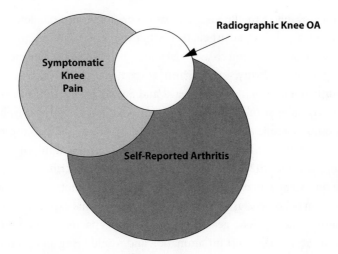

Figure 20-3. Schematic Showing Discordance Between Self-Reported Arthritis, Symptomatic Knee Pain, and Radiographic Knee Osteoarthritis (OA)

Significance

Osteoarthritis accounts for more difficulty climbing stairs and walking than any other disease (Guccione et al. 1994). In 2005, 27 million adults (> 10% of the U.S. population) had clinical OA. In 2009, OA was the fourth-most-common cause of hospitalization in the United States and was the leading indication for joint replacement surgery, with 905,000 knee and hip replacements performed in 2009 at a cost of $42.3 billion dollars (Murphy and Helmick 2012). Rapid increase in prevalence of this disease suggests increased impact on health care and public health systems in the future (Lawrence et al. 2008).

Pathophysiology

The pathogenesis of OA is incompletely understood (Bijlsma and Knahr 2007), but it is known to be multifactorial, based on both systemic and local biomechanical factors (Guccione et al. 1994). Cartilage destruction is the hallmark of disease, specifically the degradation of type II collagen. More recently, a broader view of OA places greater focus on the whole joint, rather than on cartilage only, in the pathogenesis of OA (Guccione et al. 1994).

Healthy cartilage responds to loading by increasing regional thickness; diseased or injured cartilage degenerates and decreases regional thickness.

Chondrocytes maintain the matrix components under normal, low-turnover conditions. Chondrocytes can be activated by exposure to unusual environmental conditions such as biomechanical factors (e.g., trauma or severe mechanical stress, ligamentous laxity, weight gain), altered amounts of matrix proteins, or inflammatory cytokines (Heinegard and Saxne 2011). Until recently, OA has been considered the prototypic non-inflammatory arthropathy, because there are no systemic manifestations of inflammation, and because neutrophils (a hallmark of inflammation) are typically not present in synovial fluid (Goldring and Otero 2011). However, recent studies describe pathways that activate quiescent articular chondrocytes causing a phenotypic shift, leading to disruption of homeostasis and, therefore, the abnormal expression of proinflammatory and catabolic genes. Proinflammatory factors can be produced even in the absence of overt inflammation and would bring an inflammatory aspect to OA (Goldring and Otero 2011).

Specific obesity-related mechanisms have been proposed to lead to OA pathology (Vincent et al. 2012b). They include relative loss of muscle mass and strength over time, mechanical stress, and systemic inflammation. It is known that obesity causes abnormal joint loading, resulting in adverse changes to the composition, structure, and properties of articular cartilage. Both muscle mass and fat mass increase with increased body weight; however, the volume of muscle mass remains relatively low and, therefore, inadequate to match the loads placed upon it. Low-grade systemic inflammation is now considered a hallmark of obesity, resulting in elevations of interleukin (IL)-1ß, IL-6, tumor necrosis factor-alpha (TNF-α), and acute phase reactant C-reactive protein (Schrager et al. 2007).

Descriptive Epidemiology

The prevalence of OA varies with the definition used (Hannon et al. 1993) and rates vary by joint. For instance, prevalence of radiographic hand OA has been reported to range from 27% to greater than 80% (Lawrence et al. 2008). Symptomatic hand OA according to ACR criteria, however, was 7% in the Framingham cohort and 8% in NHANES III. Hand OA rates increase with age to a peak of 13% in men and 26% in women (Litwic et al. 2013). Severe radiographic prevalence of knee OA in the United States is reported in 1% of those aged 25 to 34 years, increasing to almost 50% in persons aged 75 years and older. The Framingham Study reported 19.2% prevalence of knee OA, with an increase to 43.7% in those aged older than 80 years (Hannon et al. 1993).

NHANES III reported symptomatic knee OA prevalence was 12.1% (Litwic et al. 2013). Lifetime risk of symptomatic knee OA was 44.7% in the Johnston County Osteoarthritis Project (Murphy et al. 2008). Mean prevalence of radiographic hip OA in the United States is 7.2% (Felson et al. 1987). The Johnston County Study shows a 5.9% prevalence of symptomatic hip OA in adults aged 45 to 54 years and 17% in adults aged 75 years and older (Bijlsma and Knahr 2007). Incidence of OA has been estimated at 100 per 100,000 person-years for hand OA, 88 per 100,000 person-years for hip OA, and 240 per 100,000 person-years for knee OA (Arden and Nevitt 2006). The incidence of all types of OA increases with increasing age (Arden and Nevitt 2006).

High-Risk Populations

It is known that both systemic and local factors affect the likelihood that a joint will develop OA (Felson and Zhang 1998), and that different joints have different risk factors for incident OA. Systemic factors include age, gender, race, genetics, bone density, estrogen, nutritional, and other. Local factors include joint injury, obesity, joint deformity, and muscle weakness.

Causes

The cause of OA is known to be multifactorial, combining genetic, environmental, and local factors. Currently, malalignment (of $180° \pm 2°$ varus/valgus) is the only known risk factor for progression of knee OA (Felson et al. 2013). Genetic influence in OA is estimated to be between 35% and 65% (Cicuttini and Spector 1996). Epidemiological studies estimate that there is a 40% probability of inheritability in osteoarthritic knees and a 65% probability of inheritability in osteoarthritic hands and hips (Spector and McGregor 2004).

Age may be the greatest systemic risk factor for OA, as all forms of OA increase with increasing age (Felson and Zhang 1998; Bijlsma and Knahr 2007). Gender, another systemic factor, is often considered a risk factor for OA because the disease is more prevalent among women than men (Palazzo et al. 2016). However, there is no proof of gender as a risk factor for either incident or progressive disease (Palazzo et al. 2016). Regarding race as a potential systemic factor, there is conflicting evidence as to whether blacks have different rates of OA than whites. The higher relative weight of black women may be a confounding factor in their higher rates of knee OA (Jordan et al. 1995). A community-based study of hip OA in North Carolina did not confirm racial differences in prevalence (Jordan et al. 1995); however, prevalence of hip OA may be very low in Asians (Hoaglund et al. 1973). Common and unique environmental factors are highly significant for both genders. A Danish twin study found that, at the 50-year follow-up, the risk of OA is increased in the twin of an individual with OA. There was a discrete genetic component in women but not in men. Overall, there was an additive genetic component of 18%, a shared environmental component of 61%, and an individual environmental component of 21% (Skousgaard et al. 2016).

Joint injury has long been recognized as a local risk factor for OA. In a population-based prospective study in Finland, 840 participants were followed for 22 years to better understand the risk and disease progression of hip OA. Participants had a mean age of 63 years at the time of follow-up. It reported that heavy manual labor (odds ratio [OR]=6.7) and permanent damage attributable to hip injury (OR=5.0) were associated with developing hip OA (Juhakoski et al. 2009). Furthermore, inequality in leg length and malalignment are identified as biomechanical risk factors related to knee OA (Neogi and Zhang 2011). Obesity (body mass index [BMI] > 30 kg/m^2) is a prominent local OA risk factor that can contribute to biomechanical joint stress (Palazzo et al. 2016).

Obesity is strongly related to the prevalence of OA. Data from the first NHANES showed that women with a BMI between 30 and 35 had almost four times the risk of having OA as those with a BMI less than 25. For men in the same BMI grouping, the risk of OA was 4.8-fold greater than for men with a BMI less than 25 (Anderson and Felson 1988). Obese persons have a much greater risk of having bilateral hip and knee OA when compared with non-obese counterparts (Palazzo et al. 2016). Obesity has also been associated with hand OA (Grotle et al. 2008), suggesting that the risk from obesity is not purely mechanical, but rather, includes systemic inflammation effects.

Sarcopenia may be a risk factor in OA, but has not been shown to be conclusive for either incident or progressive disease; however, some data suggest that quadriceps weakness is attributable to arthritic inhibition of muscle contraction, contributing to incident disease (Palazzo et al. 2016).

Modifiable Risk Factors

Modifiable risk factors for incident OA include body weight, physical activity, and the strength of muscles supporting osteoarthritic joints (Table 20-1). Obesity is a key modifiable risk factor. In people who are obese or overweight,

Table 20-1. Modifiable Risk Factors for Osteoarthritis, United States

Magnitude	Risk Factor[a]
Strong (relative risk > 4)	Joint trauma
Moderate (relative risk 2–4)	Repetitive occupational usage Obesity
Weak (relative risk < 2)	Muscle weakness
	Nutritional deficiencies

Source: Reprinted from Hirsch and Hochberg (2010).
[a]Risk factors differ in their magnitude based on the site of osteoarthritis involved.

weight loss is an important factor affecting the mechanical and inflammatory disease pathway(s). For every 5% increase in BMI, the associated increased risk of developing knee OA is reported to be 35%, with the magnitude of the association stronger for women than for men (Jiang et al. 2012). It has been estimated that 24.6% of all incident knee pain is related to being overweight (Silverwood et al. 2015). Regarding obesity and hip OA, the Nurses' Health Study found that those with the highest BMI at age 18 had a five-fold increase in total hip replacement because of hip OA (Karlson et al. 2003).

Another important modifiable lifestyle risk factor is physical activity. In adults with knee OA, there is a dose–response relationship between greater levels of physical activity and the reduced development of disability and improved quality of life (Dunlop et al. 2014; Sun et al. 2014). Interventions targeting these factors may be able to achieve treatment goals of preventing or decreasing damage, reducing or preventing pain, and improving function.

Evidence-Based Interventions

Prevention

Although there is no cure for OA, managing risk factors is important in slowing or stopping disease progression. Randomized controlled trials (RCTs) have focused on lifestyle changes, targeting exercise interventions and diet for both primary and secondary prevention of OA. Messier et al. (2013) reported that, among overweight and obese adults with knee OA, with interventions including intensive diet restriction and exercise, individuals with diet only had greater reductions in knee compressive force than those in the exercise-only group. Furthermore, individuals in the group with both diet and exercise had greater weight loss and greater reductions in IL-6 levels than those in the exercise-only group (Messier et al. 2013). To date, there are no known published RCTs examining weight loss and hip OA.

In 2015, an RCT examined the use of different shoes and lateral wedge insoles on external knee adduction moment, knee adduction angular impulse, external knee flexion moment, pain, and comfort when walking in individuals with medial knee OA. The investigators found that, compared with the control shoe, lateral wedge insoles and barefoot walking significantly reduced early stance external knee flexion moment and knee adduction angular impulse (Jones et al. 2015).

In another prospective randomized multicenter trial (Petersen et al. 2016), participants were randomly assigned to six weeks of supervised physiotherapy in combination with the patellar realignment brace, or supervised physiotherapy alone. After 6 and 12 weeks of therapy, patients in the brace group had significantly better Knee Injury and Osteoarthritis Outcome Score. After one year of follow-up, this positive effect diminished (Petersen et al. 2016).

On the basis of current knowledge of risk factors, evidence supports the importance of obesity prevention, avoiding joint trauma, and modifying occupational-related joint stress for the prevention of osteoarthritis. National public health recommendations include reducing obesity (BMI > 30.0 kg/m²) to a prevalence of no more than 15% among adults, increasing the proportion of adults who perform physical activities that enhance and maintain muscular strength and endurance, and reducing the number of nonfatal unintentional injuries, especially those that are work-related (Hirsch and Hochberg 2010).

Screening

Screening and early detection of OA are not feasible at present.

Treatment

Approach to treatment of OA should be multidisciplinary. Non-pharmacological treatments include behavioral interventions, weight loss, physical therapy to maintain strength and range of motion, and occupational therapy to maximize the patient's independent ability to perform activities of daily living including dressing, feeding, bathing, toileting, and grooming. In addition, mechanical interventions such as kinesiotherapy and bracing may be useful. Some patients find acupuncture and other homeopathic remedies and spa treatments helpful, although there are no formal recommendations.

Pharmacological treatment can generally be used in conjunction with non-pharmacological treatment and includes topical treatments, oral medications, and intra-articular injections. Surgical interventions include bariatric surgery for weight loss if indicated, and joint replacement for individuals with moderate to severe pain and limitations of activities that reduce their quality of life.

In June 2013, the American Academy of Orthopedic Surgeons issued a new set of recommendations for the treatment of knee OA. On the basis of a review of 14 studies, the organization determined that hyaluronic acid does not meet the minimum clinically important improvement measures. The potential role of nutritional supplements (e.g., glucosamine, chondroitin sulfate) is still being discussed. A network meta-analysis up to June 2010, which includes 10 large trials, showed that overall pain intensity on a 10-centimeter (cm) visual analog scale compared with placebo was -0.4 cm for glucosamine, -0.3 cm for chondroitin, and -0.5 cm for combination (Wandel et al. 2010).

Physical activity is another non-pharmaceutical treatment for OA. Increasing evidence indicates that people with arthritis are less physically active and less fit than their peers. This suggests that individuals with OA could benefit from conditioning exercise programs to improve both cardiovascular and musculoskeletal fitness if they can do so without exacerbating their joint disease (Minor and Lane 1996). These exercise activities could include low-impact weight-bearing exercises (walking or resistance training for major muscle groups), water aerobics, or stationary bicycling, many of which are available in communities and through the Arthritis Foundation Exercise Program and Aquatic Program (Hirsch and Hochberg 2010). More research is needed to fully understand the direct relationship between physical activity and OA. There is currently no evidence to link physical activity with prevention of OA. In fact, large amounts of vigorous physical activity, causing high impacts or torsional loading, may serve to increase OA risk if it causes injury. However, research shows that light or moderate physical activity (low-impact and non–joint damaging) does not increase an individual's risk of OA. The most effective use of physical activity in the treatment of OA may be to use it as a rehabilitation tool and as a means to reduce other comorbidities.

Examples of Evidence-Based Interventions

A major arthritis public health initiative, The National Arthritis Action Plan: A Public Health Strategy, was developed in 1999 by the CDC, the Arthritis

Foundation, the Association of State and Territorial Health Officials, and 90 other organizations, and it outlines a national plan to reduce pain and disability and improve quality of life for people with arthritis. In 2007, CDC, the Arthritis Foundation, and other partners supported arthritis initiatives in 36 states, including arthritis public awareness efforts and evidence-based community self-management programs such as People with Arthritis Can Exercise, the Arthritis Self-Help Course, and Arthritis Foundation Aquatics Program, and a health communications campaign, Physical Activity—The Arthritis Pain Reliever.

Areas for Future Research

Research in OA presently addresses the problem of pain control and increasing function from multiple angles. In addition to continued research in exercise and diet, researchers continue to investigate the use of intra-articular platelet-rich plasma, mechanical treatments for OA, and new substances for pain control, such as low-dose radiotherapy (Minten et al. 2016), which has been found to be helpful for pain and function. However, there is no evidence available yet for the safety of this treatment. There is a need to develop chondroprotective strategies to prevent the occurrence and progression of OA. Research that is still in the animal stage includes a study that demonstrates prevention of cartilage degeneration by intra-articular treatment with recombinant lubricin (Flannery et al. 2009). An area of research that has garnered considerable interest is the issue of treatment of OA with stem cell injections. So far, literature includes only a Phase I trial with a limited number of patients without a placebo arm (Pers et al. 2016). A placebo-controlled double-blind Phase IIb study is being initiated (Pers et al. 2016).

RHEUMATOID ARTHRITIS

Rheumatoid arthritis is an autoimmune chronic inflammatory disease that affects the joints by attacking the joint lining, causing a painful swelling that can result in bone erosion and joint deformity if untreated. It can also damage other body systems, including the skin, eyes, lungs, heart, and blood vessels. The disease course can have periods of flaring and remission and final outcomes vary by individual.

Significance

Rheumatoid arthritis is common and can have a significant impact on one's ability to work and perform activities of daily living and decreases an individual's life expectancy by 10 years (Chehata et al. 2001). Although there is evidence of RA in Egyptian mummies, it is thought that the first reference to RA was around 1500 B.C. (Joshi 2012).

Including indirect costs, comprehensive U.S. societal costs of RA were estimated at $39.2 billion in 2005 (Birnbaum et al. 2010). The authors allocated 33% of the total cost to employers, 28% to patients, 20% to the government, and 19% to caregivers. They estimated intangible costs of quality-of-life deterioration at $10.3 billion and premature mortality at $9.6 billion (Birnbaum et al. 2010).

Pathophysiology

Rheumatoid arthritis is a highly debilitating chronic inflammatory immune disorder with an unknown etiology affecting mostly women and the elderly (Scott et al. 2010). It is most commonly characterized as inflammation in the joints causing pain, stiffness, and swelling, which, in turn, may lead to joint damage and disfigurement, a loss of function, and decreased quality of life (Scott et al. 2010; Lee et al. 2012). The pathophysiology of RA consists of pathways leading to the swelling and breakdown of joints, commonly in the hands and feet. In these pathways, there is an influx of lymphocytes (i.e., T cells and B cells) stimulating the production of TNF-α and IL-1. These inflammatory mediators are overproduced and overexpressed, leading to interactions with the T and B cells causing unremitting inflammation and the subsequent destruction and disfigurement of the joint (Scott et al. 2010). Recent evidence also implicates macrophages and the proliferation of synovial fibroblasts in the destructive process (Noss and Brenner 2008; Österreicher et al. 2011).

Descriptive Epidemiology

Rheumatoid arthritis is the most common form of inflammatory arthritis worldwide with a prevalence typically ranging from 0.5% to 1.0% in industrialized countries, with other estimates ranging from 0.4% to 1.3% (CDC 2015). In the United States, the prevalence is 1.1% (10.7 per 1,000; Fina-Aviles et al. 2016). However, there is significant variation among diverse populations, with RA being rarer in rural areas, a factor that may indicate the role environmental factors may play in the disease progression (Alamanos and Drosos 2004).

High-Risk Populations

Rheumatoid arthritis disproportionately affects women, who have a two- to three-fold risk compared with men; women aged older than 65 years have the highest prevalence of RA (Rindfleisch and Muller 2005; Stanaszek and Carlstedt 1999). In men, the risk of RA increases in the 60s (typical onset for both men and women occurs between the ages of 30 and 50 years; CDC 2015; Rindfleisch and Muller 2005). Furthermore, RA risk is increased in obese and overweight women. Those identified as overweight or obese had a 35% increased risk of developing RA at 18 years of age and a nearly 50% increased risk as an adult. Women with a history of 10 cumulative years of obesity had a 37% increased risk of developing RA at a younger age ($\leq$ 55 years; Lu et al. 2014).

Geographic Distribution

The geographic distribution of RA is highly variable. Prevalence of RA is greater in more industrialized countries, such as Northern Europe and North America, versus countries in the developing world (Scott et al. 2010). This geographic variability most likely points to genetic differences and environmental exposures (Scott et al. 2010). The varying prevalence may be partially attributable to urbanization (Kalla and Tikly 2003).

Time Trends

An overall decrease in RA incidence has been observed over the past four decades (Doran et al. 2002). In the disease course of RA over the past decade, trends have shown a decrease in RA activity from a high to a moderate level, presumably attributable to clinicians implementing more modern and aggressive treatment methods (Aga et al. 2015; Welsing et al. 2005).

Causes

With the etiology of RA largely unknown, current etiologic notions include family history and other genetic susceptibilities. Mounting evidence points to genetics and the environment as key factors related to the development and severity of RA (Scott et al. 2010; CDC 2015; de Hair et al. 2013). Genetic factors alone may contribute as much as 50% to 60% in the development of RA in the general population (Scott et al. 2010; MacGregor et al. 2000). A family history of RA increases an individual's risk three- to nine-fold (Karlson et al. 2016). The remaining contributions are believed to come from modifiable, environmental risk factors (CDC 2015).

Modifiable Risk Factors

Modifiable risk factors increase an individual's risk for developing RA or promote the progression of RA and are amenable to change. Many modifiable factors can be identified as environmental exposures. Smoking is a known modifiable risk factor that may significantly contribute to the development of RA, with those who smoke being twice as likely to develop RA as nonsmokers (Scott et al. 2010; de Hair et al. 2013; Karlson et al. 2016). The combination of smoking and being overweight increases an RA-prone individual's arthritis risk 60% (de Hair et al. 2013). Other potentially modifiable factors are mostly unsubstantiated (alcohol and coffee consumption, oral contraceptive use, vitamin D levels, and low socioeconomic status).

Evidence-Based Interventions

Prevention

Within one year of diagnosis, 80% of patients with RA experience some form of negative outcome (i.e., joint pain, swelling, and tenderness). Early screening and aggressive treatment hold promise for lessening the long-term burden of disease (Gibofsky 2012; Demoruelle and Deane 2012; ACR Subcommittee on Rheumatoid Arthritis 2002). There is a period of development of RA when there is no clinical RA, but individuals have elevations of disease-related biomarkers, including autoantibodies (Deane et al. 2010). This has been termed "preclinical RA." Identifying individuals at risk for RA is beneficial because of the increased efficacy of preclinical interventions resulting in better, more positive outcomes (Karlson et al. 2016). Furthermore, reducing the number of ever-smokers may have an effect on overall rates of RA incidence and prevalence. Although the link between obesity and overweight and RA rates is not fully substantiated, intervention focusing on diet modification may possibly have a long-term effect in the development and pathway of RA (Scott et al. 2010).

Screening

No clear-cut, cost-effective, pre-symptomatic screening tool is recommended for RA detection; however, early identification at the onset of RA symptoms has been shown to lead to more effective treatment and long-term positive outcomes (Karlson et al. 2016; Demoruelle and Deane 2012). However, some investigators think it is possible to identify a high-risk group with a high probability of developing clinical RA and treat them to prevent onset of the disease (Arkema et al. 2013). An NIH Clinical Trial (NCT02603146) began enrolling subjects in March 2016 to test this hypothesis.

Treatment

Our ability to treat RA has changed dramatically over the past 20 years, first with the advent of new oral disease-modifying antirheumatic drug (DMARD) therapy and then with the development of biologic agents and use of triple oral therapy (e.g., methotrexate, sulfasalazine, and hydroxychloroquine). The ACR recommendations are to start treatment early, with the ideal outcome being a reduction in RA disease activity (Gibofsky 2012; Demoruelle and Deane 2012).

Pharmacologic treatment at the onset of symptoms with analgesics and non-steroidal anti-inflammatory drugs (NSAIDs) improves function, reduces pain and lessens stiffness. In both early and established RA, a common treatment approach is the use of DMARDs (i.e., methotrexate, sulfasalazine, leflunomide; Scott et al. 2010), which reduce the disease activity of RA, allow individuals diagnosed with RA to achieve remission, and minimize joint damage and deformity (Demoruelle and Deane 2012), but can take up to 6 months to become effective. Tumor necrosis factor inhibitors (biological agents) provide effective treatment for individuals with RA (Scott et al. 2010). In addition to non-biologic and biologic treatment options, research shows the effectiveness of other, non-drug, therapies (Scott et al. 2010). Often, prednisone or an intramuscular steroid is used as a temporizing measure until the DMARD(s) become effective.

As a non-drug therapy, increased physical activity can reduce the impact of RA on symptoms (Scott et al. 2010; Lee et al. 2012). However, studies recognize difficulty in motivating patients with RA to become physically active. More data are needed to confirm if a physical activity intervention is ultimately sustainable (Scott et al. 2010; Lee et al. 2012).

Examples of Evidence-Based Interventions

Major advances include biologic agents, which have made it possible to substantially reduce joint destruction, deformity, functional limitation, and disability in a way unimaginable 20 years ago. In addition, 10 multinational evidence-based recommendations support the use methotrexate for rheumatic disorders such as RA (i.e., 9 of the 10 recommendations specifically addressed RA). These recommendations also address optimal dosage, monitoring and management, long-term safety, and single versus combined treatment (Visser et al. 2009). Additional evidence-based, non-drug therapies such as exercise, electro-physical therapy, thermotherapy, physical therapy, and self-managed care show promise, but their effectiveness varies across different studies and more research is needed (Vliet Vlieland 2007).

Areas for Future Research

In the treatment and understanding of RA, more short-term sustainable treatments, as opposed to long-term suppression, are needed to improve downstream outcomes in persons with RA (Scott et al. 2010). Research is needed to verify the effectiveness of non-drug interventions in the long-term and sustainable treatment and management of RA (Vliet Vlieland 2007). These include interventions dealing with, but not limited to, occupational therapy, physical therapy, and exercise to better understand the optimal methods for delivery of the intervention and optimal activity levels for maximum effectiveness (NCCCC 2009). Also needed are studies relating to the cost-effectiveness of many interventions available for treatment and disease management, including expanded cost-effectiveness studies in the use of DMARD treatment in advanced and moderate RA patients.

Improved pharmacologic and non-pharmacologic therapies aimed at appropriately treating an individual with RA, along with continued research focusing on RA and its etiology and disease activity, will help continue the downward trend in RA disease activity. Innovation and improved understanding may ultimately provide a long-term cure, eliminating the need for purely symptomatic treatment (NCCCC 2009). Similarly, new advances in the field may make it possible to prevent onset of this disease with existing technology.

GOUT

Gout was historically called the "disease of kings" or "rich man's disease" because of its association with obesity (Saccomano and Ferrara 2015). It is characterized by severe joint pain and can lead to irreversible joint damage if untreated (Eggebeen 2007). The symptoms of an acute gout flare (also known as gouty arthritis) include sudden onset of severe joint pain, inflammation, warmth of the affected joint, limited range of motion of the joint, and, possibly, effusion. Approximately 90% of first attacks are monoarticular; the first metatarsophalangeal joint (podagra) is the location in more than 50% of them (Harris et al. 1999).

Significance

Gout is a common form of inflammatory arthritis, affecting an estimated eight million U.S. adults and accounting for almost four million outpatient visits yearly (Zhu et al. 2011; Krishnan et al. 2008). It is the most common cause of inflammatory arthritis in men aged older than 40 years (Wijnands et al. 2015; Smith et al. 2014). Uncontrolled gout is associated with a high use of emergency care services. In the 2010 Global Burden of Disease study, gout ranked 138 of 291 conditions studied as measured by years living with disability, and 173 of 291 in terms of overall disease burden as measured by disability-adjusted life years (Smith et al. 2014). Disability-adjusted life years for gout increased from 76,000 in 1990 to 114,000 in 2010 (Smith et al. 2014). Patients with gout have an increased risk of cardiovascular disease (Roddy and Doherty 2010) and increased rates of cancer, especially urologic cancer (Chen et al. 2014).

Pathophysiology

Gout is a crystal deposition disease, caused by altered purine metabolism leading to hyperuricemia that arises when supersaturation of body tissues with urate occurs. Hyperuricemia, (serum uric acid concentration greater than 6.5 mg per dL), can be due either to increased urate production or decreased renal excretion of urine. Accumulation of uric acid leads to the formation of monosodium urate crystals in and around joints (Roddy and Choi 2014), which is the basis of an acute inflammatory reaction. When uric acid concentrations are lowered below the monosodium urate saturation point, the crystals dissolve (Richette and Bardin 2010). Asymptomatic hyperuricemia is not usually treated.

Descriptive Epidemiology

Gout has been estimated to have a 0.08% prevalence globally (Smith et al. 2014); frequency is rising both in the United States and worldwide (Mikuls and

Saag 2006; Smith et al. 2010), although it varies geographically. NHANES data from 2007 to 2008 estimate that 8.3 million Americans (3.9% of the population) have gout, with a prevalence of 5.9% in men and 2.0% in women (Singh 2013; Zhu et al. 2011). In the United States, prevalence of gout is 5.0% in blacks and 4.0% in whites (Zhu et al. 2011, Singh 2013). Information on incidence is harder to find. In 2010, the Framingham Heart Study reported an incidence of 1.4 per 1,000 person-years in women and 4.0 per 1,000 person years in men (Bhole et al. 2010). There has been an observed annual seasonal flare of gout during spring in the northern hemisphere (Kim et al. 2003).

High-Risk Populations

Primary risk factors for developing gout include enzyme deficits, decreased renal clearance of uric acid, inborn metabolic errors, gender, hyperuricemia, and family history of gout. Dietary factors in the form of a Western diet (excessive consumption of meat, seafood, sugar-sweetened soft drinks, and fructose) also increase the risk of developing hyperuricemia and gout, whereas low-fat dairy products, coffee, and vitamin C appear to be protective against these conditions (Choi et al. 2010; Roddy and Choi 2014; Choi and Curhan 2008). Risk factors also include alcohol use (especially beer), lead exposure, and diuretic use (Roddy and Doherty 2010; Kim et al. 2003). There is a linear trend of increasing prevalence of gout seen with increasing BMI (Singh 2013). A recent study on gender-specific risk factors for gout found that the serum uric acid–gout relationship had a higher impact on men than on women (Chen et al. 2012), although menopause increases gout risk in women. Association of the *ABCG2* gene (rs2231142 allele) with susceptibility to gout varied according to race and ethnicity (Phipps-Green et al. 2010). Conditions associated with (but not risk factors for) gout include hypertension, high BMI, and central obesity (Kim et al. 2003). There is a high prevalence of gout in patients with type 2 diabetes and impaired fasting glucose or impaired glucose tolerance (Liu et al. 2012).

Geographic Distribution

Historically, there have not been many studies of the epidemiology of gout. Framingham data showed a 1.5% prevalence of gout (2.8% in men and 0.4% in women; Hall et al. 1967). Prevalence was reportedly 0.26% in England in 1975 and 0.95% in a multicenter study published in 1995 (Gabriel and Michaud 2009).

Causes

Modifiable Risk Factors

For patients with gout, modifiable risk factors include obesity, diet—especially one that includes purine-rich food and high-fructose beverages, excessive alcohol intake, and lead exposure. Controlling hypertension is important, but hypertension is not a risk factor for primary gout (Roubenoff et al. 1991). Results of one study suggest use of low-dose aspirin on two consecutive days is associated with increased risk of recurrent gout attacks (Zhang et al. 2014).

Evidence-Based Interventions

Prevention

Although not every person with asymptomatic hyperuricemia will develop gout, hyperuricemia is a prerequisite to developing gout. Especially if there is a family history of gout, primary prevention should include lifestyle modifications such as weight reduction, decreasing intake of purine-rich foods and high-fructose beverages, moderating alcohol intake, and control of hypertension (without the use of thiazide diuretics) and hyperlipidemia. In addition, because of the known association of occupational lead exposure with gout, prevention efforts should also reduce such exposure in high-risk professions such as painting, plumbing, shipbuilding, and steel work.

Recurrent attacks of gout may be prevented through use of colchicine or NSAIDs, and hyperuricemia can be reversed with agents that either increase uric acid excretion or inhibit its production. The control strategies for gout should be employed in conjunction with the same strategies used for primary prevention.

Treatment

Although there are no screening recommendations for gout, it can be managed via not only pharmacological approaches, but also non-pharmacological interventions aimed at decreasing attack risk, lowering uric acid levels, and promoting general health while preventing development of comorbidities (Grassi et al. 2014). Two first-line options for prophylaxis are low-dose colchicine or low-dose NSAIDs (e.g., naproxen; Latourte et al. 2014). In those unable to take or tolerate NSAIDs, oral or intramuscular steroids can be used. Adrenocorticotropic hormone can also be used, but is more expensive and sometimes difficult to procure.

Two RCTs showed that using colchicine prophylaxis for at least six months when starting urate-lowering therapy reduces the risk of acute attacks (Seth et al. 2014; Terkeltaub et al. 2010). Recently, two RCTs showed that febuxostat is safe and efficacious to lower uric acid levels in patients with gout, with significant reduction of serum uric acid at all dosages. Febuxostat was more effective than allopurinol in lowering uric acid levels (Becker et al. 2005; Schumaker et al. 2008; Grassi et al. 2014). Canakinumab, not currently licensed for gout, has been shown to provide prophylaxis superior to colchicine when one is starting urate-lowering therapy (Seth et al. 2014).

Fibromyalgia

Pain can be classified as localized, regionalized, or generalized. Fibromyalgia is the second-most-common rheumatic disease and is in the category of generalized pain. Unlike the pain in other forms of arthritis, the pain from fibromyalgia comes from a central nervous system disturbance rather than from inflammation and nerve signals coming from the joints or muscles (Clauw 2009).

Chronic widespread pain is defined as pain above and below the waist, involving the left and right sides of the body, and also involving the axial skeleton. Once known as non-articular rheumatism (White and Harth 2001), fibromyalgia is the current term for widespread musculoskeletal pain for which no alternative cause can be identified, and is characterized by pain referred to deep tissues (Vierck 2012). Fatigue includes both central fatigue (mental exhaustion with impairment in concentration or thinking that occurs as the result of intellectually demanding activities) and physical fatigue (a sense of overall physical exhaustion or depletion of energy as a result of physical effort, which can occur with or without any medical disease; Moldofsky and MacFarlane 2009).

The ACR criteria assess fibromyalgia with the Widespread Pain Index, which divides the body into 19 regions and scores how many regions are reported as painful. A symptom severity score assesses severity of a variety of nonsomatic complaints including fatigue, sleep disturbances, and cognitive dysfunction (Chin et al. 2016; Rahman et al. 2014). Prominent diffuse musculoskeletal discomfort differentiates fibromyalgia from other chronic pain syndromes (Moldofsky and MacFarlane 2009). There is still controversy as to whether fibromyalgia is a distinct entity or a spectrum of diseases, but it is thought to be part of a group of central sensitivity syndromes, including chronic fatigue syndrome, functional dyspepsia, Gulf War syndrome, interstitial cystitis, irritable bowel syndrome, temporomandibular joint dysfunction, myofascial pain, post-traumatic stress disorder, and restless leg syndrome (Theoharides et al. 2015).

Significance

Fibromyalgia accounted for 2% to 6% of rheumatology patients in the late 1970s and early 1980s (White and Harth 2001) but has now increased to 5% to 15% of this population (Wolfe et al. 1995; Croft et al. 1993; Coster et al. 2008). It is estimated that six million people in the United States have fibromyalgia—about 2% of the entire population—accounting for 10 million patient visits annually because of pain. Patients saw an average of four doctors before being correctly diagnosed, resulting in an estimated $85 billion annually to diagnose the cause of the pain, including litigation fees (Tramer et al. 1998).

Pathophysiology

The exact cause of fibromyalgia is not known (Rahman et al. 2014), but there are many hypotheses (Abeles et al. 2007). Evidence suggests abnormal pain processing in patients with fibromyalgia (Bradley 2009). Individuals display diffuse hyperalgesia or allodynia, suggesting a fundamental problem with pain or sensory processing (Clauw 2009). Persons with fibromyalgia sense stimuli such as heat, cold, and pressure at the same level as those without the disease, but their threshold for feeling that sensation as painful is lower than average (Abeles et al. 2007). Fatigue and bodily hypersensitivity may be attributable to disturbances in central nervous system functions (Pillemer et al. 1997). Biologic abnormalities in fibromyalgia include disturbances in the neuroendocrine system and the autonomic nervous system, and sleep disturbances (Moldofsky and MacFarlane 2009; Bradley 2009).

Possible mechanisms for this difference in sensation include altered metabolism in peripheral muscle (Simms 1998), aberrant central pain mechanisms (Yunus 1992), and abnormal brain responses to pain (Abeles et al. 2007).

Of these, central sensitization is now thought to be the primary driver of fibromyalgia (Chin et al. 2016). There is an associated constellation of symptoms including pain, tenderness, fatigue, anxiety, sleep dysfunction, cognitive impairment, and mood disturbances (Chin et al. 2016).

Until recently, most pain was attributed to activation of peripheral nociceptive nerves. However, recent research into several "idiopathic" conditions suggests that the pain in these conditions is not occurring because of inflammation or damage in peripheral tissues and, thus, it is not truly nociceptive pain. Other theories for pathogenesis of fibromyalgia include involvement of infectious agents (Ablin et al. 2008) such as hepatitis B and C, HIV, and Lyme disease; stress and stress-related hormonal imbalance (Ablin et al. 2008); and activity of the hypothalamic–pituitary–adrenal axis (Carrasco and Van de Kar 2003; Goldenberg 1993). Parvovirus B19 was once thought to be associated with fibromyalgia, but this has been disproved (Ablin et al. 2008). There is also no support for leptin in the pathogenesis of fibromyalgia (Ablin et al. 2012).

Descriptive Epidemiology

Almost one in four (23%) of adults in the United States report having experienced persistent fatigue sometime during their lives (Price et al. 1992). Unexplained substantial fatigue for greater than one month occurs in approximately 8% of patients, with a range from 12% to 15% in Berlin, Germany; Santiago, Chile; and Manchester, England, to a low prevalence between 2% to 4% in Ibaden, Nigeria; Verona, Italy; Shanghai, China; Seattle, Washington; and Bangalore, India (Skapinakis et al. 2003). Fibromyalgia affects approximately 2% of the population; more than 80% of those affected are women. Debilitating fatigue affects between 76% and 81% of patients with fibromyalgia (Wolfe et al. 1996). Physicians diagnose fibromyalgia in women at a three- to six-fold rate compared with men (Marcus 2009).

High-Risk Populations

Stressors capable of triggering fibromyalgia include peripheral pain syndromes, infections, psychological stress and distress, hormonal alterations, drugs, and some catastrophic events (Clauw 2009). Genetic factors are also thought to be important. First-degree relatives of patients with fibromyalgia have an eight-fold greater risk of developing fibromyalgia than the general population (Arnold et al. 2004). Twin studies suggest that half of the risk is attributable to genetics and half of the risk is environmental (Kato et al. 2006).

Causes

It is thought that candidate genes may play a role in fibromyalgia. For instance, the *5-HTT* gene may contribute to enhanced pain sensitivity in patients with fibromyalgia and other affective spectrum disorders (Bradley 2009). In another study, significant differences in allele frequencies between fibromyalgia cases and controls were observed for three genes: *GABRB3*, *GBP1*, and *TAAR1* (Kato et al. 2006). Physical trauma (Jurell et al. 1996), either in the form of a major event or repetitive minor trauma can result in post-traumatic or reactive fibromyalgia (White and Harth 2001). Bennett (1993) suggests that, if they are going to occur, fibromyalgia symptoms develop 6 to 18 months after a traumatic event; those with traumatic fibromyalgia have a worse outcome.

Modifiable Risk Factors

Improving sleep quantity and quality, exercising, and learning stress management techniques help individuals to address aggravating factors. Avoiding cold or humid weather and noise may also help (Yunus 2009).

Evidence-Based Interventions

Prevention

The problem in preventing onset of fibromyalgia is that no markers of disease exist (Altomonte et al. 2008). Immediate care is recommended for acute pain episodes and for somatoform disturbances to prevent chronicity. Secondary prevention requires promoting early detection and treatment of known risk factors such as trauma, infection, emotional stress, catastrophic events, autoimmune diseases, or other pain conditions (Altomonte et al. 2008).

Treatment

Complete remission with complete resolution of chronic pain is rare in fibromyalgia (White and Harth 2001). There is no satisfactory effective treatment to improve sleep quality, fatigue, and debilitating somatic symptoms (Moldofsky and MacFarlane 2009). Individuals with these conditions typically do not respond to therapies that are effective when pain is caused by damage or inflammation of tissues (Clauw 2009), although those with the most favorable prognosis are children and younger women who present with milder disease. Local therapies and complementary and alternative medicines have been used with varying success for fibromyalgia (Moldofsky and MacFarlane 2009; Arnold 2009; Ernst 2009; Marcus 2009). Non-pharmacologic treatments include fitness and strengthening exercise, warm water therapy, and psychological pain management techniques (Marcus 2009).

Examples of Evidence-Based Interventions

Evidence-based guidelines recommend active physical therapy, education, and psychological and behavioral therapy (Rahman et al. 2014). Aerobic exercise, at least 20 minutes per day, two to three times per week, for at least 2.5 weeks, improves well-being, tenderness, and pain compared with no aerobic exercise (Croft et al. 1993). Acupuncture (Rahman et al. 2014) and mindfulness-based stress reduction for well-being have also been shown to help decrease pain (Grossman et al. 2007).

ANKYLOSING SPONDYLITIS

Ankylosing spondylitis is the prototypic disease of several related but phenotypically distinct disorders known as seronegative spondyloarthropathies (psoriatic arthritis, arthritis related to inflammatory bowel disease, reactive arthritis, a subgroup of juvenile idiopathic arthritis, and AS; Dougados and Baeten 2011). Diagnosis is defined by the modified New York criteria (Keat 2010) according to the following three clinical and one radiologic criteria:

- Low back pain and stiffness for more than three months that improves with exercise, but is not relieved by rest.
- Limitation of motion of the lumbar spine in the sagittal and frontal planes.
- Limitation of chest expansion relative to normal values correlated for age and sex.
- Sacroiliitis grade greater than 2 bilaterally or grade 3 to 4 unilaterally (radiologic).

A definitive diagnosis is made if the radiological criterion is associated with at least one of the clinical criteria.

Significance

Extra-articular manifestations of AS occur with varying frequency, with some being more clinically relevant than others. The most common are uveitis (pathogenesis not well understood), gastrointestinal involvement (inflammatory bowel disease), and lung abnormalities. Renal abnormalities, heart conduction disturbances, psoriasis, osteoporosis and vertebral fractures, and aortic insufficiency also occur, but less commonly (El Maghraoui 2011). Compared with the general population, patients with AS have an approximately two-fold increase in death rate attributable to an increased cardiovascular risk, and the prevalence rate for myocardial infarction is increased two- to three-fold (El Maghraoui 2011). Clinical activity can be measured by the Bath Ankylosing Spondylitis Disease Activity Index (Dougados and Baeten 2011). Clinical forms of this disease group include spinal (axial) features, peripheral arthritis, enthesopathy, and extra-articular features such as uveitis, psoriasis, and inflammatory bowel disease. Untreated, these diseases can result in structural and functional impairments and a decreased quality of life.

Pathophysiology

The most common symptom of AS is an insidious onset of low back pain. Patients may gradually develop ankylosis (abnormal stiffening and immobility of a joint due to fusion of the bones) at the entheses, which is the location where ligaments, tendons, and capsules are attached to the bone. Processes involving affected entheses are inflammation, bone erosion, and syndesmophyte (spur) formation. Tumor necrosis factor, a pro-inflammatory cytokine, is an important mediator of the inflammatory process but not of bone erosion or syndesmophyte formation (Tam et al. 2010). The arthritogenic peptide theory is the traditional pathophysiological framework for spondyloarthritis and proposes that HLA-B27 (a type of human leukocyte antigen allele) presents self-peptides that resemble pathogen-derived peptides to CD8-restricted T lymphocytes (Dougados and Baeten 2011). In patients with Reiter's syndrome and other infectious seronegative spondyloarthropathies, cross-reactive enteric organisms produce a factor, which specifically modifies the B27-positive lymphocytes of normal individuals; this factor is structurally and antigenically related to a functionally similar factor secreted by some isolates of *Klebsiella* species (Prendergast et al. 1983).

Descriptive Epidemiology

High-Risk Populations

Ankylosing spondylitis is thought to be a polygenic disease. The most well-known risk factor for AS is HLA-B27, which accounts for 20% to 50% of the total genetic risk for this disease (Vegvari et al. 2009), but it is not required for the disease to occur (Pham 2008). Only 5% to 6% of the general population with HLA-B27 develops AS. Candidate genes and cytokine expression are all thought to have a major role in AS (Dougados and Baeten 2011; Pham 2008; Hajjaj-Hassouni and Burgos-Vargas 2008).

Geographic Distribution

There is very little information on geographic distribution of AS, but a literature review from 2013 shows geographic variation. From 36 eligible studies, mean AS prevalence per 10,000 was 31.9 in North America, 23.8 in Europe, 16.7 in Asia, 10.2 in Latin American, and 7.4 in Africa (Dean et al. 2014). Incidence of AS reflects the prevalence of HLA-B27 seropositivity. HLA-B27 is highly prevalent in the circumpolar Arctic and the sub-Arctic regions of Eurasia, North America, and some parts of Melanesia. It is very high in some North American Indian populations (Saraux et al. 2005; Lawrence et al. 1996). HLA-B27 is rare among the genetic unmixed native populations of South America, Australia, and certain parts of equatorial and southern Africa (Saraux et al. 2005; Lawrence et al. 1996).

Time Trends

Available data indicate that incidence of AS has remained relatively stable, although information from Rochester, Minnesota, showed a slight decline in incidence between 1935 and 1989 (Carbone et al. 1992). Age at symptom onset remained unchanged, and overall survival was stable for up to 28 years after diagnosis (Gabriel and Michaud 2009).

Evidence-Based Interventions

Prevention

There is no known primary prevention for AS. Secondary prevention consists of exercise and taking DMARDs if applicable. Quitting smoking may have some benefit on function, but it is uncertain whether it has any effect on disease (Zochling et al. 2006). Some studies have been conducted on dietary interventions, but evidence to date is too weak for formal recommendations (Zochling et al. 2006).

Screening

There is really no way to screen patients for AS, but the Assessment in Ankylosing Spondylitis International Working Group recommends a periodic core set, which measures patient global assessment, spinal pain, spinal stiffness, spinal mobility, physical function, peripheral joints, entheses, acute phase reactants, and fatigue. The core set also contains definitions of what is considered improvement, how often to assess disease, and other information (Zochling and Braun 2007). Also, a relatively recent major improvement in diagnostic technique has been in using magnetic resonance imaging to visualize inflammatory changes in the sacroiliac joint and the axial spine, which has been especially useful given the advances in treatment (Mansour et al. 2006). Magnetic resonance imaging allows visualization of synovial fluid, synovitis within the sacroiliac joint, and subchondral bone edema (Dougados and Baeten 2011), whereas x-ray and computed tomography scan can detect only structural changes such as joint erosion and subchondral-bone sclerosis at late stage of disease (Dougados and Baeten 2011).

Treatment

There is no cure for AS. Treatment goals are to relieve pain, stiffness, and fatigue, and to prevent structural damage when possible. NSAIDs and specific cyclo-oxygenase-2 inhibitors are used to provide relief from spinal pain and peripheral joint pain and improve function over a period of approximately six weeks (Akkoc et al. 2006). Evidence supports avoiding abrupt withdrawal of NSAIDs because of possible vascular rebound effects in patients with systemic inflammatory disorders (Fischer et al. 2004).

Although DMARDs are used to mitigate stiffness and pain in other conditions, there is poor evidence for efficacy in AS (Akkoc et al. 2006). Tumor necrosis factor inhibitors are first-line treatment for axial disease. Large RCTs of infliximab and etanercept have shown short-term improvements in spinal pain, function, and inflammatory markers with therapy compared with placebo (Brandt et al. 2006). There is a large relapse rate when TNF inhibitors are discontinued (Brandt et al. 2006).

Examples of Evidence-Based Interventions

Patients with AS should be advised to exercise daily if possible, with swimming being the best exercise. A tailored therapeutic exercise program with education and disease information showed improved function without change in pain at four months compared with no intervention. Improvement was maintained with minimal treatment, consisting of 1.5 mean visits from the physiotherapist between months four and eight (Zochling et al. 2006).

Eight of eight RCTs support use of NSAIDs or cyclo-oxygenase-2 inhibitors for spinal pain in AS (Zochling et al. 2006). Intra-articular steroid injections are effective for sacroiliitis, but there has been only one RCT showing improvement in pain. There is no evidence that sulfasalazine is effective in AS. Information on methotrexate is conflicted but weakly supports use in peripheral disease (Zochling et al. 2006). Biologic agents appear to show improvement in spinal pain, peripheral joint pain, and function, but studies have so far been limited to TNF blockers and IL-1 inhibitors (Zochling et al. 2006).

Areas for Future Research

Research that has direct relevance for clinical practice is needed. Thalidomide is receiving attention as a possible treatment for severe AS. At this point, it seems that it may improve axial pain, but effects on peripheral disease are unknown and toxicity is a problem (Zochling et al. 2006). Important research areas include the development of techniques for early diagnosis, therapeutic modulation of structural damage, and induction of long-term, drug-free remission (Dougados and Baeten 2011). As with RA, biologic agents can markedly change the patient's quality of life, in addition to altering the course of the disease, if the patient's symptoms are attributable to an inflammatory spondyloarthritis.

OSTEOPOROSIS

Significance

Osteoporosis is the most common bone disease in humans, representing a major public health problem as outlined in Bone Health and Osteoporosis: A Report of the Surgeon General (USDHHS 2004). For purposes of epidemiologic studies, the World Health Organization (WHO) defines osteoporosis as a bone mineral density value measured at the femoral neck or total hip of

2.5 standard deviations below the mean for normal young white women (WHO 1994). Based on data from NHANES III, using this definition, there are an estimated 10 million women and 3 million men aged 50 years and older with osteoporosis in the United States (USDHHS 2004). According to a recommendation statement published by the U.S. Preventive Services Task Force (USPSTF) in 2011, one half of postmenopausal woman would have had fractures related to osteoporosis in their lifetime (USPSTF 2011). The annual direct costs for osteoporotic fractures ranged from $12.2 billion to $17.9 billion per year in 2002 for acute and chronic care (USDHHS 2004).

Pathophysiology

Several definitions have been proposed for osteoporosis. The classic definition is "a systemic skeletal disorder characterized by low bone mass and microarchitectural deterioration of bone tissue, with a consequent increase in bone fragility and susceptibility to fracture. At a consensus conference sponsored by the National Institutes of Health in 2000, osteoporosis was defined as a skeletal disorder characterized by compromised bone strength predisposing to an increased risk of fracture. "Bone strength" reflects the integration of two main features: bone density and bone quality. "Bone density" is expressed as grams of mineral per area or volume and "bone quality" refers to architecture, turnover, damage accumulation (e.g., micro-fractures), and mineralization (NIH 2000).

Concepts in the pathogenesis of osteoporosis have been reviewed recently with an emphasis on the complex interplay among genetics, hormones, nutrition, lifestyle, and environmental factors (Raisz 2005; Russell 2006). Bone mineral density in adulthood is determined in part by the amount of bone that is accrued by early to middle adult life, and the rate of decline in bone mass during middle to late adult life. The clinical manifestations may include fractures of the spine, hip, wrist, or other areas of the skeleton (Cummings and Melton 2002). Indeed, fractures at almost all skeletal sites, except for the fingers, toes, face, and skull, are related to low bone mineral density (Stone et al. 2003). Traditionally, fractures of the hip, spine, and wrist among older adults, especially when they occur in association with minimal or moderate trauma, have been considered osteoporotic fractures. Many epidemiologic studies have used fracture as a measure of osteoporosis because of the availability of data resources and the lack of access to technology to measure bone mineral density. However, the availability of dual x-ray absorptiometry (DXA) for measurement of bone mineral density has allowed the study of factors related to low bone mineral density. Therefore, the epidemiology of osteoporosis is a combination of both the epidemiology of low bone mineral density and the epidemiology of fracture.

Descriptive Epidemiology

High-Risk Populations

Osteoporosis is usually considered a disease of postmenopausal white women. Peak bone mass, usually achieved in the third decade, is lower in women than in men. On average, decline in bone mass occurs beginning in the fourth decade at a rate of 0.5% to 1.0% per year, with an accelerated rate of loss in the years immediately following menopause in women. Hence, the decline in bone mass in women proceeds from a lower baseline. In NHANES III, in which bone mineral density of the hip was measured as part of the examination, men had higher average bone mineral density than women in every racial group reported; consequently, the prevalence of low bone mass were higher in women than in men and in non-Hispanic whites than in blacks (Figure 20-4; Wright et al. 2014; USDHHS 2004). Not surprisingly, age-specific incidence rates for hip fracture are higher among women than among men through the ninth decade (Jacobsen et al. 1990a).

In Western populations, Hispanics and whites have lower bone mineral density, a higher prevalence of osteoporosis (Figure 20-5), a greater rate of decline in bone mineral density, and a higher rate of non-spine and hip fractures than blacks (Wright et al. 2014; USDHHS 2004). Age-specific incidence rates of hip fracture are about twice as high among white women as they are among black women, and most studies indicate a higher risk for hip fractures among white men than among black men. Mexican-American populations have lower hip fracture rates than whites but slightly higher rates than blacks (Bauer 1988). Bone mineral density is lower in Asians than in whites, but Asians may experience a lower incidence of hip fracture; this may be related to differences in geometry of the femoral neck between Asians and whites (Yano et al. 1985).

Twin and family studies suggest that genetic factors may explain as much as 85% of the variation in age-specific bone mineral density in the population (Williams and Spector 2006). Genetics play the largest role in attainment of peak bone mass and probably also have a role in the rate of bone loss with aging or after menopause. The search for single-gene effects on bone mineral density remains an active area of investigation. In genome-wide association studies, genes that

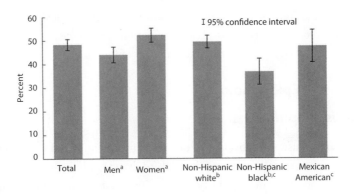

Source: Reprinted from Looker and Frenk (2015).

Note: Age-adjusted by the direct method to the year 2000 Census Bureau estimates using age groups 65-79 and 80 and over. World Health Organization diagnostic criteria were used to define low bone mass as a bone mineral density (BMD) value at the femur neck or lumbar spine that falls between 1.0 and 2.5 standard deviation units below the mean BMD for young non-Hispanic white females. BMD at the femur neck and lumbar spine was measured using dual-energy x-ray absorptiometry (DXA).

[a]Significant difference between men and women, ($p < 0.05$).

[b]Significant difference between non-Hispanic white and non-Hispanic black, ($p < 0.05$).

[c]Significant difference between non-Hispanic black and Mexican American, ($p < 0.05$).

Figure 20-4. Age-Adjusted Percentage of Adults Aged 65 and and Over with Low Bone Mass at the Femur Neck or Lumbar Spine, by Sex and Race and Hispanic Origin: United States, 2005–2010

have been identified to be associated with variation of bone mineral density are *RANKL, OPG,* and *RANK,* which are encoders of key regulation of osteoclasts. Other genes that may be associated with bone mineral density include genes that affect calcium metabolism and the estrogen receptor gene (Kumar 2010).

Other factors associated with a high risk for osteoporosis and osteoporotic fractures are older age, low body weight, weight loss, physical inactivity, a history of a previous fracture after age 50 years, current smoking, excessive alcohol consumption, and recent use of oral glucocorticoids (Espallargues et al. 2001).

Geographic Distribution

Internationally, the geographic distribution of osteoporosis has been studied principally on the basis of rates of hip fractures. The highest age-adjusted rates of hip fracture are found in the Scandinavian countries, followed by the United States and Western Europe; lower rates were reported in Latin America and

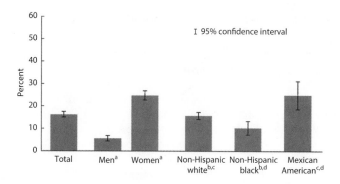

Source: Reprinted from Looker and Frenk (2015).
Note: Age-adjusted by the direct method to the year 2000 Census Bureau estimates using age groups 65-79 and 80 and over. World Health Organization diagnostic criteria were used to define osteoporosis as a bone mineral density (BMD) value at the femur neck or lumbar spine that falls more than 2.5 standard deviation units below the mean BMD for young non-Hispanic white females. BMD at the femur neck and lumbar spine was measured using dual-energy x-ray absorptiometry (DXA).
[a]Significant difference between men and women, ($p < 0.05$).
[b]Significant difference between non-Hispanic white and non-Hispanic black, ($p < 0.05$).
[c]Significant difference between non-Hispanic white and Mexican American, ($p < 0.05$).
[d]Significant difference between non-Hispanic black and Mexican American, ($p < 0.05$).

Figure 20-5. Age-Adjusted Percentage of Adults Aged 65 Years and Over with Osteoporosis at the Femur Neck or Lumbar Spine, by Sex and Race and Hispanic Origin: United States, 2005-2010

Asia (Harvey et al. 2006). The highest age-adjusted rates of spine fractures also occurred in Scandinavia with lower rates in Western European countries.

Jacobsen et al. (1990b) studied regional variations in hip fracture incidence among white women in the United States. By calculating age-specific rates of hip fracture at the county level, they identified a north–south gradient of increasing hip fracture occurrence, with a cluster of high incidence in the Southeast. An analysis of data based on hospital discharge rates for hip fracture among Medicare recipients in 2001 confirmed that the highest rates occurred in the Southeast and South-Central regions (Zingmond et al. 2004).

Time Trends

As with geographic distribution, time trends in osteoporosis have been studied on the basis of fracture rates. Hospital discharge rates for hip fractures among Medicare recipients increased during the last decade of the 20th century but

Table 20-2. Modifiable Risk Factors for Osteoporosis and Osteoporotic Fractures

Magnitude	Risk Factor
Strong (relative risk > 4)	Immobility
	Low body weight and weight loss
	Current or recent use of glucocorticoids
Moderate (relative risk 2–4)	Current smoking
	Excessive alcohol intake
	Low calcium intake or low sunlight exposure
Weak (relative risk < 2)	Current use of antidepressants
	Current use of proton-pump inhibitors

Source: Reprinted from Hirsch and Hochberg (2010).

have largely stabilized since (Zingmond et al. 2004). Data from a study in California suggest that hip fracture rates have increased in Hispanic women and men while they have declined in non-Hispanic white women from 1983 to 2000 (Zingmond et al. 2004). Also, new data from the National Center for Health Statistics show that the rate of osteoporosis and low bone density in Hispanic females is surpassing that of non-Hispanic white women (Looker et al. 2012).

Causes

Modifiable Risk Factors

A number of lifestyle factors, medical conditions, and medications are associated with osteoporosis and osteoporotic fractures (Table 20-2; USDHHS 2004; Espallargues et al. 2001). Although most of these are associated with osteoporosis as defined by low bone mineral density, some are associated only with osteoporotic fractures because of their relationship with falls (e.g., reduced visual acuity, Parkinson's disease, excessive alcohol consumption). The risk factors for osteoporosis may act by either (1) interfering with the ability to produce a skeleton of optimal mass and strength during the period of growth and development or (2) increasing the rate of bone resorption or decreasing the rate of bone formation leading to a decline in bone mineral density and deterioration of bone microarchitecture during adulthood. Recent studies have identified the molecular mechanisms involved in regulation of osteoclast and osteoblast development and function; these are the cells that are responsible for bone resorption and formation, respectively (Boyce and Xing 2007).

Table 20-3. Proportion of Hip Fractures Attributed to Modifiable Risk Factors, United States

Factor	Best Estimate, %	Range, %
Nonuse of hormone replacement	19	6–31
Thin body build	18	10.5–26
Cigarette smoking	10	4–16

Source: Reprinted from Hirsch and Hochberg (2010).

A committee of the WHO has identified a set of risk factors that, in combination with bone mineral density, can be used to predict a person's 10-year absolute risk for osteoporotic fracture (de Laet et al. 2005). These risk factors were derived from a series of meta-analyses of data from population-based longitudinal cohort studies with fracture outcomes. The risk factors include age, sex, history of clinical fracture after age 50 years, parental history of hip fracture, current smoking, use of systemic glucocorticoids within the past year, excessive alcohol intake, and presence of RA as a prototype chronic systemic inflammatory disease. When results of bone mineral density testing are not available, BMI can be used as a surrogate, as they are highly correlated. The WHO Fracture Assessment Tool is available online (http://www.shef.ac.uk/FRAX/tool.jsp) and can be used to calculate an individual's 10-year cumulative risk for osteoporotic fracture.

Population-Attributable Risk

Elimination of risk factors, especially those that are more prevalent, has the potential to reduce the occurrence of low bone density and hip fracture. Hirsch and Hochberg (2010) estimated the population attributable risks for nonuse of hormone replacement therapy, thin build, and smoking (Table 20-3). Because of the lack of definitive studies, attributable risk estimates for osteoporosis are not available.

Evidence-Based Interventions

Prevention

The prevention of osteoporosis must focus on optimizing the attainment of peak bone mass during growth and development, and slowing the rate of bone loss with aging. Measures aimed at affecting peak bone mass must begin in childhood and adolescence. These include maintaining a nutritious diet with an adequate intake of calcium and vitamin D and an active lifestyle, with an emphasis on weight-bearing physical activities. Young women, in particular, should be discouraged from smoking cigarettes or participating in overly strenuous athletics that result in the development of amenorrhea (the "female athlete triad" of amenorrhea, low body weight, and low bone mineral density; Beals and Meyer 2007). The ideal of extreme thinness, as typified by teenage actresses and models, also should be discouraged, and anorexia should be aggressively treated.

To slow bone loss, clinicians should discuss the use of hormone therapy beginning at or shortly after menopause. Again, weight-bearing exercise should be encouraged, and smoking and heavy alcohol consumption should be discouraged.

Clinicians also should consider ways of addressing the risk factors for falling, particularly in older adults with low bone mineral density. An environmental assessment to help older men and women "fall-proof" their living areas is helpful. This may include ensuring optimal lighting, installing appropriate and graspable hand rails on stairs and in the bathroom, checking throw rugs and extension cords, and placing "soft" corners on cabinets and furniture to minimize injuries if falls occur. In addition, attention to appropriate footwear to prevent tripping is important.

Screening

Current screening recommendations by the USPSTF for osteoporosis recommend screening women aged 65 years and older without previous known fractures or secondary causes of osteoporosis. The Task Force also recommends screening women aged younger than 65 years whose 10-year fracture risk is equal to or greater than that of a 65-year-old white woman without additional risk factors. The USPSTF does not recommend screening for men without previous known fractures or secondary causes of osteoporosis (USPSTF 2011).

The diagnosis of osteoporosis is currently based on results of DXA scan. There are other imaging studies that have been used to measure bone density, such as quantitative ultrasound of the calcaneus, which seems to be equivalent to DXA for predicting fractures. However, diagnostic criteria at the moment use DXA measurements as cutoffs, and there are no conversions from ultrasound results to be used as DXA equivalents. For qualitative ultrasound to be clinically relevant for diagnosis of osteoporosis, such conversion values should be developed (USPSTF 2011).

A number of algorithms and indices have been published that also can be used to identify women and men who should undergo measurement of bone mineral density (Hochberg 2006). These should complement the clinical guidelines for measurement noted previously rather than substitute for them.

Treatment

Secondary prevention involves the prevention of fractures and treatment of persons with osteoporosis, defined by low bone mineral density. There are several medications that are approved by the Food and Drug Administration for the prevention or treatment of osteoporosis; these drugs work either by decreasing the rate of bone turnover (anticatabolic or antiresorptive agents) or increasing the rate of bone formation (anabolic agents). All of these drugs have been shown to reduce the risk of spine fractures in randomized placebo-controlled clinical trials; only some have been shown to reduce the risk of non-spine fractures, including hip fractures, in these trials. A detailed discussion of these individual treatments is beyond the scope of this chapter; the reader is referred to a series of meta-analyses of osteoporosis therapies published in 2002 (Cranney et al. 2002).

Prompt treatment of fractures and aggressive rehabilitation afterward, even among older patients, could greatly decrease long-term morbidity. Public health nursing services, physical therapy services, and support services in the home often enable recovering fracture patients to stay in their own homes.

Examples of Evidence-Based Interventions

The Surgeon General's report on bone health and osteoporosis identified a number of population-based public health interventions for improving bone health in the United States (USDHHS 2004). These include programs to increase physical activity and reduce tobacco use, among others. One such program that was specifically highlighted was The National Bone Health Campaign, a multiyear national program created in 1998 by congressional mandate and conducted under the auspices of the CDC. The overall goal of the campaign is to encourage young girls to build and maintain strong bones by establishing lifelong healthy habits focused on calcium intake, physical activity, and avoidance of tobacco.

Areas of Future Research

The Surgeon General's report identified a number of key action steps as part of a National Action Plan for Bone Health. These include

- Increasing awareness of the impact of osteoporosis and how it can be prevented and treated throughout the life span.
- Changing the paradigm of preventing and treating fractures.
- Continuing to build the science base on the prevention and treatment of osteoporosis.
- Integrating health messages and programs on nutrition and physical activity relating to other chronic diseases.

Numerous areas for future research were described in the Surgeon General's report related to the epidemiology and impact of osteoporosis and fractures and the prevention and treatment of osteoporosis and related bone disease. The reader is referred to the report's sections for the individual recommendations (USDHHS 2004).

Resource

Centers for Disease Control and Prevention, http://www.cdc.gov/arthritis/data_statistics/national-statistics.html

Suggested Reading

Centers for Disease Control and Prevention. National and state medical expenditures and lost earnings attributable to arthritis and other rheumatic conditions—United States, 2003. *MMWR Weekly.* 2007;56(1):4–7. Available at: http://www.cdc.gov/mmwr/preview/mmwrhtml/mm5601a2.htm?s_cid=mm5601a2_e.

Dieppe P. The classification and diagnosis of osteoarthritis. In: Kuettner KE, Goldberg WM, eds. *Osteoarthritic Disorders.* Rosemont, IL: American Academy of Orthopaedic Surgeons; 1995: 5–12.

Felson DT. Does excess weight cause osteoarthritis and, if so, why? EULAR Workshop: Epidemiology of osteoarthritis in the peripheral joints. *J Rheum Dis.* 1996;55:668–670.

Felson DT. Weight and osteoarthritis. *Am J Clin Nutr.* 1996;63(suppl):430S–432S.

Fischer LM, Schlienger RG, Matter CM, et al. Discontinuation of nonsteroidal anti-inflammatory drug therapy and risk of acute myocardial infarction. *Arch Intern Med.* 2004;164:2472–2476.

Russell JI. Neurotransmitters, cytokines, hormones, and the immune system in chronic nonneuropathic pain. In: Fishman S, Ballantyne M, Rathmell JP, eds. *Bonica's Management of Pain.* 4th ed. Baltimore, MD: Lippincott Williams and Wilkins; 2009.

References

Abeles AM, Pillinger MH, Solitar BM, Abeles M. Narrative review: the pathophysiology of fibromyalgia. *Ann Intern Med.* 2007;146(10):726–735.

Ablin J, Neumann L, Buskila D. Pathogenesis of fibromyalgia—a review. *Joint Bone Spine.* 2008;75(3):273–279.

Ablin JN, Aronov N, Shimon I, et al. Evaluation of leptin levels among fibromyalgia patients before and after three months of treatment, in comparison with healthy controls. *Pain Res Manag.* 2012;17(2):89–92.

Aga AB, Lie E, Uhlig T, et al. Time trends in disease activity, response and remission rates in rheumatoid arthritis during the past decade: results from the NOR-DMARD study 2000–2010. *Ann Rheum Dis.* 2015;74(2):381–388.

Akkoc N, van der Linden S, Khan MA. Ankylosing spondylitis and symptom-modifying vs. disease-modifying therapy. *Best Pract Res Clin Rheumatol.* 2006; 20(3):539–557.

Alamanos Y, Drosos AA. Epidemiology of adult rheumatoid arthritis. *Autoimmun Rev.* 2004;4(3):130–136.

Altman R, Alarcon G, Appelrouth D, et al. The American College of Rheumatology criteria for the classification and reporting of osteoarthritis of the hand. *Arthritis Rheum.* 1990;33(11):1601–1610.

Altomonte L, Atzeni R, Leardini G, et al. Fibromyalgia syndrome: preventive, social, and economic aspects. *Rheumatismo.* 2008;60(suppl 1):70–78.

American College of Rheumatology (ACR) Subcommittee on Rheumatoid Arthritis Guidelines. Guidelines for the management of rheumatoid arthritis: 2002 update. *Arthritis Rheum.* 2002;46(2):328–346.

Anderson J, Felson DT. Factors associated with osteoarthritis of the knee in the First National Health and Nutrition Examination Survey (NHANES I). *Am J Epidemiol.* 1988;128(1):179–189.

Arden N, Nevitt MC. Osteoarthritis: epidemiology. *Best Pract Res Clin Rheumatol.* 2006;20(1):3–25.

Arkema EV, Goldstein BL, Robinson W, et al. Anti-citrullinated peptide autoantibodies, human leukocyte antigen shared epitope and risk of future rheumatoid arthritis: a nested case–control study. *Arthritis Res Ther.* 2013;15(5):R159.

Arnold LM. Systemic therapies for chronic pain. In: Fishman S, Ballantyne M, Rathmell JP, editors. *Bonica's Management of Pain.* 4th ed. Baltimore, MD: Lippincott Williams and Wilkins; 2009.

Arnold LM, Hudson JI, Hess EV, et al. Family study of fibromyalgia. *Arthritis Rheum.* 2004;50(3):944–952.

Bauer RL. Ethnic differences in hip fracture: a reduced incidence in Mexican Americans. *Am J Epidemiol.* 1988;127(1):145–149.

Beals KA, Meyer NL. Female athlete triad update. *Clin Sports Med.* 2007;26(1): 69–89.

Becker MA, Schumacher HR, Wortmann RL II, et al. Febuxostat, a novel nonpurine selective inhibitor of xanthine oxidase: a 28-day multi-center, phase II, randomized, double-blind, placebo-controlled dose-response clinical trial examining safety and efficacy in patients with gout. *Arthritis Rheum.* 2005;52(3):916–923.

Bedson J, Croft PR. The discordance between clinical and radiographic knee osteoarthritis: a systematic search and summary of the literature. *BMC Musculoskelet Disord.* 2008;9:116.

Bennett RM. Disabling fibromyalgia: appearance versus reality. *J Rheumatol.* 1993;20(11):1821–1824.

Bhole V, de Vera M, Rahman MM, Krishnan E, Choi H. Epidemiology of gout in women: fifty-two-year followup of a prospective cohort. *Arthritis Rheum.* 2010;62(4): 1069–1076.

Bijlsma JW, Knahr K. Strategies for the prevention and management of osteoarthritis of the hip and knee. *Best Pract Res Clin Rheumatol.* 2007;21(1):59–76.

Birnbaum H, Pike C, Kaufman R, Marynchenko M, Kidolezi Y, Cifaldi M. Societal cost of rheumatoid arthritis patients in the US. *Curr Med Res Opin.* 2010;26(1):77–90.

Boyce BF, Xing L. Biology of RANK, RANKL, and osteoprotegerin. *Arthritis Res Ther.* 2007;9(suppl 1):S1.

Bradley LA. Pathophysiology of fibromyalgia. *Am J Med.* 2009;122(12A):522–530.

Brandt J, Marzo-Ortega H, Emery P. Ankylosing spondylitis: new treatment modalities. *Best Pract Res Clin Rheumatol.* 2006;20(3):559–570.

Carbone LD, Cooper C, Michet CJ, Atkinson EJ, O'Fallon WM, Melton LJD. Ankylosing spondylitis in Rochester, Minnesota, 1935–1989. Is the epidemiology changing? *Arthritis Rheum.* 1992;35(12):1476–1482.

Carrasco GA, Van de Kar LD. Neuroendocrine pharmacology of stress. *Eur J Pharmacol.* 2003;463(1–3):235–272.

Centers for Disease Control and Prevention (CDC). Prevalence and most common causes of disability among adults—United States, 2005. *MMWR Morb Mortal Wkly Rep.* 2009;58(16):421–426.

Centers for Disease Control and Prevention (CDC). Prevalence of doctor-diagnosed arthritis and arthritis-attributable activity limitation—United States, 2007–2009. *MMWR Morb Mortal Wkly Rep.* 2010;59(39):1261–1265.

Centers for Disease Control and Prevention (CDC). Prevalence of doctor-diagnosed arthritis and arthritis-attributable activity limitation—United States, 2010–2012. *MMWR Morb Mortal Wkly Rep.* 2013;62(44):869–873.

Centers for Disease Control and Prevention (CDC), National Center for Chronic Disease Prevention and Health Promotion, Division of Population Health. Rheumatoid arthritis (RA). 2015. Available at: http://www.cdc.gov/arthritis/basics/rheumatoid.htm. Accessed September 1, 2016.

Centers for Disease Control and Prevention. About CDC's arthritis program. 2016. Available at: https://www.cdc.gov/arthritis/about/index.html. Accessed September 1, 2016.

Chehata JC, Hassell AB, Clarke SA, et al. Mortality in rheumatoid arthritis: relationship to single and composite measures of disease activity. *Rheumatology (Oxford).* 2001;40(4):447–452.

Chen CJ, Yen JH, Chang SJ. Gout patients have an increased risk of developing most cancers, especially urological cancers. *Scand J Rheumatol.* 2014;43(5):385–390.

Chen JH, Yeh WT, Chuang SY, Wu YY, Pan WH. Gender-specific risk factors for incident gout: a prospective cohort study. *Clin Rheumatol.* 2012;31(2):239–245.

Chin S, Caldwell W, Gritsenko K. Fibromyalgia pathogenesis and treatment options update. *Curr Pain Headache Rep.* 2016;20(4):25–37.

Choi HK, Curhan G. Soft drinks, fructose consumption, and the risk of gout in men: prospective cohort study. *BMJ.* 2008;336(7639):309–312.

Choi HK, Willett W, Curhan G. Fructose-rich beverages and risk of gout in women. *JAMA*. 2010;304(20):2270–2278.

Cicuttini FM, Spector TD. The genetics of osteoarthritis. *J Clin Pathol*. 1996;49(8):617–619.

Clauw DJ. Fibromyalgia. In: Fishman S, Ballantyne M, Rathmell JP, eds. *Bonica's Management of Pain*. 4th ed. Baltimore, MD: Lippincott Williams and Wilkins; 2009.

Coster L, Kendall S, Gerdle B, et al. Chronic widespread musculoskeletal pain—a comparison of those who meet criteria for fibromyalgia and those who do not. *Eur J Pain*. 2008;12(5):600–610.

Cranney A, Guyatt G, Griffith L, et al. IX: summary of meta-analyses of therapies for postmenopausal osteoporosis. *Endocr Rev*. 2002;23(4):570–578.

Croft P, Rigby AS, Boswell R, Schollum J, Silman A. The prevalence of chronic widespread pain in the general population. *J Rheumatol*. 1993;20(4):710–713.

Cummings SR, Melton LJ. Epidemiology and outcomes of osteoporotic fractures. *Lancet*. 2002;359(9319):1761–1767.

de Hair MJ, Landewe RB, van de Sande MG, et al. Smoking and overweight determine the likelihood of developing rheumatoid arthritis. *Ann Rheum Dis*. 2013;72(10):1654–1658.

de Laet C, Oden A, Johansson H, Johnell O, Jonsson B, Kanis JA. The impact of the use of multiple risk indicators for fracture on case-finding strategies: a mathematical approach. *Osteoporos Int*. 2005;16(3):313–318.

Dean LE, Jones GT, MacDonald AG, Downham C, Sturrock RD, MacFarlane GJ. Global prevalence of ankylosing spondylitis. *Rheumatology (Oxford)*. 2014;53(4):650–657.

Deane KD, Norris JM, Holers VM. Pre-clinical rheumatoid arthritis: identification, evaluation and future directions for investigation. *Rheum Dis Clin North Am*. 2010;36(2):213–241.

Demoruelle MK, Deane KD. Treatment strategies in early rheumatoid arthritis and prevention of rheumatoid arthritis. *Curr Rheumatol Rep*. 2012;14(5):472–480.

Doran MF, Pond GR, Crowson CS, O'Fallon WM, Gabriel SE. Trends in incidence and mortality in rheumatoid arthritis in Rochester, Minnesota, over a forty-year period. *Arthritis Rheum*. 2002;46(3):625–631.

Dougados M, Baeten D. Spondyloarthritis. *Lancet*. 2011;377(9783):2127–2137.

Dunlop DD, Song J, Semanik PA, et al. Relation of physical activity time to incident disability in community dwelling adults with or at risk of knee arthritis: prospective cohort study. *BMJ*. 2014;348:g2472.

Eggebeen AT. Gout: an update. *Am Fam Physician.* 2007;76(6):801–808.

El Maghraoui A. Extra-articular manifestations of ankylosing spondylitis: prevalence and therapeutic implications. *Eur J Intern Med.* 2011;22(6):554–560.

Ernst E. Complementary and alternative medicine for fibromyalgia. In: Fishman S, Ballantyne M, Rathmell JP, eds. *Bonica's Management of Pain.* 4th ed. Baltimore, MD: Lippincott Williams and Wilkins; 2009.

Espallargues M, Sampietro-Colom L, Estrada MD, et al. Identifying bone-mass related risk factors for fracture to guide bone densitometry measurements: a systematic review of the literature. *Osteoporos Int.* 2001;12(10):811–822.

Felson DT, Naimark A, Anderson J, et al. The prevalence of knee osteoarthritis in the elderly. *Arthritis Rheum.* 1987;30(8):914–918.

Felson DT, Niu J, Gross KD, et al. Valgus malalignment is a risk factor for lateral knee osteoarthritis incidence and progression: findings from the Multicenter Osteoarthritis Study and the Osteoarthritis Initiative. *Arthritis Rheum.* 2013;65(2):355–362.

Felson DT, Zhang Y. An update on the epidemiology of knee and hip osteoarthritis with a view to prevention. *Arthritis Rheum.* 1998;41(8):1343–1355.

Fina-Aviles F, Medina-Peralta M, Mendez-Boo L, et al. The descriptive epidemiology of rheumatoid arthritis in Catalonia: a retrospective study using routinely collected data. *Clin Rheumatol.* 2016;35(3):751–757.

Fischer LM, Schlienger RG, Matter CM, Jick H, Meier CR. Discontinuation of nonsteroidal anti-inflammatory drug therapy and risk of acute myocardial infarction. *Arch Intern Med.* 2004;164(22):2472–2476.

Flannery CR, Zollner R, Corcoran C, et al. Prevention of cartilage degeneration in a rat model of osteoarthritis by intraarticular treatment with recombinant lubricin. *Arthritis Rheum.* 2009;60(3):840–847.

Gabriel SE, Michaud K. Epidemiological studies in incidence, prevalence, mortality, and comorbidity of the rheumatic diseases. *Arthritis Res Ther.* 2009;11(3):229–245.

Gibofsky A. Overview of epidemiology, pathophysiology, and diagnosis of rheumatoid arthritis. *Am J Manag Care.* 2012;18(13 suppl):S295–S302.

Goldenberg DL. Fibromyalgia, chronic fatigue syndrome, and myofascial pain syndrome. *Curr Opin Rheumatol.* 1993;5(2):199–208.

Goldring MB, Otero M. Inflammation in osteoarthritis. *Curr Opin Rheumatol.* 2011;23(5):471–478.

Grassi D, Pontremoli R, Bocale R, Ferri C, Desideri G. Therapeutic approaches to chronic hyperuricemia and gout. *High Blood Press Cardiovasc Prev*. 2014;21(4): 243–250.

Grossman P, Tiefenthaler-Gilmer U, Raysz A, Kesper U. Mindfulness training as an intervention for fibromyalgia: evidence of postintervention and 3-year follow-up benefits in well-being. *Psychother Psychosom*. 2007;76(4):225–233.

Grotle M, Hagen KB, Natvig B, Dahl FA, Kvien TK. Obesity and osteoarthritis in knee, hip and/or hand: an epidemiological study in the general population with 10 years follow-up. *BMC Musculoskelet Disord*. 2008;9:132.

Guccione AA, Felson DT, Anderson JJ, et al. The effects of specific medical conditions on the functional limitations of elders in the Framingham Study. *Am J Public Health*. 1994;84(3):351–358.

Hajjaj-Hassouni N, Burgos-Vargas R. Ankylosing spondylitis and reactive arthritis in the developing world. *Best Pract Res Clin Rheumatol*. 2008;22(4):709–723.

Hall AP, Barry PE, Dawber TR, McNamara PM. Epidemiology of gout and hyperuricemia. A long-term population study. *Am J Med*. 1967;42(1):27–37.

Hannon MT, Anderson JJ, Zhang L, Levy D, Felson DT. Bone mineral density and knee osteoarthritis in elderly men and women: the Framingham study. *Arthritis Rheum*. 1993;36(12):1671–1680.

Harris MD, Siegel LB, Alloway JA. Gout and hyperuricemia. *Am Fam Physician*. 1999;59(4):925–934.

Harvey N, Earl S, Cooper C. The epidemiology of osteoporotic fractures. In: Lane NE, Sambrook PN, eds. *Osteoporosis and the Osteoporosis of Rheumatic Diseases: A Companion to Rheumatology*. 1st ed. Philadelphia, PA: Mosby Elsevier; 2006:1–13.

Heinegard D, Saxne T. The role of the cartilage matrix in osteoarthritis. *Nat Rev Rheumatol*. 2011;7(1):50–56.

Hirsch R, Hochberg MC. Arthritis and other musculoskeletal diseases. In: Remington PL, Brownson RC, Wegner MV, eds. *Chronic Disease Epidemiology and Control*. Washington, DC: American Public Health Association; 2010.

Hoaglund FT, Yau AC, Wong WL. Osteoarthritis of the hip and other joints in Southern Chinese in Hong Kong. *J Bone Joint Surg*. 1973;55(3):545–557.

Hochberg MC. Recommendations for measurement of bone mineral density and identifying persons to be treated for osteoporosis. *Rheum Dis Clin North Am*. 2006;32(4):681–689.

Hootman JM, Helmick CG, Barbour KE, Theis KA, Boring MA. Review article: updated projected prevalence of self-reported doctor-diagnosed arthritis and arthritis-attributable activity limitation among US adults, 2015–2040. *Arthritis Rheumatol.* 2016;68(7):1582–1587.

Jacobsen SJ, Goldberg J, Miles TP, et al. Hip fracture among the old and very old: a population-based study of 745,435 cases. *Am J Public Health.* 1990a;80(7):871–873.

Jacobsen SJ, Goldberg J, Miles TP, et al. Regional variation in the incidence of hip fracture. *JAMA.* 1990b;264(4):500–502.

Jiang L, Tian W, Wang Y, et al. Body mass index and susceptibility to knee osteoarthritis: a systematic review and meta-analysis. *Joint Bone Spine.* 2012;79(3):291–297.

Jones RK, Chapman GJ, Parkes MJ, Forsythe L, Felson DT. The effect of different types of insoles or shoe modifications on medial loading of the knee in persons with medial knee osteoarthritis: a randomised trial. *J Orthop Res.* 2015;33(11):1646–1654.

Jordan JM, Linder GF, Renner JB, Fryer JG. The impact of arthritis in rural populations. *Arthritis Care Res.* 1995;8(4):242–250.

Joshi VR. Rheumatology, past, present and future. *J Assoc Physicians India.* 2012;60: 21–24.

Juhakoski R, Heliovaara M, Impivaara O, et al. Risk factors for the development of hip osteoarthritis: a population-based prospective study. *Rheumatology (Oxford).* 2009; 48(1):83–87.

Jurell KC, Zanetos MA, Orsinelli A, et al. Fibromyalgia: a study of thyroid function and symptoms. *J Musculoskel Pain.* 1996;4:49–60.

Kalla AA, Tikly M. Rheumatoid arthritis in the developing world. *Best Pract Res Clin Rheumatol.* 2003;17(5):863–875.

Karlson EW, Mandl LA, Aweh GN, Sangha O, Liang MH, Grostein F. Total hip replacement due to osteoarthritis: the importance of age, obesity, and other modifiable risk factors. *Am J Med.* 2003;114(2):93–98.

Karlson EW, van Schaardenburg D, van der Helm-van Mil AH. Strategies to predict rheumatoid arthritis development in at-risk populations. *Rheumatology.* 2016;55(1):6–15.

Kato K, Sullivan PF, Evengård B, Pedersen NL. Importance of genetic influences on chronic widespread pain. *Arthritis Rheum.* 2006;54(5):1682–1686.

Keat A. Ankylosing spondylitis. *Medicine.* 2010;38(4):185–189.

Kim KY, Schumacher HR, Hunsche E, Wertheimer AI, Kong SX. A literature review of the epidemiology and treatment of acute gout. *Clin Ther.* 2003;25(6):1593–1617.

Krishnan E, Lienesch D, Kwoh CK. Gout in ambulatory care settings in the United States. *J Rheumatol.* 2008;35(3):498–501.

Kumar V. *Robbins and Cotran Pathologic Basis of Disease.* 8th ed. Philadelphia, PA: Saunders Elseiver; 2010.

Latourte A, Bardin T, Richette P. Prophylaxis for acute gout flares after initiation of urate-lowering therapy. *Rheumatology (Oxford).* 2014;53(11):1920–1926.

Lawrence RC, Everett DF, Benevolenskaya LI, et al. Spondyloarthropathies in circumpolar populations: I. Design and methods of United States and Russian studies. *Arctic Med Res.* 1996;55(4):187–194.

Lawrence RC, Felson DT, Helmick CG, et al. Estimates of the prevalence of arthritis and other rheumatic conditions in the United States. Part II. *Arthritis Rheum.* 2008;58(1):26–35.

Lee J, Dunlop D, Ehrlich-Jones L, et al. Public health impact of risk factors for physical inactivity in adults with rheumatoid arthritis. *Arthritis Care Res.* 2012;64(4): 488–493.

Litwic A, Edwards M, Dennison E, Cooper C. Epidemiology and burden of osteoarthritis. *Br Med Bull.* 2013;105:185–199.

Liu Q, Gamble G, Pickering K, Morton S, Dalbeth N. Prevalence and clinical factors associated with gout in patients with diabetes and prediabetes. *Rheumatology (Oxford).* 2012;51(4):757–759.

Looker A, Borrud L, Dawson-Hughes B, Shepperd J, Wright N. Osteoporosis or low bone mass at the femur neck or lumbar spine in older adults: United States, 2005–2008. *NCHS Data Brief.* 2012;(93):1–8.

Looker AC, Frenk SM. Percentage of adults aged 65 and over with osteoporosis or low bone mass at the femur neck or lumbar spine: United States, 2005–2010. National Center for Health Statistics, Centers for Disease Control and Prevention. 2015. Available at: http://www.cdc.gov/nchs/data/hestat/osteoporsis/osteoporosis2005_2010.htm. Accessed September 14, 2016.

Lu B, Hiraki LT, Sparks JA, et al. Being overweight or obese and risk of developing rheumatoid arthritis among women: a prospective cohort study. *Ann Rheum Dis.* 2014;73(11):1914–1922.

MacGregor AJ, Snieder H, Rigby AS, et al. Characterizing the quantitative genetic contribution to rheumatoid arthritis using data from twins. *Arthritis Rheum.* 2000;43(1):30–37.

Mansour M, Cheema GS, Naguwa SM, et al. Ankylosing spondylitis: a contemporary perspective on diagnosis and treatment. *Semin Arthritis Rheum.* 2006;36(4):210–223.

Marcus DA. Fibromyalgia: diagnosis and treatment options. *Gend Med.* 2009; 6(suppl 2):139–151.

Messier SP, Mihalko SL, Legault C, et al. Effects of intensive diet and exercise on knee joint loads, inflammation, and clinical outcomes among overweight and obese adults with knee osteoarthritis: the IDEA randomized clinical trial. *JAMA*. 2013;310(12):1263–1273.

Mikuls TR, Saag KG. New insights into gout epidemiology. *Curr Opin Rheumatol*. 2006;18(2):199–203.

Minor MA, Lane NE. Recreational exercise in arthritis. *Rheum Dis Clin North Am*. 1996;22(3):563–577.

Minten MJ, Mahler E, den Broeder AA, Leer JW, van den Ende CH. The efficacy and safety of low-dose radiotherapy on pain and functioning in patients with osteoarthritis: a systematic review. *Rheumatol Int*. 2016;36(1):133–142.

Moldofsky H, MacFarlane JG. Sleep and its potential role in chronic pain and fatigue. In: Fishman S, Ballantyne M, Rathmell JP, eds. *Bonica's Management of Pain*. 4th ed. Baltimore, MD: Lippincott Williams and Wilkins; 2009.

Murphy L, Helmick CG. The impact of osteoarthritis in the United States: a population health perspective. *Am J Nurs*. 2012;112(3):S13–S19.

Murphy L, Schwartz TA, Helmick CG, et al. A. Lifetime risk of symptomatic knee osteoarthritis. *Arthritis Rheum*. 2008;59(9):1207–1213.

National Collaborating Centre for Chronic Conditions (NCCCC). *Rheumatoid Arthritis: National Clinical Guideline for Management and Treatment in Adults*. London, England: NCCCC: 2009.

National Institutes of Health (NIH). Osteoporosis prevention, diagnosis, and therapy. *NIH Consens Statement*. 2000;17(1):1–45.

Neogi T, Zhang Y. Osteoarthritis prevention. *Curr Opin Rheumatol*. 2011;23(2):185–191.

Noss EH, Brenner MB. The role and therapeutic implications of fibroblast-like synoviocytes in inflammation and cartilage erosion in rheumatoid arthritis. *Immunol Rev*. 2008;223:252–270.

Österreicher CH, Penz-Österreicher M, Grivennikov SI, et al. Fibroblast-specific protein 1 identifies an inflammatory subpopulation of macrophages in the liver. *Proc Natl Acad Sci U S A*. 2011;108(1):308–313.

Palazzo C, Nguyen C, Lefevre-Colau MM, Rannou F, Poiraudeau S. Risk factors and burden of osteoarthritis. *Ann Phys Rehabil Med*. 2016;59(3):134–138.

Pers YM, Rackwitz L, Ferreira R, et al. Adipose mesenchynal stromal cell-based therapy for severe osteoarthritis of the knee: a phase I dose-escalation trial. *Stem Cells Transl Med*. 2016;5(7):847–856.

Petersen W, Ellermann A, Rembitzki IV, et al. Evaluating the potential synergistic benefit of a realignment brace on patients receiving exercise therapy for patellofemoral pain syndrome: a randomized clinical trial. *Arch Orthop Trauma Surg.* 2016;136(7):975–982.

Pham T. Pathophysiology of ankylosing spondylitis: what's new? *Joint Bone Spine.* 2008;75(6):656–660.

Phipps-Green AJ, Hollis-Moffatt JE, Dalbeth N, et al. A strong role for the ABCG2 gene in susceptibility to gout in New Zealand Pacific Island and Caucasian, but not Maori, case and control sample sets. *Hum Mol Genet.* 2010;19(24):4813–4819.

Pillemer SR, Bradley LA, Crofford LJ, Moldofsky H, Chrousos GP. The neuroscience and endocrinology of fibromyalgia. *Arthritis Rheum.* 1997;40(11):1928–1939.

Prendergast JK, Sullivan JS, Geczy A, et al. Possible role of enteric organisms in the pathogenesis of ankylosing spondylitis and other seronegative arthropathies. *Infect Immun.* 1983;41(3):935–941.

Price RK, North CS, Wessely S, Fraser VJ. Estimating the prevalence of chronic fatigue syndrome and associated symptoms in the community. *Public Health Rep.* 1992;107(5):514–522.

Rahman A, Underwood M, Carnes D. Clinical review. Fibromyalgia. *BMJ.* 2014;348:1224–1236.

Raisz JG. Pathogenesis of osteoporosis: concepts, conflicts, and prospects. *J Clin Invest.* 2005;115(12):3318–3325.

Richette P, Bardin T. Gout. *Lancet.* 2010;375(9711):318–328.

Rindfleisch JA, Muller D. Diagnosis and management of rheumatoid arthritis. *Am Fam Phys.* 2005;72(6):1037–1047.

Roddy E, Choi HK. Epidemiology of gout. *Rheum Dis Clin North Am.* 2014;40(2):155–175.

Roddy E, Doherty M. Epidemiology of gout. *Arthritis Res Ther.* 2010;12(6):223–234.

Roubenoff R, Klag MJ, Mead LA, Liang KY, Seidler AJ, Hochberg MC. Incidence and risk factors for gout in white men. *JAMA.* 1991;266(21):3004–3007.

Russell G. Pathogenesis of osteoporosis. In: Lane NE, Sambrook PN, eds. *Osteoporosis and the Osteoporosis of Rheumatic Diseases: A Companion to Rheumatology.* 1st ed. Philadelphia, PA: Mosby Elsevier; 2006:33–40.

Saccomano SJ, Ferrara LR. Treatment and prevention of gout. *Nurse Pract.* 2015;40(8):24–30.

Saraux A, Guillemin F, Guggenbuhl P, et al. Prevalence of spondyloarthropathies in France—2001. *Ann Rheum Dis.* 2005;64(10):1431–1435.

Schrager MA, Metter EJ, Simonsick E, et al. Sarcopenic obesity and inflammation in the InCHIANTI study. *J Appl Physiol (1985).* 2007;102(3):919–925.

Schumaker HR, Becker MA, Wortmann RL, et al. Allopurinol and placebo in reducing serum urate in subjects with hyperuricemia and gout: a 28-week, phase III, randomized, double-blind, parallel-group trial. *Arthritis Care Res.* 2008;59(11):1540–1548.

Scott DL, Wolfe F, Huizinga TW. Rheumatoid arthritis. *Lancet.* 2010;376(9746):1094–1108.

Seth R, Kydd AS, Falzon L, Bombardier C, van der eijde DM, Edwards CJ. Preventing attacks of acute gout when introducing urate-lowering therapy: a systematic literature review. *J Rheumatol Suppl.* 2014;92:42–47.

Silverwood V, Blagojevic-Bucknall M, Jinks C, Jordan JL, Protheroe J, Jordan KP. Current evidence on risk factors for knee osteoarthritis in older adults: a systematic review and meta-analysis. *Osteoarthritis Cartilage.* 2015;23(4):507–515.

Simms RW. Fibromyalgia is not a muscle disorder. *Am J Med Sci.* 1998;315(6):346–350.

Singh JA. Racial and gender disparities among patients with gout. *Curr Rheumatol Rep.* 2013;15(2):307–316.

Skapinakis P, Lewis G, Mavreas V. Cross-cultural differences in the epidemiology of unexplained fatigue syndromes in primary care. *Br J Psychiatry.* 2003;182:205–209.

Skousgaard SG, Skytthe A, Möller S, Overgaard S, Brandt LP. Sex differences in risk and heritability estimates on primary knee osteoarthritis leading to total knee arthroplasty: a nationwide population based follow up study in Danish twins. *Arthritis Res Ther.* 2016;18:46.

Smith E, Hoy D, Cross M, et al. The global burden of gout: estimates from the Global Burden of Disease 2010 study. *Ann Rheum Dis.* 2014;73(8):1470–1476.

Smith EU, Díaz-Torné C, Perez-Ruiz F, March LM. Epidemiology of gout: an update. *Best Pract Res Clin Rheumatol.* 2010;24(6):811–827.

Spector TD, McGregor AJ. Risk factors for osteoarthritis. *Osteoarthritis Cartilage.* 2004;12(suppl A):S39–S44.

Stanaszek WF, Carlstedt BC. Rheumatoid arthritis: pathophysiology. *J Pharm Pract.* 1999;12(4):282–292.

Stone KL, Seeley DG, Liu LY, et al. BMD at multiple sites and risk of fracture of multiple types: long-term results from the study of osteoporotic fractures. *J Bone Miner Res.* 2003;18(11):1947–1954.

Sun K, Song J, Manheim LM, et al. Relationship of meeting physical activity guidelines with quality-adjusted life-years. *Semin Arthritis Rheum.* 2014;44(3):264–270.

Tam LS, Gu J, Yu D. Pathogenesis of ankylosing spondylitis. *Nat Rev Rheumatol.* 2010;6(7):399–405.

Terkeltaub RA, Furst DE, Bennett K, Kook KA, Crockett RS, Davis MW. High versus low dosing for oral colchicine for early acute gout flare: 24-hour outcome of the first multi-center randomized, double-blind, placebo-controlled, parallel-group, dose-comparison colchicine study. *Arthritis Rheum.* 2010;62(4):1060–1068.

Theoharides TC, Tsilioni I, Arbetman L, et al. Fibromyalgia syndrome in need of effective treatments. *J Pharmacol Exp Ther.* 2015;355(2):255–263.

Tramer MR, Williams JE, Carroll D, et al. Comparing analgesic efficacy of non-steroidal anti-inflammatory drugs given by different routes in acute and chronic pain: a qualitative systematic review. *Acta Anaesthesiol Scand.* 1998;42(1):71–79.

US Department of Health and Human Services (USDHHS). *Bone Health and Osteoporosis: A Report of the Surgeon General.* Rockville, MD: USDHHS, Office of the Surgeon General; 2004.

US Preventive Services Task Force (USPSTF). Screening for osteoporosis: US Preventive Services Task Force Recommendation Statement. *Ann Intern Med.* 2011;154(5):356–364.

Vegvari A, Sabo Z, Szanto S, Glant TT, Mikecz K, Szekanecz Z. The genetic background of ankylosing spondylitis. *Joint Bone Spine.* 2009;76(6):623–628.

Vierck CJ. A mechanism-based approach to prevention of and therapy for fibromyalgia. *Pain Res Treat.* 2012;2012:951354.

Vincent HK, Heywood K, Connelly J, Hurley RW. Obesity and weight loss in the treatment and prevention of osteoarthritis. *PM R.* 2012a;4(5 suppl):S59–S67.

Vincent KR, Conrad BP, Fregly BJ, Vincent HK. The pathophysiology of osteoarthritis: a mechanical perspective on the knee joint. *PM R.* 2012b;4(5 suppl):S3–S9.

Visser K, Katchamart W, Loza E, et al. Multinational evidence-based recommendations for the use of methotrexate in rheumatic disorders with a focus on rheumatoid arthritis: integrating systematic literature research and expert opinion of a broad international panel of rheumatologists in the 3E Initiative. *Ann Rheum Dis.* 2009;68(7):1086–1093.

Vliet Vlieland TP. Non-drug care for RA—is the era of evidence-based practice approaching? *Rheumatology.* 2007;46(9):1397–1404.

Wandel S, Jüni P, Tendal B, et al. Effects of glucosamine, chondroitin, or placebo in patients with osteoarthritis of hip or knee: network meta-analysis. *BMJ.* 2010;341:c4675.

Welsing PM, Fransen J, van Riel PL. Is the disease course of rheumatoid arthritis becoming milder? Time trends since 1985 in an inception cohort of early rheumatoid arthritis. *Arthritis Rheum.* 2005;52(9):2616–2624.

White KP, Harth M. Classification, epidemiology, and natural history of fibromyalgia. *Curr Pain Headache Rep.* 2001;5(4):320–329.

Wijnands JMA, Viechtbauer W, Thevissen K, et al. Determinants of the prevalence of gout in the general populations: a systematic review and meta-regression. *Eur J Epidemiol.* 2015;30(1):19–33.

Williams FM, Spector TD. The genetics of osteoporosis. In: Lane NE, Sambrook PN, eds. *Osteoporosis and the Osteoporosis of Rheumatic Diseases: A Companion to Rheumatology.* 1st ed. Philadelphia, PA: Mosby Elsevier; 2006:14–21.

Wolfe F, Hawley DJ, Wilson K. The prevalence and meaning of fatigue in rheumatic disease. *J Rheumatol.* 1996;23(8):1407–1417.

Wolfe F, Ross K, Anderson J, Russell IJ. Aspects of fibromyalgia in the general population: sex, pain threshold, and fibromyalgia symptoms. *J Rheumatol.* 1995;22(1):151–156.

World Health Organization (WHO). Assessment of fracture risk and its application to screening for postmenopausal osteoporosis. *World Health Organ Tech Rep Ser.* 1994; 843:1–129.

Wright NC, Looker AC, Saag KG, et al. The recent prevalence of osteoporosis and low bone mass in the United States based on bone mineral density at the femoral neck or lumbar spine. *J Bone Miner Res.* 2014;29(11):2520–2526.

Yano K, Heilbrun LK, Wasnich RD, Hankion JH, Vogel JM. The relationship between diet and bone mineral content of multiple skeletal sites in elderly Japanese-American men and women living in Hawaii. *Am J Clin Nutr.* 1985;42(5):877–888.

Yelin E, Murphy L, Cisternas MG, Foreman AJ, Pasta DJ, Helmick CG. Medical care expenditures and earnings losses among persons with arthritis and other rheumatic conditions in 2003, and comparisons with 1997. *Arthritis Rheum.* 2007;56(5):1397–1407.

Yunus MB. Towards a model of pathophysiology of fibromyalgia: aberrant central pain mechanisms with peripheral modulation [editorial]. *J Rheumatol.* 1992;19(6):846–850.

Yunus MB. Symptoms and signs of fibromyalgia syndrome: an overview. In: Fishman S, Ballantyne M, Rathmell JP, eds. *Bonica's Management of Pain.* 4th ed. Baltimore, MD: Lippincott Williams and Wilkins; 2009.

Zhang Y, Neogi T, Chen C, Chaisson C, Hunter DJ, Choi H. Low-dose aspirin use and recurrent gout attacks. *Ann Rheum Dis.* 2014;73(2):385–390.

Zhu Y, Pandya BJ, Choi HK. Prevalence of gout and hyperuricemia in the US general populations: the National Health and Nutrition Examination Survey 2007–2008. *Arthritis Rheum.* 2011;63(10):136–3141.

Zingmond DS, Melton LJ, Silverman SL. Increasing hip fracture incidence in California Hispanics, 1983 to 2000. *Osteoporos Int.* 2004;15(8):603–610.

Zochling J, Braun J. Assessments in ankylosing spondylitis. *Best Pract Res Clin Rheumatol.* 2007;21(4):699–712.

Zochling J, van der Heijde D, Dougados M, Braun J. Current evidence for the management of ankylosing spondylitis: a systematic literature review for the ASAS/EULAR management recommendation in ankylosing spondylitis. *Ann Rheum Dis.* 2006;65(4): 423–432.

21

CHRONIC LIVER DISEASE

Adnan Said, MD, MSPH

Introduction

Liver disease is a term that encompasses a broad range of diagnoses and presentations. This includes from mild liver test abnormalities in asymptomatic
individuals at one end of the spectrum to end-stage liver disease, called cirrhosis. Liver conditions can present as acute and fulminant disease with rapid
liver failure or as chronic liver disease that slowly progresses over decades.
Commonly used liver tests include measurement of serum liver enzymes
(aspartate transaminase [AST] and alanine transaminase [ALT]) that signify
inflammation of the liver (i.e., hepatitis) and bilirubin levels that are an indicator of liver function and the severity of liver disease (Schiff et al. 1999). Complications of advanced liver disease, such as cirrhosis, can present with
complications including gastrointestinal bleeding, accumulation of fluid in
the abdominal cavity (ascites), and decreased cognitive function and neuromuscular function (encephalopathy; D'Amico et al. 1986). The causes, consequences, and populations at high risk for liver disease are summarized in
Figure 21-1 and described in detail in this chapter.

Significance

Chronic liver disease is a significant, important drain on national health care
resources with approximately 5.5 million people affected (Miller et al. 2006) in
the United States and millions globally (Shepard et al. 2005). Over the past two
decades, drastic changes in liver disease management have occurred, with
development of direct-acting antiviral therapies for chronic viral hepatitis and
liver transplantation becoming a widely accepted procedure for patients with
end-stage liver disease. The obesity epidemic in combination with metabolic

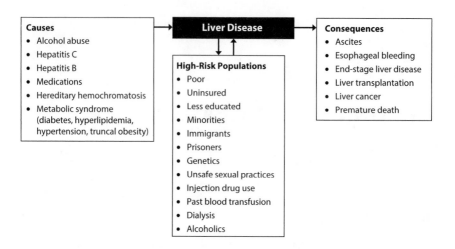

Source: Reprinted from Said and Wells (2010).

Figure 21-1. Liver Disease: Causes, Consequences, and High-Risk Groups

syndrome (diabetes, hyperlipidemia, hypertension, and truncal obesity) has led to the continued increase in non-alcoholic fatty liver disease, which is now the most common chronic liver disease in the United States and increasing worldwide as well.

Prevention of liver disease is integral to minimizing the burden of advanced liver disease. Development of the hepatitis B vaccine is one of the most important medical advances in this field. However, stigmatization of patients with alcoholism and viral hepatitis is an impediment to this goal. Patients with liver disease often are socially disadvantaged and have poor access to health care. Services to prevent and treat alcoholism and reduce the transmission of viral hepatitis have improved over the past two decades, but they need further support and dissemination. Obesity reduction through both individual practices and societal changes is needed to combat the increase in obesity-related liver disease.

Social and economic policies in the United States during the past century have played a significant role in the incidence of chronic liver disease. Liver-related mortality was high before the 1920s, plummeted during Prohibition, rose again during the Depression with persistent increases through the time of World War II, and peaked in the early 1970s (Terris 1967; Debakey et al. 1995).

Between 1981 and 2010, age-adjusted death rates from chronic liver disease and liver cancer increased significantly. From 2006 to 2010, the average annual percentage change in death rates increased 1.5% for chronic liver disease and 2.6% for liver cancer (Kim et al. 2014). In 2013, chronic liver disease and cirrhosis, based on the *International Classification of Diseases, Tenth Revision (ICD-10)*, was reported to be the 12th leading cause of death in the United States, accounting for 36,427 deaths. This represented 1.4% of the total national mortality with an age-adjusted rate of death from chronic liver disease of 10.2 per 100,000 population. In addition, liver cancer accounted for 24,000 deaths with a death rate of 7.6 per 100,000. This would indicate a decrease in liver disease death rates. When adding the impact of deaths from viral hepatitis as well as that from hepatocellular carcinoma (HCC) to these reported data, the numbers rise dramatically. In this context, liver disease accounts for approximately 68,000 deaths yearly (2.6%) thereby rising to the 8th cause of overall death (Xu et al. 2016). Trends for chronic liver disease mortality including viral hepatitis, liver cancer, and other causes from 1979 to 2005 are detailed in Table 21-1.

The morbidity from liver disease is just as important given the effects on quality of life as well as the economic consequences. Direct medical cost related to chronic liver disease and cirrhosis, excluding patients with hepatitis C virus, was estimated to be in excess of $2.4 billion in 2004 (Neff et al. 2011). The health care costs for patients with hepatitis C (including liver transplantation)

Table 21-1. Trends in Age-Adjusted Mortality Rates for Liver Diseases

Year	Liver Cancer	Viral Hepatitis	All Other Liver Disease
1980	1.2	0.4	16.5
1985	1.4	0.4	13.9
1990	1.7	0.7	12.6
1995	1.9	1.3	11.3
2000	1.9	1.9	12.0
2005	2.1	1.8	11.9
2010	2.4	2.1	12.6
2014	2.5	2.1	13.8

Source: Data from CDC WONDER (2016b).
Note: International Classification of Diseases, Ninth Revision codes were used from 1980 to 1995 and *International Classification of Diseases, Tenth Revision* codes from 2000 to 2014, when abstracting data from CDC WONDER.

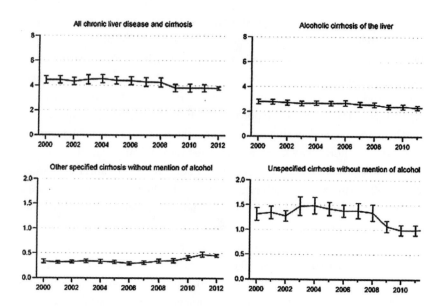

Source: Reprinted from Chiung and Chen (2013).

Figure 21-2. Trends in Liver Disease Discharges among Short-Stay Community Hospitals, United States, 2000–2012

are in excess of $21 billion annually, with $17 billion going towards hepatitis C antiviral costs, and when all aspects of liver disease are considered, the cost exceeds $3.4 billion per year (Sandler et al. 2002). Of those hospitalized, the mean length of stay is 5.9 days with an average cost of $28,703 (Kim et al. 2002). Trends in liver disease discharges in community hospitals in the United States from 1979 to 2005 are shown in Figure 21-2.

Causes

Liver disease can be attributed to a multitude of causes (Schiff and Maddrey 2011). Chronic liver disease is defined arbitrarily as liver disease that persists beyond six months from onset, and studies have demonstrated that up to 56% of persons with chronic liver disease may be completely asymptomatic (Zaman et al. 1990). This is an important factor to consider when one is studying the occurrence of new cases as well as the overall prevalence.

The most prevalent causes in the population include non-alcoholic fatty liver disease, alcoholic liver disease, viral hepatitis, hepatocellular carcinoma, and medication-related liver disease, and occasionally less common genetic conditions such as hereditary hemochromatosis, which leads to liver damage from iron overload. To investigate the epidemiology of liver disease, data from the National Health and Nutrition Examination Survey (NHANES) between 1988 and 2008 were utilized. The prevalence rate of chronic liver disease causes were examined in the 1988–1994, the 1995 to 2004, and the 2005–2008 NHANES. In this period, the prevalence of hepatitis B (0.36, 0.33%, and 0.34%, respectively), hepatitis C (2.0%, 2.0%, and 1.7%, respectively), and alcoholic liver disease (1.4%, 2.2% and 2.0%, respectively) remained stable. In contrast, the prevalence of non-alcoholic fatty liver disease increased from 5.5% to 9.8% to 11.0%, respectively. In the era from 2005 to 2008, non-alcoholic fatty liver disease accounted for 75% of chronic liver disease and its increased prevalence is related to the obesity epidemic (Younossi et al. 2011).

The Centers for Disease Control and Prevention (CDC), in collaboration with the National Institute of Diabetes and Digestive and Kidney Diseases, developed a surveillance program in which to record new instances of liver disease diagnoses made in the office of a gastroenterologist (Bell et al. 2001). Three U.S. counties were chosen: New Haven, Connecticut; Alameda (Oakland), California; and Multnomah (Portland), Oregon. Preliminary analysis of the 725 patients enrolled indicated that the etiology of these patients' chronic liver disease included

- Hepatitis C virus: 42%
- Alcohol-related liver disease: 8%
- Hepatitis C virus and alcohol combined: 22%
- Non-alcoholic fatty liver disease: 10%
- Hepatitis B virus: 4%
- Miscellaneous other liver conditions (including autoimmune hepatitis, drug-induced liver disease, hemochromatosis, primary biliary cirrhosis, sclerosing cholangitis, hepatocellular carcinoma, and granulomatous liver disease): 8%
- Unknown etiologies: 6%

On the basis of these results, it is estimated that the incidence of newly diagnosed chronic liver disease in referral practices is 67 per 100,000 in the population, and that 150,000 new cases of chronic liver disease are diagnosed in gastroenterologists' offices yearly in the United States. This does not account for those patients who are solely managed by primary care physicians (Kim et al. 2002)

Table 21-2. Primary Causes of Chronic Liver Disease

Factor	Attributable Risk for Chronic Liver Disease	Attributable Risk for Cirrhosis
Alcohol	20%	50%
Hepatitis C and alcohol	10%	10%
Hepatitis C	15%	10%
Hepatitis B	3%	5%
Non-alcoholic fatty liver disease	35%	10%
Unknown	17%	15%
Total	100%	100%

Source: Adapted from Singh and Hoyert (2000) and WHO (2016).

and the majority that have not sought medical care yet. Etiology of chronic liver disease in referral practices, non-referral practices, and the general population can vary considerably with higher attribution from alcohol and the combination of alcohol and hepatitis C. The attributable risk for chronic liver disease and cirrhosis in the U.S. population is detailed from various sources in Tables 21-2 and 21-3.

ALCOHOLIC LIVER DISEASE

Significance

Chronic heavy alcohol use can lead to liver disease that manifests as fatty liver disease, alcohol-induced hepatitis, or cirrhosis, conditions that can overlap (Schiff et al. 1999; see Chapter 10). Alcohol-induced fatty liver can be seen in up to 90% of alcoholics. It develops rapidly, in some studies after a weekend of binging. With alcohol cessation it resolves quickly as well, within two weeks in some studies (Thaler 1977). Alcohol-induced fatty liver can progress to cirrhosis in 10% to 15% of patients over long-term follow-up of 10 years or more (Sorensen et al. 1984). The risk increases with the amount of alcohol consumed over this duration.

With alcohol-induced hepatitis, the clinical spectrum ranges from a self-limited disorder to a severe life-threatening illness with liver failure. With longitudinal follow-up, the risk of developing cirrhosis can be as high as 70% in patients with alcohol-induced hepatitis (Alexander et al. 1971; Diehl 1997). With cessation of alcohol intake, the changes of alcohol-induced hepatitis can be reversible except in the most severe cases.

Table 21-3. Causes of Cirrhosis

Factor	Population Exposed	Relative Risk	Population-Attributable Risk
Alcohol	15 million	4–20	13%–50%
Hepatitis C	3.5 million	10–30	8%–25%
Hepatitis B	1 million	2.5–20	1%–7%
Metabolic syndrome	25 million	2–6	8%–20%

Note: Author's estimates are based on a review of the literature.

Descriptive Epidemiology

Alcoholic liver disease is closely linked to per capita consumption of alcohol in populations. In an examination of trends in chronic liver disease mortality and socioeconomic determinants in the United States from 1935 to 1996, alcohol use, unemployment, and minority concentration were closely linked to liver disease mortality. A 10% decrease in per capita alcohol consumption has been associated with a 2.5% reduction in cirrhosis mortality with a lag time as short as one year (Singh and Hoyert 2000). In a European study, a one-liter increase in alcohol consumption per capita was associated with a 14% increase in cirrhosis mortality for men and 8% for women (Ramstedt 2001).

Along with alcohol consumption rates, death rates from alcohol-induced cirrhosis increased after Prohibition in the United States from the 1930s to 1973, a peak of 14.9 deaths per 100,000 population (Terris 1967). Alcohol-related deaths have declined from the 1970s in the United States. From 1973 to 1997, age-adjusted death rates from cirrhosis and chronic liver disease decreased at an average annual rate of 3.0% for the entire population, by 2.6% for white men, 3.0% for white women, 4.1% for African American men, and 4.8% for African American women (Saadatmand et al. 2000).

Hospital discharges in the United States measured in short-stay community hospitals showed an upward trend in alcohol-induced liver disease and cirrhosis-related discharges between 1988 and 2005 (Chiung and Chen 2007). However, subsequently there has been a decline in hospitalizations for alcohol-induced cirrhosis (Chiung and Chen 2013; Figure 21-2). In the United States, this decreased mortality from alcoholic liver disease since the 1970s occurred despite increasing alcohol consumption rates until the 1980s. This paradox has been attributed to multiple causes including better health care, better nutrition, and increasing treatment of alcohol addiction

(Mann et al. 1991; Holder and Parker 1992; Smart and Mann 1993; Kerr et al. 2000; Ramstedt 2001).

Despite stable consumption rates, alcoholic liver disease–induced mortality has increased in the United Kingdom and other parts of Northern Europe. In England, the rate of alcohol-induced cirrhosis death increased from 2.8 per 100,000 in 1993 to 8.0 per 100,000 in 2000. These increases were seen in all ethnic groups, but the mortality rate in Asian men was 3.8 times that of white men (Fisher et al. 2002). In parts of Asia, including Japan, Korea, and China, the consumption of alcohol has increased steadily from the 1960s and the proportion of liver disease attributed to alcohol has increased commensurately (Park et al. 1998). In Japan, the proportion of all liver disease from alcohol increased from 5.1% in 1968 to 14.1% by 1986 (Hasumura and Takeuchi 1991).

Causes

The risk of alcohol-induced cirrhosis rises with the amount of alcohol consumed. The risk is increased with sustained intake of greater than 60 grams per day in men and greater than 20 grams per day in women, but the risk varies considerably (a single drink is 8 to 12 grams in the United States). Only 6% to 40% of people drinking to this level will eventually develop cirrhosis (Lelbach 1975; Bellentani et al. 1997; Corrao et al. 1997). The risk also increases with lifetime alcohol use (>100 kilograms in the Dionysos Italian population study; Bellentani et al. 1997). The risk of death after alcohol-induced cirrhosis is diagnosed is much higher with continued drinking, but improves significantly with abstinence. With continued drinking, the 5-year survival in patients with alcohol-induced cirrhosis is less than 30% but more than 60% with abstinence and more than 90% if they have compensated cirrhosis (Mandayam et al. 2004).

The wide variability in the risk of cirrhosis with alcohol intake is dependent upon poorly understood genetic factors including polymorphisms in genes that influence alcohol metabolism and absorption, coexistence of other liver injurious agents (e.g., hepatitis C), iron overload (as seen in genetic hemochromatosis), and sex differences. Although alcohol abuse and cirrhosis-related deaths predominate in men worldwide including the United States, there is a growing proportion of women among heavy drinkers (Blume 1986). Women have a higher susceptibility to alcohol compared to men. The risk of cirrhosis develops with lower rates of drinking in women (20–60 g/day) compared to men (40–80 g/day) and cirrhosis develops with shorter duration of alcohol abuse in women. Multiple mechanisms are thought to underlie this susceptibility including variations in alcohol distribution and levels in blood, gastric enzyme activity, first-pass metabolism, and sex hormone differences in endotoxin after exposure to alcohol (Frezza et al. 1990; Ikejima et al. 1998; Parlesak et al. 2000; Sato et al. 2001).

Ethnic differences in alcohol use and alcohol-induced liver disease exist, with highest rates of alcoholic liver disease in Hispanic men, followed by black men and white men (Stinson et al. 2001). Part of this may be explained by continued high rates of heavy drinking in Hispanic populations compared to other ethnic groups (Caetano and Kaskutas 1995; Stinson et al. 2001). Differences in genetic predisposition, socioeconomic status, nutrition, and access to health care may all play a role, but this has not been clarified.

Alcohol use is common in patients with hepatitis C virus infection, with some studies suggesting that as many as 60% to 70% of hepatitis C–infected individuals consume as much as 40 grams of alcohol per day (Loguercio et al. 2000). The association of alcohol abuse and hepatitis C infection is associated with higher rates of progression to cirrhosis, liver cancer, and cirrhosis-related death. Some studies suggest that the association may be synergistic (Corrao and Arico 1998). Alcoholics with hepatitis C infection are at higher risk of cirrhosis than alcoholics not infected with hepatitis C (Ostapowicz et al. 1998; Degos 1999). Conversely, of patients infected with hepatitis C, those who consume alcohol heavily (> 50 g/day) have a higher risk of progression to cirrhosis than non-drinkers (Corrao and Arico 1998). Even smaller amounts of alcohol use (30 g/day) have been shown to promote fibrosis of the liver in patients with chronic hepatitis C infection (Westin et al. 2002).

The contributing role of diabetes and obesity—which themselves are risk factors for liver disease—needs further clarification in alcohol-induced liver disease. Some studies have shown these to be independent risk factors (Naveau et al. 1997; Day 2000) whereas others have not (Bellentani et al. 1997). Obesity-related fatty liver disease may proceed along the same pathophysiologic pathways of liver injury as alcohol, and the combination may have synergistic effects on liver damage. There may also be a dose-dependent effect of alcohol on non-alcoholic fatty liver disease with small doses of alcohol being protective of progressive liver disease (Dunn et al. 2012) and increasing contribution being deleterious on development of more advanced liver disease

(Raynard et al. 2012). The association of diet, particularly of pork products, with beer drinking, has been associated with liver disease in drinkers (Nanji and French 1985; Bode et al. 1998). Other studies have found protective effects of coffee drinking (Ruhl and Everhart 2005).

Interventions

See Chapter 10, Alcohol Use.

HEPATITIS A

The hepatitis A virus is an RNA virus that spreads by fecal–oral contact from contaminated food and water as well by person-to-person contact. It occurs in both sporadic cases and in epidemic outbreaks (60% of U.S. cases). It has been spread by contaminated green onions (Dentinger et al. 2001; Wheeler et al. 2005) imported from Mexico and strawberries from Guatemala. Contaminated food, particularly shellfish, is a usual source of contamination. Susceptible individuals are at risk for epidemic outbreaks such as one that occurred in Shanghai from contaminated clams involving 290,000 people (Tang et al. 1991).

Significance

Hepatitis A causes an acute illness. The likelihood of developing symptomatic disease is age-dependent with more than 70% of children being asymptomatic and the majority of adults and adolescents (> 70%) developing symptomatic disease (Tong et al. 1995). The symptoms are nonspecific including aches, fever, abdominal pain, and jaundice. The incubation period can last from 15 to 49 days; jaundice usually lasts one to three months.

Hepatitis A does not lead to chronic hepatitis except for very rare cases of relapsing forms, which ultimately resolve as well. Development of severe acute liver failure is also rare (< 1%) but more likely to occur in adults than children and in those adults with underlying chronic liver disease such as from hepatitis C (Vento et al. 1998). Diagnosis is made by detection of serum hepatitis A antibody (hepatitis A immunoglobulin [Ig] M subtype) that is positive by the onset of symptoms and detectable up to six months after onset of illness. After recovery, the individual usually develops lifelong hepatitis A

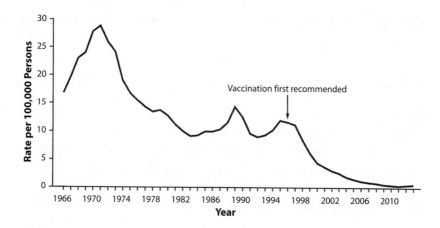

Source: Adapted from Murphy et al. (2016).
Note: The rate (no. of cases) in 1971 (peak), 1996 (first Advisory Committee on Immunization Practices recommendation for hepatitis A vaccination), and 2011 (low) were 28.9 (59,606 cases), 11.7 (31,032 cases), and 0.4 (1,398 cases), respectively.

Figure 21-3. Incidence of Reported Acute Hepatitis A by Year, United States, 1966–2013

antibody IgG subtype rendering immunity from further attacks (Koff 1992; Schiff et al. 1999).

Descriptive Epidemiology

The incidence of hepatitis A is much higher in developing countries and occurs earlier in childhood (> 95% are immune by adulthood), whereas in Europe and the United States, infection rates in children are lower and adult symptomatic infection is not uncommon, although it is decreasing. It is estimated that 33% of the U.S. population has been infected with the hepatitis A virus (ACIP et al. 2006; Brundage and Fitzpatrick 2006). There is no chronic infection, and these individuals are now immune to hepatitis A virus.

The incidence of hepatitis A in the United States has steadily decreased from the 1970s. The incidence was 28 cases per 100,000 in 1970 in the United States, decreased to 13 per 100,000 by 1980, and remained steady until 1990 (CDC et al. 2006). This decrease was likely secondary to improved food handling and processing as well as epidemic management. Since vaccination became available in 1995, hepatitis A rates have declined by 95% in the United States. In 2013 only 1,781 acute asymptomatic cases were reported in the United States with

3,473 estimated new infections occurring in the United States (CDC 2016a; Figure 21-3).

Causes

Risk factors associated with higher rates of hepatitis A included household crowding and poverty. International travel is a risk factor as well, particularly to countries where hepatitis A is endemic such as Mexico and Central or South America. Other risk factors include sexual and household contact with another person with hepatitis A, transmission in men who have sex with men, and with illicit drug use (Jacobsen and Koopman 2004).

Interventions

Hepatitis A infection can be prevented by improved sanitary conditions including treatment of water, avoidance of contaminated shellfish and food, and hand washing (Mbithi et al. 1992). In epidemics, case and source finding and vaccination of exposed susceptible individuals are key to controlling epidemics.

Eventually, vaccination of children should decrease incidence further. Immunization for hepatitis A is now recommended universally for all children aged 12 to 23 months (since 2004; ACIP et al. 2006) and those at higher risk of transmission (travelers to endemic areas, men who have sex with men, intravenous and non-intravenous drug users) since 1996. A highly effective vaccine has been available since 1996 (Wasley et al. 2006; Figure 21-4).

HEPATITIS B

Hepatitis B is a DNA virus belonging to the hepadnaviridae family and is extremely prevalent globally (Schiff and Maddrey 2011). The hepatitis B virus is spread by parenteral exposure to blood and other body fluids. Because of a large prevalence in developing countries such as China (10% to 20%), it is efficiently spread to neonates by vertical transmission, which is the main modality of transmission in the developing world (Maynard 1990; Alter et al. 1990; Beasley et al. 1982). In the United States, with a lower prevalence (estimated 730,000 million cases or 0.28% of the population) and better access to perinatal care and childhood immunization, vertical transmission is less common than adult-to-adult transmission through sexual contact or illicit

1996

1. Routine hepatitis A (HepA) vaccination for children aged ≥2 years and accelerated vaccination of older children (including children to age 10–15 years) to control ongoing outbreaks in communities that have high rates of hepatitis A and periodic hepatitis A outbreaks.
2. Vaccinate populations at increased risk for hepatitis A infection (e.g., persons traveling to or working in countries that have high or intermediate endemnicity of infection, men who have sex with men, illegal-drug users, persons who have occupational risk for infection, and persons who have clotting-factor disorders) or persons who have chronic liver disease.
3. Vaccinate any person wishing to obtain immunity.

1999

1. Routine HepA vaccination for children aged ≥2 years who live in states, counties, or communities where the average annual rate during 1987–1997 was ≥20 cases per 100,000 population (i.e., approximately twice the national average of 10.8 cases per 100,000 population) (included 11 states: Alaska, Arizona, California, Idaho, Nevada, New Mexico, Oklahoma, Oregon, South Dakota, Utah, and Washington).
2. Consider routine HepA vaccination for children aged ≥2 years living in states, counties, or

communities where the average annual rate of hepatitis A during 1987–1997 was ≥10 cases per 100,000 population but <20 cases per 100,000 population (six states: Arkansas, Colorado, Missouri, Montana, Texas, and Wyoming).
3. Vaccinate older children (e.g., up to age 10–15 years) in communities with high rates of hepatitis A to prevent epidemics.
4. Vaccinate persons at increased risk for hepatitis A and persons who have chronic liver disease (see 1996, above).
5. Vaccinate any person wishing to obtain immunity.

2006

1. Routine HepA vaccination for all children in the United States at age 12–23 months.
2. Continue HepA vaccination for children ages 2–18 months in states, counties and communities with existing vaccination programs.
3. Consider catch-up vaccination for children ages 2–18 years in areas without existing programs, especially when incidence is increasing or with ongoing outbreaks among children and adolescents.
4. Vaccinate persons at increased risk for HAV and persons who have chronic liver disease (see 1996 above).
5. Vaccinate any person wishing to obtain immunity.

Source: Adapted from Murphy et al. (2016).

Figure 21-4. Childhood Hepatitis A Vaccination Recommendations

drug use. In the era of universal vaccination in the United States (since 1991), the incidence of chronic HBV infection has declined in children, but not in adults aged older than 50 years (Wasley et al. 2010).

According to data from NHANES 1999–2006, the prevalence of markers of active or past infection from hepatitis B was higher among non-Hispanic blacks (12.2%) and persons of "other" race (13.3%) than it was among non-Hispanic whites (2.8%) or Mexican Americans (2.9%), and it was higher among foreign-born participants (12.2%) than it was among U.S.-born participants (3.5%). Prevalence among U.S.-born children aged 6 to 19 years (0.5%) did not differ by race or ethnicity. Disparities between U.S.-born and foreign-born children were smaller during 1999 to 1996 (0.5% vs. 2.0%) than during 1988 to 1994 (1.0% vs. 12.8%). Among children aged 6 to 19 years, 56.7% had markers of vaccine-induced immunity.

Significance

In children and neonates, the acute infection is clinically silent in the majority. In adults, acute infection is symptomatic in 30% to 50%. Hepatitis B virus acute infection has an incubation period of one to four months. Symptoms during the prodromal phase may be vague including fatigue, aches, malaise and abdominal pain. Jaundice can occur and can last from 4 to 12 weeks (Liaw et al. 1998).

With chronic infection, risk of developing cirrhosis and hepatocellular carcinoma increases with longer duration of infection. In endemic countries, the risk is highest in men aged older than 40 years (Fattovich et al. 1991; Liaw et al. 1998). Increased risk of progressive liver disease also depends upon the interaction between the host immune system and the virus. The risk is higher in those individuals with high levels of chronic viral replication with high levels of the virus in blood (Yang et al. 2002; Chen et al. 2006). The risk is reduced considerably in those individuals in whom the immune system successfully suppresses viral replication (Stevens et al. 1975; Tassopoulos et al. 1987).

Increased risk of progressive liver disease leading to cirrhosis and hepatocellular carcinoma also occurs with concurrent tobacco and alcohol use (Donato et al. 1997). The lifetime risk of cirrhosis and hepatocellular carcinoma is higher in individuals from endemic areas likely because of longer durations of infection (Beasley et al. 1982; Chen et al. 2006).

Descriptive Epidemiology

High rates of vertical transmission in developing countries result in high prevalence because of the high chances of developing chronic infection after exposure at this stage of life. In the United States, where most of the transmission is in adults, the lower rate of chronicity results in lower prevalence rates. The prevalence of chronic hepatitis B infection is estimated to be 0.3% (700,000 to 1.4 million individuals) in the United States (Alter and Mast 1994; Kim 2009). Prevalence rates are highest in Asians (99% born outside United States) and Alaska Natives, and are higher in incarcerated, homeless, and institutionalized individuals. According to an analysis of the national death registry, the age-adjusted mortality rate for hepatitis B–related illness increased throughout the 1980s and early 1990s from 0.2 per 100,000 to 0.8 per 100,000. This increase was followed by a relative plateau and then a decline starting in 1999. As of 2004, the mortality rate was approximately 0.6 per 100,000 (Everhart 2009). Globally, hepatitis B is a huge issue with greater than 350 million carriers and more than one million deaths from associated liver disease (Maynard 1990). The prevalence rates vary from 0.2% in the United States to 10% to 20% in Southeast Asia and China.

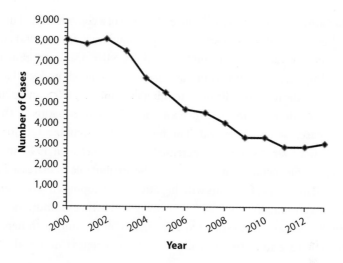

Source: Adapted from CDC (2016a).

Figure 21-5. Reported Number of Acute Hepatitis B Cases, United States, 2000–2013

The incidence of hepatitis B in the United States has decreased after peaking in the 1980s (Figure 21-5). The incidence of HBV was 4.1 per 100,000 in the United States in 1970 and peaked in 1980 to 8.4 in 100,000 and remained at 8.5 in 100,000 by 1990. Between 1995 and 2013, the incidence of acute hepatitis B declined by 79% to 1.0 in 100,000, the lowest ever reported (CDC 2016a). In the United States, 78,000 estimated new infections occurred in 2001 and this had dropped to 18,760 by 2012 (Klevens et al. 2014).

Declines were reported in all age groups but were most steep in children. In 2012, the highest rates of acute hepatitis B were in persons aged 30 to 39 years (2.2 cases per 100,000 population) and the lowest among adolescents and children aged younger than 19 years (0.03 cases per 100,000; CDC 2016a). Universal hepatitis B vaccination has resulted in these reduced rates in children. High rates for hepatitis B continue among adults, particularly men aged 25 to 44 years, emphasizing the need to identify and vaccinate high-risk adults.

The rates for hepatitis B virus infection in male individuals still predominated compared to female individuals (1.2 vs. 0.68 per 100,000 in 2012). The rates of hepatitis B declined for all races and ethnicities from 2000 to 2012. Rates were highest for non-Hispanic blacks in 2012 (1.1 cases per 100,000) followed by non- Hispanic whites (0.8 per 100,000), Hispanics (0.4 per 100,000), and Asians (0.4 per 100,000).

Reductions in incidence have occurred because of a combination of universal vaccination of neonates and adolescents (aged younger than 18 years) and recommendation of vaccination of high-risk adults. Safer needle use practices in injection drug users as well as continued screening of blood products have also contributed to the reduction in adult-to-adult transmission (CDC et al. 2006).

Despite the decrease in incidence and prevalence of hepatitis B, the burden of disease has not decreased. The number of hospitalizations for hepatitis B–related liver disease has increased four-fold between 1990 and 2006 (Kim 2009). This increased morbidity may be attributable to increased access or increased numbers of patients with hepatitis B developing cirrhosis and liver cancer from chronic infection as well as increased influx of immigrants with hepatitis B infection. It is estimated that 40,000 immigrants with hepatitis B virus infection are admitted annually to the United States (Mast et al. 2006).

Causes

Reported risk factors in the United States include sexual contact (32% multiple sex partners, 10% sexual contact with a person known to have hepatitis B, 13% men who have sex with men), and injection drug use (15%). Hemodialysis was a risk factor in 0.3%, blood transfusion in 0.2%, and occupational exposure in 0.8% (Wasley et al. 2007; Figure 21-6).

The risk of developing chronic infection is dependent upon the age at which exposure occurs. Neonatal transmission results in chronic infection in 90% of non-vaccinated children (Stevens et al. 1975). In adults, however, acute infection results in chronic infection in only 5% (Beasley et al. 1982; Tassopoulos et al. 1987; Mast et al. 2006).

Interventions

Hepatitis B is a vaccine-preventable disease. The vaccine has been available since the early 1980s and the recent vaccine is more than 95% effective (Lai et al. 1993). The World Health Organization has recommended universal childhood vaccination worldwide. So far, 158 countries have incorporated hepatitis vaccination in routine immunization, but coverage is far from universal with 60% coverage (WHO 2016). A comprehensive strategy to eliminate hepatitis B virus transmission has been introduced in the United States since 1991 and updated in 2006. Since 1991, vaccination has been recommended universally for all

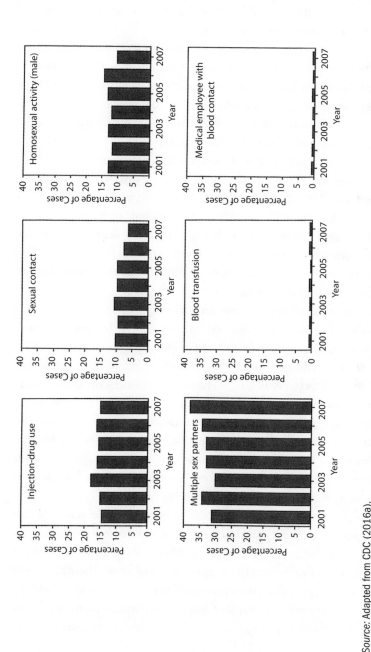

Source: Adapted from CDC (2016a).

Note: The percentage of cases among persons in which a specific risk factor was reported was calculated based on the total number of persons for whom any information for that exposure was reported. Multiple risk factors may be reported for a single case.

Figure 21-6. Trends in Selected Epidemiological Characteristics among Patients with Acute Hepatitis B by Year, United States, 2001–2007

infants born in the United States as well for children aged younger than 18 years as a catch-up program (Immunization Practices Advisory Committee 1991). The catch-up program in the United States has reached 60% of children aged between 13 and 15 years (Mast et al. 2005).

In addition, all women seeking prenatal care are screened for hepatitis B virus infection, and for women with hepatitis B, their infants are vaccinated and given prophylaxis with hepatitis B immunoglobulin at birth. Efficacy of this regimen is greater than 95%. For adults at high risk, screening and vaccination is recommended. These include users of illicit drugs, those with multiple sexual partners, sexual partners of persons with hepatitis B virus infection, solid organ recipients, dialysis patients, and health care workers, among others.

In the United States, 56% of individuals attending dialysis were vaccinated against hepatitis B virus in 2002 (47% in 1997) as well as 90% of dialysis staff. Hepatitis B incidence in 2002 was only 0.12% in dialysis center patients, compared to 1974 when the incidence of hepatitis B among dialysis patients was 6.2%, and selected hemodialysis centers reported rates as high as 30% (CDC 2001). This decline began in 1982, when hepatitis B virus vaccination was first recommended for dialysis patients.

The efficacy of childhood vaccination is already seen in countries with a high rate of vertical and early childhood transmission. In Taiwan, where universal neonatal vaccination was introduced in 1986, the prevalence of hepatitis B in children aged younger than 15 years was 9.8% before this implementation and 1.2% in 2004 (Ni et al. 2007). The rate of hepatocellular carcinoma in children in Taiwan has also decreased by a third over this time period. In the United States, where hepatitis B virus transmission occurs mostly in adults, the results of universal childhood vaccination will have a considerably longer lag time before the benefits of vaccination are seen, although the decline in acute hepatitis B rates in children born in the United States over the past 15 years is likely attributable to universal vaccination.

Hepatitis B–specific antiviral agents have been available since the late 1990s, and with high potency and low levels of resistance since 2006. The currently available agents are effective in suppressing viral replication, but are not able to eradicate the virus from the human host. As a result, these have to be taken daily and often for long durations to suppress the virus. In individuals with evidence of chronic liver damage and viral replication, these agents are used to decrease the risk of progression to cirrhosis and liver cancer (Terrault et al. 2016).

HEPATITIS C

Hepatitis C is an RNA virus belonging to the flaviviridae family that infects the liver (hepatotrophism; Schiff and Maddrey 2011). The hepatitis C virus is spread parenterally by breach of mucosal membranes and is efficiently spread by illicit drug use including injection drugs and intranasal cocaine and somewhat less efficiently by sexual transmission (Murphy et al. 2000). A surge in incidence of hepatitis C occurred in the 1970s and 1980s because of transmission of the virus by these routes as well as by blood transfusion (Alter et al. 1989). Before the discovery of the hepatitis C viral genome in 1989 (Choo et al. 1989), the safety of the blood supply was based on testing for elevated liver enzymes, and because chronic hepatitis C (called non-A non-B hepatitis before 1989) is often associated with normal liver enzymes, transfusion-associated transmission was not uncommon. With the discovery of the hepatitis C virus genome in 1989 and the development of an accurate antibody test thereafter (Kuo et al. 1989), the blood supply has become very safe, with the risk of transfusion-related hepatitis C estimated to be about 1 per 100,000 to 1 per 1,000,000 units transfused (Schreiber et al. 1996; Pomper et al. 2003; Figure 21-7).

Significance

After exposure to hepatitis C virus, chronic infection occurs in 70% to 85% with a minority clearing the virus within six months of exposure. Overall progression to cirrhosis is estimated to occur in 10% to 20% of hepatitis C virus–infected patients over their lifetime (Freeman et al. 2001). Higher rates are seen with steady alcohol intake, in male individuals, and with longer duration of infection, as well as in individuals infected at older age (>40 years; Poynard et al. 1997). On average, it takes 20 years from initial hepatitis C virus infection to develop cirrhosis in these patients. Hepatocellular carcinoma develops at the rate of 1% per year in those with cirrhosis.

It is projected that a decline in the prevalence of infection in the United States from a peak of 2.7% in the 1990s to 1% by 2030 may occur (Armstrong et al. 2000). Despite the reduced incidence, the burden of disease attributable to hepatitis C is still rising due to its chronicity and the lag time from acquisition of infection to development of clinically significant liver disease. The death rate from hepatitis C virus has increased from 0.4 deaths per 100,000 in 1982 to 2.3 per 100,000 in 2014 (CDC 2016b).

Reported Acute (New) Cases of Hepatitis C Virus (HCV)								
2005	**2006**	**2007**	**2008**	**2009**	**2010**	**2011**	**2012**	**2013**
694	802	849	878	781	853	1,230	1,778	2,138

Estimated Actual New Cases of HCV (range)		
2011 (estimated)[a]	**2012 (estimated)[a]**	**2013 (estimated)[a]**
16,500 (7,200-43,400)	24,700 (19,600-84,400)	29,700 (23,500-101,400)

Est. No. of Chronic Cases In the United States	No. of Death Certificates listing HCV as a Cause of Death			
	2010	**2011**	**2012**	**2013[b]**
2.7-3.9 million	16,627[c]	17,721[c]	18,650[c]	19,368[c]

Source: Adapted from CDC (2016a).
[a]Actual acute cases estimated to be 13.9 times the number of reported cases in any year.
[b]Underlying or contributing cause of death in most recent year available (2013).
[c]Current information indicates these represent a fraction of deaths attributable in whole or in part to chronic hepatitis C.

Figure 21-7. Burden of Hepatitis C, United States

Morbidity and health care costs for hepatitis C are also increasing. Between 1991 and 2013, the proportion of liver transplants in the United States related to hepatitis C increased from 12% to 40% (UNOS 2016). Data from the National Ambulatory Medical Care Survey, the National Hospital Ambulatory Medical Care Survey, and the Nationwide Inpatient Sample were analyzed by Galbraith et al. (2014). Individuals with hepatitis C virus infection were responsible for more than 2.3 million outpatient, 73,000 emergency department, and 475,000 inpatient visits annually. Persons in the baby boomer cohort accounted for 72%, 68%, and 71% of care episodes in these settings, respectively. Whereas the number of outpatient visits remained stable during the study period, inpatient admissions among hepatitis C virus–infected baby boomers increased by greater than 60%. Inpatient stays totaled 2.8 million days and cost more than $15 billion annually. Nonwhites, uninsured individuals, and individuals receiving publicly funded health insurance were disproportionately affected in all health care settings. Hepatitis C also has a profound effect on quality of life in patients referred to health centers (Rodger et al. 1999; Hussain et al. 2001), some of which is related to concurrent comorbid illnesses such as depression.

It is estimated that a two- to four-fold increase in numbers of persons with hepatitis C virus infection for greater than 20 years occurred between 1990 and 2015 in the United States. (Armstrong et al. 2000; Davis et al. 2003). The increase in incidence of hepatocellular carcinoma in recent years (El-Serag 2012) is in a large part attributable to the hepatitis C epidemic. As a consequence, it is projected that complications of cirrhosis will also increase (hepatocellular carcinoma up 81%, hepatic decompensation up 106%, and liver-related death up 180%; Davis et al. 2003). Even if every single hepatitis C patient is identified and treated, the number of cases with decompensated cirrhosis will decrease by only half after 20 years. Currently, most patients estimated to have hepatitis C virus infection do not know that they have the disease or do not have access to health care. As the proportion of those with cirrhosis increases and becomes clinically apparent, the burden on the health care system is expected to increase.

Descriptive Epidemiology

Hepatitis C is a reportable disease, but there is significant underreporting despite active surveillance programs (National Notifiable Disease Surveillance System; Wasley et al. 2007). The reasons for this are varied, but a large part of the problem is that acute hepatitis C is overwhelmingly asymptomatic and unnoticed. Furthermore, populations at risk for hepatitis C are socially and economically disadvantaged and often do not seek or have access to health care. Furthermore, national surveys such as NHANES exclude populations with high prevalence of the disease, such as incarcerated individuals and the homeless. Health care provider underreporting of diagnosed cases also occurs.

Hepatitis C leads to chronic disease, with spontaneous clearance occurring in only 15% to 30% of cases after exposure. As a consequence, the prevalence of the virus is high, with an estimated 3.5 million cases in the United States (Edlin et al. 2015). The highest prevalence of infection is seen in those born between 1945 and 1965 (baby boomers), with men having a higher rate of infection than women (20% more likely; Kim et al. 2002). Blacks have a higher prevalence of infection (3.2%) than whites (1.5%) with Mexican Americans

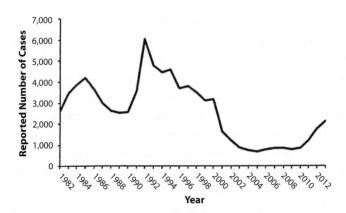

Source: Adapted from CDC (2016a).

Figure 21-8. Incidence of Reported Acute Hepatitis C by Year, United States, 1982–2013

having intermediate rates (NHANES III; Alter et al.). Hepatitis C virus prevalence is higher in certain groups including up to 18% of Veterans (Briggs et al. 2001), 40% of the homeless (Cheung et al. 2002), and 39% of incarcerated men and 54% of incarcerated women (Ruiz et al. 1999).

At the peak of the hepatitis C epidemic, in the mid-1980s, between 180,000 and 230,000 new cases were occurring yearly in the United States (Alter 1997; Williams 1999). Since then, the incidence has declined to an estimated 29,000 new infections each year in the United States (CDC 2016a; see Figure 21-8).

The decrease in hepatitis C virus incidence is multifactorial. Declines in transfusion-related hepatitis C started occurring after the introduction of the 1985 guidelines for selecting safer blood donors and sharply with the introduction of hepatitis C virus antibody testing of donated blood products starting in 1989. Safer injection drug needle practices and tattoo needle practices introduced to reduce HIV have also contributed to the reduced incidence. Declines have occurred in all groups. Persons aged 25 to 39 years have the highest incidence, but have also had the greatest declines (Wasley et al. 2007) with a 92% decline in incidence of hepatitis C infection since 1992. The incidence is higher for male (0.26 per 100,000) than female persons (0.21 per 100,000), although this gap is narrowing. Declines in the incidence of hepatitis C among racial/ethnic populations have occurred across the board. In 2005, rates were 0.36 per 100,000 in American Indians and Alaska Natives and lowest in Asians (0.02). Rates of hepatitis C virus infection were similar in Hispanics and non-Hispanics.

Causes

Several large population studies have identified risk factors for hepatitis C virus infection. The largest of these, the NHANES III study, assessed prevalence in a random sample of 21,241 U.S. participants and found a hepatitis C prevalence of 1.8% (Alter et al. 1999). Risk factors included illicit drug use and number of sexual partners, as well as weaker associations with socioeconomic markers such as poverty index, educational level, and marital status (Alter et al. 1999). Other population-based studies have found similar risk factors with injection drug use being the strongest risk factor (Garfein et al. 1996). Other risk factors include blood transfusion or organ transplant before 1992, hemodialysis, and high-risk sexual behavior (Alter et al. 1989; Pereira et al. 1991; Geerlings et al. 1994).

Dialysis remains a risk factor despite universal infection-control practices. In the national surveillance of dialysis-associated diseases in the United States in 2002, hepatitis C virus antibody was found in 7.8% of dialysis recipients with an incidence rate of 0.34%. This is a decline of 25% since 1995. Hepatitis C virus testing was done in 2002 in 64% of centers. Hepatitis C routine testing with anti–hepatitis C virus antibody was recommended routinely every six months and at entry. Using disposable equipment in the dialysis machines has been associated with lower incidence of hepatitis C as well as having a dedicated medication rooms (Finelli et al. 2005).

The incarcerated population has a high incidence and prevalence of hepatitis C virus infection. Risk factors in prison for viral hepatitis include illicit drug use in more than 50% before incarceration, but in as many as 3% to 28% during incarceration as well (Weinbaum et al. 2003). Sexual activity in jail occurs in as many as 30% of inmates and is associated with high-risk sexual practices. Hepatitis C incidence is also higher in certain populations such as the Veterans of foreign wars (5% prevalence; see Figure 21-9).

Screening for hepatitis C virus infection on the basis of these risk factors was not very effective for a multitude of reasons including both patient and provider factors. Because more than 60% of hepatitis C occurs in the baby boomer population (born between 1945 to 1965) in the United States, the CDC since 2012 has endorsed screening for this birth cohort regardless of risk factors (CDC 2016a).

Increase in progression toward severe liver disease has been shown with chronic alcohol intake, particularly moderate-to-severe alcohol intake (>50 g/day; Poynard et al. 1997; Zarski et al. 2003). Older age at infection has

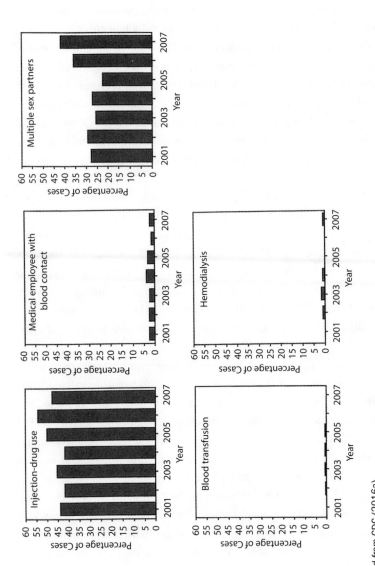

Source: Adapted from CDC (2016a).

Note: The percentage of cases among persons in which a specific risk factor was reported was calculated based on the total number of persons for whom any information for that exposure was reported. Multiple risk factors may be reported for a single case.

Figure 21-9. Trends in Selected Epidemiological Characteristics among Patients with Acute Hepatitis C by Year, United States, 2001–2007

also been associated with increased risk of progressive liver disease. Given the propensity of obesity and the metabolic syndrome to independently cause liver disease, the coexistence of obesity and the metabolic syndrome with hepatitis C has been investigated in preliminary studies. There is some evidence that with increased body mass index and features of the metabolic syndrome (diabetes, hypertension, hyperlipidemia, and truncal obesity) there is more rapid progression of liver disease in patients with hepatitis C (Zarski et al. 2003; Hourigan et al. 1999). In a large meta-analysis, steatosis (or fat in the liver) was independently associated with increased fibrosis and liver damage in hepatitis C (Leandro et al. 2006). In some analyses, male sex has been associated with increased fibrosis as well (Poynard et al. 1997; Leandro et al. 2006).

Interventions

There is no vaccine available for hepatitis C virus. National recommendations issued in 1998 for prevention and control of hepatitis C virus infection include screening and testing blood donors, viral inactivation of plasma products, risk reduction counseling to reduce transmission in injection drug users and in those at high risk of sexual transmission (multiple sexual partners), as well as in health care settings (infection control practices, dialysis).

Historically, treatment for hepatitis C was with injectable interferon and oral ribavirin, antiviral agents that are associated with an average viral clearance rate of 10% to 50% and had to be taken for 24 to 48 weeks (Manns et al. 2001; Fried et al. 2002). The treatment can be difficult to tolerate (Younossi et al. 2007) and uptake was poor. Since 2011, the therapy for hepatitis C has improved considerably with the advent of direct-acting antiviral agents. These are all oral agents that work by directly suppressing one of the viral enzymes involved in hepatitis C replication. Response "cure" rates are greater than 90% with therapies as short as 8 to 12 weeks in most patients. Therapies are also well tolerated with few drug interactions (Vachon and Dieterich 2011; AASLD 2016). Currently, given the high cost of the medications, access is limited even in those with insurance although with increased market competition pressure should improve access to these medications (Andrieux-Meyer et al. 2015).

NON-ALCOHOLIC FATTY LIVER DISEASE

Recent attention has focused on a newly recognized epidemic called non-alcoholic fatty liver disease, a chronic liver disease characterized by fat infiltration in the liver (steatosis) and consequent liver injury of varying degree and severity. By many estimates, it is the most prevalent cause of chronic liver disease worldwide (Fazel et al. 2016).

Significance

Although many patients have a benign course of bland fat deposition in the liver (fatty liver disease) there is a subset of patients who will develop inflammation and fibrosis called non-alcoholic steatohepatitis. These patients are at risk of progression to cirrhosis, liver failure, and hepatocellular carcinoma (Adams et al. 2005).

Non-alcoholic fatty liver disease is closely associated with the metabolic syndrome (truncal obesity, diabetes or insulin resistance, hyperlipidemia, hypertension; Marchesini et al. 2003). The natural history of the condition remains poorly understood. Adams et al. (2005) published accounts of 420 patients diagnosed in Olmsted County, Minnesota, between 1980 and 2000 who were followed for a mean of 7.6 years culminating in 3,192 person-years of follow-up. Five percent of these patients developed cirrhosis over this relatively short follow-up, and 3.1% developed liver-related complications. The mortality was 13% during the follow-up, significantly higher than that in the general population (standardized mortality ratio = 1.34; 95% confidence interval [CI] = 1.003, 1.76; $p = .03$). A longitudinal study describing 129 patients with biopsy-proven non-alcoholic fatty liver disease were compared with a matched reference population over 13.7 years. Those patients with more advanced proven non-alcoholic fatty liver disease (non-alcoholic steatohepatitis and fibrosis) were found to have end-stage liver disease in 5.4% as well as an increased mortality related to cardiovascular and liver-related causes. During the follow-up period, 69 of 88 patients (78%) developed diabetes or impaired glucose tolerance and 41% had progression of liver fibrosis. Those who had progressive liver damage were more likely to have had a significant amount of weight gain and were more insulin-resistant.

Although the majority of individuals with non-alcoholic fatty liver disease do not progress to end-stage liver disease, given the high prevalence and increasing incidence of non-alcoholic fatty liver disease, it now is the second-most-common indication for liver transplantation in the United States (Charlton et al. 2011) as well as the second-most-common cause of liver cancer (Younossi et al. 2015), and in the next decade is expected to surpass viral hepatitis as the most common indication for liver transplantation and cause of liver cancer in the United States. In an international study of non-alcoholic steatohepatitis–related cirrhosis, the risk of mortality was similar to that in patients with hepatitis C–related cirrhosis (Yatsuji et al. 2009).

Descriptive Epidemiology

One of the few reported studies regarding incidence is a prospective, observational study from Japan (Hamaguchi et al. 2005). Using ALT levels and ultrasonography of the liver in patients without significant alcohol use, they found that, at baseline, 812 of 4,401 (18%) participants had non-alcoholic fatty liver disease. During the mean follow-up period of 414 days, the authors observed 308 new cases (10%) of non-alcoholic fatty liver disease among 3,147 participants who were disease-free at baseline.

The determination of prevalence, while still laden with challenges, has proven more feasible. Studies have been difficult, however, because of the need for an invasive liver biopsy for definitive diagnosis. As a result, most studies have elected to use either serum liver chemistries or radiologic imaging as the surrogate diagnostic tool.

Published reports have stated non-alcoholic fatty liver disease to be present in 27% to 34% of the North American population. In a study using data from NHANES from 1988 to 1994 (Clark et al. 2003), the prevalence of non-alcoholic fatty liver disease based on elevated liver enzymes was estimated to be 4.3%. A more recent study that examined the same population from NHANES found the prevalence of non-alcoholic fatty liver disease to be 19%, based on results from ultrasonography data for fatty liver estimation (Lazo et al. 2013). Thus, the detection of non-alcoholic fatty liver disease by ultrasound increases sensitivity, as many patients with hepatic steatosis have normal liver enzymes and may be overlooked. This was also demonstrated by Browning et al. (2004) in a study of 2,287 participants of the Dallas Heart Study who were evaluated for liver steatosis (fat) by proton nuclear magnetic resonance spectroscopy and found 31% to meet their criteria for diagnosis of non-alcoholic fatty liver disease. Of these patients, 79% were found to have a normal ALT level. The prevalence of non-alcoholic fatty liver disease has been reported to vary from 8% to 45% in Europe (Blachier et al. 2013; Fazel et al. 2016) and around 15% to 20% in Asia (Farrell et al. 2013).

Increasingly, the pediatric population is being identified as part of this epidemic. There have been two population-based studies in the United States addressing this issue. Strauss et al. (2000) looked at 2,450 obese adolescents between the ages of 12 and 18 years and found 3% to have abnormal ALT levels, thought to be related to non-alcoholic fatty liver disease. More recently, a report was published by Schwimmer et al. (2006) in which autopsy specimens were reviewed in 742 pediatric victims of accidental death between the ages of 2 and 19 years. They found an astounding 9.6% rate of fatty liver in these patients with a pronounced age-related distribution of hepatic steatosis ranging from 0.7% for ages two to four years to up to 17.3% for ages 15 to 19 years. The highest rate of fatty liver was seen in obese children (38%).

Non-alcoholic fatty liver disease affects persons of all ages and sexes. Among both children and adults, non-alcoholic fatty liver disease increases with age with highest occurrences in the fifth and sixth decade (Ruhl and Everhart 2004). Data from NHANES III showed that non-alcoholic fatty liver disease based on elevated ALT levels peaked in the fifth decade among men and in the sixth decade among women (Ruhl and Everhart 2003). The comparison study of the same database by Ioannou et al. (2006) had similar findings but with an unexplained striking reduction in the ALT levels of persons with further increasing age. Early descriptions of persons with non-alcoholic fatty liver disease showed a female preponderance to the condition; however, more recent studies in Japanese, Italian, and U.S. populations have consistently found men to be at increased risk (Bellentani et al. 1994; Ruhl and Everhart 2003; Shen et al. 2003).

Ethnic variation has been demonstrated repeatedly with the Hispanic population being at the highest risk of fatty liver disease and blacks being at the lowest risk when compared to non-Hispanic whites. Asians also appear to be at decreased risk. A cross-sectional study of newly diagnosed cases of non-alcoholic fatty liver disease in the Chronic Liver Disease Surveillance Study was performed. Of the 742 persons evaluated, 159 (21.4%) had definite or probable non-alcoholic fatty liver disease with the following breakdown: whites, 45%; Hispanics, 28%; Asians, 18%; African Americans, 3%; and other races, 6%. Clinical correlates of non-alcoholic fatty liver disease (obesity, hyperlipidemia, diabetes) were similar among racial and ethnic groups, except that body mass index was lower in Asians compared with other groups. Compared with the base population, Hispanics with non-alcoholic fatty liver disease were overrepresented (28% vs. 10%) and whites were underrepresented (45% vs. 59%; Weston et al. 2005). A single nucleotide polymorphism in a gene that regulates lipid metabolism in the liver (*PNPLA3*) has been recently reported to account for a majority of the ethnic variations in the prevalence of non-alcoholic fatty liver disease (Romeo et al. 2008).

These racial and ethnic differences may be attributable to true genetic differences in risk of non-alcoholic fatty liver disease or to cultural susceptibility in diet and lifestyle patterns. However, referral patterns and health care availability may influence results. The NHANES III avoids many biases that studies in certain populations may encounter. They, too, found Hispanics to have a higher prevalence of non-alcoholic fatty liver disease independent of body mass index, demographic factors, and metabolic factors, compared with non-Hispanic whites, while blacks continued to demonstrate less non-alcoholic fatty liver disease after adjustment for these factors (Ruhl and Everhart 2003; Ruhl and Everhart 2004). Non-alcoholic fatty liver disease is also more prevalent in individuals with obesity (prevalence reported greater than 75%) and those with diabetes (prevalence reported between 60% and 70%; Williams et al. 2011; Fazel et al. 2016).

Causes

Non-alcoholic fatty liver disease is associated with the metabolic syndrome with diabetes, insulin resistance, and truncal obesity being the most closely linked correlates (Hamaguchi et al. 2005; Duvnjak et al. 2007). Secondary causes of non-alcoholic fatty liver disease include medications (such as steroids and tamoxifen), viruses, surgical procedures, rapid and excessive weight loss, and total parenteral nutrition. Gholam et al. (2007) published a paper that identified non-alcoholic fatty liver disease in 89% of severely obese patients. The presence of non-alcoholic steatohepatitis and fibrosis (signifying more-advanced liver damage from non-alcoholic fatty liver disease) was significantly less at 36% and 25%, respectively. In further subgroup analysis, hyperlipidemia, particularly low high-density lipoprotein cholesterol, hyperglycemia, and insulin resistance were strongly associated with non-alcoholic fatty liver disease (Gholam et al. 2007).

Diabetes is known to be commonly linked with central obesity. Several studies have found the risk of diabetes in causing non-alcoholic fatty liver disease to be independent of the degree of obesity (Ruhl and Everhart 2003; Ogden et al. 2007). Insulin resistance itself is believed to be centrally related to the pathogenesis of non-alcoholic fatty liver disease (Neuschwander-Tetri and Caldwell 2003). Other associations with non-alcoholic fatty liver disease include sleep apnea and hypothyroidism.

Interventions

Currently there are no U.S. Food and Drug Administration–approved thera-pies for non-alcoholic fatty liver disease, although several agents are in clinical trials. The American Association for the Study of Liver Disease (AASLD 2016) guidelines recommend weight loss of 5% to 10% of body weight (through both a hypocaloric diet and exercise) as therapy for non-alcoholic fatty liver disease. In individuals with the progressive form of non-alcoholic fatty liver disease (non-alcoholic steatohepatitis) that is biopsy-proven, agents such as vitamin E and pioglitazone can be considered, although there are no long-term trials (Chalasani et al. 2012).

As described previously, the potential for advanced liver disease in the form of cirrhosis and hepatocellular carcinoma is present in those patients with non-alcoholic fatty liver disease. Determining those at increased risk for progressive damage in non-alcoholic fatty liver disease (non-alcoholic ste-atohepatitis), as opposed to those with merely benign fatty liver disease, is the principal target for much of today's research. Noninvasive markers in the determination of these two groups are also of utmost importance given the magnitude of this condition in the otherwise healthy population. As society continues the trend toward obesity, so, too, will the trend of non-alcoholic fatty liver disease continue to rise, including the diagnosis of cirrhosis and associated hepatocellular carcinoma. Thus, many relatively new and evolving issues regarding non-alcoholic fatty liver disease will continue to be of inter-est for the coming years.

HEPATOCELLULAR CARCINOMA

Liver cancer is largely a problem of the less developed regions, where 83% (50% in China alone) of the estimated 782,000 new cancer cases world-wide occurred in 2012. It is the fifth most common cancer in men (554,000 cases, 7.5% of the total) and the ninth in women (228,000 cases, 3.4%; IARC 2016).

Significance

Hepatocellular carcinoma is rapidly fatal in the majority of patients; as a con-sequence, the prevalence, incidence, and mortality rates are very similar.

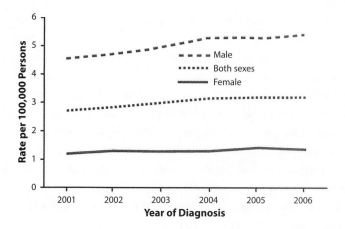

Source: Adapted from CDC (2010).
Note: Age was adjusted to the 2000 U.S. standard population. There were 48,596 cases overall.
Figure 21-10. Hepatocellular Carcinoma Incidence Rate by Sex, United States, 2001–2006

Descriptive Epidemiology

Hepatocellular carcinoma is more common in men than women worldwide. The gender disparity is noted to be more pronounced in endemic areas (2.1 to 5.7:1 male-to-female ratio) whereas intermediate- and low-incidence areas have progressively lower ratios (Bosch et al. 1999; Bosch et al. 2005). Although not fully understood, these differences are theorized to be related to variations in viral hepatitis, alcohol abuse, toxins, and the trophic effect of androgens.

The hepatocellular carcinoma incidence in the United States is low compared to that in other countries in the developing world. However, there has been an increase in the incidence over the past few decades, from 1.4 per 100,000 in 1976 to 1980 to 3.2 per 100,000 in 2006 (CDC 2010) and estimates show a continued increase (Figure 21-10).

Men are more likely to develop hepatocellular carcinoma than women in all parts of the world (two to five times more frequent in men; Jemal et al. 2011). In the United States, the incidence is highest in Asians (11 per 100,000) followed by white Hispanics (6.8 per 100,000), and then non-Hispanic whites (2.6 per 100,000; Wong and Corley 2008). In another study, the incidence rates in Asians were 7.8 per 100,000; in blacks they were 4.2 per 100,000; and in whites they were 2.6 per 100,000 (CDC 2010). Parallel to these increases in incidence, there has been a 43% increase in mortality from primary liver cancers (El-Serag 2012).

Geographic distributions are associated with significant variety among the incidence rates of this cancer, even showing variation between ethnicities and regions within the same country. The age-adjusted incidence rates for hepatocellular carcinoma in developed versus developing countries is 8.7 for males and 2.9 for females per 100,000 compared to 17.4 for males and 6.8 for females per 100,000, respectively (IARC 2016; Bosch et al. 2005). Some Asian and African regions have extraordinarily high rates, such as Mongolia (99 per 100,000) and The Gambia (39.6 per 100,000). In Australia, Europe, and the Americas, the rates are far less than 10 per 100,000 and with much less regional variability (Bosch et al. 2005).

Causes

The vast majority of hepatocellular carcinoma occurs in the setting of chronic liver disease and cirrhosis. Overall, 75% to 80% of hepatocellular carcinoma can be related to persistent viral infections with either hepatitis B virus (50% to 55%) or hepatitis C virus (25% to 30%), which is further supported by the strong geographical correlation between the incidence of hepatocellular carcinoma and known prevalence of these viral infections. The risk associated with hepatitis B appears to be more profound in endemic regions where transmission often occurs vertically (at childbirth) and, consequently, longer duration of infection is seen. In areas such as the United States, where most hepatitis B virus transmission occurs later in life by sexual transmission, the risk of hepatocellular carcinoma is much less (Sandler et al. 1983).

The risk of hepatitis C–related liver disease leading to hepatocellular carcinoma is high in the United States because of the maturing of the hepatitis C epidemic of the 1970s and 1980s leading to increased rates of hepatitis C–related cirrhosis at the current time. Any condition that can lead to cirrhosis is considered a risk for hepatocellular carcinoma. Alcohol either alone or in combination with viral hepatitis leading to cirrhosis is a risk, although it is unclear whether alcohol is itself carcinogenic in addition to increasing the risk of cirrhosis. Iron overload, autoimmune diseases, and non-alcoholic steatohepatitis are known to lead to hepatocellular carcinoma in individuals at the stage of cirrhosis. More rare and debated causes would include aflatoxin exposure in parts of Africa, a mycotoxin that may contaminate the diet; betel nut chewing, which is widespread in Asia; and tobacco use, which has been demonstrated in some studies to be a risk factor (Kuper et al. 2000).

Interventions

Protective measures include the prevention and treatment of diseases that cause cirrhosis with the goal to delay or avoid the development of cirrhosis. Recent observational studies have also suggested that coffee may be protective, and a meta-analysis performed by Larsson and Wolk (2007) showed a 43% reduction of liver cancers occurred possibly because of coffee's antioxidant properties. Association of hepatocellular carcinoma with red meat and saturated fat has been reported in epidemiologic studies (Freedman et al. 2010) and a reduced risk with consumption of fish, white meat, and vegetables (Sawada et al. 2012; Bamai et al. 2015). A remarkable decrease in hepatitis B virus infections has occurred with the introduction of the universal childhood vaccine in 1984, and the expectation is that there will be a long-term effect on the hepatocellular carcinoma rates (Chang et al. 1997). Results from Taiwan have shown that hepatocellular carcinoma incidence rate in children aged 6 to 14 years old fell from 0.52–0.54 to 0.13–0.20 per 100,000 (relative risk [RR] = 0.25–0.36; Chang 2009).

Recent advances in treatment options have brought a new perspective to this condition traditionally considered a terminal illness with very poor outcomes, few treatment options, and a life expectancy of six months or less. Such advances include surgical resection, local ablation with alcohol, radiofrequency, chemoembolization, and liver transplantation (Bruix et al. 2001). Recent studies have shown hepatocellular carcinoma to be the leading cause of mortality from cirrhosis, as opposed to liver failure or non-malignant liver-related conditions (Benvegnu et al. 2004). In response, health care providers have developed surveillance and treatment protocols that have dramatically improved survival in those patients diagnosed in the early stages of hepatocellular carcinoma (Sangiovanni et al. 2004; Bruix and Sherman 2005). Prevention of chronic liver disease, such as with hepatitis B vaccination and reducing alcoholism and transmission of hepatitis C virus, is still the most cost-effective way to deal with hepatocellular carcinoma.

HEMOCHROMATOSIS

Other causes of chronic liver disease include genetic conditions such as metabolic liver disease (increased iron deposition in the liver and organs known as hemochromatosis; copper accumulation in the liver in Wilson's disease), cholestatic disorders (primary biliary cirrhosis, primary sclerosing cholangitis), autoimmune disorders, and drug-related liver disease (Schiff et al.1999). Hereditary hemochromatosis is an autosomal recessive disorder with a prevalence of 1 in 200 to 1 in 250 in white populations in the United States and Europe. The most common genetic mutation is the *C282Y* mutation, which results in excessive absorption of iron from the gut (Steinberg et al. 2001).

Significance

Organ iron overload in time can lead to cirrhosis, heart failure, diabetes, and hypogonadism. Organ damage is delayed in women compared to men because of menstrual iron loss (Adams 2006).

Descriptive Epidemiology

Despite the presence of the mutation for hemochromatosis, the penetrance is variable. In a large study in California that used data from the Kaiser Permanente health clinic of 41,038 individuals, 152 were homozygous for the *C282Y* mutation. Of these 152, only one had clinically evident disease (Beutler et al. 2002).

The yield of severe liver disease was similarly low in the Hemochromatosis and Iron Overload Screening Study, which screened 101,168 primary care participants for iron overload (Adams et al. 2005). Three hundred thirty-three *C282Y* homozygotes were detected; 75 had been previously diagnosed. Of the 302 *C282Y* homozygotes that underwent additional testing, 16% and 12% had increased levels of ALT and AST, respectively, compared to 11% and 8%, respectively, in controls. Of the 11 centrally reviewed liver biopsies, all showed increased liver iron concentrations, but only two had stage 3 or 4 fibrosis.

Interventions

On the basis of these large population studies, the U.S. Preventive Services Task Force recommended against the use of routine genetic screening for hereditary hemochromatosis in the asymptomatic general population (Whitlock et al. 2006). Screening of family members of an individual with hemochromatosis is effective because of higher pretest probability. It should be performed with genetic testing if the proband is available.

References

Adams LA, Lymp JF, St Sauver J, et al. The natural history of nonalcoholic fatty liver disease: a population-based cohort study. *Gastroenterology*. 2005;129(1):113–121.

Adams PC. Review article: the modern diagnosis and management of haemochromatosis. *Aliment Pharmacol Ther*. 2006;23(12):1681–1691.

Adams PC, Reboussin DM, Barton JC, et al. Hemochromatosis and iron-overload screening in a racially diverse population. *N Engl J Med*. 2005;352(17):1769–1778.

Advisory Committee on Immunization Practices (ACIP), Fiore AE, Wasley A, Bell BP. Prevention of hepatitis A through active or passive immunization: recommendations of the Advisory Committee on Immunization Practices. *MMWR Recomm Rep*. 2006;55(RR-7):1–23.

Alexander JF, Lischner MW, Galambos JT. Natural history of alcoholic hepatitis. II. The long-term prognosis. *Am J Gastroenterol*. 1971;56(6):515–525.

Alter HJ, Purcell RH, Shih JW, et al. Detection of antibody to hepatitis C virus in prospectively followed transfusion recipients with acute and chronic non-A, non-B hepatitis. *N Engl J Med*. 1989;321(22):1494–1500.

Alter MJ. Epidemiology of hepatitis C. *Hepatology*. 1997;26(3 suppl 1):62S–65S.

American Association for the Study of Liver Diseases (AASLD) Guidelines. HCV guidance: recommendations for testing, managing and treating hepatitis C. 2016. Available at: http://hcvguidelines.org. Accessed September 3, 2016.

Alter MJ, Hadler SC, Margolis HS, et al. The changing epidemiology of hepatitis B in the United States. Need for alternative vaccination strategies. *JAMA*. 1990;263(9):1218–1222.

Alter MJ, Kruszon-Moran D, Nainan OV, et al. The prevalence of hepatitis C virus infection in the United States, 1988 through 1994. *N Engl J Med*. 1999;341(8):556–562.

Alter MJ, Mast EE. The epidemiology of viral hepatitis in the United States. *Gastroenterol Clin North Am*. 1994;23(3):437–455.

Andrieux-Meyer I, Cohn J, de Araujo ES, Hamid SS. Disparity in market prices for hepatitis C virus direct-acting drugs. *Lancet Glob Health*. 2015;3(11):e676.

Armstrong GL, Alter MJ, McQuillan GM, Margolis HS. The past incidence of hepatitis C virus infection: implications for the future burden of chronic liver disease in the United States. *Hepatology*. 2000;31(3):777–782.

Bamai C, Lagiou P, Jenab M, et al. Fruit and vegetable consumption in relation to hepatocellular carcinoma in a multi-centre, European cohort study. *Br J Cancer*. 2015;112(7): 1273–1282.

Beasley RP, Hwang LY, Lin CC, et al. Incidence of hepatitis B virus infections in preschool children in Taiwan. *J Infect Dis*. 1982;146(2):198–204.

Bell BP, Manos NV, Murphy RC, et al. The epidemiology of newly-diagnosed chronic liver disease in the United States: findings of population-based sentinel surveillance. *Hepatology*. 2001;34(pt 2):468A.

Bellentani S, Saccoccio G, Costa G, et al. Drinking habits as cofactors of risk for alcohol induced liver damage. The Dionysos Study Group. *Gut*. 1997;41(6):845–850.

Bellentani S, Tiribelli C, Saccoccio G, et al. Prevalence of chronic liver disease in the general population of northern Italy: the Dionysos Study. *Hepatology*. 1994;20(6):1442–1449.

Benvegnu L, Gios M, Boccato S, Alberti A. Natural history of compensated viral cirrhosis: a prospective study on the incidence and hierarchy of major complications. *Gut*. 2004;53(5):744–749.

Beutler E, Felitti VJ, Koziol JA, Ho NJ, Gelbart T. Penetrance of 845G--> A (C282Y) HFE hereditary haemochromatosis mutation in the USA. *Lancet*. 2002;359(9302):211–218.

Blachier M, Leleu H, Peck-Radosavljevic M, Valla DC, Roudot-Thoraval F. The burden of liver disease in Europe: a review of available epidemiological data. *J Hepatol*. 2013;58(3):593–608.

Blume SB. Women and alcohol. A review. *JAMA*. 1986;256(11):1467–1470.

Bode C, Bode JC, Erhardt JG, French BA, French SW. Effect of the type of beverage and meat consumed by alcoholics with alcoholic liver disease. *Alcohol Clin Exp Res*. 1998;22(8):1803–1805.

Bosch FX, Ribes J, Borràs J. Epidemiology of primary liver cancer. *Semin Liver Dis*. 1999;19(3):271–285.

Bosch FX, Ribes J, Cléries R, Díaz M. Epidemiology of hepatocellular carcinoma. *Clin Liver Dis*. 2005;9(2):191–211, v.

Briggs ME, Baker C, Hall R, et al. Prevalence and risk factors for hepatitis C virus infection at an urban Veterans Administration medical center. *Hepatology*. 2001;34(6): 1200–1205.

Browning JD, Szczepaniak LS, Dobbins R, et al. Prevalence of hepatic steatosis in an urban population in the United States: impact of ethnicity. *Hepatology*. 2004;40(6): 1387–1395.

Bruix J, Sherman M. Management of hepatocellular carcinoma. *Hepatology.* 2005;42(5): 1208–1236.

Bruix J, Sherman M, Llovet JM, et al. Clinical management of hepatocellular carcinoma. Conclusions of the Barcelona-2000 EASL conference. European Association for the Study of the Liver. *J Hepatol.* 2001;35(3):421–430.

Brundage SC, Fitzpatrick AN. Hepatitis A. *Am Fam Physician.* 2006;73(12):2162–2168.

Caetano R, Kaskutas LA. Changes in drinking patterns among whites, blacks and Hispanics, 1984–1992. *J Stud Alcohol.* 1995;56(5):558–565.

Centers for Disease Control and Prevention (CDC). Recommendations for preventing transmission of infections among chronic hemodialysis patients. *MMWR Recomm Rep.* 2001;50(RR-05):1–43.

Centers for Disease Control and Prevention (CDC), Jajosky RA, Hall PA, et al. Summary of notifiable diseases—United States, 2004. *MMWR Morb Mortal Wkly Rep.* 2006;53(53):1–79.

Centers for Disease Control and Prevention (CDC). Hepatocellular carcinoma—United States 2001–2006. 2010. Available at: http://www.cdc.gov/mmwr/preview/mmwrhtml/mm5917a3.htm. Accessed September 3, 2016.

Centers for Disease Control and Prevention (CDC). Viral hepatitis—statistics and surveillance. 2016a. Available at: http://www.cdc.gov/hepatitis/statistics/index.htm. Accessed September 3, 2016.

Centers for Disease Control and Prevention (CDC). Wide-ranging Online Data for Epidemiologic Research (WONDER). 2016b. Available at: http://wonder.cdc.gov. Accessed September 3, 2016.

Chalasani N, Younossi Z, Lavine J, et al. The diagnosis and management of nonalcoholic fatty liver disease: practice guideline by the American Association for the Study of Liver Diseases, American College of Gastroenterology, and the American Gastroenterological Association. *Hepatology.* 2012;55(6):2005–2023.

Chang MH. Cancer prevention by vaccination against hepatitis B. *Recent Results Cancer Res.* 2009;181:85–94.

Chang MH, Chen CJ, Lai MS, et al. Universal hepatitis B vaccination in Taiwan and the incidence of hepatocellular carcinoma in children. Taiwan Childhood Hepatoma Study Group. *N Engl J Med.* 1997;336(26):1855–1859.

Charlton MR, Burns JM, Pedersen RA, Watt KD, Heimbach JK, Dierkhising RA. Frequency and outcomes of liver transplantation for nonalcoholic steatohepatitis in the United States. *Gastroenterology.* 2011;141(4):1249–1253.

Chen CJ, Yang HI, Su J, et al. Risk of hepatocellular carcinoma across a biological gradient of serum hepatitis B virus DNA level. *JAMA*. 2006;295(1):65–73.

Cheung RC, Hanson AK, Maganti K, Keeffe EB, Matsui SM. Viral hepatitis and other infectious diseases in a homeless population. *J Clin Gastroenterol*. 2002;34(4):476–480.

Chiung M, Chen H-Y. Trends in alcohol related morbidity among short-stay community hospital discharges, United States, 1979–2005. Bethesda, MD: National Institute on Alcohol Abuse and Alcoholism; 2007. NIAAA Surveillance Report no. 80.

Chiung M, Chen H-Y. Trends in alcohol-related morbidity among community hospital discharges, United States, 2000–2012. Bethesda, MD: National Institute on Alcohol Abuse and Alcoholism; 2013. NIAAA Surveillance Report no. 99.

Choo QL, Kuo G, Weiner AJ, Overby LR, Bradley DW, Houghton M. Isolation of a cDNA clone derived from a blood-borne non-A, non-B viral hepatitis genome. *Science*. 1989;244(4902):359–362.

Clark JM, Brancati FL, Diehl AM. The prevalence and etiology of elevated aminotransferase levels in the United States. *Am J Gastroenterol*. 2003;98(5):960–967.

Corrao G, Arico S. Independent and combined action of hepatitis C virus infection and alcohol consumption on the risk of symptomatic liver cirrhosis. *Hepatology*. 1998;27(4):914–919.

Corrao G, Arico S, Zambon A, et al. Is alcohol a risk factor for liver cirrhosis in HBsAg and anti-HCV negative subjects? Collaborative Groups for the Study of Liver Diseases in Italy. *J Hepatol*. 1997;27(3):470–476.

D'Amico G, Morabito A, Pagliaro L, Marubini E. Survival and prognostic indicators in compensated and decompensated cirrhosis. *Dig Dis Sci*. 1986;31(5):468–475.

Davis GL, Albright JE, Cook SF, Rosenberg DM. Projecting future complications of chronic hepatitis C in the United States. *Liver Transpl*. 2003;9(4):331–338.

Day CP. Who gets alcoholic liver disease: nature or nurture? *J R Coll Physicians Lond*. 2000;34(6):557–562.

Debakey SF, Stinson FS, Grant BF, et al. *Liver Cirrhosis Mortality in the United States, 1970–92*. Bethesda, MD: National Institute on Alcohol Abuse and Alcoholism; 1995. Surveillance Report no. 37.

Degos F. Hepatitis C and alcohol. *J Hepatol*. 1999;31(suppl 1):113–118.

Dentinger CM, Bower WA, Nainan OV, et al. An outbreak of hepatitis A associated with green onions. *J Infect Dis*. 2001;183(8):1273–1276.

Diehl AM. Alcoholic liver disease: natural history. *Liver Transpl Surg*. 1997;3(3):206–211.

Donato F, Tagger A, Chiesa R, et al. Hepatitis B and C virus infection, alcohol drinking, and hepatocellular carcinoma: a case–control study in Italy. Brescia HCC Study. *Hepatology.* 1997;26(3):579–584.

Dunn W, Sanyal AJ, Brunt EM, et al. Modest alcohol consumption is associated with decreased prevalence of steatohepatitis in patients with nonalcoholic fatty liver disease (NAFLD). *J Hepatol.* 2012;57(2):384–391.

Duvnjak M, Lerotic I, Barsić N, Tomasić V, Virović Jukić L, Velagić V. Pathogenesis and management issues for non-alcoholic fatty liver disease. *World J Gastroenterol.* 2007;13(34):4539–4550.

Edlin BR, Eckhardt BJ, Shu MA, Holmberg SD, Swan T. Toward a more accurate estimate of the prevalence of hepatitis C in the United States. *Hepatology.* 2015;62(5):1353–1363.

El-Serag HB. Epidemiology of viral hepatitis and hepatocellular carcinoma. *Gastroenterology.* 2012;142(6):1264–1273.

Everhart JE. Viral hepatitis. In: Everhart JE, ed. *Burden of Digestive Diseases in the United States.* Washington, DC: US Government Printing Office; 2009:13–23.

Farrell GC, Wong WV, Chitturi S. NAFLD in ASIA—as common and important as in the West. *Nat Rev Gastroenterol Hepatol.* 2013;10(5):307–318.

Fattovich G, Brollo L, Giustina G, et al. Natural history and prognostic factors for chronic hepatitis type B. *Gut.* 1991;32(3):294–298.

Fazel Y, Koeing AB, Sayiner M, Goodman ZD, Younossi ZM. Epidemiology and natural history of non-alcoholic fatty liver disease. *Metabolism.* 2016;65(8):1017–1025.

Finelli L, Miller JT, Tokars JI, Alter MJ, Arduino MJ. National surveillance of dialysis-associated diseases in the United States, 2002. *Semin Dial.* 2005;18(1): 52–61.

Fisher NC, Hanson J, Phillips A, Rao JN, Swarbrick ET. Mortality from liver disease in the West Midlands, 1993–2000: observational study. *BMJ.* 2002;325(7359):312–313.

Freedman ND, Cross AJ, McGlynn KA, et al. Association of meat and fat intake with liver disease and hepatocellular carcinoma in the NIH-AARP cohort. *J Natl Cancer Inst.* 2010;102(17):1354–1365.

Freeman AJ, Dore GJ, Law MG, et al. Estimating progression to cirrhosis in chronic hepatitis C virus infection. *Hepatology.* 2001;34(4 pt 1):809–816.

Frezza M, di Padova C, Pozzato G, Terpin M, Baraona E, Lieber CS. High blood alcohol levels in women. The role of decreased gastric alcohol dehydrogenase activity and first-pass metabolism. *N Engl J Med.* 1990;322(2):95–99.

Fried MW, Shiffman ML, Reddy KR, et al. Peginterferon alfa-2a plus ribavirin for chronic hepatitis C virus infection. *N Engl J Med*. 2002;347(13):975–982.

Galbraith JW, Donnelly JP, Franco RA, Overton ET, Rodgers JB, Wang HE. National estimates of healthcare utilization by individuals with hepatitis C virus infection in the United States. *Clin Infect Dis*. 2014;59(6):755–764.

Garfein RS, Vlahov D, Galai N, Doherty MC, Nelson KE. Viral infections in short-term injection drug users: the prevalence of the hepatitis C, hepatitis B, human immunodeficiency, and human T-lymphotropic viruses. *Am J Public Health*. 1996;86(5):655–661.

Geerlings W, Tufveson G, Ehrich JH, et al. Report on management of renal failure in Europe, XXIII. *Nephrol Dial Transplant*. 1994;9(suppl 1):6–25.

Gholam PM, Flancbaum L, Machan JT, Charney DA, Kotler DP. Nonalcoholic fatty liver disease in severely obese subjects. *Am J Gastroenterol*. 2007;102(2):399–408.

Hamaguchi M, Kojima T, Takeda N, et al. The metabolic syndrome as a predictor of nonalcoholic fatty liver disease. *Ann Intern Med*. 2005;143(10):722–728.

Hasumura Y, Takeuchi J. Alcoholic liver disease in Japanese patients: a comparison with Caucasians. *J Gastroenterol Hepatol*. 1991;6(5):520–527.

Holder HD, Parker RN. Effect of alcoholism treatment on cirrhosis mortality: a 20-year multivariate time series analysis. *Br J Addict*. 1992;87(9):1263–1274.

Hourigan LF, Macdonald GA, Purdie D, et al. Fibrosis in chronic hepatitis C correlates significantly with body mass index and steatosis. *Hepatology*. 1999;29(4):1215–1219.

Hussain KB, Fontana RJ, Moyer CA, Su GL, Sneed-Pee N, Lok AS. Comorbid illness is an important determinant of health-related quality of life in patients with chronic hepatitis C. *Am J Gastroenterol*. 2001;96(9):2737–2744.

Ikejima K, Enomoto N, Iimuro Y, et al. Estrogen increases sensitivity of hepatic Kupffer cells to endotoxin. *Am J Physiol*. 1998;274(4 pt 1):G669–G676.

Immunization Practices Advisory Committee. Hepatitis B virus: a comprehensive strategy for eliminating transmission in the United States through universal childhood vaccination. Recommendations of the Immunization Practices Advisory Committee. *MMWR Recomm Rep*. 1991;40(RR–13):1–25.

International Agency for Research on Cancer (IARC). Liver cancer: estimated incidence, mortality and prevalence worldwide in 2012. 2016. Available at: http://globocan.iarc.fr/old/FactSheets/cancers/liver-new.asp. Accessed September 3, 2016.

Ioannou GN, Boyko EJ, Lee SP. The prevalence and predictors of elevated serum aminotransferase activity in the United States in 1999–2002. *Am J Gastroenterol*. 2006;101(1):76–82.

Jacobsen KH, Koopman JS. Declining hepatitis A seroprevalence: a global review and analysis. *Epidemiol Infect.* 2004;132(6):1005–1022.

Jemal A, Bray F, Center MM, Ferlay J, Ward E, Forman D. Global cancer statistics; CA. *Cancer J Clin.* 2011;61(2):69–90.

Kerr WC, Fillmore KM, Marvy P. Beverage-specific alcohol consumption and cirrhosis mortality in a group of English-speaking beer-drinking countries. *Addiction.* 2000;95(3):339–346.

Kim WR. The epidemiology of hepatitis B in the United States. *Hepatology.* 2009; 49(5 suppl):S28–S34.

Kim WR, Brown RS, Terrault NA, El-Serag H. Burden of liver disease in the United States: summary of a workshop. *Hepatology.* 2002;36(1):227–242.

Kim Y, Ejaz A, Tayal A, et al. Temporal trends in population-based death rates associated with chronic liver disease and liver cancer in the United States over the last 30 years. *Cancer.* 2014;120(19):3058–3065.

Klevens RM, Liu SJ, Roberts H, Jiles RB, Holmberg SD. Estimating acute viral hepatitis infections from nationally reported cases. *Am J Public Health.* 2014;104(3):482–487.

Koff RS. Clinical manifestations and diagnosis of hepatitis A virus infection. *Vaccine.* 1992;10(suppl 1):S15–S17.

Kuo G, Choo QL, Alter HJ, et al. An assay for circulating antibodies to a major etiologic virus of human non-A, non-B hepatitis. *Science.* 1989;244(4902):362–364.

Kuper H, Tzonou A, Kaklamani E, et al. Tobacco smoking, alcohol consumption and their interaction in the causation of hepatocellular carcinoma. *Int J Cancer.* 2000;85(4): 498–502.

Lai CL, Wong BC, Yeoh EK, Lim WL, Chang WK, Lin HJ. Five-year follow-up of a prospective randomized trial of hepatitis B recombinant DNA yeast vaccine vs. plasma-derived vaccine in children: immunogenicity and anamnestic responses. *Hepatology.* 1993;18(4):763–767.

Larsson SC, Wolk A. Coffee consumption and risk of liver cancer: a meta-analysis. *Gastroenterology.* 2007;132(5):1740–1745.

Lazo M, Hernaez R, Eberhardt MS, et al. Prevalence of nonalcoholic fatty liver disease in the United States: the Third National Health and Nutrition Examination Survey, 1988–1994. *Am J Epidemiol.* 2013;178(1):38–45.

Leandro G, Mangia A, Hui J, et al. Relationship between steatosis, inflammation, and fibrosis in chronic hepatitis C: a meta-analysis of individual patient data. *Gastroenterology.* 2006;130(6):1636–1642.

Lelbach WK. Cirrhosis in the alcoholic and its relation to the volume of alcohol abuse. *Ann N Y Acad Sci.* 1975;252:85–105.

Liaw YF, Tsai SL, Sheen IS, et al. Clinical and virological course of chronic hepatitis B virus infection with hepatitis C and D virus markers. *Am J Gastroenterol.* 1998;93(3):354–359.

Loguercio C, Di Pierro M, Di Marino MP, et al. Drinking habits of subjects with hepatitis C virus-related chronic liver disease: prevalence and effect on clinical, virological and pathological aspects. *Alcohol Alcohol.* 2000;35(3):296–301.

Mandayam S, Jamal MM, Morgan TR. Epidemiology of alcoholic liver disease. *Semin Liver Dis.* 2004;24(3):217–232.

Mann RE, Smart RG, Anglin L, Adlaf EM. Reductions in cirrhosis deaths in the United States: associations with per capita consumption and AA membership. *J Stud Alcohol.* 1991;52(4):361–365.

Manns MP, McHutchison JG, Gordon SC, et al. Peginterferon alfa-2b plus ribavirin compared with interferon alfa-2b plus ribavirin for initial treatment of chronic hepatitis C: a randomised trial. *Lancet.* 2001;358(9286):958–965.

Marchesini G, Bugianesi E, Forlani G, et al. Nonalcoholic fatty liver, steatohepatitis, and the metabolic syndrome. *Hepatology.* 2003;37(4):917–923.

Mast EE, Margolis HS, Fiore AE, et al. A comprehensive immunization strategy to eliminate transmission of hepatitis B virus infection in the United States: recommendations of the Advisory Committee on Immunization Practices (ACIP). Part 1: immunization of infants, children, and adolescents. *MMWR Recomm Rep.* 2005;54(RR–16):1–31.

Mast EE, Weinbaum CM, Fiore AE, et al. A comprehensive immunization strategy to eliminate transmission of hepatitis B virus infection in the United States: recommendations of the Advisory Committee on Immunization Practices (ACIP) Part II: immunization of adults. *MMWR Recomm Rep.* 2006;55(RR–16):CE1–CE4.

Maynard JE. Hepatitis B: global importance and need for control. *Vaccine.* 1990; 8(suppl):S18–S20.

Mbithi JN, Springthorpe VS, Boulet JR, Sattar SA. Survival of hepatitis A virus on human hands and its transfer on contact with animate and inanimate surfaces. *J Clin Microbiol.* 1992;30(4):757–763.

Miller ME, Everhart JE, Hoofnagle JH. Epidemiologic research and the action plan for liver disease research. *Ann Epidemiol.* 2006;16(11):861–865.

Murphy EL, Bryzman SM, Glynn SA, et al. Risk factors for hepatitis C virus infection in United States blood donors. NHLBI Retrovirus Epidemiology Donor Study (REDS). *Hepatology.* 2000;31(3):756–762.

Murphy TV, Denniston MM, Hill HA, et al. Progress toward eliminating Hepatitis A Disease in the United States. Centers for Disease Control and Prevention. *MMWR Suppl.* 2016;65(1);29–41.

Nanji AA, French SW. Relationship between pork consumption and cirrhosis. *Lancet.* 1985;1(8430):681–683.

Naveau S, Giraud V, Borotto E, et al. Excess weight risk factor for alcoholic liver disease. *Hepatology.* 1997;25(1):108–111.

Neff GW, Duncan CW, Schiff ER. The current economic burden of cirrhosis. *Gastroenterol Hepatol (N Y).* 2011;7(10):661–671.

Neuschwander-Tetri BA, Caldwell SH. Nonalcoholic steatohepatitis: summary of an AASLD Single Topic Conference. *Hepatology.* 2003;37(5):1202–1219.

Ni YH, Huang LM, Chang MH, et al. Two decades of universal hepatitis B vaccination in Taiwan: impact and implication for future strategies. *Gastroenterology.* 2007;132(4):1287–1293.

Ogden CL, Yanovski SZ, Carroll MD, Flegal KM. The epidemiology of obesity. *Gastroenterology.* 2007;132(6):2087–2102.

Ostapowicz G, Watson KJ, Locarnini SA, Desmond PV. Role of alcohol in the progression of liver disease caused by hepatitis C virus infection. *Hepatology.* 1998;27(6):1730–1735.

Park SC, Oh SI, Lee MS. Korean status of alcoholics and alcohol-related health problems. *Alcohol Clin Exp Res.* 1998;22(3 suppl):170S–172S.

Parlesak A, Schafer C, Schütz T, Bode JC, Bode C. Increased intestinal permeability to macromolecules and endotoxemia in patients with chronic alcohol abuse in different stages of alcohol-induced liver disease. *J Hepatol.* 2000;32(5):742–747.

Pereira BJ, Milford EL, Kirkman RL, Levey AS. Transmission of hepatitis C virus by organ transplantation. *N Engl J Med.* 1991;325(7):454–460.

Pomper GJ, Wu Y, Snyder EL. Risks of transfusion-transmitted infections: 2003. *Curr Opin Hematol.* 2003;10(6):412–418.

Poynard T, Bedossa P, Opolon P. Natural history of liver fibrosis progression in patients with chronic hepatitis C. The OBSVIRC, METAVIR, CLINIVIR, and DOSVIRC groups. *Lancet.* 1997;349(9055):825–832.

Ramstedt M. Per capita alcohol consumption and liver cirrhosis mortality in 14 European countries. *Addiction.* 2001;96(suppl 1):S19–S33.

Raynard B, Balian A, Fallik D, et al. Risk factors of fibrosis in alcohol-induced liver disease. *Hepatology.* 2012;35(3):635–638.

Rodger AJ, Jolley D, Thompson SC, Lanigan A, Crofts N. The impact of diagnosis of hepatitis C virus on quality of life. *Hepatology.* 1999;30(5):1299–1301.

Romeo S, Kozlitine J, Xing C, et al. Genetic variation in *PNPLA3* confers susceptibility to nonalcoholic fatty liver disease. *Nat Genet.* 2008;40(12):1461–1465.

Ruhl CE, Everhart JE. Determinants of the association of overweight with elevated serum alanine aminotransferase activity in the United States. *Gastroenterology.* 2003;124(1):71–79.

Ruhl CE, Everhart JE. Epidemiology of nonalcoholic fatty liver. *Clin Liver Dis.* 2004; 8(3):501–19,vii.

Ruhl CE, Everhart JE. Coffee and tea consumption are associated with a lower incidence of chronic liver disease in the United States. *Gastroenterology.* 2005;129(6):1928–1936.

Ruiz JD, Molitor F, Sun RK, et al. Prevalence and correlates of hepatitis C virus infection among inmates entering the California correctional system. *West J Med.* 1999;170(3):156–160.

Saadatmand F, Grant BF, Dufour M. Surveillance Report no. 54. Liver cirrhosis mortality in the United States, 1970–1997. Bethesda, MD: National Institute on Alcohol Abuse and Alcoholism; 2000.

Said A, Wells J. Chronic liver disease. In: Remington PL, Brownson RC, Wegner MV, eds. *Chronic Disease Epidemiology and Control.* Washington, DC: American Public Health Association; 2010:594.

Sandler RS, Everhart JE, Donowitz M, et al. The burden of selected digestive diseases in the United States. *Gastroenterology.* 2002;122(5):1500–1511.

Sandler DP, Sandler RS, Horney LF. Primary liver cancer mortality in the United States. *J Chronic Dis.* 1983;36(3):227–236.

Sangiovanni A, Del Ninno E, Fasani P, et al. Increased survival of cirrhotic patients with a hepatocellular carcinoma detected during surveillance. *Gastroenterology.* 2004;126(4):1005–1014.

Sato N, Lindros KO, Baraona E, et al. Sex difference in alcohol-related organ injury. *Alcohol Clin Exp Res.* 2001;25(5 suppl ISBRA):40S–45S.

Sawada N, Inoeu M, Iwasaki M, et al. Consumption of n-3 fatty acids and fish reduces risk of hepatocellular carcinoma. *Gastroenterology.* 2012;142(7):1468–1475.

Schiff ER, Sorrell MF, Maddrey WC. *Schiff's Diseases of the Liver.* Philadelphia, PA; New York, NY: Lippincott-Raven; 1999.

Schiff ER, Maddrey WC. *Schiff's Diseases of the Liver.* 11th ed. Oxford, UK: Wiley-Blackwell; 2011.

Schreiber GB, Busch MP, Kleinman SH, Korelitz JJ. The risk of transfusion-transmitted viral infections. The Retrovirus Epidemiology Donor Study. *N Engl J Med.* 1996;334(26):1685–1690.

Schwimmer JB, Deutsch R, Kahen T, Lavine JE, Stanley C, Behling C. Prevalence of fatty liver in children and adolescents. *Pediatrics.* 2006;118(4):1388–1393.

Shen L, Fan JG, Shao Y, et al. Prevalence of nonalcoholic fatty liver among administrative officers in Shanghai: an epidemiological survey. *World J Gastroenterol.* 2003;9(5): 1106–1110.

Shepard CW, Finelli L, Alter MJ. Global epidemiology of hepatitis C virus infection. *Lancet Infect Dis.* 2005;5(9):558–567.

Singh GK, Hoyert DL. Social epidemiology of chronic liver disease and cirrhosis mortality in the United States, 1935–1997: trends and differentials by ethnicity, socioeconomic status, and alcohol consumption. *Hum Biol.* 2000;72(5):801–820.

Smart RG, Mann RE. Recent liver cirrhosis declines: estimates of the impact of alcohol abuse treatment and Alcoholics Anonymous. *Addiction.* 1993;88(2):193–198.

Sorensen TI, Orholm M, Bentsen KD, Høybye G, Eghøje K, Christoffersen P. Prospective evaluation of alcohol abuse and alcoholic liver injury in men as predictors of development of cirrhosis. *Lancet.* 1984;2(8397):241–244.

Steinberg KK, Cogswell ME, Chang JC, et al. Prevalence of C282Y and H63D mutations in the hemochromatosis (HFE) gene in the United States. *JAMA.* 2001;285(17):2216–2222.

Stevens CE, Beasley RP, Tsui J, Lee WC. Vertical transmission of hepatitis B antigen in Taiwan. *N Engl J Med.* 1975;292(15):771–774.

Stinson FS, Grant BF, Dufour MC. The critical dimension of ethnicity in liver cirrhosis mortality statistics. *Alcohol Clin Exp Res.* 2001;25(8):1181–1187.

Strauss RS, Barlow SE, Dietz WH. Prevalence of abnormal serum aminotransferase values in overweight and obese adolescents. *J Pediatr.* 2000;136(6):727–733.

Tang YW, Wang JX, Xu ZY, Guo YF, Qian WH, Xu JX. A serologically confirmed, case–control study, of a large outbreak of hepatitis A in China, associated with consumption of clams. *Epidemiol Infect.* 1991;107(3):651–657.

Tassopoulos NC, Papaevangelou GJ, Sjogren MH, Roumeliotou-Karayannis A, Gerin JL, Purcell RH. Natural history of acute hepatitis B surface antigen–positive hepatitis in Greek adults. *Gastroenterology.* 1987;92(6):1844–1850.

Terrault N, Bzowej NH, Chang K-M, Hwang JP, Jonas M, Murad MH. AASLD guidelines for treatment of chronic hepatitis B. *Hepatology.* 2016;63(1):261–283.

Terris M. Epidemiology of cirrhosis of the liver: national mortality data. *Am J Public Health Nations Health.* 1967;57(12):2076–2088.

Thaler H. Alcohol consumption and diseases of the liver. *Nutr Metab.* 1977;21(1–3): 196–193.

Tong MJ, El-Farra NS, Grew MI. Clinical manifestations of hepatitis A: recent experience in a community teaching hospital. *J Infect Dis.* 1995;171(suppl 1):S15–S18.

United Network for Organ Sharing (UNOS). 2016. Available at: https://www.unos.org. Accessed September 9, 2016.

Vachon M-L, Dieterich DT. The era of direct-acting antivirals for HCV has begun: the beginning of the end for HCV? *Semin Liver Dis.* 2011;31(4):399–340.

Vento S, Garofano T, Renzini C, et al. Fulminant hepatitis associated with hepatitis A virus superinfection in patients with chronic hepatitis C. *N Engl J Med.* 1998;338(5):286–290.

Wasley A, Fiore A, Bell BP. Hepatitis A in the era of vaccination. *Epidemiol Rev.* 2006;28:101–111.

Wasley A, Kruszon-Moran D, Kuhnert W, et al. The prevalence of hepatitis B virus infection in the United States in the era of vaccination. *J Infect Dis.* 2010;202(2):192–201.

Wasley A, Miller JT, Finelli L; Centers for Disease Control and Prevention. Surveillance for acute viral hepatitis—United States, 2005. *MMWR Surveill Summ.* 2007;56(3):1–24.

Weinbaum C, Lyerla R, Margolis HS; Centers for Disease Control and Prevention. Prevention and control of infections with hepatitis viruses in correctional settings. Centers for Disease Control and Prevention. *MMWR Recomm Rep.* 2003;52(RR-1):CE1–CE4.

Westin J, Lagging LM, Spak F, et al. Moderate alcohol intake increases fibrosis progression in untreated patients with hepatitis C virus infection. *J Viral Hepat.* 2002;9(3):235–241.

Weston SR, Leyden W, Murphy R, et al. Racial and ethnic distribution of nonalcoholic fatty liver in persons with newly diagnosed chronic liver disease. *Hepatology.* 2005;41(2):372–379.

Wheeler C, Vogt TM, Armstrong GL, et al. An outbreak of hepatitis A associated with green onions. *N Engl J Med.* 2005;353(9):890–897.

Whitlock EP, Garlitz BA, Harris EL, Beil TL, Smith PR. Screening for hereditary hemochromatosis: a systematic review for the US Preventive Services Task Force. *Ann Intern Med.* 2006;145(3):209–223.

Williams CD, Stengel J, Asike MI, et al. Prevalence of nonalcoholic fatty liver disease and nonalcoholic steatohepatitis among a largely middle-aged population utilizing ultrasound and liver biopsy: a prospective study. *Gastroenterology.* 2011;140(1):124–131.

Williams I. Epidemiology of hepatitis C in the United States. *Am J Med.* 1999;107(6B): 2S–9S.

Wong R, Corley DA. Racial and ethnic variations in hepatocellular carcinoma incidence within the United States. *Am J Med.* 2008;121(8):525–531.

World Health Organization (WHO). Immunization surveillance, assessment and monitoring. 2016. Available at: http://www.who.int/immunization/monitoring_surveillance/en. Accessed September 3, 2016.

Xu J, Murphy SL, Kochanek KD, Bastian BS. Deaths. Final data for 2013. *Natl Vital Stat Rep.* 201664(2):1–119.

Yang HI, Lu SN, Liaw YF, et al. Hepatitis B e antigen and the risk of hepatocellular carcinoma. *N Engl J Med.* 2002;347(3):168–174.

Yatsuji S, Hashimoto E, Tobari M, Taniai M, Tokushige K, Shiratori K. Clinical features and outcomes of cirrhosis due to non-alcoholic steatohepatitis compared with cirrhosis caused by chronic hepatitis C. *J Gastorenterol Hepatol.* 2009;24(2):248–254.

Younossi Z, Kallman J, Kincaid J. The effects of HCV infection and management on health-related quality of life. *Hepatology.* 2007;45(3):806–816.

Younossi ZM, Otgonsuren M, Henry L, et al. Association of non alcoholic fatty liver disease (NAFLD) with hepatocellular carcinoma (HCC) in the United States from 2004 to 2009. *Hepatology.* 2015;62(6):1723–1730.

Younossi ZM, Stepanova M, Afendy M, et al. Changes in the prevalence of the most common causes of chronic liver diseases in the United States from 1988 to 2008. *Clin Gastroenterol Hepatol.* 2011;9(6):524e–530e.

Zaman SN, Johnson PJ, Williams R. Silent cirrhosis in patients with hepatocellular carcinoma. Implications for screening in high-incidence and low-incidence areas. *Cancer.* 1990;65(7):1607–1610.

Zarski JP, Mc Hutchison J, Bronowicki JP, et al. Rate of natural disease progression in patients with chronic hepatitis C. *J Hepatol.* 2003;38(3):307–314.

22

CHRONIC KIDNEY DISEASE

Sana Waheed, MD, and Jonathan B. Jaffery, MD, MS

Introduction

Chronic kidney disease (CKD) is a common but underdiagnosed health problem contributing to significant morbidity and mortality in the United States and other developed and developing countries (Rettig et al. 2008; Barsoum and Bausell 2006). Chronic kidney disease is typically a progressive disease that can ultimately lead to end-stage renal disease (ESRD), requiring maintenance dialysis treatment or kidney transplantation for survival. Moreover, it increases the risk of hospitalizations and rehospitalizations (USRDS 2015). Even more importantly, patients with CKD have a greatly increased risk of death, mainly from cardiovascular disease (Keith et al. 2004). This creates an imperative to develop strategies for prevention, early detection and slowing progression of CKD. In this chapter, we discuss the causes, high-risk populations, and consequences of CKD (Figure 22-1).

Significance

A substantial portion of the U.S. population is undergoing some form of renal replacement therapy as a result of progression of CKD. In 1973, Congress extended Medicare coverage to all Americans with ESRD regardless of age. When the ESRD program began, it provided coverage for approximately 10,000 patients to receive dialysis, a number that had grown to almost 470,000 by 2014. In 2013, the incidence of people progressing to ESRD was approximately 120,000 (Figure 22-2; USRDS 2015). In the United States, the majority of people receiving renal replacement therapy undergo in-center hemodialysis, with only 6.8% of the prevalent ESRD population undergoing peritoneal dialysis and 29.2% with a functioning renal transplant (USRDS 2015).

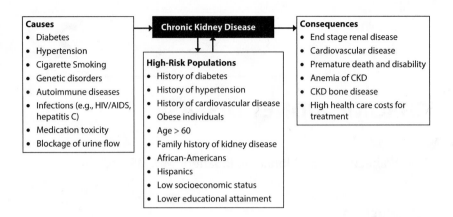

Source: Adapted from Moorthy and Jaffery (2010).

Figure 22-1. Chronic Kidney Disease: Causes, Consequences, and High-Risk Groups

It is noteworthy that recently there has been some slowing in the rate of increase in the number of patients treated for kidney failure. After a year-by-year rise in ESRD incidence over two decades from 1980 through 2000, it has been roughly stable from 2000 to 2013. Despite this, the prevalence of patients with kidney failure continues to increase. As of 2013, the ESRD prevalence had reached 1,981 per million—an increase of 1.4% since 2012 and an increase of 29% since 2000, with a further increase in prevalence anticipated as this patient population enjoys a greater life expectancy (USRDS 2015).

Despite this overall increase in patients with kidney disease, most patients with CKD do not survive to reach end stage and start renal replacement therapy (Berl and Henrich 2006; Kalantar-Zadeh et al. 2007). Mortality rates in CKD patients have decreased over time since the mid-1990s. Despite this improvement, the adjusted mortality rates in CKD patients aged older than 66 years are much higher than those of the non-CKD population (Figure 22-3; USRDS 2015), in part because of the dramatic increase in cardiovascular disease with declining kidney function (KDOQI 2004). In a review by Tonelli et al. (2006) of 39 studies with a total of 1,371,990 participants, the unadjusted relative risk for mortality in participants with CKD when compared with those without CKD ranged from 0.94 to 5.0 and was significantly more than 1.0 in 93% of cohorts. The absolute risk for death also increased exponentially with decreased kidney function in these studies.

The mechanisms for the increase in cardiovascular mortality in patients with CKD are not well understood, but both traditional and nontraditional cardiovascular risk factors play a role (Kendrick and Chonchol 2008). Some of the

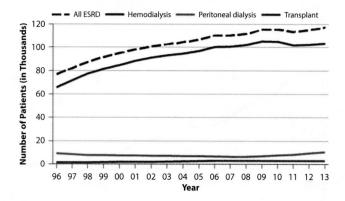

Source: Reprinted from USRDS (2015).

Figure 22-2. Trends in Patients with Incident End-Stage Renal Disease (ESRD) by Modality, 1996–2013

coexisting conditions in patients with CKD that contribute to the development of cardiovascular disease include hypertension, hyperlipidemia, smoking, malnutrition, and diabetes. Impaired kidney function may be a marker for severity of vascular disease as well as being associated with markers of chronic inflammation, itself a risk factor for cardiovascular disease (Shlipak et al. 2005).

The cost of managing patients with CKD remains high, and in 2013 alone, the Centers for Medicare and Medicaid Services (CMS) spent more than $50 billion in health care costs on patients with CKD, approximately 20% of the Medicare budget (Figure 22-4; USRDS 2015). In the United States, the average cost for a patient on dialysis varies from $69,919 to $84,500 per person per year depending on the dialysis modality. Costs to CMS for the ESRD program exceeded $30 billion in 2013, accounting for approximately 7% of the total Medicare budget to provide care for less than 1% of the total Medicare population (USRDS 2015). Despite the enormous expense, both the quality of life and the life expectancy of most patients on dialysis are low. On average, ESRD patients are admitted to the hospital nearly twice a year, and about 30% have an unplanned re-hospitalization within 30 days following hospital discharge (CMS 2014).

Pathophysiology

Chronic kidney disease is a term applied to a variety of disorders that cause progressive kidney damage resulting in decreased kidney function. These vary

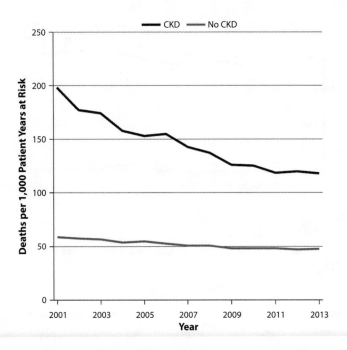

Source: Reprinted from USRDS (2015).

Figure 22-3. Adjusted All-Cause Mortality Rates for Medicare Patients Aged 66 Years and Older, by Chronic Kidney Disease (CKD) Status and Year, 2001–2013

from sequelae of chronic conditions such as diabetes mellitus, genetic disorders that may manifest at any age (such as autosomal dominant polycystic kidney disease), several types of glomerulonephritis that are generally autoimmune in nature, a variety of infections (including HIV/AIDS and hepatitis C), toxicity from medications (including non-steroidal anti-inflammatory drugs), and disorders of organs outside the kidney (e.g., prostate, urinary bladder, uterus) that result in blockage of urine flow.

The major causes of ESRD in the United States are diabetes mellitus and hypertension (Figure 22-1). Up to 40% of patients with type 1 diabetes and 5% to 10% of patients with type 2 diabetes develop kidney failure from diabetic nephropathy, and approximately 40% of patients receiving renal replacement therapy have diabetes as the underlying etiology of their ESRD (USRDS 2015). The kidney damage in patients with diabetes is a consequence of chronic elevations in blood sugar levels, which lead to advanced glycated end product formation and damage to the glomeruli. The kidney damage is one component

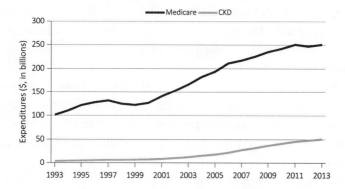

Source: Reprinted from USRDS (2015).

Figure 22-4. Overall Expenditures on Parts A, B, and D Services for the Medicare Population Aged 65 Years and Older and for Those With Chronic Kidney Disease (CKD), by Year, 1993–2013

of the widespread microvascular disease seen in patients with diabetes mellitus who develop other complications, such as diabetic retinopathy and neuropathy. Urinalysis showing increasing amounts of albumin excretion is the earliest manifestation of diabetic kidney disease. Elevation in blood pressure, which is common in patients with diabetes, compounds the kidney injury and progression of CKD.

In addition, hypertension in and of itself continues to be an important cause of CKD. In 2013, approximately 35,000 new patients required renal replacement therapy as a result of hypertension-related kidney failure (USRDS 2015). Kidneys are very sensitive to the effects of hypertension, and high blood pressure is a key pathogenic factor contributing to deterioration in kidney function. Conversely, certain pathologic processes within the kidney can result in hypertension. The prevalence of hypertension in patients is inversely related to glomerular filtration rate (GFR), and studies have shown hypertension rates increasing from 66% to 95% as the GFR drops from 85 to 12 milliliters per minute (mL/min) per 1.73 square meters (m^2; Buckalew et al. 1996). The presence of kidney disease is a common and underappreciated preexisting medical cause of resistant hypertension (Sarafidis and Bakris 2008), and an elevated serum creatinine level is noted in 10% to 20% of patients with hypertension. Moreover, multiple studies have demonstrated that poor control of blood pressure is associated with faster progression of CKD (Ravera et al. 2006). Based on the results of a meta-analysis, systolic blood pressure of 110 to 129 millimeters of mercury (mm Hg) is associated with the lowest risk of kidney disease progression (Jafar et al. 2003). The prevalence of hypertension also increases with age and leads to a much higher risk for kidney disease in this population (Lionakis et al. 2012).

Anemia is a common problem in patients with CKD and as many as 90% of patients with a GFR less than 25 to 30 mL/min/1.73 m^2 have some degree of anemia (Kazmi et al. 2001). Common symptoms include fatigue and dyspnea. Anemia is also associated with adverse cardiovascular outcomes including left ventricular hypertrophy (Levin et al. 1999).

Finally, kidney disease is an important cause of abnormalities of mineral and bone metabolism, which can manifest with abnormalities of calcium, phosphorus, parathyroid hormone, or vitamin D metabolism, or abnormalities in bone turnover. Phosphate retention because of impaired excretion by the kidney is likely the initial trigger (Martin and Gonzalez 2007).

Descriptive Epidemiology

Chronic kidney disease is a growing worldwide problem in both developed and developing countries (Levey et al. 2007). In recent years, the prevalence of CKD has been noted to be increasing, but as patients with CKD do not develop symptoms until they already have significant decline in kidney function, the epidemic of CKD is largely a silent one. Data from the National Health and Nutritional Examination Survey, 2009–2012, revealed that, in the United States, less than 10% of patients with CKD stage 1 to 3 are aware of their kidney disease (USRDS 2015; CDC 2015).

Approximately 14% of the U.S. adult population (more than 20 million patients) is affected by CKD (USRDS 2015). For an individual, lifetime risk of CKD is high, with more than half the U.S. adults aged 30 to 64 years likely to develop CKD (Hoerger et al. 2015). The prevalence of CKD is also higher in minority populations and the socially disadvantaged (Norris and Nissenson 2008; Bello et al. 2008). The number of patients at risk for developing CKD continues to be high as conditions such as diabetes and hypertension, the two leading causes of CKD in the United States, are themselves continuing to be increasingly prevalent (Mokdad et al. 2001). An aging U.S. population and an increase in the proportion of people with obesity are also factors that contribute to the high prevalence of CKD (Chen et al. 2004).

High-Risk Populations

In addition to those with diabetes mellitus and hypertension, the risk of CKD is high in patients with cardiovascular disease or obesity, those aged older than 60 years, and those with a family history of kidney disease (Figure 22-1). The decline in GFR is proportional to age and prevalence of CKD increases with age. In patients aged 65 years and older, CKD defined as an estimated GFR (eGFR) less than 60 mL/min/1.73 m² is present in more than 40% of the population (Stevens et al. 2010).

Racial and ethnic features have also been shown to have a great impact on the progression of CKD (Figure 22-5). In the United States, prevalence of early kidney disease is comparable across all racial and ethnic groups, but the progression of CKD to ESRD is much higher among minority populations (Martins et al. 2012), with the prevalent rates of ESRD in African Americans being 3.7 times higher than whites (USRDS 2015). This difference is largely attributed to higher rates and earlier onset of diabetes and hypertension in this population. Recently, this increased risk of kidney disease has also been linked to G1 and G2 high-risk alleles for a gene *APOL1* that is located on chromosome 22 (Friedman and Pollak 2011). These high-risk alleles are common and provide resistance to disease-causing trypanosomas, which may have led to their natural selection in the population. Up to 50% of African-American individuals have either one or both high-risk alleles (Genovese et al. 2010).

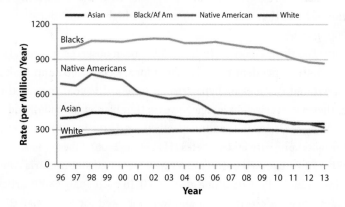

Source: Reprinted from USRDS (2015).

Figure 22-5. Adjusted End-Stage Renal Disease Incidence Rate, by Race, in the U.S. Population, 1996–2013

These high-risk alleles are associated with hypertensive-related kidney disease, focal segmental glomerulosclerosis, and HIV-associated nephropathy. The effect of carrying two *APOL1* risk alleles explains 18% of focal segmental glomerulosclerosis and 35% of HIV-associated nephropathy and eliminating this risk would reduce HIV-associated nephropathy and focal segmental glomerulosclerosis by 67% (Kopp et al. 2011). In a study of 407 African-American patients on dialysis, patients with high-risk alleles were on average significantly younger at the time of initiation of dialysis (49 years) than those without any high-risk alleles (62 years; Kanji et al. 2011).

Mexican Americans with type 2 diabetes are more likely to develop proteinuria and also more likely to progress to kidney failure than non-Hispanic whites (Pugh et al. 1988; Pugh 1996). They may share a common genetic background with Native Americans, themselves a group at high risk of developing diabetes and CKD (Benabe and Rios 2004). Hispanics are also more likely to have hypertension and obesity than the general U.S. population (Lorenzo et al. 2002; Raymond and D'Eramo-Melkus 1993). The prevalence of type 2 diabetes and the metabolic syndrome is higher in Native Americans, and in the Strong Heart study, at 9-year follow-up, the hazard ratio for CKD was 1.3 for this population (Lucove et al. 2008).

Socioeconomic factors also affect the prevalence of CKD, which is demonstrated by greater prevalence among lower-income African Americans compared with those at higher income levels (Peralta et al. 2006). Chronic kidney disease is also more prevalent among persons with less than a high-school education (22.1%) than persons with at least a high-school education (15.7%; CDC 2007).

Obesity and the metabolic syndrome have been observed in several studies as significant independent risk predictors for CKD (Wahba and Mak 2007). Patients without diabetes or hypertension have a threefold increased risk of CKD if they are overweight at age 20 years (Ejerblad et al. 2006), and higher baseline body mass index is an independent predictor for ESRD after adjustment for blood pressure and diabetes (Hsu et al. 2006). Obesity is also associated with a 70% increased risk of moderately increased albuminuria compared to lean individuals (Pinto-Sietsma et al. 2003). In more than 7,800 participants who had normal kidney function and were followed for more than 21 years, Chen et al. (2004) found that the multivariate-adjusted odds ratio for CKD was 2.6 for individuals with metabolic syndrome, compared with individuals without the metabolic syndrome.

There is also a high prevalence of CKD in individuals who have family members with kidney failure, and this is even more common among African Americans (Jurkovitz et al. 2002). Having one first-degree relative with renal disease increases the odds of ESRD by 1.3 and having two or more affected first-degree relatives increases the odds of ESRD by 10.4 (Lei et al. 1998).

Studies have shown that adults with a low birthweight face an increased risk for chronic diseases, including high blood pressure, cardiovascular disease, and renal disease (Eriksson et al. 2000; Lackland et al. 2000; Barker 1995). Low birthweight is also associated with a smaller kidney volume and lower number of nephrons and could predispose to adaptive changes that initiate and accelerate CKD (Brenner and Mackenzie 1997). In a study of more than two million children born in Norway between 1967 and 2004, births in the lowest decile had a 1.7 times increased risk for kidney failure compared with other birthweight deciles (Vikse et al. 2008).

Finally, other risk factors such as elevated levels of serum uric acid and periodontal disease have been noted as risk factors for CKD that also lead to a greater likelihood of progression to ESRD (Shultis et al. 2007; Obermayr et al. 2008). In a study by Bellomo et al. (2010), 900 healthy, normotensive adult blood donors were followed for 59 months during which the eGFR decreased from an average of 97 to 88 mL/min/1.73 m^2. Higher uric acid levels were associated with a greater likelihood of eGFR decrease with a hazard ratio of 1.13 for every 1 milligram per deciliter increase in uric acid levels.

Geographic Distribution

Because CKD is more common among African Americans and Hispanics than among whites, its geographic distribution tends to be higher in those parts of the country that have a greater proportion of racial/ethnic minorities. The prevalence of ESRD is also higher in urban areas than in rural areas and tends to be higher in Southern and Midwestern states (Figure 22-6; USRDS 2013).

Time Trends

The prevalence of ESRD in the United States has grown in recent years. As of December 31, 2013, there were 661,648 prevalent cases of ESRD in the United States—an increase of 3.5% since 2012 and an increase of 68% since 2000 (USRDS 2015). On the other hand, incident cases of ESRD have declined

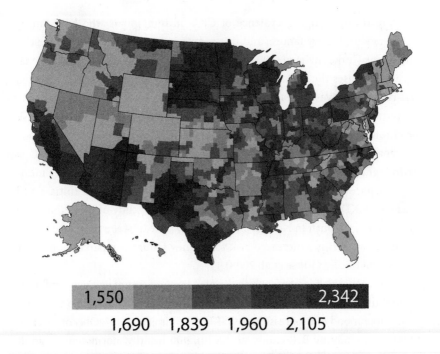

1,550					2,342

1,690   1,839   1,960   2,105

Source: Reprinted from USRDS (2013).

Figure 22-6. Geographic Variations in Adjusted Prevalent Rates of End-Stage Renal Disease per Million Population, 2011

slightly in recent years and the adjusted incidence rate of 352 per million per year in 2013 was the lowest since 1997. The incident rate of ESRD is expected to decrease in the coming years, because of increased screening and early intervention to decrease progression to CKD (USRDS 2015).

Causes

Modifiable Risk Factors

The greatest modifiable risk factors for development of CKD are diabetes, hypertension, and smoking. As stated previously, diabetes mellitus is the most common cause of CKD (USRDS 2015). Intensive glycemic control can help prevent the development of moderately increased albuminuria, and slow the progression of established diabetic nephropathy (UKPDS 1998). Hypertension is the next most common cause of CKD (USRDS 2015). The presence of inadequately controlled blood pressure in the setting of CKD from any cause has an additive impact on disease progression, and aggressive blood pressure control is recommended for all individuals with CKD, regardless of etiology. Tobacco use is also associated with the development of proteinuria and more rapid progression of CKD (Orth 2002). Aggressive tobacco cessation programs are recommended to ameliorate this modifiable risk factor.

Two other major independent risk factors for CKD progression are obesity and proteinuria. Weight loss should be helpful in decreasing risk (Pinto-Sietsma et al. 2003), and decreasing proteinuria through the use of drugs that block the renin–angiotensin system (such as angiotensin-converting enzyme [ACE] inhibitors and angiotensin-receptor blockers [ARBs]) is recommended for all individuals with proteinuric CKD, regardless of blood pressure control (KDIGO CKD Work Group 2013).

Population-Attributable Risk

In a population-based case–control study of white and African-American patients with type 1 and type 2 diabetes, the overall population-attributable risk for kidney failure was 42% (Perneger et al. 1994). Several large prospective studies (Multiple Risk Factor Intervention Trial [MRFIT] and Systolic Hypertension in the Elderly Program) have established that hypertension is an important risk factor for CKD (Pascual et al. 2005; Young et al. 2002). In a prospective study of 23,534 men and women followed for 20 years in Washington County, Maryland, 23% of the CKD cases in this population were attributable to hypertension. In addition, this study helped demonstrate the strong link between smoking and CKD, as 31% of cases of CKD in this population were attributed to cigarette smoking (Haroun et al. 2003). Therefore, efforts that successfully target diabetes, high blood pressure, and smoking would have the greatest impact on reducing the incidence of CKD in the population.

Evidence-Based Interventions

Prevention

As diabetes mellitus and hypertension together account for greater than 60% of prevalent ESRD cases in the United States (USRDS 2015), a significant proportion of cases could be prevented through aggressive risk factor modification of these identifiable and controllable diseases. Effective control of diabetes is likely to yield rich dividends in preventing the disabling and often fatal complications of diabetes such as blindness, heart disease, and peripheral vascular disease ultimately requiring amputation. Other causes of CKD, including genetic (e.g., polycystic kidney disease), immunologic (e.g., lupus nephritis), and urologic (e.g., reflux nephropathy), while modifiable, may be less preventable.

One essential first step for prevention of CKD is to increase public awareness. In a recent study of 29,144 participants with CKD, only 6,751 (23%) reported that they were aware of their disease (Shah et al. 2012). A greater emphasis should be placed on prevention of CKD in medical school curricula and by those training allied health personnel, and student clerkships in medical schools should increase the emphasis on continuity of patient care (Hirsh et al. 2007). Public health and preventive medicine programs should include training in development of community-based programs for managing the broad epidemic of CKD.

On an individual level, physicians and other health care workers need adequate training in how to diagnose CKD early in its course. Physicians and other health care providers need to stay up to date on new evidence-based measures of integrating chronic disease prevention into their practices. Greater use of web-based resources may be helpful in this endeavor. The increasing utilization of web-based education programs by organizations such as the National Kidney Foundation should be useful both to the practicing physician and the patient.

At the system level, health systems could build in appropriate screening programs, reminding health care providers to perform routine screenings, and giving them the tools to follow up the results with appropriate care. The growing epidemic of CKD has already resulted in an imbalance between the number of patients with CKD and the number of physicians who are trained specialists in treating kidney disease. One way to relieve the burden of nephrologists would be to ensure adequate training of primary care providers to deliver disease management programs that include additional innovative interventions (e.g., electronic consultation) to manage patients identified with early stages of CKD. An algorithm-based primary care management plan was implemented in the United Kingdom with a focus on patient education, medication management, dietetic advice, and optimization of clinical management to achieve clinical targets. The median decline in the eGFR in patients with various stages of CKD in the nine months before enrolling in the disease management program was 3.69 mL/min/1.73 m^2 compared with 0.32 mL/min/1.73 m^2 during the 12 months after enrollment (Richards et al. 2008).

Screening

Who to Screen

The complex care that must be provided for patients with CKD cannot be overemphasized (Choudhury and Luna-Salazar 2008). However, the ability of the current U.S. health care system to appropriately manage all of the individuals identified with CKD via effective screening programs remains unclear (McClellan et al. 2003; Thomas et al. 2008).

All patients should be assessed as a part of their health examinations to determine whether they are at increased risk of CKD. Patients with diabetes, hypertension, and cardiovascular disease are at risk for developing CKD (Levey et al. 2007). Although there are no U.S. Preventive Services Task Force recommendations on CKD screening, screening is generally recommended only for high-risk individuals (Figure 22-1), and not the general population. Mass screening of the general public for CKD is expensive, has a low yield, and is not cost-effective. However, targeted screening programs in communities with high-risk populations are effective in detecting previously unidentified persons with CKD. An example of such an approach is the Kidney Early Evaluation Program (KEEP), a free kidney disease–screening program designed to detect CKD and promote follow-up evaluation with clinicians to ultimately improve outcomes. This program screens individuals with diabetes, hypertension, or those with a first-degree relative with diabetes, hypertension, or kidney disease, and 89,552 participants were screened in 49 states from early August 2000 until end of December 2007 (Vassalotti et al. 2010). In one study, the authors concluded that limiting screening of CKD to patients with known hypertension, diabetes, aged greater than 55 years, or with a family history of CKD would have identified approximately 93% of those with CKD (Hallan et al. 2006).

Physicians are at times not aware of the need to consider CKD in patients at increased risk for this condition. In a survey of more than 400 primary care providers, although diabetes and high blood pressure were correctly identified as risk factors for CKD, more than one third did not consider family history of CKD and 22% did not consider African-American race to be risk factors (Lea et al. 2006).

How to Screen

All patients who have risk factors for CKD should be screened with a urine test for albumin and a blood test for creatinine to estimate GFR. The preferred screening strategy for albuminuria is measurement of the urine albumin-to-creatinine ratio (Levey et al. 2007). Chronic kidney disease is diagnosed in any individual who has an eGFR below 60 mL/min/1.73 m² for a period of at least three months. In addition, CKD is diagnosed in patients with any level of eGFR in the presence of structural (e.g., polycystic kidney disease) or functional (e.g., proteinuria or microalbuminuria in a patient with diabetes mellitus) damage that persists for more than three months (Stevens et al. 2006).

Serum creatinine level alone, a traditionally used blood test, is an inadequate measure of kidney function. Serum creatinine is normally produced from creatine in the muscle and is excreted by the kidney. Therefore, when kidney function declines, serum creatinine levels in the blood increase. As the muscle mass varies in patients with age, sex, and ethnicity, a given level of serum creatinine can actually reflect different levels of kidney function in different patients. Timed urine collections to measure creatinine clearance over a 24-hour period have been generally abandoned because they are time-consuming, inconvenient, and tend to be inaccurate. Formulae to estimate the creatinine clearance such as the Cockcroft–Gault equation are also inadequate in patients with CKD (Shoker et al. 2006; Poggio et al. 2005).

A more sensitive way to assess the kidney function is to estimate the GFR from the serum creatinine level by using a formula that takes into consideration the age, sex, and ethnicity of the patient. Currently, the four-variable modification of diet in renal disease (MDRD) formula for estimating the GFR is used by many clinical laboratories and is reported along with the serum creatinine results (Stevens et al. 2006).

The MDRD formula performs relatively well in populations that have CKD as it was derived from the MDRD cohort, which included patients with kidney disease. However, there are some limitations of GFR estimates by the MDRD formula that have to be kept in mind. The MDRD formula may be less reliable in persons with normal levels of kidney function, as estimates of GFR by the MDRD method are imprecise at GFR levels greater than 60 mL/min/1.73 m² (Stevens et al. 2006; Rule et al. 2004).

A newer equation derived by the CKD Epidemiology Collaboration from a larger and more diverse population (including those with normal kidney function) predicts the GFR more accurately, as it reduces the bias at higher levels of kidney function. Its use in the clinical setting is becoming more common (Florkowski and Chew-Harris 2011).

It must be pointed out that the formula for estimating GFR is unreliable in the hospitalized patient or in the setting of acute kidney injury, when serum creatinine levels can fluctuate daily because of such factors as changes in volume status and disturbances of cardiac function. The measurement of serum cystatin C level holds promise as a possible sensitive measure of kidney function. Its widespread use in clinical practice is, however, limited at the present time because of expense (Florkowski and Chew-Harris 2011; Shlipak et al. 2006).

In recent years, albuminuria has become a useful tool to detect kidney disease and the increased risk for kidney failure in patients with diabetes mellitus. In a landmark study in 609 Danish patients with diabetes, Mogensen (1984) noted that patients with albumin excretion greater than 30 micrograms per milliliter (μg/mL) in early morning urine specimens had a greater chance of progressive kidney damage with development of overt proteinuria. Healthy persons excrete less than 30 mg of albumin in 24 hours. A 24-hour urine collection is often cumbersome and may actually be inaccurate because of missed collections. Hence, it is recommended that the ratio of albumin to creatinine excreted in a random sample be used to estimate albuminuria (KDIGO CKD Work Group 2013).

Albuminuria of less than 30 milligrams per gram of creatinine is considered to be in the normal or mildly increased range of albumin excretion; moderately increased albuminuria is defined as an albumin excretion of 30 to 300 milligrams of albumin per gram of creatinine; and severely increased albuminuria is defined as an albumin excretion of greater than 300 milligrams of albumin per gram of creatinine. However, even low levels of urinary albumin excretion in patients with diabetes may be associated with an increased incidence of cardiovascular disease (Danziger 2008). In patients with proteinuria noted by a positive protein test dipstick urinalysis (which usually signifies albuminuria greater than 300 mg per g of creatinine), a protein-to-creatinine ratio in the random urine sample can be performed to assess the extent of proteinuria (Ginsberg et al. 1983).

Laboratories can greatly contribute to the efficiency of identifying CKD by instituting standard procedures of reporting the eGFR whenever an outpatient serum creatinine is checked, with a simple flag describing the appropriate CKD stage, a practice that is increasingly common. Urine tests for moderately increased albuminuria should be streamlined and results reported in a standardized manner as milligrams of albumin per gram of creatinine.

In summary, the early identification of CKD coupled with an effective intervention and management program to decrease the morbidity and mortality associated with CKD is indeed a worthy goal. However, there are pitfalls in universal screening of all patients for CKD with the laboratory tests available today (Glassock and Winearls 2008; Melamed et al. 2008). It seems prudent to pursue targeted screening of CKD in individuals at increased risk for this condition (Brown et al. 2003; Grootendorst et al. 2009). Based on this, American College of Physicians also recommends screening for CKD in patients at risk for CKD, but recommends against screening for CKD in adults without symptoms or risk factors (Saunders et al. 2015).

Treatment

Chronic kidney disease is further classified into stages depending on the eGFR (Table 22-1). Early diagnosis of the patient with CKD is the key to effective management that can prevent a progressive decline in kidney function and decrease mortality in the patient with CKD, which is indeed a worthy goal. Combining eGFR and proteinuria may improve prediction of patients with CKD who are likely to progress to kidney failure. In a multivariate analysis of

Table 22-1. Stages of Chronic Kidney Disease

CKD Category	GFR (mL/min/1.73 m²)	Terms	Detection, Evaluation, and Management[a]
Stage 1	≥ 90	Normal or high	Diagnosis and treatment of preexisting conditions
Stage 2	60–89	Mildly decreased	Estimation of progression
Stage 3a	45–59	Mild to moderately decreased	Slowing down progression
Stage 3b	30–44	Moderate to severely decreased	Management of complications
Stage 4	15–29	Severely decreased	Referral to nephrology and consideration of renal replacement therapy
Stage 5	<15	Kidney failure	Consideration for renal replacement therapy

Source: Data from Stevens (2006).
Note: CKD=chronic kidney disease; GFR=glomerular filtration rate.
[a]Recommended care at each stage of chronic kidney disease includes care for less-severe stages.

65,589 adults over a 10.3-year follow-up, Hallan et al. (2009) noted that eGFR and albuminuria were independently and strongly associated with progression to ESRD. For example, a person with an eGFR of 59 mL/min/1.73 m² with severely increased albuminuria has a higher risk of disease progression than a patient with an eGFR of 30 mL/min/1.73 m² with normal to mildly increased albuminuria (KDIGO CKD Work Group 2013).

In the patient with early stages of CKD, a greater emphasis can be placed on diagnosing and managing the conditions causing CKD, whereas in the patient with advanced stages of CKD, the care shifts to preventing and managing the complications of CKD. An early referral of the patient with advanced CKD to a kidney specialist is recommended to facilitate planning and education for transition to dialysis and kidney transplantation (Stevens et al. 2006). Despite these guidelines, in the United States, early intervention remains a challenge. A retrospective longitudinal cohort study of more than 12,500 older veterans with diabetes found that nearly half the patients had CKD, yet only 7.2% had a nephrology visit during the five-year study period. Even among those with stage 4 CKD, only 32% had been seen in the nephrology clinic (Patel et al. 2005). In a study of dialysis patients in which 428 patient surveys were returned, 36% of the patients had not seen a nephrologist for more than four months before initiation of dialysis (Mehrotra et al. 2005).

Numerous studies have shown that effective interventions such as excellent glycemic control in patients with diabetes (UKPDS 1998), aggressive blood pressure control (Ruggenenti et al. 2001), reduction in proteinuria with ACE inhibitors or ARBs (Ruggenenti et al. 2001), and appropriate diet and lifestyle modification can prevent kidney disease or delay its progression and decrease its morbidity and mortality rates (Stengel et al. 2003). In the UKPDS study, intense glycemic control was associated with a 67% risk reduction for a doubling of plasma creatinine levels at nine years (UKPDS 1998). The current KDOQI guidelines recommend a target hemoglobin A1c of 7% to prevent or delay progression of the microvascular complications, including diabetic kidney disease (National Kidney Foundation 2012). Target hemoglobin A1c can be extended above 7% in individuals with comorbidities and limited life expectancy and risk of hypoglycemia.

Blood pressure also needs to be closely monitored, as elevated blood pressure is a clear risk for progression of kidney damage in patients with CKD. Clinical guidelines have set target blood pressure values for patients with CKD at less than 130/80 mm Hg if they have moderately increased albuminuria.

A looser blood pressure target of 140/90 mm Hg is only applicable to patients with no proteinuria (KDIGO CKD Work Group 2013). Renin–angiotensin blocking agents should be the first-line drugs in patients with severely increased albuminuria.

Patients with CKD lack the drop in blood pressure at night (a phenomenon called nocturnal dipping) seen in healthy people. Several studies have shown that 24-hour ambulatory blood pressure monitoring is a stronger predictor of ESRD, cardiovascular disease, and death than office blood pressure monitoring (Agarwal and Andersen 2006; Minutolo et al. 2011). Despite that, clinical use of ambulatory blood pressure monitoring in patients with hypertension and CKD is not widespread and nearly every trial in the CKD setting has used office-based blood pressure readings as this method is most frequently used clinically.

As mentioned previously, increased urinary albumin (or protein) excretion is an important risk factor for progression of CKD. Reduction of proteinuria has been associated with a decreased risk of death and development of ESRD in patients with both diabetic and non-diabetic CKD (de Zeeuw et al. 2004). The most common treatments for albuminuria reduction are the use of drugs such as ACE inhibitors or ARBs. Studies with ARBs in patients with type 2 diabetes have shown that the reduction in albuminuria at six months strongly predicts a decrease in adverse renal and cardiovascular outcomes (de Zeeuw et al. 2004). This improvement in outcomes was independent of the blood pressure–lowering effects of these medications. African-American patients with hypertension, CKD, and cardiovascular disease also have improved cardiovascular outcomes with a reduction in proteinuria (Ibsen et al. 2005). Reducing albuminuria via treatment with drugs to block the renin–angiotensin system in patients with CKD is recommended even if the blood pressure is at goal (Tuttle 2007).

In some patients with diabetic kidney disease, proteinuria persists despite being on the maximal dosage of ACE inhibitors or ARBs. Studies looking at using a combination of both ACE inhibitors and ARBs have shown an increased risk of hyperkalemia and developing acute kidney injury (Quiroga et al. 2014). Addition of an aldosterone antagonist (e.g., spironolactone) to ACE inhibitor or ARB therapy in patients can result in a further reduction in proteinuria, but is associated with a higher risk of hyperkalemia (Navaneethan et al. 2009; Bolignano et al. 2014).

Experimental studies in animal models of CKD have shown that a decrease in protein intake results in reduced renal fibrosis and a slower decline in kidney function (Hostetter et al. 1986). Although this beneficial effect of decreased kidney scarring has not been replicated in humans, there is evidence that restriction of dietary protein to 0.6 to 0.8 grams per kilogram of body weight per day in patients with advanced CKD (eGFR between 60 and 15 mL/min/1.73 m^2) results in a less rapid decline in the kidney function (Fouque and Aparicio 2007). As such, dietary protein restriction (0.8 grams per kilogram of body weight per day) may be advised for the patient with moderately advanced CKD (Fouque and Aparicio 2007; KDIGO CKD Work Group 2013). Sodium restriction is recommended in patients with hypertension and proteinuria.

Acidemia is often seen in patients with advanced CKD and recent evidence suggests that treating such patients with bicarbonate therapy to bring their sodium bicarbonate to a level of greater than or equal to 23 milliequivalents (mEq) per liter slows the progression of CKD and decreases the risk of developing ESRD (de Brito-Ashurst et al. 2009).

Animal studies have shown a benefit to lipid lowering on the progression of kidney disease, but human studies have not been definitive, as most trials specifically looking at the impact on CKD have been small and inconclusive. A meta-analyses of 18 randomized clinical trials showed that lipid-lowering therapy in patients with CKD decreases the risk of cardiac mortality (relative risk = 0.82; Upadhyay et al. 2012). Kidney Disease: Improving Global Outcomes (KDIGO) guidelines recommend initiation of treatment with a statin in patients with CKD who are not yet on dialysis (KDIGO Lipid Work Group 2013).

Anemia is a common complication of CKD. Persistent hemoglobin levels less than 11 grams per deciliter are associated with an increased risk of death (Gilbertson et al. 2008). KDIGO guidelines recommend initiating treatment with erythropoietin-stimulating agents once the hemoglobin concentration is below 10 grams per deciliter in dialysis patients (KDIGO Anemia Work Group 2012).

These measures to limit progressive kidney damage are important, but patients diagnosed with CKD also require regular follow-up and avoidance of exposure to nephrotoxic medications and therapeutic and diagnostic agents, including non-steroidal anti-inflammatory drugs and iodinated radio-contrast agents used in diagnostic procedures (Choudhury and Luna-Salazar 2008). Another challenging area in patients with CKD is underutilization of preventive health measures (Winkelmayer et al. 2002). Preventive goals and treatment strategies specific to patients with CKD can differ from those for the general population—for example, it is recommended that all patients with CKD be vaccinated against hepatitis B (CDC 2012).

Examples of Evidence-Based Interventions

Decreasing proteinuria is the cornerstone of therapy in patients with CKD. On the basis of the results of one study, the changes in albuminuria in the first six months of therapy are roughly linearly related to the degree of long-term renal protection: every 50% reduction in albuminuria in the first 6 months was associated with a risk reduction of 45% for ESRD during follow-up (de Zeeuw et al. 2004). Patient care with multimodal intervention to decrease proteinuria in dedicated remission clinics has been noted to be very effective to prevent progression of CKD. In a median four-year follow-up of 56 patients with proteinuria greater than 3 grams, Ruggenenti et al. (2008) observed a reduction in monthly GFR in the intervention group of 0.17 mL/min/1.73 m^2 and a kidney failure rate of 3.6% as compared with a monthly decline of 0.56 mL/min/1.73 m^2 and a kidney failure rate of 30.6% in historical control patients.

Optimal blood pressure control is helpful in slowing the progression of CKD to ESRD (Jafar et al. 2003). Moreover, renin–angiotensin system blockade is associated with a decrease in the risk of CKD progression independent of its antihypertensive effects. A meta-analysis of 13 trials (n = 37,089) that compared the effect of ACE inhibitors or ARB therapy with that of other antihypertensive agents found that ACE inhibitors or ARB therapy was associated with a significant reduction in risk for ESRD (risk reduction = 0.87; 95% confidence interval = 0.75, 0.99; p = .04; Casas et al. 2005).

The recent improvement noted in the incidence of patients with ESRD in the US Renal Data System has been suggested to be attributable to better secondary prevention of kidney damage with greater glycemic control in patients with diabetes, better blood pressure control, wider use of drugs that block the renin–angiotensin system, and reduction of proteinuria (Ruggenenti and Remuzzi 2007).

Preventive strategies have been shown to preserve kidney function and prevent the development of ESRD and death in affected individuals. However, presently these preventive programs are not widely used, making CKD a prime example of a chronic health problem that may benefit from a broad-based long-term preventive health program.

Areas of Future Research

With a high prevalence, an extraordinary cardiovascular disease burden, substantial disparities in affected populations, and extreme associated costs, CKD is a major public and population health threat (DuBose 2007). Diagnosis and management of CKD needs to be a central part of future public health planning in the management of the patient with chronic non-communicable diseases.

Primary care physicians and other health care providers have an increasingly vital role to play for the patient with CKD, as it is not possible for the current number of nephrologists to directly manage the ongoing care for the expected increase in the number of patients with CKD. Appropriate guidelines and intervention programs need to be developed and a simplified and streamlined program for management must be devised to include primary care physicians as well as ancillary health care personnel. Pilot clinical programs have shown that such shared care programs are effective in caring for patients with CKD and in preserving kidney function when compared with traditional nephrology-based patient care (Jones et al. 2006).

Results of the recent Systolic Blood Pressure Intervention Trial (SPRINT) show that patients at high risk of cardiovascular events, including patients with CKD, might benefit from lower systolic blood pressure targets (< 120 mm Hg) than currently recommended targets of 130 to 140 mm Hg (Wright et al. 2015). There is a dearth of studies addressing the optimal blood pressure control in the CKD population and ideally this should be addressed in a randomized, controlled clinical trial.

For patients with diabetic nephropathy and proteinuria, the only current treatment is renin–angiotensin system blockade or aldosterone antagonists. Transforming growth factor beta (TGF-β)–blocking agents such as pirfenidone and advanced glycation end-product formation inhibitors such as pyridoxamine have been tried with variable results (Quiroga et al. 2015). Further clinical trials are needed to discover effective medications that will halt the progression of diabetic nephropathy and have beneficial effects for the degree of proteinuria.

Additional research needs to be done on the detection, management, and, most importantly, prevention of CKD. Interventions directed at the consumer level could include measures to improve the health literacy of the population, empowering patients to be responsible for their own health, and actively involving them in decision-making.

Basic research aimed at understanding the progressive nature of CKD and pathophysiologic processes responsible for tissue damage should be prioritized. Finally, the importance of translational research—applying discoveries generated during research in the laboratory and preclinical studies to studies in human participants with the disease, and methods aimed at enhancing the adoption of best practices in the community—is now being recognized. Clinical and translational science awards initiated by the National Institutes of Health and development of public–private biomedical research partnerships with the pharmaceutical industry appear to be promising (Zerhouni 2007; Bausell 2006). Clearly, easing the substantial social and economic burden that CKD imposes on both the individual and society will require a multifaceted strategy to manage the growing epidemic in the complex population that comprises those with CKD.

Resources

Kidney Disease: Improving Global Outcomes, http://www.kdigo.org

National Kidney Foundation, Kidney Disease Outcomes Quality Initiative, http://www.kidney.org/professionals/KDOQI

Suggested Reading

Kidney Disease: Improving Global Outcomes (KDIGO) CKD Work Group. 2012. KDIGO 2012 Clinical Practice Guideline for the Evaluation and Management of Chronic Kidney Disease. *Kidney Int Suppl.* 2013;(3):1–150.

Levey AS, Coresh J. Chronic kidney disease. *Lancet.* 2012;379(9811):165–180.

References

Agarwal R, Andersen MJ. Prognostic importance of ambulatory blood pressure recordings in patients with chronic kidney disease. *Kidney Int.* 2006;69(7):1175–1180.

Barker DJ. The fetal and infant origins of disease. *Eur J Clin Invest.* 1995;25(7):457–463.

Barsoum RS, Bausell RB. Chronic kidney disease in the developing world translation research: introduction to the special issue. *N Engl J Med.* 2006:354(10):997–999.

Bausell RB. Translation research: introduction to the special issue. *Eval Health Prof.* 2006;29(1):3–6.

Bello AK, Peters J, Rigby J, Rahman AA, El Nahas M. Socioeconomic status and chronic kidney disease at presentation to a renal service in the United Kingdom. *Clin J Am Soc Nephrol.* 2008;3(5):1316–1323.

Bellomo G, Venanzi S, Verdura C, Saronio P, Esposito A, Timio M. Association of uric acid with change in kidney function in healthy normotensive individuals. *Am J Kidney Dis*. 2010;56(2):264–272.

Benabe JE, Rios EV. Kidney disease in the Hispanic population: facing the growing challenge. *J Natl Med Assoc*. 2004;96(6):789–798.

Berl T, Henrich W. Kidney–heart interactions: epidemiology, pathogenesis, and treatment. *Clin J Am Soc Nephrol*. 2006;1(1):8–18.

Bolignano D, Palmer SC, Navaneethan SD, Strippoli GF. Aldosterone antagonists for preventing the progression of chronic kidney disease. *Cochrane Database Syst Rev*. 2014;(4):CD007004.

Brenner BM, Mackenzie HS. Nephron mass as a risk factor for progression of renal disease. *Kidney Int Suppl*. 1997;63(63):S124–S127.

Brown WW, Peters RM, Ohmit SE, et al. Early detection of kidney disease in community settings: the Kidney Early Evaluation Program (KEEP). *Am J Kidney Dis*. 2003;42(1):22–35.

Buckalew VM Jr, Berg RL, Wang SR, Porush JG, Rauch S, Schulman G. Prevalence of hypertension in 1,795 subjects with chronic renal disease: the Modification of Diet in Renal Disease Study baseline cohort. Modification of Diet in Renal Disease Study Group. *Am J Kidney Dis*. 1996;28(6):811–821.

Casas JP, Chua W, Loukogeorgakis S, et al. Effect of inhibitors of the renin–angiotensin system and other antihypertensive drugs on renal outcomes: systematic review and meta-analysis. *Lancet*. 2005;366(9502):2026–2033.

Centers for Disease Control and Prevention (CDC). Prevalence of chronic kidney disease and associated risk factors—United States, 1999–2004. *MMWR Morb Mortal Wkly Rep*. 2007;56(8):161–165.

Centers for Disease Control and Prevention (CDC). Guidelines for vaccinating kidney dialysis patients and patients with chronic kidney disease. 2012. Available at: http://www.cdc.gov/vaccines/pubs/downloads/dialysis-guide-2012.pdf. Accessed April 1, 2016.

Centers for Disease Control and Prevention (CDC). Chronic Kidney Disease Surveillance Project. 2015. Available at: https://nccd.cdc.gov/CKD/default.aspx. Accessed March 28, 2016.

Centers for Medicare and Medicaid Services (CMS). Report for the standardized readmission ratio. 2014. Available at: https://www.cms.gov/Medicare/Quality-Initiatives-Patient-Assessment-Instruments/ESRDQIP/Downloads/MeasureMethodologyReport-fortheProposedSRRMeasure.pdf. Accessed March 25, 2016.

Chen J, Muntner P, Hamm LL, et al. The metabolic syndrome and chronic kidney disease in U.S. adults. *Ann Intern Med.* 2004;140(3):167–174.

Choudhury D, Luna-Salazar C. Preventive health care in chronic kidney disease and end-stage renal disease. *Nat Clin Pract Nephrol.* 2008;4(4):194–206.

Danziger J. Importance of low-grade albuminuria. *Mayo Clin Proc.* 2008;83(7):806–812.

de Brito-Ashurst I, Varagunam M, Raftery MJ, Yaqoob MM. Bicarbonate supplementation slows progression of CKD and improves nutritional status. *J Am Soc Nephrol.* 2009;20(9):2075–2084.

de Zeeuw D, Remuzzi G, Parving HH, et al. Proteinuria, a target for renoprotection in patients with type 2 diabetic nephropathy: lessons from RENAAL. *Kidney Int.* 2004; 65(6):2309–2320.

DuBose TD Jr. American Society of Nephrology Presidential Address 2006: chronic kidney disease as a public health threat—new strategy for a growing problem. *J Am Soc Nephrol.* 2007;18(4):1038–1045.

Ejerblad E, Fored CM, Lindblad P, Fryzek J, McLaughlin JK, Nyren O. Obesity and risk for chronic renal failure. *J Am Soc Nephrol.* 2006;17(6):1695–1702.

Eriksson J, Forsen T, Tuomilehto J, Osmond C, Barker D. Fetal and childhood growth and hypertension in adult life. *Hypertension.* 2000;36(5):790–794.

Florkowski CM, Chew-Harris JS. Methods of estimating GFR—different equations including CKD-EPI. *Clin Biochem Rev.* 2011;32(2):75–79.

Fouque D, Aparicio M. Eleven reasons to control the protein intake of patients with chronic kidney disease. *Nat Clin Pract Nephrol.* 2007;3(7):383–392.

Friedman DJ, Pollak MR. Genetics of kidney failure and the evolving story of APOL1. *J Clin Invest.* 2011;121(9):3367–3374.

Genovese G, Friedman DJ, Ross MD, et al. Association of trypanolytic ApoL1 variants with kidney disease in African Americans. *Science.* 2010;329(5993):841–845.

Gilbertson DT, Ebben JP, Foley RN, Weinhandl ED, Bradbury BD, Collins AJ. Hemoglobin level variability: associations with mortality. *Clin J Am Soc Nephrol.* 2008;3(1):133–138.

Ginsberg JM, Chang BS, Matarese RA, Garella S. Use of single voided urine samples to estimate quantitative proteinuria. *N Engl J Med.* 1983;309(25):1543–1546.

Glassock RJ, Winearls C. Screening for CKD with eGFR: doubts and dangers. *Clin J Am Soc Nephrol.* 2008;3(5):1563–1568.

Grootendorst DC, Jager KJ, Zoccali C, Dekker FW. Screening: why, when, and how. *Kidney Int.* 2009;76(7):694–699.

Hallan SI, Coresh J, Astor BC, et al. International comparison of the relationship of chronic kidney disease prevalence and ESRD risk. *J Am Soc Nephrol.* 2006;17(8): 2275–2284.

Hallan SI, Ritz E, Lydersen S, Romundstad S, Kvenild K, Orth SR. Combining GFR and albuminuria to classify CKD improves prediction of ESRD. *J Am Soc Nephrol.* 2009;20(5):1069–1077.

Haroun MK, Jaar BG, Hoffman SC, Comstock GW, Klag MJ, Coresh J. Risk factors for chronic kidney disease: a prospective study of 23,534 men and women in Washington County, Maryland. *J Am Soc Nephrol.* 2003;14(11):2934–2941.

Hirsh DA, Ogur B, Thibault GE, Cox M. "Continuity" as an organizing principle for clinical education reform. *N Engl J Med.* 2007;356(8):858–866.

Hoerger TJ, Simpson SA, Yarnoff BO, et al. The future burden of CKD in the United States: a simulation model for the CDC CKD initiative. *Am J Kidney Dis.* 2015;65(3):403–411.

Hostetter TH, Meyer TW, Rennke HG, Brenner BM. Chronic effects of dietary protein in the rat with intact and reduced renal mass. *Kidney Int.* 1986;30(4):509–517.

Hsu CY, McCulloch CE, Iribarren C, Darbinian J, Go AS. Body mass index and risk for end-stage renal disease. *Ann Intern Med.* 2006;144(1):21–28.

Ibsen H, Olsen MH, Wachtell K, et al. Reduction in albuminuria translates to reduction in cardiovascular events in hypertensive patients: losartan intervention for endpoint reduction in hypertension study. *Hypertension.* 2005;45(2):198–202.

Jafar TH, Stark PC, Schmid CH, et al. Progression of chronic kidney disease: the role of blood pressure control, proteinuria, and angiotensin-converting enzyme inhibition: a patient-level meta-analysis. *Ann Intern Med.* 2003;139(4):244–252.

Jones C, Roderick P, Harris S, Rogerson M. An evaluation of a shared primary and secondary care nephrology service for managing patients with moderate to advanced CKD. *Am J Kidney Dis.* 2006;47(1):103–114.

Jurkovitz C, Franch H, Shoham D, Bellenger J, McClellan W. Family members of patients treated for ESRD have high rates of undetected kidney disease. *Am J Kidney Dis.* 2002;40(6):1173–1178.

Kalantar-Zadeh K, Kovesdy CP, Derose SF, Horwich TB, Fonarow GC. Racial and survival paradoxes in chronic kidney disease. *Nat Clin Pract Nephrol.* 2007;3(9):493–506.

Kanji Z, Powe CE, Wenger JB, et al. Genetic variation in APOL1 associates with younger age at hemodialysis initiation. *J Am Soc Nephrol.* 2011;22(11):2091–2097.

Kazmi WH, Kausz AT, Khan S, et al. Anemia: an early complication of chronic renal insufficiency. *Am J Kidney Dis.* 2001;38(4):803–812.

Keith DS, Nichols GA, Gullion CM, Brown JB, Smith DH. Longitudinal follow-up and outcomes among a population with chronic kidney disease in a large managed care organization. *Arch Intern Med.* 2004;164(6):659–663.

Kendrick J, Chonchol MB. Nontraditional risk factors for cardiovascular disease in patients with chronic kidney disease. *Nat Clin Pract Nephrol.* 2008;4(12):672–681.

Kidney Disease: Improving Global Outcomes (KDIGO) Anemia Work Group. 2012. KDIGO clinical practice guideline for anemia in chronic kidney disease. *Kidney Inter.* 2012;(2):279–335.

Kidney Disease: Improving Global Outcomes (KDIGO) Lipid Work Group. 2012. KDIGO clinical practice guideline for lipid management in chronic kidney disease. *Kidney Inter.* 2013;(3):259–305.

Kidney Disease: Improving Global Outcomes (KDIGO) CKD Work Group. 2012. KDIGO 2012 clinical practice guideline for the evaluation and management of chronic kidney disease. *Kidney Inter.* 2013;(3):1–150.

Kidney Disease Outcomes Quality Initiative (KDOQI). KDOQI clinical practice guidelines on hypertension and antihypertensive agents in chronic kidney disease. *Am J Kidney Dis.* 2004;43(5 suppl 1):S1–S290.

Kopp JB, Nelson GW, Sampath K, et al. APOL1 genetic variants in focal segmental glomerulosclerosis and HIV-associated nephropathy. *J Am Soc Nephrol.* 2011;22(11): 2129–2137.

Lackland DT, Bendall HE, Osmond C, Egan BM, Barker DJ. Low birth weights contribute to high rates of early-onset chronic renal failure in the Southeastern United States. *Arch Intern Med.* 2000;160(10):1472–1476.

Lea JP, McClellan WM, Melcher C, Gladstone E, Hostetter T. CKD risk factors reported by primary care physicians: do guidelines make a difference? *Am J Kidney Dis.* 2006;47(1):72–77.

Lei HH, Perneger TV, Klag MJ, Whelton PK, Coresh J. Familial aggregation of renal disease in a population-based case–control study. *J Am Soc Nephrol.* 1998;9(7):1270–1276.

Levey AS, Atkins R, Coresh J, et al. Chronic kidney disease as a global public health problem: approaches and initiatives—a position statement from Kidney Disease Improving Global Outcomes. *Kidney Int.* 2007;72(3):247–259.

Levin A, Thompson CR, Ethier J, et al. Left ventricular mass index increase in early renal disease: impact of decline in hemoglobin. *Am J Kidney Dis.* 1999;34(1):125–134.

Lionakis N, Mendrinos D, Sanidas E, Favatas G, Georgopoulou M. Hypertension in the elderly. *World J Cardiol.* 2012;4(5):135–147.

Lorenzo C, Serrano-Rios M, Martinez-Larrad MT, et al. Prevalence of hypertension in Hispanic and non-Hispanic white populations. *Hypertension.* 2002;39(2):203–208.

Lucove J, Vupputuri S, Heiss G, North K, Russell M. Metabolic syndrome and the development of CKD in American Indians: the Strong Heart Study. *Am J Kidney Dis.* 2008;51(1):21–28.

Martin KJ, Gonzalez EA. Metabolic bone disease in chronic kidney disease. *J Am Soc Nephrol.* 2007;18(3):875–885.

Martins D, Agodoa L, Norris K. Chronic kidney disease in disadvantaged populations. *Int J Nephrol.* 2012;2012:469265.

McClellan WM, Ramirez SP, Jurkovitz C. Screening for chronic kidney disease: unresolved issues. *J Am Soc Nephrol.* 2003;14(7 suppl 2):S81–S87.

Mehrotra R, Marsh D, Vonesh E, Peters V, Nissenson A. Patient education and access of ESRD patients to renal replacement therapies beyond in-center hemodialysis. *Kidney Int.* 2005;68(1):378–390.

Melamed ML, Bauer C, Hostetter TH. eGFR: is it ready for early identification of CKD? *Clin J Am Soc Nephrol.* 2008;3(5):1569–1572.

Minutolo R, Agarwal R, Borrelli S, et al. Prognostic role of ambulatory blood pressure measurement in patients with nondialysis chronic kidney disease. *Arch Intern Med.* 2011;171(12):1090–1098.

Mogensen CE. Microalbuminuria predicts clinical proteinuria and early mortality in maturity-onset diabetes. *N Engl J Med.* 1984;310(6):356–360.

Mokdad AH, Bowman BA, Ford ES, Vinicor F, Marks JS, Koplan JP. The continuing epidemics of obesity and diabetes in the United States. *JAMA.* 2001;286(10):1195–1200.

Moorthy AV, Jaffery JB. Chronic kidney disease. In: Remington PL, Brownson RC, Wegner MV, eds. *Chronic Disease Epidemiology and Control.* Washington, DC: American Public Health Association; 2010:624.

National Kidney Foundation. KDOQI clinical practice guideline for diabetes and CKD: 2012 update. *Am J Kidney Dis.* 2012;60(5):850–886.

Navaneethan SD, Nigwekar SU, Sehgal AR, Strippoli GF. Aldosterone antagonists for preventing the progression of chronic kidney disease: a systematic review and meta-analysis. *Clin J Am Soc Nephrol.* 2009;4(3):542–551.

Norris K, Nissenson AR. Race, gender, and socioeconomic disparities in CKD in the United States. *J Am Soc Nephrol.* 2008;19(7):1261–1270.

Obermayr RP, Temml C, Gutjahr G, Knechtelsdorfer M, Oberbauer R, Klauser-Braun R. Elevated uric acid increases the risk for kidney disease. *J Am Soc Nephrol.* 2008;19(12):2407–2413.

Orth SR. Smoking and the kidney. *J Am Soc Nephrol.* 2002;13(6):1663–1672.

Pascual JM, Rodilla E, Gonzalez C, Perez-Hoyos S, Redon J. Long-term impact of systolic blood pressure and glycemia on the development of microalbuminuria in essential hypertension. *Hypertension.* 2005;45(6):1125–1130.

Patel UD, Young EW, Ojo AO, Hayward RA. CKD progression and mortality among older patients with diabetes. *Am J Kidney Dis.* 2005;46(3):406–414.

Peralta CA, Ziv E, Katz R, et al. African ancestry, socioeconomic status, and kidney function in elderly African Americans: a genetic admixture analysis. *J Am Soc Nephrol.* 2006;17(12):3491–3496.

Perneger TV, Brancati FL, Whelton PK, Klag MJ. End-stage renal disease attributable to diabetes mellitus. *Ann Intern Med.* 1994;121(12):912–918.

Pinto-Sietsma SJ, Navis G, Janssen WM, de Zeeuw D, Gans RO, de Jong PE. A central body fat distribution is related to renal function impairment, even in lean subjects. *Am J Kidney Dis.* 2003;41(4):733–741.

Poggio ED, Wang X, Greene T, Van Lente F, Hall PM. Performance of the modification of diet in renal disease and Cockcroft-Gault equations in the estimation of GFR in health and in chronic kidney disease. *J Am Soc Nephrol.* 2005;16(2):459–466.

Pugh JA. Diabetic nephropathy and end-stage renal disease in Mexican Americans. *Blood Purif.* 1996;14(4):286–292.

Pugh JA, Stern MP, Haffner SM, Eifler CW, Zapata M. Excess incidence of treatment of end-stage renal disease in Mexican Americans. *Am J Epidemiol.* 1988;127(1):135–144.

Quiroga B, Arroyo D, de Arriba G. Present and future in the treatment of diabetic kidney disease. *J Diabetes Res.* 2015;2015:801348.

Quiroga B, Fernandez Juarez G, Luno J. Combined angiotensin inhibition in diabetic nephropathy. *N Engl J Med.* 2014;370(8):777.

Ravera M, Re M, Deferrari L, Vettoretti S, Deferrari G. Importance of blood pressure control in chronic kidney disease. *J Am Soc Nephrol.* 2006;17(4 suppl 2):S98–S103.

Raymond NR, D'Eramo-Melkus G. Non-insulin-dependent diabetes and obesity in the black and Hispanic population: culturally sensitive management. *Diabetes Educ.* 1993;19(4):313–317.

Rettig RA, Norris K, Nissenson AR. Chronic kidney disease in the United States: a public policy imperative. *Clin J Am Soc Nephrol.* 2008;3(6):1902–1910.

Richards N, Harris K, Whitfield M, et al. Primary care–based disease management of chronic kidney disease (CKD), based on estimated glomerular filtration rate (eGFR) reporting, improves patient outcomes. *Nephrol Dial Transplant.* 2008;23(2):549–555.

Ruggenenti P, Perna A, Remuzzi G. ACE inhibitors to prevent end-stage renal disease: when to start and why possibly never to stop: a post hoc analysis of the REIN trial results. Ramipril Efficacy in Nephropathy. *J Am Soc Nephrol.* 2001;12(12):2832–2837.

Ruggenenti P, Perticucci E, Cravedi P, et al. Role of remission clinics in the longitudinal treatment of CKD. *J Am Soc Nephrol.* 2008;19(6):1213–1224.

Ruggenenti P, Remuzzi G. Kidney failure stabilizes after a two-decade increase: impact on global (renal and cardiovascular) health. *Clin J Am Soc Nephrol.* 2007;2(1):146–150.

Rule AD, Larson TS, Bergstralh EJ, Slezak JM, Jacobsen SJ, Cosio FG. Using serum creatinine to estimate glomerular filtration rate: accuracy in good health and in chronic kidney disease. *Ann Intern Med.* 2004;141(12):929–937.

Sarafidis PA, Bakris GL. State of hypertension management in the United States: confluence of risk factors and the prevalence of resistant hypertension. *J Clin Hypertens (Greenwich).* 2008;10(2):130–139.

Saunders MR, Cifu A, Vela M. Screening for chronic kidney disease. *JAMA.* 2015;314(6): 615–616.

Shah A, Fried LF, Chen SC, et al. Associations between access to care and awareness of CKD. *Am J Kidney Dis.* 2012;59(3 suppl 2):S16–S23.

Shlipak MG, Fried LF, Cushman M, et al. Cardiovascular mortality risk in chronic kidney disease: comparison of traditional and novel risk factors. *JAMA.* 2005;293(14):1737–1745.

Shlipak MG, Katz R, Sarnak MJ, et al. Cystatin C and prognosis for cardiovascular and kidney outcomes in elderly persons without chronic kidney disease. *Ann Intern Med.* 2006;145(4):237–246.

Shoker A, Hossain MA, Koru-Sengul T, Raju DL, Cockcroft D. Performance of creatinine clearance equations on the original Cockcroft-Gault population. *Clin Nephrol.* 2006;66(2):89–97.

Shultis WA, Weil EJ, Looker HC, et al. Effect of periodontitis on overt nephropathy and end-stage renal disease in type 2 diabetes. *Diabetes Care.* 2007;30(2):306–311.

Stengel B, Tarver-Carr ME, Powe NR, Eberhardt MS, Brancati, Frederick L. Lifestyle factors, obesity and the risk of chronic kidney disease epidemiology. 2003;14(4):479–487.

Stevens LA, Coresh J, Greene T, Levey AS. Assessing kidney function—measured and estimated glomerular filtration rate. *N Engl J Med*. 2006;354(23):2473–2483.

Stevens LA, Li S, Wang C, et al. Prevalence of CKD and comorbid illness in elderly patients in the United States: results from the Kidney Early Evaluation Program (KEEP). *Am J Kidney Dis*. 2010;55(3 suppl 2):S23–S33.

Thomas MC, Viberti G, Groop PH. Screening for chronic kidney disease in patients with diabetes: are we missing the point? *Nat Clin Pract Nephrol*. 2008;4(1):2–3.

Tonelli M, Wiebe N, Culleton B, et al. Chronic kidney disease and mortality risk: a systematic review. *J Am Soc Nephrol*. 2006;17(7):2034–2047.

Tuttle KR. Albuminuria reduction: the holy grail for kidney protection. *Kidney Int*. 2007;72(7):785–786.

UK Prospective Diabetes Study (UKPDS) Group. Intensive blood-glucose control with sulphonylureas or insulin compared with conventional treatment and risk of complications in patients with type 2 diabetes (UKPDS 33). *Lancet*. 1998;352(9131): 837–853.

Upadhyay A, Earley A, Lamont JL, Haynes S, Wanner C, Balk EM. Lipid-lowering therapy in persons with chronic kidney disease: a systematic review and meta-analysis. *Ann Intern Med*. 2012;157(4):251–262.

US Renal Data System (USRDS). *Annual Data Report: Atlas of Chronic Kidney Disease and End-Stage Renal Disease in the United States*. Bethesda, MD: National Institutes of Health, National Institute of Diabetes and Digestive and Kidney Diseases; 2013.

US Renal Data System (USRDS). *Annual Data Report: Atlas of Chronic Kidney Disease and End-Stage Renal Disease in the United States*. Bethesda, MD: National Institutes of Health, National Institute of Diabetes and Digestive and Kidney Diseases; 2015.

Vassalotti JA, Li S, McCullough PA, Bakris GL. Kidney early evaluation program: a community-based screening approach to address disparities in chronic kidney disease. *Semin Nephrol*. 2010;30(1):66–73.

Vikse BE, Irgens LM, Leivestad T, Hallan S, Iversen BM. Low birth weight increases risk for end-stage renal disease. *J Am Soc Nephrol*. 2008;19(1):151–157.

Wahba IM, Mak RH. Obesity and obesity-initiated metabolic syndrome: mechanistic links to chronic kidney disease. *Clin J Am Soc Nephrol*. 2007;2(3):550–562.

Winkelmayer WC, Owen W, Glynn RJ, Levin R, Avorn J. Preventive health care measures before and after start of renal replacement therapy. *J Gen Intern Med*. 2002;17(8): 588–595.

Wright JT Jr, Williamson JD, Whelton PK, et al. A randomized trial of intensive versus standard blood-pressure control. *N Engl J Med*. 2015;373(22):2103–2116.

Young JH, Klag MJ, Muntner P, Whyte JL, Pahor M, Coresh J. Blood pressure and decline in kidney function: findings from the Systolic Hypertension in the Elderly Program (SHEP). *J Am Soc Nephrol*. 2002;13(11):2776–2782.

Zerhouni EA. Translational research: moving discovery to practice. *Clin Pharmacol Ther*. 2007;81(1):126–128.

CONTRIBUTORS

Alexandra Adams, MD, PhD
Center for American Indian and Rural
Health Equity
Montana State University
Bozeman, MT
Chapter 8: Diet and Nutrition

Henry A. Anderson, MD
Department of Population Health Services
School of Medicine and Public Health
University of Wisconsin
Madison, WI
Chapter 17: Chronic Respiratory Diseases

**Barbara E. Ainsworth, PhD, MPH,
FACSM**
School of Nutrition and Health Promotion
College of Health Solutions
Arizona State University
Phoenix, AZ
Chapter 9: Physical Activity

Benjamin J. Apelberg, PhD, MHS
Center for Tobacco Products
Food and Drug Administration
Silver Spring, MD
Chapter 7: Tobacco Use

Karina A. Atwell, MD, MPH
School of Medicine and Public Health
University of Wisconsin
Madison, WI
*Chapter 5: The Role of Health Care
Systems in Chronic Disease Prevention
and Control*

John Auerbach, MBA
Centers for Disease Control and Prevention
Atlanta, GA
Foreword

Julie A. Baldwin, PhD
Center for Health Equity
Northern Arizona University
Flagstaff, AZ
Chapter 4: Community-Based Interventions

Ursula E. Bauer, PhD, MPH
National Center for Chronic Disease
Prevention and Health Promotion
Centers for Disease Control and
Prevention
Atlanta, GA
*Chapter 1: Current Issues and Challenges
in Chronic Disease Prevention and Control*

Leonelo E. Bautista, MD, DrPH, MPH
Department of Population Health Sciences
University of Wisconsin
Madison, WI
Chapter 13: High Blood Pressure

Donald B. Bishop, PhD
Center for Health Promotion
Minnesota Department of Health
St. Paul, MN
Chapter 12: Diabetes

Peter A. Briss, MD, MPH, CAPT USPHS
National Center for Chronic Disease
Prevention and Health Promotion
Centers for Disease Control and
Prevention
Atlanta, GA
*Chapter 1: Current Issues and Challenges
in Chronic Disease Prevention and
Control*

Heidi M. Blanck, PhD, CAPT USPHS
Division of Nutrition, Physical Activity,
and Obesity
National Center for Chronic Disease
Prevention and Health Promotion
Centers for Disease Control and
Prevention
Atlanta, GA
Chapter 11: Obesity

Randall Brown, MD, PhD, FASAM
School of Medicine and Public Health
University of Wisconsin
William S. Middleton Memorial
Veterans Hospital
Madison, WI
Chapter 10: Alcohol Use

Ross C. Brownson, PhD
Prevention Research Center
Brown School and Washington University
School of Medicine,
St. Louis, MO
Preface
Chapter 2: Chronic Disease Epidemiology
Chapter 16: Cancer

Carol A. Bryant, PhD
Florida Prevention Research Center
College of Public Health University of
South Florida Tampa, FL
Chapter 4: Community-Based Interventions

Huan J. Chang, MD, MPH
University of Illinois at Chicago
Jesse Brown VA Hospital
Chicago, IL
*Chapter 20: Arthritis and Other
Musculoskeletal Diseases*

Rowland W. Chang, MD, MPH
Feinberg School of Medicine
Northwestern University
Chicago, IL
*Chapter 20: Arthritis and Other
Musculoskeletal Diseases*

Karly Christensen, BS
School of Medicine and Public Health
University of Wisconsin
Madison, WI
Chapter 10: Alcohol Use

Brienna Deyo, MPH
School of Medicine and Public Health
University of Wisconsin
Madison, WI
Chapter 10: Alcohol Use

Ousmane Diallo, MD, PhD
Wisconsin Division of Public
Health
Department of Health Services
Madison, WI
*Chapter 3: Chronic Disease
Surveillance*

Dorothy D. Dunlop, PhD
Feinberg School of Medicine
Northwestern University
Chicago, IL
*Chapter 20: Arthritis and Other
Musculoskeletal Diseases*

Daniel J. Finn, MPH
Feinberg School of Medicine
Northwestern University
Chicago, IL
*Chapter 20: Arthritis and Other
Musculoskeletal Diseases*

Deborah A. Galuska, PhD, MPH
Division of Nutrition, Physical
Activity, and Obesity
National Center for Chronic
Disease Prevention and Health
Promotion
Centers for Disease Control and
Prevention
Atlanta, GA
Chapter 11: Obesity

Cassandra Greenwood, BS
School of Medicine and Public
Health
University of Wisconsin
Madison, WI
Chapter 8: Diet and Nutrition

Debra Haire-Joshu, PhD
Center for Obesity Prevention and
Policy Research
Washington University in St. Louis
St. Louis, MO
Chapter 12: Diabetes

Brittany Hayes, MA
School of Medicine and Public Health
University of Wisconsin
Madison, WI
Chapter 10: Alcohol Use

Carlyn M. Hood, MPA, MPH
OCHIN (Oregon Community Health
Information Network)
Portland, Oregon
*Chapter 6: The Social Determinants of
Chronic Disease*

Corinne G. Husten, MD, MPH
Center for Tobacco Products
Food and Drug Administration
Silver Spring MD
Chapter 7: Tobacco Use

Jonathan B. Jaffery, MD, MS
School of Medicine and Public
Health
University of Wisconsin
Madison, WI
Chapter 22: Chronic Kidney Disease

Corinne Joshu, PhD, MPH, MA
Department of Epidemiology
Bloomberg School of Public Health
Johns Hopkins University
Baltimore, MD
Chapter 16: Cancer

Renée S.M. Kidney, PhD, MPH
Health Promotion and Chronic
Disease Division
Minnesota Department of Health
St. Paul, MN
Chapter 12: Diabetes

Paula Lantz, PhD, MS
Gerald R. Ford School of Public
Policy University of Michigan
Ann Arbor, MI
*Chapter 6: The Social Determinants of
Chronic Disease*

Longjian Liu, MD, PhD, MSc
Department of Epidemiology and
Biostatistics
Dornsife School of Public Health
Drexel University
Philadelphia, PA
Chapter 15: Cardiovascular Disease

Fleetwood Loustalot, PhD, FNP
Division for Heart Disease and Stroke
Prevention
National Center for Chronic
Disease Prevention and Health
Promotion
Centers for Disease Control and
Prevention
Atlanta, GA
Chapter 14: Dyslipidemia

Caroline A. Macera, PhD, FACSM
Graduate School of Public Health
San Diego State University
San Diego, CA
Chapter 9: Physical Activity

Ron Manderscheid, PhD
National Association of County
Behavioral Health
Washington, DC
Chapter 18: Mental Disorders

James S. Marks, MD, MPH
Robert Wood Johnson Foundation
Princeton, NJ
Foreword

Mary P. Martinasek, PhD, MPH
College of Natural and Health Sciences
University of Tampa
Tampa, FL
Chapter 4: Community-Based Interventions

Alyssa B. Mayer, PhD, MPH
Center for Health Equity
Northern Arizona University
Flagstaff, AZ
*Chapter 4: Community-Based
Interventions*

Robert J. McDermott, PhD
School of Medicine and Public Health
University of Wisconsin
Madison, WI
Chapter 4: Community-Based Interventions

Carla I. Mercado, PhD, MS
Division for Heart Disease and Stroke
Prevention
National Center for Chronic Disease
Prevention and Health Promotion
Centers for Disease Control and
Prevention
Atlanta, GA
Chapter 14: Dyslipidemia

Jordan Mills, DO, PhD
School of Medicine and Public Health
University of Wisconsin
William S. Middleton Memorial
Veterans Hospital
Madison, WI
Chapter 10: Alcohol Use

Julianne Nelson, MPH
Department of Epidemiology and
Biostatistics
Dornsife School of Public Health
Drexel University
Philadelphia, PA
Chapter 15: Cardiovascular Disease

Craig J. Newschaffer, PhD
Department of Epidemiology and
Biostatistics
Dornsife School of Public Health
Drexel University
Philadelphia, PA
Chapter 15: Cardiovascular Disease

Patrick J. O'Connor, MD, MA, MPH
HealthPartners Institute
Center for Chronic Care
Innovation
Minneapolis, MN
Chapter 12: Diabetes

Parvathy Pillai, MD, MPH
School of Medicine and Public
Health
University of Wisconsin
Madison, WI
*Chapter 6: The Social Determinants of
Chronic Disease*

Maria Mora Pinzon, MD, MS
School of Medicine and Public Health
University of Wisconsin
Madison, WI
Chapter 16: Cancer

Robert Redwood, MD, MPH
School of Medicine and Public
Health
University of Wisconsin
Madison, WI
*Chapter 2: Chronic Disease
Epidemiology*

Patrick L. Remington, MD, MPH
School of Medicine and Public Health
University of Wisconsin
Madison, WI
Preface
Chapter 2: Chronic Disease Epidemiology
Chapter 3: Chronic Disease Surveillance

Adnan Said, MD, MSPH
Division of Gastroenterology and
Hepatology
Department of Medicine
School of Medicine and Public
Health
University of Wisconsin
Madison, WI
Chapter 21: Chronic Liver Disease

Rachel Sippy, MPH
Department of Population Health
Sciences
University of Wisconsin
Madison, WI
Chapter 8: Diet and Nutrition

Maureen A. Smith, MD, PhD, MPH
School of Medicine and Public Health
University of Wisconsin
Madison, WI
Chapter 5: The Role of Health Care Systems in Chronic Disease Prevention and Control

Elizabeth Stein, MD, MS
School of Medicine and Public Health
University of Wisconsin
Madison, WI
Chapter 18: Mental Disorders

Diego Tamez, MD
School of Medicine and Public Health
University of Wisconsin
Madison, WI
Chapter 20: Arthritis and Other Musculoskeletal Disorders

Matthew Thomas, MD
School of Medicine & Public Health
University of Wisconsin
William S. Middleton Memorial Veterans Hospital
Madison, WI
Chapter 10: Alcohol Use

Carrie Tomasallo, PhD, MPH
Wisconsin Division of Public Health
Department of Health Services
Madison, WI
Chapter 17: Chronic Respiratory Diseases

Edwin Trevathan, MD, MPH
Division of Pediatric Neurology
Vanderbilt Institute for Global Health
Vanderbilt University Medical Center
Nashville, TN
Chapter 19: Neurological Disorders

Sandra D. Vamos, EdD
School of Public Health and Social Policy
University of Victoria
Victoria, BC (Canada)
Chapter 4: Community-Based Interventions

Sana Waheed, MD
School of Medicine and Public Health
University of Wisconsin
Madison, WI
Chapter 22: Chronic Kidney Disease

Mark V. Wegner, MD, MPH
Wisconsin Division of Public Health
Department of Health Services
Madison, WI
Preface
Chapter 3: Chronic Disease Surveillance

Bethany Weinert, MD, MPH
Children's Medical Group
Children's Hospital of Wisconsin
Milwaukee, WI
Chapter 8: Diet and Nutrition

Mark A. Werner, PhD
Wisconsin Division of Public Health
Department of Health Services
Madison, WI
Chapter 17: Chronic Respiratory Disease

INDEX

A

abortion and breast cancer, 59
ACA. *See* Patient Protection and Affordable
　Care Act
acamprosate (Campral), 466
access to health care. *See* disparities in health
　care
accountable care organizations (ACOs),
　170–171
　Chronic Care Model, 178–179
Accountable Health Communities Model,
　173–174
Active for Life, 418
Active Living Every Day, 410, 968
activity dose definition, 393, 394
acupuncture
　fibromyalgia, 989
　osteoarthritis, 974
acute stroke. *See also* stroke
　recombinant tissue plasminogen activator,
　　707–708
　significance, 695
　state-based registries, 87, 708
addiction to tobacco, 243. *See also* substance
　use disorders
　cigarettes, 243
　cigars, 253
　electronic cigarettes, 256
　hookahs, 254
　pipes, 254
　smokeless tobacco, 243, 251, 252
　withdrawal from nicotine, 263–264
ADHD. *See* attention-deficit/hyperactivity
　disorder
adherence to prescribed care
　communication by care provider, 126
　dyslipidemia, 634, 656
　mental health, 612, 881–882

administrative data collection systems, 82, 89–90
adolescents. *See* youths
advertising. *See* media influence
Affordable Care Act (ACA). *See* Patient
　Protection and Affordable Care Act
Afterschool Snacks, 361
age differences, controlling for, 47–48
aging population
　alcohol consumption, 442–443
　arthritis
　　osteoarthritis, 971
　　rheumatoid arthritis, 977
　cancer
　　breast cancer, 762
　　cervical cancer screening, 772
　　colorectal cancer, 758, 760
　　lung cancer, 753
　　significance, 743
　diabetes, 530
　expenditures for health care, 7
　heart failure, 711, 713
　high blood pressure, 587, 596
　　kidney disease and, 1070
　kidney disease, 1066, 1068, 1070, 1071
　liver disease
　　hepatitis C, 1036, 1037, 1039
　　non-alcoholic fatty liver, 1044
　mental health
　　anxiety disorders, 867
　　depression, 869
　neurological disorders
　　Alzheimer's disease, 910
　　epilepsy, 903–904
　　Parkinson's disease, 906–907
　　spinal cord injuries, 935
　nutrition, 339
　　salt intake, 333
　　Senior Farmer's Market Nutrition
　　　Program, 361

obesity and mortality, 489
osteoporosis, 994, 996, 999, 1000, 1001
peripheral arterial disease, 719
physical activity, 392, 402, 418
respiratory diseases
  asthma, 808
  chronic obstructive pulmonary
    disease, 813
  sleep apnea, 821
significance, 4, 7, 20
  health system interventions, 165
agricultural policy, 361, 363
AIDS and Hodgkin's lymphoma, 775
Alcohol Related Disease Impact
  System, 455
alcohol use
  alcohol-based hand sanitizer, 442
  analytic epidemiology
    causes, 456–457, 468
    interventions, 457–468
    population-attributable risk, 457
  as behavioral determinant, 111
  caloric density, 433
  cancer and, 750
    breast cancer, 763, 764
    colorectal cancer, 759
    oral cavity, 779
    pharyngeal cancer, 436, 779
  coronary heart disease and, 433, 686–687
  costs of, 111, 433, 437
  definitions of terms, 434–435
  dementias and, 912
  descriptive epidemiology, 437–441
    adolescents, 440, 441–442, 448,
      449–452
    binge drinking, 448, 449–451, 452
    college drinking, 446
    gender, 440, 443–444
    genetics, 447
    geographic distribution, 447–453
    older adults, 440, 442–443
    social stigma, 446–447
    race/ethnicity, 440, 444–446
    surveillance, 439–441, 448, 452–453,
      454–455
    time trends, 453–456, 1023–1024
  diabetes and, 539
  Dietary Guidelines, 333
  dyslipidemia and, 648, 649
  future research, 468–469
  gout and, 983, 984
  guidelines for consumption, 432, 437
  hepatitis B and, 1030
  hepatitis C and, 1035
  high blood pressure and, 457, 599–600, 604,
    605, 607, 686
  interventions

examples, 465–468
prevention, 457–458
screening, 459–462
treatment, 462–465, 466
liver disease and, 1021, 1022. See also
  alcoholic liver disease
  cirrhosis, 1022, 1023
  hepatitis C, 1039, 1041
  hepatocellular carcinoma, 1048, 1049
mental illness and, 874
osteoporosis and, 999
pathophysiology, 435–437
  vehicle crashes, 435, 457, 466
price and, 458
protective effects of, 433, 686–687
significance, 433–435
  alcohol-induced deaths, 455–456
  overview, 7, 111
sleep apnea and, 821
socioeconomic status and, 447
use vs. misuse, 431–432
withdrawal, 436, 463–464
Alcohol Use Disorders Identification Test
  (AUDIT), 459–460, 461
Alcohol Use Disorders Identification
  Tool, 460
alcohol-based hand sanitizer ingestion, 442
alcoholic liver disease
  descriptive epidemiology, 1023–1024
    as attributable risk, 1021, 1022
    time trends, 1023–1024
  interventions for alcohol use
    examples, 465–468
    prevention, 457–458
    screening, 459–462
    treatment, 462–465, 466
  significance, 1022, 1024–1026
allostatic load, 210–211
Alzheimer's disease
  causes, 896, 911–912
    aluminum ingested, 912
  definition, 909–910
  dementia absent, 912
  descriptive epidemiology, 911
  diabetes and, 524
  future research, 913
  interventions, 912–913
  as mental disorder, 865
  pathophysiology, 911
  significance, 910
    high-risk groups, 896
ambulatory blood pressure monitoring,
  584–585, 613
  kidney disease, 1082
amenorrhea and osteoporosis, 1000
American Community Survey (ACS), 91
American Diabetes Association (ADA), 544

American Psychiatric Association (APA), 434, 435
American Stop Smoking Intervention Study (ASSIST), 289, 756
American Travel Survey. *See* National Household Travel Survey
Amigos en Salud diabetes education, 362
amputations
  diabetes, 521, 522–523, 528
    geographic distribution, 532
  peripheral arterial disease, 717, 722
amyotrophic lateral sclerosis (ALS)
  causes, 897, 921–922
  definition, 920
  descriptive epidemiology, 920–921
    high-risk groups, 897
  future research, 922–923
  interventions, 922–923
  pathophysiology, 920
  significance, 920
analytic epidemiology. *See also* determinants of disease
  chronic disease continuum, 38
  definition, 36–37, 40
  overview, 38, 49–52
    attributable risk, 62
    causality of associations, 59–62
    population-attributable risk, 63–65
    relative risk, 45, 56–57
    series of studies, 68–72
    single study insufficiency, 66–68
    study designs, 52–56
    validity of study results, 57–59
  relative risk, 45, 56–57
    population-attributable risk versus, 64
anemia and kidney disease, 1070
ankle–brachial index (ABI), 718, 722
ankylosing spondylitis (AS)
  Bath Ankylosing Spondylitis Disease Activity Index, 990
  definition, 989
  descriptive epidemiology, 991
  diagnosis, 989, 993
  future research, 993
  interventions, 991–993
    examples, 993
    prevention, 991–992
    screening, 992
    treatment, 992
  pathophysiology, 990
  significance, 990
ankylosis definition, 990
Annual Social and Economic Supplement (CPS), 214–217
Antabuse (disulfiram), 466
antisocial personality disorder and violent crimes, 861

anxiety
  alcohol use, 456, 874
  attention-deficit/hyperactivity disorder, 936
  coronary heart disease, 687
  fibromyalgia, 987
  as intervention side effect, 69
  medication adherence, 612
  mental health
    descriptive epidemiology, 870
    mortality, 861
    pathophysiology, 866–867
    screening, 877
  social anxiety
    pathophysiology, 866–867
    prevalence, 870
    youth alcohol use for, 456
  Tourette syndrome, 930
apnea definition, 820. *See also* sleep apnea
  apnea–hypopnea index, 820–821, 822
applied epidemiology definition, 37
arthritis
  ankylosing spondylitis
    definition, 989
    descriptive epidemiology, 991
    future research, 993
    interventions, 991–993
  descriptive epidemiology, 965–966, 967
  diabetes and, 524
  fibromyalgia
    causes, 988
    definition, 985–986
    descriptive epidemiology, 965
    interventions, 988–989
    pathophysiology, 986
    significance, 986
  gout
    causes, 984
    definition, 981–982
    descriptive epidemiology, 982–983
    interventions, 984–985
    pathophysiology, 982
    significance, 982
  interventions, 966–968
    social cognitive theory, 121
  osteoarthritis
    causes, 971–973, 975
    definition, 968
    descriptive epidemiology, 970–971
    future research, 976
    interventions, 973–976
    pathophysiology, 969–970
    significance, 969
  rheumatoid arthritis
    causes, 978–979
    definition, 976
    descriptive epidemiology, 977–978
    future research, 981

interventions, 979–981
pathophysiology, 977
significance, 976–977
smoking and, 262, 979
seronegative spondyloarthropathies, 989,
990
significance, 6, 965–966
Arthritis Foundation Aquatics Program, 976
Arthritis Foundation Exercise Program, 968
Arthritis Self-Help Course, 976
artificial sunlamps and melanoma, 780
asbestosis
causes, 834
descriptive epidemiology, 833–834
interventions, 835
lung cancer and asbestos, 65, 754, 826
significance, 832–833
aspartate transaminase (AST), 1017
Asperger's syndrome, 917
aspirin
cardiovascular impact, 288
colorectal cancer, 759, 760
diabetes, 529, 549
gout, 984
peripheral arterial disease, 721
stroke, 709
Assertive Community Treatment (ACT), 881
Assessment in Ankylosing Spondylitis
International Working Group, 992
asthma
analytic epidemiology
causes, 805–807
interventions, 807–810
modifiable risk factors, 805–807
population-attributable risk, 807
as chronic obstructive pulmonary disease,
796, 797
definition, 798
descriptive epidemiology
geographic distribution, 804
high-risk populations, 801–804
time trends, 804–805
future research, 810–811
hospitalization duration, 795
ICD-10 code, 798
interventions
community health workers, 125
examples, 809–810
prevention, 807–808
screening, 799, 808–809
treatment, 809
obesity and, 488, 489, 806
occupational asthma, 836–839
pathophysiology, 797–798, 800–801
significance, 800
socioeconomic status and, 205
tobacco use pathophysiology, 260

atherosclerosis
atherosclerotic cardiovascular disease
(ASCVD) risk scores, 657
ASCVD, 635, 650, 654, 655
cerebral thrombosis, 696
coronary heart disease, 677
CVD underlying disease process, 676
definition, 676
plaque buildup, 634, 652
peripheral arterial disease, 718
Pooled-Cohort ASCVD risk equation,
650–651
Atherosclerosis Risk in Communities (ARIC)
B-mode ultrasound screening, 677
heart failure, 710, 712
high blood pressure, 591
alcohol and, 600
peripheral arterial disease, 719
attention-deficit/hyperactivity disorder
(ADHD)
causes, 898, 938
definition, 936
descriptive epidemiology, 937
high-risk groups, 898
interventions, 938
as neurodevelopmental disorder, 864
pathophysiology, 937
significance, 936–937
Tourette syndrome and, 930
attributable risk definition, 62
audience of communication, 98
auras of seizures, 902
autism spectrum disorders
causes, 897, 918–919
definition, 916–917
descriptive epidemiology, 917–918
high-risk groups, 897
future research, 919
interventions, 919
as neurodevelopmental disorder, 864
pathophysiology, 917
significance, 917
automobile crashes. See motor vehicle crashes

B

back pain. See low back pain
Balance after Baby online intervention, 554
bariatric surgery and type 2 diabetes, 527
Bath Ankylosing Spondylitis Disease Activity
Index, 990
A Beautiful Mind (movie), 866
behavioral control perception, 119
behavioral determinants
cervical cancer, 771
lifestyle behaviors, 5–6.
overview, 110–112

parent education and child behavior, 879–880
physical activity, 404
significance, 187
as social over individual, 113–114, 120, 201
socioeconomic status and, 206–208
Theory of Planned Behavior, 118–119
Behavioral Risk Factor Surveillance System (BRFSS)
alcohol use, 448
chronic obstructive pulmonary disease, 811
nutritional data, 339, 351
physical activity, 398–399
smoking trends data, 83
stroke, 697
surveillance data, 17, 81, 88
Beijing Fangshan cardiovascular prevention program (BFCP), 692–693
benign rolandic epilepsy, 900, 904
benign tumors, 747–748
melanoma of the skin, 780
Best Practices for Comprehensive Tobacco Control (CDC), 756
beverages with sugar, 338
diabetes and, 338, 538
Dietary Guidelines, 333
gout and, 984
obesity and, 495
bias in studies, 58–59
bilirubin levels, 1017
binge drinking
definition, 452
descriptive epidemiology, 448, 449–451, 452
biomarkers
alanine transaminase as, 1017
alcohol use, 462
aspartate transaminase as, 1017
bilirubin levels as, 1017
chronic obstructive pulmonary disease, 816, 817
C-reactive protein as, 487, 684, 720, 970
diabetes strategies, 559
interleukin 6 as, 720, 970, 972–973
liver disease, 1017
nicotine biomarker, 251
obesity, 970
peripheral arterial disease, 720
prostate-specific antigen as, 773, 774
rheumatoid arthritis, 979
tumor necrosis factor-alpha as, 720, 970, 977
biopsychosocial model of mental health, 863, 880–881
bipolar disorder
attention-deficit/hyperactivity disorder and, 936
descriptive epidemiology, 869
homelessness and, 862

pathophysiology, 866
treatment, 880–881
violent crime and, 861
birth certificates, 84
birthweight. *See* low birthweight
Black Lung Compensation Program, 827
black lung disease. *See* coal workers' pneumoconiosis
bladder cancer
causes, 778
descriptive epidemiology, 777
induction period, 748
interventions, 778
significance, 744, 777
smoking and, 243, 252, 259, 778
blaming the victim, 114, 115, 138
blindness from diabetes, 521, 523, 528
blood alcohol concentration (BAC)
driving and, 457, 466
health care intervention, 467
as indicator of impairment, 437, 438
blood pressure monitoring. *See also* high blood pressure
ambulatory, 584–585, 613
kidney disease, 1082
home monitoring, 585, 613
measurement of blood pressure, 583–587
blood transfusions
hepatitis B, 1032, 1033
hepatitis C, 1035, 1038, 1040, 1041
Blueprint for Health (Vermont), 191
B-mode ultrasound, 677
body mass index (BMI)
arthritis
gout, 983
osteoarthritis, 972–973
as bone mineral density surrogate, 999
cancer, 750
colorectal cancer, 758, 759
coronary heart disease, 676, 686
diabetes
adult obesity, 487, 488, 528, 531, 533, 537
obesity pathophysiology, 490–491
obesity treatment, 501
type 2 diabetes pathophysiology, 526
youth obesity, 489
dyslipidemia, 644–645
health outcome and, 488
high blood pressure, 597–598, 604
kidney disease, 1072
liver disease, 1041
mortality and, 489
as obesity assessment, 485, 686
obesity screening, 500
sleep apnea, 821
youth, 485

bone density definition, 994
  measuring, 994
bone quality definition, 994
bone strength definition, 994
Boston Area Community Health (BACH) study,
  532–533
Brain Attack Surveillance in Corpus Christi
  (BASIC) Project, 696, 697–698
Breast and Cervical Cancer Mortality Prevention
  Act (1990), 772
breast cancer
  abortion and, 59
  age of first birth and, 45, 46
  alcohol use and, 436, 457
  analytic epidemiology
    causes, 763–764
    interventions, 765–768
    modifiable risk factors, 763–764
    population-attributable risk, 763, 764
  case-control study, 56
  chest x-rays and, 55
  chronic disease continuum, 39
  cumulative incidence, 44
  descriptive epidemiology
    geographic distribution, 762
    high-risk populations, 762
    introduction to, 42
    time trends, 762–763
  future research, 768
  information bias, 59
  interventions
    examples, 767–768
    Health Belief Model, 116–117
    prevention, 765
    screening, 112, 116, 762, 765–767,
      767–768
    treatment, 767
  mortality rates, 50
  pathophysiology, 761–762
  physical activity and, 392
  racial differences, 95, 96, 213–214
  significance, 45, 744, 761
  prevalence, 44
breast-feeding. See lactation
brief intervention
  alcohol use, 460, 462–463
  definition, 126–127
  for education, 140
  tobacco use, 287–288
bronchiectasis, 798
bronchitis
  as chronic obstructive pulmonary disease,
    796, 797, 811
  definition, 798
  hospitalization duration, 795
  ICD-10 code, 798
  pathophysiology, 797

buddy systems as interpersonal interventions,
  123–124
Building on Existing Tools to Improve Chronic
  Disease Prevention and Screening in
  Family Practice (BETTER), 186
bundled payment, 172–173
byssinosis
  causes, 836
  descriptive epidemiology, 836
  interventions, 836
  significance, 835

C

CAGE questionnaire, 459
Calgary Charter on Health Literacy, 150
Campral (acamprosate), 466
cancer. See also cancer and cigarette smoking;
    specific cancer
  alcohol use and, 436
  analytic epidemiology
    causes, 747, 749–750
    interventions, 750, 751
    risk assessment, 71
  classification, 748
    ICD-10 codes, 744, 748
  definition, 747–748
  depression from, 860
  descriptive epidemiology
    geographic distribution, 776
    time trends, 15, 743, 745
  gout and, 982
  induction period, 748
  interventions, 751
    prevention, 749–750
  nutrition
    dietary fat, 336
    dietary fiber, 335–336
    fruits and vegetables, 335
    red meat, 337
  obesity and, 488, 489, 490
  pathophysiology, 747–749
  physical activity and, 392, 396, 397
  significance, 743–747
    mortality, 15, 743, 745, 746, 747
    overview, 6, 15
  surveillance
    disease registries, 45, 86–87, 748–749
    evaluation of programs, 751
  tobacco use and, 749, 750
    cigar smoking, 252
    cigarette smoking. See cancer and
      cigarette smoking
    hookah smoking, 254
    pathophysiology, 258–259
    pipe smoking, 253
    relative risk, 247

secondhand smoke, 245, 246, 252, 258
smokeless tobacco, 251, 252
cancer and cigarette smoking, 749, 750
bladder cancer, 243, 778
cervical cancer, 770, 771
leukemia, 243, 259, 777
lung cancer, 243, 244, 245, 248, 254, 752, 754, 755
oral cavity cancer, 243, 252, 253, 259, 779
pathophysiology, 258–259
pharyngeal cancer, 243, 253
prostate cancer, 773
relative risk, 247
secondhand smoke, 245, 246, 249, 252, 258
tongue cancer, 779
Cancer Control P.L.A.N.E.T., 751
Capital Steel and Iron Company Cardiovascular Intervention Program (CSICIP), 692–693
car crashes. See motor vehicle crashes
cardiovascular disease (CVD). See also coronary heart disease; heart failure; peripheral arterial disease; stroke
ACA and screening charges, 112
alcohol use, 436, 468
chronic obstructive pulmonary disease, 813
definition, 673
depression from, 860
descriptive epidemiology
time trends, 673, 675
diabetes, 520–521, 522, 539–540
dyslipidemia as risk factor, 633, 635
diabetes type 2 and, 649–650
diverse populations, 639
familial hypercholesterolemia, 636
socioeconomic status and, 640
global health, 22
gout as risk factor, 982
high blood pressure, 595–596, 607, 609–610
prehypertension, 613
interventions
aspirin, 759
coalitions in health promotion, 136–137
information delivery, 19, 126
screening, 112
social cognitive theory, 121, 125
kidney disease, 1065, 1066–1067, 1071
anemia, 1070
nutrition
Dietary Approaches to Stop Hypertension (DASH), 351
dietary fat, 336–337
dietary fiber, 335–336
fruits and vegetables, 334–335
milk, 337
sugar, 338
obesity, 487, 488, 489, 490, 644
pathophysiology, 676

physical activity, 395, 396
significance, 673–675
mortality, 633, 640, 673–674, 675
sleep apnea, 821
tobacco use
cigar smoking, 252
cigarette smoking, 243, 245, 246, 248
pathophysiology, 256–258
pipe smoking, 253
relative risk, 247
secondhand smoke, 245, 246, 249, 252
Career Academies, 221
carpal tunnel syndrome
causes, 898, 938, 939
definition, 938–939
descriptive epidemiology, 939
high-risk groups, 898
interventions, 939
significance, 939
Cartesian dichotomy of mind and body, 858–859
case-control studies, 54, 55–56
bias, 58, 59
systematic reviews, 69–70
causes of chronic disease. See also analytic epidemiology; determinants of disease
causality checklist, 59–62
definition, 40, 49
Centers for Medicare and Medicaid Services Innovation Center, 169–170
accountable care organizations, 170–171
Accountable Health Communities Model, 173–174
bundled payment, 172–173
Diabetes Prevention Program, 556
State Innovation Models Initiative, 170
central fatigue of fibromyalgia, 985
central sensitivity syndromes, 986
fibromyalgia, 986, 987
cerebral embolism, 696
cerebral palsy
causes, 896, 915
definition, 913
descriptive epidemiology, 914–915
high-risk groups, 896
future research, 916
interventions, 915–916
significance, 914
coexisting morbidities, 914
cerebral thrombosis, 696
cerebrovascular disease. See stroke
cervical cancer
analytic epidemiology
causes, 770–771
interventions, 771–772
modifiable risk factors, 770
population attributable risk, 771

descriptive epidemiology
    geographic distribution, 770
    high-risk populations, 769
    time trends, 770
future research, 772
interventions
    examples, 772
    prevention, 771
    screening, 112, 769, 771–772
    treatment, 772
pathophysiology, 769
significance, 744, 768–769
challenges facing health care
    aging population, 20
    climate change and nutrition, 343
    disease origin complexity, 109
    diversity of population, 20
    health information technology
        incorporation, 180
    health literacy, 147–148
    mental health disorders
        connecting with treatment, 857–858
        integrated with primary care, 10–11,
            858–859, 881–882
    physical activity barriers, 404–405
    substance use disorders, 10–11
    training health workers, 22–24
channel of communication, 98–99
CHD. See coronary heart disease
chest radiograph
    asbestosis, 833
    interstitial lung disease, 823
    pneumoconioses, 825–826
        coal workers' pneumoconiosis, 826,
            827, 829
    respiratory diseases, 799
    silicosis, 830
chewing tobacco. See smokeless tobacco
child. See youths
Child and Adult Care Food Program, 347, 361
child care subsidies, 223
Child Nutrition Reauthorization Act, 363
Child Parent Centers (Chicago), 221
child support, 223
childhood absence epilepsy, 904
Childhood Obesity Intervention Cost-
    Effectiveness Study (CHOICES), 507
children. See youths
Children's Health Insurance Program, 170
Chinese Da Qing IGT and Diabetes Study, 542
cholesterol
    coronary heart disease and, 684
    dyslipidemia pathophysiology, 634–636
    gender differences, 637–638
    lipid profile, 633
    physical activity and, 395
    screening, 652–654

sources of, 634
stroke and, 702–703
treatment, 654–655, 657
Chronic Care Model, 175–184, 180–181
    actionable, 184
    Expanded Chronic Care Model, 189–191
Chronic Disease Indicators website
    alcohol use, 452–453
    surveillance data, 83
chronic diseases
    continuum of, 37–41
    definition, 5
    disease latency period, 825
    induction periods of cancers, 748
    infectious causes of death versus, 3–4, 5, 22
    mental illness and, 858–860
    registries of chronic diseases, 81, 85–87.
        See also surveillance
    top-10 causes of death, 6
        cancer, 743
        cardiovascular disease, 633
        chronic respiratory diseases, 795
        coronary heart disease, 678, 679
        stroke, 695
        suicide, 871
chronic fatigue syndrome, 986
Chronic Liver Disease Surveillance Study, 1044
chronic obstructive pulmonary disease
        (COPD)
    analytic epidemiology
        causes, 814–815
        interventions, 815–817
            modifiable risk factors, 814–815
            population-attributable risk, 815
    cigar smoking, 252
    cigarette smoking, 244, 246, 247, 248
    coal workers' pneumoconiosis, 827, 828–829
    definition, 796, 797, 811
    descriptive epidemiology
        geographic distribution, 814
        high-risk populations, 813
        time trends, 814
    future research, 817
    interventions
        examples, 816–817
        prevention, 815
        screening, 816
        treatment, 816
    pathophysiology, 797–798, 812–813
    pipe smoking, 253
    significance, 811–812
Chronic Renal Insufficiency Cohort, 719
cigar smoking
    diabetes and, 528
    oral cavity cancer, 779
    prevalence, 266
    secondhand smoke, 252

significance, 252–253
time trends, 267–271
cigarette smoking. *See also* tobacco use
　ankylosing spondylitis, 991–992
　cancer, 749, 750
　　bladder cancer, 243, 778
　　cervical cancer, 770, 771
　　leukemia, 243, 259, 777
　　lung cancer, 243, 244, 245, 248, 254, 752,
　　　754, 755
　　oral cavity cancer, 243, 252, 253, 259, 779
　　pharyngeal cancer, 243, 253
　　prostate cancer, 773
　costs of, 111
　depression, 860
　descriptive epidemiology
　　time trends, 683
　diabetes
　　dementia and, 524
　　macrovascular complications, 528
　　relative risk, 537, 538
　dyslipidemia, 648–649
　hepatitis B, 1030
　interventions
　　minor access to products, 274–275, 284,
　　　300–301
　　multilevel approach, 140
　　Not-On-Tobacco, 129
　　prevention, 281–285
　　screening, 285–286, 287–288
　　smoke-free policies, 296–297
　　telephone cessation quitlines, 286–287,
　　　288–289, 301–302
　　tobacco regulation, 302–304
　　treatment, 286–289
　　treatment insurance coverage, 297–300
　kidney disease, 1074, 1075
　Master Settlement Agreement, 290–291,
　　292, 294–295, 305
　neurological disorders
　　attention-deficit/hyperactivity disorder,
　　　936
　　dementias, 912
　　low back pain, 940
　　multiple sclerosis, 926
　osteoporosis, 999, 1000, 1001–1002
　peripheral arterial disease, 720, 721
　relative risk, 246–247
　reproductive disorders, 244, 245, 261
　respiratory diseases, 244, 245, 246, 247,
　　248–249
　　asthma, 808
　　chronic obstructive pulmonary disease,
　　　813, 814, 815, 829
　　interstitial lung disease, 824
　　pneumoconiosis, 826
　　sleep apnea, 821

secondhand smoke
　death rate, 99, 243
　environmental interventions, 13
　lung cancer and, 245, 246, 249, 754, 755
　significance, 245, 246
　stroke, 245, 246, 702
significance, 246–250
　mortality, 246, 248–249
　overview, 6, 15, 111, 243–246
smoking as reportable, 243
socioeconomic status and, 202, 206, 250,
　265, 281, 447, 679
stroke, 244, 245, 701–702
cirrhosis
　causes
　　alcoholic liver disease, 1022, 1023,
　　　1024–1025
　　attributable risks, 1022, 1023
　　hepatitis B, 1030, 1032
　　hepatitis C, 1035, 1037
　　non-alcoholic fatty liver, 1042, 1046
　as end-stage liver disease, 1017
　hepatocellular carcinoma and, 1048, 1049
　pathophysiology, 1017
　significance
　　mortality rates, 1019
clinical information systems, 180–181
Clubhouse Model of mental health, 880–881
coal rank, 828
coal workers' pneumoconiosis (CWP)
　causes, 828–829
　descriptive epidemiology, 827, 828
　interventions, 829
　significance, 826–827
coalitions
　alcohol use, 467–468
　arthritis interventions, 966–968, 975–976
　cancer, 751
　cardiovascular disease, 136–137
　　coronary heart disease, 694
　community coalitions, 136–137
　community health business model, 188–189
　diabetes prevention, 555, 561
　"health in all policies" framework, 227–229
　housing efforts, 226–227
　mental health, 10–11, 858–859, 881–882
　nutrition, 354–355, 367
　obesity, 188–189
　overview, 24
　physical activity, 407, 410, 412, 416
　spinal cord injury, 936
Cochrane reviews as systematic, 69
coffee
　bean grinding exposure, 824
　gout protective effect, 983
　liver disease protective effect, 1026
　　cirrhosis, 1049

cognitive health
    alcohol use, 436, 438
    dementias, 909–910
    diabetes, 524
    fibromyalgia, 987
    memory
        alcohol use, 436, 437, 438
        dementias, 909–910
        hippocampus, 211
        insulin resistance, 911–912
        post-traumatic stress disorder, 867
        recall bias, 59
        seizure auras, 902
        sleep apnea, 821
    obesity, 489
    Parkinson's disease, 906, 908
    post-traumatic stress disorder, 867
    traumatic brain injury, 932
collaborations and patient confidentiality, 468.
        See also coalitions
college alcohol use, 446
college enrollment programs, 222
colorectal cancer
    analytic epidemiology
        causes, 758–759
        interventions, 760
    descriptive epidemiology
        high-risk populations, 758
        time trends, 758
    interventions
        aspirin, 759
        prevention, 759, 760
        screening, 112, 760
        treatment, 760
    obesity and, 488
    pathophysiology, 757–758
    red meat and, 337
    significance, 744, 757
    smoking and, 253
Commodity Food Assistance Program, 363
communicable diseases. See infectious diseases
communication
    audience, 98
    autism spectrum disorders, 897, 916–917
    Chronic Care Model, 178
    collaboration and patient confidentiality, 468
    data dissemination, 95–99
    disorders as neurodevelopmental, 864
    lifestyle counseling
        pharmacists, 186–187
        physical activity, 411
        sun exposure, 781
    multiple sclerosis, 923
    organization of health systems, 176
    patient adherence and, 126
    translation by community health
        workers, 125

Communities Mobilizing for Change on
        Alcohol, 467
community
    academic achievement and health, 124
    alcohol outlet density, 456, 467
    American Community Survey, 91
    applied epidemiology definition, 37
    clinic-community link
        Accountable Health Communities Model,
            173–174
        Chronic Care Model, 183
        community health business model,
            188–189
        community health workers, 189–191.
            See also community health workers
        as prevention strategy, 14, 16–20
    coalitions, 136–137. See also coalitions
    Community Guide, 71–72, 306, 467, 505
    community-based participatory research,
        134–135, 146, 147
        weight status program, 362
    engagement of, 134
        participatory research, 134–135, 146,
            147, 362
        prevention marketing, 145–147
    health workers. See community health
        workers
    hospitals and community benefit, 174
    interventions
        alcohol use, 467–468
        arthritis, 976
        autism spectrum disorders, 919
        community-level, 132–139
        coronary heart disease, 690–694
        examples, 141–147
        kidney disease, 1076
        media advocacy, 137–139
        mental health. See community mental
            health treatment
        nutrition, 346–348, 358–359
        obesity, 499–500
        physical activity, 406, 407, 409, 410,
            416–418
        prevention marketing, 145–147
        Prevention Research Centers, 128–129
        skin cancer, 781
    Community Coalition Action Theory (CCAT),
        136–137
    community health workers
        coronary heart disease intervention,
            691, 692
        health care–community liaisons, 189–191
        interpersonal interventions, 124–125
        nutrition interventions, 362
        promotores, 124, 125, 189–191
    Community Mental Health Centers and Mental
        Retardation Act (1963), 872

community mental health treatment
  biopsychosocial models, 880–881
  depression prevention, 879–880
  recovery-oriented model, 876, 878–879
  transition from state institutions
    Assertive Community Treatment, 881
    homeless or incarcerated population,
      857, 860, 862, 872
    time trends, 872
Community Preventive Services Task Force
  Community Guide, 71–72, 306, 467, 505
  diabetes prevention, 545, 550
  obesity prevention, 499
Community Transformation Grants, 173
community-based participatory research
  (CBPR), 134–135, 146, 147
  weight status program, 362
commuting as physical activity, 395, 400, 403
  walking to school, 410
complex care management, 175, 178–179
Comprehensive Primary Care Initiative, 171
confidentiality in collaboration, 468
confounding in studies, 57–58
consequences. See significance
continuous positive airway pressure
  (CPAP), 822
contraceptives
  breast cancer, 764
  cervical cancer, 770
  multiple sclerosis, 926
contributing cause of death, 84
"control of chronic disease" meaning, 39
Coordinated Approach to Child Health
  (CATCH), 129, 357
coronary artery disease registry, 722
Coronary Artery Risk Development in (Young)
  Adults (CARDIA), 600
coronary heart disease (CHD). See also heart
  disease
  alcohol protective effects, 433, 686–687
  analytic epidemiology
    causes, 681–688
    interventions, 688–694
    modifiable risk factors, 681–687
    population-attributable risk, 682,
      687–688
  descriptive epidemiology
    geographic distribution, 679
    high-risk populations, 677–679
    smoking-related ratios, 46, 47
    time trends, 15, 675, 679–681
  diabetes, 685–686
  dyslipidemia, 633, 676, 684
  future research, 694–695
  high blood pressure
    cardiovascular mortality, 588
    CHD attributable to, 595, 596, 601, 681

definition of high blood pressure, 581
    as predictor of CHD, 594, 596
    treatment and CHD risk, 610, 681
  interventions
    examples, 690–694
    prevention, 688
    screening, 677, 688–689
    treatment, 689–690
  lung cancer mortality versus, 46, 47
  nutrition, 335, 336
  obesity, 487, 488, 676, 686
  pathophysiology, 677
  physical inactivity, 392, 395, 686
  risk factors, 676
  significance, 676–677
    mortality rates, 15, 676–677, 678,
      679–681
  smoking and, 243, 247, 248, 256, 682–683
    cigars, 252
    secondhand smoke, 245, 249, 683
  socioeconomic status and, 209–210,
    679, 688
Costa Rica life expectancy, 5
costs of health care
  aging population, 20
  alcohol use, 111, 433, 437
  Alzheimer's disease, 910
  arthritis, 966
    fibromyalgia, 986
    rheumatoid arthritis, 977
  behavioral determinants, 111–112
  cancer, 747
  cardiovascular disease, 674–675
    heart disease, 111
    heart failure, 710
    peripheral arterial disease, 717
    stroke, 695
  diabetes, 525–526, 529
    cost-effectiveness, 559–561
  dyslipidemia, 529, 634
  high blood pressure, 529, 591, 613
  joint replacements, 969
  kidney disease, 1067, 1069
  liver disease, 1019–1020
    hepatitis C, 1036
  noncommunicable diseases, 7, 333
  obesity related, 111, 489–490
    cost-effectiveness, 507
  osteoporosis, 994
  patient characteristics, 166–167
  physical activity, 393
  respiratory diseases
    chronic obstructive pulmonary
      disease, 812
    occupational lung exposures, 825
  spinal cord injury, 935
  tobacco use, 111

smoking-attributable, 247, 250
tobacco-use treatment, 288
United States
Medicare spending, 112
noncommunicable diseases, 7
others versus, 5
wellness promotion returns, 131, 187
"cotton washing," 836
Council of State and Territorial Epidemiologists
(CSTE), 80, 83
County Health Rankings Model of Population
Health, 169
cow's milk. See milk
C-reactive protein (CRP), 681, 682, 684–685
Cuba life expectancy, 5
cumulative incidence
comparing across groups, 45
definition, 42, 44
Current Population Survey (CPS), 214–217
CVD. See cardiovascular disease
cystic fibrosis
causes, 819
definition, 796, 798, 817
descriptive epidemiology
high-risk populations, 819
time trends, 818
ICD-10 code, 798
interventions
prevention, 819–820
screening, 820
pathophysiology, 818–819
significance, 817–818

D

Da Qing IGT and Diabetes Study, 542
dairy product nutrition, 337–338
Dietary Guidelines, 333
Dallas Heart Study, 1043
DASH diet. See Dietary Approaches to Stop
Hypertension
data dissemination, 95–99
death certificates, 83–84. See also
mortality rates
decision support
Chronic Care Model, 179–182
clinical information systems, 180–181
information sources, 16, 17–18
media advocacy, 138
self-management support, 181–183
degenerative joint disease. See osteoarthritis
delivery system design, 178–179
Expanded Chronic Care Model, 189–191
dementias. See also Alzheimer's disease
amyotrophic lateral sclerosis (ALS), 920, 921
causes, 896, 911–912
definition, 909–910

descriptive epidemiology, 911
diabetes, 524
future research, 913
interventions, 912–913
as mental disorder, 865
obesity, 489
Parkinson's disease, 906
pathophysiology, 911
significance, 910
high-risk groups, 896
depression (mental health)
alcohol use, 874
anxiety disorders, 867
attention-deficit/hyperactivity disorder,
936, 937
bipolar disorder, 866
cancer causing, 860
cardiovascular disease causing, 860
descriptive epidemiology, 869
diabetes, 523, 525, 537
epilepsy, 901
hepatitis C, 1037
immune system, 859–860
income inequality, 874
interventions
preventing, 879–880
screening, 877
medication adherence and, 612
migraine headaches, 942, 943
mortality, 861
obesity, 487, 491
Parkinson's disease, 906
pathophysiology, 866
post-traumatic stress disorder, 867
primary care integration, 881–882
smoking comorbidity, 860
traumatic brain injury, 932
descriptive epidemiology
chronic disease continuum, 38
definition, 36, 40
overview, 38, 41–42
age differences across groups, 47–48
calculating rates in groups, 43–44, 73
comparing rates across groups, 44–47
measuring burden of disease, 42–43
surveillance, 92–95
determinants of disease. See also analytic
epidemiology
behavioral
cervical cancer, 771
lifestyle behaviors, 5–6.
overview, 110–112
parent education and child behavior,
879–880
physical activity, 404
significance, 187
as social over individual, 113–114, 120, 201

socioeconomic status and, 206–208
Theory of Planned Behavior, 118–119
definition, 36–37
environmental, 112–113. *See also* environmental determinants
health care, 112
social. *See also* socioeconomic status
behavioral determinants as, 113–114, 120, 201
future research, 229–232
"health in all policies" framework, 227–229
mental health, 871, 874, 876
mental health treatment, 879
overview, 113–114, 201–202
significance, 201
suicide, 871
detoxification from alcohol, 463–464
diabetes. *See also* metabolic syndrome
analytic epidemiology
causes, 519, 529, 536–540
population-attributable risk, 538–540
cardiovascular disease
coronary heart disease, 685–686
heart failure, 713, 716
carpal tunnel syndrome, 939
"control" meaning, 39
descriptive epidemiology
geographic distribution, 531–533
high-risk populations, 529–531
lifetime risk, 536
time trends, 519–520, 533–536
future research, 557–561
gestational diabetes mellitus, 527, 534–535
high blood pressure and stroke, 700
impaired fasting glucose, 528
impaired glucose tolerance, 527–528
interventions
Amigos en Salud, 362
Diabetes Prevention Program, 504
examples, 554–556
family-based, 122
Fit Body and Soul, 358
high-risk vs. population-wide, 556
prevention, 540–546
research into practice, 551–554
screening, 529, 546–548
treatment, 548–551
WORD, 362
kidney disease, 1070, 1071, 1074, 1075
end-stage renal disease, 1068–1069
prevention, 1075–1076
liver disease, 1025
alcoholic, 1025
non-alcoholic fatty liver, 1042, 1045
mental health

post-traumatic stress disorder, 867
psychiatric medication as risk factor, 860
microbiome and, 342
obesity and
adult obesity, 487, 488, 528, 531, 533, 537
lifespan obesity, 538
obesity pathophysiology, 490–491
obesity treatment, 501
type 2 diabetes pathophysiology, 526
youth obesity, 489
pathophysiology, 526–529
peripheral arterial disease, 719, 720
physical activity, 392, 395, 397
prediabetes, 6, 527–528
Diabetes Prevention Program, 19
pregnancy and, 521–522, 534
Balance after Baby, 554
gestational diabetes mellitus, 527, 534–535
prevalence, 534–535
screening, 548
significance
economic costs, 525–526, 529
morbidity, 521–525
mortality, 520–521
overview, 6, 519–520
sugar and, 338, 538
tobacco use
cigarette smoking, 244, 245
pathophysiology, 262
relative risk, 247
smokeless tobacco, 251
type 1
causes, 519
multifactorial therapy, 528
pathophysiology, 526
percentage of cases, 519
prevention, 540–542
screening, 547
treatment, 548–549
type 2
bariatric surgery remission, 527
causes, 519, 529, 536–540
depression and, 525
dyslipidemia and, 649–650, 656
gout, 983
multifactorial therapy, 528–529
pathophysiology, 526–527
percentage of cases, 519
prevention, 542–546
prevention in youth, 545–546
screening, 112
treatment, 549–551
Diabetes Control and Complications Trial, 548–549

A Diabetes Outcome Progression Trial
(ADOPT), 545
Diabetes Prevention Act (2009), 554–555
Diabetes Prevention Program (DPP), 19, 501,
504, 543–544, 554–556
DPP Outcomes Study, 543–544
research into practice, 551–554
Diabetes Prevention Recognition
Program, 555
Diabetes Prevention study (Finnish), 542–543
Diabetes Training and Technical Assistance
Center, 555
Diagnostic and Statistical Manual of Mental
Disorders, 5th Edition (APA)
alcohol abuse, 442
alcohol dependence, 442
alcohol use disorder, 434, 435
range of diagnostic criteria, 454
attention-deficit/hyperactivity disorder, 936
ICD-10 codes versus, 864–865
mental health criteria, 863, 864–865
dialysis
costs of, 1067
end-stage renal disease, 523, 595, 1065
as hepatitis B risk factor, 1032
hepatitis B vaccination during, 1034
as hepatitis C risk factor, 1039, 1040
diet. See food; nutrition; obesity; weight loss
Dietary Approaches to Stop Hypertension
(DASH), 351
coronary heart disease, 691
high blood pressure, 604, 606
dietary fat, 336–337, 338
breast cancer, 763, 764
hepatocellular carcinoma, 1049
dietary fiber, 335–336
colorectal cancer, 759
Dietary Guidelines, 333
insulin resistance, 336
Dietary Guidelines for Americans (USDHHS &
USDA), 333–334
alcohol use, 648
dyslipidemia, 647
nutrition, 349–351
obesity, 494–495
differential misclassification, 59
diplegia in cerebral palsy, 913
disabilities
arthritis as most common, 6, 965
activity limitations, 965, 966
Child and Adult Care Food Program, 347
diabetes causing, 523–525, 531
fetal alcohol exposure, 437
mental health
anxiety risk, 870
global burden, 859
neurological disorders

low back pain, 940
migraine headaches, 941
spinal cord injury, 934
traumatic brain injury, 932
osteoporosis, 965
physical inactivity from, 402, 405
diabetes and arthritis, 524
smoking cessation assistance, 298
socioeconomic status and, 20–21, 203
as high-risk population, 214, 215, 217
disability-adjusted life years (DALYs)
alcohol use, 433
cardiovascular disease, 675
gout, 982
high blood pressure, 587–588
mood disorders, 866
nutritional deficit, 333
Parkinson's disease, 907
traumatic brain injury, children, 932
disaster and emergency preparedness, 121
discrimination
obesity, 486
racial and stress, 212–214
disease latency period. See latency period
disease registries. See patient registries
disease-modifying antirheumatic drug
(DMARD), 980, 991, 992
disparities in health care
asthma, 804
cancer
mammography, 95
significance, 744–745
diabetes mortality rates, 520
mental health treatment and
mortality, 861
overview, 20–22
social determinants, 114
socioeconomic status, 202–209
distribution of disease. See descriptive
epidemiology
disulfiram (Antabuse), 466
downstream consequences. See also
significance
overview of book figures, 40, 41
drinking. See alcohol use
dropout prevention programs, 221
duration of a physical activity, 393, 394
dyslipidemia. See also metabolic syndrome
analytic epidemiology
causes, 644–649
comorbidities, 649–650
interventions, 651–657
population-attributable risk, 651
risk scores, 650–651
as cardiovascular disease risk factor, 633
definition, 633
descriptive epidemiology

geographic distribution, 640–641, 642
high-risk populations, 636–640
time trends, 641, 643–644
diabetes, 528
Dietary Approaches to Stop Hypertension (DASH), 351
future research, 657
gout, 984
interventions
examples, 655–657
patient medication adherence, 634, 656
prevention, 651–652
screening, 112, 652–654, 657
treatment, 654–655
mixed dyslipidemia, 633
non-alcoholic fatty liver, 1045
obesity, 487
pathophysiology, 634–636
familial hypercholesterolemia, 636
peripheral arterial disease, 720
physical activity, 395, 396
psychiatric medication risk factor, 860
significance, 6, 633–634
dyspnea, 795–796
anemia, 1070
chronic obstructive pulmonary disease, 812, 816
coal workers' pneumoconiosis, 827
grain dust exposure, 840
heart failure, 710, 714, 715
interstitial lung disease, 823
kidney disease and anemia, 1070
treatment, 816

E

Early Head Start, 221
Earned Income Tax Credit, 223, 225
economic factors. *See* socioeconomic status (SES)
educating clients. *See also* training health workers
arthritis
ankylosing spondylitis, 993
fibromyalgia, 989
brief intervention
alcohol use, 460, 462–463
definition, 126–127
for education, 140
tobacco use, 287–288
cancer
breast cancer screening, 767–768
cervical cancer, 772
community health workers, 189–191
diabetes, 548, 550
Amigos en Salud, 362
ergonomics, 939–940, 941
high blood pressure, 602

kidney disease, 1076
mental health, 877
migraine headaches, 942
nutrition
Amigos en Salud on diabetes, 362
Dietary Guidelines, 349–351
MyPlate, 348, 350–351
obesity prevention, 498–500
osteoporosis, 1002
parent education and child behavior, 879–880
physical activity, 411
respiratory diseases
asthma, 809, 810
occupational asthma, 839
silicosis, 832
self-management, 182
tobacco use, 283
educational attainment
alcohol use and, 447
behavioral determinants, 202
cancer and, 744–745
diabetes and, 531, 532, 534, 538
dyslipidemia and, 640, 653
educational achievement programs, 221–223
health status influencing, 208
hepatitis C and, 1039
kidney disease and, 1072
nutrition and, 341
obesity and, 492
physical activity and, 402
socioeconomic status and, 204, 220–223, 224–225
poverty rate, 215–216, 217
tobacco use and, 265, 281
vocational training, 223
effect modification definition, 64
electronic cigarettes
pathophysiology, 259
prevalence, 266
significance, 255–256
time trends, 267–271
electronic health records (EHRs)
decision support tools, 180, 181
"meaningful use" concept, 79
patient registries, 181, 186
social determinants to be captured, 230, 231
surveillance data, 82, 90
nutrition surveillance, 352
Emergency Food Assistance Program, 363
emergency preparedness, 121
Emerging Risk Factors Collaboration, 690
emphysema
as chronic obstructive pulmonary disease, 796, 797, 811
definition, 798

ICD-10 code, 798
pathophysiology, 812
significance, 811
employer programs. *See* workplaces
employment status
  health status affecting, 208
  pathophysiology of, 209–210
  socioeconomic status
    interventions, 223, 225
    poverty rate, 215, 217
    significance, 203–204, 205
end-stage renal disease (ESRD)
  ambulatory blood pressure
    monitoring, 1082
  descriptive epidemiology
    geographic distribution, 1074
    time trends, 1073–1074
  diabetes and, 521, 523, 528, 1068–1069
  dialysis, 523, 595, 1065
  intervention examples, 1084
  periodontal disease, 1073
  race, 1071
Engel, George, 863
EnhanceFitness program, 968
environmental determinants
  alcohol use, 456, 458
  amyotrophic lateral sclerosis (ALS), 921, 922
  arthritis
    fibromyalgia, 988
    osteoarthritis, 971, 972
    rheumatoid arthritis, 977, 978
  autism spectrum disorders, 917, 919
  coronary heart disease, 691
  diabetes, 530, 553–554
  epilepsy, 904
  gene–environment interactions, 904
    autism spectrum disorders, 917, 919
    epilepsy, 904, 906
    multiple sclerosis, 925
    osteoarthritis, 971, 972
    Parkinson's disease, 908
  housing, 225–227
  mental health
    anxiety disorders, 867
    schizophrenia, 866
  neurological disorders
    amyotrophic lateral sclerosis (ALS), 921, 922
    autism spectrum disorders, 917, 919
    epilepsy, 904
    multiple sclerosis, 924–925
    Parkinson's disease, 908
  obesity, 112–113
  osteoporosis, 994
  overview, 112–113
  physical activity, 113, 402–403, 405
  respiratory diseases

asbestosis, 832–833
  asthma, 800, 801, 805–807, 808, 809–810, 811
  byssinosis, 836
  chronic obstructive pulmonary disease, 815, 817
  coal workers' pneumoconiosis, 827, 828–829
  interstitial lung disease, 823, 824
  occupation-related, 799
  occupational asthma, 836–839
  organic dust–related lung disease, 839–841
  silicosis, 830
  smoking initiation, 272–275
  socioeconomic status, 204, 207–208, 226
    coronary heart disease, 679
EPIC-Norfolk study, 702
Epidemiologic Catchment Area Study, 861, 868
epidemiology
  analytic epidemiology
    attributable risk, 62
    causality of associations, 59–62
    definition, 36–37, 40
    introduction to, 38, 49–52
    population-attributable risk, 63–65
    relative risk, 45, 56–57
    series of studies, 68–72
    single study insufficiency, 66–68
    study designs, 52–56
    validity of study results, 57–59
  causal factors vs. associated, 49
  chronic disease continuum, 37–41
  definition, 36–37
  "control" meaning, 39
  descriptive epidemiology
    age differences across groups, 47–48
    calculating rates in groups, 43–44, 73
    comparing rates across groups, 44–47
    definition, 36, 40
    introduction to, 38, 41–42
    measuring burden of disease, 42–43
    surveillance, 92–95
  prevention strategy overview, 12–13, 18–19
epilepsy
  attention-deficit/hyperactivity disorder, 936
  autism spectrum disorders, 917
  causes, 896, 904–905
  cerebral palsy, 914, 916
  definition, 899
  descriptive epidemiology, 903–904
    high-risk groups, 896
  future research, 906
  interventions, 905–906
  migraine headaches, 942
  pathophysiology, 902
  significance, 900–901

comorbidities, 900–901
  sudden death, 901, 903
erectile dysfunction, smoking-induced, 245, 262
ergonomics
  carpal tunnel syndrome, 939–940
  low back pain, 941
ethnic differences. *See* race/ethnicity
evaluation
  community-based prevention
    marketing, 147
  data dissemination evaluation, 99
  intervention program effects, 51–52
    cancer interventions, 751
    high blood pressure treatment, 611
    mental illness prevention programs, 876
  National 5 a Day Program, 354–355
  National Physical Activity Plan, 412
  Secondary Prevention of Coronary
    Events After Discharge from Hospital
    (SPREAD), 692
evidence-based interventions. *See*
  interventions
exercise
  arthritis interventions, 967–968, 976
    ankylosing spondylitis, 991, 993
    fibromyalgia, 988, 989
    osteoarthritis, 973–974, 975
    rheumatoid arthritis, 980, 981
  low back pain, 941
    ankylosing spondylitis, 989
  osteoporosis, 1000
  peripheral arterial disease, 721
  physical activity versus, 393, 394, 395
Exercise and Nutrition Interventions for
  Cardiovascular Health (ENCORE), 691
Exercise Is Medicine, 411
Expanded Chronic Care Model (ECCM),
  189–191
expectancy and locus of control, 119–120
experimental studies
  bias, 58–59
  community-based participatory research,
    134–135, 146, 147
    weight status program, 362
  confounding, 57–58
  definition, 52–53, 54
  quasi-experimental studies, 52–53, 54
  systematic reviews, 69–70
extreme obesity, 485

F

faith-based venues for interventions, 132
  nutrition, 358, 362
falls
  cerebral palsy causing, 913
  osteoporosis and, 998, 1000

Parkinson's disease causing, 907, 909
seizures causing, 901
spinal cord injury caused by, 934, 935
traumatic brain injury caused by, 933–934
familial hypercholesterolemia (FH), 636–637
Families and Schools Together, 221
family history
  arthritis
    fibromyalgia, 987–988
    gout, 984
    rheumatoid arthritis, 978–979
  asthma, 804–805, 806
  cancer
    breast cancer, 762, 767
    colorectal cancer, 758
    prostate cancer, 773
  cardiovascular disease
    coronary heart disease, 678
    stroke, 698
  diabetes, 527, 529, 530–531
    screening, 547
  hemochromatosis, 1050
  high blood pressure, 597, 607
  kidney disease, 1073
  mental health
    depression, 869
    schizophrenia, 869
    suicide, 871
  migraine headaches, 942
  neurological disorders
    amyotrophic lateral sclerosis (ALS),
      921, 922
    multiple sclerosis, 925
    Tourette syndrome, 931
family-based interventions, 122
Farm Bill, 361, 363
farmers' lung, 840
Farmer's Market Nutrition Program, 361
farmers' markets, 365
fat from diet, 336–337, 338
  breast cancer, 763, 764
  hepatocellular carcinoma, 1049
fatigue
  depression, 866
  diabetes, 547
  fibromyalgia, 986, 987, 989
    central and physical fatigue, 985
  globally, 987
  heart failure, 710, 714
  hepatitis B, 1030
  kidney disease and anemia, 1070
  as migraine trigger, 942
  physical fitness and, 393, 394
  sleep quality and obesity, 496
febrile seizures, 905, 906
Federal Coal Mine Health and Safety Act
  (1969), 829

fiber from diet, 335–336
  colorectal cancer, 759
  Dietary Guidelines, 333
  insulin resistance, 336
fibrinogen and coronary heart disease, 685
fibromyalgia
  causes, 988
  definition, 985–986
  descriptive epidemiology, 965, 987–988
  interventions
    examples, 989
    prevention, 988
    treatment, 988–989
  pathophysiology, 986
  significance, 986
firearms
  suicide and access to, 868, 871, 875
  traumatic brain injury, 933
fish nutrition
  cirrhosis prevention, 1049
  DASH diet, 351
  Dietary Guidelines, 333
  geographic distribution, 342
  Mediterranean diet, 351, 647
  obesity risk and, 495
  omega-3 fatty acids, 336
  as Western diet, 983
Fit Body and Soul, 358
flexible scheduling of employment, 223
focal seizures, 902
food. *See also* nutrition
  disappearance data, 352
  farmers' markets, 365
  food deserts, 19, 208, 333
    disease rates and, 342
  food frequency questionnaires (FFQs),
    352–353
  food insecurity, 333, 341
    diabetes prevalence, 532
    smoking and, 250
    socioeconomic status and, 203, 205, 207
  gardening, 365–366
  gout, 983, 984
  hepatitis A, 1026, 1028
  hepatocellular carcinoma, 1049
  liver disease, 1026
  migraine headaches, 942
  obesity, 494–495. *See also* obesity
  sustenance and beyond, 331
Food Stamp Program. *See* Supplemental
  Nutrition Assistance Program (SNAP)
forced expiratory volume, first second
  (FEV1), 799
  chronic obstructive pulmonary disease, 815
  cystic fibrosis, 819
forced vital capacity (FVC), 799
  interstitial lung disease, 823

Fountain House (New York City), 881
Fracture Assessment Tool (WHO), 999
framing of issues, 138
Framingham Heart Study
  arthritis
    gout, 983
    osteoarthritis, 970
  cardiovascular disease
    heart failure, 714
    risk equations, 650
  high blood pressure, 590–591
  stroke, 697, 703, 704–705
  smoking and, 701–702
frequency of an activity, 393, 394
Fresh Fruit and Vegetable Snack Program, 361
fruit nutrition, 334–335
  amyotrophic lateral sclerosis (ALS)
    and, 922
  cancer and, 749, 750
    breast cancer, 764
    lung cancer, 754, 755
    oral cavity cancer, 779
  Dietary Guidelines, 333
Fruits & Veggies—More Matters, 354–355
full-day kindergarten, 221
functional dyspepsia, 986

G

gastroesophageal reflux, 798
generalized seizures, 902
genetics
  alcohol use, 447, 468
  arthritis
    ankylosing spondylitis, 991
    fibromyalgia, 987–988
    osteoarthritis, 971, 972
    rheumatoid arthritis, 978
  cancer
    breast cancer, 761, 762, 767
    colorectal cancer, 758
    leukemia, 776
    lung cancer, 752
  cardiovascular disease
    coronary heart disease, 678, 694
    peripheral arterial disease, 720–721
  diabetes, 530
  familial hypercholesterolemia, 636–637
  gene–environment interactions, 904
    autism spectrum disorders, 917, 919
    epilepsy, 904, 906
    multiple sclerosis, 925
    osteoarthritis, 971, 972
    Parkinson's disease, 908
  high blood pressure, 597
  kidney disease, 1071–1072, 1073, 1076
  liver disease

cirrhosis, 1024
   hemochromatosis, 1050
   non-alcoholic fatty liver, 1044–1045
mental health, 863, 874
   anxiety disorders, 867
   bipolar disorder, 869
   depression, 869
   post-traumatic stress disorder, 870
   schizophrenia, 866, 869
neurological disorders
   Alzheimer's disease, 911
   amyotrophic lateral sclerosis (ALS), 922
   attention-deficit/hyperactivity
      disorder, 938
   autism spectrum disorders, 917, 918, 919
   epilepsy, 904–905, 906
   low back pain, 940
   migraine headaches, 942
   multiple sclerosis, 925
   Parkinson's disease, 908, 909
   Tourette syndrome, 931
nutrition, 341–342
osteoporosis, 994, 995–996
respiratory diseases
   asthma, 804, 805, 807, 810
   chronic obstructive pulmonary disease,
      813, 816, 817
   cystic fibrosis, 818, 819–820
geographic distributions
   alcohol use, 447–453
   arthritis
      ankylosing spondylitis, 991
      gout, 983
      rheumatoid arthritis, 978
   cancer
      breast cancer, 762
      cervical cancer, 770
      leukemia clusters, 776
      lung cancer, 753
   cardiovascular disease
      coronary heart disease, 679
      heart failure, 712
   descriptive epidemiology identifying, 42
   diabetes, 531–533
      diabetes belt, 532
   disease clusters, 94–95
   dyslipidemia, 640–641, 642
   high blood pressure, 592
   kidney disease, 1073, 1074
   mental health, 871
   neurological disorders
      amyotrophic lateral sclerosis (ALS),
         920–921
      cerebral palsy, 915
      multiple sclerosis, 924–925
   nutrition, 342–343
   obesity, 493

osteoporosis, 996–997
physical activity, 402–403, 405
poverty rate, 217–218
respiratory diseases
   asthma, 804
   chronic obstructive pulmonary
      disease, 814
   coal workers' pneumoconiosis, 828
stroke, 697, 698
   Reasons for Geographic and Racial
      Differences in Stroke, 697, 702
   stroke belt, 342
surveillance data analysis, 93–95
tobacco use, 267
Germany life expectancy, 5
gestational diabetes mellitus (GDM), 527,
   534–535
   Balance after Baby, 554
   diabetes relative risk, 537
      reducing, 538
   lifestyle factors and, 539
   screening, 548
Global Burden of Disease study
   cardiovascular disease, 675
   as data source, 17
   gout, 982
   mental illness, 859
global health and chronic diseases
   alcohol use
      Alcohol Use Disorders Identification
         Tool, 460
      significance, 433
      youth access, 467
   arthritis
      gout, 982–983
      osteoarthritis, 972
      rheumatoid arthritis, 977, 978
   cancer
      breast cancer, 762
      cervical cancer, 768–769, 770
      hepatocellular carcinoma, 1047–1048
      lung cancer, 753
   cardiovascular disease, 675
      coronary heart disease, 679, 692–693
      heart failure, 716
      REACH Registry, 722
   climate change and nutrition, 343
   diabetes, 535
   dyslipidemia, 640
   fatigue, 987
   Global Burden of Disease study
      cardiovascular disease, 675
      as data source, 17
      gout, 982
      mental illness, 859
   "health in all policies" framework, 228–229
   high blood pressure, 587–588, 612

International Study of Salt and Blood Pressure, 598, 599, 600
Identification and Prevention of Dietary- and Lifestyle-Induced Health Effects in Children and Infants, 357
kidney disease, 1070, 1073
    interventions, 1076
    Kidney Disease: Improving Global Outcomes, 1083
life expectancy by country, 5
liver disease, 1017, 1042
    alcoholic, 1023, 1024
    hemochromatosis, 1050
    hepatitis A, 1027, 1028
    hepatitis B, 1028, 1030, 1034
    hepatocellular carcinoma, 1047–1048
    non-alcoholic fatty liver, 1042, 1043, 1044
mental health, 859
    firearm ownership and suicide, 875
    schizophrenia treatment, 878
neurological disorders
    Alzheimer's disease, 910
    amyotrophic lateral sclerosis (ALS), 920
    autism spectrum disorders, 918
    cerebral palsy, 914
    epilepsy, 899–900, 901, 903
    epilepsy diagnosis, 902
    migraine headaches, 941
    multiple sclerosis, 924, 926
    Parkinson's disease, 906–907
    significance, 895
    spinal cord injury, 934–935
    Tourette syndrome, 930
    traumatic brain injury, 932
obesity and diabetes, 531
osteoporosis, 996–997
peripheral arterial disease, 720
physical activity, 392–393, 416
    Exercise Is Medicine, 411
prevention initiatives overview, 22, 23
respiratory diseases
    asbestosis, 833, 835
    asthma, 800
    byssinosis, 836
    chronic obstructive pulmonary disease, 815
    coal workers' pneumoconiosis, 826–827
    cystic fibrosis, 819
    occupational asthma, 836
    silicosis, 829–830
    significance, 22
    stroke, 695
gout
    causes, 984
    definition, 981–982
    descriptive epidemiology, 965, 982–983

geographic distribution, 983
    high-risk populations, 983
    time trends, 982, 983
interventions
    prevention, 984
    screening, 984
    treatment, 984–985
pathophysiology, 982
significance, 982
grain dust, 840
grain-handlers' disease, 840
The Guide to Clinical Preventive Services (USPSTF), 406
The Guide to Community Preventive Services (USPSTF), 406, 409
    asthma prevention, 810
    lung cancer prevention, 756
    skin cancer prevention, 781
Guillain-Barré syndrome
    causes, 897, 928–929
    definition, 927
    descriptive epidemiology, 928
        high-risk groups, 897
    future research, 929
    interventions, 929
    pathophysiology, 928
    significance, 927–928
Gulf War syndrome, 986
Gynecologic Cancer Education and Awareness Act (2005), 772

H

hand sanitizer ingestion, 442
headaches. *See* migraine headaches
Health Belief Model, 116–117
health career recruitment, 221
Health Impact Pyramid, 7–11, 219–220
health information exchanges, 181
Health Information Technology for Economic and Clinical Health Act (HITECH; 2009)
    decision support, 180
    "meaningful use" concept, 79
health literacy
    Chronic Care Model, 178
    enhancement of, 147–150
Health Locus of Control Model, 119–120
health policy
    ACA health care reform, 169–174
    alcohol use, 458, 465–466
    cancer, 749
        breast and cervical, 772
        lung cancer, 756–757
    diabetes, 554–555
    "health in all policies" framework, 227–229
    as intervention, 139
    liver disease, 1018

media advocacy, 138
    tobacco advertising, 283–284,
        294–295, 296
mental health, 858, 872, 873
nutrition, 347, 363–365, 499
    Farm Bill, 361, 363
obesity, 139
physical activity, 406–408, 415–416
respiratory diseases
    asbestosis, 835
    asthma, 808
    byssinosis, 836
    chronic obstructive pulmonary
        disease, 817
    coal workers' pneumoconiosis, 829
socioeconomic status, 227–229
spinal cord injury, 936
surveillance of, 91–92
technology, 79, 180
tobacco use
    advertising restrictions, 283–284,
        294–295, 296
    health warnings, 295–296
    Master Settlement Agreement, 290–291,
        292, 294–295, 305
    minor access, 300–301
    smoke-free policies, 296–297
    tobacco regulation, 302–304, 305
traumatic brain injury, 933, 934
Health Professionals Follow-up Study, 539
health survey surveillance systems, 81, 87–89
health system interventions
    ACA health care reform, 169–174
    Chronic Care Model, 175–184
        Expanded Chronic Care Model, 189–191
    complex care management, 175,
        178–179
    multiple chronic conditions, 165–166
    organization of health systems, 176
    overview, 13–14, 126–127
    patient characteristics, 166–167
    population health, 167–169
    screening approaches, 126, 127, 184–187
    wellness promotion, 187–191
Healthcare Effectiveness Data and Information
    Set (HEDIS), 90
Healthier Worksite Initiative, 356
Healthy, Hunger-Free Kids Act (2010), 347,
    364, 499
Healthy Eating Index, 353–354
Healthy Hearts program, 690
Healthy People 2020 (USDHHS)
    alcohol use, 434
    cardiovascular health, 703, 706
    physical activity, 405–406
HEALTHY Study on diabetes, 546
heart disease. See also cardiovascular disease

alcohol protective effects, 433, 686–687
cigar smoking, 252
    secondhand smoke, 252
cigarette smoking, 243, 244, 245
    secondhand smoke, 245, 246, 249
coronary. See coronary heart disease
costs of, 111
diabetes and, 521, 522, 528
dyslipidemia and, 633
heart failure. See heart failure
high blood pressure and, 594, 595, 597,
    601, 610
infectious diseases overtaken by, 3
mental health
    depression, 874
    post-traumatic stress disorder, 867
nutrition
    dietary fat, 336–337
    dietary fiber, 335–336
obesity and, 487, 488
physical activity and, 392, 395, 396
significance, 6, 15
smokeless tobacco, 251
smoking relative risks, 247
smoking-related ratios, 46, 47
social cognitive theory, 121
socioeconomic status and, 209–210
heart failure
    analytic epidemiology
        causes, 713–714
        interventions, 714–716
        modifiable risk factors, 713–714
        population-attributable risk, 714
    classification of, 714, 715–716
    coronary heart disease, 678, 680–681
    CVD risk factors, 676
    descriptive epidemiology
        geographic distribution, 712
        high-risk populations, 711–712
        time trends, 712–713
    diabetes and, 713, 716
    dyslipidemia and, 651
    future research, 716–717
    high blood pressure and, 595, 596, 610, 716
    interventions
        classification of heart failure, 714,
            715–716
        examples, 716
    metaformin and congestive, 550
    obesity and, 490
    pathophysiology, 710–711
    significance, 710
    stroke and, 707
Helping Patients Who Drink Too Much:
    A Clinician's Guide (NIAAA), 460
Hemachromatosis and Iron Overload
    Screening Study, 1050

hemochromatosis
 descriptive epidemiology, 1050
 interventions, 1050
 significance, 1050
hemodialysis. *See* dialysis
hemorrhagic strokes, 695, 696, 702
hepatitis
 alcohol-induced, 1022
  cirrhosis, 1022
 biomarkers, 1017
 definition, 1017
hepatitis A
 causes, 1028
 definition, 1026
 descriptive epidemiology, 1027–1028
  time trends, 1027–1028
 diagnosis, 1026
 interventions, 1028
 significance, 1026–1027
  incubation period, 1026
 transmission, 1026, 1028
hepatitis B
 causes, 1032, 1033
 definition, 1028
 descriptive epidemiology, 1030–1032
  time trends, 1030–1032
 interventions
  prevention, 1032, 1034
  screening, 1034
  treatment, 1034
 liver disease and, 1021, 1022
  cirrhosis, 1022, 1023
  hepatocellular carcinoma, 1030, 1032, 1034, 1048
 significance, 1029–1030
  incubation period, 1030
 transmission, 1028–1029
hepatitis C
 alcohol use and, 1025
 causes, 1035, 1039–1041
 definition, 1035
 descriptive epidemiology, 1037–1038
  time trends, 1035, 1037, 1038
 hepatitis A and, 1026
 interventions
  prevention, 1041
  screening, 1039, 1041
  treatment, 1041
 liver disease and, 1021, 1022, 1025, 1040, 1041
  cirrhosis, 1022, 1023, 1025
  hepatocellular carcinoma, 1037, 1048
 significance, 1035–1037
  morbidity, 1036–1037
 transmission, 1035
hepatocellular carcinoma
 causes, 1048–1049
  hepatitis B, 1030, 1032, 1034, 1048, 1049
  hepatitis C, 1035, 1037, 1048, 1049
  non-alcoholic fatty liver, 1042, 1046
 descriptive epidemiology, 1021, 1047–1048
  time trends, 1047, 1049
 interventions, 1049
  coffee, 1049
 significance, 1046, 1047
  mortality rates, 1019, 1046, 1047
high blood pressure. *See also* metabolic
  syndrome
 alcohol use and, 457, 599–600, 604, 605, 607, 686
 ambulatory blood pressure monitoring, 584–585, 613
 kidney disease, 1082
 analytic epidemiology
  causes, 597–601
  interventions, 601–612
  population-attributable risk, 594, 596, 600, 601
  relative risk, 594, 599
 coronary heart disease
  cardiovascular mortality, 588
  CHD attributable to, 595, 596, 601, 681
  definition of high blood pressure, 581
  as predictor of CHD, 594, 596
  treatment and CHD risk, 610, 681
 definition, 581, 585, 586
 diagnosis of, 583–587
 descriptive epidemiology
  geographic distribution, 592
  high-risk population, 589–592, 593
  time trends, 587, 588, 591, 592–593
 diabetes and, 521, 528, 537
  dementia and, 524
 dyslipidemia and, 650
 future research, 612–613
 gout and, 983, 984
 heart failure, 595, 596, 610, 716
 interventions
  Dietary Approaches to Stop
   Hypertension (DASH), 351
  individual vs. population levels, 601
  lifestyle modifications, 602, 603–606
  measurement, 583–587
  prevention at population level, 606–612
  prevention in individuals, 601–606
  screening, 112, 606–607
  treatment, 607–612
  Trials of Hypertension Prevention,
   Phase II, 504
 kidney disease, 1069–1070, 1071, 1074–1075
  interventions, 1082, 1084, 1085
 measurement of, 583–587
 obesity, 487, 593
 pathophysiology, 581–587

peripheral arterial disease, 719, 720
physical activity, 395, 396
prehypertension, 587
    cardiovascular health and, 613
    lifestyle modifications, 603–606, 607–608
    screening, 607
significance, 587–588
    morbidity and mortality, 594–597
    overview, 6
smokeless tobacco, 251
socioeconomic status and, 679
stroke
    blood pressure reduction, 601, 607,
        609–610, 700
    cardiovascular disease risk factors, 676
    stroke strongest risk factor, 594–595,
        596, 699
white coat hypertension, 584
high cholesterol. *See* dyslipidemia
high-density lipoprotein cholesterol (HDL-C)
    alcohol use, 648, 649
    body mass index and, 644–645
    coronary heart disease, 684
    descriptive epidemiology
        diverse populations, 639–640
        gender differences, 637–638
        geographic distribution, 641
        time trends, 641, 643–644
    dietary intake and, 645–647
    dyslipidemia pathophysiology, 635–636
    lipid profiles, 633, 636
    physical activity and, 395
    smoking and, 648–649
    socioeconomic status and, 640
    youth, 652
high-risk populations
    book epidemiology summary figures, 40, 41
    community-clinic link, 14
    descriptive epidemiology identifying, 40,
        42, 47
    high-risk vs. population-wide, 15, 556
Hill causality checklist, 60–62
historical cohort studies definition, 55
Hodgkin's lymphoma
    causes, 775
    descriptive epidemiology, 774–775
    interventions, 775
    significance, 744, 774
home blood pressure monitoring, 585, 613
homelessness
    hepatitis B and, 1030
    hepatitis C and, 1038
    mental health and, 860, 882
        bipolar disorder, 862
        community treatment transition, 857, 872
        schizophrenia, 862, 866, 869
    NHANES excluded population, 1037

homocysteine and coronary heart
    disease, 685
hookah tobacco smoking, 254, 266
Hooked on Nicotine Checklist (HONC), 277
hormones
    Alzheimer's and hormone replacement, 912
    autism spectrum disorders, 919
    breast cancer, 761, 764
    cholesterol in, 634
    lipid profiles and, 638
    multiple sclerosis, 926
    osteoporosis, 994, 999, 1000
    physical activity and, 395, 396
    stress hormones, 211
    tobacco use and, 263
hospitals and community benefit, 174
housing
    asthma and, 804
    cancer and, 744–745
    hepatitis B and homelessness, 1030
    hepatitis C and homelessness, 1038
    homelessness
        hepatitis B and, 1030
        hepatitis C and, 1038
        mental health and, 857, 860, 862, 869,
            872, 882
        NHANES excluded population, 1037
    interventions, 223–224, 225–227
    mental health and
        bipolar disorder, 869
        depression, 871
        homelessness, 857, 860, 862, 869, 872, 882
        National Alliance to End Homelessness, 862
Housing First, 223
human papillomavirus (HPV)
    cervical cancer cause, 769, 770, 771
    oral cavity cancer, 779
    race/ethnicity and cancer prevalence, 745
    vaccines against, 771
hypersensitivity pneumonitis. *See* organic
    dust–related lung disease
hypertension. *See* high blood pressure
hypomanic episodes, 866
hypopneas, 820–821
hypothalamic–pituitary–adrenal (HPA) axis
    fibromyalgia and, 987
    stress and, 210–211
hypothyroidism
    carpal tunnel syndrome, 939
    non-alcoholic fatty liver, 1045
    sleep apnea, 822

I

ICD-10 codes, 89
    cancers, 744, 748
    death certificates, 84

DSM-5 categories versus, 864–865
  mental health, 863, 864–865
  respiratory diseases, 796, 798
Identification and Prevention of Dietary- and
    Lifestyle-Induced Health Effects in
    Children and Infants (IDEFICS), 357
immigrant populations
  diet changes, 343
  hepatitis B, 1032
  multiple sclerosis risk, 925
  schizophrenia, 869
  socioeconomic status, 217
immune system
  autism spectrum disorders, 919
  autoimmune hepatitis, 1021
  diabetes type 1 autoimmunity, 526
    prevention, 540–541
  Guillain-Barré syndrome, 928–929
  hepatitis A, 1026–1027
  hepatitis B, 1030
  kidney disease, 1076
  mental health and, 859
  multiple sclerosis, 925–926
  physical activity and, 396
  rheumatoid arthritis, 977
  smoking and, 262
immunizations
  autism spectrum disorders caused by,
    918–919
  cervical cancer HPV infection, 771
  clinical information systems, 180
  epilepsy
    caused by, 905
    prevention, 905
  Guillain-Barré syndrome and, 928–929
  Health Impact Pyramid, 8, 9
  health policy, 139
  heart failure and, 715
  hepatitis A, 1027, 1028, 1029
  hepatitis B, 1018, 1028–1029, 1031–1032,
    1034, 1049
    kidney disease, 1083
  impact of, 288
  influenza and asthma, 808
  interstitial lung disease prevention, 824
  surveillance of, 83
impaired fasting glucose (IFG), 528
impaired glucose tolerance (IGT), 527–528
  diabetes type 2 prevention, 542–543
impaired pressure natriuresis, 582–583
incarceration
  hepatitis C and, 1039
  of mentally ill, 857, 860, 862, 872, 882
  NHANES excluded population, 1037
incidence rates
  breast cancer example, 45
  definition, 42, 43–44, 73

difference in, 45–46
  mortality rates as substitute, 42, 44
income. *See also* socioeconomic status
  asthma and, 804
  cancer and, 744–745
  diabetes and, 531, 532, 535, 537, 538
  dyslipidemia and, 640
  epilepsy and, 904
  hepatitis C and, 1039
  interventions, 223, 225
  kidney disease and, 1072
  mental health and
    depression, 869, 871, 874
    post-traumatic stress disorder, 871
    suicide, 875
  nutrition and, 340
  obesity and, 486–487, 492
  physical activity and, 402
Income, Housing, Education, Legal Status,
    Literacy, Personal Safety tool, 230
Incredible Years, 221
incubation period
  hepatitis A, 1026
  hepatitis B, 1030
indoor tanning and melanoma, 780
induction periods of cancers, 748
infantile spinal muscular atrophy, 922
infectious diseases
  chronic diseases versus, 3–4, 5, 22
  surveillance definition, 77–78, 79
influenza and asthma, 808
information bias, 58–59
Inside Knowledge: Get the Facts about
    Gynecologic Cancer Campaign, 772
insulin resistance. *See also* metabolic syndrome
  Alzheimer's disease, 911–912
  diabetes type 2, 526–527
  dietary fiber, 336
  high blood pressure, 597
  non-alcoholic fatty liver, 1042, 1045
  obesity, 262, 487, 491
  physical activity, 600
  smoking, 262
  socioeconomic status, 212
  weight loss, 501
integrated pest management for housing, 224
intellectual disability
  autism spectrum disorders, 917
  cerebral palsy, 914
  as neurodevelopmental disorder, 864
intensity of an activity, 393, 394
interleukin 1 (IL-1), 970, 977, 993
interleukin 6 (IL-6), 720, 970, 972–973
International Agency for Research on
    Cancer, 759
*International Classification of Diseases for
    Oncology* (WHO), 748

International Statistical Classification of Diseases and Related Problems, Tenth Revision (WHO)
 ICD-10 codes, 89
  cancers, 744, 748
  death certificates, 84
  DSM-5 categories versus, 864–865
  mental health criteria, 863, 864–865
  respiratory diseases, 796, 798
 liver disease, 1019
International Study of Salt and Blood Pressure (INTERSALT), 598, 599, 600
interstitial cystitis, 986
interstitial lung disease
 causes, 824
 definition, 822–823
 descriptive epidemiology, 823
 interventions, 824
interventions
 analytic epidemiology for, 50–52
 brief interventions, 126–127
  alcohol use, 460, 462–463
  for education, 140
  tobacco use, 287–288
 chronic disease continuum, 38
 Community Guide, 71–72, 306
 community-level, 132–139
  examples, 141–147
  media advocacy, 137–139
 data dissemination, 99
 educational attainment, 221–223
 employment and income, 223
 faith-based venues, 132
  nutrition, 358, 362
 health literacy enhancement, 147–150
 health policy for, 139
 health system interventions
  ACA health care reform, 169–174
  Chronic Care Model, 175–184
  complex care management, 175, 178–179
  Expanded Chronic Care Model, 189–191
  multiple chronic conditions, 165–166
  organization of health systems, 176
  overview, 13–14, 126–127
  patient characteristics, 166–167
  population health, 167–169
  screening approaches, 126, 127, 184–187
  wellness promotion, 187–191
 housing, 223–224
 interpersonal approaches, 120–126
  buddies and friends, 123–124
  community health workers, 124–125
  examples, 125–126
  family-based, 122
  social cognitive theory, 120–121, 125–126
  social support, 122–123

 intervention mapping, 144–145
 intrapersonal approaches, 116–120
 levels of intervention
  overview, 109–110
  primary to tertiary, 140–141, 174–175
  social-ecological perspective, 114–116
 models
  Chronic Care Model, 175–184
  Health Belief Model, 116–117
  Health Impact Pyramid, 7–11, 219–220
  Health Locus of Control Model, 119–120
  Mobilizing Action through Planning and Partnerships, 143–144
  PRECEDE-PROCEED Framework, 142–143
  Stages of Change Model, 117–118
  Theory of Planned Behavior, 118–119
  Total Worker Health, 130–131
  Transtheoretical Model, 117–118
 National Registry of Evidence Based Practices and Programs, 879
 school venues, 127–129
  educational achievement, 221–223
 workplace venues, 129–132
iron overload and hemochromatosis, 1049–1050
irritable bowel syndrome, 986
ischemic heart disease. *See* coronary heart disease
ischemic strokes, 695–696

J

Japan life expectancy, 5
jaundice from hepatitis, 1026, 1030
job site exposures. *See* workplaces
Johnston County Osteoarthritis Project, 971
juvenile myoclonic epilepsy, 904

K

kidney disease
 causes
  modifiable risk factors, 1074–1075
  population-attributable risk, 1075
 definition, 1067–1068
 descriptive epidemiology, 1070–1074
  geographic distribution, 1073, 1074
  high-risk populations, 1071
  time trends, 1065–1066, 1067, 1068, 1071, 1073–1074
 diabetes and
  dementia, 524
  end-stage renal disease, 521, 523, 528, 1068–1069
  microvascular complications, 528
 future research, 1084–1086
 high blood pressure and

chronic kidney disease, 594, 595, 597
    impaired pressure natriuresis, 582–583
    nocturnal dipping, 1082
    salt intake, 598
    interventions
        examples, 1084
        prevention, 1075–1076, 1084
        screening, 1076, 1077–1080
        screening how, 1077–1080
        screening who, 1077, 1079–1080
        treatment, 1075, 1080–1083
    pathophysiology, 1067–1070
    peripheral arterial disease, 719
    significance, 1065–1067
    stages of, 1080
Kidney Disease: Improving Global
    Outcomes, 1083
Kidney Early Evaluation Program (KEEP), 1077
kindergarten, full-day, 221
knee pain from osteoarthritis, 968, 969
    shoes and, 974
    treatment, 975
Knowledge Is Power Program, 221
Korsakoff's syndrome, 437

L

lactation
    asthma and, 806
    breast cancer and, 763, 764, 768
    duration and social support, 768
    support for breastfeeding, 356
latency period
    definition, 825
    incubation period
        hepatitis A, 1026
        hepatitis B, 1030
    occupational lung diseases, 825
        asbestosis, 834
        occupational asthma, 837
        reactive airways dysfunction syndrome,
            837
    study design and, 54
leisure definition, 393–395
Lennox-Gestaut syndrome, 900
leukemia
    causes, 776–777
    cigarette smoking and, 243, 259
    descriptive epidemiology, 776
    interventions, 777
    significance, 744, 776
life expectancy
    by country, 5
    disparities in health care, 21
    United States
        lifestyle behaviors, 6
        other countries versus, 5

lipid profile measures, 633, 636, 641
    dietary intake and, 645–647
    lifestyle modifications, 652
    physical activity and, 647–648
    youth, 652
lipoproteins in dyslipidemia pathophysiology,
    635–636
liver cancer. *See* hepatocellular carcinoma
liver disease
    alcohol use, 436, 447
    alcohol-induced
        descriptive epidemiology, 1021, 1022,
            1023–1024
        interventions for alcohol use, 457–468
        significance, 1022, 1024–1026
    causes, 1020–1022
    definition, 1017, 1020
    descriptive epidemiology
        time trends, 1017–1019, 1020
    hemochromatosis
        descriptive epidemiology, 1050
        interventions, 1050
        significance, 1050
    hepatitis, 1017, 1022
    hepatitis A
        causes, 1028
        definition, 1026
        descriptive epidemiology, 1027–1028
        interventions, 1028
        significance, 1026–1027
        transmission, 1026, 1028
    hepatitis B
        causes, 1032, 1033
        definition, 1028
        descriptive epidemiology, 1030–1032
        significance, 1029–1030
        transmission, 1028–1029
    hepatitis C
        causes, 1039–1041
        definition, 1035
        descriptive epidemiology, 1037–1038
        interventions, 1039, 1041
        significance, 1035–1037
        transmission, 1035
    hepatocellular carcinoma
        causes, 1048–1049
        descriptive epidemiology, 1021,
            1047–1048
        interventions, 1049
        significance, 1046, 1047
    interventions
        prevention, 1018
        treatment, 1017
    non-alcoholic fatty liver
        causes, 1045
        definition, 1041–1042
        descriptive epidemiology, 1022, 1043–1045

interventions, 1046
  obesity and, 1017–1018
  significance, 1042–1043
obesity, 488
  non-alcoholic fatty liver disease,
    1017–1018
  significance, 1017–1020
    morbidity, 1019–1020
    mortality, 1018–1019
Locus of Control Model, 119–120
Lou Gehrig's disease. *See* amyotrophic lateral
  sclerosis (ALS)
low back pain
  ankylosing spondylitis, 989, 990
  causes, 899, 940
  descriptive epidemiology, 940
    high-risk groups, 899
  interventions, 941
  significance, 940
low birthweight
  cardiovascular disease, 1073
  cerebral palsy, 896
  chronic diseases, 1073
  chronic obstructive pulmonary disease, 813
  diabetes, 537
  high blood pressure, 597, 1073
  kidney disease, 1073
  mental illness, 874
  tobacco use, 244, 251, 254
low-density lipoprotein cholesterol (LDL-C)
  alcohol use, 648
  atherosclerotic CVD risk, 654
  body mass index, 644–645
  coronary heart disease, 684
  descriptive epidemiology
    diverse populations, 639–640
    gender differences, 637–638
    geographic distribution, 641
    time trends, 641, 643–644
  dietary intake and, 645–647
  dyslipidemia pathophysiology, 635–636
  familial hypercholesterolemia, 636–637
  lipid profiles, 633, 636
  smoking and, 649
  youth, 652
lower-limb amputations
  diabetes, 521, 522–523, 528
    geographic distribution, 532
  peripheral arterial disease, 717, 722
lung cancer
  analytic epidemiology
    causes, 754–755
    interventions, 755–757
    modifiable risk factors, 754–755
    population-attributable risk, 755
  asbestos and, 65, 754, 826
  cigar smoking, 252

secondhand smoke, 252
cigarette smoking, 243, 244, 245, 248,
  254, 752
  secondhand smoke, 245, 246, 249,
    754, 755
  as strongest risk factor, 754, 755
coronary heart disease mortality versus,
  46, 47
descriptive epidemiology
  geographic distribution, 753
  high-risk populations, 753
  smoking-related ratios, 46, 47, 752
  time trends, 753
future research, 757
hookah tobacco smoking, 254
interventions
  examples, 756–757
  prevention, 755–756
  screening, 112, 756
  treatment, 756
pathophysiology, 752
pipe smoking, 253, 254
relative risk
  age and smoking status, 247
  asbestos and smoking, 65
  smokers vs. non-, 56
significance, 744, 752
  mortality rates, 51
smokeless tobacco, 251
lymphoma
  causes, 775
  definition, 774
  descriptive epidemiology, 774–775
  interventions, 775
  significance, 744, 774

M

macrovascular diabetic complications, 528
magnetic fields and leukemia, 777
major depressive disorder. *See* depression
  (mental health)
malignant tumors, 748. *See also* cancer
mammography
  breast cancer
    mortality, 765
    time trends, 762
  disparity, 95
  false positives, 39, 765, 767
  Health Belief Model, 116–117
  health literacy and, 148
  recommendations, 116, 766, 768
mania from bipolar disorder, 866
manner of death, 84
Master Settlement Agreement, 290–291, 292,
  294–295, 305
meat nutrition

Dietary Guidelines, 333
fish
    cirrhosis prevention, 1049
    DASH diet, 351
    geographic distribution, 342
    Mediterranean diet, 351, 647
    obesity risk and, 495
    omega-3 fatty acids, 336
red meat, 337
    colorectal cancer and, 759
    hepatocellular carcinoma, 1049
    pork, beer, and liver disease, 1026
as Western diet, 983
white meat
    cirrhosis and, 1049
    DASH diet, 351
    Mediterranean diet, 647
media influence
    alcohol use, 456
    community-level interventions, 137–139
    food advertising, 348, 364–365
    tobacco industry promotion, 272–274,
        280, 294
        advertising restrictions, 283–284,
            294–295, 296
    Youth Media Campaign for physical
        activity, 399
Medicaid
    Centers for Medicare and Medicaid Services
        Innovation Center, 169–170
    health homes, 172
    Incentives for the Prevention of Chronic
        Diseases Model Grants, 173
    preventive services, 187
    smoking Master Settlement
        Agreement, 292
    tobacco-use treatment, 297–300
medical homes, 171–172
    Blueprint for Health, 191
    Chronic Care Model, 178
    as screening venue, 185
Medicare
    Centers for Medicare and Medicaid Services
        Innovation Center, 169–170
    Diabetes Prevention Program, 556
    federal budget percentage, 112
    kidney disease, 1067, 1069
        end-stage renal disease coverage,
            1065, 1067
    multiple chronic conditions, 165–166
    payment reform goal, 173
    Shared Savings Program, 170–171
    smoking Master Settlement Agreement, 292
    tobacco-use treatment, 297–300
medication adherence. *See* adherence to
    prescribed care
Mediterranean diet

Dietary Guidelines, 351
    dyslipidemia, 646, 647
    obesity, 502
    stroke, 702
melanoma of the skin
    causes, 780
    descriptive epidemiology, 780
    interventions, 781
    significance, 744, 780
memory
    alcohol use, 436, 437, 438
    dementias, 909–910
    hippocampus, 211
    insulin resistance, 911–912
    post-traumatic stress disorder, 867
    recall bias, 59
    seizure auras, 902
    sleep apnea, 821
menopause
    alcohol use and, 436
    breast cancer, 56, 488, 762, 763, 764
    coronary heart disease, 678
    gout, 983
    lipid profiles, 638
    low back pain, 940
    migraine headaches, 942
    osteoporosis, 994, 995, 1000
    smoking and, 263
mental health. *See also* alcohol use;
    Alzheimer's disease; anxiety; depression;
    schizophrenia
    analytic epidemiology
        causes, 873–875
        interventions, 875–881
        modifiable risk factors, 873–874
        population-attributable risk, 875
    biopsychosocial model, 863
    Chronic Care Model, 179
    "common cold of mental illness," 869. *See*
        also depression
    criteria for disorders, 863
    descriptive epidemiology
        geographic distribution, 871
        psychiatric epidemiological surveys, 868
        time trends, 872–873
    diabetes and, 523, 525, 537
    future research, 881–883
    homelessness or incarceration, 860, 882
        bipolar disorder, 862
        community treatment transition, 857, 872
        schizophrenia, 862, 866, 869
    immune system and, 859–860
    interventions
        examples, 879–881
        preventing depression, 879–880
        preventing illness, 875–876, 877, 879–880
        recovery promotion, 876, 878–879

screening, 877–878, 882
Strategic Plan of NIMH, 882–883
treatment, 878–879
treatment biopsychosocial model, 863, 880–881
treatment reaching people, 857, 861, 878, 881
medications as chronic disease risks, 860
mind–body dualism, 10–11, 858–859
mood disorders. *See also* bipolar disorder; depression
descriptive epidemiology, 869
fibromyalgia mood disturbance, 987
pathophysiology, 866
obesity and, 487, 491
obsessive–compulsive disorder
attention-deficit/hyperactivity disorder, 936
causes, 931
Tourette syndrome, 930
overview, 858–859
pathophysiology, 862–868
post-traumatic stress disorder (PTSD)
as central sensitivity syndrome, 986
comorbid disease risk, 860
descriptive epidemiology, 870–871
pathophysiology, 867
resilience traits and, 870, 874
violence and, 870–871, 874
significance, 857, 862
morbidity, 859–860
mortality, 861
social burden, 857, 860, 862
social anxiety
pathophysiology, 866–867
prevalence, 870
youth alcohol use for, 456
suicide
attention-deficit/hyperactivity disorder, 936–937
descriptive epidemiology, 871
mental illness comorbid diseases versus, 859
pathophysiology, 868
population-attributable risk, 875
violence and, 861
Mental Health Parity and Addiction Equity Act (2008), 858, 872, 873
mentoring programs, 221
meta-analyses of studies, 69–70
metabolic syndrome
C-reactive protein biomarker, 684
diabetes, 537. *See also* diabetes
features of, 1041, 1042. *See also* diabetes; dyslipidemia; high blood pressure; obesity
kidney disease, 1072
liver disease, 1041

cirrhosis, 1023
non-alcoholic fatty liver, 1042, 1045
obesity, 487, 489. *See also* obesity
METs of an activity, 394
mHEALTH intervention, 692
microbiome, 342, 496
microvascular diabetic complications, 528
migraine headaches
causes, 899, 942
descriptive epidemiology, 941–942
high-risk groups, 899
interventions, 942–943
significance, 941
migrant populations
diet changes, 343
hepatitis B, 1032
multiple sclerosis risk, 925
promotores, 124, 125, 189–191
schizophrenia, 869
socioeconomic status, 217
military veterans and hepatitis C, 1038, 1039
milk
diabetes type 1 prevention, 541
Dietary Guidelines, 333
nutrition, 337–338, 355
mind–body dualism, 858–859
"ministrokes," 696
Minnesota Heart Health Program, 656
mixed dyslipidemia, 633
mobile phone–based intervention
coronary heart disease, 692
physical activity, 417
Mobilizing Action through Planning and Partnerships (MAPP), 143–144
Mobilizing Action Toward Community Health, 141
"Monday morning syndrome," 835
mood disorders. *See also* depression
bipolar disorder
attention-deficit/hyperactivity disorder and, 936
descriptive epidemiology, 869
homelessness and, 862
pathophysiology, 866
treatment, 880–881
violent crime and, 861
descriptive epidemiology, 869
fibromyalgia mood disturbance, 987
pathophysiology, 866
mortality data, 83–84
mortality rates
alcohol use, 455–456
anxiety untreated, 861
cancer, 15, 743, 745, 746, 747
bladder cancer, 777
breast cancer, 50, 762, 763
colorectal cancer, 757, 758

lung cancer, 51, 752, 753, 755
    lymphoma, 774, 775
    oral cavity cancer, 778
    prostate cancer, 773
cardiovascular disease, 633, 640,
        673–674, 675
    coronary heart disease, 15, 676–677, 678,
        679–681
    globally, 675
    heart failure, 710
    stroke, 695, 696–697
diabetes, 520–521, 528
    youth, 521, 536
dyslipidemia, 651
high blood pressure, 588, 591
incidence rate substitute, 42, 44
kidney disease, 1066, 1068
lifestyle behaviors, 6
liver disease, 1019
    alcoholic, 1023, 1024
    hepatitis B, 1030
    hepatitis C, 1035, 1036
    hepatocellular carcinoma, 1019,
        1046, 1047
    non-alcoholic fatty liver, 1043
mental health
    depression untreated, 861
    suicide, 871
neurological disorders
    epilepsy, 901
    Guillain-Barré syndrome, 928
    traumatic brain injury, 931–933
obesity, 489
respiratory diseases, 795
    asbestosis, 833, 834
    asthma, 805
    byssinosis, 835
    chronic obstructive pulmonary disease,
        811, 813, 814
    coal workers' pneumoconiosis, 826
    pneumoconioses, 826
    silicosis, 831
smoking-attributable mortality, 246,
        248–249
    cigars, 252
    pipes, 253–254
stroke, 695, 696–697
motor vehicle crashes
    alcohol use causing, 435, 457, 466
    sleep apnea causing, 821
    spinal cord injury from, 934, 935
    traumatic brain injury from, 933, 934
mouth cancer. See oral cavity cancer
Moving to Opportunity, 224, 227
Multiethnic Cohort Study, 539
Multi-Ethnic Study of Atherosclerosis (MESA),
        533, 694, 712

Multilevel Approach to Community Health
        (MATCH) model, 693
Multiple Risk Factor Intervention Trial, 690
multiple sclerosis (MS)
    causes, 897, 924–926
    definition, 923
    descriptive epidemiology, 924
        high-risk groups, 897
    future research, 927
    interventions, 923, 926–927
    pathophysiology, 923–924
    significance, 923
musculoskeletal disorders. See arthritis;
        osteoporosis
myofascial pain, 986
MyPlate nutrition guide, 348, 350–351

N

naltrexone
    alcohol use, 466
    obesity, 503
Nash, John, Jr., 866
National 5 a Day Program, 354–355
National Action Plan for Bone Health, 1002
National Alliance to End Homelessness, 862
National Ambulatory Medical Care
        Survey, 1036
National Arthritis Action Plan, 975–976
National Bone Health Campaign, 1001–1002
National Cancer Institute–Kellogg's
        Campaign, 354
National Cancer Moonshot Initiative, 750
National Center for Health Statistics (NCHS)
    alcohol use, 455–456
    blood pressure, 589
    death certificates, 84
    physical activity, 398
    respiratory diseases, 795
National Coalition for Promoting Physical
        Activity, 412
National Comorbidity Survey on mental illness,
        862, 868
    anxiety, 870
National Comorbidity Survey Replication, 868
National Epidemiologic Survey on Alcohol and
        Related Conditions, 439–441, 454–455
    mental health and violence, 861
National Health and Nutrition Examination
        Survey (NHANES), 89, 338–339, 352
    high blood pressure, 589–592, 593
    kidney disease, 1070
    liver disease, 1021
        hepatitis C, 1037, 1039
        non-alcoholic fatty liver, 1043, 1044, 1045
    obesity, 489
    osteoarthritis, 970–971, 972

peripheral arterial disease, 718, 719
physical activity, 398
respiratory diseases
asbestosis, 833–834
chronic obstructive pulmonary disease,
811, 815
National Health Interview Survey (NHIS), 87
arthritis, 966
asthma, 800, 801–802, 804
mental health, 860
physical activity, 398
National Heart Disease and Stroke Prevention
Program, 706, 708–709
National Hospital Ambulatory Medical Care
Survey, 1036
National Household Travel Survey (NHTS), 400
National Institute of Mental Health (NIMH)
Strategic Plan, 882–883
National Institute on Alcohol Abuse and
Alcoholism (NIAAA), 454, 460, 463
National Institutes of Health Stroke Scale
(NIHSS), 706
National Kidney Foundation, 1076
National Longitudinal Alcohol Epidemiologic
Survey, 454–455
National Nutrition Monitoring System, 351
National Physical Activity Plan, 411–412
National Physical Activity Society, 413–414
National Poison Data System
alcohol-based hand sanitizer
consumption, 442
National Prevention, Health Promotion, and
Public Health Council, 24
National Program of Cancer Registries
(NPCR), 749
National Registry of Evidence Based Practices
and Programs, 879
National Resource Center for Health and Safety
in Child Care and Early Education, 499
National Safe Routes to School Task Force, 410
National School Lunch Program, 347,
359–360, 364
National Survey of Children's Health, 351
National Survey on Drug Use and Health
alcohol use, 439, 454–455
geographic distribution, 448–452
race/ethnicity, 444
National Tobacco Control Program, 289, 756
National Weight Loss Registry, 504
Nationwide Inpatient Sample, 1036
Nationwide Personal Transportation Survey. See
National Household Travel Survey
neurological disorders. See also Alzheimer's
disease; amyotrophic lateral sclerosis
(ALS); autism spectrum disorders;
cerebral palsy; dementias; epilepsy;
Parkinson's disease

attention-deficit/hyperactivity disorder
causes, 898, 938
definition, 936
descriptive epidemiology, 898, 937
interventions, 938
as neurodevelopmental disorder, 864
pathophysiology, 937
significance, 936–937
Tourette syndrome and, 930
carpal tunnel syndrome
causes, 898, 938, 939
definition, 938–939
descriptive epidemiology, 898, 939
interventions, 939
significance, 939
causes and consequences, 896–899
Guillain-Barré syndrome
causes, 897, 928–929
definition, 927
descriptive epidemiology, 897, 928
future research, 929
interventions, 929
pathophysiology, 928
significance, 927–928
high-risk groups, 895–899
low back pain
ankylosing spondylitis, 989, 990
causes, 899, 940
descriptive epidemiology, 899, 940
interventions, 941
significance, 940
migraine headaches
causes, 899, 942
descriptive epidemiology, 899,
941–942
interventions, 942–943
significance, 941
multiple sclerosis
causes, 897, 924–926
definition, 923
descriptive epidemiology, 897, 924
future research, 927
interventions, 923, 926–927
pathophysiology, 923–924
significance, 923
significance, 895
spinal cord injury
causes, 898, 934, 935
descriptive epidemiology, 898, 935
interventions, 936
significance, 934–935
Tourette syndrome. See also tic disorders
causes, 897, 931
definition, 929–930
descriptive epidemiology, 897, 930
future research, 931
interventions, 931

pathophysiology, 930
significance, 930
traumatic brain injury
causes, 898, 933
descriptive epidemiology, 898, 932–933
interventions, 933–934
post-traumatic stress disorder and, 870
registries for surveillance data, 87
significance, 931–932
surveillance, 87
neuropathy from diabetes, 521, 522–523
newborn screening statistics, 85
nicotine
addiction to, 263–264, 277, 278–279
pathophysiology, 263–264
reproductive disorders, 256, 261
withdrawal from, 263–264
youth dependence, 263–264, 277
effects on brain, 256, 263, 277
No Excuses charter school model, 222
non-alcoholic fatty liver disease
causes, 1045
definition, 1041–1042
descriptive epidemiology, 1043–1045
future research, 1046
interventions, 1046
screening, 1043
as liver disease attributable risk, 1022
cirrhosis, 1022
hepatocellular carcinoma, 1048
obesity and, 1017–1018
significance, 1042–1043
non-articular rheumatism. See fibromyalgia
non-Hodgkin's lymphoma
causes, 775
descriptive epidemiology, 775
interventions, 775
significance, 744, 774
normative beliefs, 119
North Karelia Project, 656
Northern Manhattan Stroke Study, 702
Norway life expectancy, 5
notifiable disease systems data, 80, 81, 83
Not-On-Tobacco (N-O-T), 129
Nurses' Health Study
diabetes population-attributable risk, 539
hip replacements and BMI, 973
stroke, 702
nutrition
alcohol use
caloric density, 433
nutritional deficiencies, 437
amyotrophic lateral sclerosis (ALS) and, 922
analytic epidemiology
causes, 344–349
interventions, 349–365
population-attributable risk, 349

ankylosing spondylitis and, 992
as behavioral determinant, 111
cancer and, 749
breast cancer, 763, 764
colorectal cancer, 759
hepatocellular carcinoma, 1049
lung cancer, 754, 755
significance, 744–745
descriptive epidemiology, 338–344
geographic distribution, 342–343
time trends, 343–344
diabetes
dietary fiber and, 336
glycemic load, 537, 538
healthier diets, 538
Dietary Guidelines, 333–334
alcohol use, 648
dyslipidemia, 647
nutrition, 349–351
obesity, 494–495
dyslipidemia and, 645–647
environmental determinants, 113
future research, 365–367
gout and, 983, 984
high blood pressure
Dietary Approaches to Stop
Hypertension (DASH), 351, 604, 606
salt and blood pressure, 598, 599,
603–604
interventions
large-scale initiatives, 354–355
Nutrition and Physical Activity Self-
Assessment for Child Care, 505
policy approaches, 363–365
population-based, 358–362
prevention, 349–351
Reading, Writing, and Reducing
Obesity, 129
screening, 351–352
site-based, 356–358
treatment, 352–354
kidney disease restrictions, 1082–1083
liver disease and, 1026
hepatocellular carcinoma, 1049
neurological disorders
cerebral palsy, 916
multiple sclerosis, 927
obesity and, 494–495, 538. See also obesity
dietary modification, 501–502. See also
weight loss
osteoporosis and, 994, 1000
pathophysiology, 334–338
potassium and blood pressure, 599,
604, 605
salt
blood pressure, 598, 599, 603–604
cancer, 750

Dietary Guidelines, 333
  kidney disease, 1083
significance, 111, 331–334
socioeconomic status and, 202, 205,
  208, 340
stroke and, 336, 702
Nutrition and Physical Activity Self-Assessment
  for Child Care, 505

O

obesity. *See also* metabolic syndrome
  alcohol use
    caloric density, 433
    liver disease, 1025
  analytic epidemiology
    causes, 494–497
    interventions, 497–505
    population-attributable risk, 497
  arthritis
    gout, 981, 983, 984
    osteoarthritis, 970, 972–973, 974
    rheumatoid arthritis, 978, 979
  asthma, 488, 489, 806
  body mass index assessment, 485
  cancer, 750
    breast cancer, 763, 764
    colorectal cancer, 758, 759
    prostate cancer, 773
  cardiovascular disease, 487, 488, 489,
    490, 644
    coronary heart disease, 487, 488, 676, 686
  carpal tunnel syndrome, 939, 940
  costs of, 111, 489–490
    cost-effectiveness, 507
  definition, 485, 686
  descriptive epidemiology
    geographic distribution, 493
    high-risk populations, 491–493
    time trends, 494, 593
  diabetes
    adult obesity, 487, 488, 528, 531, 533, 537
    lifespan obesity, 538
    obesity pathophysiology, 490–491
    obesity treatment, 501
    type 2 pathophysiology, 526
    youth obesity, 489
  dyslipidemia and, 644–645
  environmental determinants, 112–113
  future research, 505–507
  health policy, 139
  high blood pressure and, 597–598, 599, 607
    obesity-related hypertension, 582–583
  interventions
    Childhood Obesity Intervention Cost-
      Effectiveness Study, 507
    coalitions, 188–189

    examples, 504–505
    family-based, 122
    policy based, 365
    prevention, 497–500
    prevention in children, 367
    Project SMART, 125–126
    Reading, Writing, and Reducing
      Obesity, 129
    school-based, 357
    screening, 112, 500–501
    treatment, 501–504
    weight-loss maintenance, 504
  kidney disease and, 1070, 1071, 1072, 1075
  liver disease and, 1025, 1041
    alcoholic, 1025
    non-alcoholic fatty liver, 1044, 1045
  low back pain and, 940
  microbiome and, 342
  pathophysiology, 490–491
  physical activity and, 395
  significance, 485–491
    economic, 489–490
    metabolic chronic disease, 487, 489
    morbidity, 487–489
    mortality, 489
    overview, 111
    prevalence, 93, 94
    psychosocial, 486–487, 491
    reproductive, 487, 490
  sleep apnea and, 821
  socioeconomic status and, 208, 486–487,
    492, 679
  sugar and, 338
observational studies
  bias, 58–59
  confounding, 57–58
  definition, 53–56
  systematic reviews, 69–70
obsessive–compulsive disorder
  attention-deficit/hyperactivity disorder, 936
  causes, 931
  Tourette syndrome, 930
obstructive sleep apnea, 796–797, 820
  conditions stemming from, 821
  high-risk populations, 821
occupational asthma
  causes, 838–839
  descriptive epidemiology, 837–838
  interventions, 839
  significance, 836–837
occupational exposures. *See* workplaces
occupational lung diseases, 825–826
occupational safety *promotores* programs, 125
1% or Less Campaign, 355
oral cavity cancer
  alcohol use, 436
  causes, 779

definition, 778
descriptive epidemiology, 778, 779
interventions, 779
significance, 744, 778
smokeless tobacco and, 251, 252, 259, 779
smoking and, 243, 252, 253, 259, 779
organic dust–related lung disease
causes, 841
descriptive epidemiology, 840
interventions, 841
significance, 839–840
osteoarthritis
causes, 971–973, 975
modifiable risk factors, 972–973
definitions, 968
descriptive epidemiology, 965, 970–971
future research, 976
interventions
examples, 975–976
prevention, 973–974, 976
screening, 974
treatment, 974–975
pathophysiology, 969–970
significance, 969
high-risk populations, 971
osteoporosis
causes
modifiable risk factors, 998–999
population-attributable risk, 999
definition, 993–994
descriptive epidemiology, 965
geographic distribution, 996–997
high-risk populations, 995–996
time trends, 997–998
diagnosis, 993–994, 1000–1001
future research, 1002
interventions
examples, 1001–1002
prevention, 999–1000
screening, 112, 1000–1001
treatment, 1001
nutrition and, 332, 337
pathophysiology, 994–995
physical activity and, 396, 397
significance, 993–994

P

PAD. See peripheral arterial disease
pancreatic cancer
significance, 744
smoking and, 252
panic disorder, 866–867, 870
Pap (Papanicolaou) test, 769, 771–772
health literacy and, 148
high-risk populations, 772
Parkinson's disease

amyotrophic lateral sclerosis (ALS) and, 921
causes, 896, 907–908
definition, 906
descriptive epidemiology, 907
high-risk groups, 896
future research, 909
interventions, 909
melanoma risk factor, 780
pathophysiology, 907
significance, 906–907
Partnership for an Active Community
Environment, 691
partnerships. See coalitions
pathophysiology definition, 40
patient confidentiality during
collaboration, 468
Patient Protection and Affordable Care Act
(ACA; 2010)
Chronic Care Model and, 176
"culture of health," 16, 18
employee wellness initiatives, 131, 331
funding for community-clinic coalitions, 189
health care access and, 139
health care reform, 169–174
mental health treatment access, 858,
872–873
National Prevention, Health Promotion, and
Public Health Council, 24
nutrition right-to-know, 364
population health, 167, 169
prevention and management activities,
173–174
preventive services coverage, 112, 187, 653
surveillance need, 79
tobacco-use treatment, 297–300
patient registries, 180–181, 185–186
acute stroke, 87, 708
cancer, 748–749
National Program of Cancer
Registries, 749
cardiovascular disease, 722
chronic diseases, 81, 85–87
coronary artery disease, 722
electronic health records, 181, 186
weight loss, 504
patient-centered medical homes (PCMH),
171–172
Blueprint for Health, 191
as screening venue, 185
Paul Coverdell National Acute Stroke Registry
(PCNASR), 708
Pawtucket Heart Health Program, 656
payment to providers
accountable care organizations, 170–171
bundled payment, 172–173
Centers for Medicare and Medicaid Services
Innovation Center, 169–170

fee-for-service shifts, 174
    medical homes, 171–172
Pediatric Nutrition Surveillance, 351
peer groups in interventions, 124
peer review of studies, 71–72
People with Arthritis Can Exercise, 976
periodontal disease
    diabetes, 521
    kidney disease, 1073
    smoking, 262
peripheral arterial disease (PAD)
    analytical epidemiology
        causes, 719–721
        interventions, 721–722
    as cardiovascular disease, 655, 673
    descriptive epidemiology, 718–719
    diabetes and, 522, 676
    interventions, 721–722
        screening, 718, 722
    pathophysiology, 718
    physical activity, 721
    REACH Registry, 722
    risk factors, 676
    significance, 717–718
    smoking and, 676
pest management for housing, 224
pharmacists for screening, 186–187
pharyngeal cancer
    alcohol use, 436
    causes, 779
    descriptive epidemiology, 778, 779
    interventions, 779
    significance, 778
    smokeless tobacco and, 779
    smoking and, 243, 253, 779
physical activity
    Alzheimer's disease, 912–913
    analytic epidemiology
        causes, 403–405
        interventions, 405–414
        population-attributable risk, 405
    arthritis
        ankylosing spondylitis, 991, 993
        fibromyalgia, 988, 989
        interventions, 967–968
        limitations, 965, 966
        osteoarthritis, 973, 974, 975
        rheumatoid arthritis, 980, 981
    as behavioral determinant, 111
    cancer, 749, 750
        breast cancer, 763, 764
        colorectal cancer, 759
    coronary heart disease, 392, 395, 686
    definitions of terms, 393–395
    descriptive epidemiology
        geographic distribution, 402–403, 405
        high-risk populations, 400–402

surveillance, 397–400, 411, 415
    time trends, 403, 404
    diabetes, 538
    dyslipidemia, 647–648
    environmental determinants of, 113,
        402–403, 405
    exercise versus, 393, 394, 395. See also
        exercise
    future research, 414–418
    high blood pressure, 599, 600–601, 604,
        605–606
    importance of, 391
    interventions
        behavioral, 405–406, 407
        Coordinated Approach to Child
            Health, 129
        environmental, 406–408, 415–416
        examples, 408–414
        health-enhancing physical activity, 414
        Nutrition and Physical Activity Self-
            Assessment for Child Care, 505
        Physical Activity Guidelines, 398, 648
        policy, 406–408, 415–416
        social cognitive theory, 121
    minimum level of, 391, 648
        dyslipidemia and, 648
        meeting the Guidelines, 400, 401,
            403, 404
        Physical Activity Guidelines, 398, 648
    obesity, 495, 501, 502
    osteoporosis, 1000, 1001–1002
    pathophysiology, 393–397
    peripheral arterial disease, 721
    SAID principle, 397
    significance, 111, 392–393
    socioeconomic status and, 202, 208
    stroke, 396, 702
Physical Activity Guidelines for Americans,
    398, 648
Physical Activity Policy Research Network,
    415–416
physical fatigue of fibromyalgia, 985
physical fitness definitions, 393, 394
Physicians' Health Study, 702
pipe smoking
    oral cavity cancer, 779
    significance, 253–254
plaque and atherosclerosis, 634
pneumoconioses, 798, 825–841
    ICD-10 code, 798
    work exposure, 799
policy surveillance, 91–92
Pooled-Cohort atherosclerotic cardiovascular
        disease (ASCVD) risk equation, 650–651
Population Assessment of Tobacco and Health
        (PATH), 266, 274–275
population health

ACA provisions, 167, 169
County Health Rankings Model of
    Population Health, 169
definition, 167, 168
medicalization of, 231
social determinants, 114
wellness promotion, 187–191
population-attributable risk, 63–65, 73, 538
populations
    age differences across, 47–48
    comparing rates across, 44–47
    standard population, 48
pork, beer, and liver disease, 1026
post-traumatic stress disorder (PTSD)
    as central sensitivity syndrome, 986
    comorbid disease risk, 860
    descriptive epidemiology, 870–871
    pathophysiology, 867
    resilience traits and, 870, 874
    violence and, 870–871, 874
potassium intake and blood pressure, 599,
    604, 605
poverty rate, 214–219. See also socioeconomic
    status (SES)
PRECEDE-PROCEED Framework, 142–143
prediabetes, 6, 527–528
    Diabetes Prevention Program, 19, 501
    diagnosis of, 547
    reducing diabetes risk, 538
    screening, 546–547
pregnancy. See also low birthweight
    birth certificate data, 84
    breast cancer risk, 45, 46
    carpal tunnel syndrome, 939
    cervical cancer risk, 770
    diabetes, 521–522, 534
        Balance after Baby, 554
        gestational diabetes mellitus, 527,
            534–535
        prevalence, 534–535
        screening, 548
    Dietary Guidelines, 350
    hepatitis B, 1034
    mental health of child, 874
    multiple sclerosis, 926
    nutrition assistance, 359
    obesity and, 496
    prematurity and cerebral palsy, 915–916
    screening
        diabetes, 548
        hepatitis B, 1034
        mental illness, 877
        newborns, 85
        substance use disorder, 877
    smoking
        decline in, 290, 298
        underreporting, 286

Zika virus during, 915
prehypertension, 587
    cardiovascular health and, 613
    lifestyle modifications, 603–606, 607–608
    screening, 607
preschool
    attention-deficit/hyperactivity disorder, 936
    education programs, 222
    Nutrition and Physical Activity Self-
        Assessment for Child Care, 505
    nutrition programs, 357–358
    obesity prevention, 498–499
    skin cancer prevention, 781
President's Council on Fitness, Sports, and
    Nutrition, 413
prevalence definition, 42, 44
Prevent online social network, 554
Prevention and Public Health Fund, 173
prevention of chronic disease
    ACA and preventive services charges, 112
    Chronic Care Model, 178
        Expanded Chronic Care Model, 189–191
    chronic disease continuum, 38
    definition, 12
    Health Impact Pyramid, 7–11, 219–220
    strategies in four domains
        community-clinic link, 14, 16–20
        environmental approaches, 13
        epidemiology and surveillance, 12–13,
            18–19
        interventions, 13–14
    wellness promotion, 187–191
"Prevention of Mental Disorders" (WHO),
    873–874, 879
Prevention Research Centers (PRCs), 128–129
price
    alcohol use and, 458
    tobacco use and, 280–281, 282
        tobacco excise taxes, 292–293, 756–757
primary care
    community health business model,
        188–189
    kidney disease interventions, 1076, 1085
    medical homes, 171–172
    as screening venue, 185, 186
privacy of communication in collaboration, 468
processed meat and colorectal cancer, 759
Project Active, 409–410
Project SMART for weight loss, 125–126
promotores (community health workers), 124,
    125, 189–191
Prospective Cardiovasular Münster (PROCAM)
    study, 687
prospective cohort studies, 53–55
prostate cancer
    causes, 773
    descriptive epidemiology, 773

false positives, 39, 773
interventions
    prevention, 773
    screening, 773, 774
    significance, 744, 773
prostate-specific antigen (PSA) screening,
    773, 774
proteinuria and kidney disease, 1072, 1075,
    1082, 1084, 1085
provider payment. *See* payment to providers
psychiatric issues. *See* mental health
psychosocial issues
    alcohol use stigma, 446–447, 1018
    breast cancer, 762
    Chronic Care Model, 179
    coronary heart disease, 687
    epilepsy, 901
    liver disease and immunization, 1018
    mental health
        biopsychocial model, 863, 880–881
        recovery despite stigma, 876
        stigma, 858, 861, 876, 878
        suicide, 871
        treatment, 878–879
        treatment access, 858
        violence and mental illness, 861
    obesity, 486–487, 491
    socioeconomic status, 207, 211–214
Public Health Accreditation Standards, 80
public health policy. *See* health policy
public health professionals
    community health workers
        coronary heart disease intervention,
            691, 692
        health care–community liaisons,
            189–191
        interpersonal interventions, 124–125
        nutrition interventions, 362
        promotores, 124, 125, 189–191
    global training needs, 22–23
    skills required, 23–24
public health surveillance. *See* surveillance
pulmonary fibrosis, 840

Q

quasi-experimental studies, 52–53, 54

R

race/ethnicity
    alcohol use, 440, 444–446, 1025
        Alcohol Use Disorders Identification
            Tool, 460
    arthritis
        gout, 983
        osteoarthritis, 971–972

cancer
    bladder cancer, 777
    breast cancer, 95, 96, 762, 763
    cervical cancer, 769
    colorectal cancer, 744, 758
    leukemia, 776
    lymphoma, 774
    melanoma of the skin, 780
    oral cavity cancer, 778
    prostate cancer, 773
    significance, 744–747
cardiovascular disease
    coronary heart disease, 678, 680,
        691, 694
    heart failure, 712
    mortality, 674
    peripheral arterial disease, 719
    stroke, 697–698
challenges of health care, 20
Chronic Care Model, 178
diabetes
    arthritis, 524
    cardiovascular disease, 540
    end-stage renal disease, 523
    geographic distribution, 532–533
    lower-limb amputations, 522–523
    mortality rates, 520
    Multiethnic Cohort Study, 539
    prevalence, 530, 532, 534
    youth, 535–536
discrimination and stress, 212–213
dyslipidemia
    descriptive epidemiology, 639–640
    screening, 653
food insecurity, 341
high blood pressure
    alcohol use and, 600
    descriptive epidemiology, 589–592
    Dietary Approaches to Stop
        Hypertension (DASH), 606
    medication non-persistence, 612
    morbidity and mortality, 594–596
    physical activity and, 600–601, 606
    screening, 607
    treatment outcome, 611
kidney disease, 1071–1073, 1075
liver disease
    alcoholic, 1023, 1024, 1025
    hepatitis B, 1029
    hepatitis C, 1037–1038
    hepatocellular carcinoma, 1047
    non-alcoholic fatty liver, 1044–1045
mental health, 868
    bipolar disorder, 869
    post-traumatic stress disorder,
        870–871, 874
neurological disorders

Alzheimer's disease, 911
amyotrophic lateral sclerosis (ALS), 921
cerebral palsy, 915
Guillain-Barré syndrome, 928
multiple sclerosis, 924
Parkinson's disease, 907
nutrition, 339–340
interventions, 361–362
obesity, 93, 491–493
osteoporosis, 995, 996, 997, 998
physical activity, 402
poverty rate, 214–217
promotores, 124, 125, 189–191
respiratory diseases
asthma, 801–804
byssinosis, 836
cystic fibrosis, 819
tobacco use, 264–266, 267
time trends, 270
radiograph of chest
asbestosis, 833
coal workers' pneumoconiosis, 826, 827, 829
interstitial lung disease, 823
pneumoconioses, 825–826
respiratory diseases, 799
silicosis, 830
radon and lung cancer, 754, 755
randomized controlled trials (RCTs)
definition, 52–53
meta-analyses, 69–70
randomized clinical trial, 54
randomized community trial, 54
Reach Out and Read, 222
REACH Registry, 722
Reach to Recovery Program, 767
reactive airways dysfunction syndrome, 837
Reading, Writing, and Reducing Obesity, 129
Reasons for Geographic and Racial Differences
in Stroke (REGARDS), 697, 702
recall bias, 59
recombinant tissue plasminogen activator
(rtPA), 707–708
Recombinant t-PA Stroke Study Group,
707–708
recruitment for health careers, 221
red meat nutrition, 337
colorectal cancer, 759
Dietary Guidelines, 333
hepatocellular carcinoma, 1049
as Western diet, 983
regional analyses. *See* geographic distributions
reimbursement. *See* payment to providers
Reiter's syndrome, 990
relative risk, 45, 56–57
cigarettes, 246–247
definition, 45, 56, 73
population-attributable risk versus, 64

renal disease. *See* kidney disease
reproductive disorders
alcohol use, 436–437
obesity and, 487, 490
tobacco use
cigarette smoking, 244, 245, 261
nicotine, 256, 261
pathophysiology, 261
smokeless tobacco, 251, 261
resilience traits
mental health and, 874, 876
post-traumatic stress disorder and, 870, 874
socioeconomic status and, 207
respiratory diseases. *See also* asthma; chronic
obstructive pulmonary disease (COPD);
respiratory diseases from cigarette
smoking; sleep apnea
asbestosis
causes, 834
descriptive epidemiology, 833–834
interventions, 835
lung cancer and asbestos, 65, 754, 826
significance, 832–833
bronchiectasis, 798
bronchitis
as chronic obstructive pulmonary
disease, 796, 797, 811
definition, 798
hospitalization duration, 795
ICD-10 code, 798
pathophysiology, 797
byssinosis
causes, 836
descriptive epidemiology, 836
interventions, 836
significance, 835
coal workers' pneumoconiosis
causes, 828–829
descriptive epidemiology, 827, 828
interventions, 829
significance, 826–827
cystic fibrosis
causes, 819
definition, 796, 798, 817
descriptive epidemiology, 818, 819
ICD-10 code, 798
interventions, 819–820
pathophysiology, 818–819
significance, 817–818
definitions, 795, 796
dyspnea, 795–796
anemia, 1070
chronic obstructive pulmonary disease,
812, 816
coal workers' pneumoconiosis, 827
grain dust exposure, 840
heart failure, 710, 714, 715

interstitial lung disease, 823
  kidney disease and anemia, 1070
  treatment, 816
interstitial lung disease
  causes, 824
  definition, 822–823
  descriptive epidemiology, 823
  interventions, 824
"Monday morning syndrome," 835
obesity and, 488, 489
occupational asthma
  causes, 838–839
  descriptive epidemiology, 837–838
  interventions, 839
  significance, 836–837
occupational lung disease significance,
  825–826
organic dust–related lung disease
  causes, 841
  descriptive epidemiology, 840
  interventions, 841
  significance, 839–840
pathophysiology, 797–800
physical activity, 396
reactive airways dysfunction syndrome, 837
screening, 799
significance, 795–797
silicosis
  causes, 831–832
  coal workers' pneumoconiosis, 828
  descriptive epidemiology, 830–831
  interventions, 832
  significance, 829–830
tobacco use
  cigar smoking, 252
  cigarette smoking. See respiratory
    diseases from cigarette smoking
  pathophysiology, 259–260
  pipe smoking, 253
  relative risk, 247
  secondhand smoke, 245, 246
respiratory diseases from cigarette smoking
asthma, 808
chronic obstructive pulmonary disease, 813,
  814, 815, 829
interstitial lung disease, 824
overview, 244, 245, 246, 247, 248–249
pneumoconiosis, 826
sleep apnea, 821
restless leg syndrome, 986
retrospective cohort studies definition, 55
reverse causality of SES, 208–209
Revia (naltrexone), 466
rheumatism. See fibromyalgia
rheumatoid arthritis (RA)
  causes, 978–979
    modifiable risk factors, 979

  definition, 976
  descriptive epidemiology, 977–978
    geographic distribution, 978
    high-risk populations, 978
    time trends, 978
  future research, 981
  interventions
    examples, 980–981
    prevention, 979
    screening, 979–980
    treatment, 980, 981
  osteoporosis and, 999
  pathophysiology, 977
  significance, 976–977
  smoking and, 262, 979
risk assessment definition, 70–71
risk factors. See also analytic epidemiology
  attributable risk, 62
  comparing across groups, 44–47
  high-risk vs. general population, 15
  population-attributable risk, 63–65
risk ratio. See relative risk

S

SAID principle (Specific Adaptations to
  Imposed Demands), 397
salt intake
  blood pressure, 598, 599, 603–604
  cancer, 750
  Dietary Guidelines, 333
  kidney disease, 1083
San Diego Healthy Weight Collaborative,
  188–189
schizophrenia
  A Beautiful Mind (movie), 866
  descriptive epidemiology, 868–869
  homelessness, 862, 866, 869
  immune system and mental health,
    859–860
  pathophysiology, 865–866
  treatment, 878
    biopsychosocial approach, 880–881
  violent crime and, 861
School Breakfast Program, 347, 361
School Health Policies and Practices Study, 351
schools as intervention venues
  community health business model, 188–189
  diabetes prevention, 545–546
  dropout prevention, 221
  education programs, 221–223
  No Excuses charter school model, 222
  nutrition, 347, 356–358, 364
  obesity prevention, 498–499
  obesity screening, 500–501
  overview, 127–129
  physical activity, 410

Prevention Research Centers, 128–129
skin cancer prevention, 781
technology-enhanced classroom
    instruction, 223
tobacco use prevention, 284–285
truancy interventions, 223
School-Wide Positive Behavioral Interventions
    and Supports (SWPBIS), 222
screening for chronic diseases
    ACA and charges for, 112, 187, 653
    alcohol use, 459–462
    arthritis
        ankylosing spondylitis, 992
        gout, 984
        osteoarthritis, 974
        rheumatoid arthritis, 979–980
    brief interventions, 127
    cancer
        breast cancer, 112, 116, 762, 765–768
        cervical cancer, 112, 769
        colorectal cancer, 112, 760
        leukemia, 777
        lung cancer, 112, 756
        lymphoma, 775
        melanoma of the skin, 781
        oral cavity cancer, 779
        prostate cancer, 773, 774
    cardiovascular disease, 112
        coronary heart disease, 677, 688–689
        peripheral arterial disease, 718, 722
        stroke, 703, 704–705, 706–707
    diabetes, 112, 529, 546–548
    dyslipidemia, 652–654, 657
    faith-based venues, 132
    Health Impact Pyramid, 8, 9
    health literacy and, 148, 149
    health system interventions, 126, 127,
        184–187
    high blood pressure, 606–607
        measurement, 583–587
        prehypertension, 607
    information campaigns, 53, 69
    kidney disease, 1076, 1077–1080
    liver diseases
        hemochromatosis, 1050
        hepatitis B, 1034
        hepatitis C, 1039, 1041
        non-alcoholic fatty liver, 1043
    mental health, 877–878, 882
    nutrition, 351–352
    obesity, 112, 500–501
    osteoporosis, 112, 1000–1001
    peripheral arterial disease, 718, 722
    pharmacists for, 186–187
    pregnancy
        diabetes, 548
        hepatitis B, 1034

    maternal and birth screening, 85
    mental illness, 877
    substance use disorder, 877
    as prevention, 12, 50–51
    respiratory diseases, 799
        asthma, 799, 808–809
        chronic obstructive pulmonary
            disease, 816
        cystic fibrosis, 820
        sleep apnea, 822
        spirometric testing, 799
    school venues, 127
    sleep apnea, 822
    stroke, 703, 704–705, 706–707
        NIH Stroke Scale, 706
    tobacco use, 285–286
    ultrasound
        breast cancer, 767
        coronary heart disease, 677
        non-alcoholic fatty liver, 1043
    workplace venues, 129–132
seafood. See fish nutrition
SEARCH for Diabetes in Youth Study
    (SEARCH), 535
Secondary Prevention of Small Subcortical
    Strokes trial, 700
secondhand smoke
    coronary heart disease, 245, 249, 683
    lung cancer, 245, 246, 249, 754, 755
    pathophysiology, 258, 260
    respiratory diseases
        asthma, 806, 808, 810
        chronic obstructive pulmonary
            disease, 814
    significance, 245, 246
        death rate, 99, 243, 246
        lost productivity, 250
    smoke-free policies, 13, 285, 296–297
    stroke, 245, 246, 702
Section 8 voucher program, 223, 227
sedentary behavior, 391
    diabetes, 538
    food insecurity and, 532
    dyslipidemia, 647
    high blood pressure, 607
    modifying sedentary activities, 417
    television viewing and obesity, 496, 537, 538
seizure pathophysiology, 902–903
Selected Metropolitan/Micropolitan Area Risk
    Trends (SMART), 399
selection bias, 58
self-efficacy of patient. See also self-
    management by patient
    Chronic Care Model, 179, 181–183
    educational attainment and, 204
    Health Belief Model, 116, 117
    nutrition and, 345

physical activity and, 404
social cognitive theory, 121
socioeconomic status and, 207
self-management by patient. *See also* self-
    efficacy of patient
    adherence to prescribed care
        communication by care provider, 126
        dyslipidemia, 634, 656
        mental health, 612, 881–882
    arthritis interventions, 976
        rheumatoid arthritis, 981
    asthma, 810
    Chronic Care Model, 181–183
    diabetes, 548, 549, 550
    dyslipidemia, 634
    high blood pressure, 612
    patient wellness portals, 186
Senior Farmer's Market Nutrition
    Program, 361
sentinel surveillance, 81, 85, 87
seronegative spondyloarthropathies,
    989, 990
SES. *See* socioeconomic status
sexual assault and alcohol, 446
sexual transmission
    hepatitis A, 1028
    hepatitis B, 1028, 1032, 1033, 1034
    hepatitis C, 1035, 1039, 1040
    human papilloma virus, 770, 771
        cervical cancer, 770, 771
Shape Up Somerville, 357, 505
significance
    behavioral determinants, 187
    definition, 40
    descriptive epidemiology identifying, 42
    social determinants, 201, 202–209
silicosis
    causes, 831–832
    coal workers' pneumoconiosis, 828
    descriptive epidemiology, 830–831
    interventions, 832
    significance, 829–830
skin cancer
    counseling, 112, 781
    melanoma
        causes, 780
        descriptive epidemiology, 780
        interventions, 781
        significance, 744, 780
    significance, 744
    sunlight exposure, 750
sleep
    diabetes relative risk, 537, 538
    disorders and ADHD, 936
    fibromyalgia, 986, 987, 989
        prevention, 988
    obesity and, 488, 490, 496

sleep apnea
    causes, 821–822
    definition, 796–797, 798
    high-risk populations, 821
    ICD-10 code, 798
    interventions
        examples, 822
        screening, 822
    non-alcoholic fatty liver and, 1045
    obesity and, 111, 489, 490
    obstructive, 796–797, 820
        conditions stemming from, 821
        high-risk populations, 821
        pathophysiology, 820–821
        significance, 820
    smokeless tobacco and, 261
"Smart Snacks in School" guidelines, 347
smokeless tobacco
    definition, 251
    oral cavity cancer, 251, 252, 259, 779
    prevalence, 266
    reproductive disorders, 251, 261
    significance, 251–252
    time trends, 267–271
smoking tobacco
    ankylosing spondylitis, 991–992
    as behavioral determinant, 111
    cancer, 749, 750
        bladder cancer, 243, 778
        cervical cancer, 770, 771
        leukemia, 243, 259, 777
        lung cancer, 243, 244, 245, 248, 254, 752,
            754, 755
        oral cavity cancer, 243, 252, 253, 259, 779
        pharyngeal cancer, 243, 253
        prostate cancer, 773
    costs of, 111
    depression, 860
    diabetes
        dementia and, 524
        macrovascular complications, 528
        relative risk, 537, 538
    dyslipidemia, 648–649
    hepatitis B, 1030
    interventions
        minor access to products, 274–275, 284,
            300–301
        multilevel approach, 140
        Not-On-Tobacco, 129
        prevention, 281–285
        screening, 285–286, 287–288
        smoke-free policies, 13, 285, 296–297
        telephone cessation quitlines, 286–287,
            288–289, 301–302
        tobacco regulation, 302–304
        treatment, 286–289
        treatment insurance coverage, 297–300

kidney disease, 1074, 1075
neurological disorders
    attention-deficit/hyperactivity
        disorder, 936
    dementias, 912
    low back pain, 940
    multiple sclerosis, 926
osteoporosis, 999, 1000, 1001–1002
peripheral arterial disease, 720, 721
respiratory diseases, 244, 245, 246, 247,
        248–249
    asthma, 808
    chronic obstructive pulmonary disease,
        813, 814, 815, 829
    interstitial lung disease, 824
    pneumoconiosis, 826
    sleep apnea, 821
risk factors, 64
significance, 6, 15, 111, 243–246
    cigarettes vs. other, 245
smoking as reportable, 243
smoking-attributable mortality, 246,
        248–249
socioeconomic status and, 202, 206, 250,
        265, 281, 447, 679
stroke, 701–702
surveillance of, 83
    as reportable, 243
snuff. See smokeless tobacco
social anxiety
    pathophysiology, 866–867
    prevalence, 870
    youth alcohol use for, 456
social cognitive theory
    definition, 120–121
    example uses, 121, 125–126
social determinants. See also psychosocial
        issues; socioeconomic status (SES)
    behavioral determinants as, 113–114,
        120, 201
    future research, 229–232
    "health in all policies" framework, 227–229
    mental health, 874, 876
        suicide, 871
        treatment, 879
    overview, 113–114, 201–202
    significance, 201, 202–209
Social Security Disability Survey, 837
social support, 122–123
    lactation, 356
        duration and, 768
    lifestyle behaviors, 123
social-ecological perspective on intervention,
        114–116
    coronary heart disease intervention, 693
    nutrition, 344–348
    physical activity, 408

socioeconomic status (SES)
    alcohol use and, 447
    analytic epidemiology, 219–229
        causes, 219–227
        education, 204, 220–223, 224–225
        employment and income, 225
        housing, 225–227
        interventions, 220, 221–224, 226,
            227–229
    asthma and, 804
    cancer and
        breast cancer, 762
        cervical cancer, 769, 771, 772
        lung cancer, 753
        significance, 744–745
    coronary heart disease and, 209–210,
        679, 688
    descriptive epidemiology, 214–219
    diabetes and, 531, 532, 535, 537, 538
    disparities in health care, 20–22, 209. See
        also disparities in health care
    dyslipidemia and, 640, 653
    global chronic disease, 22
    Health Impact Pyramid, 8, 9, 11, 12, 219–220
    high blood pressure and, 679
    interventions
        educational, 221–223
        employment and income, 223
        health homes for low-income patients,
            172, 185
        Health Impact Pyramid, 219–220
        housing, 220, 223–224
        policy, 227–229
    kidney disease and, 1072
    liver disease and, 1018
        hepatitis A, 1028
        hepatitis B, 1030
        hepatitis C, 1037, 1039
    mental health and, 871
        bipolar disorder, 869
        depression, 869, 874
        post-traumatic stress disorder, 871
        suicide, 875
    neurological disorders and
        epilepsy, 903, 904
        low back pain, 940
        migraine headaches, 942
        multiple sclerosis, 924
        traumatic brain injury, 932
    nutrition and, 202, 205, 208, 340
    obesity and, 208, 486–487, 492, 679
    pathophysiology, 209–214
    significance, 202–209
        health behaviors, 206–208
        health status influencing SES,
            208–209, 531
        material living conditions, 203–205

neighborhood factors, 207–208, 226
psychosocial risk factors, 207, 211–214
as social determinant, 114, 201, 202
tobacco use and, 206, 250, 265, 281, 447, 679
U.S. Census surveillance data, 82, 90–91
poverty rate, 214–219
sodium chloride. *See* salt intake
spasticity of cerebral palsy, 913
double hemiplegia, 914
spastic diplegia, 913
spastic hemiplegia, 913–914
spastic quadriplegia, 914
Special Supplemental Nutrition Program for
Women, Infants, and Children (WIC), 348,
351, 359
Farmer's Market Nutrition Program, 361
spending for health care. *See* costs of health care
spinal cord injury (SCI)
causes, 898, 934, 935
descriptive epidemiology, 935
high-risk groups, 898
interventions, 936
significance, 934–935
Spinal Cord Injury Information Network, 934
spirometric testing, 799
chronic obstructive pulmonary disease,
811, 816
occupational asthma, 837
Stages of Change Model, 117–118
physical activity, 408–409
standard population, 48
Stanford Chronic Disease Self-Management
Program, 182
Stanford Five-City Project, 656
State Governor's Council on Physical
Fitness, 413
State Heart Disease and Stroke Prevention
Programs, 706
State Vital Records Systems, 84–85
status epilepticus
cerebral palsy, 914
epilepsy, 905, 906
stereotypic seizures, 902
stomach cancer
significance, 744
smoking and, 252
STOP-Bang questionnaire, 822
Strategic Framework on Multiple Chronic
Conditions, 184
stress
coronary heart disease, 687
discrimination and, 212–214
fibromyalgia stress management, 988, 989
good from physical activity, 397
headaches and, 942, 943
nutrition and, 345
socioeconomic status

pathophysiology, 210–213
significance, 207
stress-related hypertension, 582–583
stroke
alcohol use, 436
analytic epidemiology
causes, 698–703
interventions, 703, 706–709
modifiable risk factors, 699–703
population-attributable risk, 703, 704–705
definition, 695–696
descriptive epidemiology
geographic distribution, 697, 698
high-risk populations, 696–698
time trends, 675
diabetes and, 521, 522, 528, 701
direct medical costs, 111
future research, 709–710
high blood pressure and
blood pressure reduction, 601, 607,
609–610, 700
cardiovascular disease risk factors, 676
stroke strongest risk factor, 594–595,
596, 699
interventions
ABCs of prevention, 709
examples, 708–709
NIH Stroke Scale, 706
screening, 703, 704–705, 706–707
stroke system of care, 706
treatment, 707–708
nutrition, 702
dietary fat, 336
obesity and, 487, 488
pathophysiology, 695–696
physical activity, 396, 702
REACH Registry, 722
registries for surveillance data, 87
risk factors, 676
significance, 695
mortality rates, 695, 696–697
tobacco use
cigar smoking, 252
cigarette smoking, 244, 245, 701–702
pipe smoking, 253
secondhand smoke, 245, 246, 702
smokeless tobacco, 251
Studies to Treat or Prevent Pediatric Type 2
Diabetes, 546
study designs, 52–56
subarachnoid hemorrhagic stroke, 696
subjective norm, 119
substance use disorders
alcohol
medications for abstinence, 466
use vs. misuse, 431–432
withdrawal, 436, 463–464

attention-deficit/hyperactivity disorder, 936
as behavioral determinant, 111
as health care challenge, 10–11
interventions
    family-based, 122
    preventing development of, 877
liver disease
    hepatitis B, 1032, 1033, 1034
    hepatitis C, 1035, 1038, 1039, 1040
mental health, 874
    suicide, 871
tobacco as addicting, 243
    cigarettes, 243
    cigars, 253
    electronic cigarettes, 256
    hookahs, 254
    nicotine dependence, 263–264, 277,
        278–279
    pipes, 254
    smokeless tobacco, 243, 251, 252
violent crime and, 861
withdrawal from substances
    alcohol, 436, 463–464
    nicotine, 263–264
sugar-sweetened beverages, 338
    diabetes and, 338, 538
    Dietary Guidelines, 333
    gout and, 984
    obesity and, 495
suicide
    attention-deficit/hyperactivity disorder,
        936–937
    descriptive epidemiology, 871
    mental illness comorbid diseases versus, 859
    pathophysiology, 868
    population-attributable risk, 875
Summer Food Service Program, 361
summer learning programs, 222
sun exposure and melanoma, 750, 780, 781
SuperMICAR coding software, 84
Supplemental Nutrition Assistance Program
    (SNAP), 348, 351, 360–361, 363
surgery
    joint replacements, 969, 973, 975
    obesity, 503, 975
        bariatric and type 2 diabetes, 527
surveillance
    acute stroke, 87, 708
    alcohol use, 439–441, 448, 452–453,
        454–455
    cancer, 45, 86–87, 748–749, 751
        hepatocellular carcinoma, 1049
    cardiovascular disease, 722
    chronic disease, 81, 85–87
        national system, 78–79
    coal workers' pneumoconiosis, 827
    data analysis, 92–95

data dissemination, 95–99
data sources, 80, 81–82
    administrative data collection systems,
        82, 89–90
    electronic health records, 82, 90
    health surveys, 81, 87–89
    National Center for Health Statistics, 84,
        398, 455, 589, 795
    notifiable disease systems, 80, 81, 83
    patient registries, 180–181, 185–186
    sentinel surveillance, 81, 85, 87
    U.S. Census, 82, 90–91
    vital statistics, 81, 83–85
definition, 77–78, 79
diabetes, 533–534, 535
electronic health records, 181, 186
health policy, 91–92
immunizations, 83
infectious diseases, 77–78, 79
liver disease, 1021
    hepatitis C, 1036, 1037, 1039
    hepatocellular carcinoma, 1049
    non-alcoholic fatty liver, 1044
mental health, 868
nutrition, 351–354
physical activity, 397–400, 411, 415
poverty rate, 214–217
as prevention strategy, 12–13, 18–19
social determinant health indicators, 230
traumatic brain injury, 87
weight loss, 504
Surveillance, Epidemiology, and End Results
    (SEER)
    cancer, 748–749
        breast cancer, 45
    surveillance data, 86–87
Surveillance, Prevention, and Management of
    Diabetes Mellitus (SUPREME-DM), 534
Swedish Trial in Old Patients with
    Hypertension, 716
sympathetic nervous system and blood
    pressure, 582–583
systematic reviews of studies, 69–70
Systolic Blood Pressure Intervention Trial, 609

T

taxes
    Earned Income Tax Credit, 223, 225
    lung cancer intervention, 756–757
    tobacco excise taxes, 292–293
Technical Development in Health Agencies
    Program, 751
technology
    coronary heart disease intervention, 692
    Health Information Technology for
        Economic and Clinical Health Act, 79, 180

patient wellness portals, 186
physical activity promotion, 417–418, 545
technology-enhanced classroom
  instruction, 223
television viewing
  diabetes relative risk, 537, 538
  obesity and, 496
temporal analysis. *See* time trends
temporomandibular joint dysfunction, 986
tension headaches
  causes, 899, 942
  descriptive epidemiology, 941–942
    high-risk groups, 899
  interventions, 942–943
  significance, 941
Theory of Planned Behavior, 118–119
thiamine and alcohol use, 437
tic disorders
  attention-deficit/hyperactivity disorder, 936
  causes, 897, 931
  definition, 929–930
  descriptive epidemiology, 930
    high-risk groups, 897
  future research, 931
  interventions, 931
  as neurodevelopmental disorders, 864
  pathophysiology, 930
  significance, 930
time trends
  alcohol use, 453–456, 1023–1024
  arthritis, 965, 966
    ankylosing spondylitis, 991
    gout, 982, 983
    osteoarthritis, 969
    rheumatoid arthritis, 978
  cancer, 15, 743, 745
    bladder cancer, 777
    breast cancer, 762–763
    cervical cancer, 770
    colorectal cancer, 758
    hepatocellular carcinoma, 1047, 1049
    leukemia, 776
    lung cancer, 753
    lymphoma, 775
    melanoma of the skin, 780
    oral cavity cancer, 778
    prostate cancer, 773
  cardiovascular disease, 673, 675
    coronary heart disease, 15, 675, 679–681
    heart failure, 712–713
    stroke, 675
  descriptive epidemiology identifying, 42
  diabetes, 519–520, 533–536
    lifetime risk, 536
  dyslipidemia, 641, 643–644
  high blood pressure, 587, 588, 591,
    592–593

kidney disease, 1065–1066, 1067, 1068,
    1071, 1073–1074
liver disease, 1017–1019, 1020
  alcoholic, 1023–1024
  hepatitis A, 1027–1028
  hepatitis B, 1030–1032
  hepatitis C, 1035, 1037, 1038
  hepatocellular carcinoma, 1047, 1049
mental health, 872–873
neurological disorders
  amyotrophic lateral sclerosis (ALS), 921
  attention-deficit/hyperactivity
    disorder, 937
  carpal tunnel syndrome, 939
  multiple sclerosis, 924
  spinal cord injuries, 935
  traumatic brain injury, 932–933
nutrition, 343–344
obesity, 494, 593
osteoporosis, 997–998
physical activity, 403, 404
poverty rate, 218–219
respiratory diseases
  asbestosis, 833
  asthma, 804–805
  chronic obstructive pulmonary
    disease, 814
  coal workers' pneumoconiosis,
    826, 827
  cystic fibrosis, 818
  occupational asthma, 836
  silicosis, 831
stroke, 675
surveillance data analysis, 95
tobacco use, 83, 267–271, 305, 683
tissue plasminogen activator (t-PA), 707–708
Tobacco Control Act (2009), 295–296
tobacco use
  as addicting, 243
    cigarettes, 243
    cigars, 253
    electronic cigarettes, 256
    hookahs, 254
    nicotine dependence, 263–264, 277,
      278–279
    pipes, 254
    smokeless tobacco, 243, 251, 252
  analytic epidemiology
    interventions, 289–297
    smoking continuation, 278–281
    smoking initiation, 271–278
  ankylosing spondylitis, 991–992
  as behavioral determinant, 111
  cancer, 749, 750
    bladder cancer, 243, 778
    cervical cancer, 770, 771
    leukemia, 243, 259, 777

lung cancer, 243, 244, 245, 248, 254, 752, 754, 755
oral cavity cancer, 243, 252, 253, 259, 779
pharyngeal cancer, 243, 253
prostate cancer, 773
cigars
    prevalence, 266
    secondhand smoke, 252
    significance, 252–253
depression and, 860
descriptive epidemiology
    geographic distribution, 267
    high-risk populations, 264–267
    time trends, 83, 267–271, 305, 683
diabetes, 528
    dementia and smoking, 524
    macrovascular complications, 528
    relative risk, 537, 538
dyslipidemia, 648–649
electronic cigarettes, 255–256, 259, 266
future research, 304–307
heart disease, 46, 47
hepatitis B, 1030
hookah, 254, 266
interventions
    minor access to products, 274–275, 284, 300–301
    multilevel approach, 140
    Not-On-Tobacco, 129
    prevention, 281–285
    screening, 285–286, 287–288
    smoke-free policies, 296–297
    telephone cessation quitlines, 286–287, 288–289, 301–302
    tobacco regulation, 302–304
    treatment, 286–289
    treatment insurance coverage, 297–300
kidney disease, 1074, 1075
Master Settlement Agreement, 290–291, 292, 294–295, 305
neurological disorders
    attention-deficit/hyperactivity disorder, 936
    dementias, 912
    low back pain, 940
    multiple sclerosis, 926
osteoporosis, 999, 1000, 1001–1002
pathophysiology
    cancer, 258–259
    cardiovascular disease, 256–258
    lung cancer, 46, 47. See also lung cancer
    nicotine dependence, 263–264
    other adverse effects, 261–263
    reproductive disorders, 261
    respiratory diseases, 259–260

peripheral arterial disease, 720, 721
pipe smoking, 253–254
price and, 280–281, 282
    tobacco excise taxes, 292–293
relative risk
    cigarettes, 246–247
    overview, 56
reproductive disorders
    cigarette smoking, 244, 245, 261
    nicotine, 256, 261
    pathophysiology, 261
    smokeless tobacco, 251, 261
respiratory diseases
    asthma, 808
    chronic obstructive pulmonary disease, 813, 814, 815, 829
    interstitial lung disease, 824
    pneumoconiosis, 826
    sleep apnea, 821
risk factors, 64
secondhand smoke, 99, 243, 246. See also secondhand smoke
significance, 243–246
    overview, 6, 15
smokeless tobacco
    definition, 251
    oral cavity cancer and, 251, 252, 259, 779
    prevalence, 266
    reproductive disorders, 251, 261
    significance, 251–252
    time trends, 267–271
smoking as reportable, 243
smoking-attributable mortality, 246, 248–249
socioeconomic status and, 202, 206, 250, 265, 281, 447, 679
stroke
    cigar smoking, 252
    cigarette smoking, 244, 245, 701–702
    pipe smoking, 253
    secondhand smoke, 245, 246, 702
    smokeless tobacco, 251
    waterpipe, 254, 266
tolerance to alcohol, 436
tongue cancer, 779
total cholesterol (TC), 633, 635
    alcohol use, 648
    dietary intake and, 645–647
    diverse populations, 639–640
    gender differences, 637–638
    geographic distribution, 640–641
    smoking and, 648–649
    time trends, 641, 643–644
    youth, 652
Total Worker Health, 130–131
Tourette syndrome
    causes, 897, 931
    definition, 929–930

descriptive epidemiology, 930
  high-risk groups, 897
future research, 931
interventions, 931
pathophysiology, 930
significance, 930
traffic crashes. *See* motor vehicle crashes
training health workers
  alcohol intervention, 467
  Diabetes Prevention Program, 555
  global improvements needed, 22–23
  kidney disease, 1076, 1077, 1085
  multiple sclerosis, 926
  PAD and future cardiovascular events,
    721–722
  physical activity promotion, 411
  skills required, 23–24
  social determinants of health, 231
transfusions of blood. *See* blood transfusions
transient ischemic attacks (TIAs), 696
transitional jobs, 223
Transtheoretical Model, 117–118
  physical activity, 408–409
traumatic brain injury (TBI)
  causes, 898, 933
  descriptive epidemiology, 932–933
    high-risk groups, 898
  interventions, 933–934
  post-traumatic stress disorder and, 870
  significance, 931–932
  surveillance, 87
trends. *See* time trends
Trials of Hypertension Prevention, 603, 604
Trials of Hypertension Prevention, Phase II, 504
triglycerides (TGs), 633
  alcohol use, 648
  body mass index and, 644–645
  coronary heart disease, 684
  dietary intake and, 645–647
  diverse populations, 639–640
  dyslipidemia pathophysiology, 635–636
  gender differences, 637–638
  physical activity and, 395
  smoking and, 649
  time trends, 641, 643–644
truancy interventions, 223
tumor necrosis factors (TNFs)
  ankylosing spondylitis, 990, 993
  as biomarkers, 720, 970, 977
  inhibitors
    ankylosing spondylitis, 992
    rheumatoid arthritis, 980
  rheumatoid arthritis, 977
type 1 diabetes
  causes, 519
  multifactorial therapy, 528
  pathophysiology, 526

percentage of cases, 519
prevention, 540–542
screening, 547
treatment, 548–549
type 2 diabetes
  bariatric surgery remission, 527
  causes, 519, 529, 536–540
  depressive disorders and, 525
  dyslipidemia and, 649–650, 656
  gout, 983
  multifactorial therapy, 528–529
  pathophysiology, 526–527
  percentage of cases, 519
  prevention, 542–546
  prevention in youth, 545–546
  screening, 112
  treatment, 549–551
Type 2 Diabetes in Adolescents and Youth
  (TODAY), 545

U

ultrasound screening
  breast cancer, 767
  coronary heart disease, 677
  non-alcoholic fatty liver, 1043
"underlying cause of death," 84
unemployment. *See* employment status
United Kingdom
  life expectancy, 5
  Prospective Diabetes Study Group, 716
United States (U.S.). *See also* Patient Protection
    and Affordable Care Act (ACA)
  aging population, 4, 20
  Census for surveillance, 82, 90–91
    poverty rate, 214–219
  diversity of population
    health care challenges, 20
    poverty rate disparities, 214–217
  Environmental Protection Agency, 71
  life expectancy
    by country (2015), 5
    lifestyle behaviors, 6
  Medicare budget percentage, 112
  "multiple chronic conditions," 7
  obesity and immigrants, 343
  spending on health care
    Medicare, 112
    noncommunicable diseases, 7
    others versus, 5
U.S. Department of Agriculture (USDA)
  Continuing Survey of Food Intakes by
    Individuals, 352
  Dietary Guidelines for Americans,
    349–351
  Economic Research Service, 352
  nutrition assistance programs, 359–361

Afterschool Snacks, 361
Child and Adult Care Food Program, 347, 361
Commodity Food Assistance Program, 363
Emergency Food Assistance Program, 363
Farm Bill and, 361, 363
Farmer's Market Nutrition Program, 361
Fresh Fruit and Vegetable Snack Program, 361
National School Lunch Program, 347, 359–360, 364
School Breakfast Program, 347, 361
Senior Farmer's Market Nutrition Program, 361
Special Supplemental Nutrition Program for Women, Infants, and Children (WIC), 348, 351, 359
Summer Food Service Program, 361
Supplemental Nutrition Assistance Program (SNAP), 348, 351, 360–361, 363
U.S. Department of Health and Human Services (USDHHS)
ACA mental health marketplaces, 873
Dietary Guidelines for Americans, 349–351
Healthy People 2020
alcohol use, 434
cardiovascular health, 703, 706
physical activity, 405–406
U.S. Renal Data System, 523
universal pre-kindergarten, 223
upstream causes
overview of book figures, 40, 41
population attributable risk, 63
U.S. Preventive Services Task Force (USPSTF), 406
uterine (corpus) cancer, 744. See also cervical cancer

V

vaccines. See also immunizations
autism spectrum disorders caused by, 918–919
cervical cancer HPV infection, 771
epilepsy
caused by, 905
prevention, 905
Guillain-Barré syndrome and, 928–929
hepatitis A, 1027, 1029
hepatitis B, 1018, 1028–1029, 1031–1032, 1034, 1049
kidney disease, 1083
hepatitis C, 1041
validity of study results, 57–59
vegetable nutrition, 334–335

amyotrophic lateral sclerosis (ALS) and, 922
cancer and, 749, 750
breast cancer, 764
hepatocellular carcinoma, 1049
lung cancer, 754, 755
oral cavity cancer, 779
cirrhosis prevention, 1049
Dietary Guidelines, 333
vegetarian diet, 351
veterans of military and hepatitis C, 1038, 1039
victim blaming, 114, 115, 138
violence
mental illness and, 861
post-traumatic stress disorder and, 870–871, 874
spinal cord injury, 935
vital statistics as surveillance data, 81, 83–85
vitamin B1 and alcohol use, 437
Vivitrol (naltrexone), 466
vocational training, 223

W

Walk with Ease Program, 968
Walking School Bus, 410
waterpipe tobacco smoking, 254, 266
weight loss
fruit and vegetable consumption, 335
high blood pressure, 603, 604
insulin resistance, 501
interventions
Fit Body and Soul, 358
Project SMART, 125–126
WORD, 362
kidney disease, 1075
maintenance, 504
non-alcoholic fatty liver, 1046
obesity treatment, 501–504
osteoarthritis, 973–974
physical activity, 397
Wernicke–Korsakoff syndrome, 437
Western diet, 983
What We Eat in America, 352
white coat hypertension, 584
white meat nutrition
cirrhosis prevention, 1049
DASH diet, 351
Dietary Guidelines, 333
Mediterranean diet, 647
as Western diet, 983
Whole School, Whole Community, Whole Child (WSCC), 127–128
WIC. See Special Supplemental Nutrition Program for Women, Infants, and Children
Widespread Pain Index and fibromyalgia, 985
withdrawal from substances

alcohol, 436, 463–464
nicotine, 263–264
WORD (Wholeness, Oneness, Righteousness,
    Deliverance), 362
workforce. *See* public health professionals
workplaces
    arthritis
        gout and lead exposure, 981, 983, 984
        osteoarthritis, 974
    cancer
        carcinogens in workplace, 754, 755,
            777, 778
        costs of, 747
        melanoma of the skin, 781
        skin cancer, 781
    intervention venues, 129–132
        physical activity, 412
        promotores programs, 125
    neurological disorders
        carpal tunnel syndrome, 938–939
        low back pain, 940
        Parkinson's disease, 908
        traumatic brain injury, 933
    nutrition and, 347–348, 356
    obesity
        costs of, 490
        prevention, 499
    respiratory diseases, 799
        asbestosis, 832–835
        asbestosis carried home, 834
        byssinosis, 835–836
        chest radiograph, 799
        chronic obstructive pulmonary disease,
            812, 814–815, 817
        interstitial lung disease, 823, 824
        occupational asthma, 836–839
        occupational lung diseases, 825–841
        organic dust–related lung disease,
            839–841
        silicosis, 829–832
        sleep apnea, 821, 822
    smoke-free policies, 296–297
    smoking-attributable costs, 250
    Total Worker Health, 130–131

Y

YMCA Diabetes Prevention Program (YDPP),
    552–553, 555, 556
Youth Media Campaign Longitudinal Survey
    (YMCLS), 399
Youth Risk Behavior Surveillance System
    (YRBSS), 88
    physical activity, 399
Youth Risk Factor Behavioral Surveillance
    System, 351
youths

alcohol use
    access to alcohol, 456, 465–466, 467
    age of onset, 456
    binge drinking, 448, 449–451, 452
    college drinking, 446
    descriptive epidemiology, 438, 440,
        441–442, 448, 449–452
    geographic distribution, 448–452
    significance, 433
cancer
    hepatocellular carcinoma, 1049
    leukemia, 776
    lung cancer prevention, 755
    melanoma of the skin, 781
    oral cavity cancer, 779
    significance, 743–744
college enrollment programs, 222
diabetes
    mortality, 521, 536
    prevalence, 535–536
    prevention of type 1, 540–542
    prevention of type 2, 545–546
dyslipidemia
    body mass index and, 645
    descriptive epidemiology, 638, 652
    diverse populations, 639–640
    lifestyle modifications, 652
    physical activity and, 648
    screening, 654
    time trends, 643–644
fibromyalgia, 989
kidney disease, 1073
liver disease
    hepatitis A, 1026, 1028
    hepatitis B, 1028, 1029, 1031,
        1032, 1034
    hepatocellular carcinoma, 1049
    non-alcoholic fatty liver, 1043–1044
mental health
    anxiety disorders, 456, 867
    childhood and risk, 874
    depression, 869
    preventing illness, 875–876
    schizophrenia, 865–866, 869
    screening, 877
    suicide, 871
mentoring programs, 221
neurological disorders
    amyotrophic lateral sclerosis (ALS), 921
    attention-deficit/hyperactivity disorder,
        936, 937, 938
    autism spectrum disorders, 917–919
    cerebral palsy, 914–915
    epilepsy, 899–900, 903, 904, 905
    epilepsy diagnosis, 906
    Guillain-Barré syndrome, 927
    migraine headaches, 941–942

spinal cord injuries, 935
tic disorders, 929–930
traumatic brain injury, 932, 933–934
obesity
body mass index as relative, 485
Childhood Obesity Intervention
Cost-Effectiveness Study, 507
morbidities, 489
mortality and, 489
prevalence, 492–493
prevention, 497–499
screening, 500–501
spending for health care, 490
osteoporosis, 1000, 1001–1002
peer group interventions, 124
physical activity, 400–401, 403, 415
respiratory diseases
asthma, 800, 801, 802, 805–806, 807,
808–809, 810
chronic obstructive pulmonary disease,
814, 816
sleep apnea, 489
smoking
access to tobacco products, 274–275,
284, 300–301

advertising targeting, 294–295, 296
causes of smoking initiation, 271–278
cigarettes, 246–247
cigars, 253
descriptive epidemiology, 264–267
education campaigns, 283
lung growth and, 260
movies showing smoking, 56, 63–64,
273, 274
nicotine dependence, 263–264, 277
nicotine effects on brain, 256, 263, 277
Not-On-Tobacco, 129
personal characteristics, 276
population-attributable risk, 63–64
risk perception, 277–278, 279–280
social influences, 275–276
time trends, 269–271
tobacco product design, 276–277
treatment, 288

Z

Zika virus
Guillain-Barré syndrome, 928
pregnancy and, 915